Applied Radiological Anatomy

This profusely illustrated text will provide trainee radiologists with a unique overview of normal anatomy as illustrated by the full range of modern radiological procedures. The theme throughout is not only to illustrate the appearance of normal anatomical features as visualized by radiology, but also to provide a comprehensive text which describes, explains and evaluates the most current imaging practice for all the body systems and organs. Where necessary, the images are supplemented with line drawings, to illustrate essential anatomical features. This combination of a wealth of high-quality images, fully supported by an authoritative text, will give all radiologists an insight into normal anatomy, which is such a vital prerequisite for interpreting abnormal radiological images.

It will be an essential illustrated text for trainee radiologists studying Part 1 of the examination of the Fellowship of the Royal College of Radiologists, and also for trainees elsewhere in the world studying for their specialist examinations in radiology.

Applied

Radiological Anatomy

Edited by

PAUL BUTLER
Royal Hospitals of St Bartholomew, The London and the London Chest

ADAM W·M·MITCHELL
Charing Cross Hospital, London

HAROLD ELLIS
King's College (Guy's Campus), London

23/8/09

To cool Herb,

This is to let you know how proud I am of you

Enjoy!

I love u Maitu

CAMBRIDGE
UNIVERSITY PRESS

PUBLISHED BY THE PRESS SYNDICATE OF THE UNIVERSITY OF CAMBRIDGE
The Pitt Building, Trumpington Street, Cambridge, United Kingdom

CAMBRIDGE UNIVERSITY PRESS
The Edinburgh Building, Cambridge CB2 2RU, UK   www.cup.cam.ac.uk
40 West 20th Street, New York, NY 10011-4211, USA   www.cup.org
10 Stamford Road, Oakleigh, Melbourne 3166, Australia
Ruiz de Alarcón 13, 28014 Madrid, Spain

First South Asian edition 2001
Reprinted 2005, 2009

Printed and bound by Replika Press Pvt. Ltd., India

Typefaces Swift (8.5/11.5pt *and* Vectora   *System* QuarkXPress   [SE]

A catalogue record for this book is available from the British Library

Library of Congress Cataloguing in Publication data available

ISBN 978 0 521 68324 1

Special edition for sale in South Asia only, not for export elsewhere.

*Every effort has been made in preparing this book to provide
accurate and up-to-date information which is in accord with accepted
standards and practice at the time of publication. Nevertheless,
the authors, editors and publisher can make no warranties that the
information contained herein is totally free from error, not least
because clinical standards are constantly changing through research
and regulation. The authors, editors and publisher therefore
disclaim all liability for direct or consequential damages resulting
from the use of material contained in this book. Readers are
strongly advised to pay careful attention to information provided by
the manufacturer of any drugs or equipment that they plan to use.*

Contents

List of contributors VII
Foreword IX
Preface XI
Acknowledgements XII

1 **Surface anatomy** 1
H. ELLIS

2 **The skull and brain** 17
P. BUTLER *and* M. A. JEFFREE

3 **The orbit and visual pathways** 61
I. MOSELEY

4 **The ear and auditory pathways** 85
P. BUTLER *and* I. G. WYLIE

5 **The extracranial head and neck** 95
J. BHATTACHARYA *and* P. BUTLER

6 **The chest** 121
R. R. PHILLIPS *and* P. ARMSTRONG

7 **The heart and great vessels** 153
B. J. KENNY *and* P. WILDE

8 **The breast** 173
J. A. HANSON *and* N. M. PERRY

9 **Embryology of the gastrointestinal tract and its adnexae** 185
H. ELLIS

10 **The anterior abdominal wall and peritoneum** 189
J. C. HEALY *and* R. H. REZNEK

11 **The gastrointestinal tract** 207
S. E. ROBBINS *and* J. VIRJEE
Vascular anatomy of the gastrointestinal tract 223
J. E. JACKSON

12 **Liver, gall bladder, pancreas and spleen** 239
A. W. M. MITCHELL *and* R. DICK

13 **The renal tract and retroperitoneum** 259
J. CROSS *and* A. K. DIXON

14 **The pelvis** 279
S. J. VINNICOMBE *and* J. E. HUSBAND

15 **The vertebral column and spinal cord** 301
S. A. A. SOHAIB *and* P. BUTLER

16 **The musculoskeletal system 1 · The upper limb** 331
A. W. M. MITCHELL *and* C. W. HERON

17 **The musculoskeletal system 2 · The lower limb** 351
A. NEWMAN-SANDERS *and* A. L. HINE

18 **The limb vasculature and the lymphatic system** 381
M. EASTY *and* O. CHAN

19 **Obstetric anatomy** 399
A. D. G. WOOD *and* K. C. DEWBURY

20 **Paediatric anatomy** 415
R. A. L. BISSET, B. WILSON *and* N. WRIGHT

Index 431

Contributors

PETER ARMSTRONG FRCR
Professor of Radiology, The Medical College of The Royal Hospitals of St Bartholomew and the London

JO BHATTACHARYA MRCP FRCR
Consultant Neuroradiologist, Institute of Neurological Sciences, Glasgow (formerly Specialist (Senior) Registrar in Radiology, The Royal Hospitals of St Bartholomew, the London and the London Chest, London)

ROBERT A. L. BISSET MB BS FRCR Cert MHS
Consultant Radiologist, Booth Hall and The Royal Manchester Children's Hospitals, Manchester

PAUL BUTLER MRCP FRCR
Consultant Neuroradiologist, The Royal Hospitals of St Bartholomew, the London and the London Chest, London

OTTO CHAN FRCS, FRCR
Consultant Radiologist, The Royal Hospitals of St Bartholomew, the London and The London Chest, London

JUSTIN CROSS MRCP FRCR
Senior Registrar in Radiology, Addenbrooke's Hospital, Cambridge

KEITH C. DEWBURY BSc MB BS FRCR
Consultant and Honorary Clinical Senior Lecturer in Radiology, Southampton University Hospitals Trust

ROBERT DICK FRCR FRACR
Consultant Radiologist, The Royal Free Hospital, London

ADRIAN K. DIXON MD FRCP FRCR
Professor of Radiology, University of Cambridge, Honorary Consultant Radiologist, Addenbrooke's Hospital, Cambridge

MARIAN EASTY MRCP FRCR
Consultant Paediatric Radiologist, The Royal Hospitals of St Bartholomew, the London and the London Chest, London

HAROLD ELLIS CBE DM MCh FRCS
Emeritus Professor of Surgery, University of London, Clinical Anatomist, King's College (Guy's Campus), London

JULIAN A. HANSON MRCP FRCR
Research Fellow, Harborview Medical Center, Seattle, Washington, USA (formerly Specialist (Senior) Registrar in Radiology, The Royal Hospitals of St Bartholomew, the London and the London Chest, London)

JEREMIAH C. HEALY MA MB BChir MRCP FRCR
Consultant Radiologist, Department of Diagnostic Radiology, Chelsea and Westminster Hospital, London (formerly Clinical Lecturer, St Bartholomew's Hospital, London)

CHRISTINE W. HERON MRCP FRCR
Consultant Radiologist, St George's Hospital, London

ANDREW L. HINE MB BS MRCP FRCR
Consultant Radiologist,
Central Middlesex Hospital, London

JANET E. HUSBAND FRCP FRCR
Professor of Diagnostic Radiology,
The Royal Marsden NHS Trust (London and Surrey)

JAMES E. JACKSON MRCP FRCR
Senior Lecturer and Honorary Consultant Radiologist,
Department of Imaging, Hammersmith Hospital, London

MARTIN A. JEFFREE MRCP FRCR
Consultant Neuroradiologist, King's Healthcare, London

BRYAN J. KENNY MB FFR(RSCI) FRCR
Radiology Fellow, McMaster University Medical Center,
Hamilton, Ontario (formerly Senior Registrar in
Radiology, Bristol Royal Infirmary)

ADAM W. M. MITCHELL MB BS FRCS FRCR
Consultant Radiologist, Charing Cross Hospital, London
(formerly Lecturer in Radiology, Department of Imaging,
Hammersmith Hospital, London)

IVAN MOSELEY BSc MD PhD
Director, Department of Radiology,
Moorfields Eye Hospital, London

ANTHONY P. G. NEWMAN-SANDERS
MB BS MRCP FRCR
Consultant Radiologist, Mayday Hospital, Croydon,
Surrey (formerly Specialist (Senior) Registrar in
Radiology, St Mary's Hospital, London)

N. M. PERRY FRCR
Consultant Radiologist,
St Bartholomew's Hospital, London

RACHEL R. PHILLIPS MRCP DCH FRCR
Consultant Radiologist, The Whittington Hospital,
London (formerly Research Fellow in Magnetic
Resonance Imaging, St Bartholomew's Hospital, London)

RODNEY H. REZNEK FRCP FRCR
Professor of Academic Radiology, The Medical College of
The Royal Hospitals of St Bartholomew and the London

SIAN E. ROBBINS MB BS MRCP FRCR
Specialist (Senior) Registrar in Radiology,
Bristol Royal Infirmary, Bristol

S. ASLAN A. SOHAIB MRCP FRCR
Specialist (Senior) Registrar in Radiology,
The Royal Hospitals of St Bartholomew,
the London and the London Chest, London

SARAH J. VINNICOMBE MRCP FRCR
Consultant Radiologist, The Royal Hospitals of
St Bartholomew, the London and the London Chest,
London (formerly Senior Registrar in Radiology,
St George's Hospital, London)

JIM VIRJEE MB ChB FRCR
Consultant Radiologist, Bristol Royal Infirmary, Bristol

PETER WILDE BM BCh MRCP FRCR
Consultant Cardiac Radiologist,
United Bristol Healthcare Trust

BRENNAN WILSON MA MB BS LRCP MRCS
FRCR MRCP Cert MHS
Consultant Radiologist, Booth Hall and
The Royal Manchester Children's Hospitals,
Manchester

ANGUS D. G. WOOD MB BS MRCP FRCR
Consultant Radiologist, Poole Hospital, Dorset,
(formerly Lecturer in Magnetic Resonance Imaging,
The Royal Hospitals of St Bartholomew,
the London and the London Chest, London)

NEVILLE WRIGHT MB ChB DMRD FRCR
Consultant Radiologist, Booth Hall and
The Royal Manchester Children's Hospitals,
Manchester

IAN G. WYLIE FRCS FRCR
Consultant Neuroradiologist, formerly of
The Royal Hospitals of St Bartholomew,
the London and the London Chest, London)

Foreword

DAVID J·ALLISON

In the past two decades the nature of radiology has changed almost beyond recognition. The fundamental nature of this change is reflected in the increasing use of the term 'imaging' to encompass all those activities that now lie within the ambit of the radiologist and to which the somewhat restrictive term 'radiology' seems ever more inappropriate.

The continuing burgeoning in the number and variety of imaging methods available to us has been engendered in no small part by the technological advances that have taken place in physics, electronics, engineering, the structural and material sciences and, of course, computer science; these advances have not only improved existing techniques beyond recognition, but have also actually spawned entirely new modalities of investigation. It is no exaggeration to say that the changes that the application of these new modalities have wrought have revolutionized the practice of medicine in terms of both the diagnosis and subsequent management of patients. One consequence of these changes, however, is the perplexing array of imaging sub-specialities that now exists and which creates problems for the young and old radiologist alike. The former has to get to grips with the fundamental principles of not just one or two but a dozen imaging modalities, learn their appropriate applications in a diagnostically effective, safe and economic manner, and learn a variety of interventional techniques that are little different in their complexity and potential risk from what was formerly a large tranche of conventional surgery. The older radiologist, while often possessed of good general ability in radiology, has to grapple with the complexities of new and increasingly computer-dependent methods of investigation, without which his or her diagnostic capabilities begin to look extremely patchy. The best plain-film reader in the country is now likely to be of considerably less value in practice than a fourth-year registrar who has mastered the basic principles of ultrasound, CT and MRI, and can also undertake some core interventional procedures.

Radiology training has adapted, and continues to adapt remarkably quickly, to the new situation in which we find ourselves, and there is widespread recognition of the fact that each new method of investigation that comes along may offer unique benefits in some aspect of diagnosis, replace some previous techniques and assume a complementary role in respect of already extant techniques. There has also been an impressive willingness on the part of our clinical colleagues to explore the clinical benefits of new imaging techniques and to embrace them where appropriate; the willingness to reject outdated radiological methods in favour of the new has also been remarkable (in most cases!).

One of the most striking aspects of all these changes has, however, been less appreciated in general terms than the immediate clinical diagnostic advantages they confer. This has been the fundamental manner in which our knowledge and appreciation of anatomy has been irrevocably altered by the new modalities. We now see living anatomy in ways which have hitherto been simply impossible. Never mind the whiff of formalin surrounding the dehydrated and stiffened dissection cadaver or even the disposition of the living viscera as viewed by the surgeon at laparotomy, distorted as they are by the opening of the abdominal wall and their subsequent deformation by gravity and the retractor. The exquisite and anatomically perfect images we can now see in vivid three-dimensional image reconstructions of organs and systems in the living subject have radically altered our appreciation both of normal living anatomy and pathophysiology of the disorders we investigate. With this facility, however, has come an educational problem: the anatomy we learnt (and continue to learn) at medical school simply does not equip us to appreciate and exploit the anatomy daily presented to us on our wonderful machines.

The present work seems to redress this problem for the practising radiologist and clinician and does so brilliantly. Drs Butler and Mitchell, and that doyen of anatomy teaching, Professor Harold Ellis, have achieved a quite remarkable fusion between the long-established skills of anatomy teaching and the refined imaging techniques that present the anatomy to us in ever more comprehensive (and potentially confusing) ways. The team that has been assembled to address this task at individual organ and system level is formidable and includes some of the great names in radiology.

With the rapid changes taking place in electronic image transfer and presentation, the teaching of anatomy at all levels is undergoing far-reaching changes; this book will be at the forefront of a new generation of books and electronic teaching systems that will revolutionize the way in which we teach and learn anatomy in a manner that is more relevant to the clinical diagnosis and management of patients than has ever previously been the case.

DAVID J·ALLISO
MD BSc DMRD FRCR FRC
*Professor and Director of Im
Imperial College School of M
and Hammersmith Hospital
NHS Trust, London*

Preface

Diagnostic imaging is an indispensable part of modern practice, and few important clinical decisions in hospital are made without it. Interpretation of these images is the responsibility, primarily, of the radiologist and, in the search for what is abnormal, he or she must have a sound knowledge of normal anatomy and the range of normal variation. CT and MRI, in particular, provide exquisite examples of living anatomy. In many institutions this contribution of imaging is recognized, and radiologists and anatomists collaborate in the teaching of anatomy to doctors at various stages of their training. *Applied Radiological Anatomy* attempts both to describe radiological anatomy and to promote the understanding of anatomy by means of imaging. In each chapter, those techniques featured most prominently reflect current imaging practice for that organ or system. Traditional plain radiography is not neglected where appropriate, but obsolete investigations have not been included. The numerous illustrations are accompanied by a comprehensive text and, where possible, normal 'ranges' are given, notably in children.

This book is designed to fulfil the requirements of the Part 1 examination for the Fellowship of the Royal College of Radiologists of the United Kingdom (the FRCR Diploma). It is expected, nevertheless, that all radiologists, radiographers studying for higher diplomas and others with an interest in anatomy will also find it useful.

The editors are grateful to their artists, Mr Jack Barber and Dr Jo Bhattacharya, for their skilful production of so many, often very complex, illustrations. The staff of Cambridge University Press provided patient advice and encouragement. We would also like to thank the staff of all the radiology departments involved in this project, for their diligence and forebearance in providing the necessary images.

PAUL BUTLER
ADAM MITCHELL
HAROLD ELLIS
London 1999

Acknowledgements

The editors and publisher wish to acknowledge with thanks the excellent work of Mr Jack Barber and Dr Jo Bhattacharya in the preparation of the line drawings which illustrate the radiology images. Some of these line drawings have been redrawn and adapted from originals which appeared in *Grant's Atlas of Anatomy* © Williams & Wilkins and from *Langman's Medical Embryology* © Williams & Wilkins and we are grateful for the permission of the publisher to allow their adaptation in this work.

Surface anatomy

H. ELLIS

Introduction

Surface anatomy, to the radiologist, is principally concerned with bony landmarks, anatomical levels and vascular access. Bony landmarks
allow for accurate positioning of the patient
and provide convenient points of reference for
adjacent soft tissue structures. Anatomical levels facilitate structure localization; for example, the coeliac axis origin from the aorta lies
at the level of the twelfth thoracic vertebra.
The anatomy of vascular access, in this modern
era of invasive radiology, is of obvious practical
importance. It is these three topics that will
therefore be highlighted in this chapter.

The head and neck

Because the skull and mandible are covered,
for the most part, only by skin, cutaneous tissues and a thin layer of muscle, their bony landmarks can be easily palpated and many of them
in a thin subject, are actually visible (Fig. 1).

Anteriorly, the depression at the root of the
nose is termed the nasion, which overlies the
suture between the frontal and nasal bones.
Above the nasion is felt the elevation on the
frontal bone termed the glabella which, traced
laterally, continues as the superciliary arch,
which lies above and parallel with the supraorbital margin. The whole of the orbital border is
readily felt by a finger run round the deeper
aspect of its edge. Usually the supraorbital
notch can be felt along the upper margin
about 2.5 cm from the midline. This transmits
the supraorbital branch of the ophthalmic
division of the trigeminal nerve. Not infrequently, however, the notch is replaced by a
foramen. Laterally, the suture between the
frontal and zygomatic bones can be felt as a
slight but distinct depression (the frontozygomatic suture).

The posterior border of the zygomatic process of the frontal bone can be traced upwards
from the level of the frontozygomatic suture
into the temporal line, which curves upwards
and backwards on the parietal bone. The parietal eminence lies above the posterior part of
the temporal line. A line joining the parietal
eminence on each side forms the greatest
transverse diameter of the skull.

The prominence of the cheek is formed by
the zygomatic bone, whose lateral surface can
be readily palpated. It can be traced upwards
into the frontal process, backwards into the
zygomatic arch and forwards and downwards
into the maxilla.

Posteriorly, the external occipital protuberance can be felt and often seen at the upper end
of the median nuchal furrow, which is plainly
visible at the back of the neck and overlies the
ligamentum nuchae. The inion is the term
given to the point situated on the tip of the protuberance in the midline and is used in skull

Fig. 1.
Surface anatomy features
of the skull.

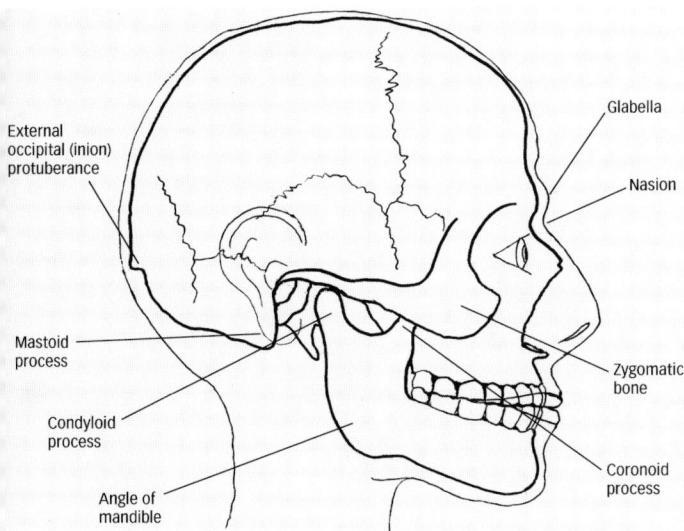

External
occipital (inion)
protuberance

Mastoid
process

Condyloid
process

Angle of
mandible

Glabella

Nasion

Zygomatic
bone

Coronoid
process

measurements. Above the protuberance, the skull presents a backward convexity and the point of greatest curvature is named the maximum occipital point. Above, and in front of this, can be felt an irregular depression in the midline, the lambda. This corresponds to the posterior fontanelle in the newborn, at the junction of the sagittal and lambdoid sutures. Extending laterally from the external occipital protuberance the superior nuchal line can be felt.

The mastoid process is hidden by the lobule and lower part of the concha of the external ear. Its lateral aspect and anterior border are readily palpated but its tip and posterior border are obscured by the attachments of the sternocleidomastoid and splenius capitis muscles.

Almost the whole of the outer aspect of the mandible is readily palpable, including its body, angle and ramus. The condyloid process lies in front of the tragus of the external ear and can be felt to move forwards and downwards if the mouth is opened. It can also be felt to move with a finger placed within the external auditory meatus. The coronoid process can be identified by a finger placed in the angle between the zygomatic arch and the masseter muscle with the mouth opened. Its anterior border can also be palpated within the mouth. The overlying masseter muscle is readily appreciated with the teeth clenched, and the parotid duct can be rolled across its anterior border just below the zygomatic bone. The orifice of this duct can be seen within the mouth at the level of the second upper molar tooth. Here, it can be intubated to perform a parotid sialogram.

The mental foramen can be represented by a point midway between the upper and lower borders of the body of the mandible at the level of the interval between the two premolar teeth. It marks the point of egress of the mental branch of the inferior alveolar nerve.

The neck

The prominent landmark on the lateral side of the neck is the sternocleidomastoid (Fig. 2). This passes from the mastoid process and lateral half of the superior nuchal line of the occipital bone obliquely downwards and forward to a medial (or sternal) head, which is tendinous, and attached to the upper part of the anterior surface of the manubrium and a lateral (or clavicular) head, of fleshy fibres, which attaches to the superior border and anterior surface of the medial one-third of the clavicle. The depression between these two heads is easily felt and is an important landmark to the internal jugular vein (see below). The sternocleidomastoid on one side is tensed by pressing the chin against the examiner's

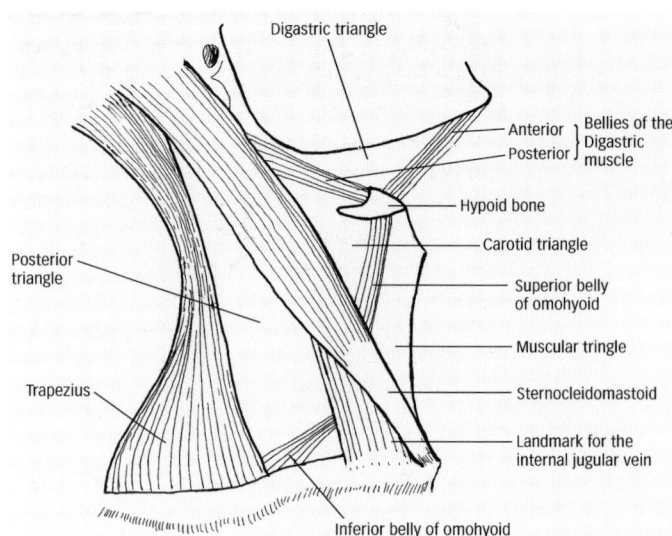

Fig. 2.
The triangles of the neck. The anterior triangle is further subdivided into digastric, carotid and muscular triangles.

hand towards the opposite side. This is a useful test for the eleventh cranial nerve (accessory nerve) which supplies this muscle. The anterior edge of trapezius can be seen and felt as it inserts along the lateral one third of the clavicle.

The sternocleidomastoid divides the lateral aspect of the neck into the anterior and posterior triangles, which are useful for descriptive purposes. The posterior triangle lies between the posterior border of sternocleidomastoid, the anterior border of trapezius and the clavicle. The anterior triangle is formed by the midline anteriorly, the sternocleidomastoid behind and the base above is formed by the lower border of the body of the mandible and a line from its angle to the mastoid process.

In the midline of the neck, from above downwards, the following can be palpated (Fig. 3):

Fig. 3.
Palpable structures in the front of the neck and their vertebral levels.

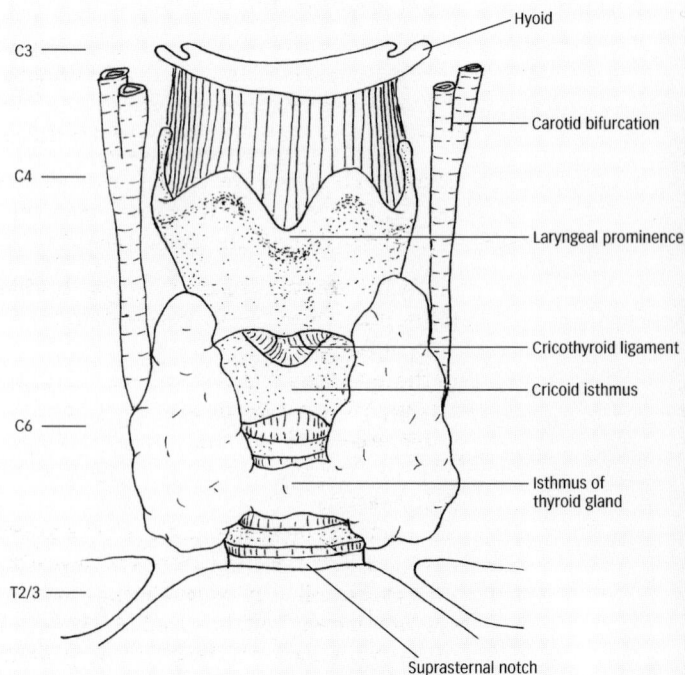

The hyoid bone can be felt immediately below the mandible and can be moved between the thumb and finger from side to side.

The laryngeal prominence of the thyroid cartilage is the midline point of fusion of the upper borders of the thyroid lamina. In the post-pubertal male, the laryngeal prominence, or 'Adam's apple' is usually visible because of the considerable enlargement that takes place in the male larynx at puberty. In the female and pre-pubescent male the prominence is easily palpable but not visible.

The thyroid cartilage isthmus can be felt in the midline running downwards from the laryngeal prominence.

The cricothyroid ligament is represented by a gap between the inferior border of the thyroid cartilage and the cricoid cartilage. This ligament is the site of puncture for emergency access to the trachea.

Below the cricoid can be felt the trachea with its characteristic rings. This extends down to the suprasternal notch of the manubrium.

Often the isthmus of the thyroid gland can be felt to cross, usually, the second to fourth tracheal rings.

Vertebral levels

The following vertebral levels are readily identified in the cervical region:

- The atlas and the dens of the axis: lie in the horizontal plane of the open mouth. (It is through the open mouth that a satisfactory radiograph of these structures can be obtained in the AP position.)
- The third cervical vertebra: lies at the level of the hyoid bone.
- The fourth cervical vertebra: lies at the level of the upper border of the thyroid lamina.
- The sixth cervical vertebra: lies at the level of the lower border of the cricoid cartilage.

The lower border of the cricoid cartilage, the level of the sixth cervical vertebra, is an important landmark since this demarcates:

(a) the junction of the larynx with the trachea.
(b) the junction of the pharynx with the oesophagus.
(c) the level at which the vertebral artery usually passes into the foramen transversarium of the cervical vertebra.

Blood vessels

The course of the carotid artery can be marked out by a line connecting the sternoclavicular joint to the hollow between the mastoid process and the angle of the mandible. At the level of the upper border of thyroid cartilage (fourth cervical vertebra) the common carotid artery divides into its external and internal branches. The carotid pulse can be felt throughout its course but is most readily felt lateral to the thyroid cartilage. Inferiorly, the artery can be compressed by a direct backward pressure as it passes in front of the transverse process of the sixth cervical vertebra. This is sometimes performed during carotid arteriography when the contralateral carotid artery is injected with contrast medium in order to assess 'cross flow' through the circle of Willis (see Chapter 2).

The external jugular vein lies in the superficial fascia covered by the platysma muscle. Its surface marking is a line which joins the angle of the jaw to the midpoint of the clavicle (Fig. 4).

The vein can be made visible by performing the Valsava manoeuvre (forcibly blowing with the mouth closed and nose gripped between the fingers). It passes obliquely across the sternocleidomastoid muscle and then the posterior triangle, pierces the deep fascia immediately above the clavicle and drains into the subclavian vein. Not infrequently, it is double.

The surface marking for the internal jugular vein is just lateral and parallel to the line described for the carotid artery (see above). The vein can be cannulated using either a high or low approach. The patient is tilted head downwards (in order to distend the vein) with the neck extended and the head turned to the opposite side. Catheterization of the right side is preferred as the internal jugular vein, right brachiocephalic vein and superior vena cava are nearly in a straight line. In the anaesthetized patient under complete muscular relaxation, the internal jugular vein can be palpated

Fig. 4.
The veins of the head and neck.

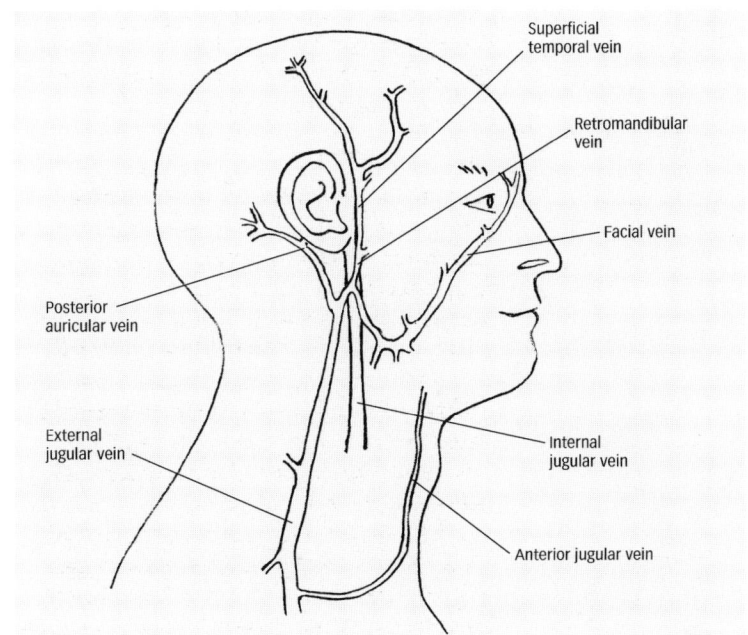

Superficial temporal vein

Retromandibular vein

Facial vein

Posterior auricular vein

External jugular vein

Internal jugular vein

Anterior jugular vein

deep to the sternocleidomastoid muscle about midway along a line joining the mastoid process and the sternoclavicular joint immediately lateral to the carotid pulse. The vein is punctured deep to the muscle and the needle advanced at an angle of 30 to 40 degrees to the skin surface. The low approach is used in the conscious patient or in an emergency situation where muscular relaxation is not obtained. The patient is positioned in a similar manner. The triangular gap between the sternal and clavicular heads of the sternocleidomastoid is identified immediately above the clavicle. The needle is inserted near the apex of this triangle at an angle of 30 to 40 degrees to the skin and is advanced caudally towards the inner border of the anterior end of the first rib behind the clavicle. A reflux of blood confirms successful venepuncture. The use of ultrasound to locate the internal jugular vein is now standard practice.

Thorax

Bony landmarks and levels

In the midline of the thorax, the sternum can be felt throughout its length (Fig. 5). Superiorly, the suprasternal (jugular) notch is obvious and lies between the sternoclavicular joint on each side. Immediately above the notch can be felt the cartilages of the trachea. A finger running down in the midline from the suprasternal notch then identifies the sternal angle of Louis, which marks the junction of the manubrium with the body of the sternum. This angle marks the medial end of the second costal cartilage on each side, which can be identified by placing the index and middle fingers, respectively, in the intercostal space above and below the cartilage at the manubriosternal junction. From this landmark,

successive ribs can be palpated and enumerated from above downwards.

Continuing to palpate along the sternum in the midline, the finger reaches, at its lower end, the xiphisternal joint and the xiphoid process. From the lower end of the sternum, the costal margin can be palpated from the seventh costal cartilage downwards. The lowermost extremity of the costal margin is formed by the tenth costal cartilage and rib. Posteriorly, the free end of the eleventh costal cartilage is usually palpable, as may be the twelfth. However, frequently the twelfth rib is very short and may not be felt.

Vertebral levels

(a) The suprasternal notch corresponds to the level between the second and third thoracic vertebrae (Fig. 5).

(b) The angle of Louis is at the level of the junction between the fourth and fifth thoracic vertebrae.

(c) The manubrium therefore, lies in front of the bodies of the third and fourth thoracic vertebrae.

(d) The junction of the body of the sternum and the xiphoid process lies at the level of the eighth thoracic vertebra.

(e) The body of the sternum therefore lies in front of the fifth to eighth thoracic vertebral bodies.

(f) The tip of the xiphoid process usually lies at the level of the ninth thoracic vertebra.

(g) A line drawn across the inferior costal margin on each side transects the third lumbar vertebra.

Note that the manubriosternal junction (angle of Louis), as well as marking the level of the second costal cartilage and also the junction of the fourth and fifth thoracic vertebral bodies, also marks the junction between the superior and inferior mediastina, the origin and termination of the aortic arch, the level at which the azygos vein enters the superior vena cava and the point at which the right and left pleura come into contact with each other (see below).

In the preserved cadaver, the trachea bifurcates at this level, but in the living subject in the erect position the lower end of the trachea can be seen in oblique radiographs of the chest to extend to the level of the fifth or, in full inspiration, the sixth thoracic vertebra.

Posteriorly, the thoracic cage is covered by muscles and obscured by the scapula, but note that there are two useful landmarks to the rib levels (see Fig. 9):

The easily felt transversely running spine of the scapula lies at the level of the third thoracic vertebra and at the level of the third rib.

Fig. 5.
The mediastinal compartments and the angle of Louis.

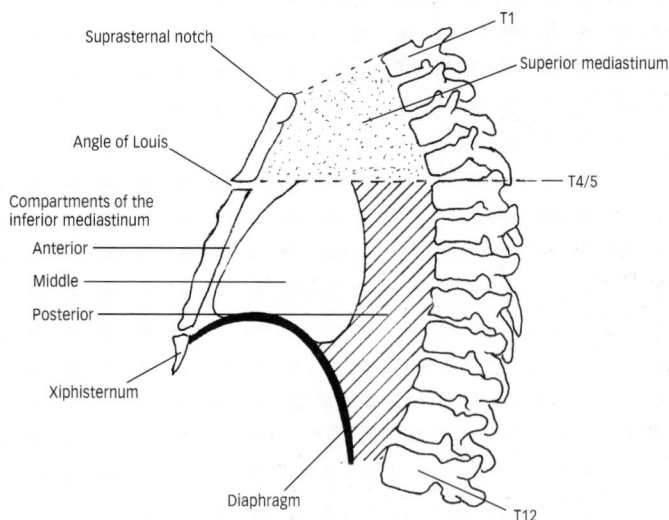

Suprasternal notch
T1
Superior mediastinum
Angle of Louis
T4/5
Compartments of the inferior mediastinum
Anterior
Middle
Posterior
Xiphisternum
Diaphragm
T12

The lower pole of the scapula overlies the seventh rib.

Although the thoracic viscera are completely enclosed within the bony cage of the chest, their positions are quite constant and can therefore be marked out with a fair degree of accuracy from the bony landmarks.

The lines of pleural reflection

The outline of the pleural margins can be marked out on the chest wall as follows (Fig. 6):

- The apex of the pleura extends about 3 cm above the medial third of the clavicle.
- The pleura then passes downwards and medially behind the sternoclavicular joint to meet the opposite pleura behind the sternum at the level of the sternal angle of Louis.
- At the fourth cartilage, the left pleural margin deflects to the lateral edge of the sternum. This corresponds to the cardiac notch of the underlying lung produced by the bulging to the left of the heart and pericardium. This deflection then descends to the sixth costal cartilage.
- On the right side, however, the pleural edge continues vertically downwards and projects somewhat below the right costo-xiphoid angle.

The pleural margin then descends on each side to lie at:

- the level of the eighth rib in the mid-clavicular line;
- the level of the tenth rib at the mid-axillary line;
- at the twelfth rib at the paravertebral level posteriorly.

Note that the pleural edge is at its lowest level in the mid-axillary line and also that posteriorly the margin extends slightly below the costal margin at the costo-vertebral angle.

From the practical point of view, the pleura is at risk of damage as it projects above the clavicle during operations on the neck, stab wounds in this region and, most especially, in attempts at subclavian venepuncture. Inferiorly, the pleura may be opened in resection of the twelfth rib during surgical access to the kidney or suprarenal gland.

The lungs

The surface projection of the lungs is somewhat less extensive than that of the parietal pleura (Fig. 6). Moreover, the lower border of the lung varies quite considerably with the phase of respiration.

The apex of the lung closely follows the line of the cervical pleura and the surface marking of the anterior border of the right lung corresponds to that of the right mediastinal pleura. However, on the left side the anterior border of the lung has a distinct notch, termed the cardiac notch, which passes behind the fifth and sixth costal cartilages.

The lower border of the lung has an excursion of between 5 to 8 cm in the extremes of respiration, but in the neutral position it lies along a line which may be marked out as crossing the sixth rib in the mid-clavicular line, the eighth rib in the mid-axillary line and which reaches the tenth rib adjacent to the vertebral column posteriorly. It will be noted that the lower border thus lies about two rib-breadths above the corresponding lower border of the parietal pleura.

The lung fissures

Each lung is divided by a deep oblique fissure and the right lung is further divided by a transverse fissure. Thus, the right lung is trilobed and the left bilobed.

The right oblique fissure can be marked out by a line which leaves the vertebral column posteriorly at the level of the fifth rib and then follows the rough direction of this rib, tending to lie slightly lower than this landmark, to end near the costo-chondral junction, either in the

Fig. 6(a).
Surface markings of the lungs and pleura (anterior aspect).

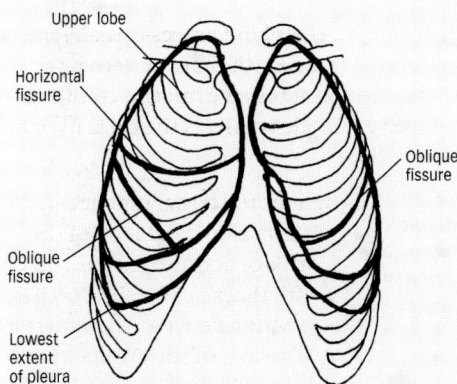

Fig. 6(b).
Surface markings of the lungs and pleura (posterior aspect).

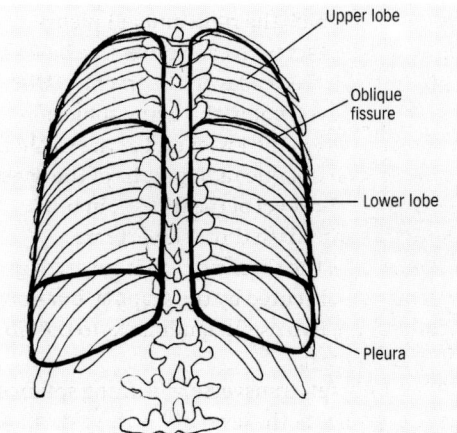

fifth space or at the level of the sixth rib. The left oblique fissure has a more variable origin, anywhere from the third to the fifth rib level, but its subsequent course is similar to that of the right side. A useful and quite accurate surface marking is to ask the subject to hold the arm above the head; the vertebral (medial) border of the scapula corresponds to the line of the oblique fissure.

The transverse fissure can be marked out by a horizontal line which runs backwards from the fourth right costal cartilage to reach the oblique fissure in the mid-axillary line at the level of the fifth rib or interspace.

These fissures are far from constant and more often than not the transverse fissure is either incomplete (about the half the specimens) or absent, in about 10% of cases.

The heart
The outline of the heart can be represented on the chest wall by an irregular quadrangle bounded by the following four points (Fig. 7):

(a) The lower border of the second left costal cartilage a finger's breadth from the edge of the sternum.
(b) The upper border of the third right costal cartilage a finger's breadth from the sternal edge.
(c) The sixth right costal cartilage a finger's breadth from the sternum.
(d) The fifth left intercostal space 9 cm from the midline.

The left border of the heart, which is indicated by the curved line which joins points (a) and (d), is formed almost entirely by the left ventricle, apart from superiorly, where the apex of the auricular appendage of the left atrium peeps round the left border. The lower border (the horizontal line joining points (c) and (d), corresponds to the right ventricle and the

Fig. 7. **Surface markings of the heart**.

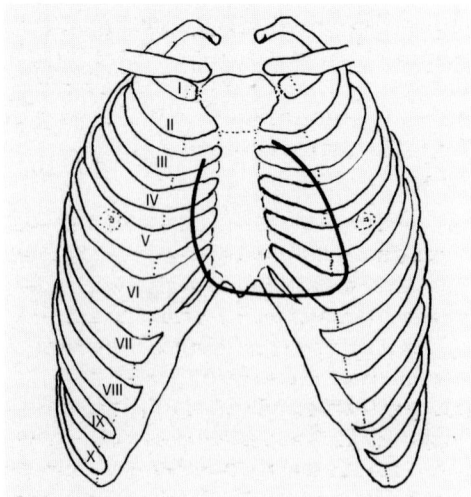

apical part of the left ventricle, while the right border demarcated by the line (which joins points (b) and (c)), is formed entirely by the right atrium.

To outline the heart as described above is something of an academic exercise. In practice, it is sufficient to note that the boundaries of the heart are demarcated above and below by the body of the sternum, whereas the great vessels lie behind the manubrium. A useful approximation to the surface markings of the heart is for the subject to place his closed right fist, palmar surface against the chest, over the body of the sternum. The fist corresponds closely to what should be the normal heart outline of the subject. Note that the fist projects over to the left side along its inferior (ulnar) border to mimic the projection of the heart apex to the left.

The great vessels
The aortic arch can be marked out by a curved line which commences behind the manubrium at the level of the second right costal cartilage (the sternal angle of Louis) arches upwards to the midpoint of the manubrium sterni, then passes downwards to the level of the second left costal cartilage to become the descending aorta. The brachiocephalic artery on the right side and the common carotid artery on the left can be marked out by lines which arise behind the midpoint of the manubrium and ascend to the right and left sternoclavicular joints respectively.

The right brachiocephalic vein commences behind the medial end of the clavicle, just lateral to the right sternoclavicular joint, where it is formed by the junction of the right internal jugular and right subclavian veins, to pass vertically downwards behind the superior portion of the manubrium. The longer left brachiocephalic vein passes almost horizontally from behind the medial end of the left clavicle to join the right brachiocephalic vein behind the superior portion of the manubrium at the level of its junction with the first costal cartilage. Both join to form the superior vena cava at this point.

The superior vena cava then descends as a 2 cm wide band along the right sternal margin to enter the right atrium at the level of the third right costal cartilage. The azygos vein enters the superior vena cava at the level of the sternal angle of Louis.

The vessels of the thoracic wall
The surface markings of the vessels of the thoracic wall are of importance if these structures are to be avoided in the performance of aspiration of the chest.

The internal thoracic (internal mammary) vessels run vertically downwards behind the costal cartilages half an inch (1.5 cm), or approximately a finger's breadth, from the lateral border of the sternum. The intercostal vessels lie immediately below their corresponding ribs (the vein above the artery). It is therefore safe to pass a needle immediately above a rib while it is more dangerous to pass it immediately below.

Abdomen

The bony margins of the abdomen (Fig. 8) are bounded above centrally by the xiphoid and flanked by the costal margin on either side. The tip of the lower border of the ninth costal cartilage can usually be defined as a distinct step along this border.

Inferiorly, the midline limit is marked by the upper border of the pubic symphysis. Laterally from this extends the pubic crest which ends at the pubic tubercle, about 2.5 cm from the midline. This tubercle can be identified by direct palpation in a thin subject but can be detected, even in the obese, by running the fingers along the tendon of adductor longus, which is tensed by flexion, abduction and external rotation of the thigh, to its origin immediately below the tubercle.

For the purpose of description, the abdomen can be divided by a number of imaginary horizontal and vertical lines. The horizontal planes are also used to define approximate vertebral levels and the position of some relatively fixed intra-abdominal viscera.

Horizontal planes

(a) The xiphisternal plane passes through the xiphoid at the level of the ninth thoracic vertebra. This plane marks the level of the upper border of the liver, the central part of the diaphragm and the lower margin of the heart. Note, however, that the position of these structures varies with the position of the body, the phase of respiration and the body habitus.

(b) The transpyloric plane. This was defined by Addison as a point midway between the suprasternal notch of the manubrium and the upper border of the symphysis pubis. In clinical practice it corresponds to the hand's breadth of the subject below the xiphoid. This plane passes through the body of the first lumbar vertebra and laterally passes through the costal margin at the ninth costal cartilage (usually marked by a distinct step at the costal margin).

Structures demarcated by this plane include:

- the fundus of the gall bladder at the costal margin on the right side;
- the origin of the superior mesenteric artery from the aorta; the neck of the pancreas;
- the junction of the superior mesenteric and splenic veins to form the origin of the portal vein;
- the hila of both kidneys together with their vascular pedicle; posteriorly, the termination of the spinal cord.

In spite of its name, the plane does not typically correspond with the pylorus of the stomach. Indeed, the position of the pylorus, together with the rest of the stomach, depends on body type, extent of gastric filling and the position of the subject. In the erect position and with the stomach full and with a stomach of the J-shape the pylorus may descend to the level of the third lumbar vertebra or even below.

(c) The subcostal plane passes across the lower margins of the thoracic cage formed by the tenth costal cartilage on each side. It transects the third lumbar vertebral body. This indicates the level of origin of the inferior mesenteric artery from the aorta.

(d) The supracristal plane joins the highest point of the iliac crest on each side. It transects the body of the fourth lumbar vertebra and corresponds to the level of bifurcation

8.
abdominal zones.

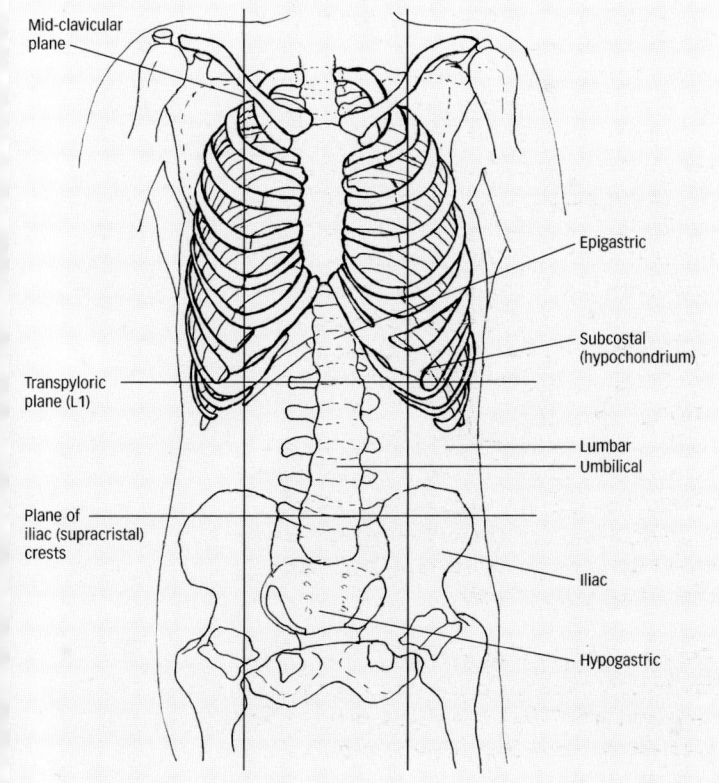

Mid-clavicular plane

Transpyloric plane (L1)

Plane of iliac (supracristal) crests

Epigastric

Subcostal (hypochondrium)

Lumbar
Umbilical

Iliac

Hypogastric

of the aorta. It is a useful landmark in the performance of a lumbar puncture. This procedure should be carried out below this level, when the spinal theca will be punctured at an intervertebral space safely below the termination of the spinal cord (see p. 9).

(e) The plane of the pubic crest passes through the termination of the sacrum.

Vertical planes

(a) The midline passes from the xiphoid to the pubic symphysis (Fig. 8). It passes through the umbilicus which is an obvious but somewhat inconstant landmark. In the normal recumbent adult, it lies at the level of the disc between the third and fourth lumbar vertebrae so that the aorta bifurcates 2 cm distal to it. However, in the erect position, in subjects with a pendulous abdomen and in the child, the umbilicus is at a lower level. The median groove of the linea alba can readily be seen in the thin subject when the abdominal muscles are tensed. It is wide and obvious above the umbilicus but almost linear and invisible below this level.

(b) The mid-clavicular line passes vertically downwards through the midpoint of the clavicle. It is sometimes termed the lateral, or the mammary, line. Inferiorly it passes through a point midway between the anterior superior iliac spine and the symphysis pubis.

The abdominal regions

The abdomen is divided into nine regions, which are used for descriptive localization. The regions are constructed of a combination of the two mid-clavicular lines with two transverse lines constructed by dividing the distance between the xiphoid and the symphysis pubis into thirds.

The nine regions thus formed are termed (Fig. 9):

(a) The epigastrium, or epigastric region.
(b) The right and left hypochondrium, or subcostal region.
(c) The umbilical or periumbilical region.
(d) The right and left lumbar region.
(e) The hypogastrium or suprapubic region.
(f) The right and left iliac region or fossa.

Palpable abdominal organs

In normal subjects, the abdominal aorta can be felt by deep palpation. Its pulsations can be felt by pressing firmly in the midline downwards on to the vertebral column with the subject recumbent. It bifurcates at the level of the fourth lumbar vertebra in the supracristal plane just below the level of the umbilicus. The other abdominal organs or viscera are often totally impalpable. However, the lower border of the normal liver may be felt below the right costal margin, the lower pole of the normal right kidney may sometimes be felt by bimanual palpation of the right flank during deep inspiration, especially in a thin female subject. It is not rare to palpate a soft gurgling caecum in the right iliac fossa in thin females. The sigmoid colon may be felt as a sausage-shaped swelling in the left iliac fossa, particularly if the bowel is loaded with faeces.

The introduction of imaging of the abdominal viscera has shown that considerable variations occur in what was once believed to be 'normal' anatomy. Little emphasis is now placed on specific definition of the surface outlines of the intra-abdominal structures.

The back

In the midline a median furrow extends from the external occipital protuberance downwards to the natal cleft. In the cervical region, the tips of the spines of the cervical vertebrae are obscured by the overlying tough, fibrous ligamentum nuchae. This terminates inferiorly at the spine of the seventh cervical vertebra, which can be felt and may be visible as the highest projection in this region (the vertebra prominens). Immediately below this, the spine of the first thoracic vertebra can be felt and is usually more prominent than the seventh cervical spine. From here downwards the successive spines can be felt (Fig. 9).

Fig. 9.
Anatomical landmarks: posterior trunk.

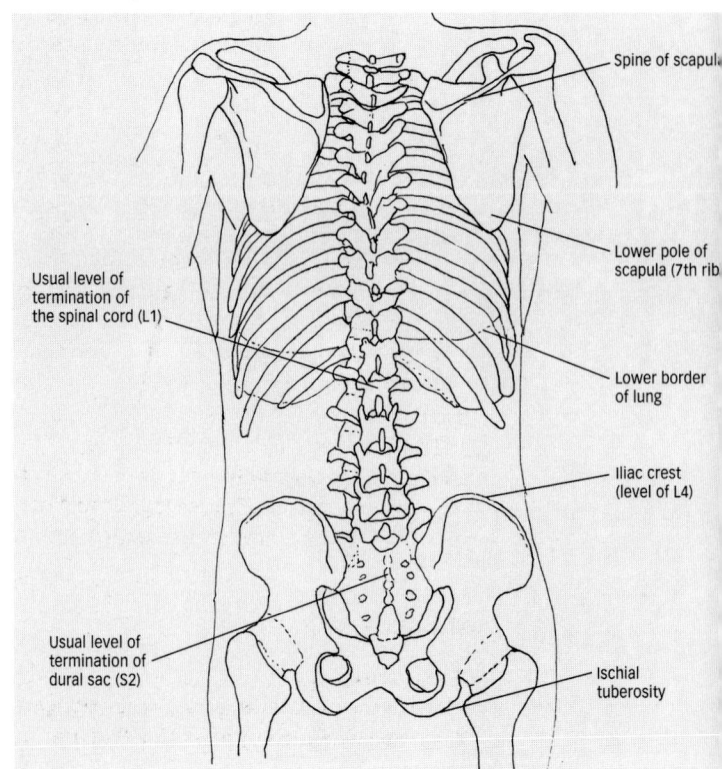

Spine of scapula
Lower pole of scapula (7th rib)
Lower border of lung
Iliac crest (level of L4)
Ischial tuberosity
Usual level of termination of the spinal cord (L1)
Usual level of termination of dural sac (S2)

At the sides of the lower part of the back, the iliac crest can be palpated through its whole length downwards and medially to the posterior superior iliac spine. This lies 5 cm from the midline. This corresponds to the position of the obviously visible sacral dimple. A line joining the dimple of each side passes through the second sacral spine and marks the level of the centre of the sacroiliac joint. This is also the level of the termination of the dural sac.

The spinal cord

The surface markings of the spinal cord and its membranes are of obvious clinical relevance.

Up to the third fetal month, the spinal cord extends the length of the vertebral column. As a result of more rapid differential growth of the vertebrae compared with the cord, at birth the spinal cord terminates at the lower border of the third lumbar vertebra. In the adult, the termination of the cord is usually found at the level of the disc between the first and second lumbar bodies. However, there is considerable variation in this level which ranges frequently from the body of the first to the body of the second lumbar vertebra. Rarely the range extends to the twelfth thoracic vertebra above down to the third lumbar vertebra.

The differential growth between the spinal cord and the vertebral column results in the lumbar and sacral nerve roots becoming considerably elongated in their passage to their corresponding intervertebral foramina. This results in the formation of the cauda equina. In contrast, the cervical roots pass almost laterally in their intraspinal course and the upper thoracic roots incline only slightly. As an approximate guide, there is one segment difference in the cervical cord between the cord segment and the vertebral body level, two in the upper thoracic region, three in the lower thoracic zone and four to five in the region of the lumbar and sacral cord.

The lower limit of the spinal cord (the conus medullaris) lies a little above the level of the elbow joint when the arm is by the side and is approximately demarcated anteriorly by the transpyloric plane.

The dural sac and its contained subarachnoid space usually extends to the level of the second segment of the sacrum. This corresponds to the line joining the sacral dimples.

The upper limb

Bony landmarks
Much of the skeletal anatomy of the upper limb can be defined by palpation (Fig. 10).

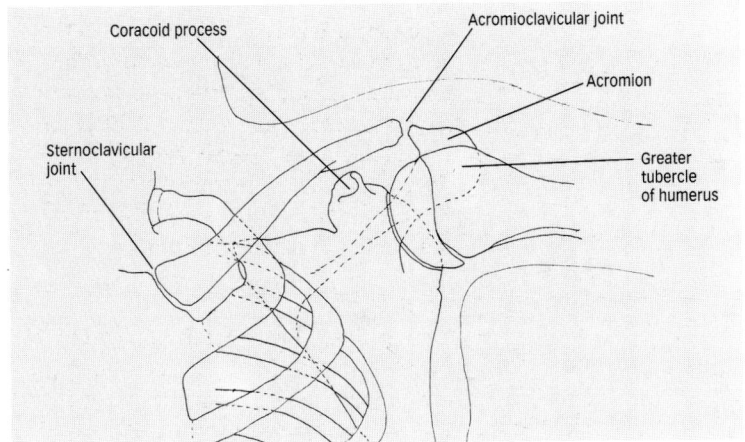

Fig. 10.
Bony landmarks: left shoulder.

The clavicle is visible and palpable throughout its course. Its outline can be traced from the expanded sternal end, at the lateral boundary of the suprasternal notch, to its flattened acromial extremity. Its medial two-thirds is convex forwards, while its lateral one-third is concave anteriorly. Medially, it forms the sternoclavicular joint, which is a ball and socket joint and which can be felt to move in a reciprocal direction from the movements of the shoulder joint.

Laterally, the line of the acromioclavicular joint can be felt as a distinct transversely placed step. The acromion process of the scapula can then be traced from this joint to its lateral extremity and then backwards until it meets the crest of the spine of the scapula which can be palpated across the scapula to reach the medial (vertebral) scapular border. The spine is easily visible in a thin subject. Below, the medial border of the scapula ends at the inferior angle, which overlies the seventh rib.

Inferior to the clavicle, at the junction of its medial convex and lateral concave portions can be seen a small depression which lies between the origins of pectoralis major and the deltoid. This is the infraclavicular fossa (or deltopectoral triangle). In this groove lies the cephalic vein as it passes up the lateral aspect of the upper arm on its way to drain into the subclavian vein. Just to the lateral side of this fossa, about 2.5 cm below the clavicle, and under cover of the fibres of the deltoid can be felt the coracoid process of the scapula and indeed this can be seen in a very thin subject. Confirm that this is part of the scapula and not the humerus because it will not move when the humerus is rotated. Palpation lateral to the coracoid process reveals another bony swelling; this is the lesser tubercle of the humerus and this, in contrast, will be felt to move as the humerus is rotated laterally or medially. The most lateral extremity of the shoulder is the greater tubercle of the humerus. The head of the humerus is palpated on deep pressure in the apex of the axilla when the arm is raised and can be felt to rotate on movement of the upper limb.

The shaft of the humerus can be felt rather vaguely throughout its course since it is obscured by overlying muscles. At the elbow (Fig. 11) the medial, and less prominent, lateral epicondyle are easily felt and each can be traced upwards as the medial and lateral supracondylar ridge on either side. The ulnar nerve can be rolled posteriorly as it runs behind the medial epicondyle. Distal to the lateral epicondyle, and in the floor of a depression that can be seen posteriorly with the elbow extended can be felt the head of the radius. This can be felt to rotate as the forearm is pronated and supinated. Between the lateral epicondyle and the radial head can be felt a distinct transverse depression, which is the humeroradial section of the elbow joint.

The olecranon is obvious at the tip of the elbow. Its posterior surface is subcutaneous and forms a triangle apex downwards. From this apex, the posterior border of the ulna is subcutaneous and can be felt throughout its whole extent to the styloid process of the ulna inferiorly. This projects distally from the postero-medial aspect of the rounded head of the ulna, which forms the obvious elevation on the posterior aspect of the ulnar side of the pronated wrist.

In contrast, the shaft of the radius can only be felt indistinctly because of its covering of muscles. Its expanded lower end forms a slight elevation on the radial side of the wrist and can be traced downwards into the styloid process of the radius (Fig. 12). This is easily felt in the most proximal part of the obvious anatom-

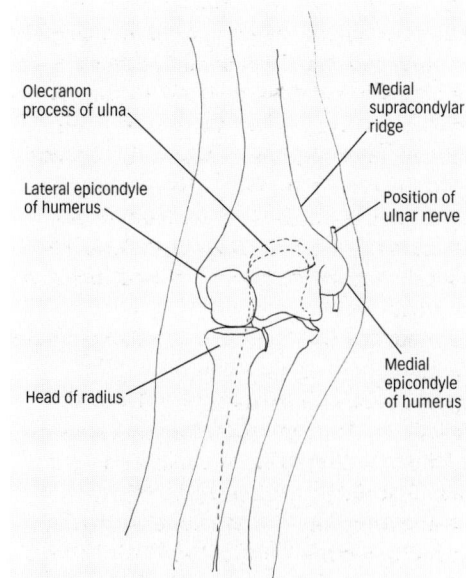

Fig. 12.
Palpable landmarks: wrist and hand.

ical snuffbox. The expanded distal end of the posterior aspect of the radius is somewhat obscured by the overlying extensor tendons, but in spite of this can be both seen and felt.

Note that the styloid process of the ulna projects less distally than that of the radius. This allows a greater degree of adduction than of abduction of the wrist joint.

The anterior line of the wrist joint is demarcated by the proximal of the two transverse skin creases at the wrist. The more distal crease, in fact, lies superficial to the proximal carpal bones. Four of the bones of the carpus can be palpated and positively identified. The tubercle of the scaphoid lies at the base of the thenar eminence; it can often be seen as a small elevation. Immediately distal to it, the crest of the trapezium can be identified on deep pressure. Both these bones can also be palpated in the anatomical snuffbox immediately distal to the radius and the wrist joint. The pisiform can be felt, and usually seen, at the proximal extremity of the hypothenar eminence. On flexing the wrist the tendon of flexor carpi ulnaris can be felt, and often seen, to insert into it. The hook of the hamate lies 2.5 cm distal to the pisiform and can be felt on deep pressure. This is uncomfortable because the superficial division of the ulnar nerve lies over the bone at this point.

Fig. 11.
Bony landmarks: right elbow.

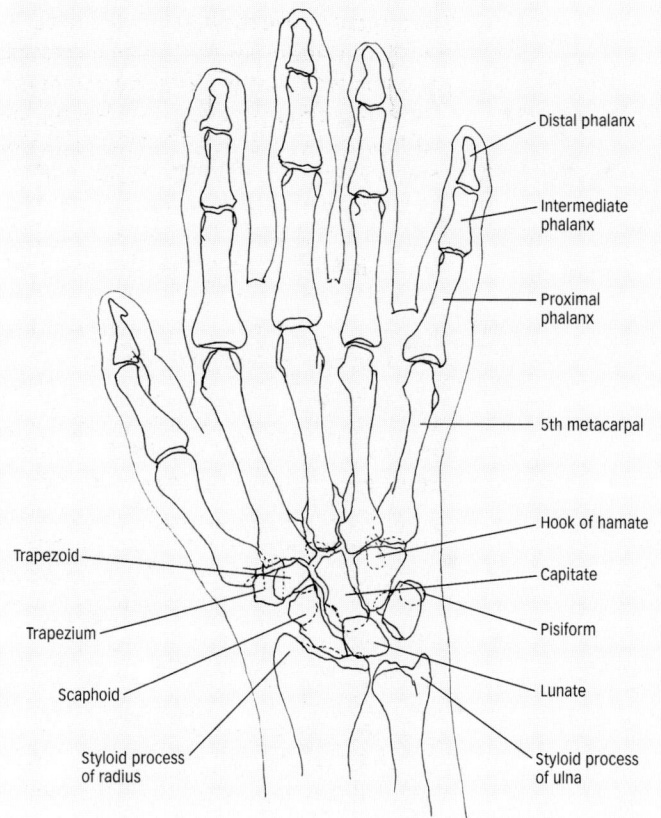

Pulses

The arterial tree in the upper limb can be traced from above downwards by successive palpation of the pulses. The third part of the subclavian artery can be felt by pressing downwards onto the first rib behind the midpoint of the clavicle with the head deviated to the same side in order to relax the neck muscles. This palpation is uncomfortable because of pressure against the adjacent trunks of the brachial plexus.

The axillary artery can be felt by pressing against the upper shaft of the humerus in front of the posterior axillary fold. It will usually be accompanied by paraesthesiae along the radial side of the palm of the hand due to pressure on the subjacent median nerve.

The brachial artery pulse can be felt in the furrow along the medial side of the biceps muscle and can be felt more distally adjacent to, and on the medial side of, the biceps tendon immediately above the elbow where the artery lies directly in front of the lower end of the shaft of the humerus.

The radial artery is readily felt at the wrist in the interval between the tendon of flexor carpi radialis and the lower part of the anterior border of the distal radius on the lateral side. Its pulsation can be picked up again in the anatomical snuffbox.

The ulnar artery can be felt less easily at the wrist immediately to the radial side of the tendon of flexor carpi ulnaris. Here it lies on the radial side of the adjacent ulnar nerve.

The superficial veins

The irregular plexus of the dorsal venous arch is visible on the back of the hand and its arrangement is highly variable. The cephalic vein arises from the radial extremity of the arch and can be both seen and felt, if a venous tourniquet is applied, as it lies immediately posterior to the styloid process of the radius at the wrist. This is a common site for intravenous cannulation. The cephalic vein then ascends along the radial border of the forearm to the lateral side of the antecubital fossa and then lies in a groove along the lateral border of the biceps. In a well-developed subject it may be visible throughout its course before it dives beneath the deep fascia at the distal border of pectoralis major. The vein then lies in a groove between this muscle and the deltoid, then finally pierces the clavipectoral fascia to enter the axillary vein. The groove between pectoralis major and deltoid is a conveniently identifiable site for a cutdown if no other superficial vein can be found. A catheter inserted into the cephalic vein, however, frequently fails to enter the axillary vein because of the sharp curve as it passes through the clavipectoral fascia and because a valve commonly guards this junction.

The basilic vein originates from the ulnar side of the dorsal venous arch and ascends along the ulnar side of the forearm. Its position in the forearm is quite variable and there are usually other minor superficial veins ascending along the anterior aspect of the forearm. The basilic vein then ascends along the medial border of the biceps before piercing the deep fascia at the middle of the upper arm. Near the lower border of the axilla, it is joined by the venae comitantes of the brachial vein to form the axillary vein.

The median cubital vein (which may also be termed the median basilic or median cephalic vein) usually arises from the cephalic vein about 2.5 cm distal to the lateral epicondyle of the humerus. It then runs upwards and medially to join the basilic vein about 2.5 cm above the transverse crease of the elbow to give a rather drunken H-shaped arrangement. The median cubital vein receives a number of tributaries from the veins running along the front of the forearm, as well as giving off a deep median vein, which pierces the deep fascia roofing the antecubital fossa to join the venae comitantes of the brachial vein. A frequent variation is for a median forearm vein to bifurcate just distal to the antecubital fossa. One limb then passes to the cephalic and the other to the basilic vein, to give an M-shaped pattern.

In a plump upper limb, the median cubital vein may be the only superficial vein which can be made obvious. It is quite safe to use this for venepuncture but there is a danger in employing this vein for an intravenous injection. This is because the brachial artery lies immediately deep to the vein and may be inadvertently punctured. Fortunately a sheet of deep fascia, termed the bicipital aponeurosis, which arises from the medial border of the lower end of the biceps muscle and its tendon, is placed between the two. This was much appreciated by the Barber–Surgeons of old who used the antecubital vein for blood-letting; they named it the 'grâce à Dieu' (praise be to God) fascia.

The surface markings for cannulation of the subclavian vein are important. It may be approached either from below or above the clavicle. The patient is tipped head downwards and the head turned to the opposite side. For infraclavicular puncture, the needle is inserted below the midpoint of the clavicle and is directed medially and upwards behind the clavicle towards the tip of the index finger of the operator placed deeply into the suprasternal notch. Supraclavicular puncture is achieved by inserting the needle through a point which joins the medial one-third and lateral two-thirds of the clavicle about 2 cm above the clavicle. This corresponds to the lateral border of the clavicular head of the sterno-cleidomastoid muscle. The needle is then inserted medially and upwards towards the subclavian vein, which lies about 2.5 cm behind the sternoclavicular joint.

The lower limb

The upper bony landmarks of the lower limb, the iliac crest, its anterior termination at the anterior superior iliac spine and its posterior termination, at the posterior superior iliac spine, have already been described (p. 9). The ischial tuberosity is readily palpated in the inferior portion of the buttock. In the standing position, the tuberosity is covered by the fleshy fibres of gluteus maximus, but when the hip is flexed, this muscle slips above the tuberosity so that, when we sit, the tuberosity adopts a subcutaneous position, separated from the skin only by fat and a bursa.

The greater trochanter of the femur lies a hand's breadth below the midpoint of the iliac crest. It can be felt and usually seen as the prominence in front of a hollow on the side of the hip. It is the only part of the proximal femur which can be palpated distinctly and it can be felt to move as the hip is rotated. The shaft of the femur can only be vaguely felt on deep palpation through the muscles of the thigh. Distally, the medial aspect of the medial condyle and the lateral aspect of the lateral condyle of the femur can be palpated, and part of the femoral articular surface can be felt on either side of the lower part of the patella (Fig. 13).

The patella is subcutaneous and readily palpated. When the knee is fully extended, the patella can be moved from side to side over the lower articular surface of the femur because the quadriceps femoris is relaxed. The lower limit of the patella terminates in the ligamentum patellae, which can be felt to descend and insert into the tibial tuberosity.

It is important to note that the knee joint extends a handsbreadth above the upper border of the patella as the suprapatellar pouch. This becomes obviously distended when there is a significant effusion of fluid into the knee joint. The tibial condyles are visible and palpable on either side of the ligamentum patellae. When the knee is in the flexed position, their anterior margins can be felt in the depression on either side of this ligament. Above them,

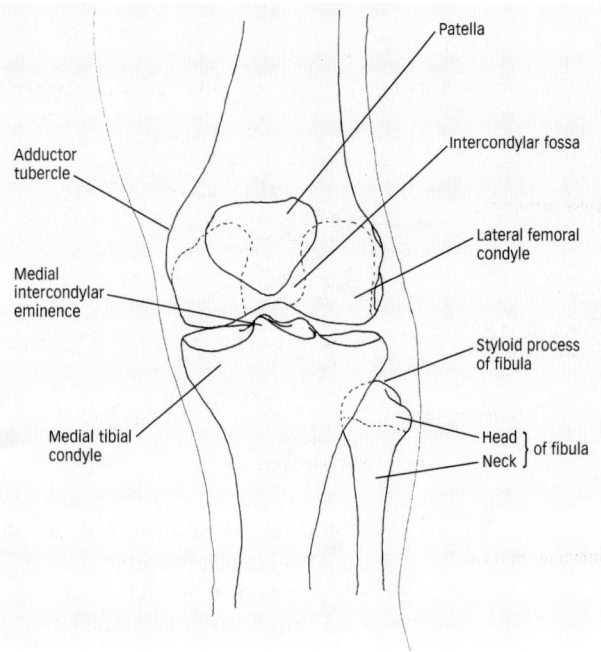

Fig. 13.
Bony landmarks: knee.

a distinct groove can be felt, which demarcates the line of the knee joint.

The head of the fibula can be felt as a projection on the upper part of the postero-lateral aspects of the leg. Below the head can be felt the neck of the fibula, around which passes the common peroneal nerve, which can be felt indistinctly at this point. The shaft of the fibula can only be felt indistinctly through its overlying muscles but inferiorly the lateral malleolus of the fibula forms a conspicuous projection on the lateral side of the ankle. This lateral aspect of the lateral malleolus continues superiorly with an elongated triangular area of the lower shaft of the fibula which is also subcutaneous. The subcutaneous medial surface of the tibia can be felt throughout its course from the medial condyle of the tibia above to the visible prominence of the medial malleolus below. It is crossed only by the great saphenous vein and the accompanying saphenous nerve immediately in front of the medial malleolus and here the vein is easily visible when the leg is dependent. The medial malleolus descends less than the lateral malleolus and is placed on a more anterior plane. It is the more extensive projection of the lateral malleolus that accounts for the fact that eversion of the angle is more limited than inversion. Much of the bony anatomy of the foot is palpable (Fig. 14). The conspicuous tendo calcaneus (Achilles tendon) is obvious on the posterior aspect of the lower leg and can be followed downwards into its insertion into the posterior aspect of the calcaneus. On the dorsum of the foot, the upper anterior part of the calcaneus can be palpated in front of the lateral

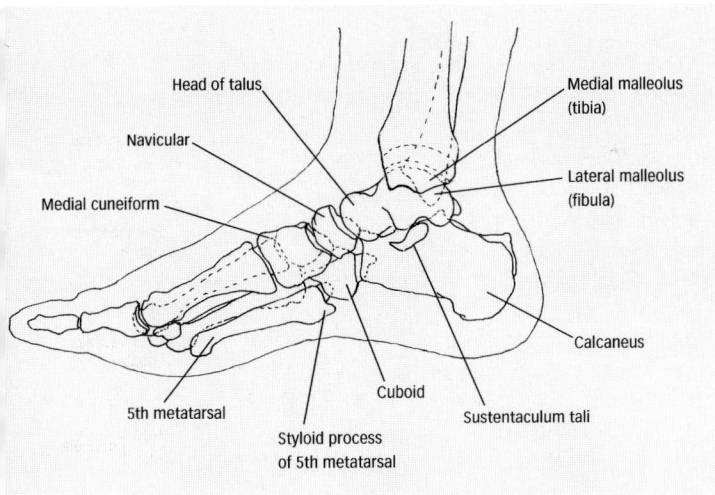

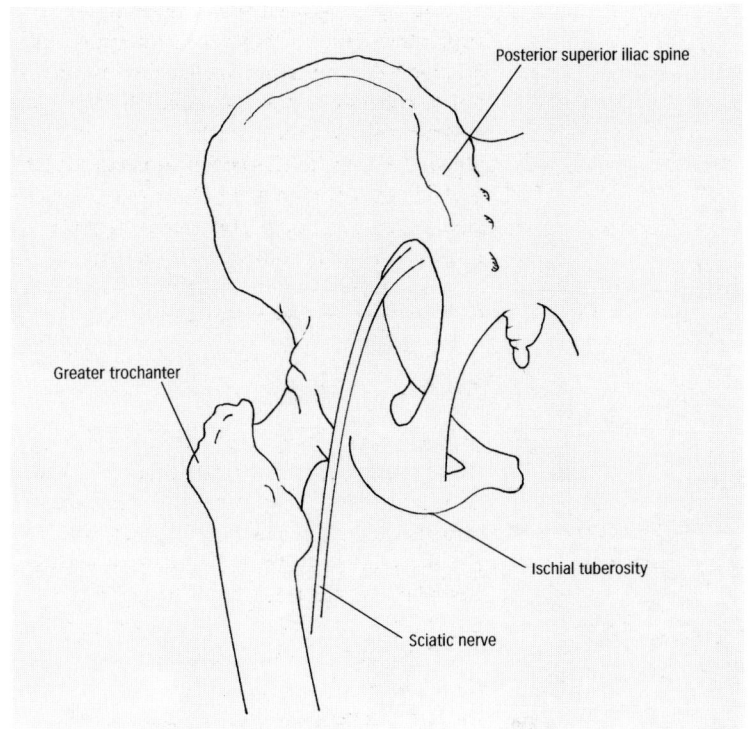

malleolus. The lateral surface of the calcaneus can be felt on the lateral aspect of the heel and usually its peroneal tubercle can be felt 2 cm below the tip of the lateral malleolus. Medially, the sustentaculum tali of the calcaneus can be felt 2 cm below the medial malleolus. With the foot inverted, the upper part of the head of the talus can be felt and usually seen about 3 cm anterior to the distal end of the tibia. The tuberosity of the navicular can be felt and is often visible 2.5 cm in front of the sustentaculum tali. Anterior to this, the medial cuneiform can be identified by tracing the tendon of tibialis anterior into it when the foot is inverted and extended. The styloid process at the base of the fifth metatarsal is palpable on the lateral side of the foot and marks the insertion of peroneus brevis.

In the standing position, the foot rests on the posterior part of the inferior surface of the calcaneus, on the heads of the metatarsal bones and, to a lesser extent, on the lateral border of the foot, which forms the lateral longitudinal arch of the foot. The instep, which corresponds to the medial longitudinal arch, is elevated from the ground.

The sciatic nerve

Because of the risk of damage to the sciatic nerve from intramuscular injections, its exact surface markings are of considerable importance. The course of the nerve (Fig. 15) can be represented by a line which commences at a point midway between the posterior superior iliac spine (shown by the lumbar dimple) and the ischial tuberosity and which then curves outwards and downwards through a point midway between the greater trochanter of the femur and the ischial tuberosity. Continue the line vertically downwards in the midline of the posterior aspect of the thigh to the upper angle of the popliteal fossa.

Arteries

The femoral artery (Fig. 16) enters the thigh at a point midway between the anterior superior iliac spine and the midline pubic symphysis. Its course down the leg can be represented by the upper two-thirds of the line which joints that point to the adductor tubercle when the thigh is flexed, abducted and laterally rotated. The adductor tubercle itself is felt by sliding the hand down the medial side of the thigh until it hits the first bony prominence immediately above the medial condyle of the femur.

At its origin, the pulsations of the femoral artery can be felt as this vessel emerges from under the inguinal ligament to lie in front of the tendon of psoas major as this crosses the superior ramus of the pubis. The pulse is a useful landmark to the position of the head of the femur. A finger's breadth lateral to the femoral pulse marks the position of the femoral nerve and immediately medial to the pulse is the surface marking of both the femoral vein and great saphenous vein (see below). The popliteal artery can be represented by a line which begins at the junction of the middle and lower one-third of the thigh along the line drawn from the femoral pulse at the groin to the adductor tubercle. The artery then runs downwards and laterally in the popliteal fossa to reach the midline at the level of the knee joint. It then descends to the level of the tibial tubercle, where it bifurcates into the anterior and posterior tibial arteries. The popliteal pulse is often difficult to feel.

Fig. 15.
The surface markings of the sciatic nerve. The midpoint between the ischial tuberosity and the posterior superior iliac spine is joined to the midpoint between the ischial tuberosity and the greater trochanter by a curved line which is continued vertically down the back of the leg. This line represents the course of the sciatic nerve.

Fig. 16.
The surface markings of the
femoral artery; the upper
two-thirds of a line joining
the mid-inguinal point
(halfway between the
anterior superior iliac spine
and the symphysis pubis),
to the adductor tubercle.

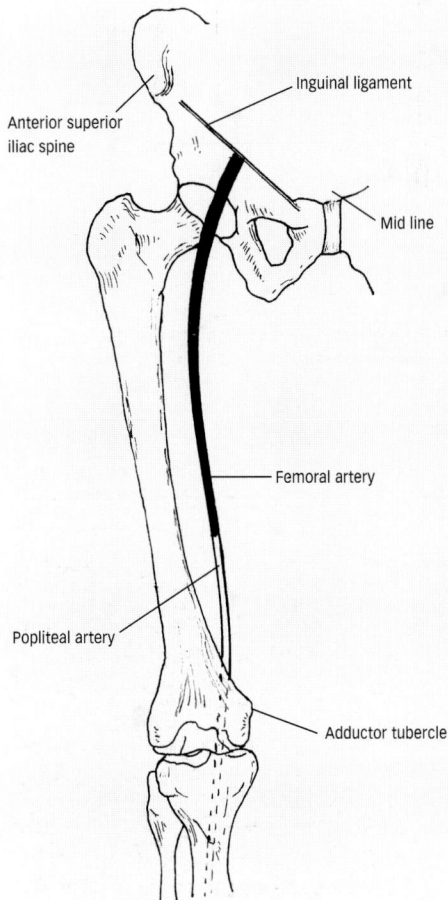

Fig. 16.
The surface markings of the femoral artery; the upper two-thirds of a line joining the mid-inguinal point (halfway between the anterior superior iliac spine and the symphysis pubis), to the adductor tubercle.

Anterior superior iliac spine

Inguinal ligament

Mid line

Femoral artery

Popliteal artery

Adductor tubercle

It is usually palpated with the patient lying on his back and with the knee bent to a right angle, the foot resting on the bed. This relaxes the tense popliteal fascia, which roofs the fossa. The pulse is felt by deep pressure over the midline of the fossa against the popliteal surface of the femur. An alternative method is to lie the subject face downwards with the knee bent to a right angle and supported by the examiner so that the muscles are relaxed.

The pulse of dorsalis pedis, the termination of the anterior tribial artery, is felt immediately lateral to the tendon of extensor hallucis longus against the underlying tarsal bones. That of the posterior tibial artery is sought by palpation behind the medial malleolus as the artery runs between the tendons of flexor hallucis longus and flexor digitorum longus.

The superficial veins
The dorsal venous arch, together with its tributaries, forms a conspicuous feature of the dorsum of the foot and curves, convex forwards, across the metatarsal bones. From its medial end, the great saphenous vein arises and runs upwards and backwards immediately in front of the medial malleolus to cross the subcutaneous surface of the tibia. It is accompanied by the saphenous nerve (which arises from the femoral nerve at the groin and which runs down to supply the medial side of the leg to the base of the great toe), and which usually lies in front of the vein. This nerve is a occasionally damaged in varicose vein surgery. The small saphenous vein arises from the lateral extremity of the dorsal venous arch. It then passes posterior to the lateral malleolus and drains into the popliteal vein in the popliteal fossa.

The surface marking of the great saphenous vein can be indicated by a line passing from the obviously visible vein in front of the medial malleolus to a point a hand's breadth behind the patella at the level of the knee joint and then upwards to a point a finger's breadth medial to the femoral pulse, where the vein drains into the femoral vein at the groin.

The anatomy of surgical access in upper respiratory obstruction

In an acute emergency, with the patient dying of laryngeal obstruction, intubation of the trachea can be carried out via the cricothyroid ligament or through the trachea itself.

Cricothyroid puncture (laryngotomy)

To perform a tracheostomy does require a modicum of surgical skill and is not a particularly easy operation. In an acute emergency, a cricothyroid puncture may be a life-saving temporary procedure, which has the merit of requiring little prowess on behalf of the operator. The head of the patient is firmly held in the midline position with the neck fully extended. The operator grasps the larynx between the thumb and little finger of the left hand and palpates the groove between the cricoid and the thyroid cartilages with the left index finger. Any available cutting instrument is used to make a 2.5 cm transverse incision over this groove through skin, deep fascia and the avascular cricothyroid ligament to open into the larynx (Fig. 17). The knife handle then levers open a space through which any suitable tube is passed downwards into the trachea. Even if nothing at all is to hand, direct mouth-to-larynx artificial respiration can be applied through the opening.

The procedure is made even easier if a special trocar and cannula in a sterile pack specially designed for cricothyroid puncture is available in the department.

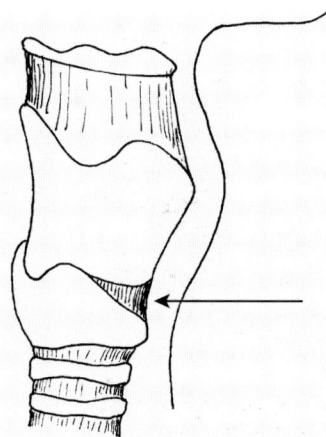

Fig. 17.
Site for cricothyroid puncture (arrowed). The soft area between the cricoid and thyroid cartilages is easily palpated in the midline and is relatively avascular.
(Redrawn from Ellis & Feldman, 1996)

Tracheostomy

Anterior relations of the cervical portion of the trachea are naturally of importance in performing a tracheostomy. The head is kept fully extended with a sand bag or firm pillow placed between the patient's shoulders. The head must be maintained absolutely straight with the chin and the sternal notch in a straight line. From the cosmetic point of view, it is better to use a short transverse incision placed mid-way between the cricoid cartilage (which is easily felt), and the suprasternal notch. The tyro may find in an emergency that it is safer to use a vertical incision which passes from the lower border of the thyroid cartilage to just above the suprasternal notch.

The great anatomical and surgical secret of the operation is to keep exactly in the midline. In doing so, the major vessels of the neck are out of danger. The skin incision is deepened to the investing layer of deep fascia, which is split and held apart by retractors. The first ring of the trachea now comes into view and the position of the trachea is carefully checked by

palpation of its rings. It is usually possible to push the isthmus of the thyroid gland downwards to expose the upper rings of the trachea. Occasionally, the isthmus is enlarged and, under these circumstances,
it must be lifted up by blunt dissection and divided vertically between artery forceps. The trachea is opened by a small transverse incision between the second and third rings. This alone will suffice to insert a tube, but it is advisable to make a small window by removing portions of the second and third, or third and fourth rings, using a fine scalpel or scissors. (Fig. 18). A tracheostomy tube of the largest size that will fit the tracheostome comfortably is inserted. The trachea is aspirated through it, and the wound loosely closed with two or three skin sutures.

The introduction of the mini-tracheostomy tube had made construction of a small tracheostomy possible as a temporary emergency procedure with a minimum of dissection.

Reference
Ellis, H. & Feldman, S. (1996,
Anatomy for Anaesthetists,
7th edn. Oxford: Blackwell
Scientific.

Fig. 18(a).
Tracheostomy. The incision is placed midway between the cricoid cartilage and the suprasternal notch

Fig. 18(b).
The investing layer of fascia covering the pretracheal muscles is exposed.

Fig. 18(c).
The isthmus of the thyroid is cleared. This must either be divided between artery forceps or displaced downwards.

Fig. 18(d).
A tracheal window is fashioned by resecting a circular area through the second and third, or third and fourth cartilaginous rings. A vertical incision alone is inadequate.

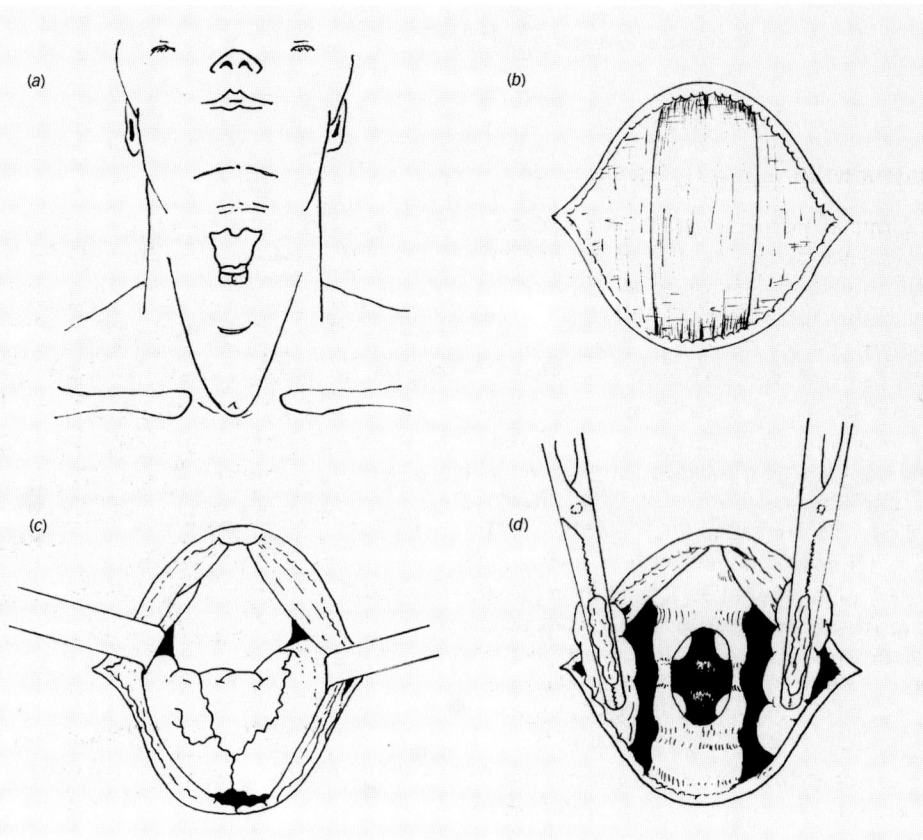

(a) (b) (c) (d)

2

The skull and brain

P. BUTLER
and M. A. JEFFREE

Introduction and imaging methods

Computed tomography (CT) and magnetic resonance imaging (MRI) are the most commonly performed imaging investigations of the brain. Skull radiography remains the investigation of choice for the detection of fractures but it is a relatively insensitive indicator of cerebral pathology.

Anatomical detail is far better displayed by MRI than by CT, although both are valuable in clinical practice. The contrast sensitivity of MRI is superior to that of CT and MRI can also provide images in multiple planes without the need to alter the patient's position in the scanner. In most cases it is usual to rely on imaging in the three orthogonal planes (axial, coronal and sagittal), although other scan planes are utilised, for example, in imaging the hippocampus.

The contents of the middle and posterior fossae are better visualized using MRI because it does not suffer from the streak artefacts arising from bone, in CT, which may mask soft tissue detail.

On T1-weighted (T1W) MR images, grey matter is of lower signal intensity (i.e. darker), than white matter. On T2-weighted (T2W) images, the reverse is true. Cerebrospinal fluid is grey-black (low signal or hypointense), on T1W images and white (high signal or hyperintense) on T2W images. MR images are also acquired in which contrast between structures is based on differences in their proton density. In such proton density (PD) images, grey matter is also hyperintense in comparison to white matter (Fig. 1).

With CT, white matter, somewhat paradoxically, is depicted as darker grey than grey matter since lipid-containing material is relatively radiolucent. The demonstration of myelinated tracts with MRI is more complex. Heavily myelinated fibre tracts such as the fornix

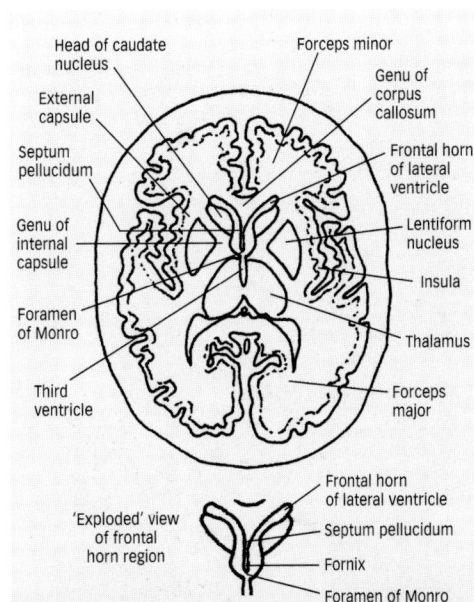

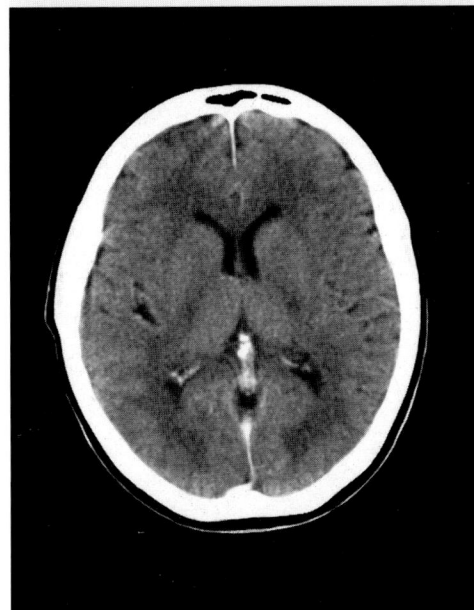

Fig. 1.
(*a*) Axial images at level of the basal ganglia (*a*) CT (*b*) TIW MRI (*c*) T2W MRI (*d*) PD MRI. Note the superior demonstration of anatomy by MRI.

(b)

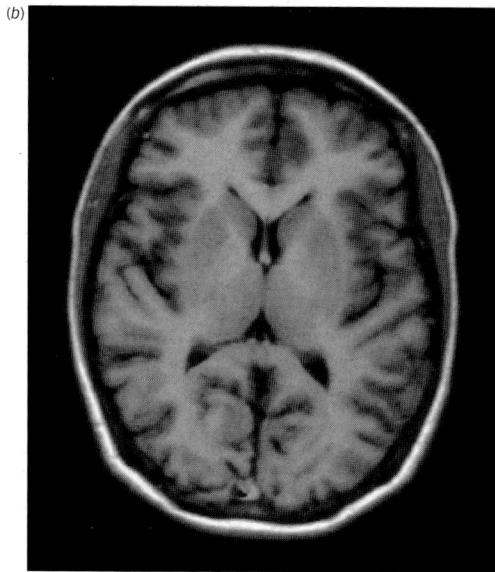

(d)

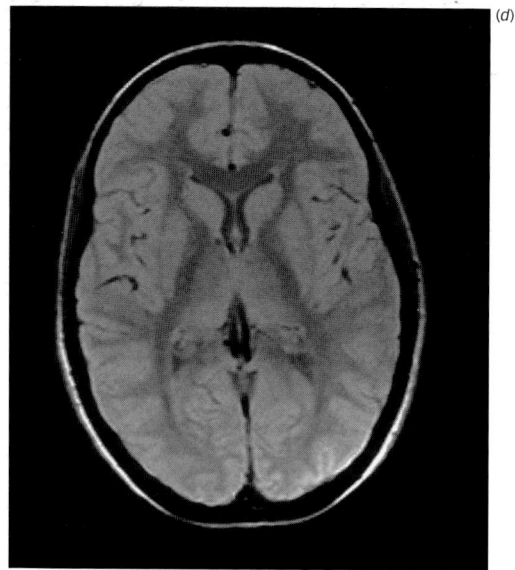

(c)

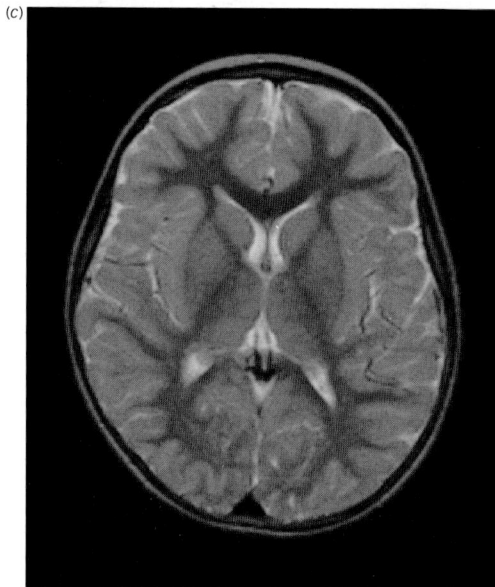

and anterior commissure have an hypointense appearance on T2W MR images, whereas the increased signal intensity of the corticospinal tracts within the internal capsules on T2W images is thought to be due to lower myelin density (Fig. 2).

Hypointensity on both T1W and particularly T2W images can result from iron deposition, which is prominent in the globus pallidus, substantia nigra and red nucleus (Fig. 3.) Interestingly, the brain is free of iron at birth.

So-called 'axial' CT and MRI scans are not usually obtained strictly in that anatomical plane but are usually taken parallel to a line tangential to the orbital roofs running to the anterior margin of the foramen magnum. This reduces the radiation dose to the lens of the eye but increases streak artefact within the middle cranial fossa. This scan plane approximates to the line joining anterior and posterior commissures (the 'AC–PC' line: see p. 40), which is the usual reference plane for MRI. For temporal lobe studies, some centres advocate MRI scanning parallel to the long axis of the lobe with coronal sections obtained perpendicular to that axis. Usually, however, coronal and sagittal scans approximate more closely to the respective anatomical planes. Optimal images of the skull base result from scanning parallel to a straight line passing anteriorly from the posterior lip of the foramen magnum and tangential to the floor of the sphenoid sinus.

Iodinated contrast medium administered intravenously enhances blood within cranial arteries, veins and dural venous sinuses on CT. Enhancement is also seen in the highly vascular choroid plexuses and in those structures outside the blood–brain barrier such as the pituitary gland and infundibulum. With MRI, the mechanism of contrast enhancement with intravenous gadolinium DTPA is quite different, but on T1W images those structures which enhance become hyperintense (i.e. whiter) in much the same way as with CT. There are important differences, however. Rapidly flowing blood is displayed as a 'signal void' and arteries and veins in which flow is rapid remain hypointense even after gadolinium. A combination of calcification and blood flowing rapidly within them often cause the choroid plexuses to remain hypointense on MRI. Veins in which flow is sluggish may enhance and there is also the MR phenomenon of 'flow-related' enhancement in which even rapidly flowing blood can appear hyperintense in the absence of contrast administration. The pituitary gland, infundibulum,

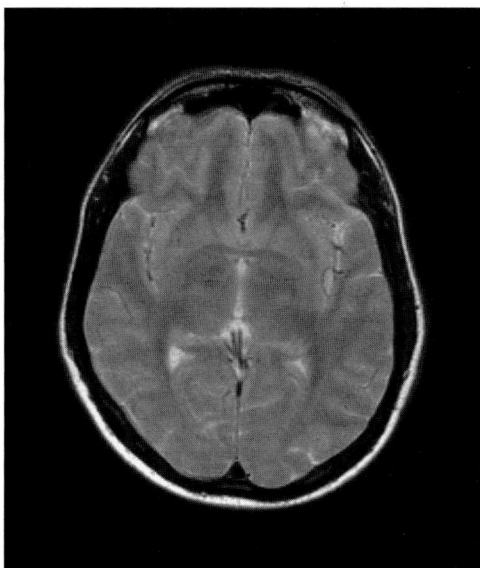

Fig. 2.
T2W Axial MRI showing the anterior commissure and corticospinal tracts.

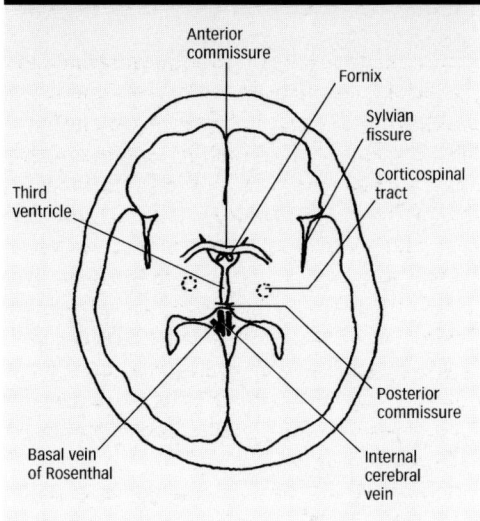

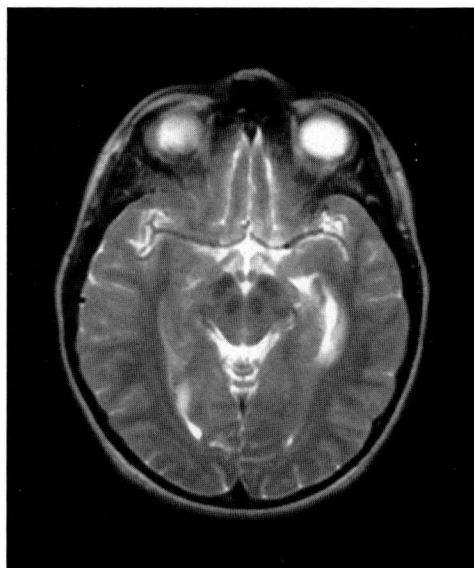

Anterior commissure
Fornix
Sylvian fissure
Corticospinal tract
Third ventricle
Posterior commissure
Basal vein of Rosenthal
Internal cerebral vein

Fig. 3.
T2W Axial MRI showing the substantia nigra and red nucleus. Their hypo-intensity is due to iron deposition.

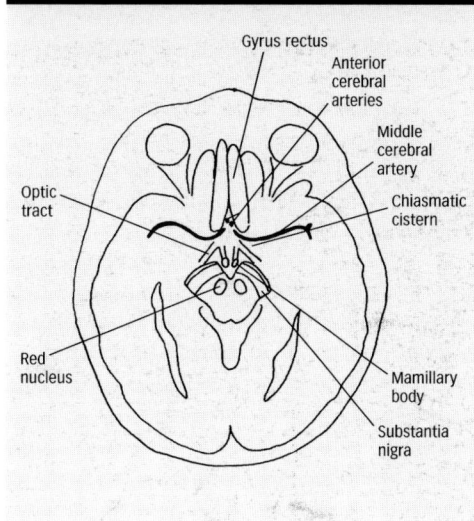

Gyrus rectus
Anterior cerebral arteries
Middle cerebral artery
Chiasmatic cistern
Optic tract
Red nucleus
Mamillary body
Substantia nigra

cavernous sinuses and dura enhance with gadolinium. The degree and extent of dural enhancement is influenced by the MRI pulse sequence and the field strength of the magnet.

The role of angiography is primarily in the diagnosis and, in some cases, the treatment of vascular lesions. Catheter angiography remains the gold standard for the demonstration of the cerebral vasculature but magnetic resonance angiography (MRA) and CT angiography are making significant progress towards the goal of non- or minimally invasive angiography. Both may show vasculature in relation to the cerebral parenchyma. MRA is non-invasive and usually requires no contrast agent. CT angiography requires an intravenous injection of contrast medium.

Conventional catheter angiography without subtraction shows bone detail in addition to the vasculature; digital subtraction angiography (DSA) shows the vasculature in near isolation. Imaging over 7–8 seconds following

the injection of contrast medium into carotid or vertebral arteries will display arterial, capillary and venous phases of the circulation. The cervical carotid and vertebral arteries are usually cannulated via the femoral artery, although a brachial or radial arterial approach can be used. In a similar manner, the femoral vein may be punctured to obtain access to the jugular veins and dural venous sinuses. In the presence of severe occlusive peripheral arterial disease the cervical carotid artery can be punctured directly, although this approach is rarely used.

The skull

Osteology of the skull

The brain is supported by the skull base and enclosed in the vault or calvarium (Fig. 4). The skull base develops in cartilage, the vault in membrane. The central skull base consists of the occipital, sphenoid and temporal bones.

(a)

Frontal diagram labels:

Sagittal suture

Lambdoid suture

Dural calcification

Frontal sinus

Lesser wing of sphenoid

Crista galli

Cribriform plate

Floor of the anterior cranial fossa

Greater wing of sphenoid

Innominate line

Anterior clinoid process

Superior orbital fissure

Zygomatic bone

Maxilla

Lateral diagram labels:

Pterion

Anterior clinoid process

Orbital roof

Dorsum sellae

Habenular commissure (calcifed)

Frontal sinus

Frontal

Parietal

Pineal gland calcification

Floor of the anterior cranial fossa

Cribriform plate

Temporal

Occipital

Sphenoid sinus

Calcified choroid plexus

Lamina dura of pituitary fossa

Normal temporal bone 'thinning'

Clivus (basiocciput and basisphenoid)

Zygomatic recesses of the maxillary antra

Mandibular condyle

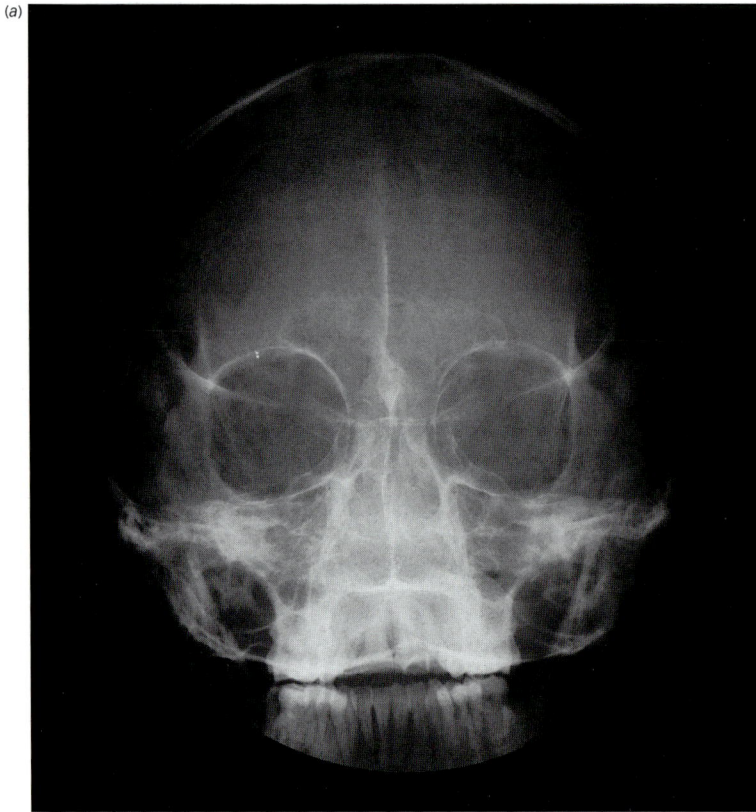

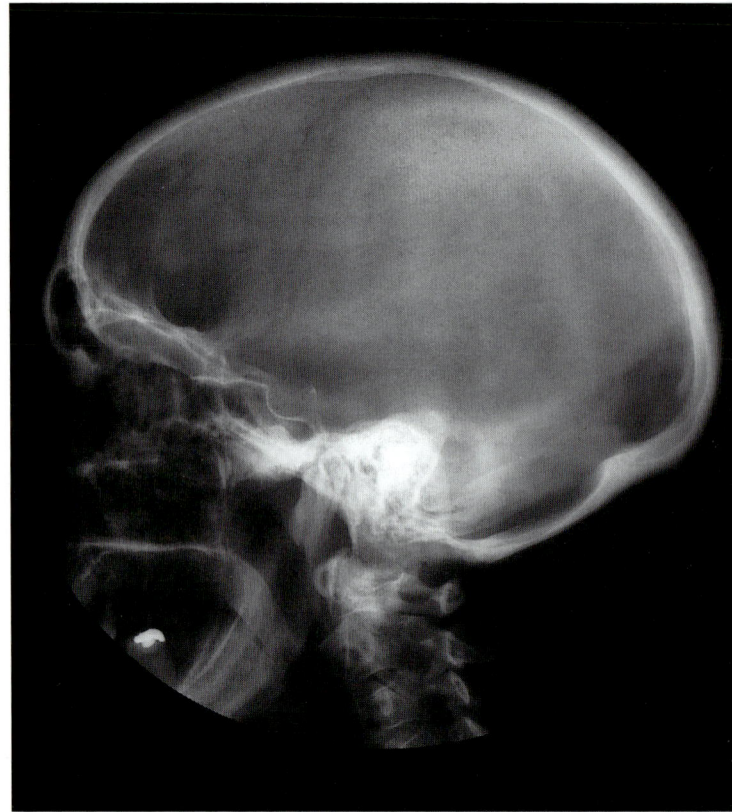

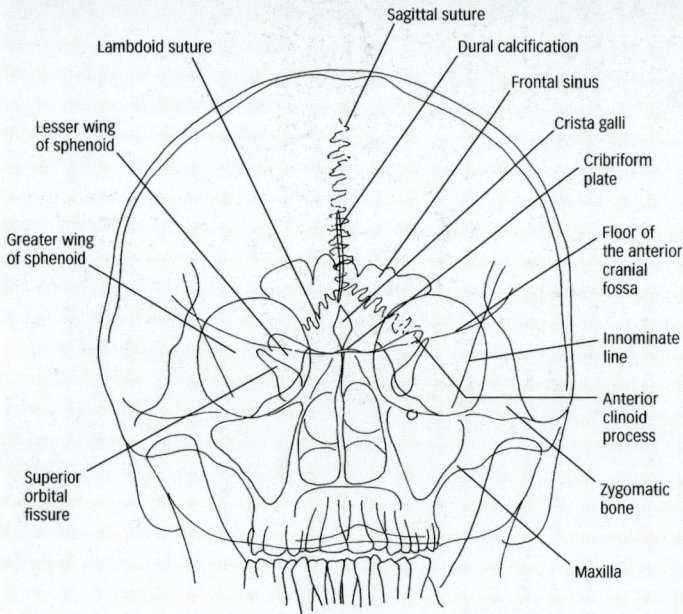

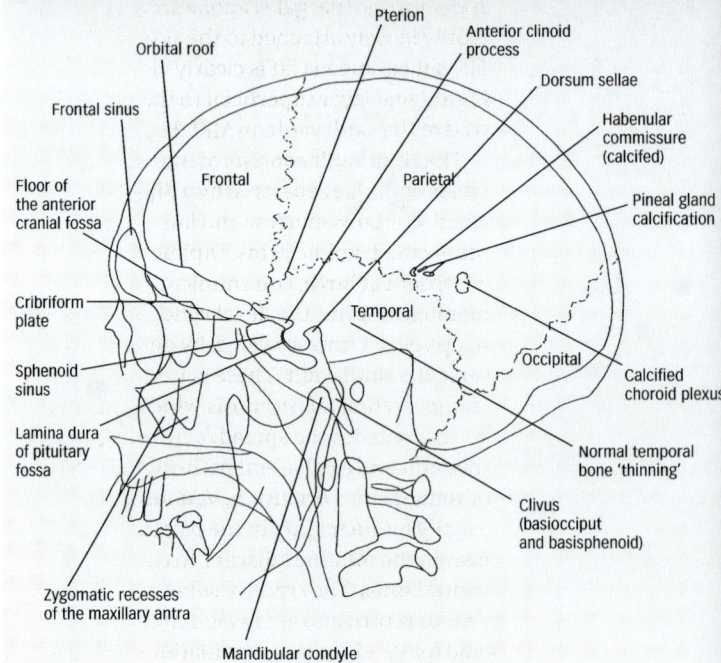

Fig. 4.
(a) Frontal, (b) lateral skull radiographs.

The frontal and ethmoidal bones complete the five bones of the skull base.

Skull sutures are located between bones formed by membranous ossification and consist of dense connective tissue (Fig. 5). In the neonate they are smooth but through childhood interdigitations develop followed by perisutural sclerosis, prior to fusion in the third or fourth decades or even later. For practical purposes sutural fusion occurs in adolescence, since only in children does raised intracranial pressure present with head enlargement. The anterior fontanelle or bregma is located between frontal and parietal bones at the junction of sagittal and coronal sutures. The bregma closes in the second year. The lambda is closed by the second month after birth and the pterion (see below) usually closes by 3–4 months of age.

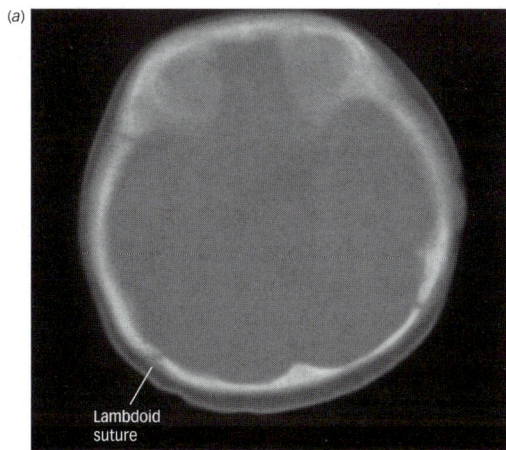

Fig. 5.
Axial CT showing the skull sutures. (*a*) The lambdoid sutures. (*b*) The coronal and sagittal sutures.

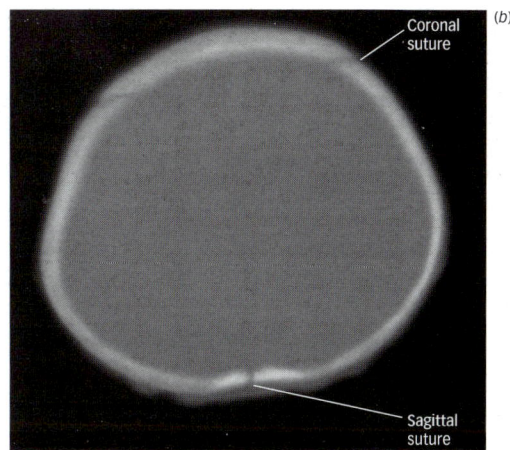

The skull is invested by periosteum both externally (the pericranium) and internally (the endosteum). The endosteum is the outer of the two dural layers and is continuous with the connective tissue of the sutures and fontanelles. Both extradural and subdural haematomas may cross sutures although, in principle at least, this anatomical boundary should prevent the spread of extradural collections.

The skin and subcutaneous tissue of the scalp are firmly adherent to the epicranial aponeurosis (the 'galea aponeurotica') which is only loosely attached to the skull vault. The subcutaneous fat is clearly visible as a high signal layer superficial to the signal void of the skull vault on MRI (Fig. 17).

The skull vault consists of inner and outer tables or diploe separated by a diploic space which contains marrow and large, valveless, thin-walled diploic veins. Diploic veins, which are absent at birth, communicate with meningeal veins, the dural venous sinuses and scalp veins. Emissary veins, by definition, traverse the skull vault. These veins form a rich craniocerebral anastomosis which provides both a route for the spread of infection across the vault and a collateral pathway in the event of venous sinus occlusion. Venous lacunae are usually found mainly in the parietal bone, near to the midline adjacent to the superior sagittal sinus. They receive some of the cerebral venous return and are invaginated by arachnoid (or Pacchionian) granulations which are the sites of reabsorption of cerebrospinal fluid into the venous system. Lacunae cause localized thinning of the inner table (Fig. 6).

The frontal bone forms in two halves which normally fuse at five years. The intervening suture is known as the metopic suture. Occasionally the halves remain separate and this suture may persist, wholly or in part, into adult life in 5–10% of individuals (Figs. 7, 11). The orbital plates of the frontal bone

contribute most of the anterior fossa floor, with the cribriform plate of the ethmoid bone interposed between them in the midline. The crista galli, to which the falx is attached, ascends vertically from the cribriform plate (Fig. 4(*a*)). The two parietal bones are separated from each other by the sagittal suture and from the frontal bone by the coronal suture (Fig. 5). Posteriorly, each parietal bone articulates with the occipital bone. Anteriorly, it articulates with the frontal bone and the

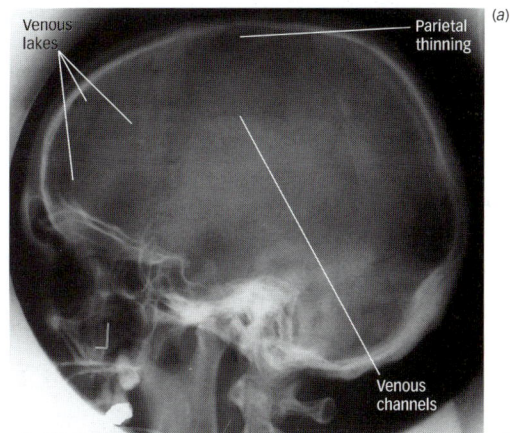

Fig. 6.
(*a*) Lateral skull radiograph showing multiple lucencies due to venous lakes and arachnoid granulations (arrowed). Note also normal thinning of the parietal bone. (*b*) Diagram of venous lacunes (lakes) and arachnoid granulations.

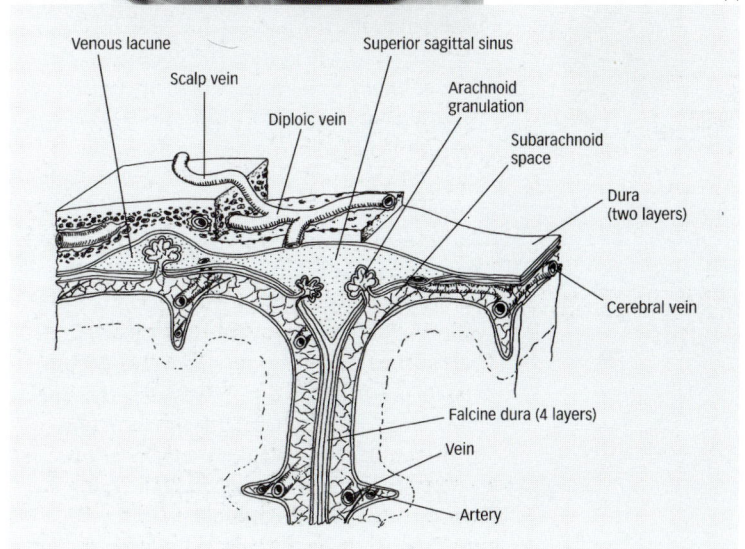

(a)

(b)

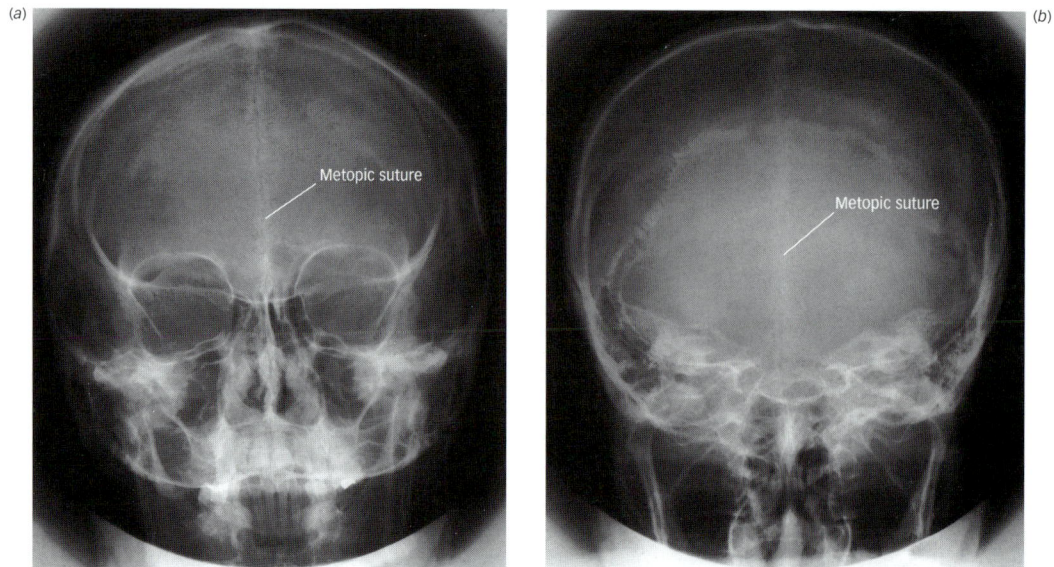

Metopic suture

Metopic suture

Metopic suture

Fig. 7.
(a) PA, (b) Towne's skull radiographs of the metopic suture (arrows). In (b) the midline suture is seen below the posterior lip of the foramen magnum, indicating that it must be within the frontal bone rather than the occipital bone.

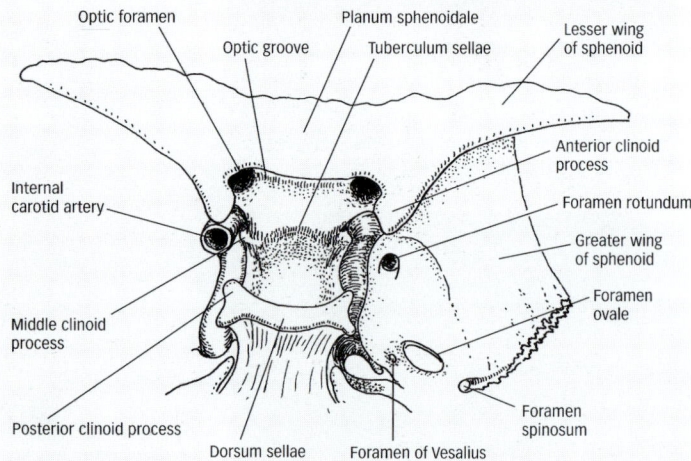

Optic foramen

Optic groove

Planum sphenoidale

Tuberculum sellae

Lesser wing of sphenoid

Internal carotid artery

Anterior clinoid process

Foramen rotundum

Greater wing of sphenoid

Foramen ovale

Middle clinoid process

Posterior clinoid process

Dorsum sellae

Foramen of Vesalius

Foramen spinosum

Fig. 8.
The bony anatomy of the sellar region.

greater wing of the sphenoid bone and inferiorly with the temporal bone. The frontal, sphenoidal, parietal and temporal bones meet at the pterion.

The sphenoid bone consists of a body (the basisphenoid), the greater and lesser wings and the pterygoid plates. The body encloses the sphenoid air sinuses, which are paired and usually asymmetrical. The pituitary fossa and posterior clinoid processes are borne on its superior surface (Fig. 8) and the planum sphenoidale articulates with the cribriform plate. The anterior clinoid processes are part of the lesser wing and the tuberculum sellae dips anteriorly between them into the optic groove. The lesser wing forms the posterior part of the floor of the anterior cranial fossa and its posterior border constitutes the sphenoid 'ridge'. Meningiomas of the skull base may arise from these sphenoidal locations.

The greater wing of the sphenoid bone forms the floor of the middle cranial fossa, which extends posteriorly to the petrous ridge

and dorsum sella. The dorsum sella is the posterior boundary of the pituitary fossa and merges laterally with the posterior clinoid processes. The greater wing also separates the temporal lobe of the brain from the infratemporal fossa below. The medial and lateral pterygoid plates of the sphenoid bone pass inferiorly behind the maxilla.

The foramina ovale, rotundum and spinosum are within the greater wing of the sphenoid bone (Fig. 9). The foramina ovale and spinosum are often asymmetrical, the foramen rotundum rarely so.

The foramen rotundum travels from Meckel's cave to the pterygopalatine fossa and transmits the maxillary division of the trigeminal (Vth) nerve. On coronal CT the foramina are demonstrated inferior to the anterior clinoid processes.

The foramen ovale transmits the mandibular division of the trigeminal nerve and the accessory meningeal artery. It runs anterolaterally from Meckel's cave to emerge near to the lateral pterygoid plate. The foramina may be identified on coronal CT scans inferolateral to the posterior clinoid processes.

The foramen spinosum is situated posterolateral to the larger foramen ovale and transmits the middle meningeal artery and vein between the infratemporal and middle cranial fossae. Other foramina are sometimes encountered. The Vidian or pterygoid canal is found inferior to the sphenoid sinus, medial to the foramen rotundum. It transmits the artery of the pterygoid canal (the Vidian artery) which is a branch of the maxillary artery and which runs posteriorly through the canal towards the foramen lacerum. The foramen of Vesalius transmits an emissary vein and is medial to the foramen ovale (Fig. 9(f)).

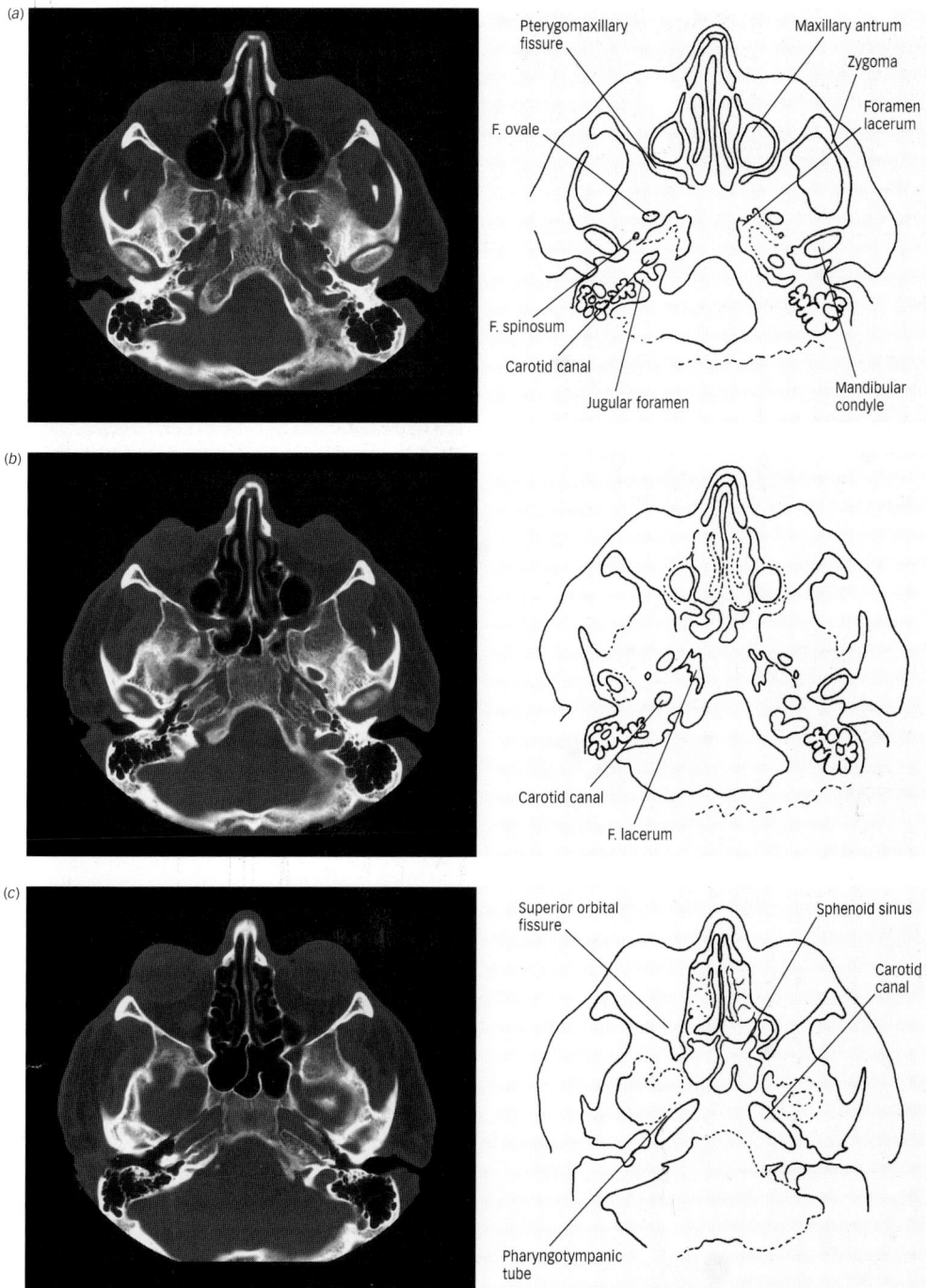

Fig. 9.
CT of the skull base: *(a)*–*(c)* **are contiguous axial images,** *(a)* **the most inferior. Coronal image** *(d)* **is anterior to** *(e)***. Axial image** *(f)* **shows the foramen of Vesalius. This is inconstant and, when present, carries an emissary vein.**

The foramen lacerum contains cartilage and is traversed only by small veins and nerves. It separates the petrous apex, the body of the sphenoid and basiocciput. The internal carotid artery crosses its cranial part.

The larger basal foramina can be recognized on the submentovertical (basal) skull radiograph (Fig. 10).

The temporal bone has four parts. The squamous part forms the lateral wall of the middle cranial fossa and is separated from the parietal bone by the squamosal suture. Its zygomatic process contributes to the zygomatic arch and the squamous portion also bears the mandibu-

lar condylar fossa. The petromastoid portion forms part of the middle and posterior fossa floors. The curved tympanic portion forms part of the external auditory canal and the non articular posterior part of the mandibular fossa. The styloid process passes inferiorly from the base of the petrous bone and calcification of the stylohyoid ligament may be seen on a lateral radiograph. The stylomastoid foramen lies behind the styloid process and transmits the facial (VIIth cranial) nerve.

The occipital bone forms most of the walls and floor of the posterior cranial fossa, which is the largest of the three cranial fossae. The

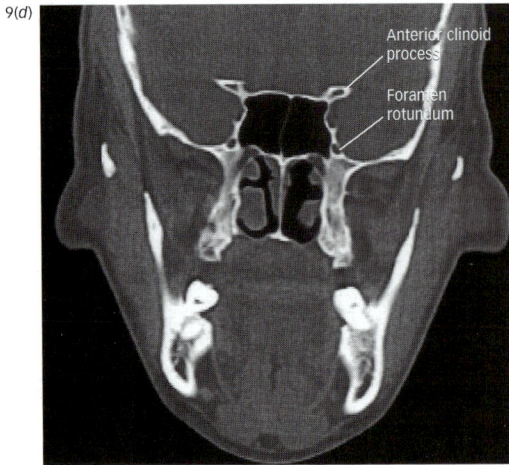

9(d)

Anterior clinoid process

Foramen rotundum

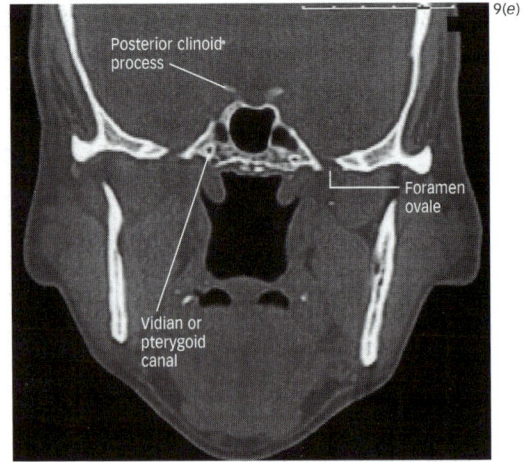

9(e)

Posterior clinoid process

Foramen ovale

Vidian or pterygoid canal

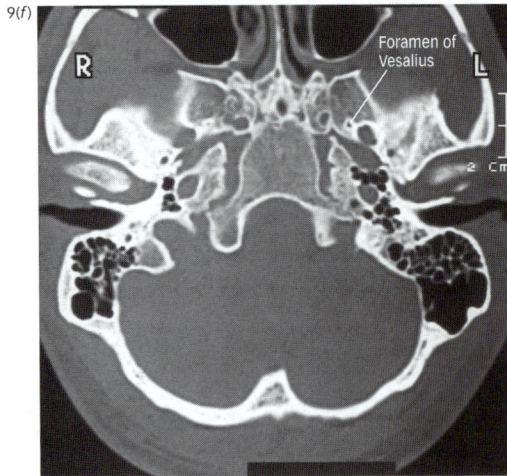

9(f)

R   L

Foramen of Vesalius

2 Cm

lambdoid suture separates the parietal and occipital bones. The occipital bone consists of a squamosal segment, the basiocciput and two lateral or exoccipital portions. The squamous part lies posterior to the foramen magnum and is further divided into the interparietal portion superiorly and the supraoccipital part from which arises the external occipital protuberance. The mendosal suture separates these subdivisions. The basiocciput articulates anteriorly with the basisphenoid to form the clivus. The articulation is known as the basisphenoid synchondrosis (Figs. 11, 53(c)) and is also the site at which the petrous apex joins the clivus. In the adult the clivus is hyperintense on T1W MR images due to replace-

Fig. 10.
Skull radiograph, the bas or submentovertical projection.

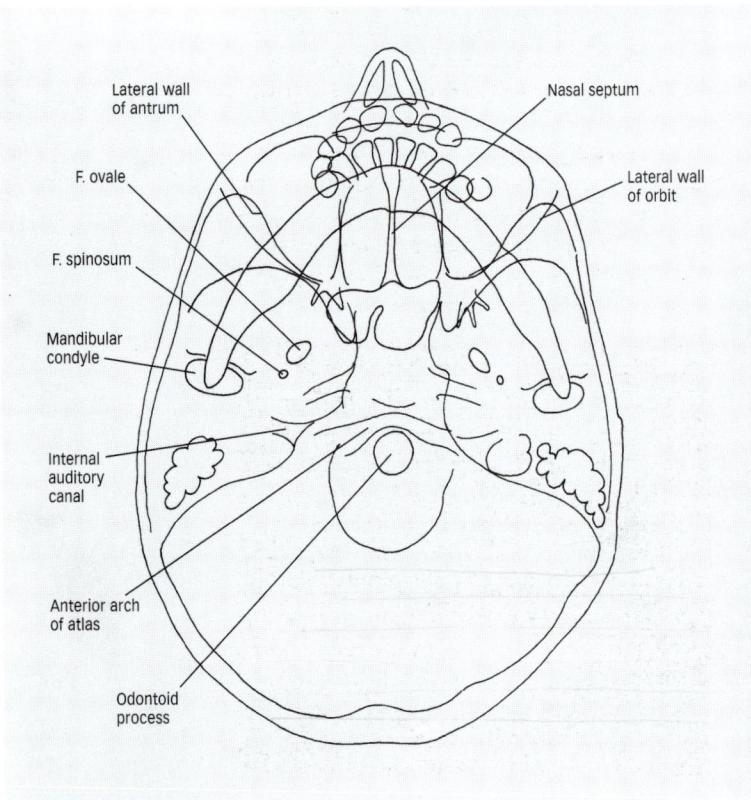

Lateral wall of antrum

Nasal septum

F. ovale

Lateral wall of orbit

F. spinosum

Mandibular condyle

Internal auditory canal

Anterior arch of atlas

Odontoid process

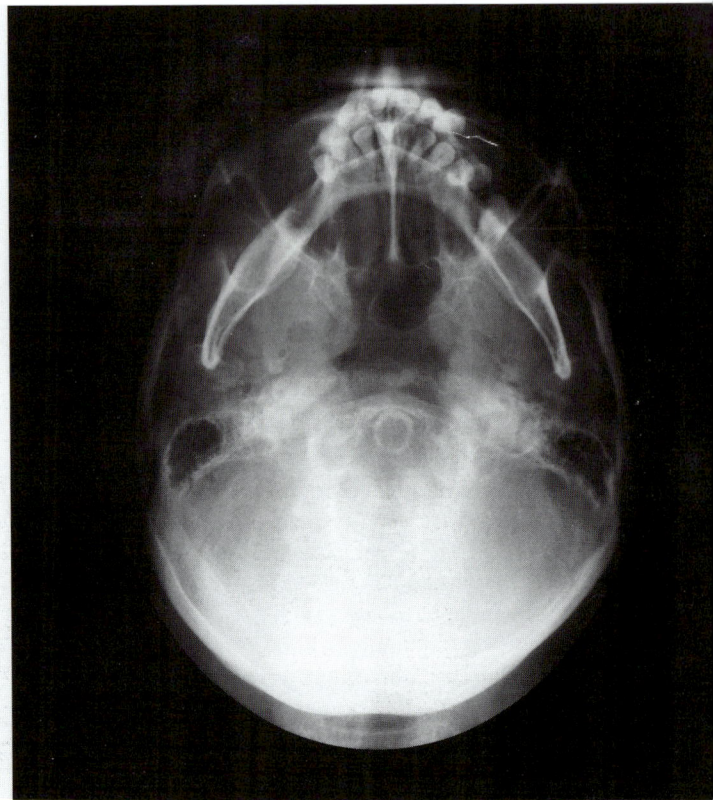

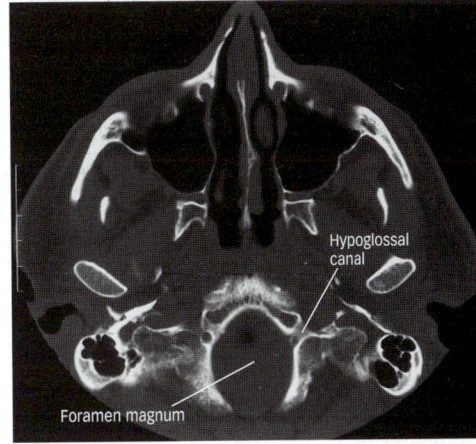

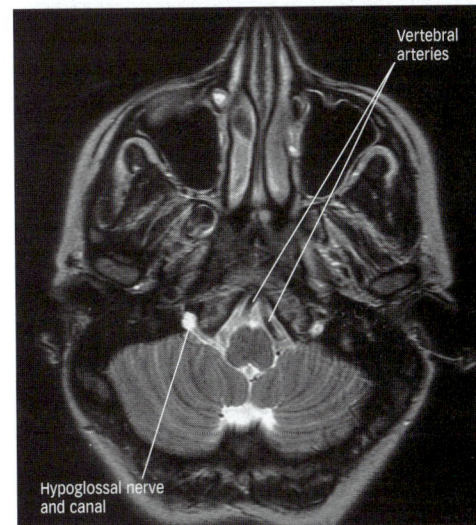

(a)

(b)

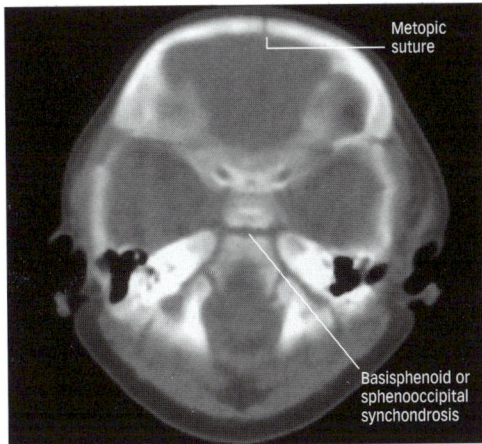

ment of red marrow with fat. The transition from hypointensity occurs at around 7 years. Immature red marrow in children can enhance with intravenous gadolinium.

The lateral condylar (or exoccipital) portions have the occipital condyles and contain the hypoglossal (anterior) condylar canals lying medial to the jugular foramina on each side (Fig. 12). The occipital bone is often devoid of a diploic space inferiorly. This accounts for the sparing of the occipital squame in thalassaemia major, where marrow hyperplasia in response to chronic haemolysis causes reactive change ('hair-on-end' appearance), elsewhere in the skull vault.

The jugular foramen lies between the temporal and occipital bones (see Chapter 4).

The normal skull radiograph

Convolutional markings are absent at birth, most prominent at between two and five years and absent after about 12 years of age. Vascular markings similarly do not develop until the postnatal period but then persist through life. They are less radiolucent than fractures with indistinct margins and often branch. Diploic veins are responsible for the majority of these impressions, although the dural venous sinuses (superior sagittal, lateral and sigmoid), cause depressions on the inner table, visible on plain radiographs. There is a vein running along the coronal suture of sufficient size to be labelled the sphenobregmatic sinus, which gives rise to a prominent vascular impression (Fig. 13). Venous impressions on the vault are larger than those due to arteries and vary in

(a)

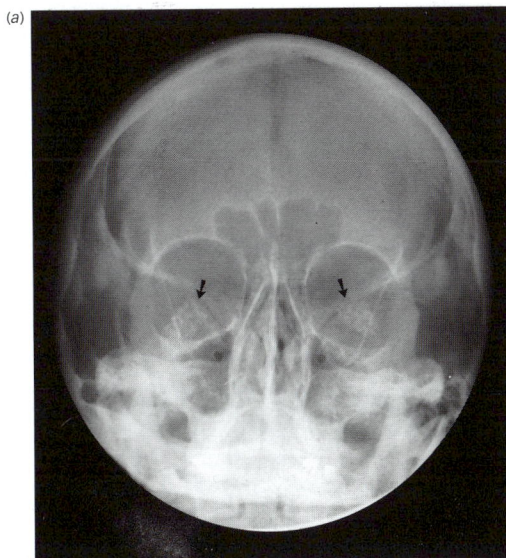

(b)

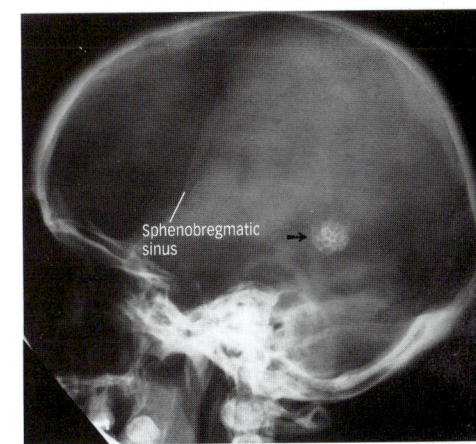

TABLE 1

Lucencies within the vault seen on skull radiography

Sutures (see Figs 4, 6)
Vascular impressions (see Fig 6)
Normal thinning, e.g. of the temporal squame, and parietal bone (see Figs. 4, 6)
Parietal foramina (see below)
Pacchionian depressions (Fig. 6)
Pneumatisation (Fig. 14)

Calcifications within the vault seen on skull radiography

Pineal gland (see Fig. 4)
Habenular commissure (see Fig. 4)
Choroid plexuses (see Fig. 13)
Petroclinoid and interclinoid 'ligaments' (see below) (Fig. 15)
Dura (see Fig. 4)

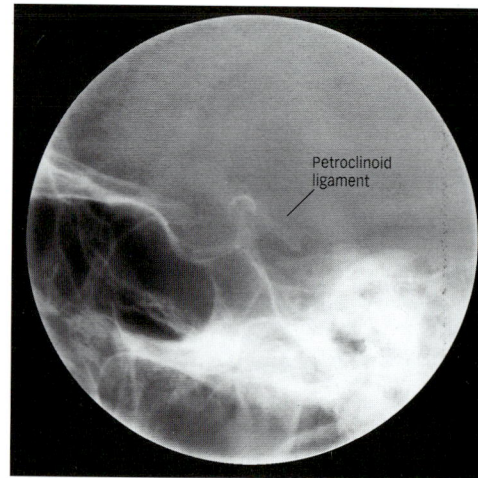

(a) Fig. 15.
Lateral skull radiographs showing calcification of the (a) petroclinoid and (b) interclinoid ligaments (indicated).

Fig. 14.
Frontal skull radiograph showing pneumatization of the right anterior clinoid process (arrow).

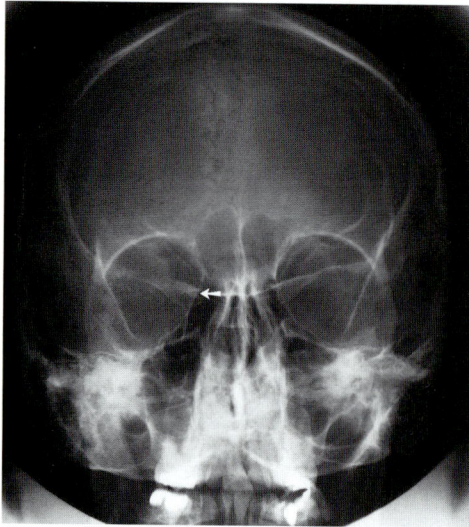

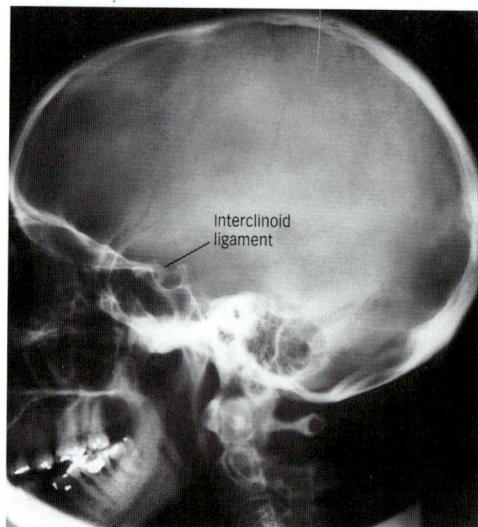

(b)

calibre. Arterial impressions have parallel walls and reduce in calibre only after branching.

Normal vault lucencies and calcifications are listed in Table 1.

Parietal foramina are paired, symmetrical lucencies also near the midline and transmit the emissary vein of Santorini. Large foramina (several centimetres in diameter), are not classed as normal variants as they arise from defects in membranous ossification.

Intrasutural, or Wormian, bones occur most often as normal variants but are also associated with a number of pathological conditions, particularly when multiple. These are usually conditions in which there is defective ossification such as cleidocranial dysostosis, osteogenesis imperfecta and hypophosphatasia.

Petroclinoid ligament calcification results in a linear calcific density passing obliquely inferiorly and posteriorly from the posterior clinoid processes on a lateral radiograph. On axial CT it is identified as calcification running posterolaterally from the clinoid processes along the tentorial edge. Interclinoid ligament

calcification involves the diaphragma sellae and appears to bridge the sella on the lateral radiograph. This 'ligamentous' calcification is thus strictly dural in origin (Fig. 15).

The cerebral envelope

The meninges invest the brain and spinal cord. The three constituent parts are the outer, fibrous dura mater, the avascular, lattice-like arachnoid mater and the inner, vascular layer, the pia mater. Although the dura and arachnoid are applied closely, there is a potential space, known as the subdural space between them into which haemorrhage may occur or pus form. Its existence in the normal individual is controversial. The subarachnoid space contains the cerebrospinal fluid, which surrounds the cerebral arteries and veins. It is situated between the arachnoid and the pia which is closely applied to the cerebral surface. The cranial dura has two layers which separate to enclose the dural venous sinuses (Fig. 16).

The outer layer is the periosteum of the inner table of the skull (endosteum). The inner

Fig. 16.
The cranial dura.

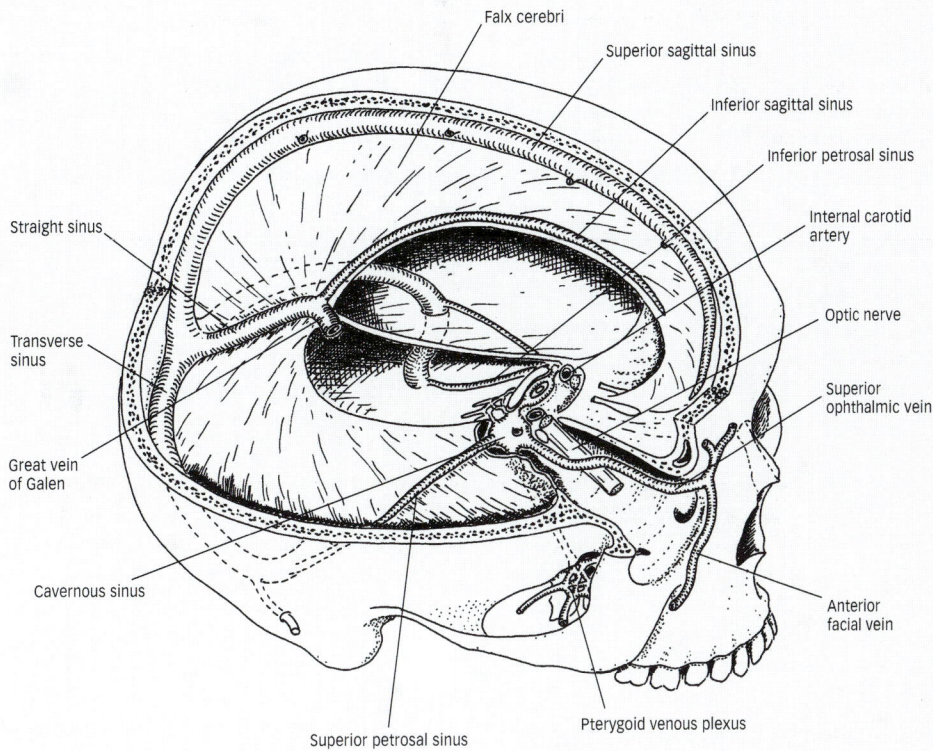

Falx cerebri
Superior sagittal sinus
Inferior sagittal sinus
Inferior petrosal sinus
Internal carotid artery
Optic nerve
Superior ophthalmic vein
Anterior facial vein
Straight sinus
Transverse sinus
Great vein of Galen
Cavernous sinus
Superior petrosal sinus
Pterygoid venous plexus

layer covers the brain and gives rise to the falx and tentorium. Dura is hyperdense on CT images and relatively hypointense on MRI. It shows contrast enhancement on both modalities and since the falx may calcify or ossify, MRI may demonstrate focal regions of signal void due to calcification or of hyperintensity due to fat within marrow (Fig. 17). The falx cerebri is a sickle-shaped fold of dura, comprising two layers, which forms an incomplete partition between the cerebral hemispheres. It extends from the crista galli to the internal occipital protuberance, where it joins the tentorium and is thinner anteriorly. The falx is displayed as a midline linear density on axial CT scans near to the vertex, but inferiorly

and posteriorly assumes a triangular shape conforming to the superior sagittal sinus in cross-section.

The tentorium cerebelli, another double dural fold, is attached from the posterior clinoid processes along the petrous ridges to the internal occipital protuberance. Its upper, free, medial border surrounds the midbrain, which passes anteriorly through the opening, known as the tentorial hiatus or incisura (Fig. 18). The uncus of the hippocampus and the posterior cerebral artery lie above the free edge of the tentorium and both are at risk of compression against the tentorial edge when there is raised intracranial pressure in the supratentorial compartment ('coning'). The

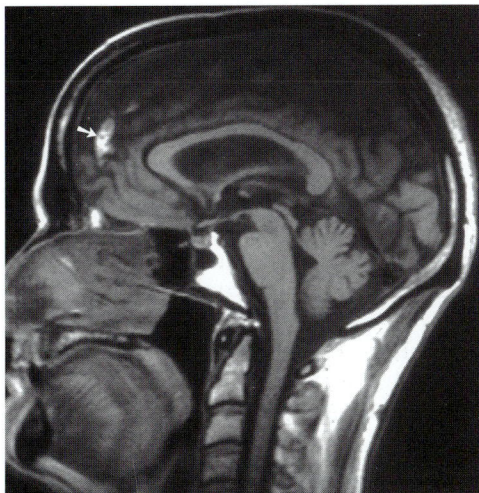

Fig. 17.
Cranial MRI. Midline TIW sagittal image showing hyperintense (yellow) marrow within an ossified region of the falx (arrow).

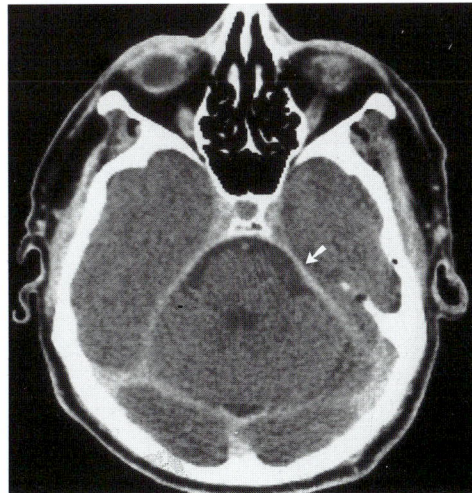

Fig. 18.
Axial CT with intravenous contrast showing the enhancing tentorial margins (arrow). Note that the dura continues anteriorly to form the lateral wall of the cavernous sinus.

free border anteriorly encloses the cavernous sinus on each side of the pituitary fossa before attaching to the anterior clinoid processes.

For diagnostic purposes it is important to identify in which intracranial compartment a lesion is situated. On axial CT, structures medial to the line of the tentorial edge are within the infratentorial compartment; those lateral to that line are within the supratentorial compartment.

The falx cerebelli is a small fold of dura attached superiorly to the posterior part of the tentorium in the midsagittal plane which encloses the occipital sinus posteriorly. It terminates just above the foramen magnum and its free anterior border projects into the cerebellar notch. The diaphragma sellae is an incomplete dural roof over the pituitary gland and is pierced by the pituitary stalk. There is no subarachnoid space in the sella since the meningeal layers fuse. On both CT and MRI meningeal enhancement following intravenous contrast is a normal feature.

Meningeal blood supply and innervation

The middle meningeal artery (Fig. 19) is the main arterial supply to the meninges but there are contributions from the cavernous carotid, the ophthalmic and vertebral arteries . There is also an accessory meningeal artery, which arises either from the maxillary or middle meningeal artery and enters the skull through the foramen ovale. The middle meningeal artery is extradural and both it and the meningeal veins groove the inner table of the skull. Branches of the external carotid artery may often supply the lower cranial nerves. The middle meningeal artery supplies branches to both the trigeminal and the facial ganglia. The occipital artery (Fig. 19) gives branches which pass via the jugular foramen and condylar canal to supply glossopharyngeal (IXth), vagal (Xth), accessory (XIth) and hypoglossal (XIIth) nerves. Innervation of the dura is primarily from the trigeminal nerve (Vth) but also from the lower cranial nerves and the first three cervical segments. This may account for cervical pain in cranial subarachnoid haemorrhage. (See also Chapter 5.)

Normal development of the brain

During the fourth week of intrauterine development the neural tube expands to form the three vesicles of the forebrain, midbrain and hindbrain. The surface of the brain is smooth up to 18 weeks and although the Rolandic fissure appears at 20 weeks, relatively few gyri are present before 28 weeks.

The cerebral ventricles are recognized on CT at about 24 weeks and both they and the cortical subarachnoid spaces may appear prominent in both the premature and term neonate. Towards the end of normal gestation, brain growth and gyration proceed rapidly, along with myelination.

Owing to the relatively high water content, poorly myelinated white matter, particularly of the normal preterm infant, will appear hypodense in comparison to the older child. It should not be mistaken for ischaemia.

The embryonic brain is supplied exclusively by the internal carotid artery, a situation which may persist in the adult when usually one of the two posterior cerebral arteries is supplied only via the ipsilateral posterior communicating artery.

The germinal matrix is subependymal in location and overlies the head and body of the caudate nucleus on each side. It is supplied mainly by Heubner's artery (see p. 53) and involutes between 32 weeks and term.

Cerebral myelination

MRI is used to assess the progress of myelination. T1W inversion recovery (IR) images are particularly sensitive to myelination in the first six months. T2W images are used thereafter. On IR images, unmyelinated white matter is hypointense to grey matter reflecting its relatively high water content. Myelination causes the white matter to become hyperintense (whiter) (Fig. 20). Conversely on T2W images, myelinated white matter is represented as low signal relative to grey matter (Fig. 21). The 'adult' patterns for both IR and T2W MRI are shown in Figs. 22 and 23.

Fig. 19.
External carotid angiogram, lateral projection. There is faint opacification of the internal carotid artery.

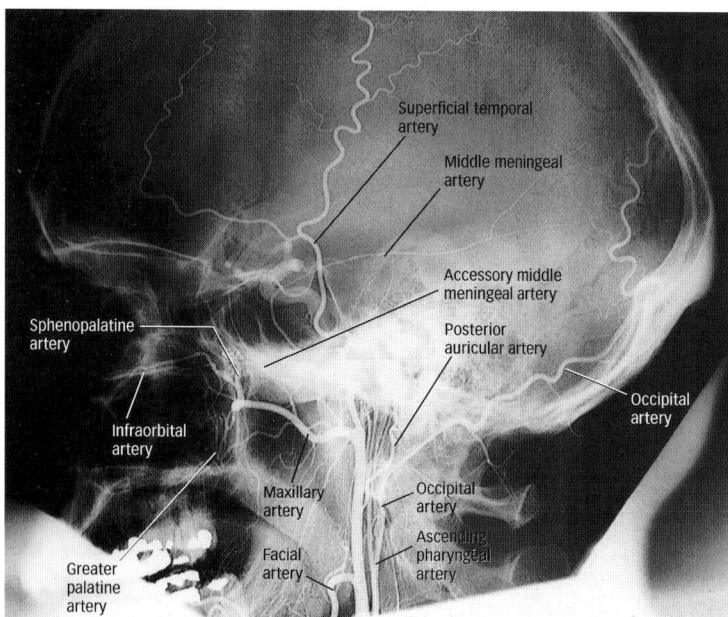

Superficial temporal artery

Middle meningeal artery

Accessory middle meningeal artery

Posterior auricular artery

Occipital artery

Sphenopalatine artery

Infraorbital artery

Maxillary artery

Occipital artery

Ascending pharyngeal artery

Facial artery

Greater palatine artery

On IR MR images, the term infant demonstrates myelination within the brainstem (but not the ventral pons) and the cerebellar white matter. Myelination is also evident in the posterior limb of the internal capsule, extending through the corticospinal tracts superiorly to the parasagittal areas. Soon after birth the optic radiation becomes myelinated, followed by the ventral pons at 2 to 3 months. Myclination proceeds from the splenium of the corpus callosum, beginning at three months, towards the genu at 5 to 6 months. At 4 months myelination begins in the anterior limb of the internal capsule.

IR images indicate that myelination is complete during the last half of the first year, as evidenced by uniform hyperintensity of the white matter. T2W images, however, still show a heterogeneity of white matter signal intensity at this time and thus reliance is placed on this sequence after 6 months.

On T2W MR images, the splenium of the corpus callosum is myelinated between 6 and 8 months and the genu at 8 to 11 months. The

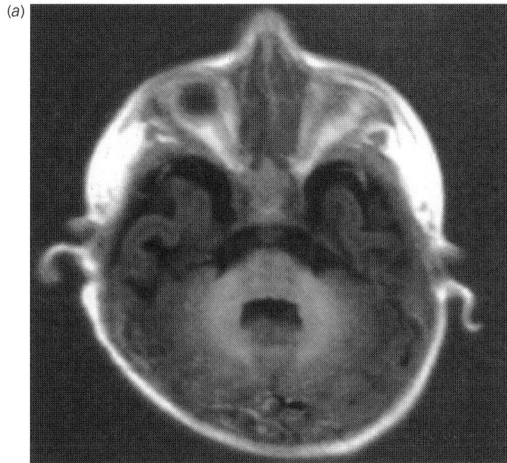

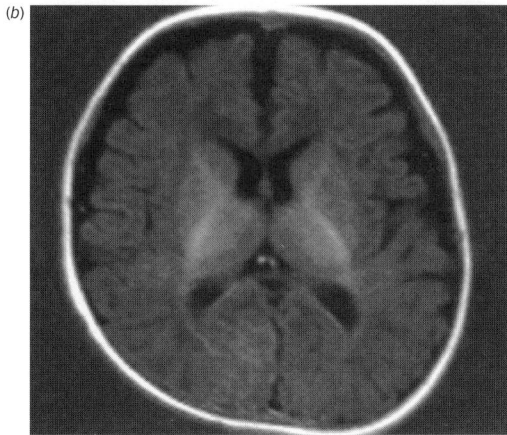

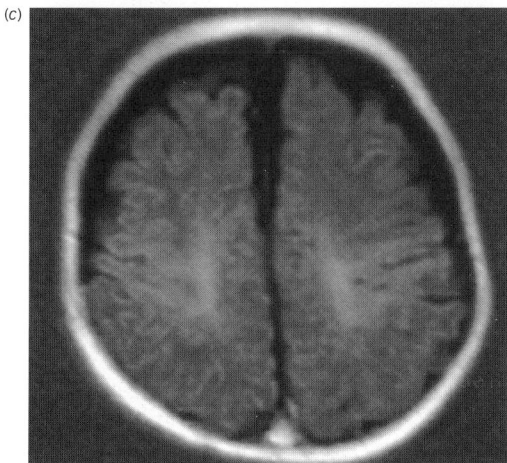

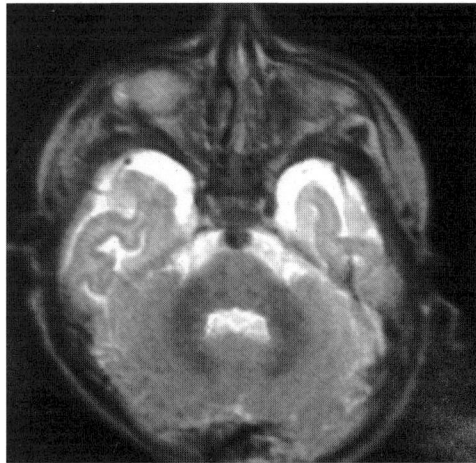

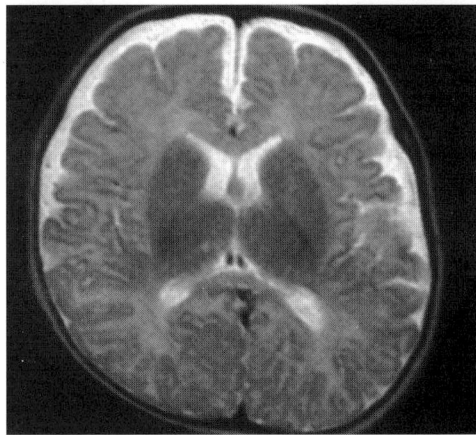

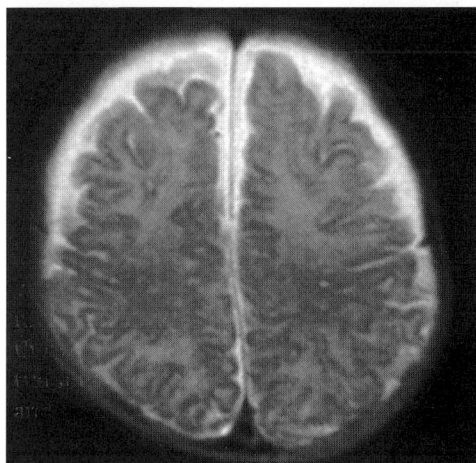

Fig. 20.
Axial IR (T1W) MRI. Normal term neonate.

Fig. 21.
Axial T2W MRI.
Normal term neonate.

anterior limb of the internal capsule myelinates between 11 and 14 months and myelination of the frontal white matter should be nearly complete at 14 months. The temporal white matter is the last to myelinate between 14 and 18 months. The normal 'adult' MRI pattern is attained at about 2 years, although some subtle differences may persist beyond this time.

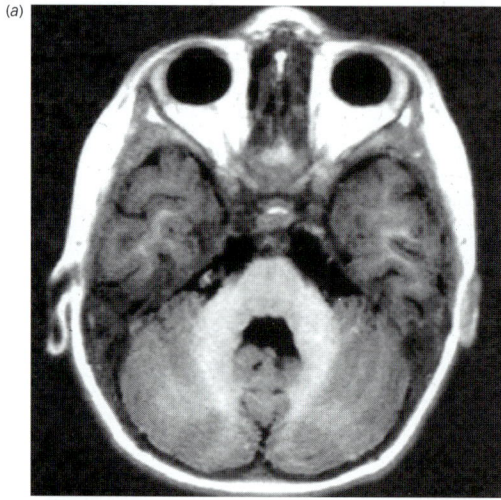

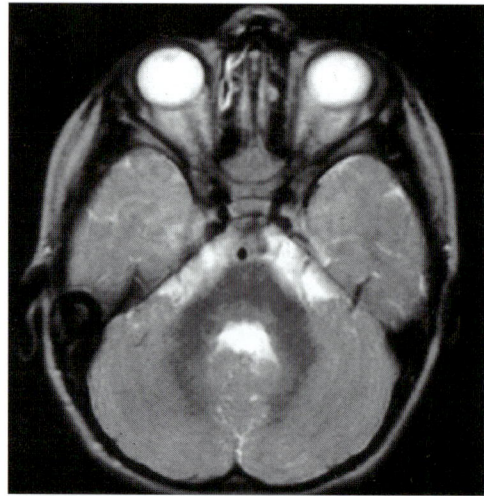

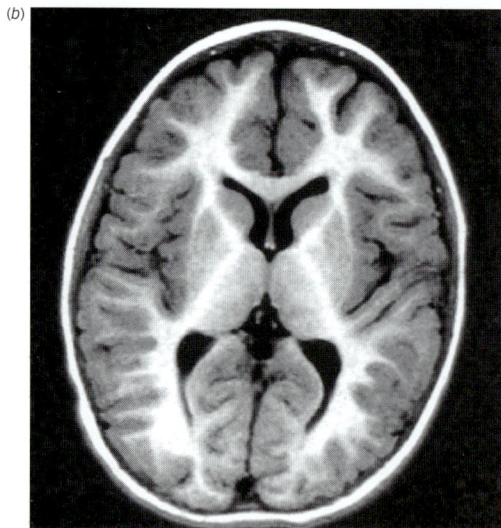

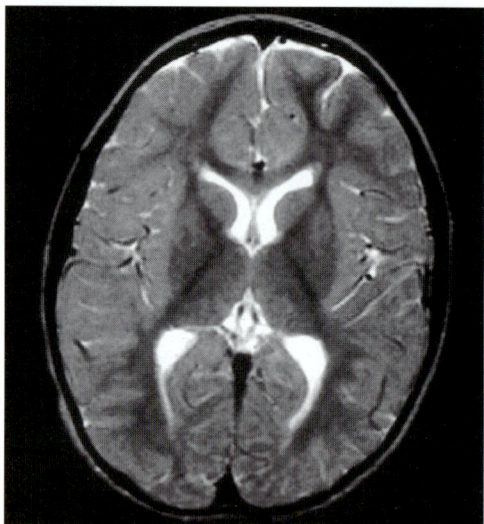

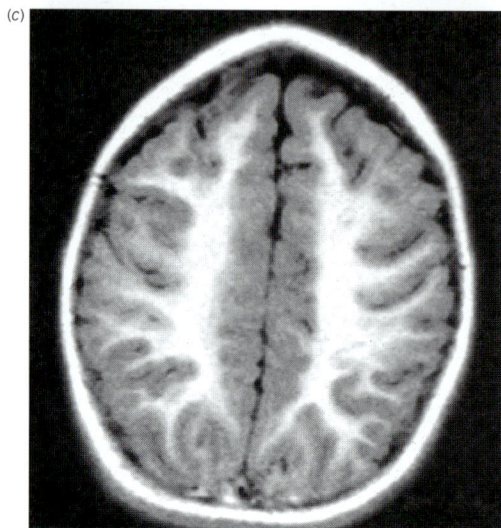

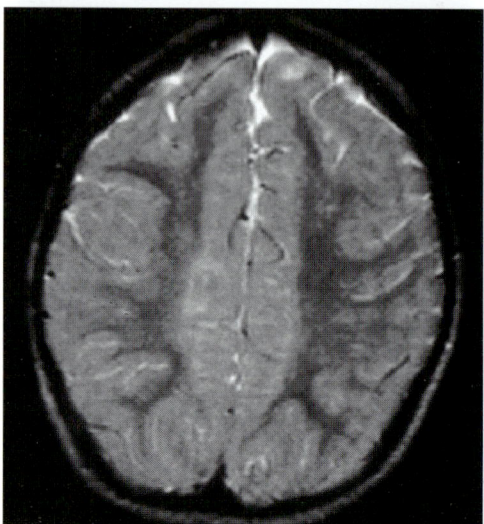

Fig. 22.
Axial IR (T1W) MRI.
Normal child of 4 years.

Fig. 23.
Axial T2W MRI. Normal child of 4 years. Fig. 23(c) shows some heterogeneity of the signal from the centrum ovale, indicating that some unmyelinated fibres remain.

(a)

Pyramid

Central canal

Vertebral artery

Dorsal columns

(c)

Basilar artery

Inferior cerebellar peduncle

Foramen of Luschka

Floor of IVth ventricle

Tonsil

Nodulus

(b)

Vertebral arteries

Pyramid

Preolivary sulcus

Olive

Post-olivary sulcus

Foramen of Magendie

(d)

Basilar artery

Inferior cerebellar peduncle

Foramen of Luschka

Floor of IVth ventricle

Tonsil

Nodulus

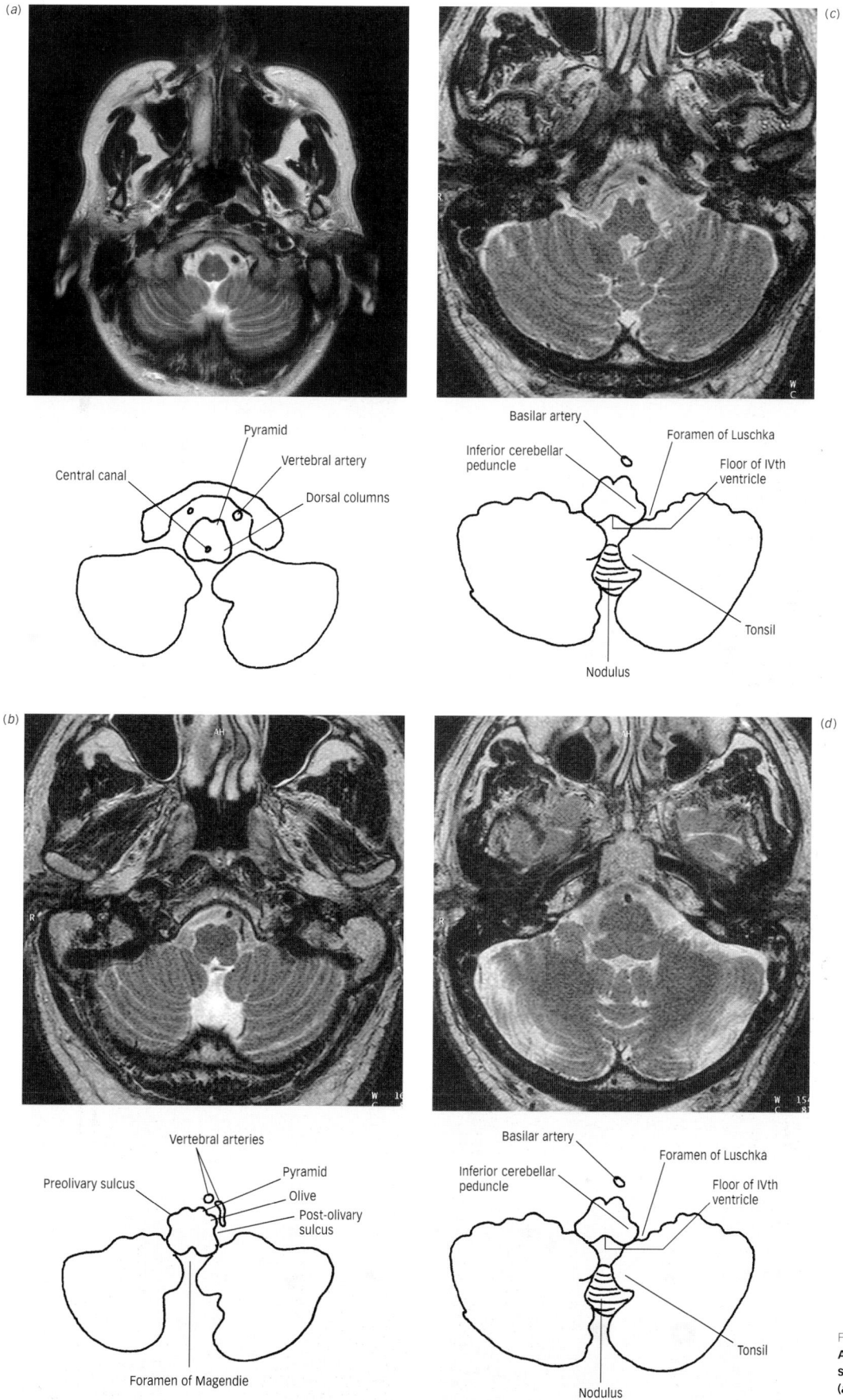

Fig. 24.
Axial MRI scans (inferior to superior) of the brainstem (a)–(e) T2W, (f)–(i)-T1W images. (After Mawad et al., 1983.)

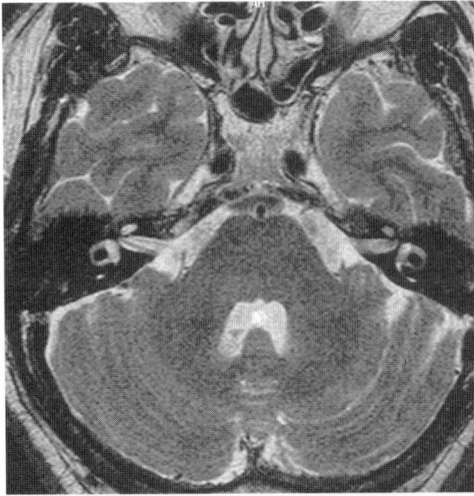

24(e)

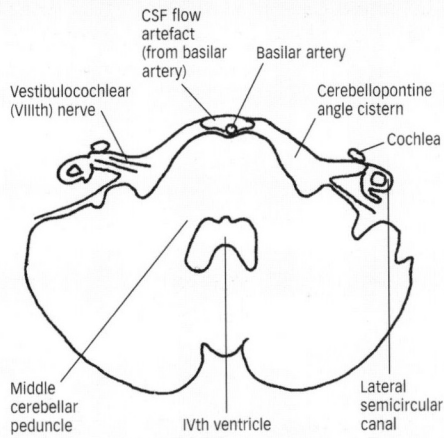

CSF flow
artefact
(from basilar
artery)

Basilar artery

Vestibulocochlear
(VIIIth) nerve

Cerebellopontine
angle cistern

Cochlea

Middle
cerebellar
peduncle

IVth ventricle

Lateral
semicircular
canal

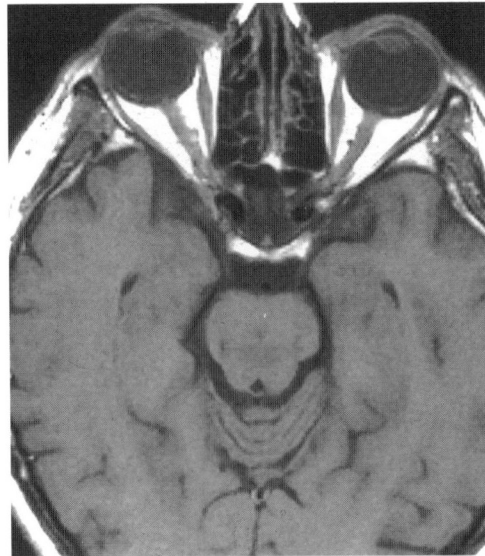

24(g)

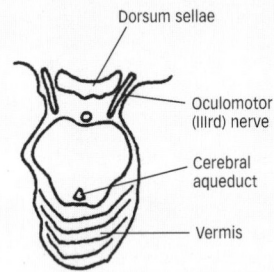

Dorsum sellae

Oculomotor
(IIIrd) nerve

Cerebral
aqueduct

Vermis

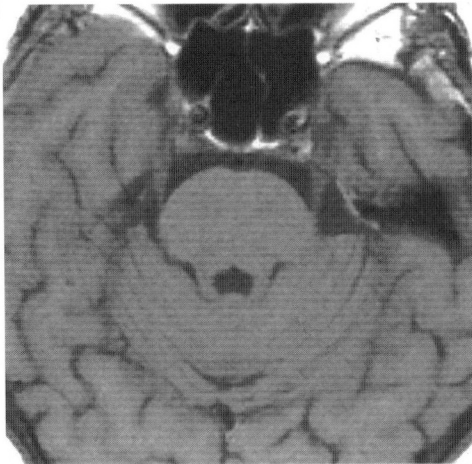

24(f)

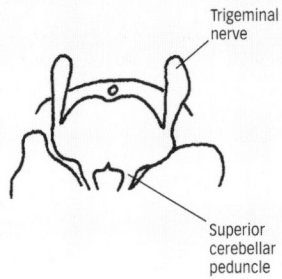

Trigeminal
nerve

Superior
cerebellar
peduncle

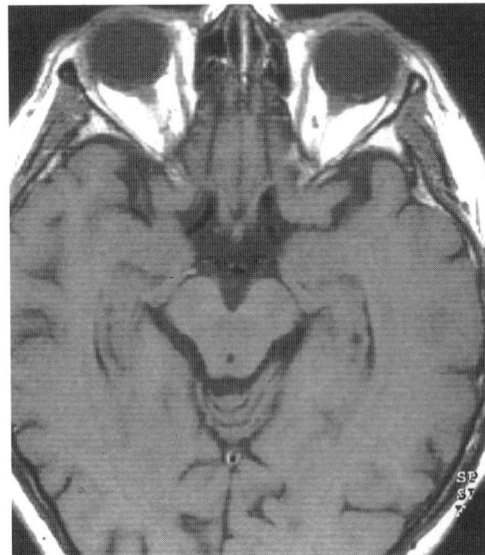

24(h)

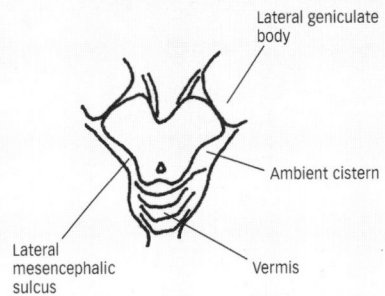

Lateral geniculate
body

Ambient cistern

Lateral
mesencephalic
sulcus

Vermis

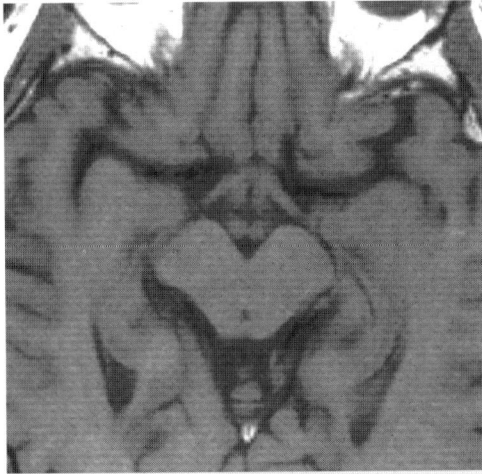

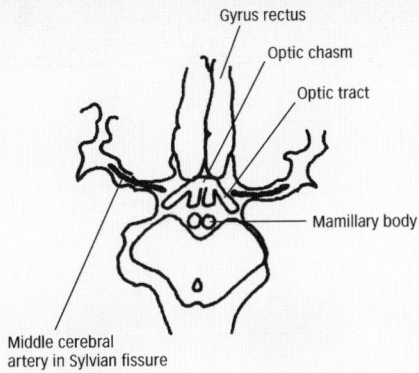

The cerebral parenchyma

The brainstem and cranial nerves

The brainstem consists of the medulla, pons and midbrain (Fig. 24). The hindbrain or rhombencephalon comprises the medulla, pons and cerebellum with the midbrain or mesencephalon classed separately.

A number of decussations occur within the brainstem where both motor and sensory fibres cross the midline in accordance with the general principle that functional control of one half of the body is largely exercised by the contralateral cerebral hemisphere.

The medulla is 'closed' inferiorly around a central canal continuous with that of the spinal cord and 'open' superiorly where it is related to the lower part of the fourth ventricle. The closed medulla extends from the point of emergence of the C1 spinal roots at the level of the foramen magnum to the obex. The obex is a small curved margin covering the inferior angle of the fourth ventricle anterior to which is the commencement of the central canal. On the ventral surface between the anterior median fissure and the anterolateral sulcus on each side is the pyramid. Lateral to this is another elevation, the olive.

24(*i*)

Gyrus rectus
Optic chasm
Optic tract
Mamillary body
Middle cerebral artery in Sylvian fissure

Fig. 24. line illustrations (*a*)–(*i*) represent the levels of the MRI scans in Fig. 24.

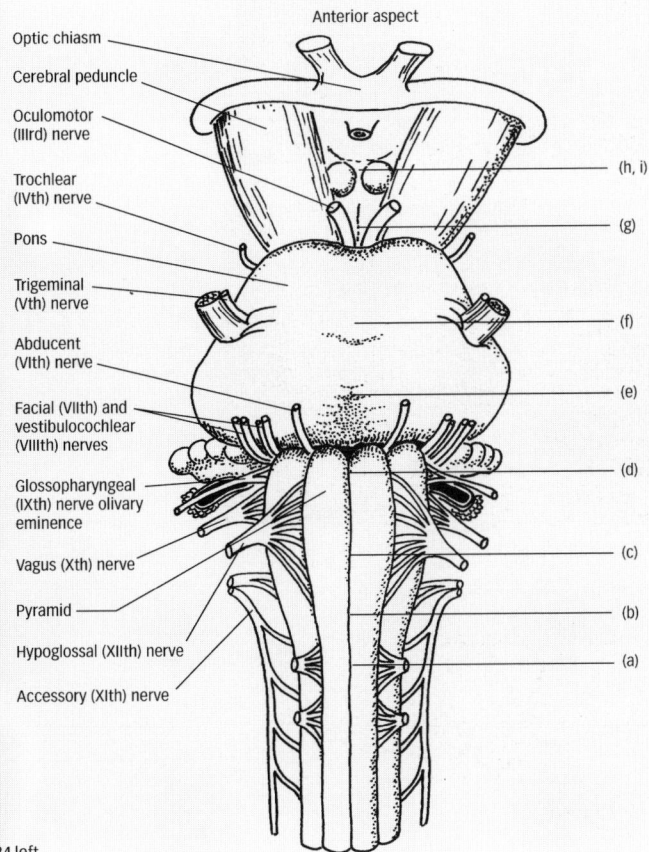

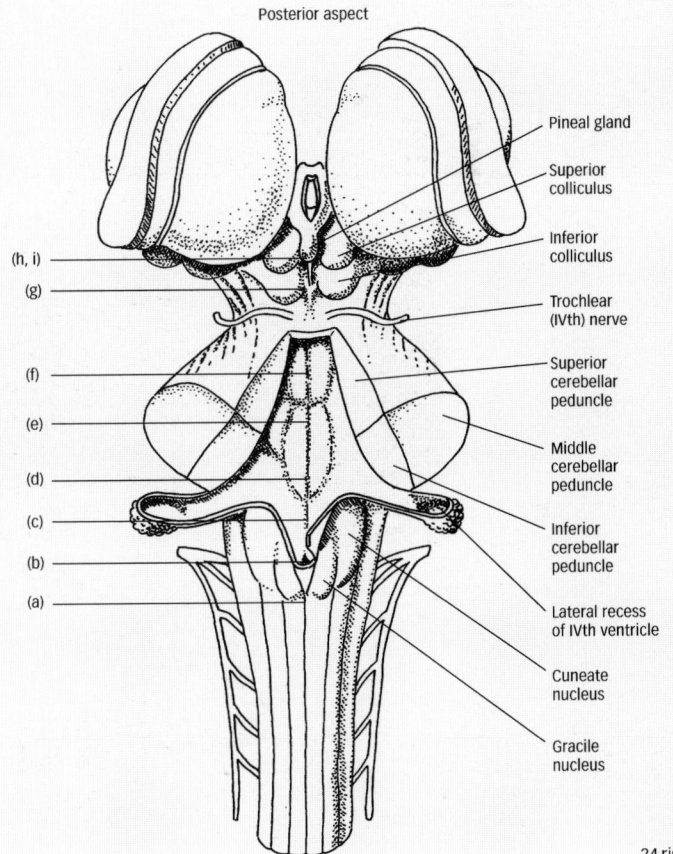

Anterior aspect

Optic chiasm
Cerebral peduncle
Oculomotor (IIIrd) nerve
Trochlear (IVth) nerve
Pons
Trigeminal (Vth) nerve
Abducent (VIth) nerve
Facial (VIIth) and vestibulocochlear (VIIIth) nerves
Glossopharyngeal (IXth) nerve olivary eminence
Vagus (Xth) nerve
Pyramid
Hypoglossal (XIIth) nerve
Accessory (XIth) nerve

(h, i)
(g)
(f)
(e)
(d)
(c)
(b)
(a)

24 left

Posterior aspect

Pineal gland
Superior colliculus
Inferior colliculus
Trochlear (IVth) nerve
Superior cerebellar peduncle
Middle cerebellar peduncle
Inferior cerebellar peduncle
Lateral recess of IVth ventricle
Cuneate nucleus
Gracile nucleus

(h, i)
(g)
(f)
(e)
(d)
(c)
(b)
(a)

24 right

33

(a)

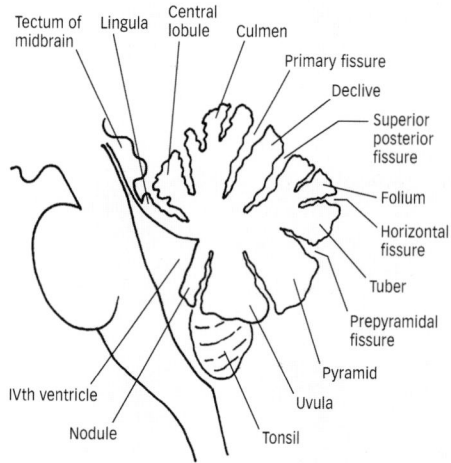

(c)

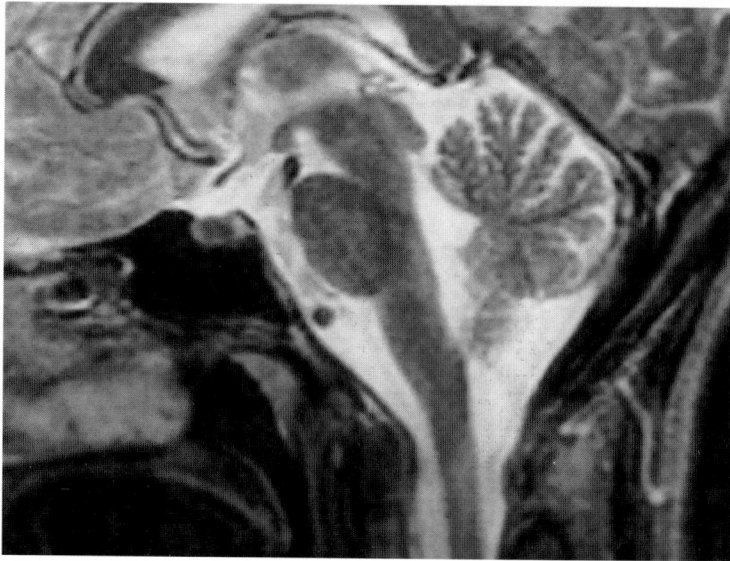

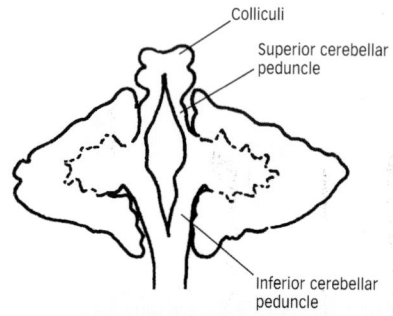

Fig. 25.
The cerebellum (a) T2W sagittal, (b), (c), (d) coronal T1W and (e) T2W MRI scans ((b)–(e), anterior to posterior).

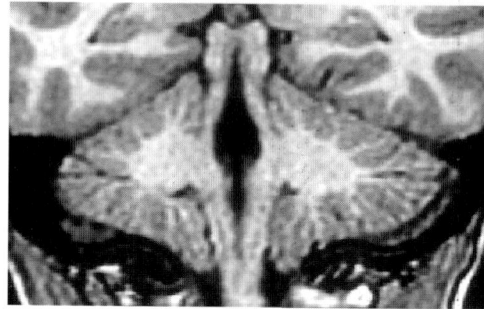

(b)

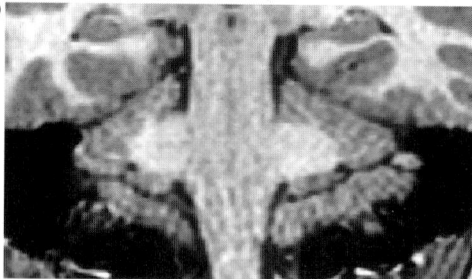

(d)

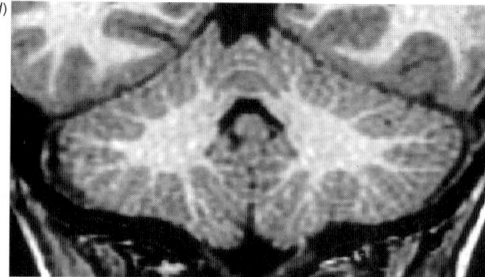

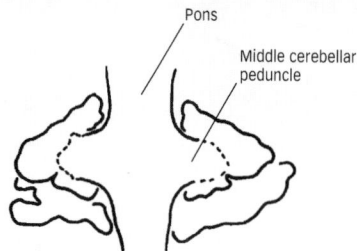

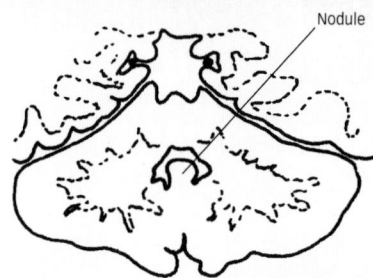

25(e)

Superior
posterior
fissure

Horizontal
fissure

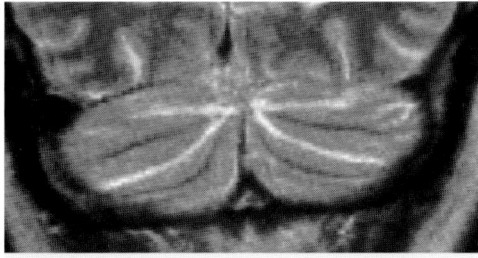

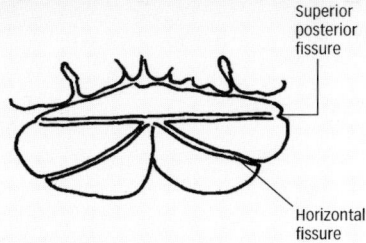

On the dorsal surface of the medulla, on each side of the posterior median sulcus, is the fasciculus gracilis which carries posterior column fibres from the lower part of the body, and lateral to this, the fasciculus cuneatus transmitting posterior column fibres from the upper body. These synapse in the gracile and cuneate nuclei from which arise internal arcuate fibres which pass medially to decussate and ascend in the medial lemnisci. This sensory decussation is craniad and dorsal to the pyramidal decussation but both occur in the closed medulla. The closed medulla on axial scanning is pear-shaped and may be rotated (Fig. 24(a)). The pyramids are seen anteriorly either side of the ventral fissure. The posterior columns form the large posterior eminences. Further craniad, at the foramen of Magendie, the medulla takes on a square shape (Fig. 24(b)) with an indentation on each lateral wall corresponding to the post-olivary sulcus. Above this, the dorsal surface becomes the floor of the fourth ventricle which opens into the cerebellopontine angle on each side through the foramen of Luschka around the inferior cerebellar peduncle. This is a route by which intraventricular tumours may spread into the subarachnoid space (see p. 49, 'fourth ventricle').

The anterior eminences now consist of the pyramids medially and the olives laterally separated by the pre-olivary sulcus. The inferior medullary velum can also be seen and the posterior eminences become more prominent as the inferior cerebellar peduncles. The diamond shaped floor of the fourth ventricle, the rhomboid fossa, is formed from the posterior surfaces of both the pons and upper medulla. Two swellings either side of a median groove are known as the facial colliculi and are due to the intramedullary facial nerves looping in a

medial to lateral direction dorsally over the abducent nuclei. Inferior to the striae medullares three triangular areas are identified on each side. The vagal, the hypoglossal and the less well-defined vestibular areas overlie their respective nuclei. The pontomedullary junction on axial MRI is denoted by a prominent pontomedullary sulcus on each lateral wall and the ventral fissure is replaced by a broader basilar sulcus (Fig. 24(d)).

The cranial nerves which arise from the medulla are, from above down, the glossopharyngeal (IXth), the vagus (Xth), the spinal accessory (XIth) and the hypoglossal (XIIth) nerves. The glossopharyngeal and vagus nerves emerge from a sulcus posterolateral to the olive and are in line with the dorsal spinal nerve roots.

The glossopharyngeal (IXth) nerve carries sensory fibres from the pharynx, carotid sinus and body and transmits taste from the posterior third of the tongue. It also supplies the stylopharyngeus muscle.

The vagus (Xth) nerve provides a motor supply to the intrinsic muscles of the larynx, the pharynx and soft palate. Its parasympathetic supply extends to the heart, the airways and the gastrointestinal tract. The meninges of the posterior fossa, part of the external auditory canal and pinna and tympanic membrane also receive a vagal sensory supply.

The accessory (XIth) nerve has a nucleus in the upper medulla and receives contributions from the anterior horn cells of the upper five or six cervical segments which coalesce and pass upwards through the foramen magnum (the 'spinal root'). The cranial root of the accessory nerve conveys fibres which join the vagus nerve to be distributed in the recurrent laryngeal nerve. The cranial root is thus 'accessory' to the vagus nerve. The accessory nerve also supplies the sternocleidomastoid and trapezius muscles.

The glossopharyngeal and spinal accessory nerves as well as the vagus have substantial parasympathetic components and the three together form a bundle which leaves the cranium via the jugular foramen; the glossopharyngeal nerve entering the pars nervosa, the other two the pars vascularis in a common dural sheath. It is not normally possible to identify the ninth, tenth or eleventh cranial nerves by MRI or CT cisternography. The hypoglossal (XIIth) nerve emerges more anteriorly in the pre-olivary sulcus between the olive and the pyramid and is thus in line with the ventral spinal roots. It supplies all the intrinsic and extrinsic muscles of the tongue except the

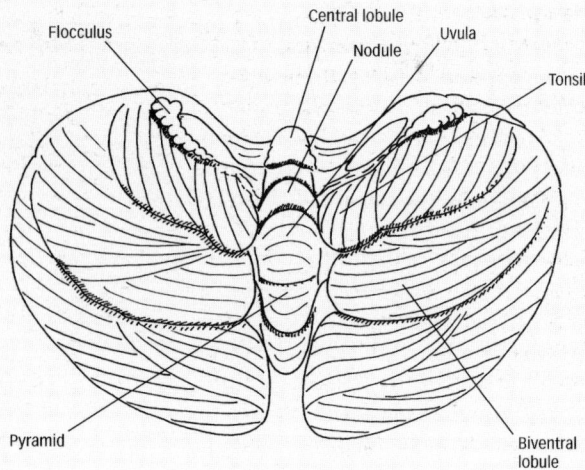

Fig. 26.
**The inferior aspect
of cerebellum.**

palatoglossus. Before entering the hypoglossal canal in the occipital bone, the hypoglossal nerve lies posterolateral to the vertebral artery, the two thus being closely related (Fig. 12).

The pons
The pons has a convex bulbous ventral portion containing mainly transverse fibres which pass posterolaterally as the middle cerebellar peduncle on each side. This ventral portion also transmits corticosopinal fibres and is continuous with the cerebral peduncles of the midbrain above.

The dorsal tegmentum of the pons contains, amongst other nuclei, the main nuclei of the trigeminal (Vth) cranial nerve in the upper portion and the abducent (VIth), facial (VIIth) and vestibulocochlear (VIIIth) cranial nerves in the lower part.

On axial imaging the lower pons (Fig. 24(*e*)) is dominated by the posterolaterally directed middle cerebellar peduncles, lateral to which are the cerebellopontine angle cisterns limited posteriorly by the flocculi.

The trigeminal nerves arise from the mid pons to pass anteriorly into Meckel's cave. The superior cerebellar peduncles are also identified, forming the lateral borders of the fourth ventricle (Fig. 24(*f*)).

The trigeminal nerve innervates those structures derived from the first branchial arch and consists of a large sensory root and a smaller motor root which has a separate fascial sheath but which cannot be resolved separately with imaging. The nerve arises at the junction of the pons and the more laterally placed middle cerebellar peduncle and passes directly forwards to the trigeminal ganglion.

There are four trigeminal nuclei: two in the pons, a mesencephalic nucleus and a spinal nucleus in the medulla which extends caudally into the upper cervical cord.

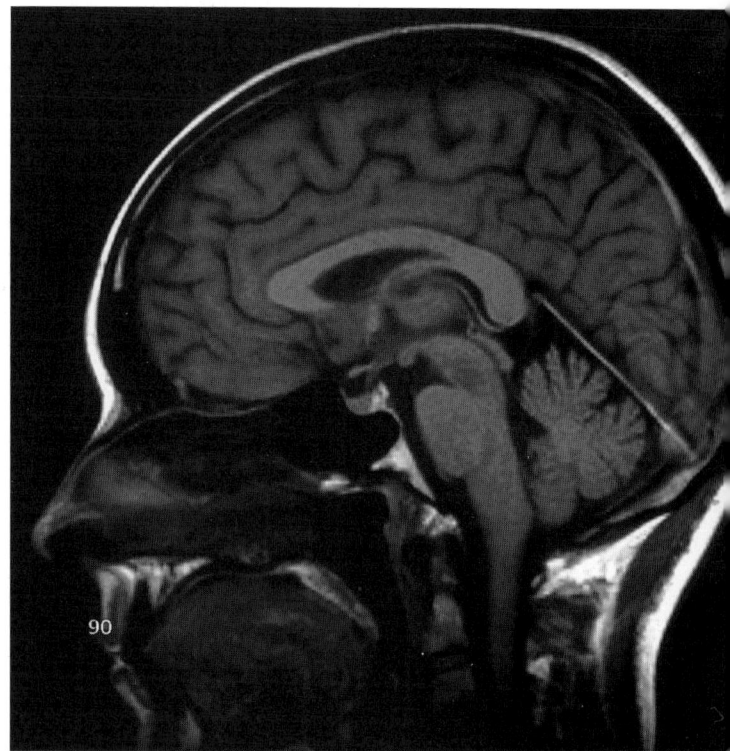

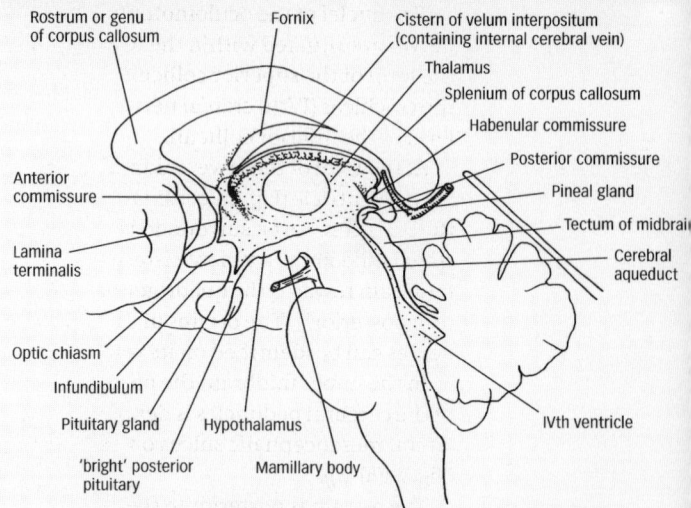

The abducent (VIth) nerve has a long intracranial course and may thus be damaged in a fracture of the skull base. It runs in an anterolateral direction to bend over the petrous apex, and pierces the dura covering the sphenoid bone (Dorello's canal) to enter the cavernous sinus.

The facial (VIIth) nerve has a motor root supplying the muscles of facial expression, stapedius, platysma, stylohyoid and the posterior belly of the digastric. The motor nucleus is in the lower pons. Its sensory root, the intermediate nerve, transmits secretomotor fibres to the lacrimal, submandibular and sublingual glands and fibres conveying taste from the anterior two-thirds of the tongue.

Fig. 27.
**T1W sagittal MRI scan to
show the diencephalon.**

36

The two roots pass from the inferior pontine border laterally in the cerebellopontine angle cistern, closely related to the vestibulocochlear nerve.

The dorsal and ventral cochlear nuclei are in the lower pons close to the inferior cerebellar peduncle. The vestibular nuclei are located at the pontomedullary junction lying beneath the lateral part of the floor of the fourth ventricle (see Chapter 4).

The midbrain

The midbrain comprises the dorsal tectum and the paired cerebral peduncles. Each peduncle consists of the crus cerebri, which contains the motor corticospinal tracts and the tegmentum, which lies ventral to the cerebral aqueduct and contains cranial nerve and other nuclei. Of these, the red nuclei, at the level of the superior colliculi, are well shown by MRI. The substantia nigra, a pigmented grey matter tract, separates the crus and tegmentum.

The cavity of the midbrain is the cerebral aqueduct (of Sylvius) which connects the third and fourth ventricles.

The nuclei of the oculomotor (IIIrd) cranial nerves are situated within the tegmentum at the level of the superior colliculi and those of the trochlear (IVth) cranial nerves are at the level of the inferior colliculi.

At the level of the lower midbrain, above the fourth ventricle (Fig. 24(*g*)), axial images show the brainstem to be surrounded by cerebrospinal fluid in the ambient cisterns circling the midbrain towards the quadrigeminal plate cistern posteriorly. The origins of the oculomotor nerves can be identified on its ventral aspect.

In the upper midbrain the posterior limit of the cerebral peduncles is denoted by the lateral mesencephalic sulcus on each side (Fig. 24(*h*), (*i*)).

The tectum is posterior to the cerebral aqueduct and consists of four colliculi or quadrigeminal bodies. The superior pair are concerned with visual reflexes, the inferior pair with auditory reflexes (Fig. 25(*a*)).

The oculomotor (IIIrd) nerve arises from the anterior surface of the midbrain, on the medial side of the cerebral peduncle, and passes between the posterior cerebral and superior cerebellar arteries (Fig. 51(*a*)). It then runs lateral to the posterior communicating artery to enter the cavernous sinus (Fig. 28). Parasympathetic fibres travel in the periphery of the nerve and are vulnerable to pressure from an expanding aneurysm at the origin of the posterior communicating artery, which may thus be responsible for an oculomotor palsy 'without pupil sparing', i.e. with pupillary dilatation on the affected side.

The trochlear (IVth) nerve is a small motor nerve which supplies the superior oblique muscle and is the only cranial nerve to emerge from the dorsal aspect of the brainstem, arising just below the inferior colliculus to course anteriorly around the midbrain. Fibres from the nucleus loop around the aqueduct and then cross to the opposite side within the superior medullary velum – another unique feature. The trochlear nerve passes forwards lateral to the superior cerebellar peduncle and inferior to the oculomotor nerve. It then turns superiorly to the lateral aspect of the third nerve as both pass between the posterior cerebral and superior cerebellar arteries, (Fig. 51(*a*)). The trochlear nerve assumes a position inferior to the oculomotor nerve in the lateral wall of the cavernous sinus.

The cerebellum

The cerebellum lies posterior to the brainstem to which it is connected by the cerebellar peduncles. The cortical mantle of the cerebellum overlies the white matter core as in the cerebral hemispheres but the cerebellar cortical ridges, known as folia, and the intervening sulci are approximately parallel to one another. In section, the grey matter has a tree-like configuration and is therefore described as the 'arbor vitae'.

The cerebellum consists of the narrow midline vermis separated by a paramedian sulcus on each side from two hemispheres. Deep transverse fissures divide the vermis and hemispheres into three lobes, each comprising a number of lobules which, since the fissures are orientated perpendicular to the midline, are shown on sagittal MRI sections. Seen from above, each of the fissures describes an arc extending into the hemispheres.

Fig. 28.
The pituitary and perisellar region: (*a*) diagram, (*b*)–(*d*) coronal CT, (*e*), T1W coronal and (*f*), (*g*) axial MRI scans, all after intravenous contrast administration.

(*a*)

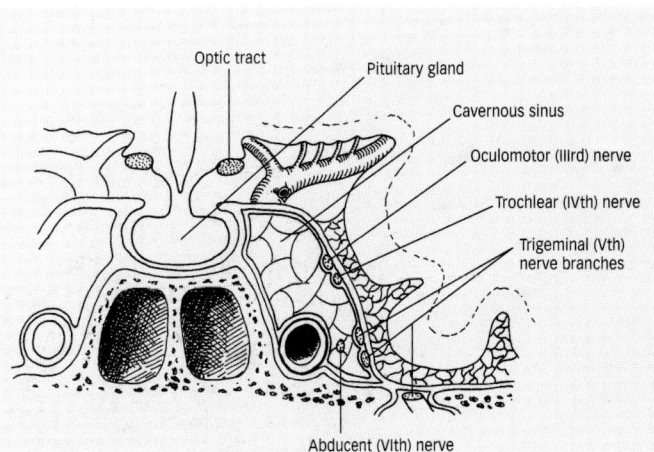

Optic tract

Pituitary gland

Cavernous sinus

Oculomotor (IIIrd) nerve

Trochlear (IVth) nerve

Trigeminal (Vth) nerve branches

Abducent (VIth) nerve

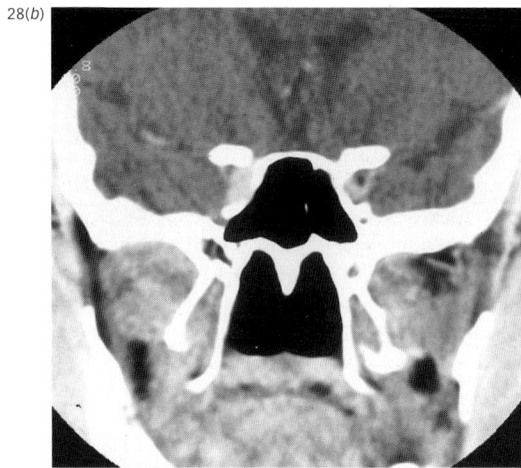

28(*b*)

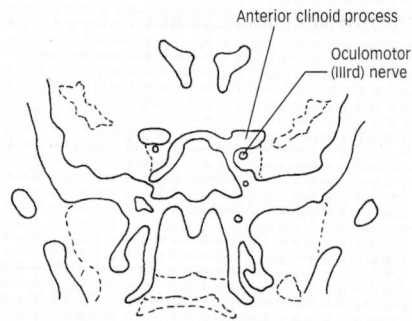

Anterior clinoid process

Oculomotor
(IIIrd) nerve

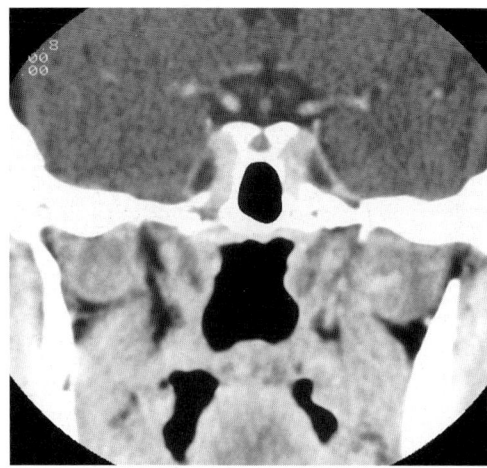

28(*c*)

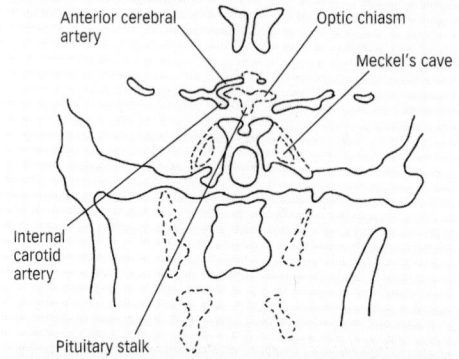

Anterior cerebral
artery

Optic chiasm

Meckel's cave

Internal
carotid
artery

Pituitary stalk

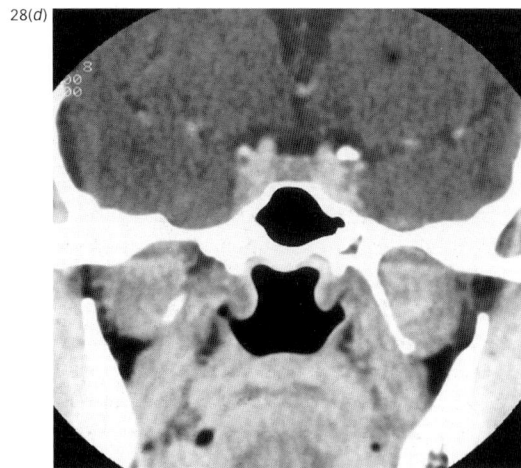

28(*d*)

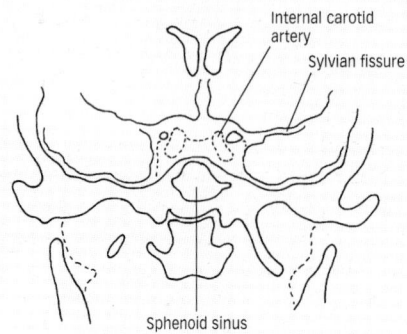

Internal carotid
artery

Sylvian fissure

Sphenoid sinus

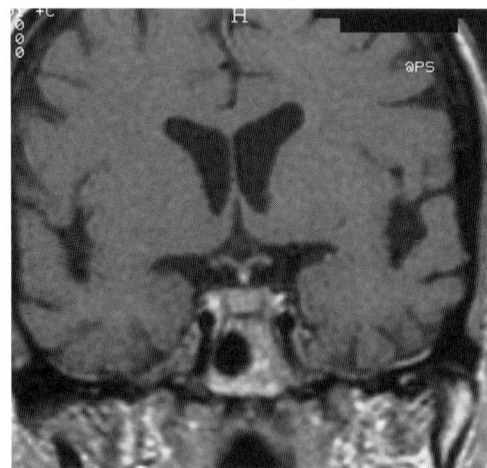

28(*e*)

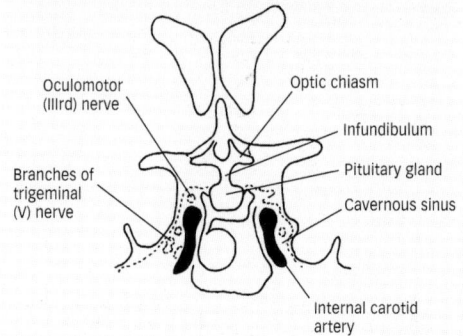

Oculomotor
(IIIrd) nerve

Optic chiasm

Infundibulum

Pituitary gland

Branches of
trigeminal
(V) nerve

Cavernous sinus

Internal carotid
artery

28(f)

Pituitary gland

Internal carotid
artery within
cavernous sinus

Petrosal vein
of Dandy

28(g)

Infundibulum

Middle cerebral
artery

Suprasellar
cistern

Posterior
cerebral artery

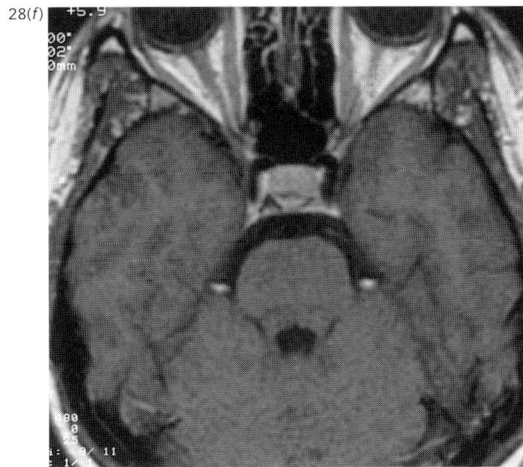

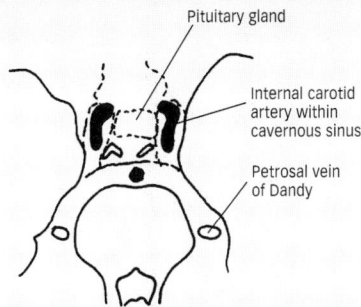

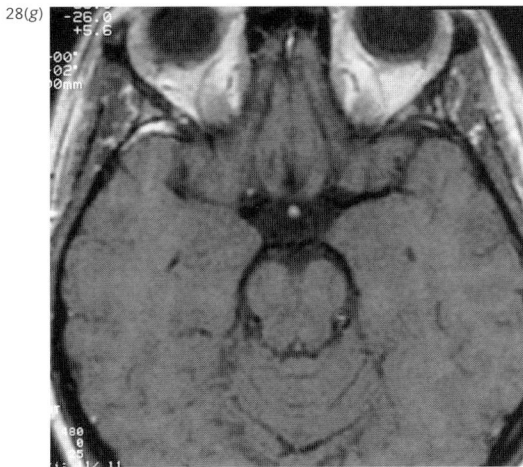

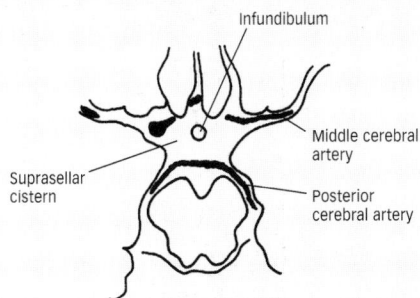

The primary fissure separates the anterior
lobe from the larger posterior lobe. The smallest lobe, the flocculonodular lobe, is separated
from the posterior lobe by the posterolateral

sulcus. The lobules are identified in Fig. 25.
The lingula, central lobule and culmen are
part of the anterior lobe. The declive, folium,
tuber, pyramid and uvula are part of the posterior lobe and the nodule is the only lobule of
the flocculonodular lobe.

The vermis is slender and anatomical detail,
particularly of the inferior portions, may be
obscured due to partial volume averaging on
MR scans. The flocculus is largely separate
from the rest of the cerebellum and extends
laterally inferior to the vestibulocochlear
nerve. The normal flocculus enhances more
than the rest of the cerebrum after intravenous iodinated contrast medium because
of its proximity to the choroid plexus and
anterior inferior cerebellar artery. It can therefore be mistaken for an acoustic neurinoma
on CT but the recognition that it is posterior to
the porus acousticus should avoid this pitfall.

The nodule is the most ventral structure on
the inferior vermian surface and is frequently
identified on axial scans lying posterior to the
fourth ventricle (Fig. 24).

The biventral lobule forms the anterior surface of the inferior cerebellar hemisphere and
its medial part is at the level of the foramen
magnum. The cerebellar tonsils are smaller
and more medial, lying posterior to the
medulla. Since both may descend to the foramen magnum, they may be confused (Fig. 26).

Three cerebellar peduncles arise from the
white matter core on each side and are demonstrated on both axial and coronal MR scans
(Figs. 24, 25). The superior cerebellar peduncle
(brachium conjunctivum) passes to the midbrain, the middle cerebellar peduncle
(brachium pontis) to the pons and the inferior
cerebellar peduncle (restiform body) to the
medulla.

The middle cerebellar peduncles are the
largest and pass horizontally whereas the
superior and inferior peduncles are orientated
vertically. The superior cerebellar peduncles
form the lateral border of the upper part of the
fourth ventricle. The inferior cerebellar peduncles border the inferior part but are separated
from the ventricle by the vestibular nuclei.

The diencephalon

The diencephalon lies between the cerebral
hemispheres and brainstem and includes the
thalamus, hypothalamus, pineal gland and
habenula, all of which are structures border-
ing the third ventricle (Fig. 27). The pineal
gland and habenular complex are together
known as the epithalamus. There is a close
association between the diencephalon and
the limbic system.

The ovoid pineal gland lies between the two superior colliculi in the posterior wall of the third ventricle. Pineal gland calcification can be detected in 50–70% of adult lateral skull radiographs but it is almost invariable on CT scans. It is rarely present below 10 years. In a midline sagittal MRI scan, two laminae can be seen arising anteriorly from the pineal gland. The superior of the two is the habenular commissure, which describes a 'reversed' C shape (with the open part posteriorly) corresponding to the calcification seen on lateral skull radiographs (Fig. 4). The inferior lamina is the posterior commissure (Fig. 27).

The anterior commissure (Fig. 2) consists of myelinated fibres embedded in the lamina terminalis, the anterior limit of the diencephalon. It can be seen on MRI scans as a convex arc of fibres and is a useful location to identify prominent perivascular spaces, found along its lateral aspects. A line joining the anterior and posterior commissures on midline sagittal MRI scans (the 'AC–PC' line) is a standard reference in image-guided sterotactic surgery. The thalami are paired, olive-shaped nuclear masses, extending anteriorly as far as the interventricular foramen and forming most of the lateral walls of the third ventricle.

Laterally, the posterior limb of the internal capsule separates it from the lentiform nucleus. Medially the two thalami are apposed (not in continuity) at the interthalamic adhesion or massa intermedia. The posterior end or pulvinar projects over the midbrain and beneath it are the medial and lateral geniculate bodies (Fig. 24). The lateral geniculate body is concerned with the visual pathway and the medial geniculate body, which is part of the midbrain, is concerned with the auditory pathway.

The hypothalamus forms the floor and part of the walls of the third ventricle. Posterior to the optic chiasm, the infundibulum (or pituitary stalk), a hollow, conical structure, descends to the pituitary gland. The tuber cinereum extends posteriorly from the infundibulum towards the mamillary bodies and thence to the midbrain.

The pituitary gland

The pituitary gland and the perisellar region are frequently imaged in cases of endocrine disturbance or visual failure. The gland is situated within the pituitary fossa, above the sphenoid sinus with the cavernous sinuses on each side (Fig. 28). The suprasellar cistern is a superior relation, containing the optic pathways and circle of Willis.

The pituitary gland varies in size. In some normal individuals the gland may simply

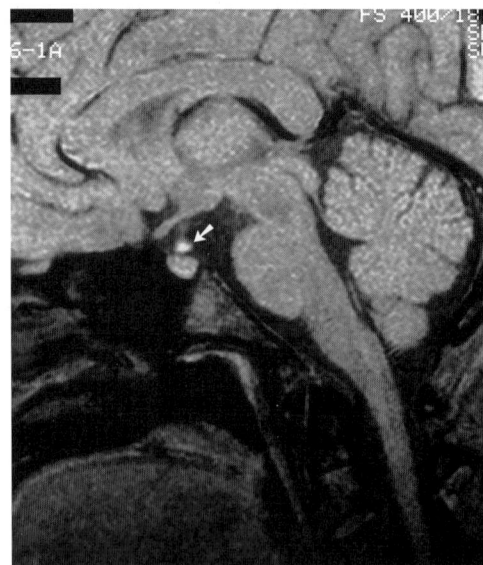

Fig. 29.
Ectopic posterior pituitary gland within the pituitary stalk (arrow); T1W sagittal MRI scan.

appear as a thin rim of tissue at the base of the sella (partially empty sella). Conversely, particularly in females of childbearing age, the pituitary gland will fill the sella and have a superior margin which is convex. The infundibulum is larger in girls than in boys but in neither sex should it exceed the diameter of the basilar artery, which will be included in axial scans of this region. The normal pituitary gland should be no greater than 9 mm in height and both it and the infundibulum enhance on CT and T1W MRI following intravenous contrast medium. The anterior and posterior lobes of the pituitary gland may be identified separately on MR scans. In some individuals, the posterior pituitary returns a high signal on T1W images (Fig. 27). The 'bright' signal is thought to be due to neurosecretary granules in the pituitary and it is not surprising therefore that its presence may be variable in sequential scans of the same individual. The pituitary gland may be uniformly bright in the neonate.

Ectopic pituitary tissue, usually originating from the posterior lobe, may be found as a rounded high signal soft tissue 'mass' expanding the infundibulum (Fig. 29).

The basal ganglia

The basal ganglia are part of the extrapyramidal system and consist of the caudate and lentiform nuclei, together known as the corpus striatum, the amygdala and claustrum. The amygdala is associated with the limbic system (Figs. 1, 30).

The caudate nucleus is C-shaped with the concavity facing inferiorly. The head indents the anterior horn and its shape is similar on both axial and coronal images. The body can be seen lying alongside the body of the lateral

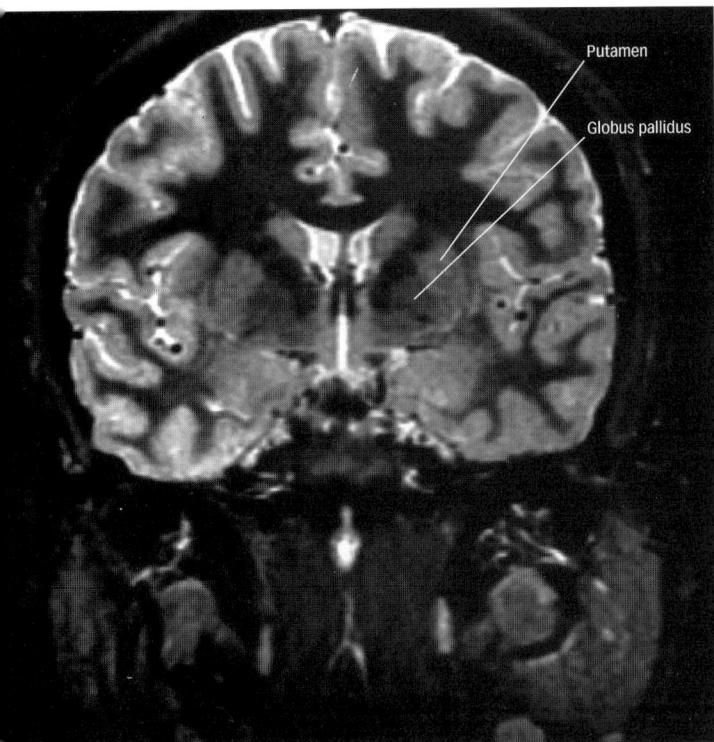

(d)

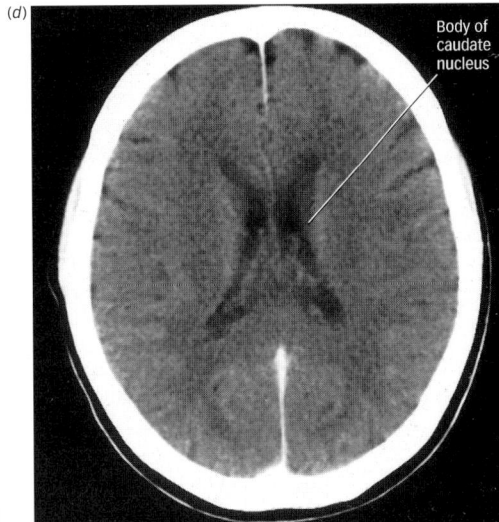

Body of caudate nucleus

Putamen

Globus pallidus

Fig. 30.
e basal ganglia: (*a*) TW, (*b*)
TW coronal and (*c*) T1W
xtended axial MRI and (*d*)
CT scan.

(b)

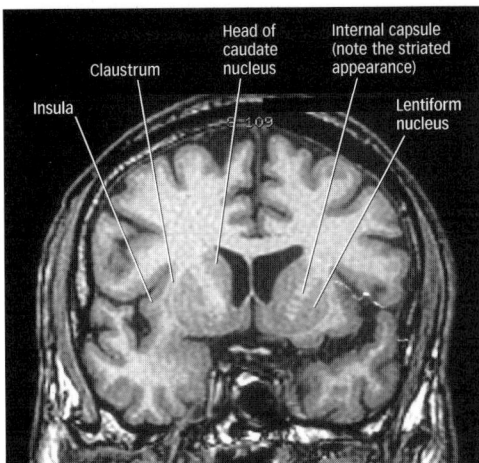

Insula

Claustrum

Head of caudate nucleus

Internal capsule (note the striated appearance)

Lentiform nucleus

(c)

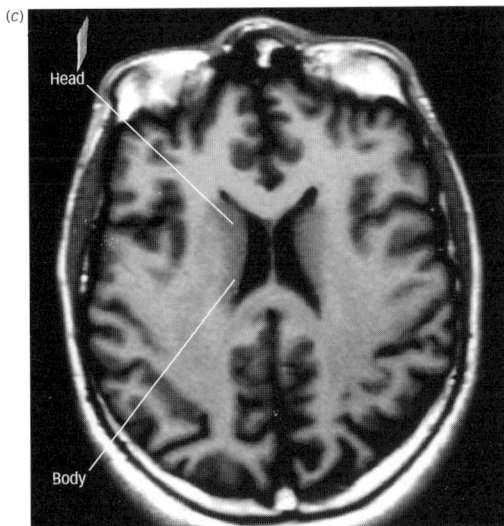

Head

Body

ventricle on CT and MR. The tail of the caudate nucleus comes to lie above the temporal horn and is not readily seen on MRI. The lentiform nucleus is divided into two by a sheet of white matter lying in the parasagittal plane. The larger lateral component is the putamen. The smaller medial component is the globus pallidus. They are both well demonstrated on axial and coronal images (Fig. 30). The claustrum is a thin sheet of grey matter interposed between the grey matter of the putamen and the insula. It is separated from the putamen by the white matter of the external capsule and from the insular cortex by the extreme capsule. The lentiform nucleus is bounded on its medial aspect by the internal capsule which is traversed by connecting fibres between thalamus and lentiform nucleus which can be appreciated on MR scans (Fig. 30(*a*)).

The motor pathways
Voluntary movement is controlled by the motor pathways which descend from the cerebral cortex to motor nuclei in the brain stem (corticobulbar tracts) and the spinal cord (corticospinal tracts). The upper motor neurones arise in the precentral gyrus of the frontal lobe, the primary motor cortex and join the corona radiata which converges on the internal capsule.

The internal capsule (Fig. 1) is a myelinated tract of projection fibres which, by definition, pass to or from the more caudal parts of the central nervous system. It is V-shaped when viewed in the axial plane. The genu points medially and separates the anterior limb and larger posterior limb. Corticobulbar fibres are present at the genu. Corticospinal fibres are found in the posterior limb and their relatively large fibres, with thick myelin sheaths but low overall myelin density, can be shown as rounded high signal foci on T2W images in about 50% of normal individuals (Fig. 2).

The lenticulostriate arteries supply the region of the genu; the artery of Heubner (from the anterior cerebral artery), the anterior limb and the anterior choroidal artery, the posterior limb. The white matter above the lateral ventricles is known as the centrum ovale (Fig. 31).

The cerebral hemispheres

The cerebral hemispheres lie above the tentorium cerebelli and are divided conventionally into frontal, parietal, occipital and temporal lobes by fissures and sulci.

The cerebral hemispheres are linked by the corpus callosum the largest of the commissural tracts which interconnect paired structures across the midline. In sagittal view it is a curved structure. The most anterior portion is the rostrum, or genu which blends inferiorly with the anterior commissure (Figs. 27, 46). More superiorly, the genu curves posteriorly towards the body. The posterior part of the corpus callosum, which is also the bulkiest, is the splenium. The corpus callosum is a myelinated tract with the appropriate CT and MRI appearances.

Fibres of the corpus callosum sweep anteriorly into the frontal white matter as the forceps minor and posteriorly into the occipital lobes as the larger forceps major (Fig. 1).

(a)

(b)

Fig. 32.
The cortical gyri: (a) medial and (b) lateral aspects.

Fig. 31.
The centrum ovale: axial PD MRI scan

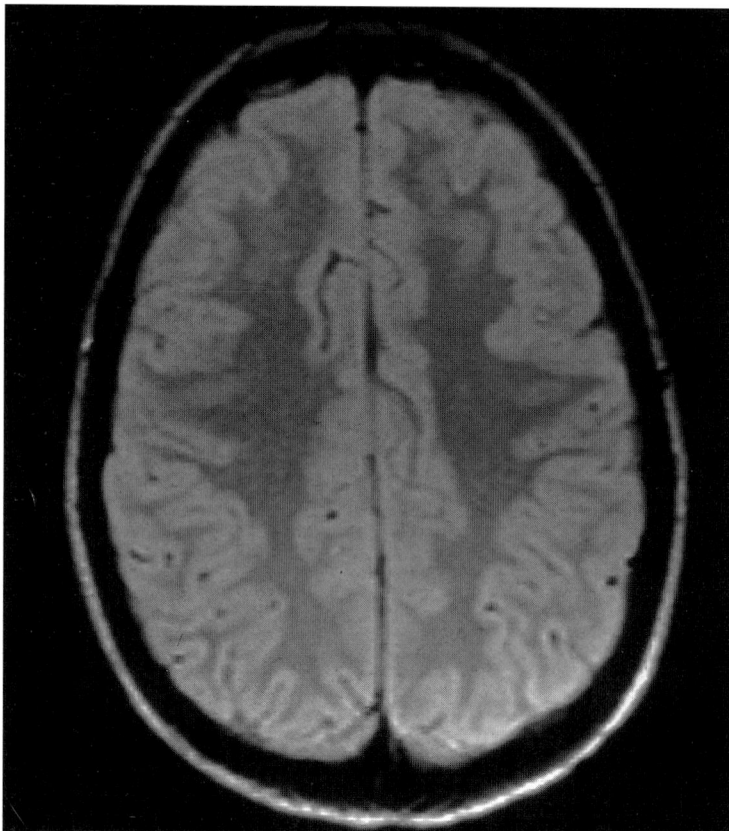

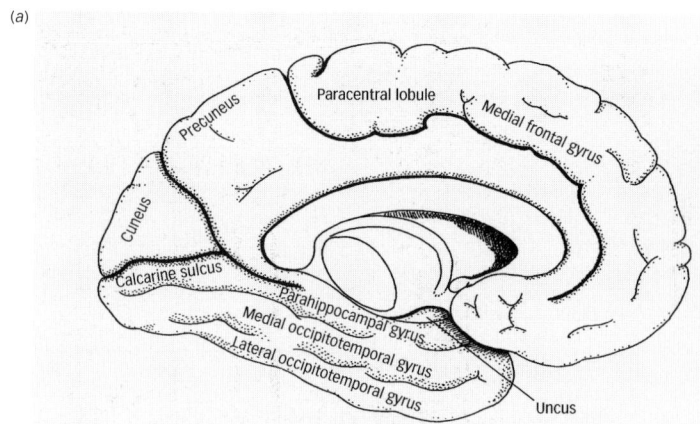

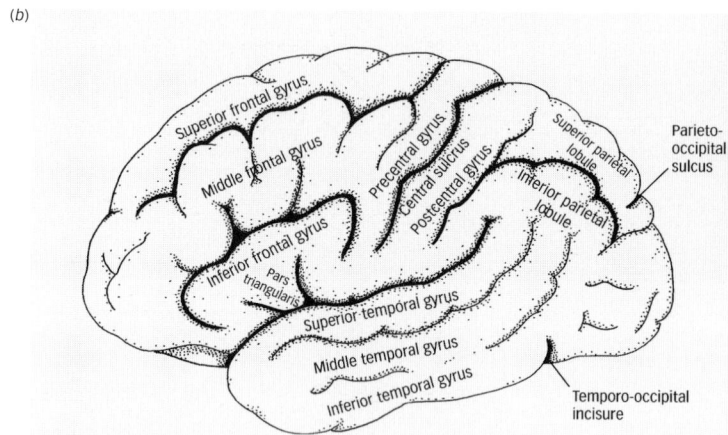

The central sulcus (or Rolandic fissure) which runs in the near coronal plane on the lateral surface of each hemisphere separates the frontal and parietal lobes. The parieto-occipital fissure, which runs obliquely on the medial aspect of each hemisphere, separates the parietal and occipital lobes and can be seen on midline sagittal MR sections (Fig. 46). The temporo-occipital incisure is a short fissure on the inferior and lateral aspects of each hemisphere and demarcates the division between the posterior aspect of the temporal

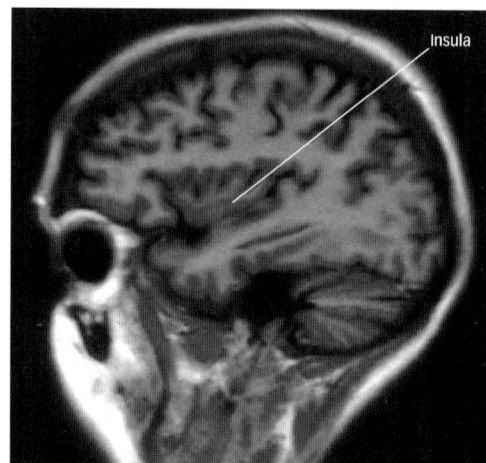

Fig. 33.
Parasagittal T1W MRI scan to show the triangular shaped insula (arrow).

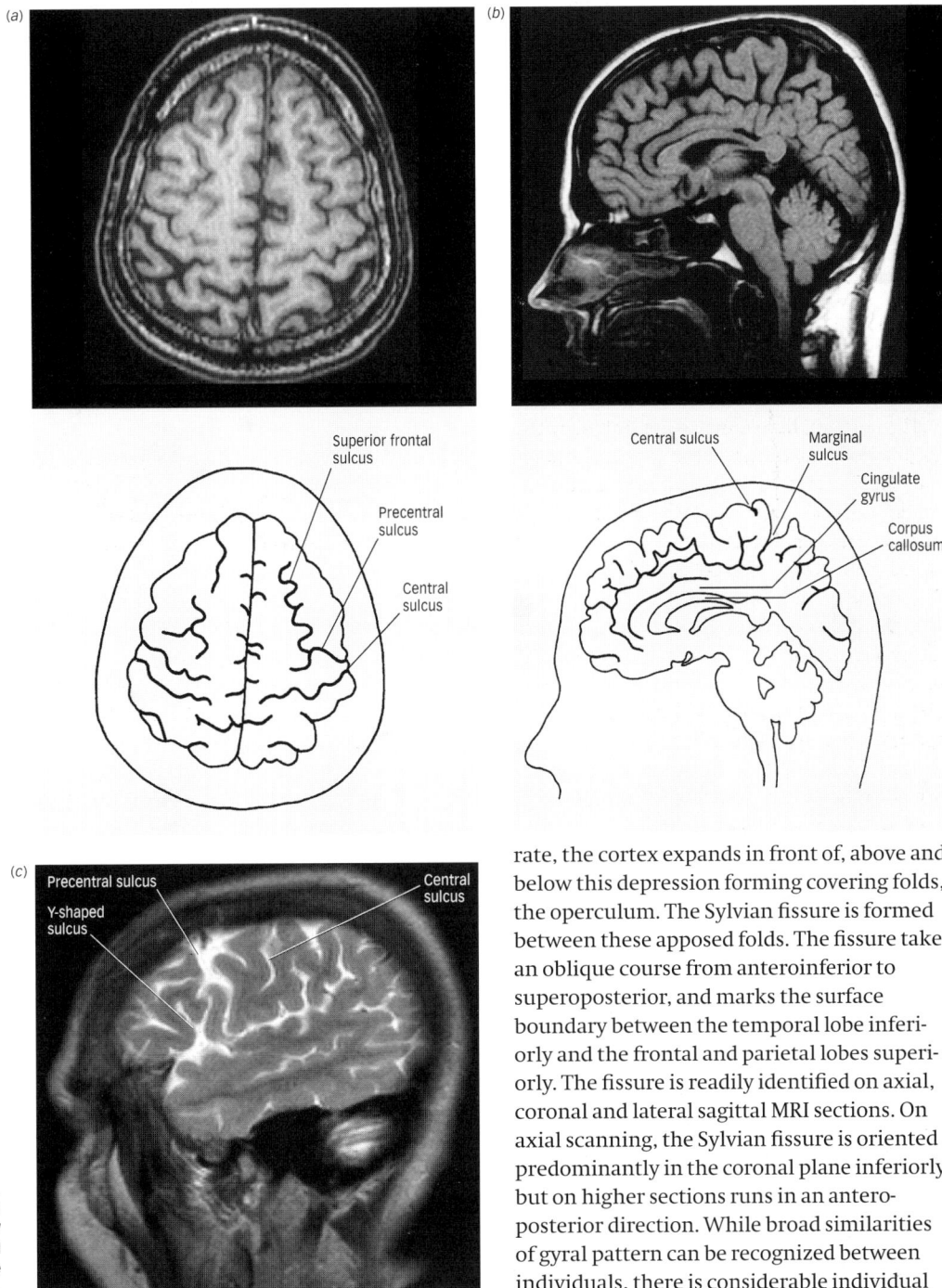

(a)

(b)

Superior frontal
sulcus

Precentral
sulcus

Central
sulcus

Central sulcus   Marginal
sulcus

Cingulate
gyrus

Corpus
callosum

(c)

Precentral sulcus   Central
sulcus
Y-shaped
sulcus

Fig. 34.
MRI scans of the central
sulcus (a) T1W axial, (b) T1W
midline sagittal images and
(c) T2W parasagittal image
through the Sylvian fissure.

and anterior aspect of the occipital lobes (Fig. 32). The demarcation between the posterior aspect of the temporal lobe and the parietal lobe on the lateral aspect of each hemisphere is ill-defined. The Sylvian or lateral fissure separates the superior surface of the temporal lobe from the inferior surface of the frontal lobe and the anterior aspect of the parietal lobe (Figs. 1, 34(c)). During development the cortex overlying the corpus striatum is invaginated to form the insula or 'island of Reil' which comes to form the floor of a deep depression (Figs. 1, 30, 33). Due to a differential growth rate, the cortex expands in front of, above and below this depression forming covering folds, the operculum. The Sylvian fissure is formed between these apposed folds. The fissure takes an oblique course from anteroinferior to superoposterior, and marks the surface boundary between the temporal lobe inferiorly and the frontal and parietal lobes superiorly. The fissure is readily identified on axial, coronal and lateral sagittal MRI sections. On axial scanning, the Sylvian fissure is oriented predominantly in the coronal plane inferiorly but on higher sections runs in an antero-posterior direction. While broad similarities of gyral pattern can be recognized between individuals, there is considerable individual variation. The more constant cortical gyri and sulci are illustrated in Fig. 32. With a few exceptions, such as the gyri recti, the cingulate gyri and the parahippocampal gyri, it is difficult to identify named gyri with certainty on orthogonal MR images of the cortical mantle. Surface rendering techniques, in which the image data is manipulated to produce a three-dimensional representation of the cortical surface, are now available on many MRI scanners. These provide a better means of identifying individual gyri and their relationship to cortical lesions.

The central sulcus

The identification of the precise location of the central sulcus is of great importance when surgery in the vicinity of the motor cortex is planned. Besides forming the boundary between the frontal and parietal lobes, the sulcus separates the motor cortex anteriorly in the precentral gyrus and the sensory 'strip' lying immediately posteriorly in the postcentral gyrus. Although at the vertex, these gyri and thus the central sulcus have their long axes in the coronal plane, the location of the sulcus may not always be readily determined and this is compounded by the fact that its position on axial images of the vertex, taken parallel to the canthomeatal line, is more posterior than would be expected intuitively.

Because of the ability of MRI to image in multiple planes, methods have been described for locating the central sulcus on sagittal and parasagittal as well as axial sections.

On axial sections, parallel to the canthomeatal line (Fig. 34(*a*)) the superior frontal sulcus is first identified running in the sagittal plane and separating the superior and middle frontal gyri. At its posterior end it forms a right angle with the precentral sulcus. The next sulcus posterior to this, running in the coronal plane, is the central sulcus. If the right angle formed between the superior frontal sulcus and the precentral sulcus is difficult to identify, the right angle formed between the superior frontal gyrus and the precentral sulcus can be used instead.

On medial sagittal sections, (Fig. 34(*b*)) the cingulate sulcus is identified above the cingulate gyrus. Near its posterior limit, almost vertically above the splenium of the corpus callosum, it divides and one segment, known as the marginal sulcus, ascends towards the vertex. The surface notch in the cortex immediately anterior to the marginal sulcus is the central sulcus.

On lateral sagittal sections (Fig. 34(*c*)) through the Sylvian fissure, the anterior horizontal ramus of the inferior frontal gyrus and the ascending ramus of the Sylvian fissure form a Y-shaped sulcus above the anterior aspect of the Sylvian fissure. The next major fissure posterior to the Y is the precentral sulcus with the central sulcus being the next major fissure posterior to this.

Despite using these techniques, the central sulcus is only identified with certainty in approximately 75% of cases. MR images can however be acquired as a 'block' of tissue and, with reformatting and cross-referencing, it is possible to mark the central sulcus in one plane and transfer this location to scans in other planes.

The limbic system

The limbic system has a complex structure and function. It includes the limbic lobe, olfactory apparatus and the septal areas, but its clinical and radiological importance arises principally in patients with temporal lobe epilepsy.

The limbic lobe is a complex three-dimensional structure which cannot be completely visualized in any one section or indeed any one plane. It can be divided into a large limbic gyrus and two slender intralimbic gyri. These are three concentric C-shaped structures in the near sagittal plane with the C rotated in each case by 90 degrees so that their concavities face inferiorly (Figs. 32(*a*), 35).

The limbic gyrus comprises the subcallosal gyrus, the cingulate gyrus, the isthmus (frontal and parietal lobes), the parahippocampal gyrus, and the anterior segment of the uncus (temporal lobe).

The outer intralimbic gyrus comprises the hippocampus and the dentate gyrus together with their posterior extensions which include the indusium griseum (or supracallosal gyrus). The indusium griseum curves around the splenium of the corpus callosum to lie on its superior surface, below the callosal sulcus.

The inner intralimbic gyrus consists of the fimbria and the fornix, which arises from the posterior aspect of the fimbria.

The parahippocampal gyrus forms the medial aspect of the temporal lobe. It is continuous posteriorly with the isthmus of the cingulate gyrus which follows the curve of the corpus callosum, separated from it by the callosal sulcus. Anteriorly the parahippocampal gyrus turns upwards and backwards on itself to form the uncus and to become continuous with the head of the hippocampus

Fig. 35.
(*a*) Medial aspect of cerebral hemisphere showing the limbic system (*b*) The hippocampus viewed from above.

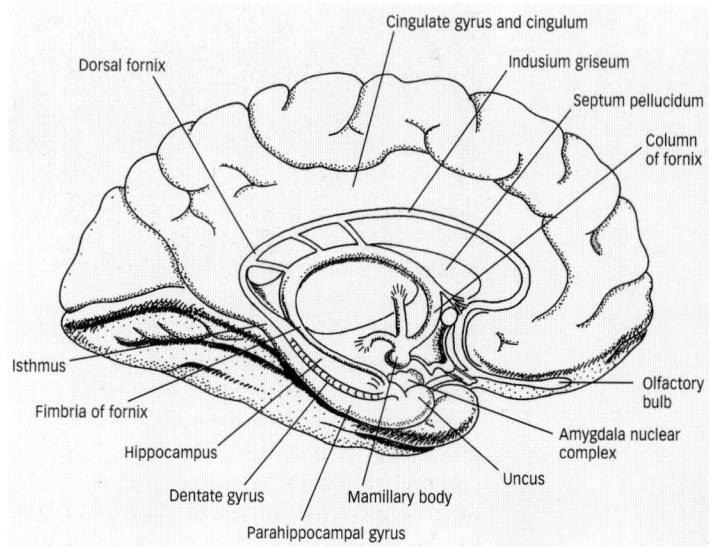

Cingulate gyrus and cingulum
Dorsal fornix
Indusium griseum
Septum pellucidum
Column of fornix
Isthmus
Olfactory bulb
Fimbria of fornix
Amygdala nuclear complex
Hippocampus
Uncus
Dentate gyrus
Mamillary body
Parahippocampal gyrus

35(*b*)

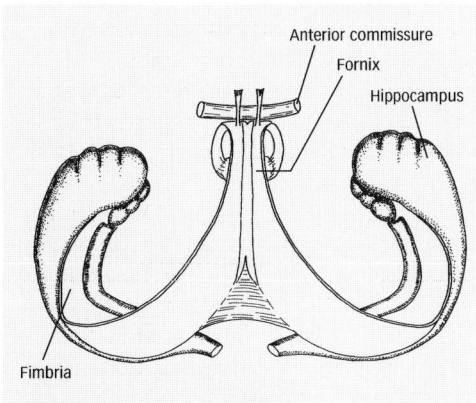

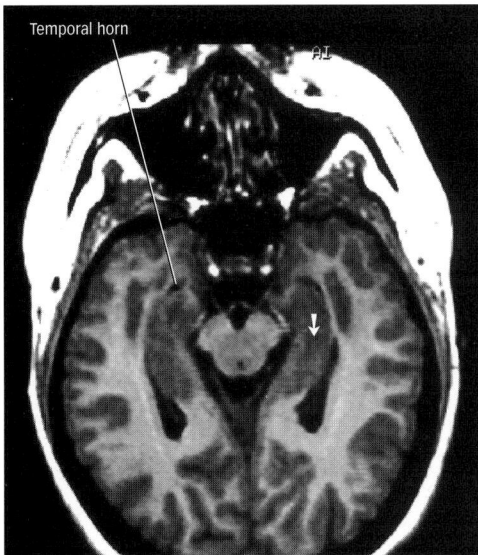

(*a*) Fig. 38.
Diagrammatic representation, (*a*) and MRI scans of the limbic lobe, (*b*) T1W, (*c*) T2W coronal images.

Fig. 36.
The hippocampus shown on an extended axial T1W MRI scan (3D volume acquisition). The pes hippocampi is arrowed.

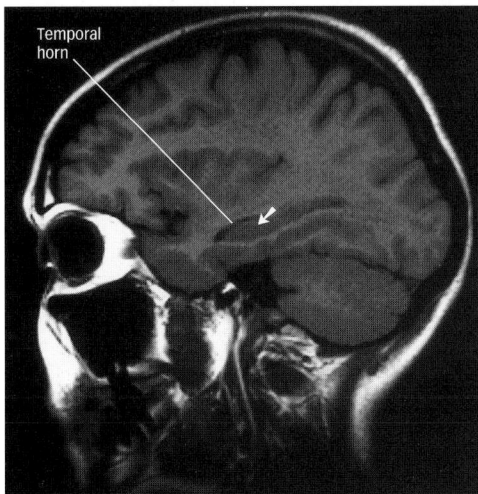

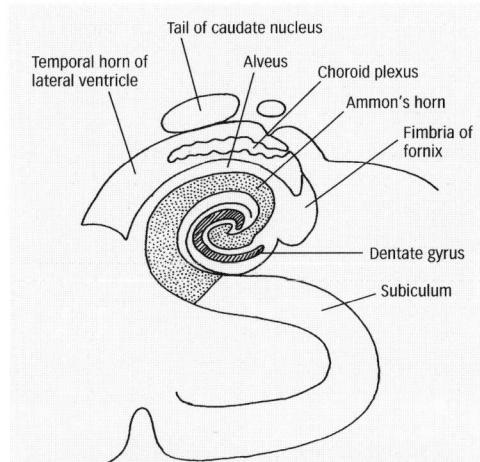

(*b*)

Fig. 37.
T1W parasagittal MRI hippocampus (arrow).

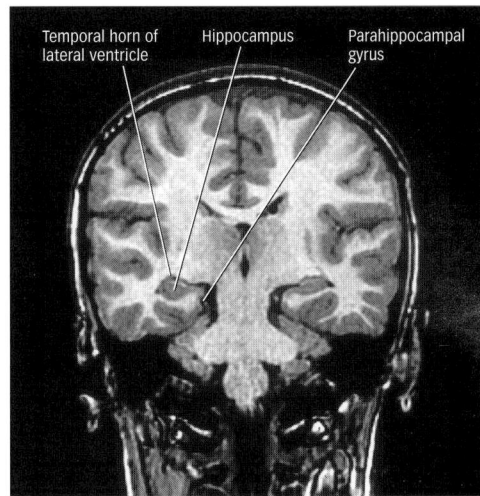

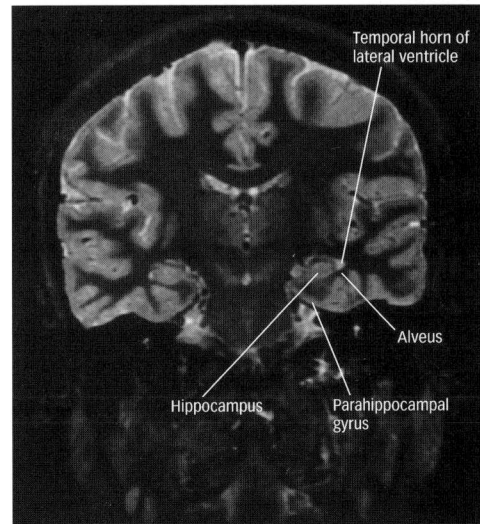

(*c*)

posteriorly. The parahippocampal gyrus is limited inferolaterally by the collateral sulcus and superiorly by the transverse fissure and hippocampal sulcus above which lies the hippocampus.

The hippocampus lies in the floor of the temporal horn of the lateral ventricle and is so called because of its supposed resemblance to a sea horse when viewed from above through the opened temporal horn (Fig. 36). It widens progressively from posterior to anterior.

The body of the hippocampus lies in the parasagittal plane (Fig. 37) and both its head, (the pes hippocampi indentatus), and tail curve medially.

In coronal section the hippocampus has a rolled construction (Fig. 38). There are two

Fig. 39. (a)
The fornix (arrows); T1W (a),
(b) coronal MRI scans.

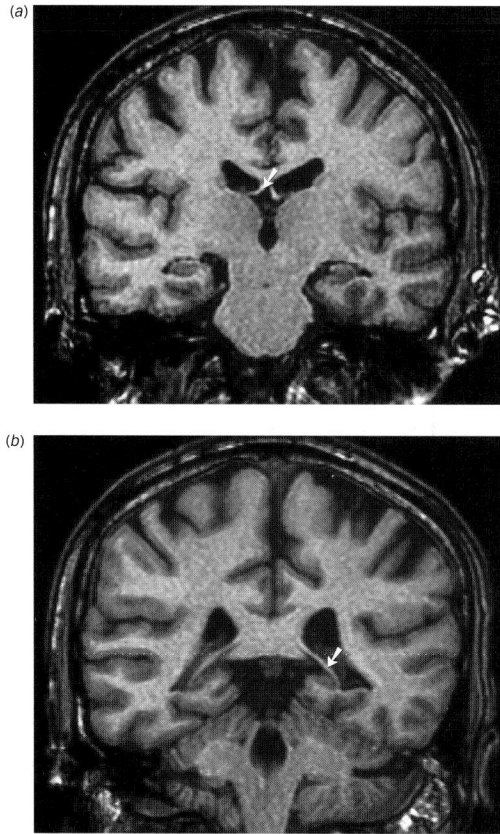

(b)

Fig. 40.
T1W coronal MRI scan
showing the olfactory
bulbs (arrows).

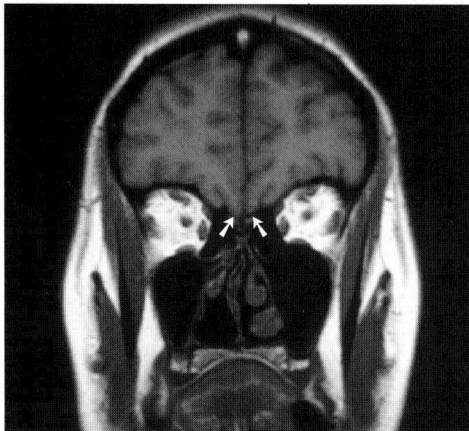

Fig. 41.
The olfactory pathways.

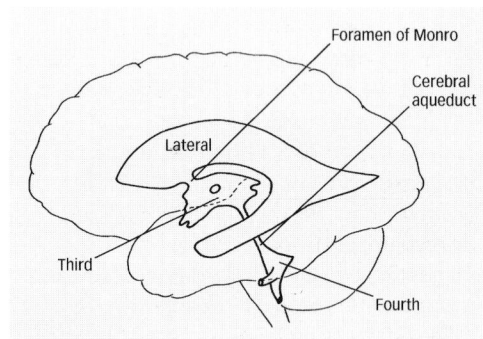

Olfactory bulb
Medial olfactory stria
Olfactory trigone
Lateral olfactory stria
Anterior perforated substance
Uncus

Fig. 42.
The cerebral ventricles.

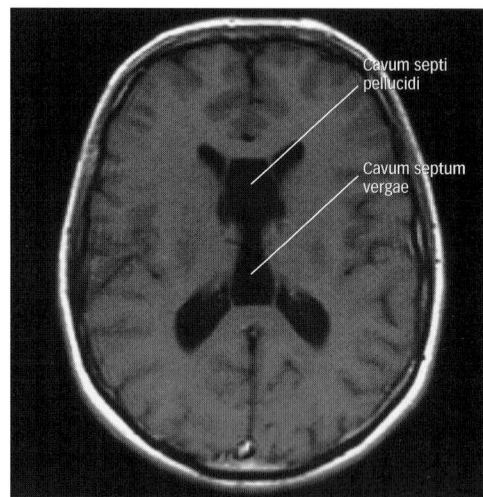

Foramen of Monro
Cerebral aqueduct
Lateral
Third
Fourth

Fig. 43.
T1W axial MRI scan to
show the cavum septi
pellucidi et vergae.

Cavum septi pellucidi
Cavum septum vergae

cortical components, the cornua ammonis (Ammon's horn) and the dentate gyrus. Ammon's horn is continuous with the subiculum of the parahippocampal gyrus and is convex laterally. The dentate gyrus is C-shaped in coronal section. It is also convex laterally and curves around the in-curved edge of Ammon's horn, although the degree of in-rolling is variable. The hippocampal sulcus separates the lateral aspect of the dentate gyrus and the lateral part of Ammon's horn. Overlying Ammon's horn and separating it from the temporal horn of the lateral ventricle is the alveus, a layer of white matter. The alveus is thickened medially with a thin upward pointing edge, the fimbria.

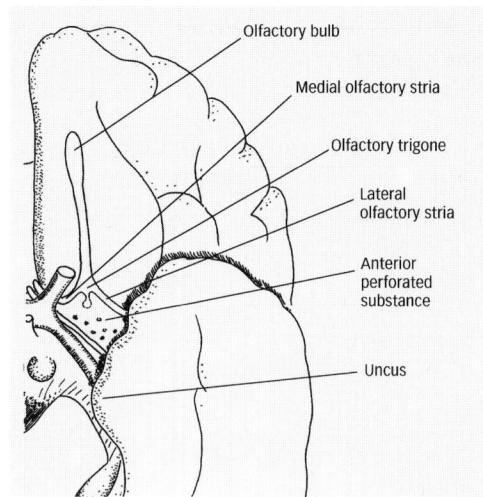

The temporal horn of the lateral ventricle lies immediately above and lateral to the hippocampus. The tail of the caudate nucleus lies superior to the temporal horn where it overlies the body of the hippocampus. Superior to the tail of the caudate nucleus, where it overlies the head of the hippocampus, is the amygdala nuclear complex which is situated just anterior to the temporal horn.

Ammon's horn is particularly susceptible to hypoxia and is the region involved in mesial temporal sclerosis, a surgically resectable cause of temporal lobe epilepsy.

Figs. 36 and 38 show the MRI appearance of the temporal lobe in axial and coronal section. The hippocampal gyrus is well displayed in the axial plane and its rolled configuration can be appreciated on the coronal scan. Axial MR images of the hippocampus are obtained parallel to the long axis of the temporal lobe with coronal sections perpendicular to these. The fornix (Figs. 1, 2, 39) which is the posterior extension of the fimbria, diverges from the posterior extensions of Ammon's horn and the dentate gyrus. The crus of the fornix sweeps backwards, upwards and medially, anterior to the splenium of the corpus callosum. The two crura then pass forwards and converge to form the body in the midline where it is suspended from the septum pellucidum. The body passes forwards and downwards to separate, just above the foramina of Monro, into the columns of the fornices. These are well recognized on axial MR and CT images posterior to the septum pellucidum forming the anteromedial margins of the foramina. Only the columns of the fornices are readily recognized on axial CT but the columns, body and crura are recognized on axial and sagittal MRI images (Fig. 27), and the bodies and crura are recognized on coronal MR images.

The olfactory bulb lies beneath the inferior surface of the ipsilateral frontal lobe, just lateral to the gyrus rectus (Fig. 40). The olfactory tract runs posteriorly from the bulb to the olfactory trigone, a small pyramidal mass on the inferior aspect of the hemisphere just in front of the anterior perforated substance. Olfactory pathways are distributed from the olfactory trigone into and around the anterior perforated substance. The medial olfactory stria pass to the septal area, the lateral olfactory stria pass to the temporal pole. The lateral olfactory stria is located on the surface of the lateral olfactory gyrus at the ventral border of the insula (Fig. 41).

The cerebral ventricles, subarachnoid cisterns and related structures

The cerebral ventricular system contains between 20 and 25 ml of cerebrospinal fluid in the young adult.

The lateral ventricles are C-shaped cavities within the hemispheres, which are roofed by the corpus callosum. Each lateral ventricle has a frontal (anterior) horn, anterior to the interventricular foramen of Monro which projects into the frontal lobe. Posterior to this foramen is the body of the ventricle. The temporal (inferior) horn is within the temporal lobe and the occipital (posterior) horn within the occipital

lobe (Fig. 42). In many normal individuals, one lateral ventricle may be larger than the other and the occipital horn in particular may not be well developed.

The lateral ventricles dilate with age due to cerebral involution and it may be important to distinguish this from dilatation due to obstructive hydrocephalus. Despite the existence of various measurements, this is often based on qualitative, and therefore subjective, criteria. In hydrocephalus, the anterior horns may become bulbous with their long axes oriented more towards the sagittal plane. The most reliable indicators of hydrocephalus appear to be cortical sulcal effacement and ventricular dilatation with proportionate dilatation of the temporal horns. In cortical atrophy the temporal horns are minimally dilated if at all. With modern generation CT scanners and MRI the temporal horns may be seen normally but they are slit-like. Their dilatation can be a sensitive indicator of early or mild hydro-

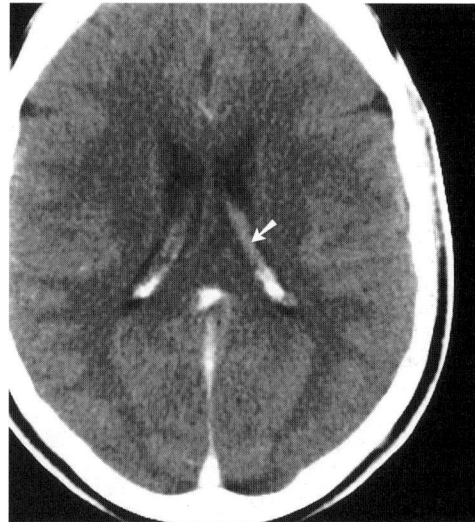

Fig. 44.
Axial and diagram CT scan after intravenous contrast showing the calcified enhancing choroid plexuses (arrow).

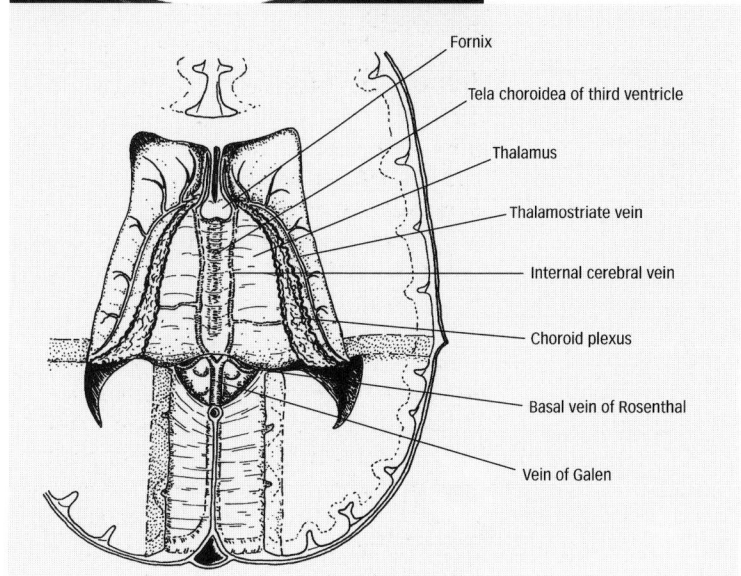

Fornix
Tela choroidea of third ventricle
Thalamus
Thalamostriate vein
Internal cerebral vein
Choroid plexus
Basal vein of Rosenthal
Vein of Galen

cephalus. The septum pellucidum separates the anterior horns and bodies of the lateral ventricles (Fig. 1). It is a midline triangular sheet, attached above and anteriorly to the corpus callosum and posteriorly to the fornix. The septum consists of two laminae and a narrow intervening cavity which is an extrapial space and thus not in continuity with the subarachnoid space.

The cavum septi pellucidi results from the separation of the two laminae of the septum pellucidum. The cavum vergae is the continuation of the cavum septi pellucidi beneath the splenium and superior to the fornix. The cava are present in virtually all neonates but close from posterior to anterior very rapidly thereafter. Persistence of the cavum septi pellucidi into adulthood is not uncommon (10%) and because of the direction of closure a cavum vergae should not occur in isolation (Fig. 43).

The choroid plexuses are invaginated into the medial walls of the lateral ventricles and into the roofs of the third and fourth ventricles through the choroidal fissure. Two layers of fused pia which cross the midline constitute the tela choroidea which is a triangular fold, the lateral edges of which are the choroid plexuses (Fig. 44). Here the pia and ependymal linings of the ventricles are in direct contact and are the sites at which most of the cerebrospinal fluid is secreted at a rate of 500 ml every 24 hours.

The choroid plexuses of the lateral ventricle are located in its trigonal region, at the confluence of the body, posterior and temporal horns, and are almost invariably calcified on CT.

Calcification is less commonly seen on the lateral skull radiograph and, like the pineal gland, is rare before 10 years of age. The choroid plexus of the fourth ventricle is occasionally calcified on CT but not sufficiently to be seen on skull radiography. The velum interpositum is a cisternal space created by an infolding of the tela choroidea beneath the fornix. It is limited anteriorly by the foramen of Monro with the choroid plexuses of the lateral ventricles laterally. Posteriorly the cistern opens into the quadrigeminal plate cistern. The cistern of the velum interpositum

(a)

Fig. 45.
Cistern of the velum interpositum: (a) sagittal diagram. Arrow shows the position of the foramina of Monro, (b) T2W axial MRI scan. Arrow shows cistern of the velum interpositum.

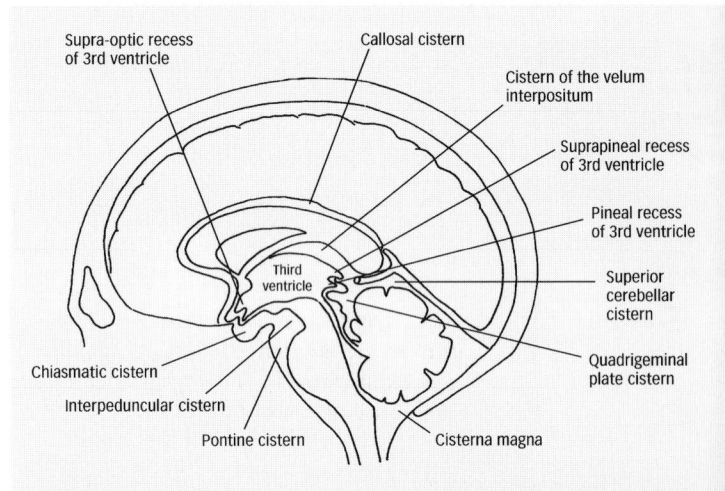

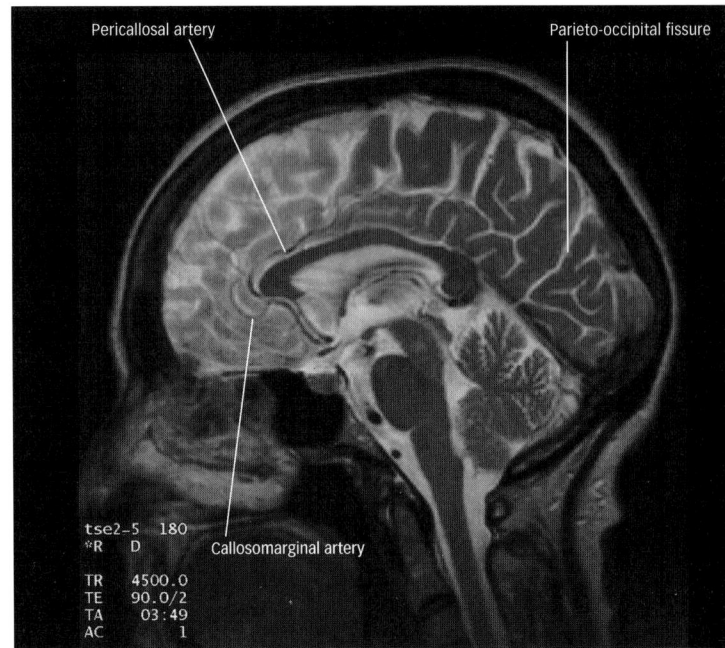

Septum pellucidum — Fornix — Cistern of the velum interpositum

3rd ventricle

(b)

Fig. 46.
The subarachnoid cisterns (a) diagram (b) T2W sagittal MRI.

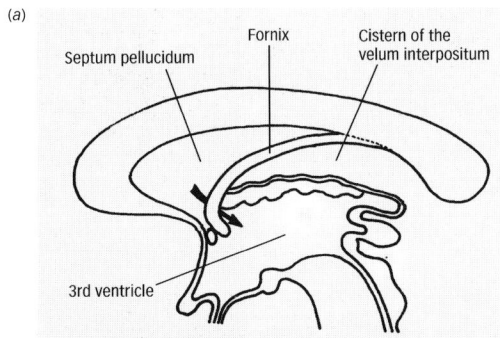

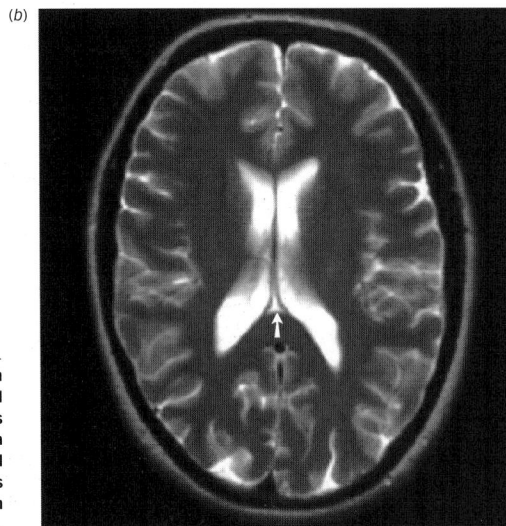

Supra-optic recess of 3rd ventricle — Callosal cistern — Cistern of the velum interpositum — Suprapineal recess of 3rd ventricle — Pineal recess of 3rd ventricle — Superior cerebellar cistern — Quadrigeminal plate cistern

Third ventricle

Chiasmatic cistern — Interpeduncular cistern — Pontine cistern — Cisterna magna

Pericallosal artery — Parieto-occipital fissure

tse2–5 180
*R   D   Callosomarginal artery

TR   4500.0
TE   90.0/2
TA   03:49
AC   1

contains the internal cerebral veins and is distinguished from the cavum vergae in that the latter extends anterior to the foramen of Monro and is above the fornix (Figs. 27, 45).

The third ventricle

This is narrow in the axial plane and lies in the midline. Its diencephalic relations are described on p. 39, 40. Although ventriculography of the third ventricle is now rarely performed, the contrast agent, either air or iodinated medium, outlines a number of recesses which are illustrated in Fig. 46. The flow of cerebrospinal fluid through the cerebral aqueduct between the third and fourth ventricles may be sufficiently rapid to cause a flow-void on MRI scans.

The fourth ventricle

This lies between the cerebellum posteriorly and the pons and upper medulla anteriorly (Figs. 24, 25, 27). In sagittal section, it appears triangular with an anterior floor and a roof with two sides converging to a posteriorly directed apex. The floor of the fourth ventricle is described on p. 35.

The upper part of the roof is formed by the superior cerebellar peduncles and an intervening glial sheet, the superior medullary velum. The roof below the apex is formed by an ependymal sheet, the inferior medullary velum, which is situated between the inferior cerebellar peduncles. The inferior medullary velum has a median aperture, the foramen of Magendie, which, along with the paired foramina of Luschka at the tips of the lateral recesses, constitute the only three outlets connecting the cerebral ventricles with the extracerebral subarachnoid spaces. Cerebrospinal fluid produced within the lateral ventricles flows caudally through the third and fourth ventricles. Most then flows into the basal cisterns (see below) and thence into the cortical subarachnoid space overlying the cerebral hemispheres to be absorbed into the venous system via the arachnoid villi. A small amount of cerebrospinal fluid circulates around the spinal cord.

The subarachnoid cisterns

Where the brain and skull are not closely applied, the arachnoid and pia separate and a number of subarachnoid cisterns are defined. They are situated at the base of the brain and around the brainstem, the free edge of the tentorium and the major arteries. The subarachnoid cisterns connect freely with one another and their patency is essential for the normal circulation of cerebrospinal fluid

(Figs. 25, 46). It can thus be appreciated that the definition of a particular cistern is a result of the arbitrary division of a single space.

The cisterna magna lies between the medulla and the posteroinferior surface of the cerebellum and is triangular in sagittal section. It is continuous below with the spinal subarachnoid space and receives cerebrospinal fluid from the fourth ventricle via the foramina of Magendie and Luschka. It is sometimes punctured percutaneously in the midline to obtain cerebrospinal fluid for examination when spinal puncture is inappropriate. The vertebral and posterior inferior cerebellar arteries travel through the lateral parts of the cistern, which also contains the glossopharyngeal (IXth), vagus (Xth) and spinal accessory (XIth) nerves. In some, other-

Fig. 47.
An arch aortogram:
(*a*) subtraction mask to show LAO projection,
(*b*) DSA arch aortogram.

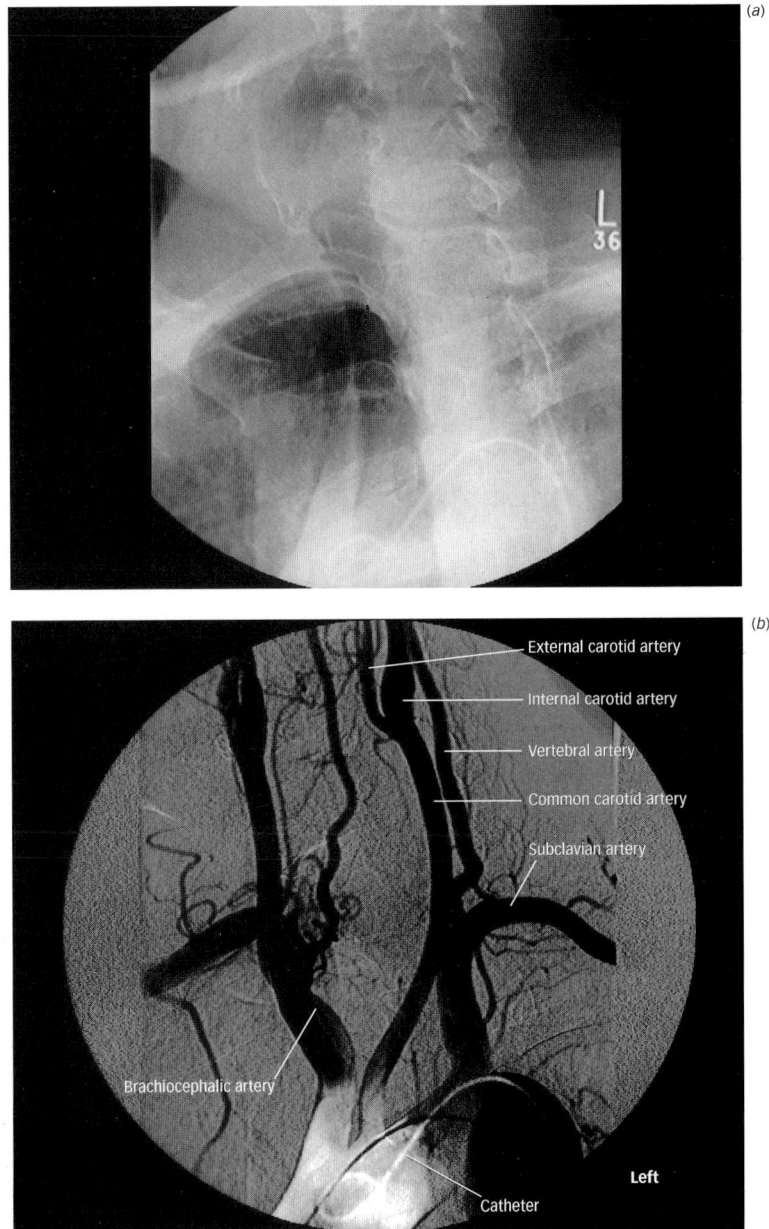

(*a*)

(*b*)

External carotid artery

Internal carotid artery

Vertebral artery

Common carotid artery

Subclavian artery

Brachiocephalic artery

Left

Catheter

wise normal, individuals the cistern is very large and described as a megacisterna magna.

The pontine cistern is anterior to both the pons and medulla and contains the basilar artery and cranial nerves V to XII. It is continuous around the brainstem with the quadrigeminal plate cistern posteriorly and the interpeduncular cistern superiorly.

The ambient cistern (Fig. 24) surrounds the midbrain and transmits the posterior cerebral and superior cerebellar arteries, the basal veins of Rosenthal and the trochlear nerves. The 'wings' of the ambient cistern are lateral extensions, posterior to the thalami.

The chiasmatic or suprasellar cistern extends from the infundibulum to the posterior surface of the frontal lobes and lies between the uncus on either side. It includes the proximal parts of the Sylvian fissures and contains the circle of Willis. Since the majority of berry aneurysms are borne on the circle of Willis, it can be appreciated that their rupture results in subarachnoid haemorrhage.

The chiasmatic cistern leads posteriorly to the interpeduncular or intercrural cistern, which contains the terminal basilar artery and its branches and the oculomotor nerves. Blood within this cistern may be the only evidence of subarachnoid haemorrhage. Superior to the chiasmatic cistern is the cistern of the lamina terminalis which contains the anterior communicating artery and the callosal cistern through which the pericallosal artery travels. The quadrigeminal cistern (cistern of the great cerebral vein) lies adjacent to the superior surface of the cerebellum and extends superiorly around the splenium of the corpus callosum. It contains the posterior cerebral, posterior choroidal and superior cerebellar arteries, and the trochlear nerves. It is also the location of the venous confluence where the vein of Galen joins the inferior sagittal and straight dural venous sinuses. The cistern of the velum interpositum is described on pp. 48 and 49. The cerebello-pontine angle cistern is described in Chapter 4.

The intracranial circulation

The brain is supplied with blood by four arteries and their branches, the paired internal carotid and vertebral arteries (Fig. 47). The carotid arteries enter the cranial cavity towards the rostral end of the brainstem whereas the vertebral arteries enter towards the caudal end.

There are several embryonic connections between the carotid and basilar arteries which may rarely persist into adulthood. The com-

monest is the trigeminal artery, which arises from the internal carotid artery just before it enters the cavernous sinus and passes lateral to the dorsum sellae to the upper basilar artery (Fig. 48).

The internal carotid artery

The internal carotid artery is the larger of the two terminal branches of the common carotid artery. It arises at approximately C3 level. A fusiform dilatation at its origin, the carotid sinus, is concerned with the regulation of blood pressure. No constant branches arise from the cervical segment of the internal carotid artery. There may be tortuosity in the cervical segment leading to the so-called tonsillar loop (Fig. 49(a) arrow). The artery enters the cranial cavity via the carotid canal in the petrous bone. Here it runs an approximately horizontal course, passing anteromedially, to cross the upper half of the foramen lacerum where it turns upwards and medially to enter the posterior part of the cavernous sinus (Fig. 9). It then turns forwards within the cavernous sinus as far as its anterior wall, where it turns upwards again to pierce the dura and arachnoid mater and enters the subarachnoid space just inferomedial to the anterior clinoid process. It turns posteriorly, just below the optic nerve before bearing laterally, between the optic and oculomotor nerves and again superiorly to terminate, just lateral to the optic chiasm, in its major branches the anterior and middle cerebral arteries. Its relations within the cavernous sinus are shown in Fig. 28. The U-shaped loop formed by the cavernous and immediately supracavernous portions of the internal carotid artery is called the carotid siphon.

It should be noted that there are no angiographic indicators of the precise limits of the intracavernous portion of the internal carotid artery.

The meningo-hypophyseal trunk arises from the posterior surface of the internal

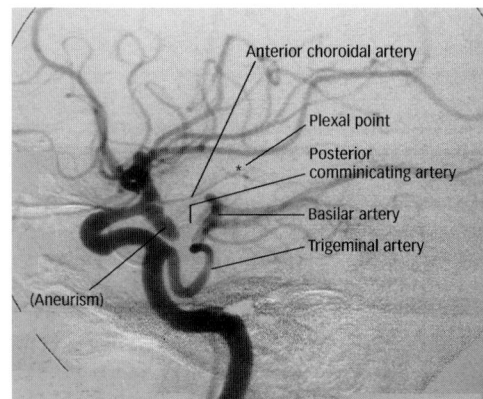

Anterior choroidal artery
Plexal point
Posterior comminicating artery
Basilar artery
Trigeminal artery
(Aneurism)

Fig. 48.
Internal carotid angiogram lateral projection, showing the trigeminal artery, an embryonic variant. There is an aneurysm at the origin of the posterior communicating artery and above this is the anterior choroidal artery.

carotid artery just before it enters the cavernous sinus. It supplies the posterior pituitary gland and adjacent meninges but is not shown at angiography unless hypertrophied.

The ophthalmic artery is the first supraclinoid branch of the internal carotid artery. It arises in the subarachnoid space and runs forward to pass through the optic foramen within the optic nerve sheath (see Chapter 5).

The posterior communicating artery (Fig. 49) is the second intracranial branch of the internal carotid artery and connects it to the ipsilateral posterior cerebral artery about 1 cm from its origin. It is not, however, just a simple

anastomotic link as it also gives off small branches to the diencephalon and to the genu of the internal capsule.

The anterior choroidal artery arises from the posterior aspect of the internal carotid artery lateral to the optic chiasm and distal to the posterior communicating artery (Figs. 49, 50). It has an extensive supply involving the optic pathways, the posterior limb of the internal capsule immediately above the basis pedunculi, the diencephalon, basal ganglia, hippocampus and midbrain. The first or cisternal part of the anterior choroidal artery lies between the optic tract and the uncus. It then passes across the medial wing of the ambient cistern to enter the choroidal fissure where it

Fig. 49. (a) Digital subtraction angiograms of the internal carotid artery: (a) lateral cervical. A tonsillar loop is arrowed in (a). (b), (c), frontal (d) frontal oblique and (e), (f) lateral cranial projections.

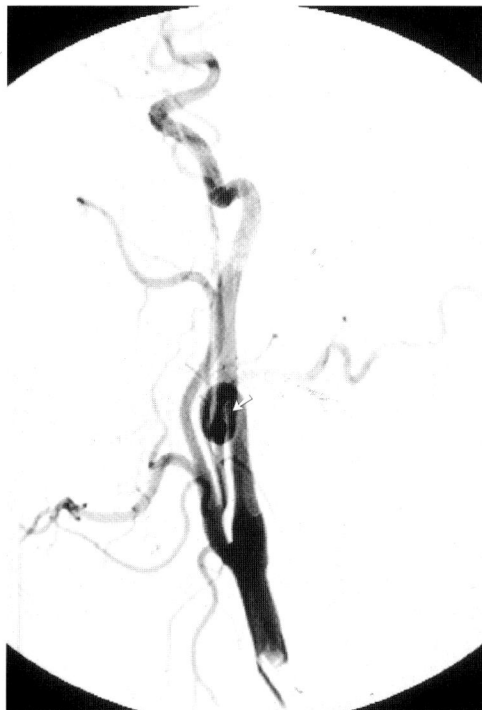

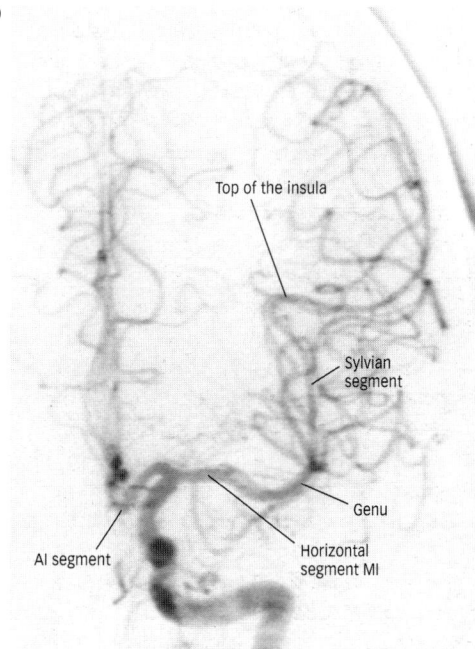

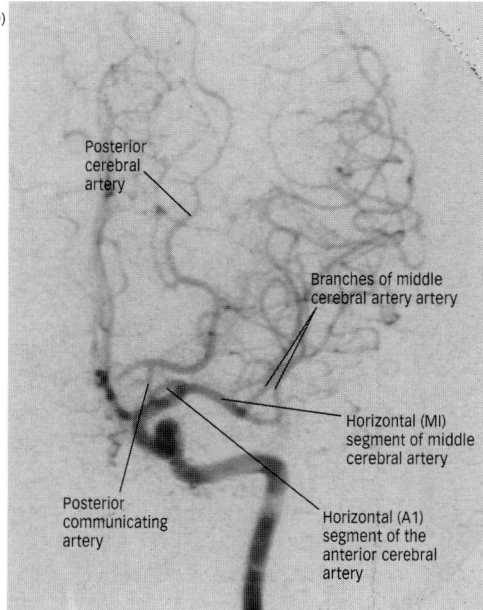

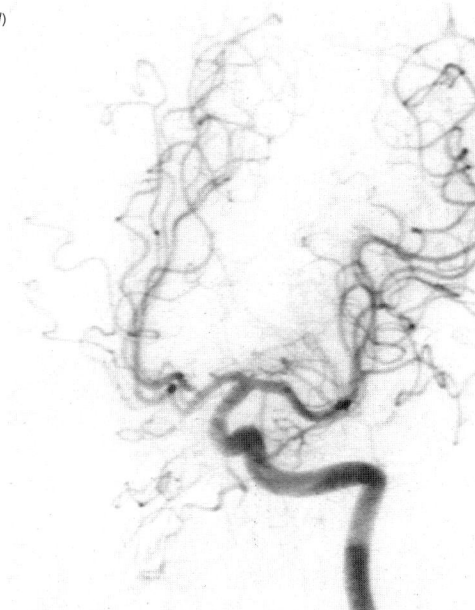

49(e)

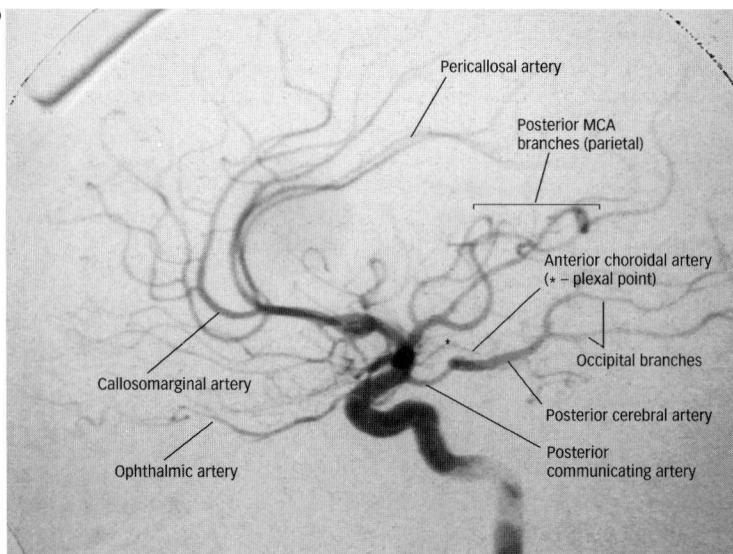

49(f)

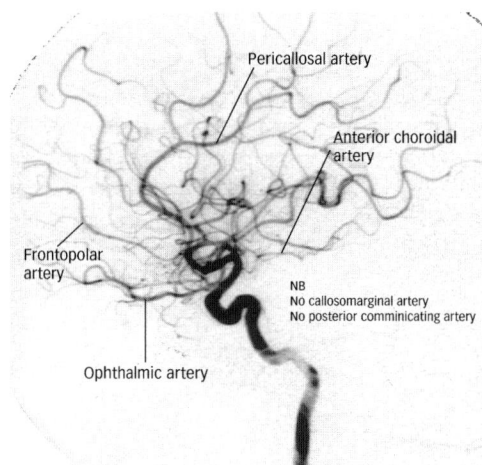

Fig. 50. below
The choroidal arteries.

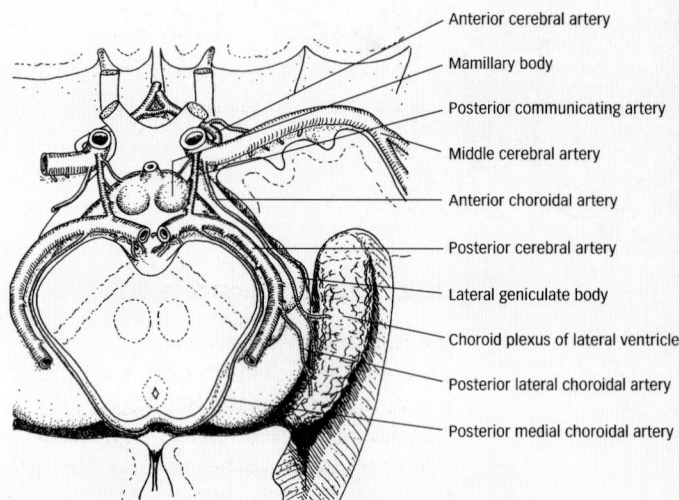

becomes the plexal segment. This runs within the choroid plexus of the temporal horn and continues around the trigone of the lateral ventricle (the confluence of the body, posterior and inferior horns), into the choroid plexus of the posterior horn and body, sometimes as far anteriorly as the foramen of Monro.

On the lateral angiogram it is seen to run almost horizontally backwards, the proximal cisternal segment having a downward convexity and the distal plexal segment a more gentle upward curve. It accompanies the optic tract, arising from the internal carotid artery and it follows the optic tract as far as the lateral side of the lateral geniculate body, where it enters and supplies the choroid plexus of the temporal horn of the lateral ventricle. The plexal or choroidal point is denoted on both frontal and lateral angiographic projections by a 'kink' in the vessel and is the position where the artery enters the choroidal fissure (Figs 48, 49(e)). The internal carotid artery terminates below the anterior perforated substance by dividing into the anterior and middle cerebral arteries. The T-shaped bifurcation is not normally in the coronal plane since the middle cerebral artery is directed posterolaterally. This necessitates an oblique projection to display 'the tuning-fork' like arrangement of the anterior and middle cerebral arteries en face (compare Figs. 49(c) and (d)).

The circle of Willis
Branches of the internal carotid and basilar arteries form an anastomotic circle on the ventral surface of the brain known as the circle of Willis, which affords limited protection against cerebral infarction in the event of arterial occlusion. The participating arteries are the terminal internal carotid arteries, the

first part of the anterior cerebral arteries, the anterior communicating artery, the posterior communicating arteries, the first parts of the posterior cerebral arteries and the basilar artery termination (Fig. 51). In the axial plane the 'circle' can be seen to have a stellate configuration within the suprasellar cistern. Hypoplasia and aplasia of its component parts are common and the circle is complete in only a minority of individuals. The integrity of the circle of Willis can be tested angiographically. A cross-compression study involves the manual compression of one cervical carotid artery whilst the other is injected with contrast medium to demonstrate whether there is intracranial 'cross-flow' of contrast medium in the distribution of the compressed carotid artery. If there is a high flow lesion such as a caroticocavernous fistula, it may be valuable to inject contrast medium into a vertebral artery while compressing the affected carotid artery. The fistulous connection may be identified more easily by a relatively small amount of contrast medium entering by way of the posterior communicating artery.

(a)

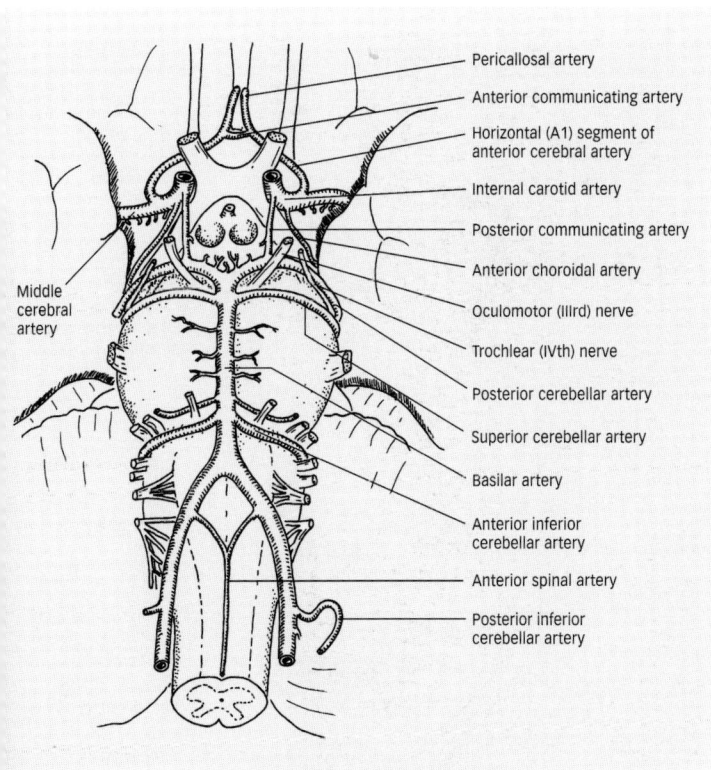

Pericallosal artery
Anterior communicating artery
Horizontal (A1) segment of anterior cerebral artery
Internal carotid artery
Posterior communicating artery
Anterior choroidal artery
Oculomotor (IIIrd) nerve
Trochlear (IVth) nerve
Posterior cerebellar artery
Superior cerebellar artery
Basilar artery
Anterior inferior cerebellar artery
Anterior spinal artery
Posterior inferior cerebellar artery

Middle cerebral artery

(b) Fig. 51.
The circle of Willis shown (a) diagrammatically, by (b) digital subtraction angiography, (c) CT angiography and (d), magnetic resonance angiography (MRA).

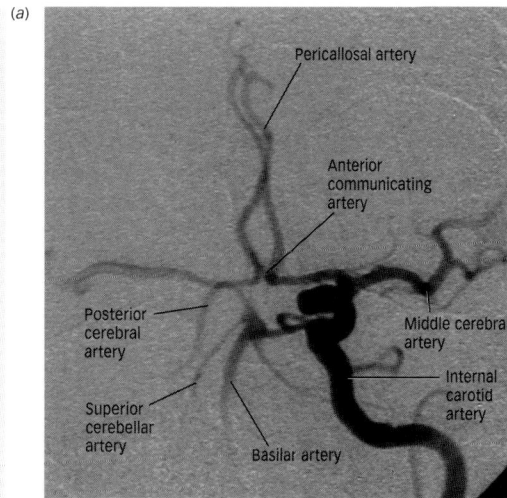

Pericallosal artery
Anterior communicating artery
Posterior cerebral artery
Middle cerebral artery
Internal carotid artery
Superior cerebellar artery
Basilar artery

(c)

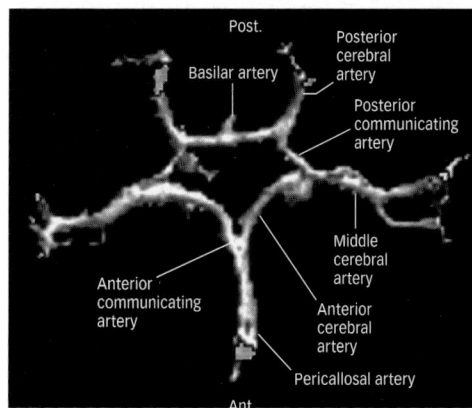

Post.
Basilar artery
Posterior cerebral artery
Posterior communicating artery
Middle cerebral artery
Anterior communicating artery
Anterior cerebral artery
Pericallosal artery
Ant.

(d)

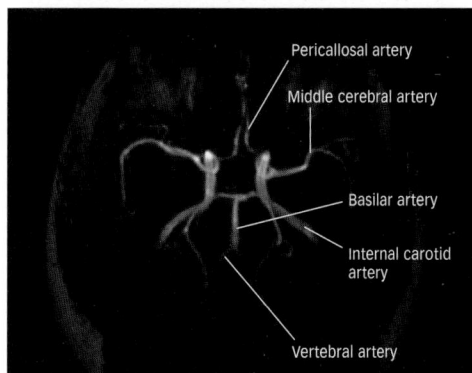

Pericallosal artery
Middle cerebral artery
Basilar artery
Internal carotid artery
Vertebral artery

The anterior cerebral artery

The anterior cerebral artery is the smaller terminal branch of the internal carotid artery and it runs anteromedially, approximately in the midline, below the anterior perforated substance and above the optic nerve on to the medial surface of the hemisphere in the interhemispheric fissure where both anterior cerebral arteries lie in close proximity. They are usually linked by a short bridging vessel, the anterior communicating artery, within the cistern of the lamina terminalis. The precommunicating, horizontal or 'AI' segment of the anterior cerebral artery may occasionally be hypoplastic and its distal territory be supplied by the contralateral anterior cerebral artery via the anterior communicating artery. Heubner's recurrent artery is the largest of the perforating medial lenticulostriate branches which course posterosuperiorly. It usually arises from the proximal A2 segment but may instead originate from the AI segment along with the majority of the medial striate branches. It runs laterally above and behind the anterior cerebral artery and the proximal part of the middle cerebral artery to the base of the olfactory trigone to supply the anterior limb of the internal capsule and parts of the caudate nucleus and globus pallidus.

The anterior communicating artery, although short, gives rise to several branches which course superiorly to supply the optic chiasm and other anterior midline structures. The A2 segment of the anterior cerebral artery extends from the anterior communicating artery to the origin of the callosomarginal artery close to the genu of the corpus callosum. The orbitofrontal artery is usually the first cortical branch of the A2 segment, arising from the subcallosal segment to supply the inferior and inferomedial surfaces of the frontal lobe including the gyri recti.

The frontopolar artery runs from the genu of the corpus callosum to the frontal pole and supplies the orbital gyri, olfactory bulb and tract and the anterior part of the superior frontal gyrus.

(a)

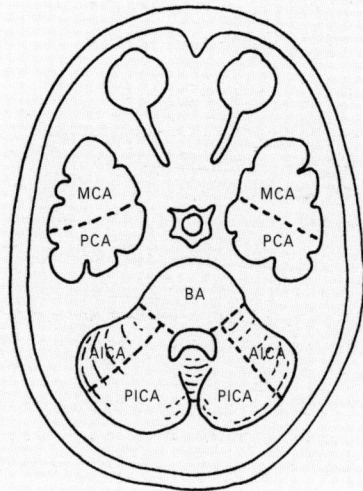

(b)

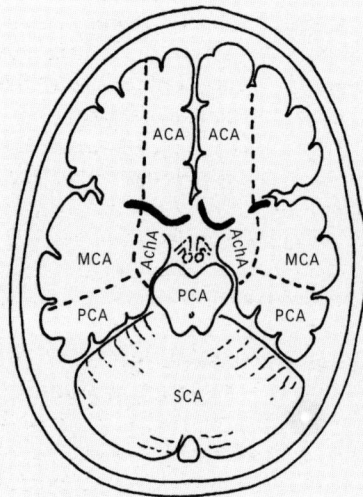

(c)

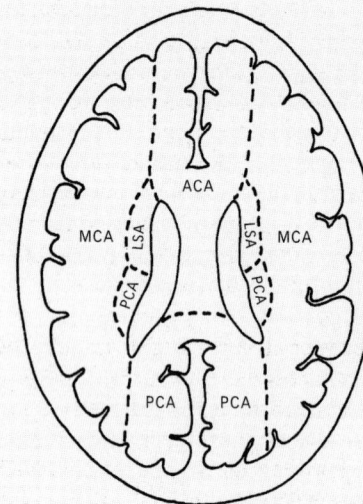

(d)

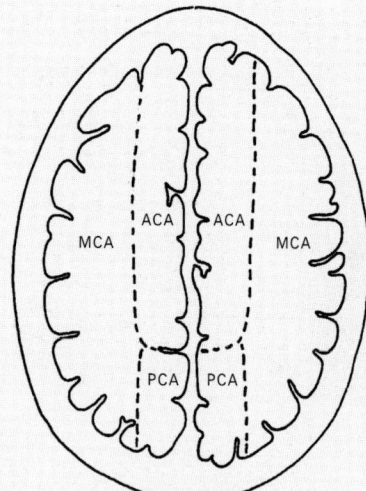

(e)

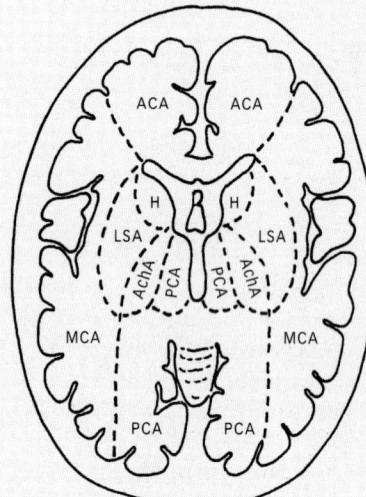

Fig. 52.
The vascular territories. Brain arterial distribution. *ACA*=anterior cerebral artery, *H*=recurrent artery of Heubner, *MCA*=middle cerebral artery, *LSA*=lenticulostriate artery, *AChA*=anterior choroidal artery, *PCA*=posterior cerebral artery, *BA*=basilar artery, *SCA*=superior cerebellar artery, *AICA*=anterior inferior cerebellar artery, *PICA*=posterior inferior cerebellar artery.

The callosomarginal artery is present in approximately half of all cases. It runs through the cingulate sulcus (Fig. 46(b)) and gives rise to anterior, middle and posterior internal frontal branches. These supply the superior frontal gyrus.

The pericallosal artery is the continuation of the anterior cerebral artery beyond the origin of the callosomarginal artery (Fig. 46(b)). It arches posteriorly over the genu of the corpus callosum to lie on its superior surface as far as the splenium.

The pericallosal arteries give off major branches which extend obliquely to the margins of the hemispheres and on to their orbital and superior surfaces. Each supplies a strip of medial cortex almost as far posteriorly as the parietooccipital fissure. The main branch, the superior internal parietal artery, passes upwards to the precuneus and superior parietal lobule. Smaller branches supply the

(a)

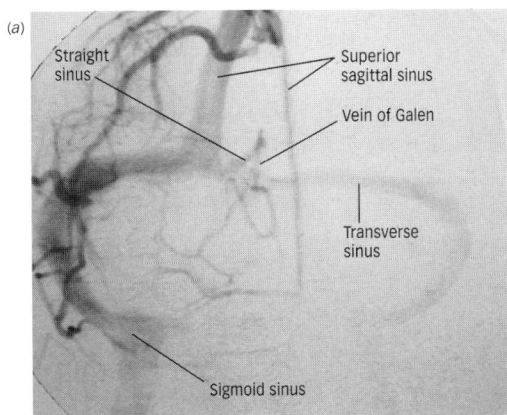

Straight sinus

Superior sagittal sinus

Vein of Galen

Transverse sinus

Sigmoid sinus

Fig. 53.
The dural venous sinuses:
(a) frontal, (b) lateral
projections of a digital
subtraction angiogram,
(c) T1W sagittal MRI scan
after intravenous
gadolinium DTPA.

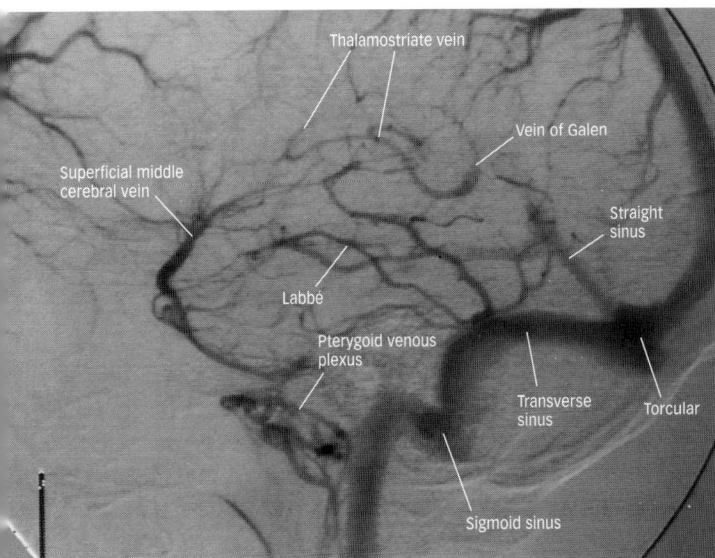

Thalamostriate vein

Vein of Galen

Superficial middle
cerebral vein

Straight sinus

Labbé

Pterygoid venous plexus

Transverse sinus

Torcular

Sigmoid sinus

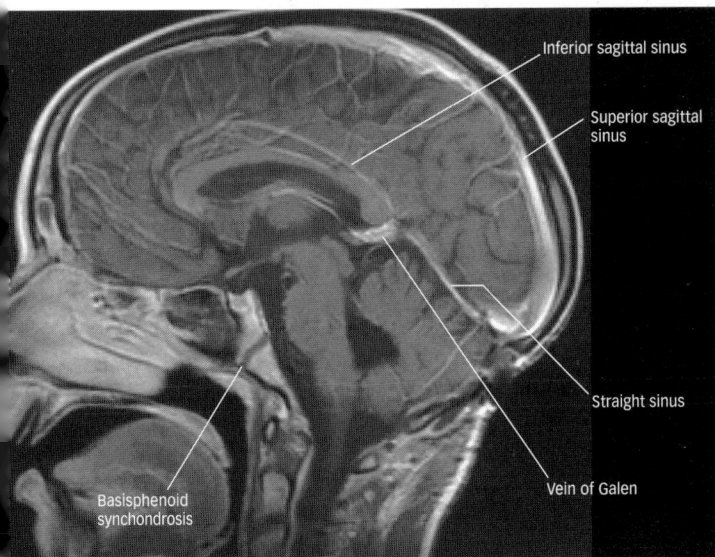

Inferior sagittal sinus

Superior sagittal sinus

Straight sinus

Vein of Galen

Basisphenoid synchondrosis

frontal and parietal regions near to the midline, the corpus callosum and the cingulate gyrus.

Cortical branches of the anterior cerebral arteries anastomose with those of the middle and posterior cerebral arteries.

The anterior cerebral arteries are sometimes fused proximally to form a single trunk

or azygos artery which arises between the hemispheres before dividing near the genu of the corpus callosum.

The middle cerebral artery

This is the larger terminal branch of the internal carotid artery (Fig.49). Its proximal portion, the so-called MI segment, runs laterally through the horizontal limb of the Sylvian fissure between the frontal and temporal lobes. A variable number of lateral striate branches arise from the MI segment which supply the basal ganglia, internal capsule and caudate nucleus.

At the anteroinferior aspect of the insula the middle cerebral artery turns upwards forming its genu (the distal limit of the MI segment), and its branches then run over the surface of the insula in the depths of the Sylvian fissure. At the superior limit of the insula they turn inferiorly and then laterally under the frontoparietal opercula to emerge from the lateral aspect of the Sylvian fissure and spread out over the cortical surfaces of the frontal, parietal, occipital and temporal lobes.

The anterior temporal artery usually arises from the MI segment and courses over the anterior pole of the temporal lobe.

At the bifurcation the middle cerebral artery usually divides into groups of anterior and posterior branches although its cortical branches are variable.

The anterior group includes the orbitofrontal, operculofrontal (the 'candelabra' group) and central sulcus arteries. They supply the inferolateral parts of the frontal lobe, the middle and inferior frontal gyri and the motor and sensory strips.

The posterior group generally comprises three major branches which arise in the Sylvian fissure. The posterior parietal artery supplies the parietal lobe behind the sensory strip. The angular artery is usually the largest cortical branch. It emerges from the apex of the Sylvian fissure and supplies the posterior parietal and lateral occipital lobes and the superior temporal gyri. The posterior temporal artery descends over the lateral aspect of the temporal lobe to supply a variable amount of its posterolateral aspect.

The posterior cerebral artery (see pp. 59, 60)
The vascular territories are shown in Fig. 52. The anatomy of the intracerebral arteries and the territory supplied by them are variable. It may therefore be necessary to undertake functional testing during superselective angiography to determine whether embolization of a particular artery might result in disability.

55

Fig. 54.
Digital subtraction
angiogram of the dural
venous sinuses showing a
cavernous nodule (arrow).

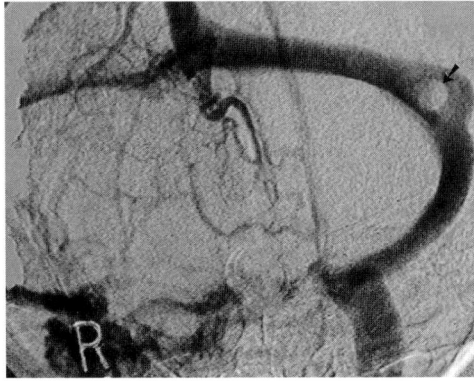

(a)

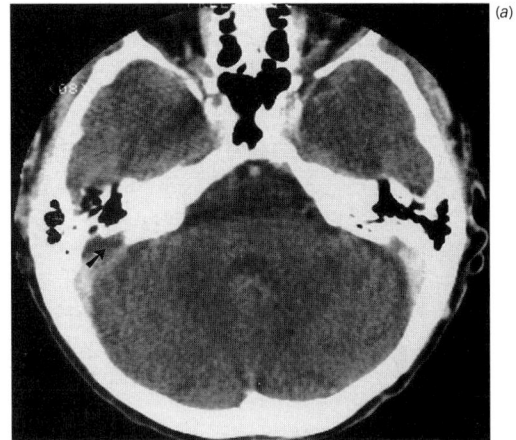

Fig. 55.
Axial CT showing
pseudoerosive vault
change (arrows); (*a*) soft
tissue, (*b*) bony algorithm

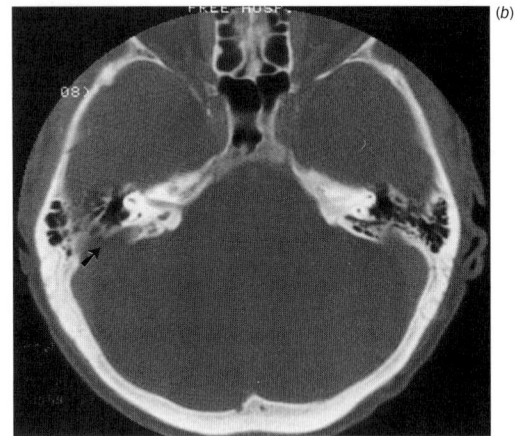

(b)

The dural venous sinuses

The dural sinuses are valveless, trabeculated venous channels and may conveniently be divided into a superior group related to the vault and a basal group found at the skull base (Fig. 53). The sagittal, transverse and straight sinuses are the main components of the superior group. The basal group comprises the cavernous, petrosal and sphenoparietal sinuses.

The superior sagittal sinus, which is triangular in cross-section, increases in size from before backwards and usually begins near the crista galli, although it may not develop anterior to the coronal suture. In the majority of individuals, most of its flow is directed to the right transverse sinus with the straight sinus draining to the left transverse sinus. Cortical veins enter perpendicular to the superior sagittal sinus anteriorly but the angle becomes shallower more posteriorly with the veins entering against the direction of flow. As with venous systems elsewhere, normal anatomical variants are common. The superior sagittal sinus may bifurcate well above its normal termination at the internal occipital protuberance. This early separation may lead to an erroneous diagnosis of sagittal sinus thrombosis on CT if the intervening space is mistaken for non-enhancing thrombus (a false positive 'empty triangle' or 'empty delta' sign).

The inferior sagittal sinus, lying in the free margin of the falx cerebri, is seen only rarely in adult angiography but more commonly in children. It is not recognized on CT nor usually on unenhanced MR images.

The transverse sinuses commence at the torcular and lie within the outer margins of the tentorium. The right is usually 'dominant' and larger than that on the left, receiving almost the entire output of the superior sagittal sinus. The sinus on one side can be poorly developed or even absent. In order to distinguish such a normal variant from sinus occlusion, it is often helpful to examine with CT the bony depressions in the vault in which the sinus runs, and the jugular foramen, both of which will be correspondingly underdeveloped in the congenital variant.

The transverse sinuses become the sigmoid sinuses at the posterior petrous edge continuing towards the jugular bulb. The transverse and sigmoid sinuses are together known as the lateral sinus. Occasionally one encounters intraluminal filling defects in the transverse sinus due either to prominent arachnoid granulations or larger 'cavernous nodules' (Fig. 54). Where the sigmoid sinus is adjacent to the petrous bone, there can be pseudo-erosive changes in the bone margin. Normal petromastoid aeration is a useful guide to this variant (Fig. 55).

The straight sinus lies at the juntion of the falx and the tentorium and the torcular herophili is where the straight, transverse and superior sagittal sinuses meet. The vein of Galen (the great cerebral vein), joins the inferior sagittal and straight sinuses at the 'venous confluence' within the quadrigeminal plate cistern (Fig. 53).

An occipital sinus is not usually identified at angiography but may occasionally be seen coursing superiorly in the midline from the foramen magnum towards the torcular. At the foramen magnum it anastomoses with the marginal sinuses.

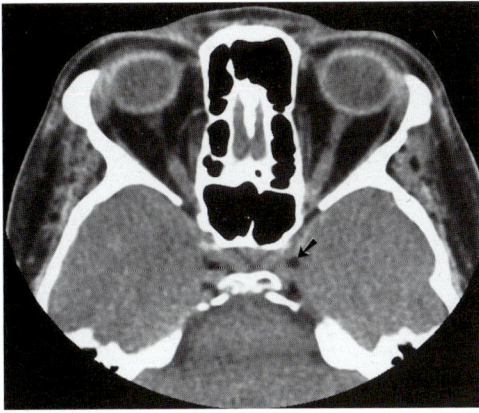

Fig. 56.
Axial CT showing intracavernous fat deposits (arrow).

The paired cavernous sinuses (Fig. 28) are situated either side of the pituitary fossa and receive the superior and inferior ophthalmic veins and the sphenoparietal sinuses. They connect with each other through the inter-cavernous sinuses and posteriorly they communicate with the transverse sinuses, via the superior petrosal sinus on each side. Each is a trabeculated, extradural venous channel lying on the body of the sphenoid bone. The internal carotid artery pursues an S-shaped course through the sinus before piercing its dural roof, medial to the anterior clinoid. The abducent nerve lies free within the sinus applied to the lateral wall of the artery. From above down, the oculomotor, trochlear, ophthalmic and maxillary nerves run in a common dural tunnel in the lateral wall of the sinus to reach the superior orbital fissure. The cavernous sinus enhances with intravenous contrast on both CT and MRI. Fat deposits can occur normally within the sinus and are demonstrated by CT as hypodense foci (Fig. 56). The normal sinus has a concave lateral wall and the two sinuses should be symmetrical. Inferiorly, the ophthalmic division of the trigeminal nerve, also embedded into the lateral wall, courses towards the trigeminal (Gasserian) ganglion.

The trigeminal ganglion contains the cell bodies of the sensory root of the trigeminal nerve. It is crescentric in shape and occupies a dural recess in the medial wall of the middle fossa at the petrous apex posterior to the cavernous sinus. This recess, known as Meckel's cave, is in continuity with the prepontine cistern and is of cerebrospinal fluid density and signal intensity on CT and MRI, respectively (Fig. 28(c)). It will also be opacified during CT cisternography (see Chapter 4, Fig. 1).

The petrosal and sphenoparietal sinuses all drain the cavernous sinuses on each side. The superior petrosal sinuses are situated at the junction of the tentorium and the petrous bone. They drain to transverse sinuses. The

inferior petrosal sinuses lie between the clivus and petrous apex and run medial to the superior sinus joining the jugular bulb (Figs. 16, 61). The sphenoparietal sinus is a medial extension of the Sylvian vein and courses around the greater sphenoid wing.

The supratentorial venous system

Blood within the superficial cerebral veins flows in a centrifugal direction radially towards the dural venous sinuses or adjacent lacunae. Almost all of superficial veins are unnamed and inconstant, with three exceptions.

The superficial middle cerebral (or Sylvian) vein forms an arc along the surface of the Sylvian fissure and is convex anteriorly on a lateral projection. It is continuous with the sphenoparietal sinus (Fig. 53 (b)).

The anastomotic veins of Trolard, superiorly, and Labbe, inferiorly, connect the superficial middle cerebral vein with the superior sagittal and transverse sinuses, respectively. It is uncommon for both anastomotic veins to be well developed in an individual (Figs. 53 (b) and 57).

Fig. 57.
Digital subtraction angiogram, lateral projection, showing the cerebral veins.

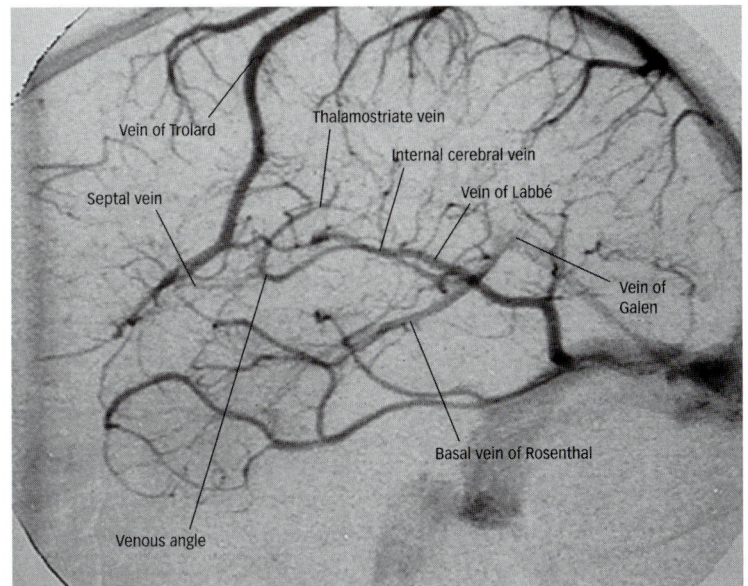

Fig. 58.
Axial CT showing the deep cerebral veins.

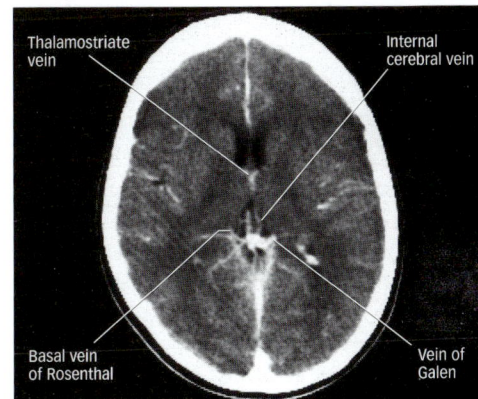

(a)

(b)

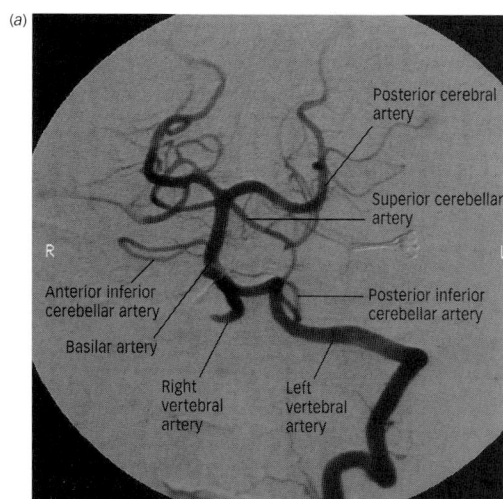

Fig. 59.
The vertebrobasilar arterial
system: digital subtraction
angiograms (a), (b) frontal,
(c), (d) lateral projections.

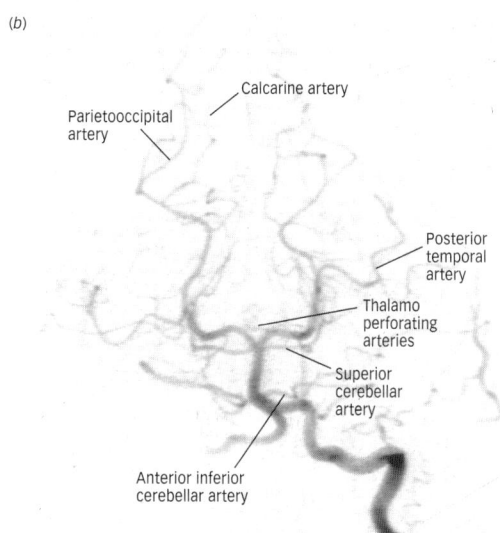

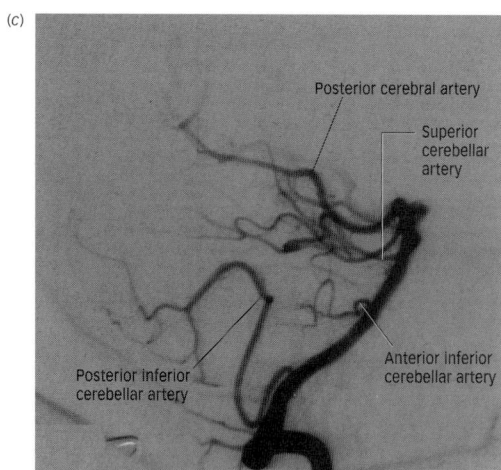

(c)

Blood in the deep cerebral veins flows centripetally (i.e. centrally). Medullary veins drain into subependymal veins along the walls of the lateral ventricles (Fig. 44). The thalamostriate vein is a member of the subependymal group and runs across the floor of the lateral ventrical over the thalamus to enter the internal cerebral vein behind the foramen of

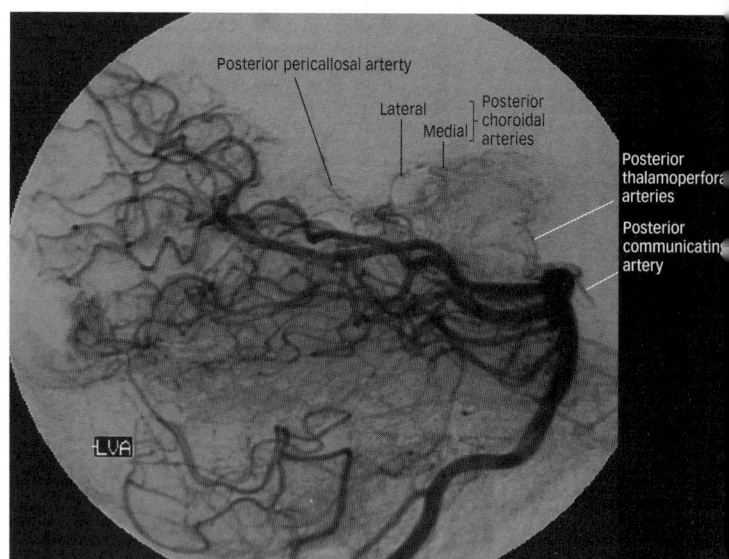

Monro. The septal vein, another subependymal vein, passes around the head of the caudate nucleus and travels posteriorly in the septum pellucidum. It too enters the internal cerebral vein behind the foramen of Monro. The venous angle, at the confluence of the thalamostriate and septal veins, denotes the posterior margin of the foramen on the lateral angiogram (Fig. 57).

The basal vein of Rosenthal forms in the Sylvian fissure and travels in the ambient cistern around the midbrain to enter the Vein of Galen, along with the internal cerebral vein. Both the basal vein and internal cerebral vein are paired structures, the latter running along the roof of the third ventricle, from the Foramen of Monro in the cistern of the velum interpositum. The vein of Galen is a short (1–2 cm) single midline vessel and originates under the splenium of the corpus callosum, curving posteriorly and superiorly towards the straight sinus. Elements of the deep cerebral venous system can be identified on intravenous contrast-enhanced CT (Fig. 58).

The vertebrobasilar arterial system
The normal anatomy of the intracranial vertebrobasilar arterial system is subject to some individual variation in the origins, course and distribution of the component arteries (Fig. 59). There is also a well-developed network of anastomoses between those arteries. Vascular territories are shown in Fig. 52.

The posterior inferior cerebellar artery (PICA) arises from the vertebral artery as its largest and most distal branch. It usually arises well above the foramen magnum but may arise below it. There is a reciprocal arrangement with the anterior inferior cerebellar artery such that if one is hypoplastic then the

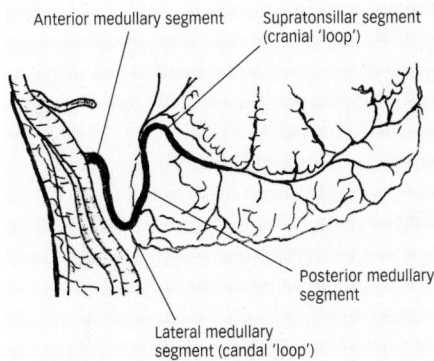

Fig. 60.
The course of the posterior inferior cerebellar artery.

other will be well developed. In a small proportion of cases, one, usually hypoplastic, vertebral artery will terminate as the PICA.

The PICA first winds around the olive of the medulla and comes near to the biventral lobule of the cerebellum (Fig. 60). This is the anterior medullary segment. The vessel then courses around the brainstem as the lateral medullary segment which corresponds to the caudal loop seen on the lateral projection at angiography. This curves around the inferior margin of the cerebellar tonsil. The posterior medullary segment ascends to the superior part of the tonsil and, at the apex of the cranial loop, gives off branches which supply the choroid plexus of the fourth ventricle. The PICA then proceeds to supply the undersurface of the cerebellar hemisphere. Meningeal branches may also arise from it. The basilar artery forms from the confluence of the vertebral arteries at the pontomedullary junction. It ascends approximately in the midline in the pontine cistern and grooves the surface of the anterior pons. Superiorly, it curves a little posteriorly before dividing into the posterior cerebral arteries. Throughout the length of the basilar artery, small penetrating branches pass posteriorly into the brainstem which are at risk during vascular interventional procedures. The anterior inferior cerebellar artery (AICA) passes laterally from the basilar artery closely related to the abducent nerve. It traverses the cerebellopontine angle cistern usually anterior and medial to the neural bundle. A lateral branch then courses around the flocculus and a medial branch supplies the biventral lobule and cerebellar hemisphere. A labyrinthine artery supplies the inner ear. The superior cerebellar artery arises from the basilar artery near to its terminal division. It runs laterally around the brainstem and comes to lie inferior to the oculomotor nerve which separates it from the posterior cerebral artery (Fig. 51(*a*)). At the lateral border of the pons it turns posteriorly over the middle

cerebellar peduncle as the ambient segment and the tentorium may come into contact with the artery. The ambient segment parallels the course of the trochlear nerve and it is notable that the basal vein of Rosenthal, the posterior cerebral artery and the free edge of the tentorium are also in this plane.

In the quadrigeminal cistern both superior cerebellar arteries approach the midline. They supply the hemispheres and superior vermis.

The posterior cerebral artery

Each posterior cerebral artery can be divided into a number of segments (Fig. 59). The P1 or pre-communicating segment, extends from the basilar bifurcation to the origin of the posterior communicating artery. It lies within the interpeduncular fossa and thalamic perforating arteries arise from both this P1 segment and from the posterior communicating artery. These branches have an extensive distribution to the thalamus, hypothalamus, the

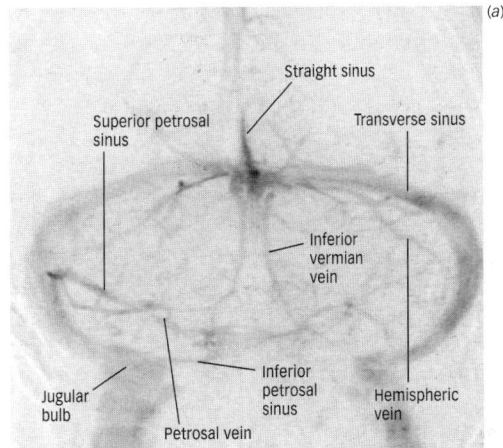

(*a*)

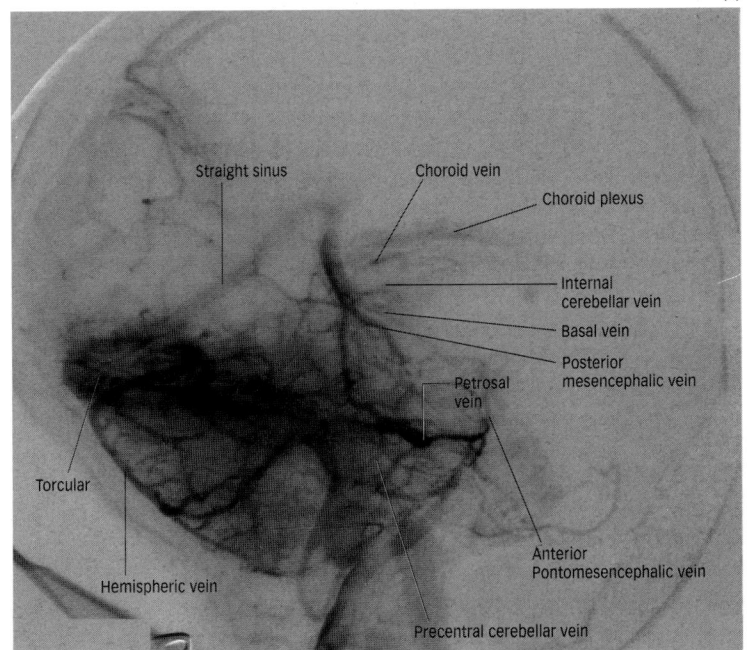

Fig. 61.
The veins of posterior fossa: (*a*) frontal and (*b*) lateral digital subtraction angiograms.

(*b*)

oculomotor (IIIrd) and trochlear (IVth) nerves and to the internal capsule.

The P2, or ambient segment, runs around the brainstem in the ambient cistern, parallel to the basal vein of Rosenthal and to the optic tract. It courses around the cerebral peduncles to lie above the tentorium. The P2 segment may be compressed against the tentorial edge when there is uncal pressure on the mid-brain in the presence of raised intracranial pressure. Infarction of the occipital lobe is thus a recognized consequence. The P2 segment usually gives rise to the inferior temporal artery and to a single medial and multiple lateral posterior choroidal arteries.

The P3 segment extends from the quadrigeminal plate cistern to the calcarine fissure. The two major terminal branches of the posterior cerebral artery are the parietooccipital and calcarine arteries. The smaller calcarine artery is seen angiographically to pursue a straight course, running between the parieto-occipital branch posteriorly and the posterior temporal branch inferiorly on the lateral projection. The posterior pericallosal arteries arch over the splenium and arise either from the posterior cerebral or parieto-occipital arteries. There is some variation between individuals as to the origin of the posterior cerebral artery branches. It is not uncommon to encounter the so-called fetal origin of the posterior cerebral artery. In this case, the pre-communicating (P1) segment is undeveloped and the posterior cerebral artery fills exclusively from the internal carotid artery and not from the basilar artery.

The veins of the posterior fossa
These can be divided into three groups: a superior group, draining towards the vein of Galen, an anterior group, draining to the petrosal vein of Dandy, and a posterior group, draining to the venous sinuses in the vicinity of the torcular (Fig. 61).

The prominent veins of the superior group, the precentral cerebellar, superior vermian and anterior pontomesencephalic veins are close to the midline.

The petrosal vein of Dandy forms in the cerebellopontine angle from numerous tributaries and runs anterolaterally below the trigeminal nerve to join the superior petrosal sinus just above the pons. It can be seen on axial images (Fig. 28).

Reference
Mawad, M.E., Silver, A.J., Hilal, S.K. & Ganti, S.R. (1983). Computed tomography of the brainstem with intrathecal Metrizamide. Part 1: The normal brainstem. *American Journal of Neuroradiology*, **4**, 1–11.

Further reading
Barkovich, A.J. (ed.) (1995). Normal development of the neonatal and infant brain. In *Pediatric Neuroimaging*. 2nd edn. pp. 9–38. New York: Raven.
Daniels, D.L., Haughton, V.M., Williams, A.L. *et al.* (1981). The flocculus in computed tomography. *American Journal of Neuroradiology*, **2**, 227–30.
Duvernoy, H. (1995). Brain anatomy. In *Magnetic Resonance in Epilepsy*, ed. R.I. Kuzniecky & G.D. Jackson. New York: Raven Press.
Kline, L.B., Acker, J.D., Post, M.J.D. *et al.* (1981). The cavernous sinus: a computed tomographic study. *American Journal of Neuroradiology*, 299–305.
Mark, L.P., Daniels, D.L. & Naidich, T.P. (1993). The fornix. *American Journal of Neuroradiology*, **14**, 1355–8.
Mark, L.P., Daniels, D.L., Naidich, T.P. *et al.* (1993). Hippocampal anatomy and pathologic alterations on conventional MR images. *American Journal of Neuroradiology*, **14**, 1237–40.
Mark, L.P., Daniels, D.L., Naidich, T.P. *et al.* (1993). Limbic system anatomy: an overview. *American Journal of Neuroradiology*, **14**, 349–52.
Mark. L.P., Daniels, D.L., Naidich, T.P., Yetkin, Z. & Borne, J.A. (1993). The hippocampus. *American Journal of Neuroradiology*, **14**, 709–12.
Manelfe, C., Clanet, M., Gigaud, M. *et al.* (1981). Internal capsule: normal anatomy and ischemic changes demonstrated by computed tomography. *American Journal of Neuroradiology*, **2**, 149–55.
Sobel, D.F., Gallen, C.C., Schwartz, B.J. *et al.* (1993). Locating the central sulcus: comparison of MR anatomic and magnetoencephalographic functional methods. *American Journal of Neuroradiology*, **14**, 915–25.
Yagashita, A., Nakano, I., Oda, M. *et al.* (1994). Location of corticospinal tract in the internal capsule at MR imaging. *Radiology*, **191**, 455–60.

3

The orbit and visual pathways

I. MOSELEY

Imaging methods

Eye

Satisfactory images of the normal eye can be obtained by sonography, computed X-ray tomography (CT) or magnetic resonance imaging (MRI). At present, the most satisfactory technique is sonography, but improvements in MRI, with separation of the coats of the eye on contrast-enhanced images, may supersede sonography. At present, the latter is the only technique which yields dynamic information, such as the mobility of a detached retina.

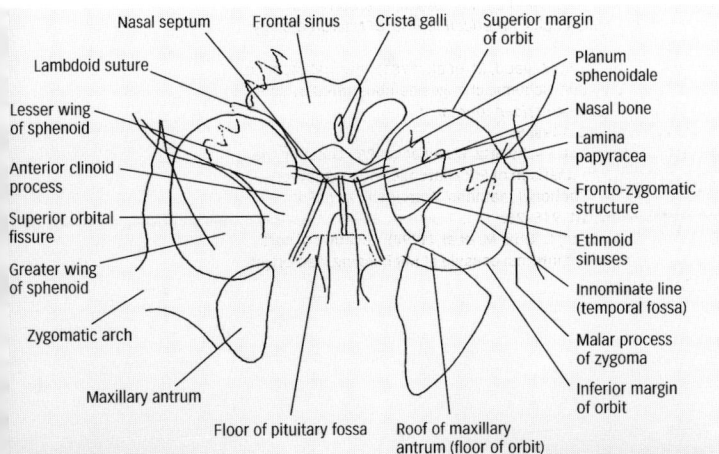

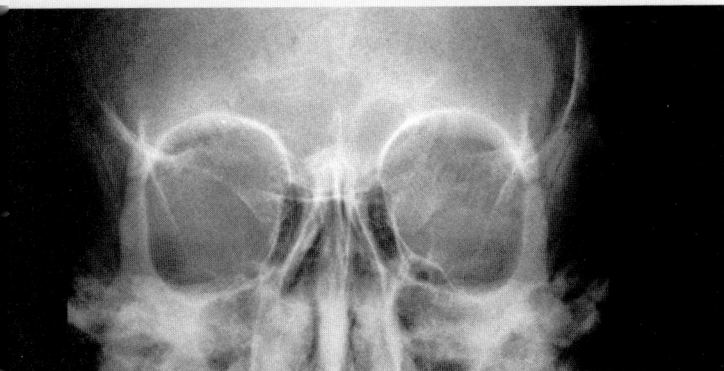

Orbit

The bony orbit and optic canal, together with the adjacent osseous structures, are best shown by fine-section, bone-algorithm CT, although plain films may show major fractures, for example. The contents of the optic canal, however, can be shown only by MRI.

The soft tissue structures of the orbit are demonstrated with great clarity by CT, thanks to the high contrast afforded by bone, air, orbital fat and soft tissues. However, technical advances in MRI, especially faster imaging, may well make this the method of choice for these anatomical areas. When MRI contrast media are employed, the bright signal given by the orbital fat on T1-weighting can complicate analysis of the images; a fat-suppression sequence is therefore particularly helpful.

Optic nerve

The anterior part of the optic nerve/sheath complex can be shown by sonography, but CT or MRI is required for adequate demonstration, particularly of the more posterior segments. The only technique which reliably gives information about the internal structure of the non-expanded nerve and sheath is MRI.

Labels for diagram: Nasal septum, Frontal sinus, Crista galli, Superior margin of orbit, Lambdoid suture, Planum sphenoidale, Lesser wing of sphenoid, Nasal bone, Anterior clinoid process, Lamina papyracea, Superior orbital fissure, Fronto-zygomatic structure, Greater wing of sphenoid, Ethmoid sinuses, Zygomatic arch, Innominate line (temporal fossa), Maxillary antrum, Malar process of zygoma, Inferior margin of orbit, Floor of pituitary fossa, Roof of maxillary antrum (floor of orbit)

Fig. 1.
(a) Occipitofrontal plain radiograph of the bony orbits. Note the normal asymmetry of the superior orbital fissures. In this case the right maxillary antrum is mildly hypoplastic, a normal variant. (b) Diagram of the osseous anatomy of the orbit.

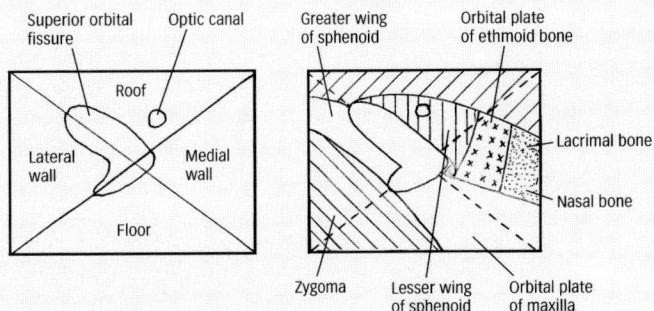

(b)

Labels: Superior orbital fissure, Optic canal, Greater wing of sphenoid, Orbital plate of ethmoid bone, Roof, Lateral wall, Medial wall, Lacrimal bone, Nasal bone, Floor, Zygoma, Lesser wing of sphenoid, Orbital plate of maxilla

(a)

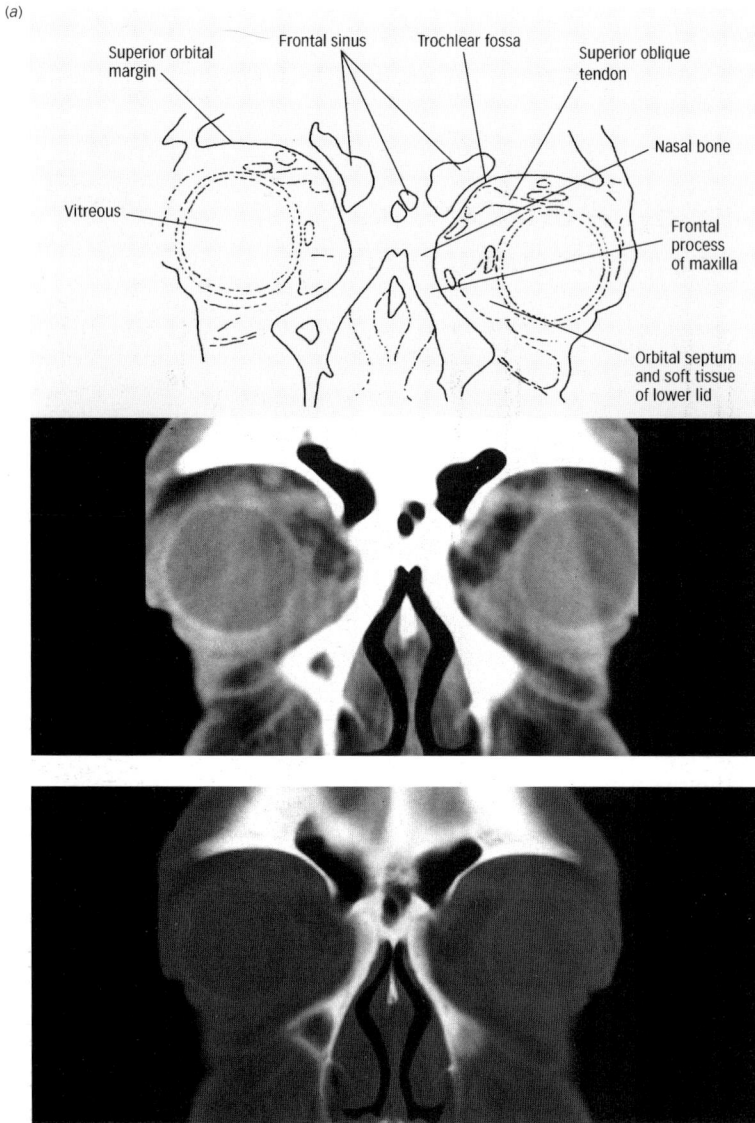

Fig. 2.
Direct coronal CT sections of the orbits, from anterior to posterior, imaged on soft-tissue (top) and bone (below) windows. (a) At level of reflected portion of superior oblique tendon. (b) 9 mm more posteriorly, at level of inferior oblique muscle and bony nasolacrimal duct. (c) 10 mm further back, at posterior pole of eye; note that the optic nerve, which emerges medial (and therefore anterior) to the posterior pole of the globe, may be seen on the same section as the latter. (d) 5 mm further back, showing normal disposition of extraocular muscles. (e) 10 mm further back, just anterior to apex of orbit.

Lacrimal pathways

The most widely used method for demonstrating the lacrimal pathways is positive contrast dacryocystography, with injection of contrast medium into one of the canaliculi, usually the inferior. Radionuclide studies may give more physiological information, but lack anatomical detail.

Intracranial visual pathways

MRI is once again the technique of choice, especially for the intracranial optic nerves, chiasm and tracts. Sellar region masses and large cerebral lesions can, of course, be shown by CT, but in most cases MRI is distinctly superior.

Vascular imaging

The blood supply to the orbit and visual pathways is described below. This is currently demonstrated by intra-arterial digital subtrac-

tion angiography (DSA), but this role will increasingly be assumed by magnetic resonance angiography (MRA), particularly as far as the intracranial vessels are concerned.

Orbital phlebography was used in the past for investigation of orbital masses. There are now no firm indications for its use; a transvenous approach via the orbit is, however, sometimes employed in interventional treatment of lesions around the cavernous sinus.

Radiological anatomy

Orbit
Osseous anatomy

The orbit is a more or less pyramidal cavity whose apex is continued posteriorly as the optic canal, and whose rectangular base opens on to the face.

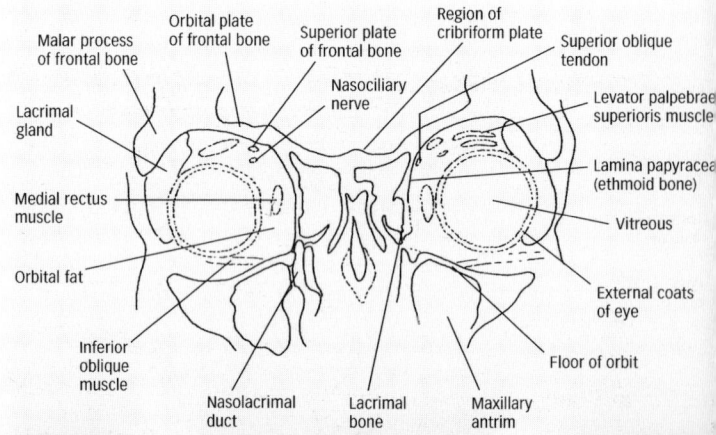

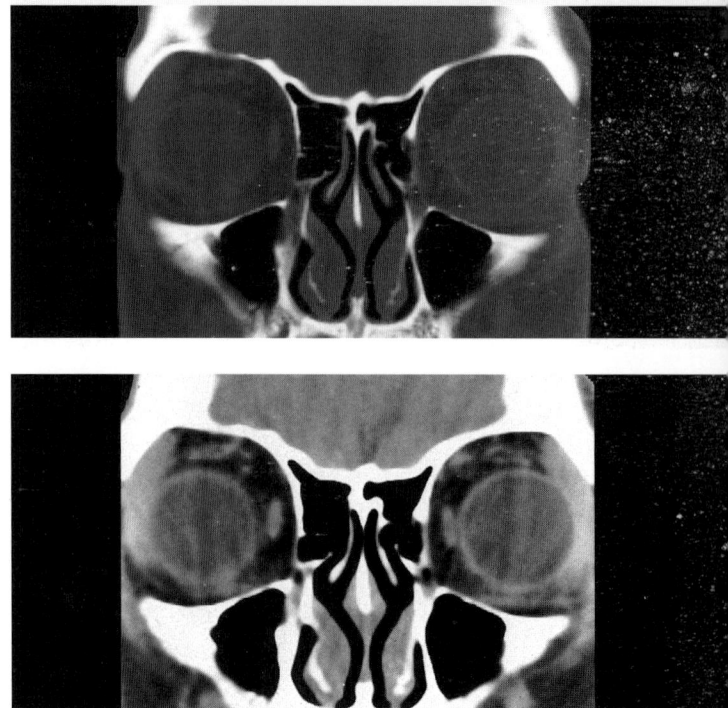

The bony structure of the orbit is very complex. It is convenient to consider the medial wall, floor, lateral wall and roof, in turn. Coronal imaging shows that the medial and lateral walls are essentially vertical, and the roof, while convex upwards, is horizontal. However, the floor of the orbit slopes downwards from the medial to the lateral side (Fig. 1).

The medial wall is formed, from before backwards, by the frontal process (the antero-superior angle) of the maxilla, which abuts the nasal bone anteriorly, the lacrimal bone with anterior and posterior lacrimal crests, between which lies the lacrimal sac, and behind this the orbital plate of the maxilla below, with the ethmoid bone and frontal bone above it. At the apex, the sphenoid bone contributes a small portion. The main component of the rectangular medial wall, formed by the usually convex lateral surface of the

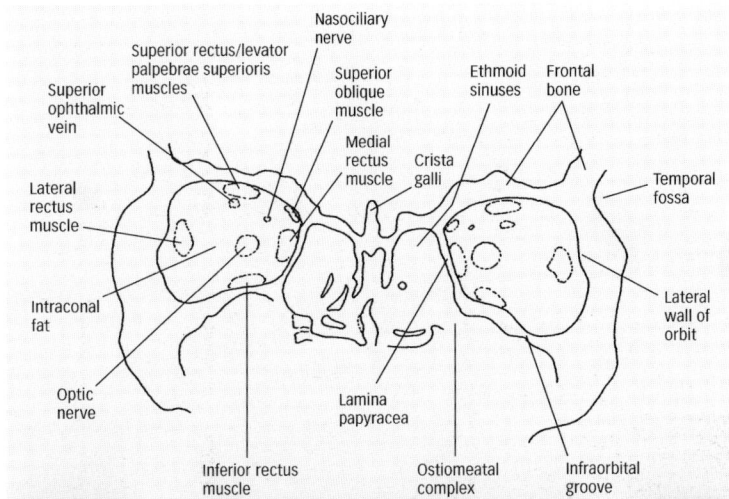

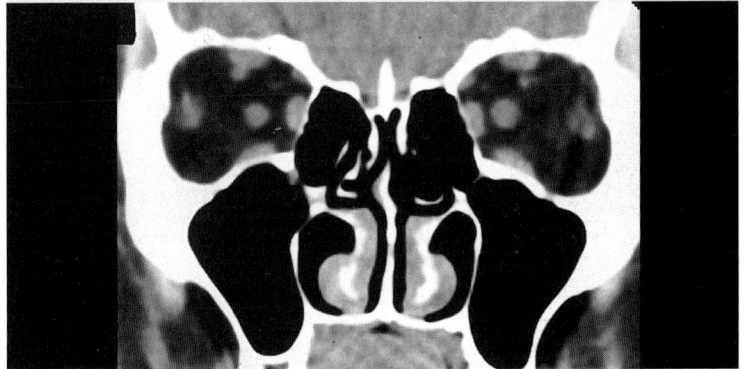

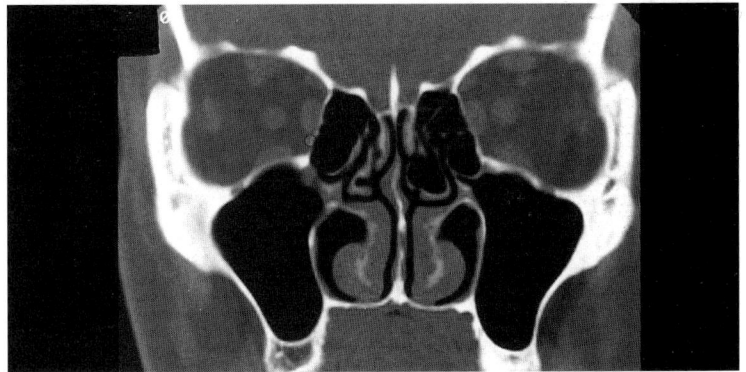

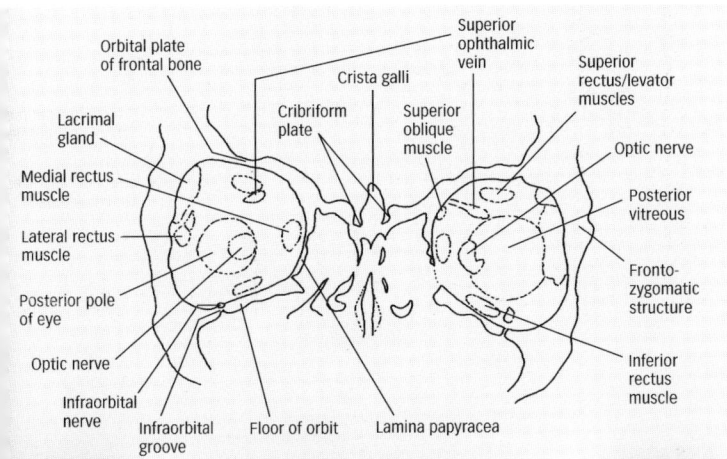

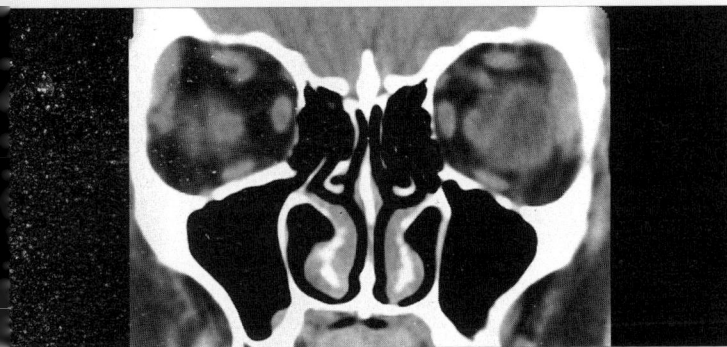

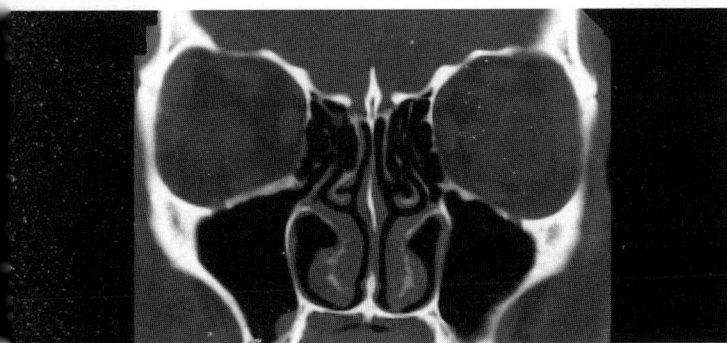

(d)

ethmoid labyrinth, is thin and fragile, hence its name: the lamina papyracea (Fig. 2).

The triangular floor is formed, from medial to lateral, by the orbital plate of the maxilla, and the zygomatic bone. Near the apex, a small portion of the palatine bone, the orbital plate, separates the maxilla and ethmoid bone. The thin floor, between the orbit and the maxillary antrum, slopes downwards and laterally, and is separated by the inferior orbital fissure from the lateral wall. It is grooved by the infraorbital groove, which, in its anterior half, becomes the infraorbital canal, closed above by the infraorbital suture. The groove and canal form a relatively weak area, prone to give way in blow-out fractures.

2(e)

Labels: Optic nerve, Planum sphenoidale, Frontal lobes, Rectus muscles

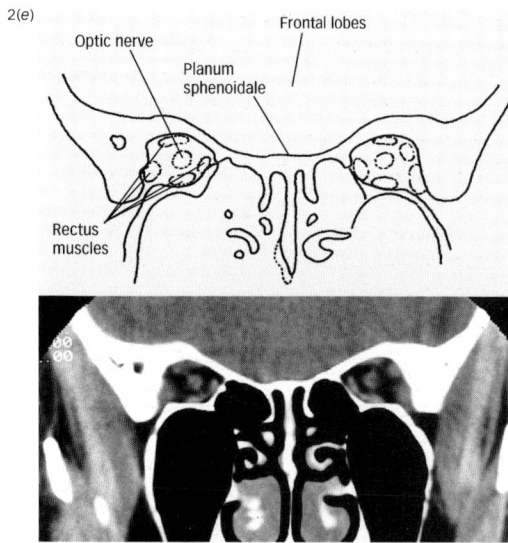

Fig. 3.
Axial CT 1.5 mm section through optic canals and superior orbital fissures, imaged on bone window. Note that the fissure, which has virtually no anteroposterior extent, lies anteroinferior to the longer optic canal.

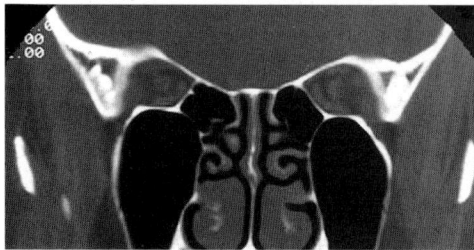

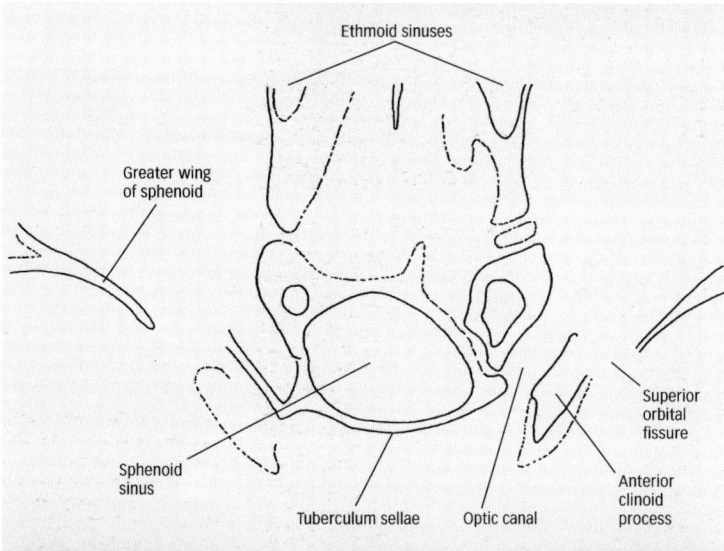

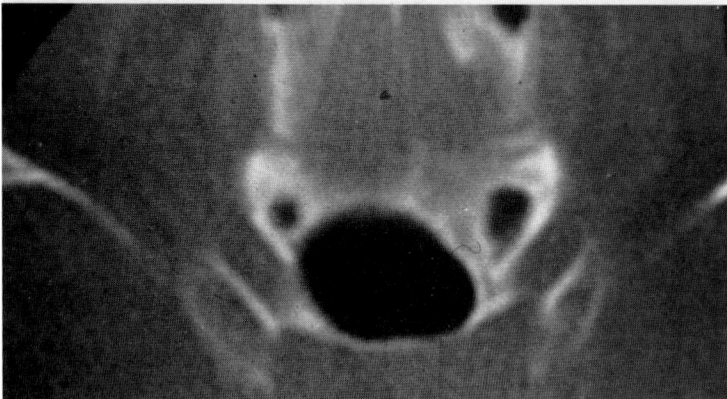

Labels: Ethmoid sinuses, Greater wing of sphenoid, Sphenoid sinus, Tuberculum sellae, Optic canal, Anterior clinoid process, Superior orbital fissure

On coronal images, the canal is seen as a circle of bone close to the midpoint of the floor.

The lateral wall, also triangular, is largely composed of the zygomatic bone, which has an anterior condensation forming the lower half of the lateral margin of the orbit; above the frontozygomatic suture this is continued by the frontal bone. The suture is often visible on plain radiographs, and should not be mistaken for a fracture. More posteriorly, the greater wing of the sphenoid lies posterosuperior to the inferior orbital fissure and is separated by the superior orbital fissure from the lesser wing of the sphenoid and optic canal.

Apart from a small posteromedial contribution from the lesser wing of the sphenoid, almost all the triangular roof of the orbit is formed by the frontal bone which, at the

Fig
Postero-anterior obliq plain radiograph of rig optic can

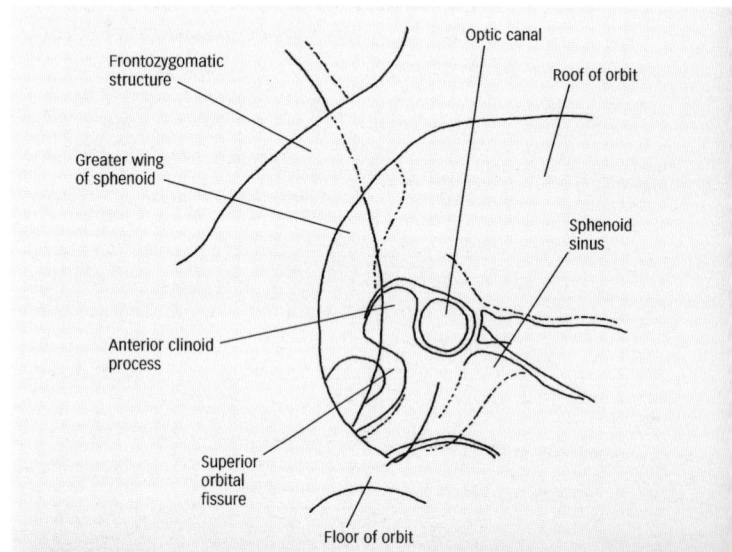

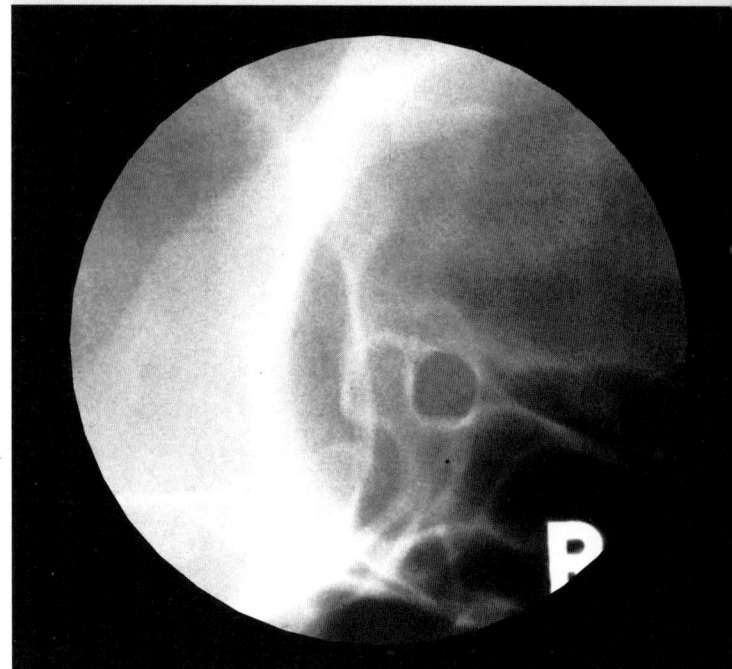

Labels: Frontozygomatic structure, Greater wing of sphenoid, Anterior clinoid process, Superior orbital fissure, Optic canal, Roof of orbit, Sphenoid sinus, Floor of orbit

superolateral angle of the orbit, shows a depression for the lacrimal gland. Its anterior margin is thick, but the orbital plate of the frontal bone, which separates the orbital from the cranial cavity, varies markedly in thickness, because of the convolutional impressions corresponding to the frontal lobe. In some areas, particularly in the elderly, it is very thin. The roof may be further attenuated by extensive frontal sinus air cells. Near the superomedial border of the orbit, the trochlea, around which the tendon of the superior oblique muscle passes, shows a variable degree of ossification.

The approximately rectangular thickened anterior orbital margin is thus formed by the frontal bones, maxilla and zygoma.

Optic canal The term 'optic canal' is preferred to 'optic foramen' because it underlines the fact that this opening is longer than it is wide. The orbital end, where the vertical dimension is slightly greater than the width, is also slightly wider than the cranial end; the mean diameter is 5 mm, whereas its roof is 10–12 mm long (Fig. 3). It is formed by the two roots of the lesser wing of the sphenoid bone. A strut of bone separates it from the superior orbital fissure (Fig. 4). It is intimately related to the sphenoid sinus and the posterior ethmoid air cells, and most or even all of its circumference may rarely be pneumatized.

The long axis of the canal is directed superomedially as well as posteriorly. It forms an angle of about 35 degrees with the sagittal plane, and the plane of its lateral wall is more or less a continuation of that of the lateral wall of the orbit. On axial cross-sectional imaging, therefore, this narrow, elongated canal, forming an angle of approximately 45 degrees with the lamina papyracea, should not be confused with the irregular defect in the sphenoid wings which lies inferolateral to it, the superior orbital fissure (Fig. 3).

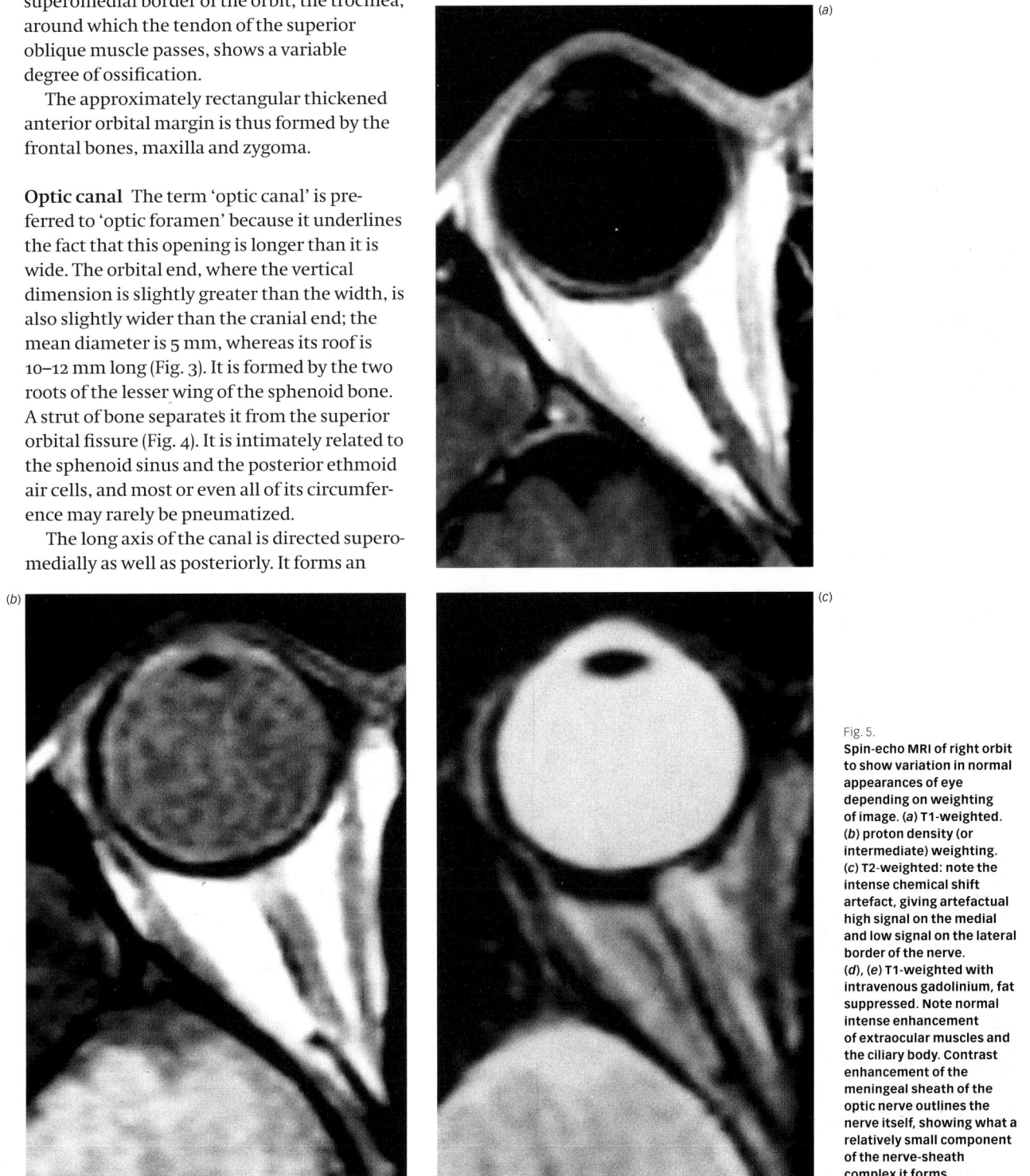

Fig. 5.
Spin-echo MRI of right orbit to show variation in normal appearances of eye depending on weighting of image. (a) T1-weighted. (b) proton density (or intermediate) weighting. (c) T2-weighted: note the intense chemical shift artefact, giving artefactual high signal on the medial and low signal on the lateral border of the nerve. (d), (e) T1-weighted with intravenous gadolinium, fat suppressed. Note normal intense enhancement of extraocular muscles and the ciliary body. Contrast enhancement of the meningeal sheath of the optic nerve outlines the nerve itself, showing what a relatively small component of the nerve-sheath complex it forms.

Soft tissues

The soft tissue structures of the orbit are embedded in the orbital fat, which fills all the orbital cavity. It is limited anteriorly by the orbital septum, and can be divided into intraconal and extraconal components. These are subdived by fine septa which run parallel with the optic nerve, and which are better developed in young people than in the elderly. The fat extends posteriorly into the very apex of the orbit, and may extend, particularly in the elderly, into the anterior part of the superior orbital fissure and even the cavernous sinus.

Eye The ocular globe lies at the anterior base of the orbit; it is approximately 25 mm in diameter, while its anterior portion, the cornea, has a visibly smaller radius of curvature. Myopia is so common as to be regarded as a normal variant; when marked, it is associated with increase in the anteroposterior diameter of the globe, while the transverse diameter is normal.

The coats which form the covering of the globe are, from outside inwards, the tough, fibrous sclera, the finer, pigmented choroid and the light-sensitive retina. Near the anterior pole of the eye, a circumferential soft tissue structure, the ciliary body, supports the lens and, anterior to it, the iris. The lens, containing only 65–70% water, is one of the least

(d)

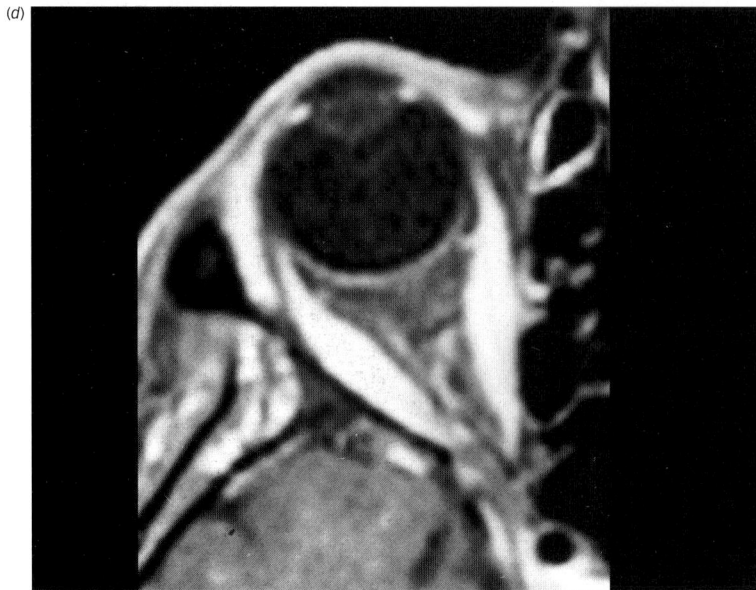

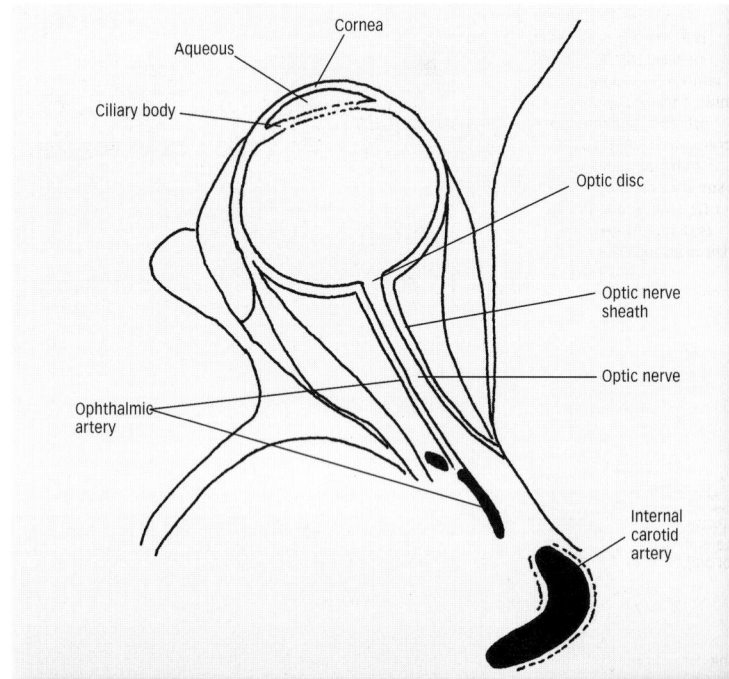

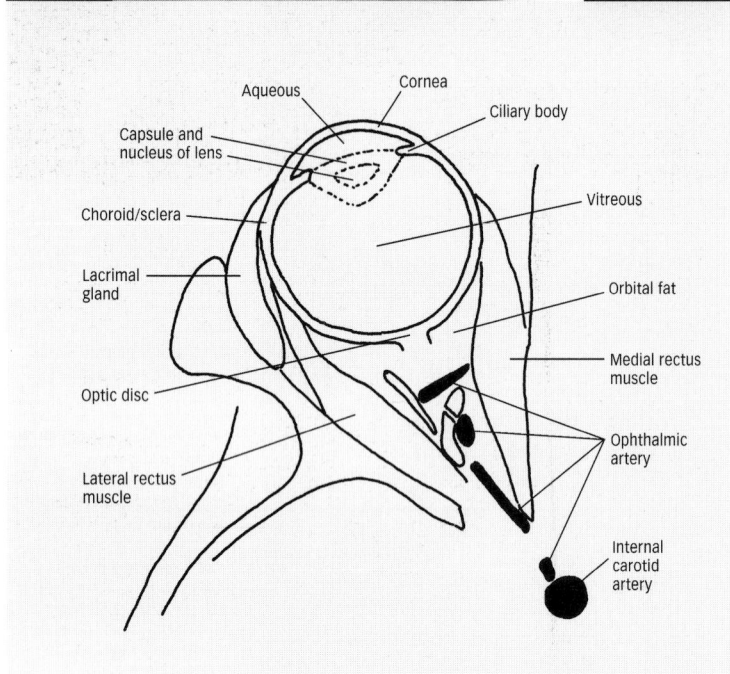

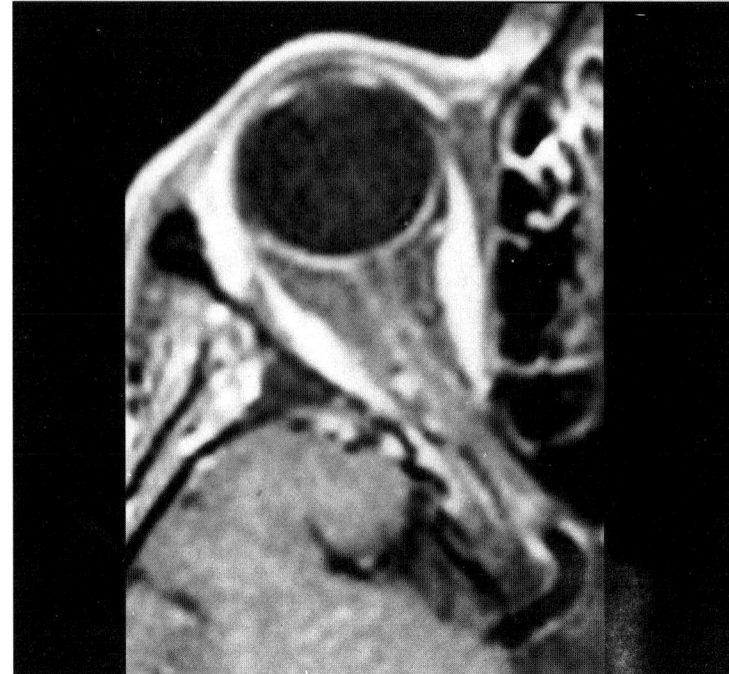

Fig. 6.
CT of orbits, from below
upwards, imaged at soft-
tissue windows. (a) Through
inferior orbital fissure and
bony nasolacrimal ducts.
(b) 1.5 mm more craniad
(bone window). (c) 3 mm
more craniad, through
inferior oblique muscle.
(d) 4 mm more craniad,
through lacrimal crests.
(e) 4 mm more craniad,
through annulus of Zinn.
Note asymmetrical position
of lenses, as patient
looks to right; this is
accompanied by
contraction of the left
medial rectus, which
appears thicker than its
fellow (f) 4 mm more
craniad, through optic
nerves. (g) as (f) (bone
window). (h) 3 mm more
craniad, through ophthalmic
arteries. (i) 3 mm more
craniad, through superior
ophthalmic veins and
superior rectus muscles.
(j) 3 mm more craniad.
(k) 3 mm more craniad,
through superior oblique
tendons.

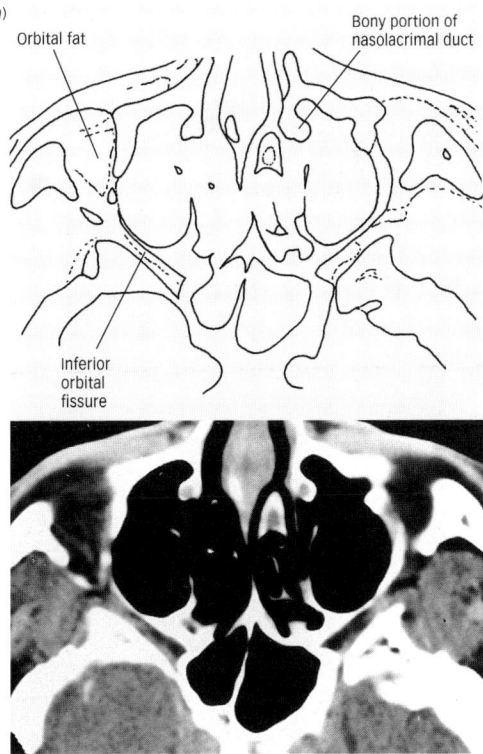

water-laden tissues in the body, and appears
homogeneously dense on CT. It has a relatively
long T1 but a short T2. The nucleus, which has
the lowest water content, has the shortest T2
relaxation time, and T1-weighted MRI shows
the capsule to give higher signal than the
nucleus (Fig. 5).

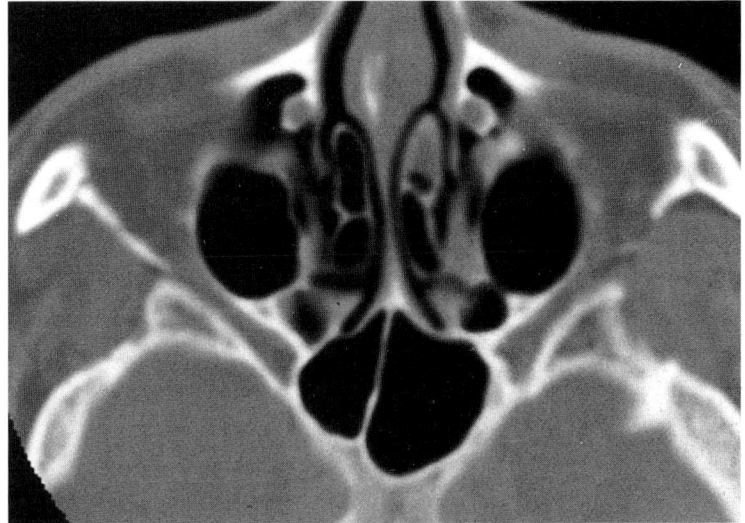

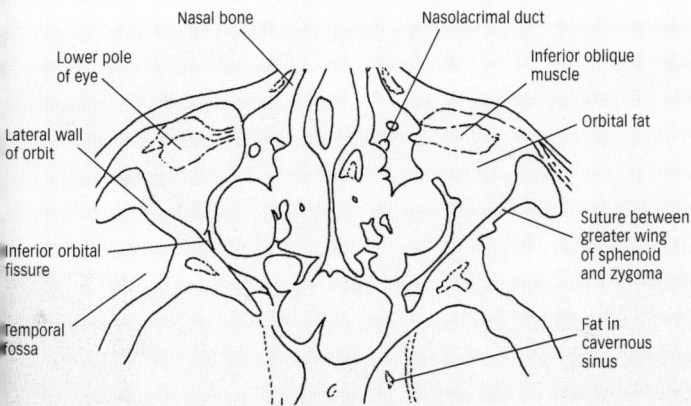

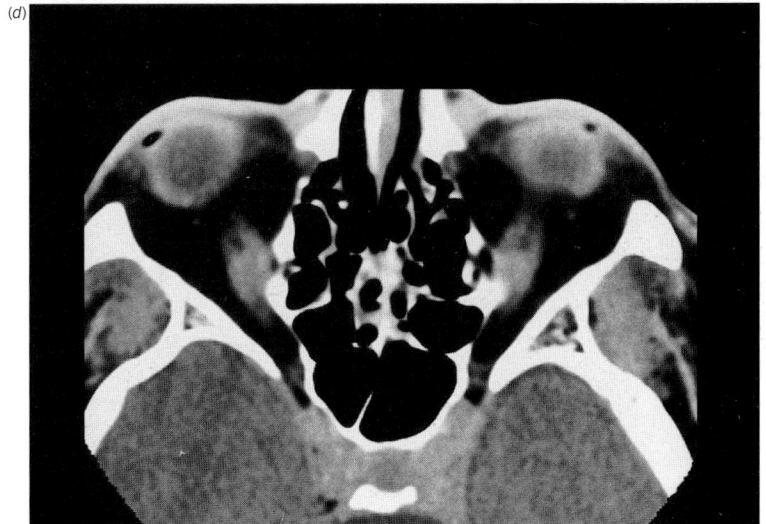

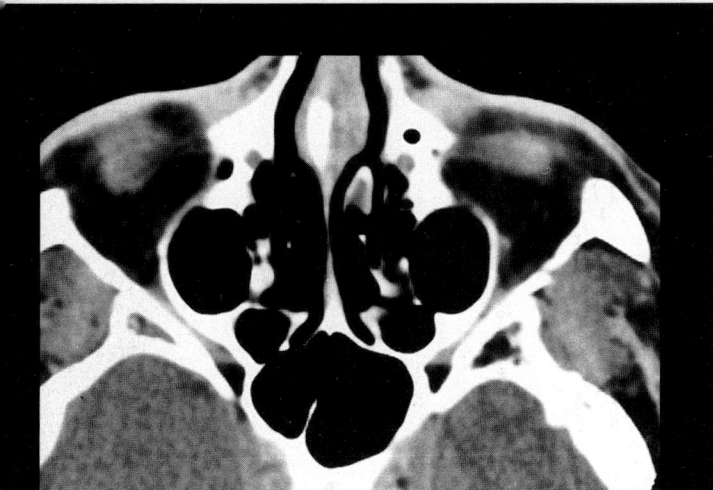

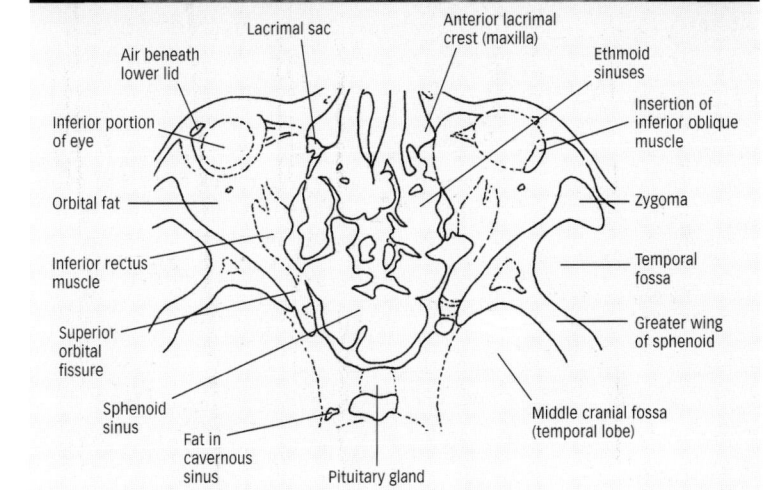

(a)

Orbital fat

Bony portion of
nasolacrimal duct

Inferior
orbital
fissure

(b)

(d)

Nasal bone

Lower pole
of eye

Lateral wall
of orbit

Inferior orbital
fissure

Temporal
fossa

Nasolacrimal duct

Inferior oblique
muscle

Orbital fat

Suture between
greater wing
of sphenoid
and zygoma

Fat in
cavernous
sinus

Air beneath
lower lid

Lacrimal sac

Anterior lacrimal
crest (maxilla)

Ethmoid
sinuses

Inferior portion
of eye

Insertion of
inferior oblique
muscle

Orbital fat

Zygoma

Inferior rectus
muscle

Temporal
fossa

Superior
orbital
fissure

Greater wing
of sphenoid

Sphenoid
sinus

Fat in
cavernous
sinus

Pituitary gland

Middle cranial fossa
(temporal lobe)

67

(e)

Labels: Orbital vessels, Lacrimal sac, Orbital septum, Lids, Outer coats of eye, Vitreous, Orbital fat, Lateral rectus muscle, Annulus of Zinn, Lamina papyracea, Ethmoid sinuses, Superior orbital fissure, Dorsum sellae, Infundibulum, Medial rectus muscle

Labels: Orbital septum, Medial rectus muscle, Cornea, Aqueous, Lens, Vitreous, Outer coats of eye, Optic disc (intraocular optic nerve), Lateral rectus muscle, Ophthalmic artery, Optic nerve (intraorbital) in meningeal sheath, Inferior pole of lacrimal gland, Extraconal fat, Intraconal fat, Superior orbital fissure, Anterior clinoid process, Sphenoid sinus, Optic nerve (intracranial), Optic nerve (intracanalicular)

(g)

Labels: Medial rectus muscle, Lacrimal gland, Optic nerve, Ophthalmic artery, Superior orbital fissure, Lateral rectus muscle

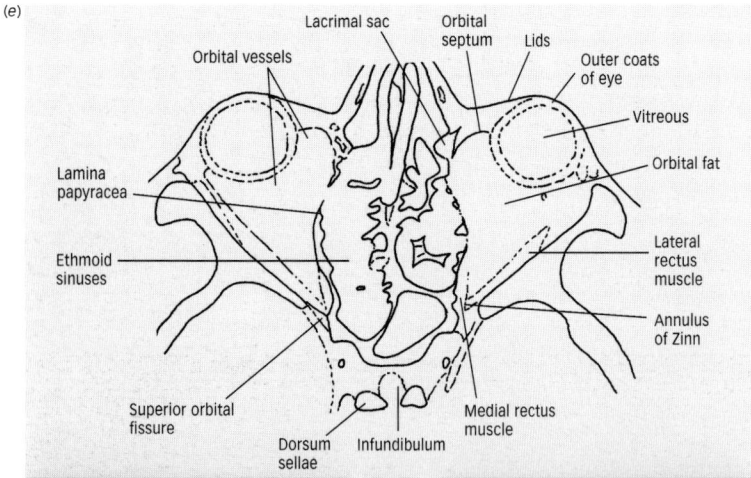

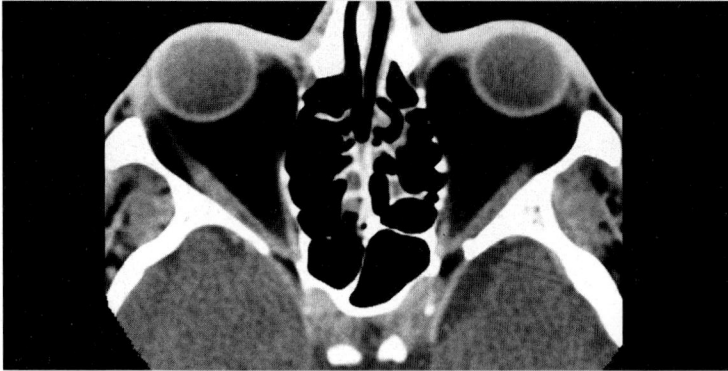

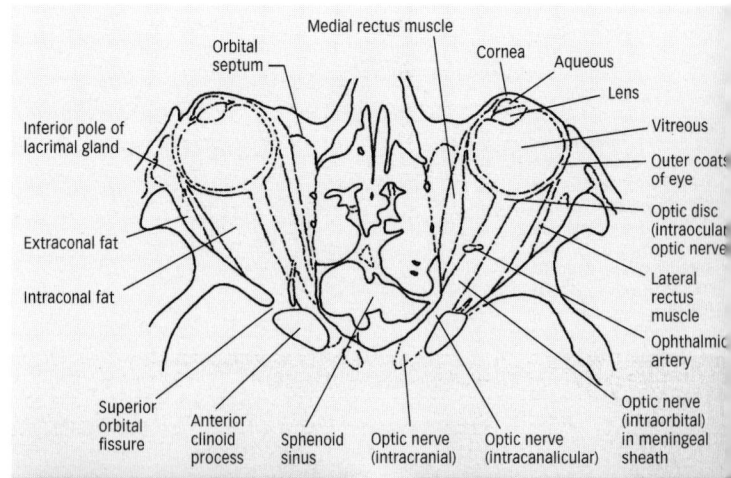

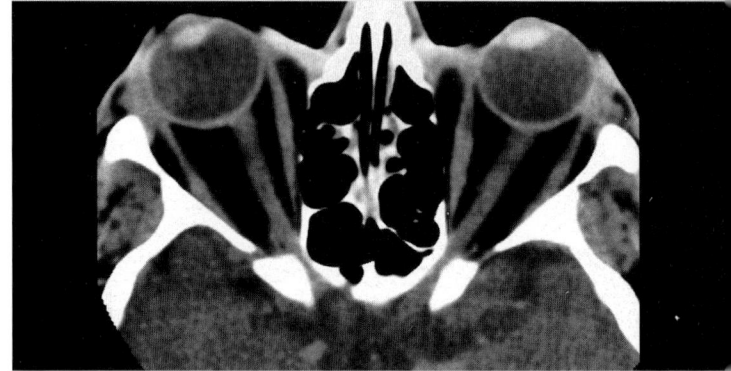

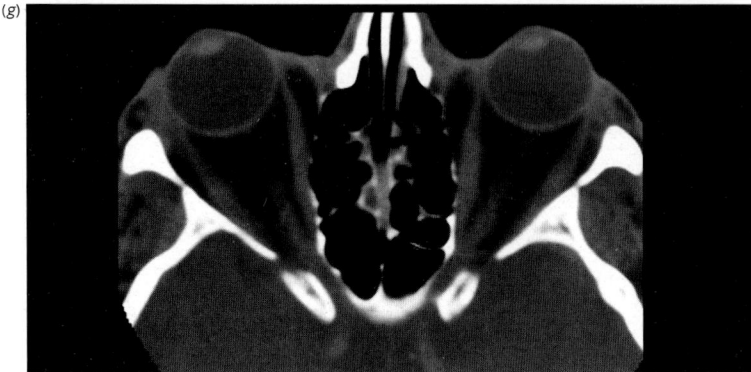

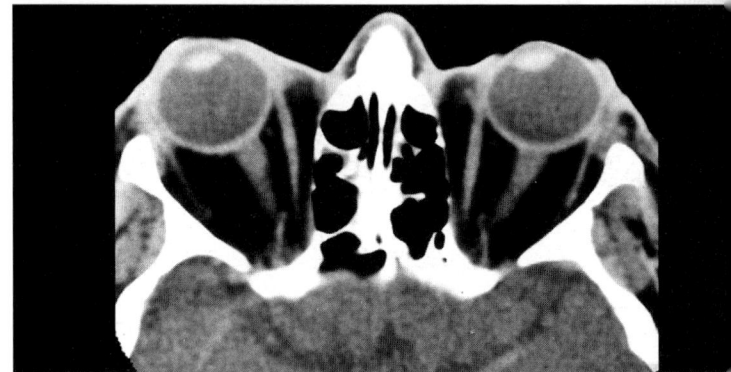

The lens separates the interior of the globe into two cavities, named after the nature of their contents: the vitreous posteriorly and the aqueous anteriorly. The space containing the watery aqueous is incompletely divided into anterior and posterior chambers by the iris. The shallow posterior chamber is poorly shown on radiological images. On CT, the normal aqueous and vitreous humours are similar in density to the intracranial cerebrospinal fluid, although streak artefacts across the eye frequently produce slightly more dense areas. The very high water content of not only the aqueous but also the vitreous gives them a long T1 and an exceptionally long T2. They therefore give homogeneously low signal on heavily T1-weighted images, and increase in intensity with T2-weighting. However, on T1-weighted STIR images, commonly used for the orbit, they also give high signal. These extreme variations in signal render the vitreous of questionable use as a reference signal.

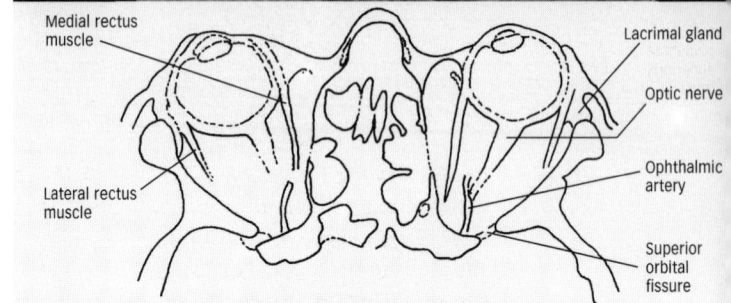

The optic disc lies to the medial side of the posterior pole of the globe, abutting the vitreous. The meningeal sheath of the optic nerve surrounds this attachment.

(j)

Upper lid — Orbital veins — Upper part of eye

Orbital fat

Top of lacrimal gland

Superior ophthalmic vein

Superior rectus muscle

Superior oblique muscle

Orbital fat — Position of trochlea — Upper part of eye

Minor orbital veins

Superior oblique muscle

Superior ophthalmic vein

Superior rectus/levator palpebrae superioris muscles

Upper lid (tarsal plate) — Frontal sinus — Upper lid (skin)

Top of eye

Superior oblique tendon

Levator palpebrae superioris muscle

Orbital fat

Superior ophthalmic vein

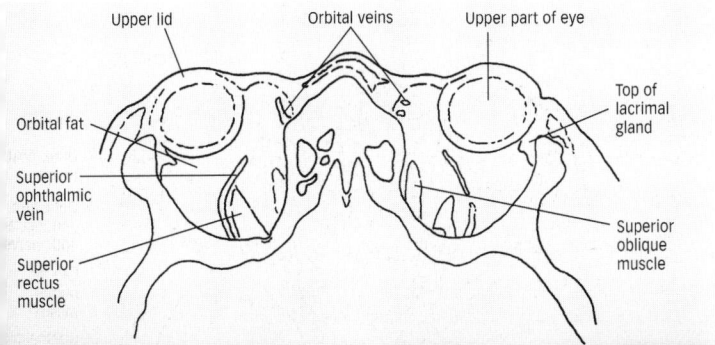

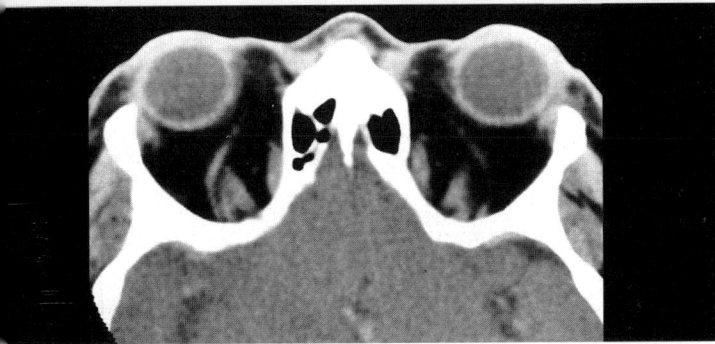

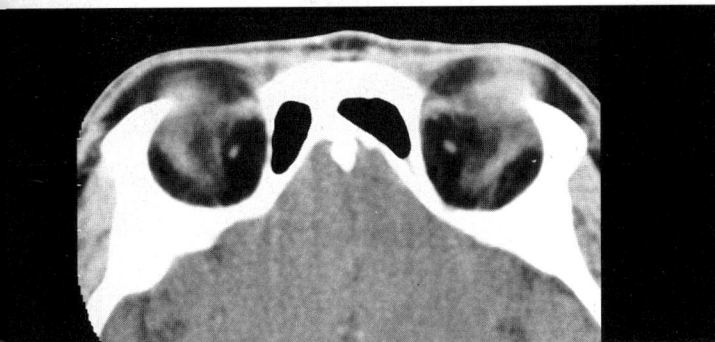

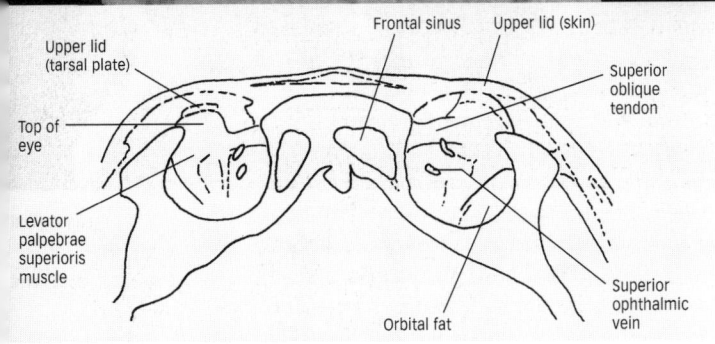

Optic nerve With the eye looking straight forward (the primary position), the optic nerve runs diagonally back from its attachment at the globe to the medially lying optic canal at the apex. However, the nerve is of necessity mobile, since the normal and constant movements of the eye must be accommodated (Fig. 6). Thus, in abduction, the nerve abuts the medial rectus muscle, and in adduction lies close to the lateral rectus, while in upgaze it lies just above the inferior rectus and in downgaze just below the superior. The only portion of the orbit the nerve does not enter in the normal range of eye movements is the most inferolateral, but this is quite capacious. The somewhat sigmoid shape of the nerve in either downward or lateral gaze may be related to the fact that its posterior portion is rather less flexible than the anterior, and/or that it enters the orbit running in an inferolateral direction. On images showing its long axis in the vertical plane, the nerve in the primary position frequently appears to take a sinusoidal course, as it dips below the encircling ophthalmic artery. The nerve tends to be more tortuous in high myopia, where the globe is elongated in the anteroposterior plane.

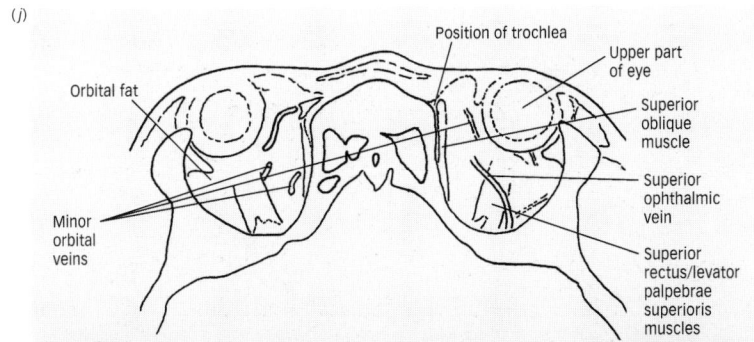

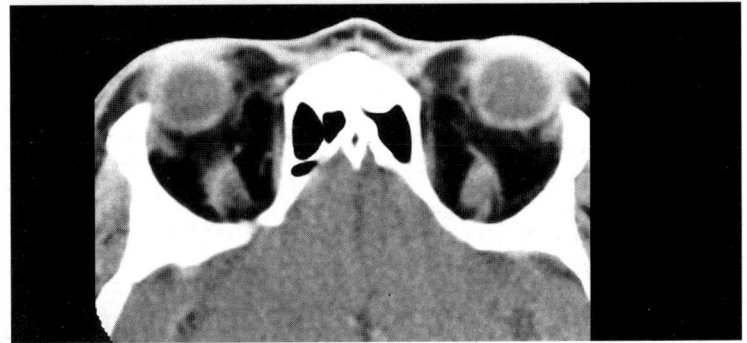

The term 'optic nerve' is a misnomer, because the 'nerve', in fact, is a white matter tract of the cerebrum. As such, it is surrounded by all the normal layers of the meninges, the pia, arachnoid and dura mater, the first two being separated by the cerebrospinal fluid in the subarachnoid space, in continuity with the intracranial subarachnoid space. This space is normally widest just behind the globe, so that the 'nerve' often appears to expand just behind at its anterior end. On MRI it is frequently possible to identify the normal-sized nerve within this more patulous segment (see Fig. 10). High-resolution coronal MRI will demonstrate the cerebrospinal fluid (CSF) surrounding the nerve within the sheath, often as far as the posterior orbit, but not usually within the optic canal. The dura mater of the sheath blends with the sclera of the eye anteriorly and with the periorbita around the optic canal posteriorly; it is continuous with the intracranial dura mater.

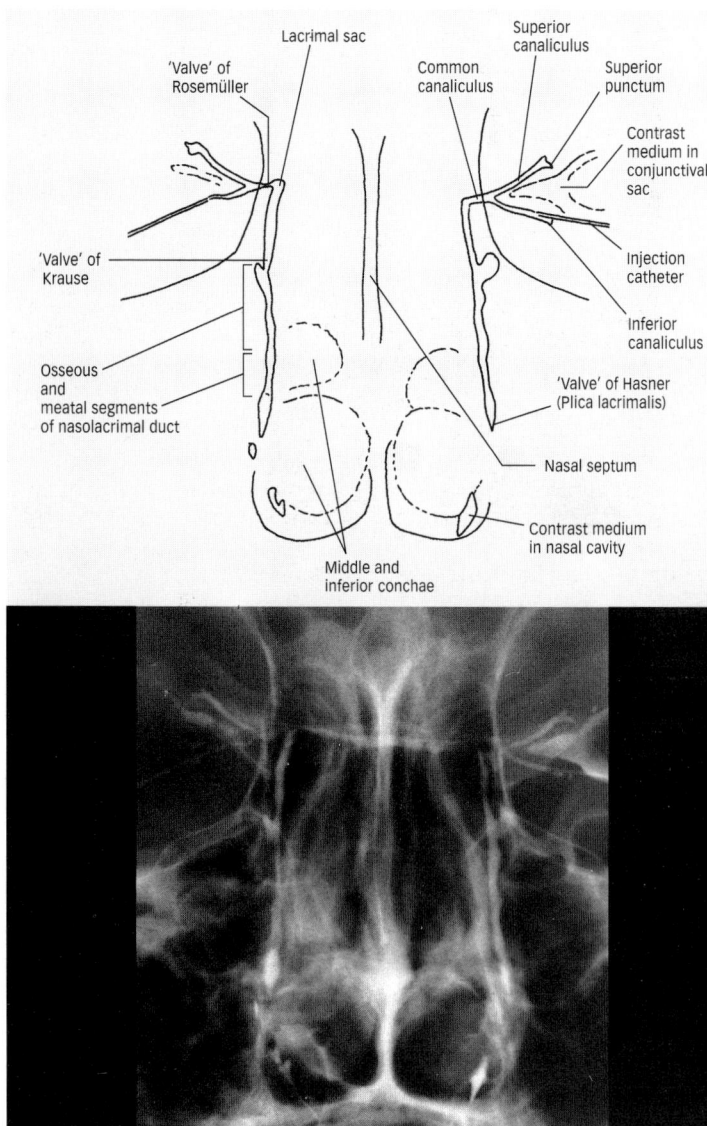

than its width. The opposing lateral rectus muscle is much smaller. It arises from the common tendon both above and below the superior orbital fissure, and runs along the lateral wall of the orbit to insert about 7 mm behind the cornea. In coronal sections, the lower border of its more posterior portion is seen to lie more medially than the upper, because of the obliquity of the lateral wall.

The superior rectus muscle arises from the annulus of Zinn above the optic nerve, and from the adjacent upper surface of its dural sheath. It runs anteriorly and at about 25 degrees laterally, to insert on the sclera about 8 mm from the cornea. Its breadth is greater than its height. Directly above this muscle, and separating it from the roof of the orbit, lies the levator palpebrae superioris, which takes origin from the lesser wing of the sphenoid and the adjacent fibrous origin of the superior rectus. It is broader than the latter, particularly anteriorly, where it fans out to insert on the upper lid. However, on imaging studies it is often difficult to distinguish the two muscles.

The origin of the inferior rectus lies below the orifice of the optic canal. Its anterolateral course is parallel with that of the opposing superior rectus. It inserts mainly on to the sclera, about 7 mm behind the cornea, but a slip runs forward to the lower lid.

The superior oblique, the longest and thinnest of the extraocular muscles, takes origin superomedial to the optic canal. It initially runs forward above the medial rectus, from which its belly may not be distinguishable on axial images. About 1 cm from the trochlea, it becomes a rounded tendon, which is reflected around the trochlea before fanning out posterolaterally at an angle of 55 degrees over the upper surface of the eye, inferior to the superior rectus muscle. The inferior oblique is, by contrast, short and rather thick. It arises from the orbital plate of the maxilla, just lateral to the orifice of the bony portion of the nasolacrimal duct, and runs posterolaterally, separating the inferior rectus from the floor of the orbit, to end deep to the lateral rectus.

The superior oblique is supplied exclusively by the IVth cranial (trochlear) nerve, and the lateral rectus by the VIth (abducens) nerve. All the other striated extraocular muscles are innervated by the IIIrd (oculomotor) nerve.

Change in size and shape of the striated extraocular muscles occur normally with eye movements; the contracting muscle, e.g. the left medial rectus on right gaze (adduction), becomes thicker (Fig. 6(e)), while the lateral rectus relaxes and becomes thinner. In the

Fig. 7.
Dacryocystogram, anteroposterior supine projection.

At this point it is also intimately related with the annulus of Zinn, from which the extraocular muscles arise.

Extraocular muscles There are striated and unstriated extraocular muscles. The former comprise four rectus muscles: medial, inferior, lateral and superior, two oblique muscles: inferior and superior, and the levator palpebrae superioris. These muscles show normal soft tissue density and intensity characteristics on CT and MRI respectively (Fig. 6). Fat-suppressed, contrast-enhanced MRI reveals intense contrast enhancement of these structures, which have no blood–tissue barrier, as a normal finding (Fig. 5).

The medial rectus is the largest single muscle. It arises from the inferomedial part of the annulus of Zinn and the sheath of the optic nerve, to run forwards along the medial wall of the orbit and insert on the sclera about 5 mm behind the sclera. Its height is greater opposite orbit, the appearances are reversed, since the eye is abducted. The position of the eyes during imaging, often best appreciated by looking at the lens or optic nerve, should always be taken into account when assessing the relative sizes of the muscles. If the patient falls asleep during imaging, the eyes may normally diverge.

The unstriated muscles are involved mainly with movements of the lids. The largest, the capsulopalpebral muscle of Hessel and Muller's muscle, can be shown by very high resolution MRI, but cannot be identified clearly with conventional imaging.

Lacrimal pathways The tears are formed in the lacrimal gland, whence they diffuse across the conjunctiva to drain via the tear ducts.

The orbital portion of the lacrimal gland lies at the superolateral angle of the orbit, in a bony fossa. It also extends forwards into the upper lid, as the smaller palpebral lobe. The gland is often said to be almond-shaped, but its inferomedial surface is frequently concave, moulded to the globe. Its size is variable, but the glands are usually the same size, so that asymmetry may be a better indication of pathology than actual size. On CT and MRI the gland shows non-specific soft-tissue density and intensity characteristics.

Tear ducts run in the medial portions of the margins of the upper and lower lids. About 6

mm from the inner canthus, small upper and lower puncta open into the superior and inferior canaliculi, turning through 90 degrees to run parallel with the free edge of the lid. They then join to form a common canaliculus of variable length before discharging into the lacrimal sac (Fig. 7). The latter lies in the lacrimal fossa, between the anterior and posterior lacrimal crests, at the medial canthus. The sac can sometimes be identified as a soft-tissue density structure at the medial canthus, but is usually not prominent. It drains inferiorly into the almost vertical nasolacrimal duct, which lies in a bony canal formed by the maxilla, the lacrimal bone and the lacrimal process of the inferior turbinate, opening into the inferior meatus of the nasal cavity. Although a number of 'valves' are described along the lacrimal pathways, they are of little or no functional significance. The bony portion of the nasolacrimal duct is clearly seen, often with a slightly sclerotic border, on CT (Figure 6(b)), and its mucosal lining may give higher signal than the adjacent bone on MRI. However, it is not infrequent for one or both of the ducts to contain air.

Arteries and veins of the orbit

The orbit receives a dual arterial supply, from the ophthalmic artery, the first principal branch of the internal carotid artery, and from various branches of the external carotid artery.

The ophthalmic artery usually arises just after the internal carotid exits the cavernous sinus, at which point it is deep to the optic nerve, and covered by the anterior clinoid process. It runs through the optic canal within the dural sheath of the nerve, usually lying inferior to the latter, and pierces the sheath near the apex of the orbit. It commonly crosses over the nerve (often appearing to groove it), lying

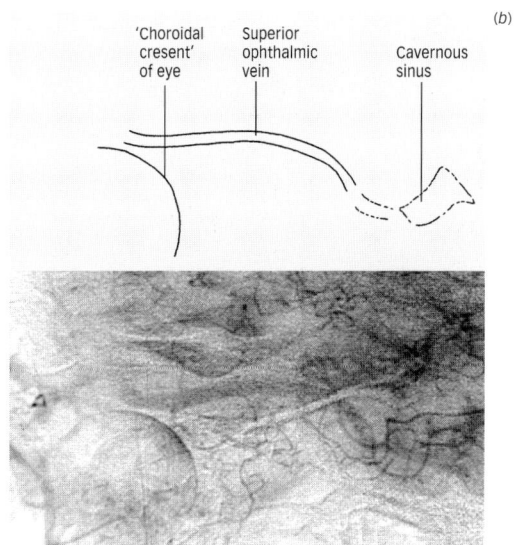

(b)

'Choroidal crescent' of eye — Superior ophthalmic vein — Cavernous sinus

Fig. 8. Selective injection of internal carotid artery; digital subtraction angiography, lateral projection: (a) arterial and (b) venous phases.

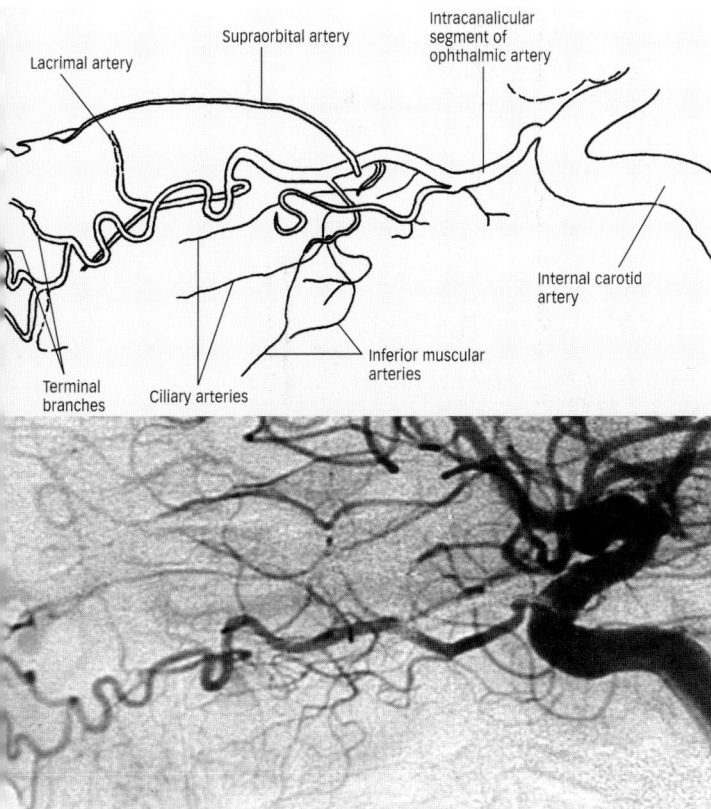

Lacrimal artery — Supraorbital artery — Intracanalicular segment of ophthalmic artery — Internal carotid artery — Inferior muscular arteries — Terminal branches — Ciliary arteries below the superior rectus muscle, and running anteromedially to divide into terminal nasal and frontal branches. While in the orbit, it has the following branches:

(a) the central artery of the retina;
(b) the long and short posterior ciliary arteries;
(c) muscular arteries (which also give off the anterior ciliary arteries);
(d) the lacrimal artery;
(e) posterior and anterior ethmoidal arteries;
(f) supraorbital artery;
(g) palpebral arteries.

It is not rare for the lacrimal artery to give rise to a recurrent branch, which passes back into the cranial cavity to communicate with the mdidle meningeal artery. The significance of this potential anastomosis is that embolization of the middle meningeal artery can endanger the territory of the ophthalmic artery.

Fig. 9.
Selective injection of external carotid artery; digital subtraction angiography, lateral projection, arterial phase.

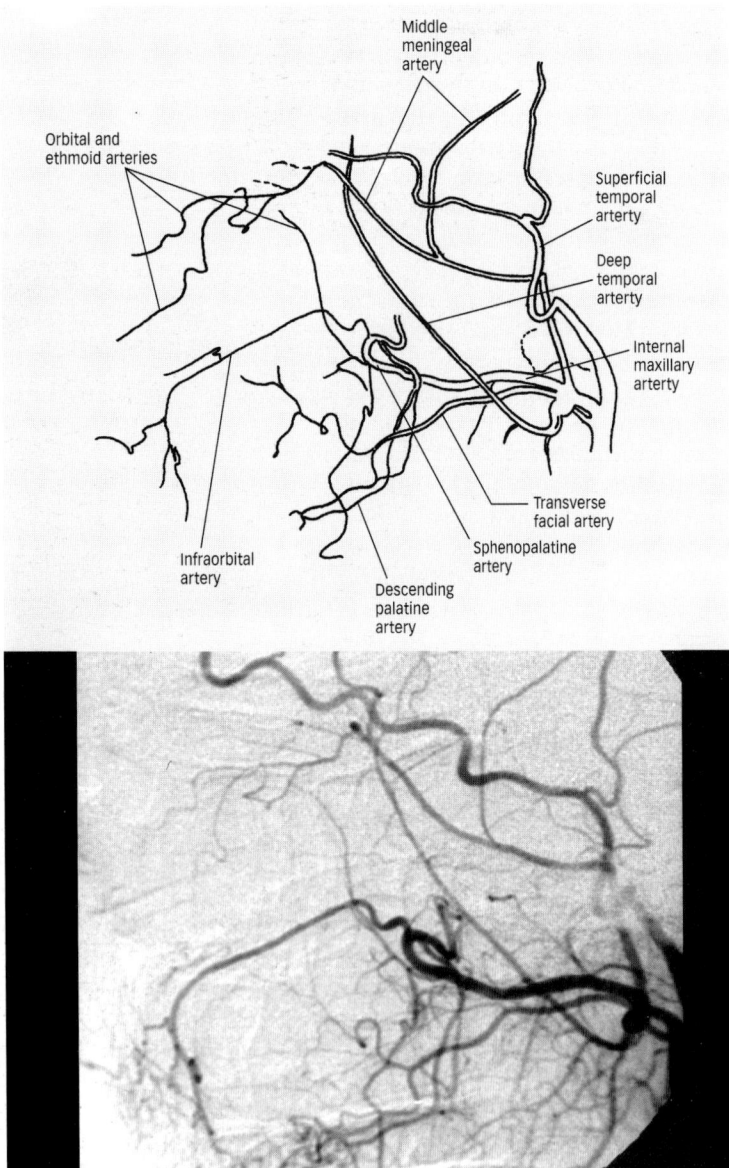

Because of their tortuosity, the ophthalmic artery and its branches are often only incompletely seen on CT or MRI. The angiographic appearances are shown in Fig. 8.

The external carotid arterial system also gives branches to the orbit (Fig. 9). Small branches of the superficial temporal artery and the anterior temporal branch of the internal maxillary artery give transosseous branches to the lateral wall of the orbit. Anastomoses also exist around the floor of the orbit between the anterior deep temporal and infraorbital arteries and the muscular branches of the ophthalmic artery. The infraorbital artery may also have a relatively large lacrimal branch. The lids have a rich arterial anastomosis derived both from the ophthalmic artery branches and the transverse facial, zygomaticomalar, facial and infraorbital arteries. In all of these anastomotic areas, the relative importance of the internal and external carotid artery contribution varies from person to person.

The major orbital vein, the superior ophthalmic vein, is formed near the junction of the angular and supraorbital veins at the superomedial angle of the orbit. It runs posterolaterally between the superior rectus muscle and optic nerve, turning medially once it approaches the lateral wall of the orbit, and discharges into the cavernous sinus via the superior orbital fissure. The superior ophthalmic veins are usually more or less symmetrical, but minor asymmetry is not uncommon (Fig. 6). Much of the blood flowing in them comes from the superficial tissues rather than from the orbital structures themselves, so that they are better seen after injection of the external carotid artery than during internal carotid arteriography (Fig. 8). The veins often fill before the intracranial veins, and this should not be mistaken for pathologically early drainage.

The inferior ophthalmic vein arises near the anterior border of the orbit, and runs backwards in relation to the inferior rectus muscle. It may drain into the much larger superior vein, or directly into the cavernous sinus.

The remaining orbital veins are much smaller and inconstant. The veins anastomosing between the inferior and superior ophthalmic systems are sometimes referred to as the 'vortex' veins.

Intracranial optic pathways

The visual pathways comprise the optic nerves, the optic chiasm, the optic tracts, the lateral geniculate bodies, the optic radiations and the primary and secondary visual ares of the cerebral cortex.

Optic nerve

The optic nerve has four segments: intra-ocular, intraorbital, intracanalicular and intra-cranial (Fig. 10). The first of these is very short, being less than 1 mm in length, and difficult to identify specifically on imaging studies other than very high definition MRI, except when it is pathological, e.g. bulging towards the vitreous as a result of chronic disc swelling, or calcified due to the presence of drusen.

The intraorbital segment of the nerve has been described above. It is the longest portion, measuring usually about 3 cm in length.

The intracanalicular segment is also short, having a length of 6 mm (Fig. 10). It is encircled by its dural sheath, which blends with the periosteum of the canal. Strands of collagen from the sheath pierce this part of the nerve, as do blood vessels, explaining why trauma to this portion can produce irreversible visual loss even in the absence of a fracture. Fine dissection shows that the bony wall of the optic canal may be defective in some areas, so that its periosteum may be in direct contact with that of the sphenoid sinus. The significance in terms of spread of infection or tumours from the sinus is evident.

The intracranial segment of the optic nerve is very variable, depending on the position of the optic chiasm; its length may be a centimetre or more with a 'post-fixed' chiasm or only a few millimetres when the chiasm is 'pre-fixed'. The internal carotid and anterior cerebral arteries may be intimately related to this part of the nerve, but vascular compression is rare.

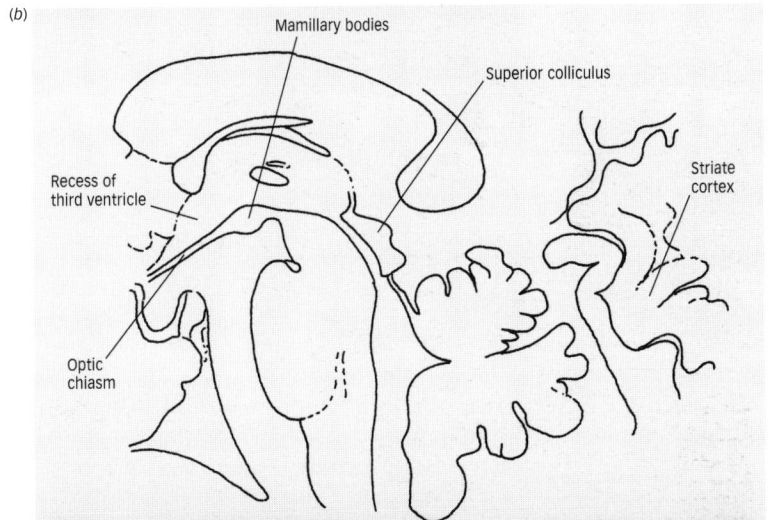

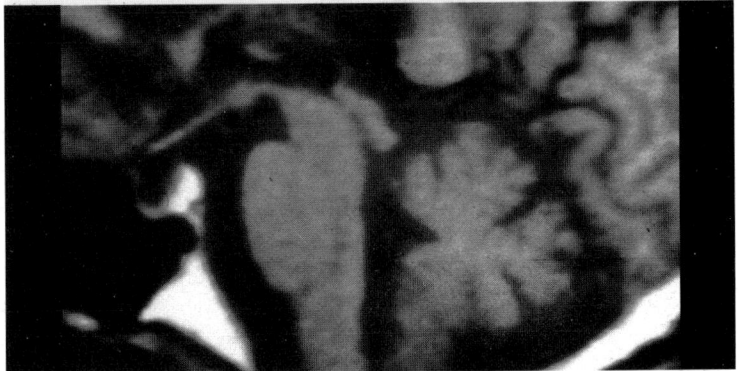

Fig. 10.
T1-weighted inversion-recovery MRI, reformatted from 1.5 mm coronal sections, to show intracanalicular and intracranial portions of optic nerves.

Fig. 11.
Optic chiasm. T1-weighted MRI, sagittal images from different individuals, to show how normal variations in position relative to the pituitary fossa. (a) The chiasm lies virtually on top of the dorsum, and the mamillary bodies just a few millimetres behind it. The plane of the chiasm is more or less perpendicular to that of the clivus. (b) The chiasm lies several millimetres above the dorsum sellae, angling upwards relative to the clivus as it passes backwards, and the mamillary bodies lie both higher and more posteriorly.

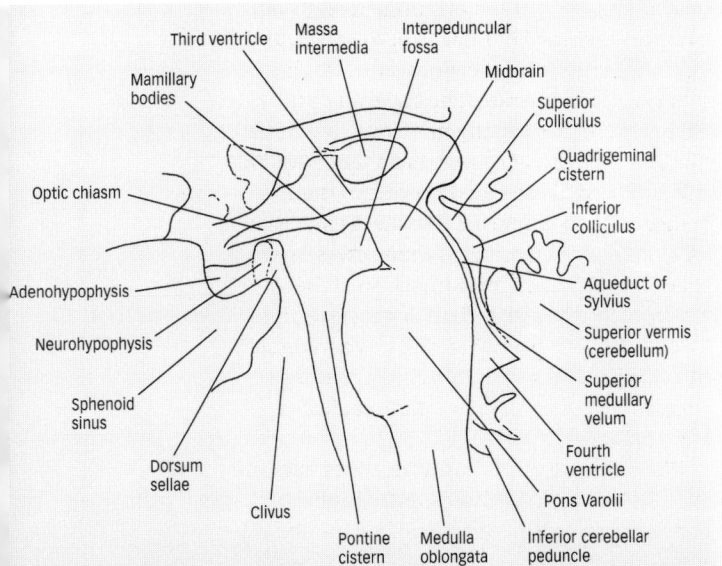

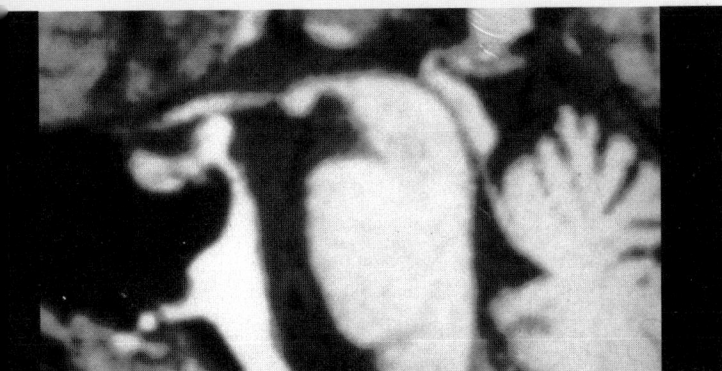

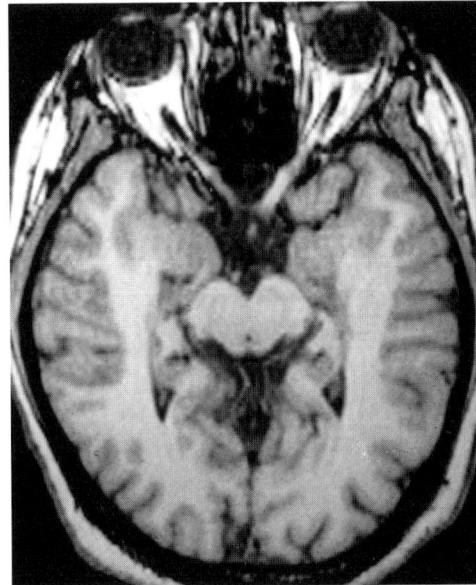

(a)

(b)

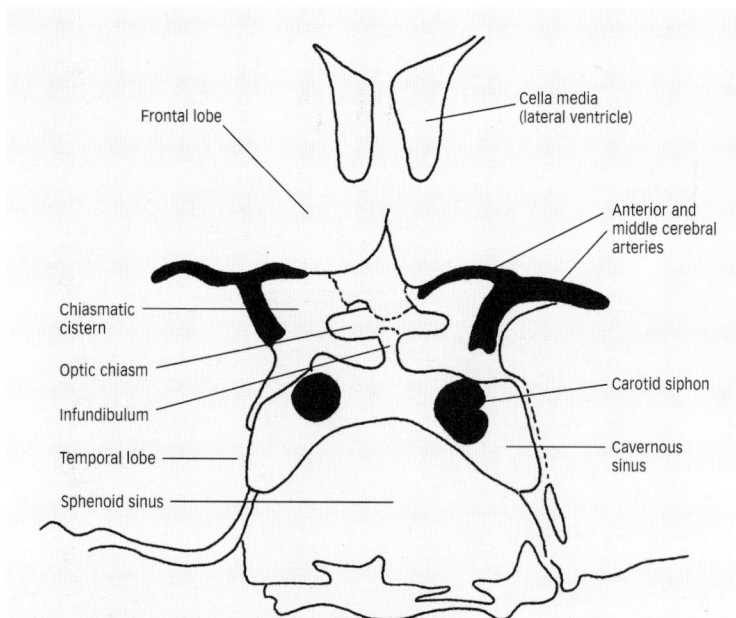

Frontal lobe

Cella media (lateral ventricle)

Anterior and middle cerebral arteries

Chiasmatic cistern

Optic chiasm

Infundibulum

Temporal lobe

Sphenoid sinus

Carotid siphon

Cavernous sinus

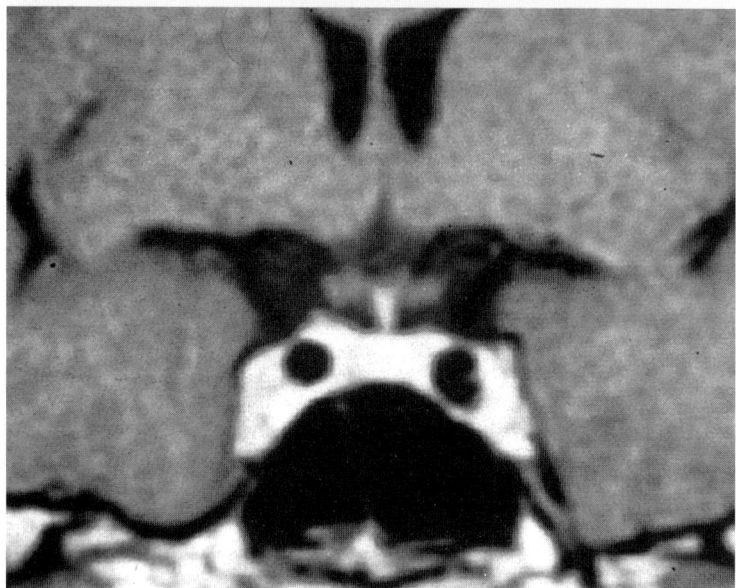

(a)

Fig. 12.
Optic chiasm. Coronal MRI sections. (a) Contrast-enhanced T1-weighted image through the infundibulum of the pituitary. (b) T2-weighted image slightly further posteriorly. (c) T2-weighted image slightly behind b, showing the chiasm beginning to divide into the tracts.

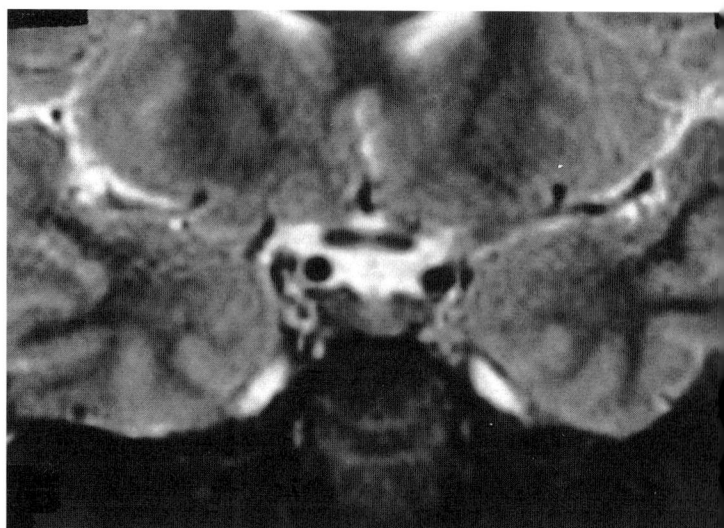

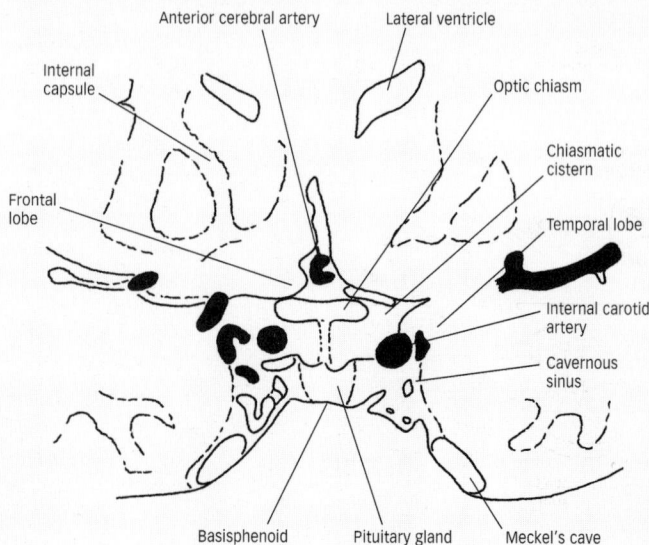

Anterior cerebral artery

Lateral ventricle

Internal capsule

Optic chiasm

Chiasmatic cistern

Frontal lobe

Temporal lobe

Internal carotid artery

Cavernous sinus

Basisphenoid

Pituitary gland

Meckel's cave

of the gyrus rectus anteriorly, the uncus of the temporal lobe laterally and the anterior surface of the midbrain (indented by the interpeduncular fossa) posteriorly (Fig. 13).

Optic tracts

Posteriorly, the chiasm divides into the optic tracts, which run posterolaterally, between the cerebral peduncle and the uncus of the temporal lobe, beneath the anterior perforated substance. On coronal images, they appear to blend with the brain above them as they pass posteriorly (Fig. 14). Here they lie lateral to the cerebral peduncles and above the hippocampal formation. They end in the lateral geniculate bodies; it is debated whether some fibres go to the superior colliculus.

Lateral geniculate body & superior colliculus

Both the form and internal structure of the lateral geniculate body are complex; the former has been described as resembling a 'Moorish

Optic chiasm

The optic chiasm is an X-shaped plate of white matter, which lies more or less above the pituitary fossa, although its exact position is very variable, as noted above (Fig. 11). It is distinctly unusual for it to lie so far anterior that it occupies the chiasmatic sulcus on the superior surface of the body of the sphenoid. The posterior border, which is higher than the anterior, forms part of the anterior wall of the third ventricle, with the optic recess above it and the infundibular recess below. The pituitary stalk descends posterior to it. A cerebrospinal fluid-containing space, the chiasmatic cistern (often referred to as the 'suprasellar cistern'), is usually visible all round the chiasm (Fig. 12). It is bounded by the base of the frontal lobe above, the diaphragma sella below, the posterior end saddle' or 'fireman's helmet'. However, little of this detail is visible on images, and so need not concern us. The lateral geniculate body is seen on CT, and rather better on MRI, as a slightly raised area of grey matter on the posterior surface of the thalamus, lateral to the pulvinar (Fig. 15). It extends into the substance of the thalamus, although remaining functionally separate.

Some fibres, the superior brachium, pass from the lateral geniculate body to the superior colliculus. The two superior colliculi form the superior corpora quadrigemina, sitting on the tectum of the midbrain (Fig. 16). They project further but are smaller in volume than the inferior corpora quadrigemina.

Optic radiations

The geniculocalcarine pathway arises in the lateral geniculate body as a new set of nerve fibres, the optic radiations, which run in the

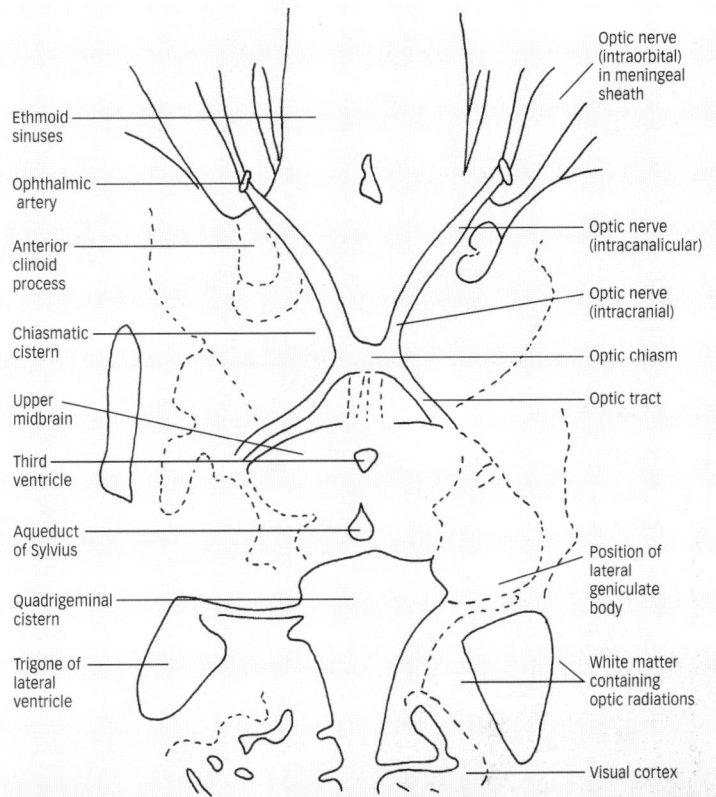

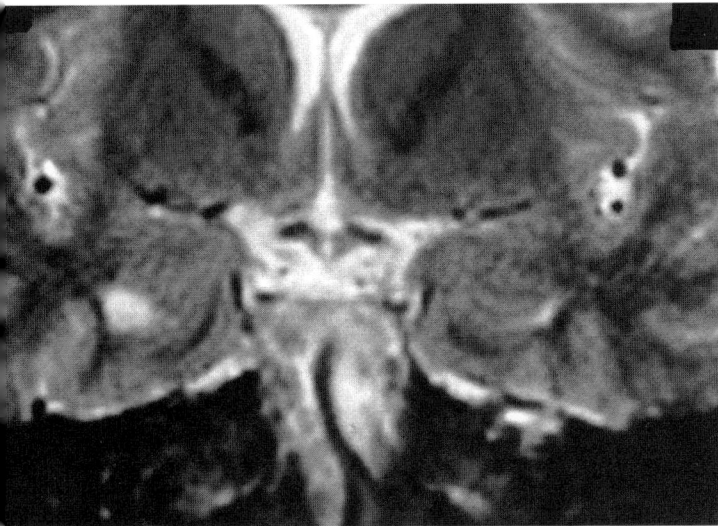

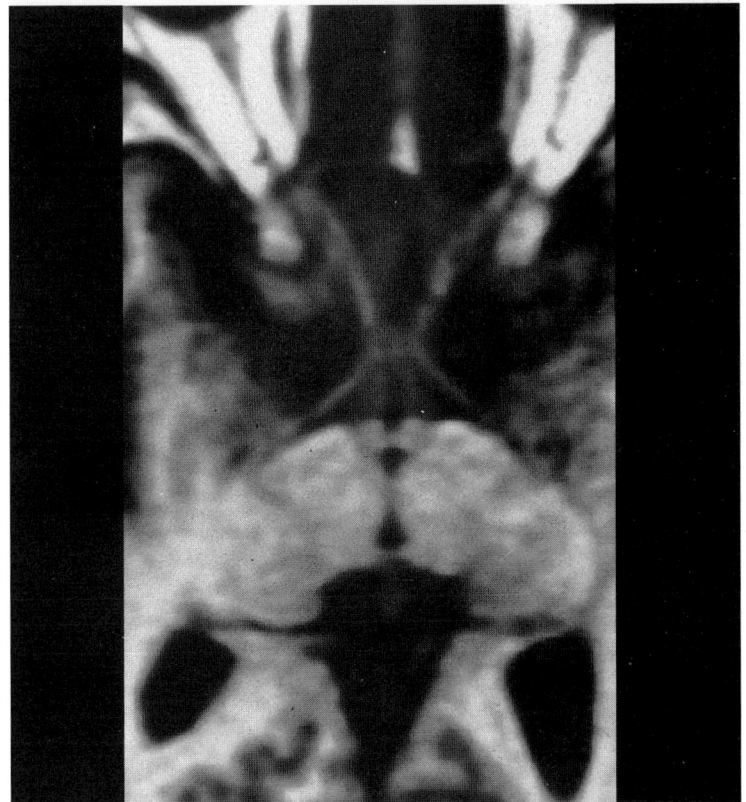

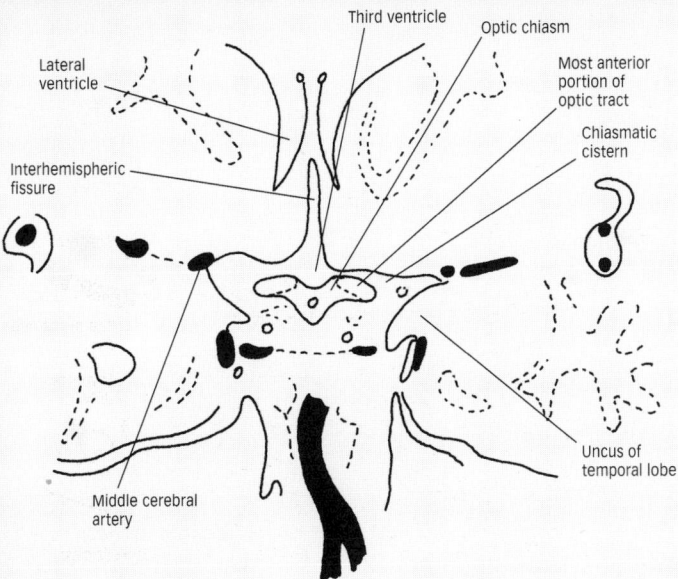

Fig. 13.
Optic chiasm. T1-weighted axial MRI showing the intracranial optic nerves, chiasm and tracts. Note the difference in shape of the normal chiasm between this individual and that in Fig. 10.

(a)

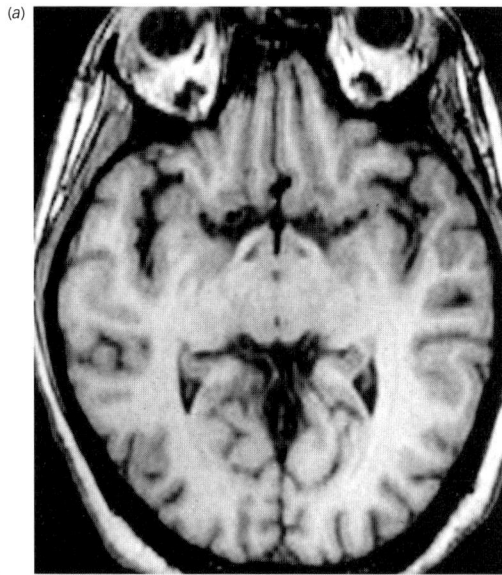

Fig. 14.
Optic tracts. (a) Axial reformatted inversion-recovery MRI showing tracts and position of lateral geniculate bodies. (b) Coronal contrast-enhanced T1-weighted spin-echo image.

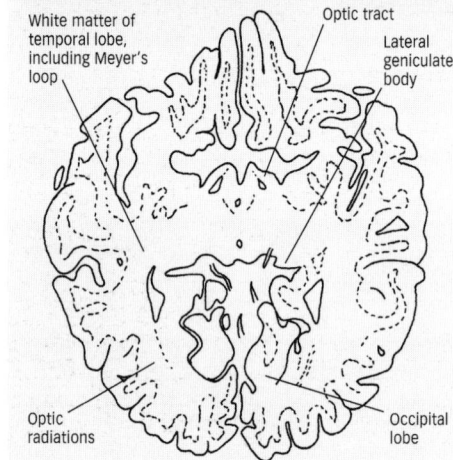

mined largely by the angle of the upper surface of the tentorium, on which the occipital lobe lies. The straight sinus, which forms the superomedial limit of the tentorium, at the falcotentorial junction, is nearly vertical in some normal individuals, while at the other extreme it can be almost horizontal; any intermediate position may be seen. It should be emphasised that the occipital lobe is relatively small, and the visual cortex lies inferiorly on coronal sections (Fig. 19). On cross-sectional imaging, the angle at which the sections pass through the visual cortex is extremely variable, since variations in radiographic positioning may compound a wide range of normal angulation. Even so, when the CT gantry is angulated so as to avoid excessive radiation to the orbits, the plane of section is often parallel

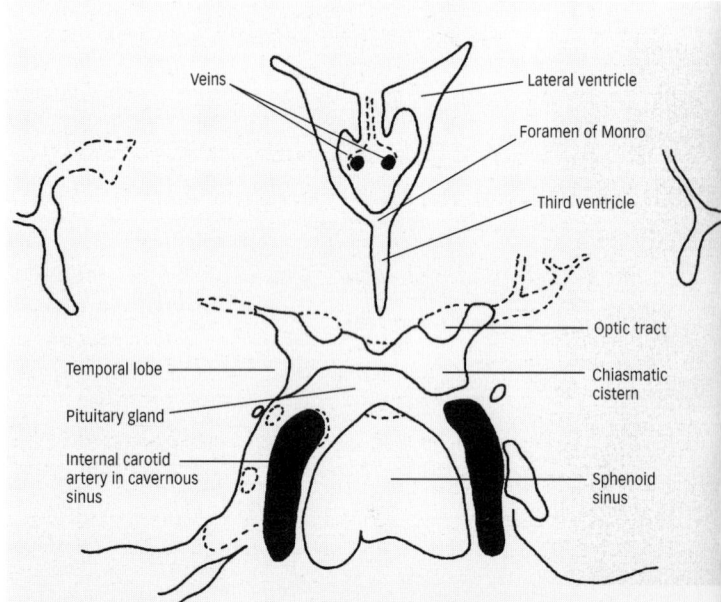

white matter of the temporal and occipital lobes to the primary visual cortex, situated on either side of the calcarine fissure. On their way, they pass through Wernicke's area and the posterior limb of the internal capsule. Inferiorly placed fibres sweep into the temporal lobe, around the temporal horn of the lateral ventricle, forming Meyer's loop. The main group of fibres passes lateral to the occipital horn and deep to the middle temporal gyrus (Fig. 17).

Visual cortex

The visual or striate cortex (so-called because a thin white line, Gennari's line or the line of Vicq d'Azir, can be identified running parallel with its surface on gross anatomical sections) lines the lips of the deep calcarine fissure (Fig. 18). This is on the medial surface of the occipital lobe, although it may extend round the posterior pole just onto the lateral surface. Its position on the medial surface is somewhat variable, but it is usually near the inferomedial angle. Much more variable is its inclination to the horizontal plane, which is deter-

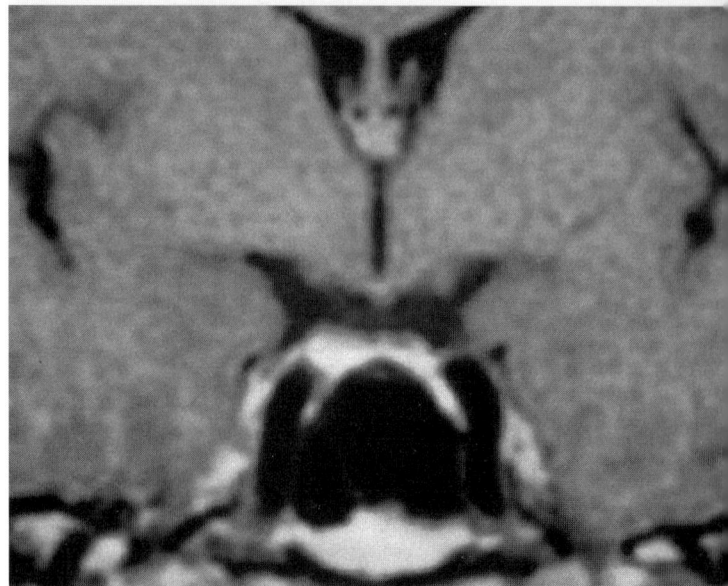

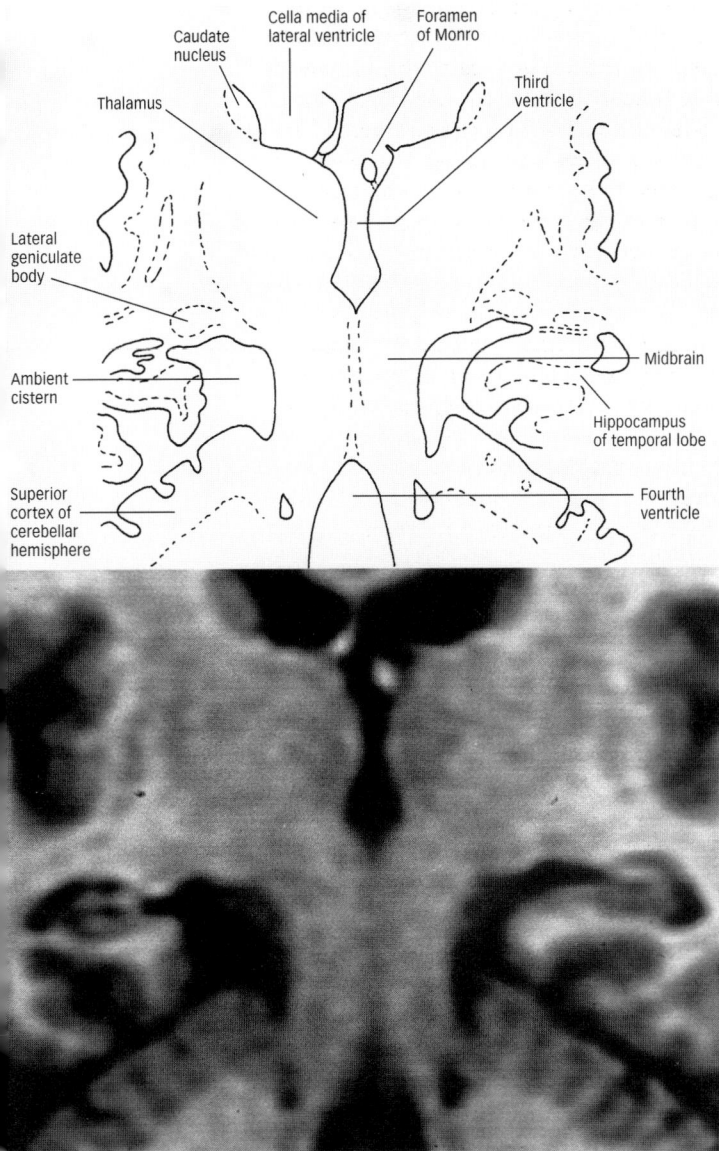

Fig. 15.
Lateral geniculate bodies. Coronal T1-weighted MRI.

(labels on figure: Caudate nucleus; Cella media of lateral ventricle; Foramen of Monro; Thalamus; Third ventricle; Lateral geniculate body; Ambient cistern; Midbrain; Hippocampus of temporal lobe; Superior cortex of cerebellar hemisphere; Fourth ventricle)

where more posteriorly the posterior communicating artery and anterior choroidal artery, especially the latter, make important contributions. The anterior choroidal artery, a direct branch of the internal carotid artery, also supplies most of the blood to the lateral geniculate body, to which the posterior cerebral artery also contributes.

From before backwards the optic radiations are supplied by the anterior choroidal, middle

Fig. 16.
Superior corpora quadrigemina. (*a*) Axial T1-weighted inversion-recovery MRI through midbrain. (*b*) Sagittal T1-weighted image showing plane of section used for (*c*) coronal T1-weighted image through quadrigeminal plate.

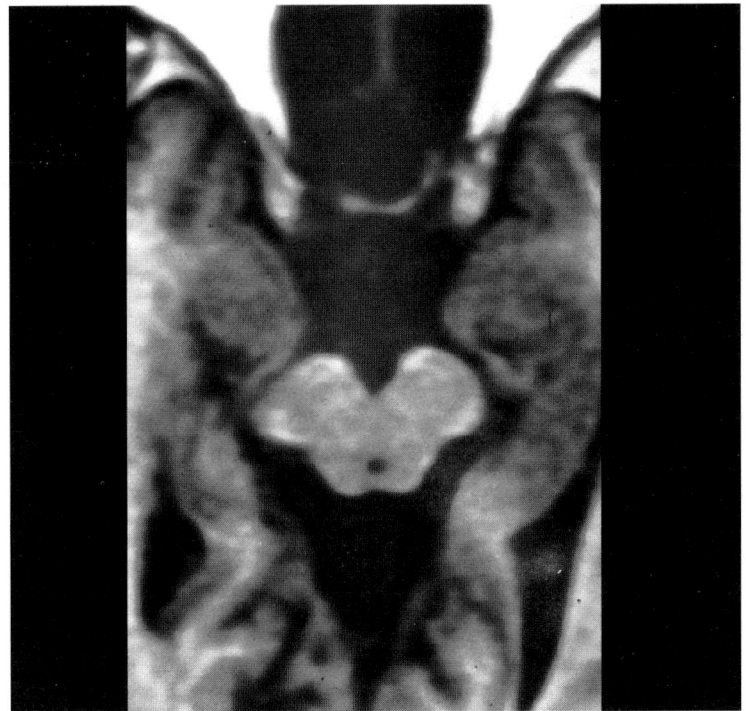

(a)

with the long axis of the fissure, and it is most commonly to be found on the section(s) passing through the pineal gland (Fig. 20).

There are a number of cortical areas other than the primary visual cortex, described here, which subserve vision, the visual association areas (Fig. 21). However, although the gyri responsible, such as the angular gyrus, can be recognised on CT and to a greater extent on MRI, they are not dedicated exclusively to visual function and will not be described further here.

Blood supply of the visual pathways

The blood supply to the eye and optic nerve, from the branches of the ophthalmic artery, has already been described. The optic chiasm has a rich pial anastomotic supply from the internal carotid artery and its major terminal branches, particularly the anterior cerebral. This pial network continues on the optic tract,

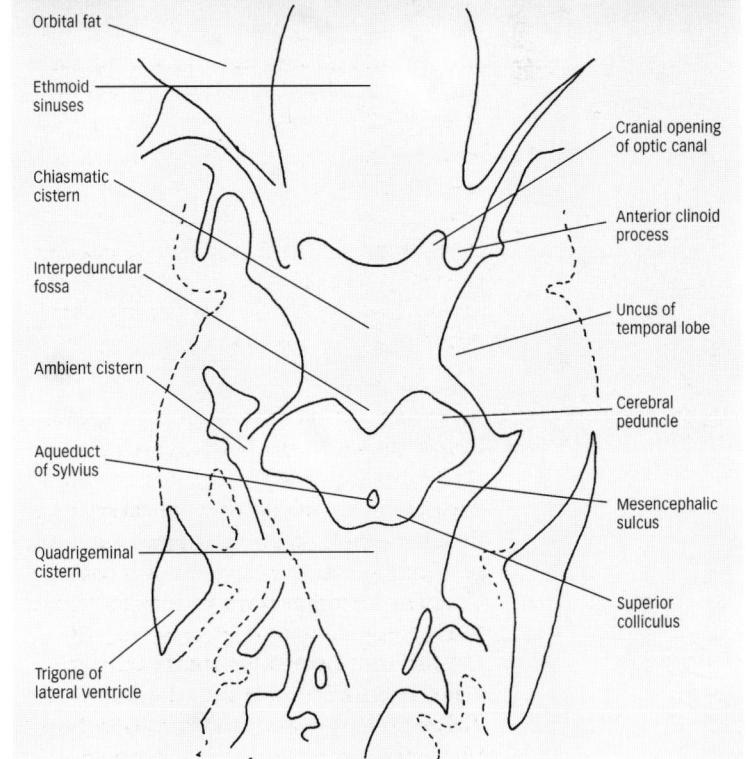

(labels on figure: Orbital fat; Ethmoid sinuses; Chiasmatic cistern; Interpeduncular fossa; Ambient cistern; Aqueduct of Sylvius; Quadrigeminal cistern; Trigone of lateral ventricle; Cranial opening of optic canal; Anterior clinoid process; Uncus of temporal lobe; Cerebral peduncle; Mesencephalic sulcus; Superior colliculus)

Splenium of corpus callosum

Quadrigeminal cistern

Superior and inferior colliculi

Superior medullary velum

Optic chiasm

Mamillary bodies

Interpeduncular fossa

Pons Varolii

Medulla oblongata

Fourth ventricle

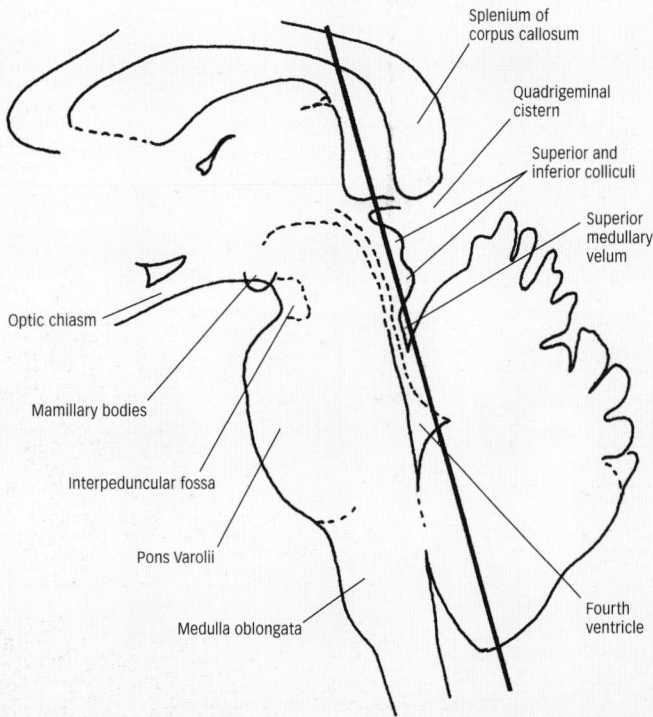

enable clinical localization of lesions affecting the optic pathways. The fine details are not usually relevant to imaging, but a general idea is essential (Fig. 23).

Monocular visual defects obviously indicate a lesion anterior to the optic chiasm. In the retina there is no overlap between the upper and lower halves, so that a superior or inferior altitudinal field defect generally indicates ocular disease. As soon as they enter the optic nerve, the fibres are arranged in a retinotopic fashion; towards the posterior end of the nerve the macular fibres are at the centre of the nerve, and a central scotoma usually indicates a lesion in this region.

Just anterior to their decussation in the chiasm, the nasal fibres actually loop into the most posterior part of the contralateral nerve, forming 'Wilbrand's knee'. For this reason, a lesion involving the intracranial segment of one optic nerve can produce not only ipsilateral visual loss, but a contralateral 'junctional scotoma'.

From this point on, lesions of the optic pathways produce binocular visual defects.

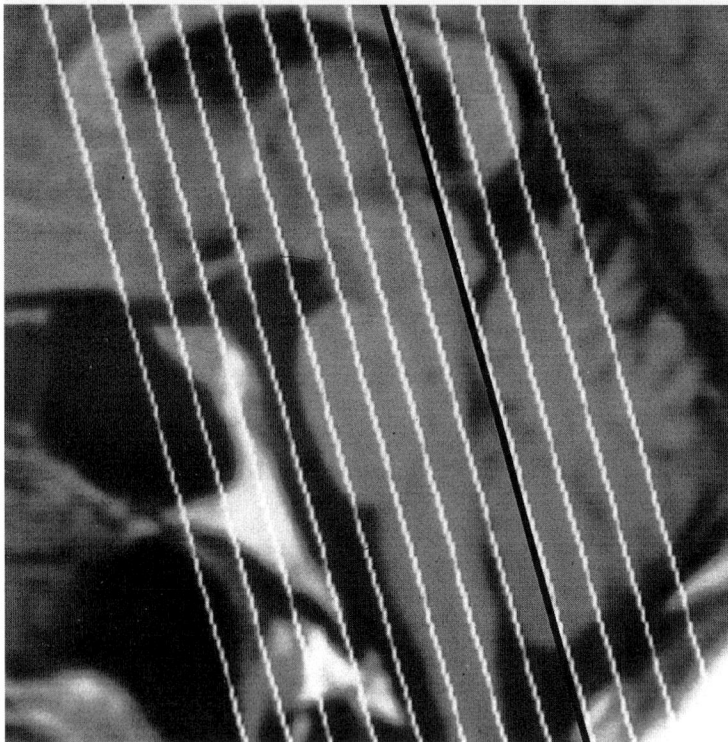

(b)

cerebral and posterior cerebral arteries (Fig. 22). The posterior cerebral artery is the major nutrient vessel to the visual cortex, but the middle cerebral artery shares to a variable extent in the supply of the occipital pole.

Organization of the fibres in the visual pathways

The retinotopic organization of the fibres shows certain characteristic features which

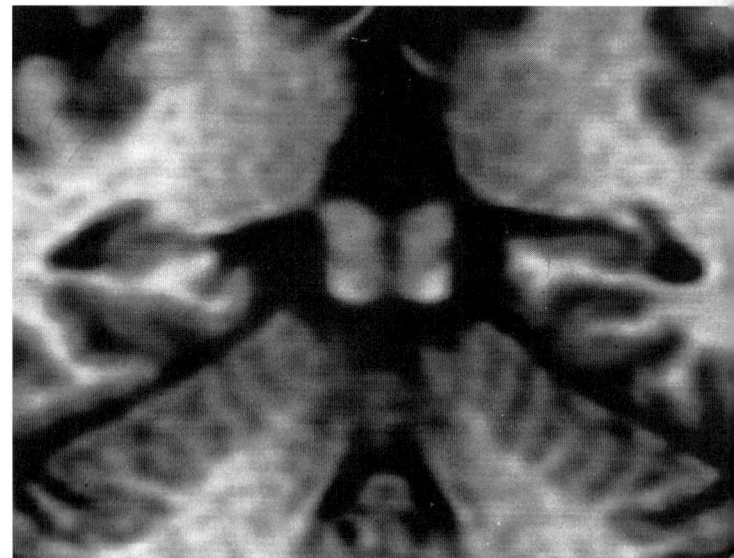

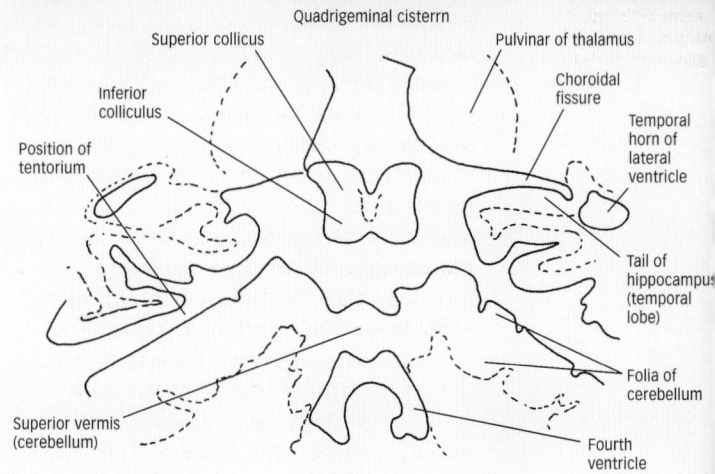

Quadrigeminal cisterrn

Superior collicus

Pulvinar of thalamus

Choroidal fissure

Inferior colliculus

Temporal horn of lateral ventricle

Position of tentorium

Tail of hippocampus (temporal lobe)

Folia of cerebellum

Superior vermis (cerebellum)

Fourth ventricle

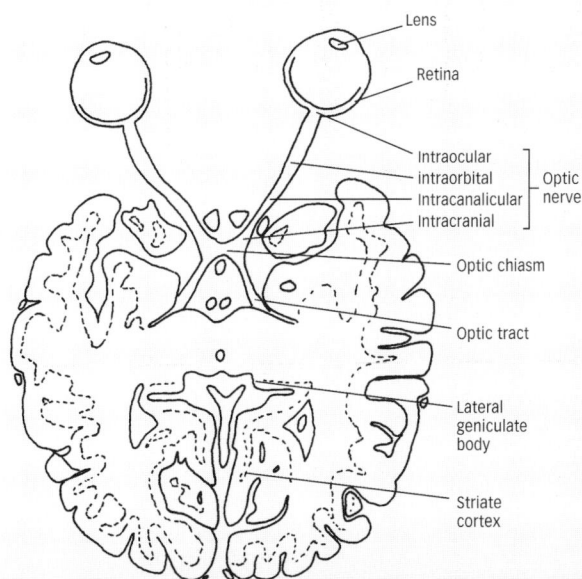

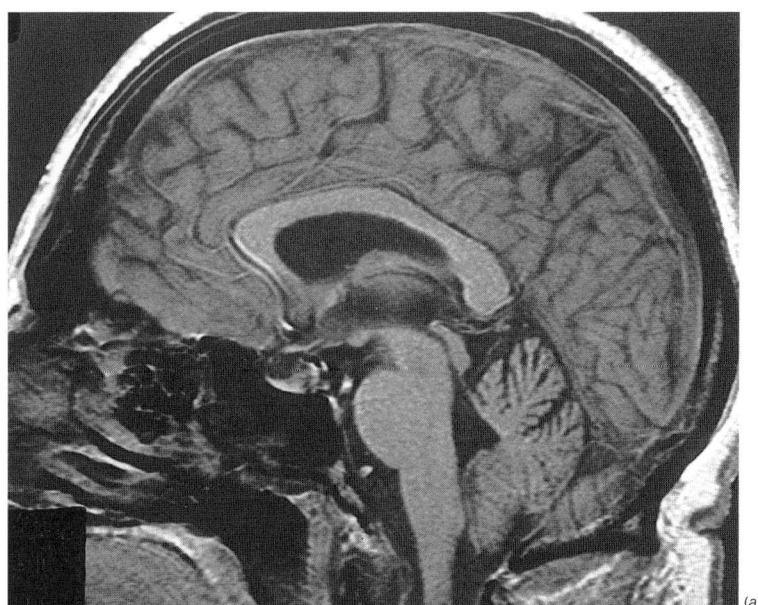

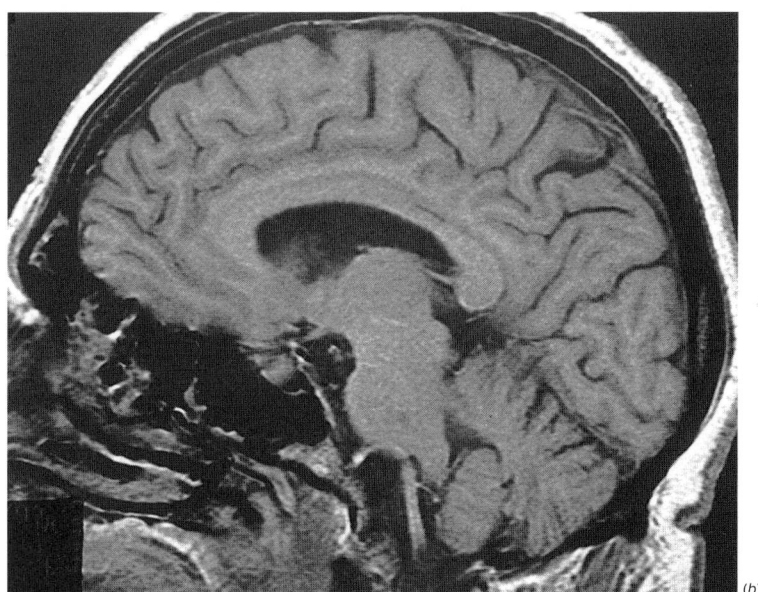

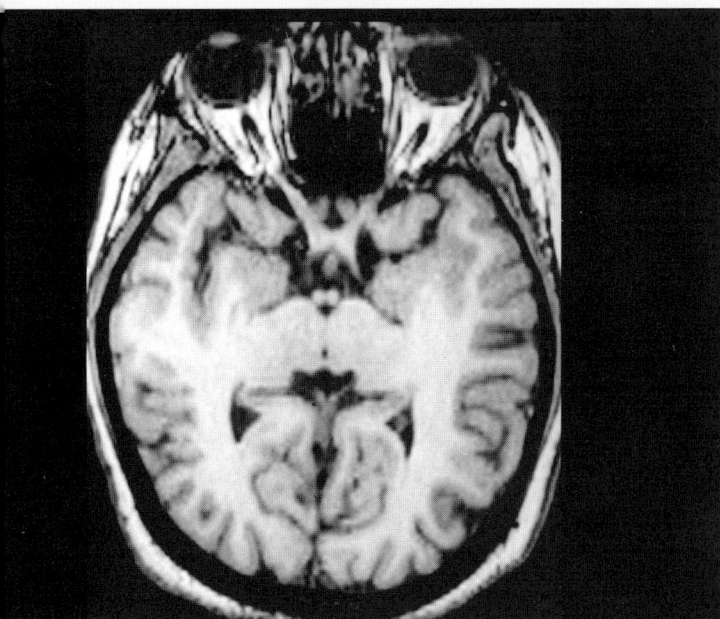

Fig. 17.
Retrochiasmal optic pathways. Reformatted T1-weighted inversion recovery image showing optic pathways from lateral geniculate body to visual cortex.

Compression of the optic chiasm classically gives rise to a bitemporal defect. From the optic tracts posteriorly, the field loss takes the form of a homonymous hemianopia, i.e. loss of the left half of both visual fields with a lesion in the right retrochiasmal visual pathways. The retinotopic organization may not, however, be fully developed in the optic tract, so that the defect may be similar but not symmetrical ('incongruous') in the two eyes. A characteristic pattern of visual loss indicating a lateral geniculate body lesion may be revealed only by sophisticated mapping of the visual fields (campimetry).

Because the optic radiations are so extensive, some of the fibres may be involved while others are spared, and this is classically the case when Meyer's loop is injured in the temporal lobe, giving a homonymous upper quadrantanopia. Cerebral infarcts can also involve either predominantly the upper or lower lips of the calcarine fissure, giving an inferior or superior quadrantic defect, respectively. The macular area is represented at the occipital pole, and this may or may not be spared depending on how far posteriorly the territories of the middle and posterior cerebral arteries extend, and how adequate the collateral supply is, in the individual case. Thus, when there is an infarct of the posterior cerebral artery territory, an individual whose occipital pole is supplied by the middle cerebral artery will retain central vision ('macular sparing'). Lastly, the extreme temporal field has unilateral cortical representation, so that a 'temporal crescent' may also be spared.

Fig. 18.
Visual cortex in the sagittal plane. (a) Midline sagittal T1-weighted gradient-echo image. (b) Similar section 5 mm from midline; note greater clarity of demonstration of calcarine fissure.

(a)

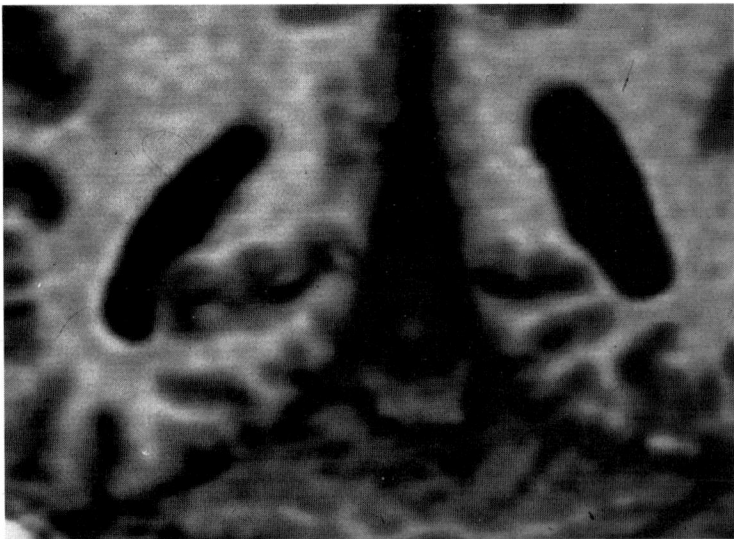

Fig. 19.
Visual cortex in coronal plane. (a) T2-weighted image through cranium, showing position of visual cortex. (b) T1-weighted inversion-recovery image through occipital lobes. Note the marked, complex infolding of the cortex lining the calcarine fissure, as compared with adjacent areas. The deep fissure and the grey matter lining it indent the occipital horns, especially on the right side, producing the so-called *calcar avis*.

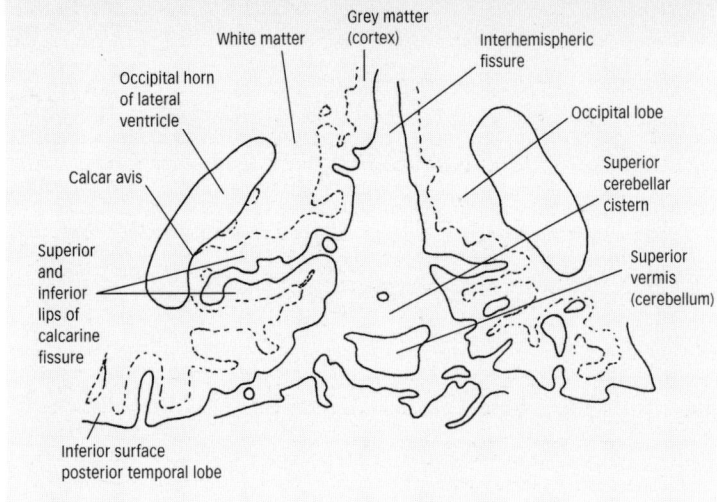

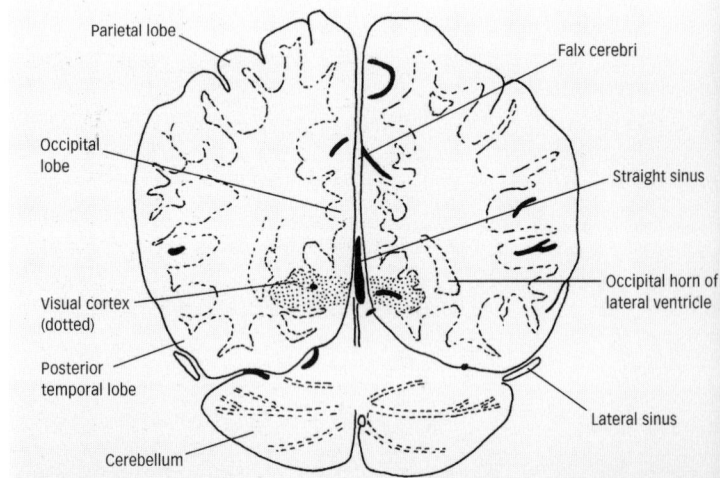

(b)

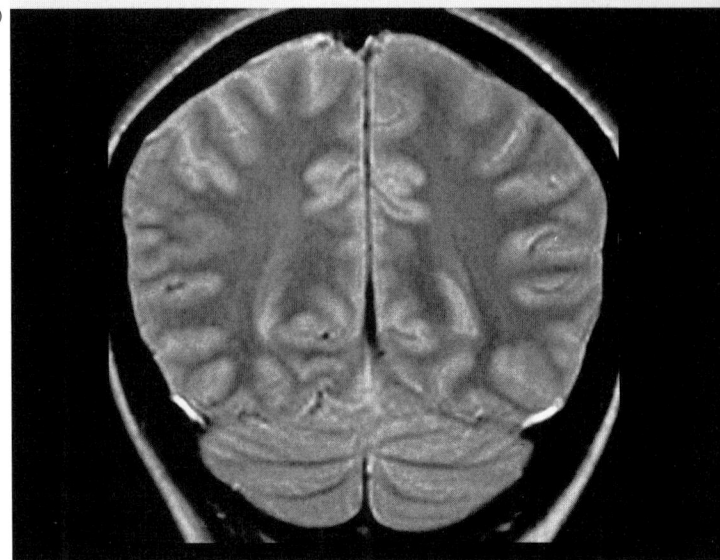

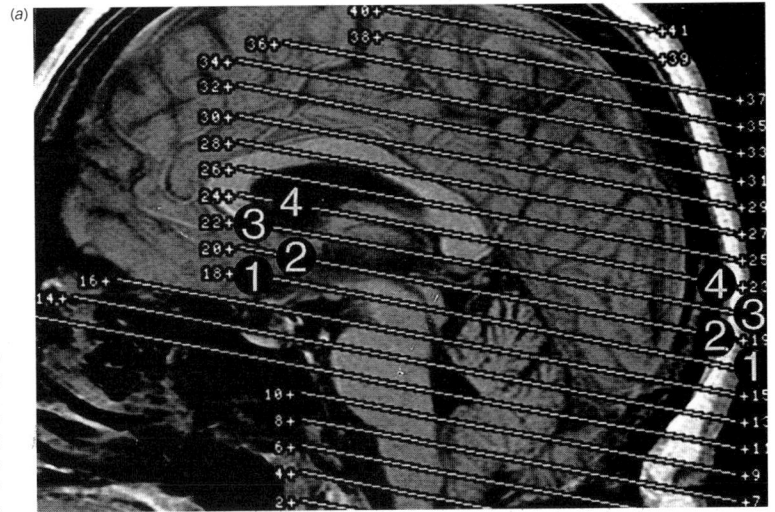

Fig. 20.
Visual cortex in the axial plane. (a) T1-weighted image corresponding to Figure 18(a), indicating levels of axial section. (b)–(e) Sections indicated by 1–4 in (a). The visual cortex is stippled. Note how it lies more anteriorly as the sections ascend.

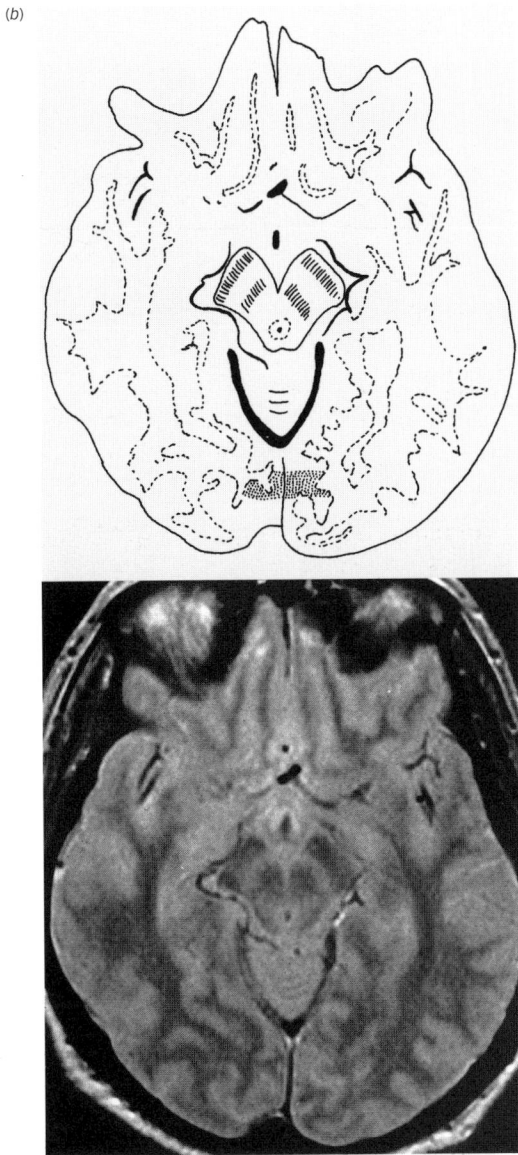

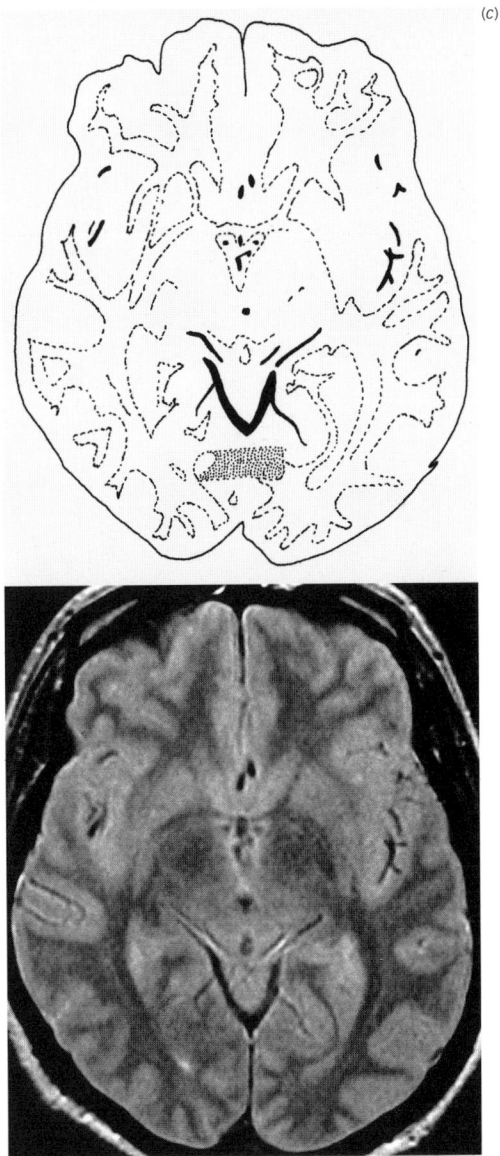

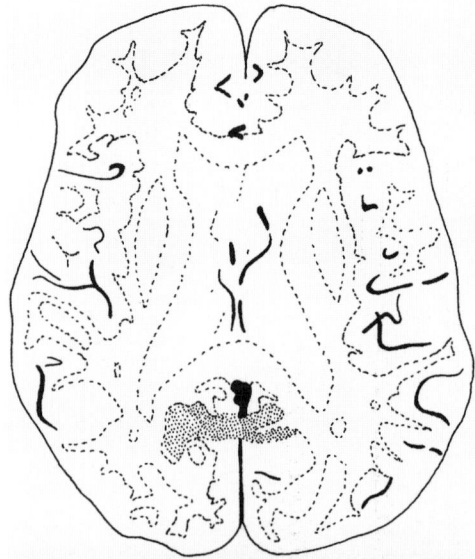

20(d)

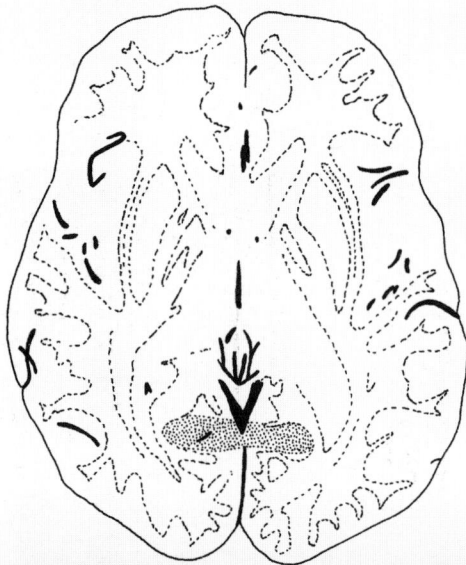

20(e)

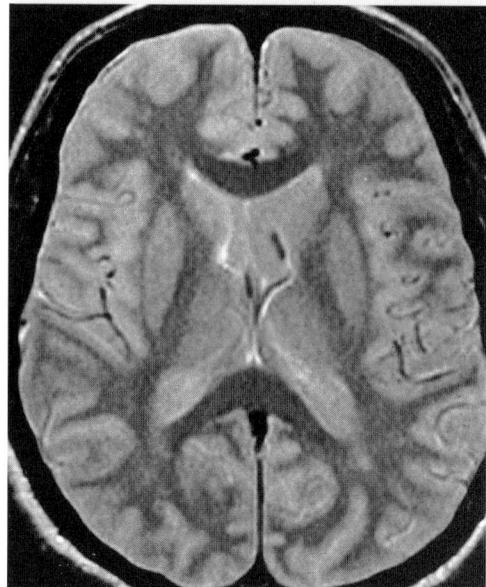

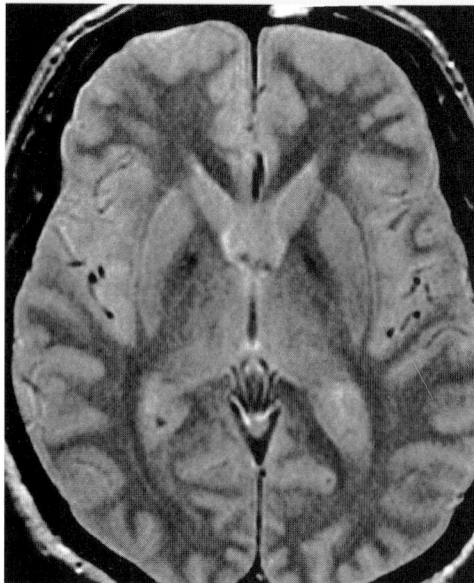

Angular
gyrus

Visual
association
cortex

Occipital pole
(macular area)

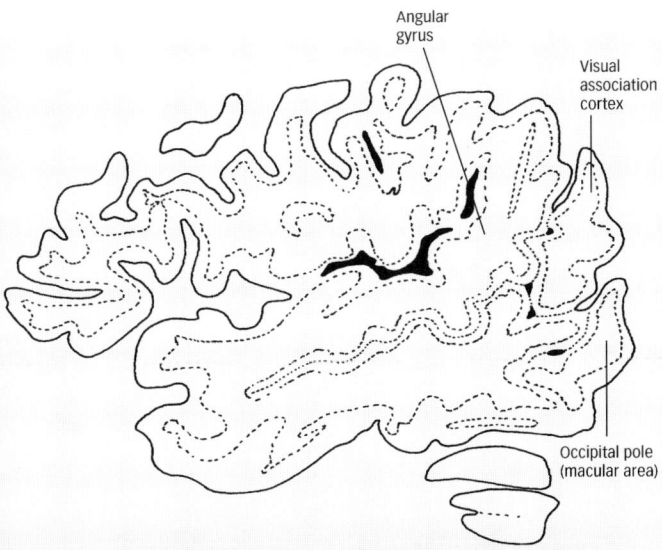

Fig. 21.
Lateral surface of cerebral
hemisphere. T1-weighted
sagittal section (anterior to
left), showing primary
(macular) and secondary
visual cortex.

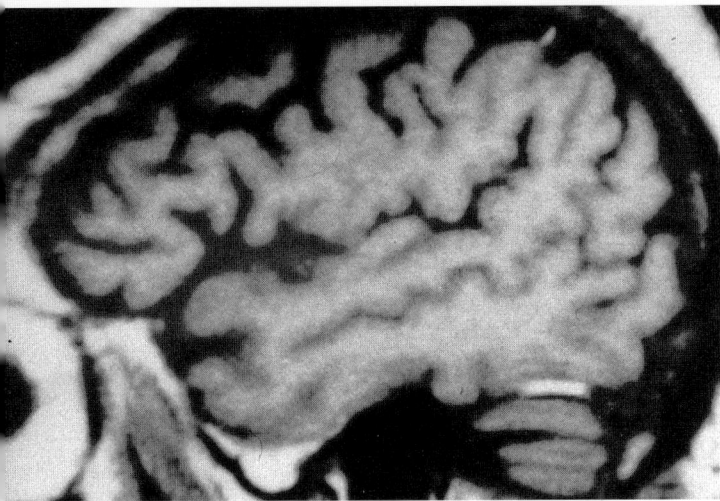

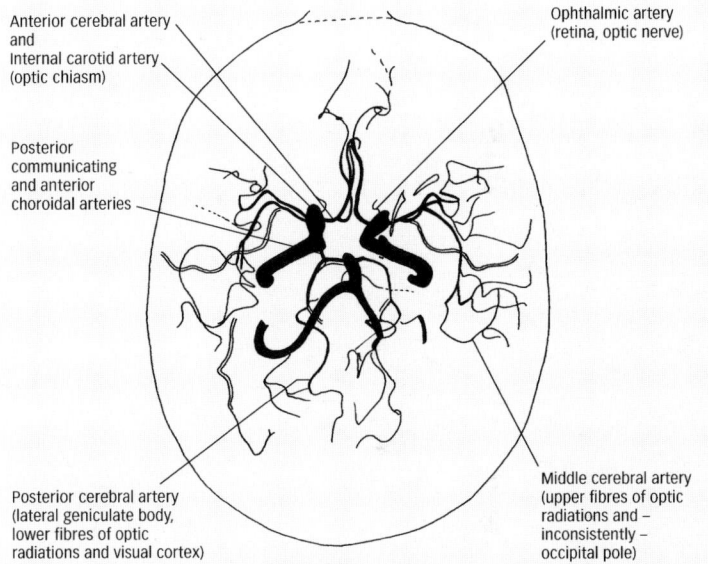

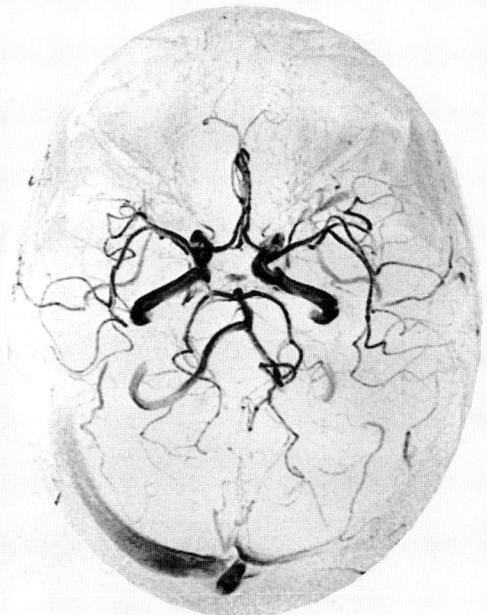

Anterior cerebral artery
and
Internal carotid artery
(optic chiasm)

Posterior
communicating
and anterior
choroidal arteries

Ophthalmic artery
(retina, optic nerve)

Middle cerebral artery
(upper fibres of optic
radiations and –
inconsistently –
occipital pole)

Posterior cerebral artery
(lateral geniculate body,
lower fibres of optic
radiations and visual cortex)

Fig. 22.
Blood supply of visual
pathways. 'Collapsed' axial
magnetic resonance
angiogram, showing main
intracranial vessels and
vascular territories.

83

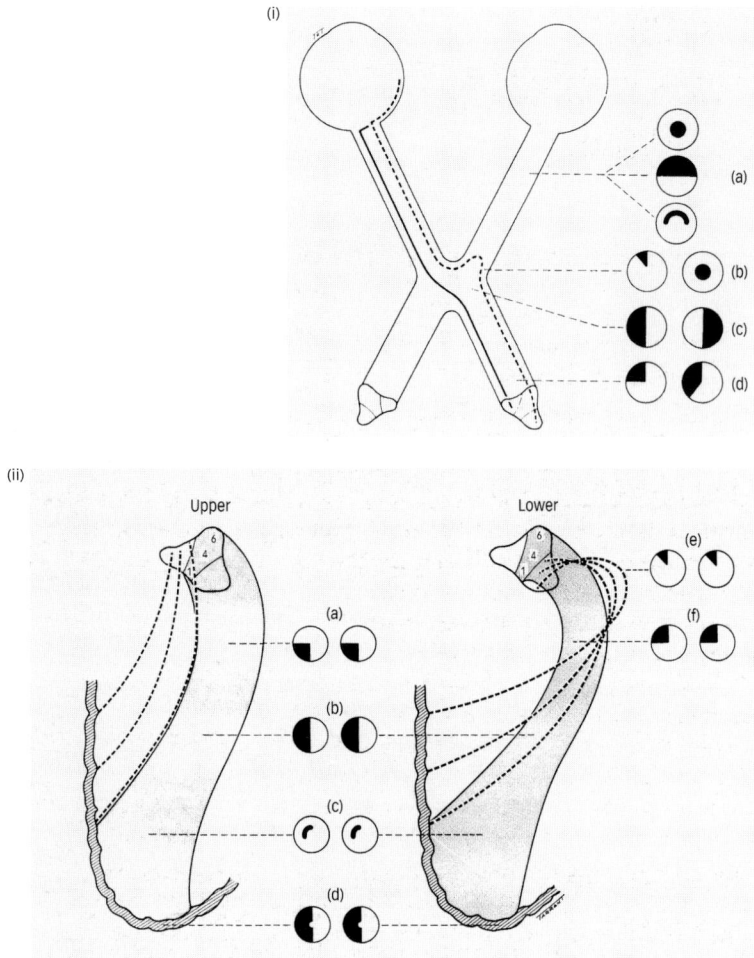

Reference

Moseley, I.F. & Sanders, M.D. (1982). *Computerized Tomography in Neuro-oph-thalmology*. London: Chapman and Hall.

Further reading

Gonzalez, C.F., Becker, M.H. & Flanagan, J.C. (1986). *Diagnostic Imaging in Ophthalmology*. Berlin: Springer-Verlag.

Guillot, P., Sariaux, J. & Sedan, J. (1966). *L'Exploration Neuroradiologique en Ophtalmologie*. Paris: Masson.

Newton, T.H. & Bilaniuk, L.T. (1990). *Radiology of the Eye and Orbit*. New York: Raven Press.

Wolff, E. (1954). *The Anatomy of the Eye and Orbit*. London: Lewis.

Fig. 23.
Diagram showing the effects on vision of lesions at various points in the visual pathways. (i) *a*, Intraorbital optic nerve: central scotoma, altitudinal defect, arcuate scotoma. *b*, Intracranial optic nerve: central scotoma and contralateral 'junctional scotoma'. *c*, Optic chiasm: bitemporal hemianopia. *d*, Optic tract: incongruous homolateral hemianopia. (ii) *a*, Optic radiations (upper fibres): homonymous inferior quadrantanopia. *b*, Optic radiations (posterior fibres): homonymous hemianopia. *c*, Optic radiations (small lesion): homonymous scotoma. *d*, Visual cortex, with sparing of occipital pole: homonymous hemianopia with macular sparing. *e*, Lateral geniculate body: homonymous segmental defect. *f*, Meyer's loop: homonymous superior quadrantopia. (From Moseley, I.F. & Sanders, M.D., 1982, with permission.)

4

The ear and auditory pathways

P. BUTLER
I. G. WYLIE

Imaging methods

High resolution computerized tomography (HRCT) and magnetic resonance imaging (MRI) provide complementary information on the anatomy of the petrous temporal bone. HRCT, with sections as thin as 1 mm, can display the bone anatomy in fine detail, whereas MRI is able to show the intrapetrous soft-tissue structures, including the facial and auditory nerves, directly and essentially free of surrounding bone. MRI has consequently become the examination of choice for the contents of the internal auditory meatus and cerebellopontine angle cistern.

Intravenous contrast enhanced CT cannot resolve these cranial nerves in the normal individual and it is necessary to resort to cisternography if CT is used for this purpose. In positive-contrast CT cisternography, an iodinated contrast medium such as iohexol or iopamidol is introduced into the subarachnoid space by lumbar puncture and allowed to mix uniformly with cerebrospinal fluid (Fig. 1). In negative-contrast CT cisternography, a small amount (about 5 ml) of air or carbon dioxide is injected, again by lumbar puncture, to provide a more focused study of the internal meatus and adjacent cistern (Fig. 2).

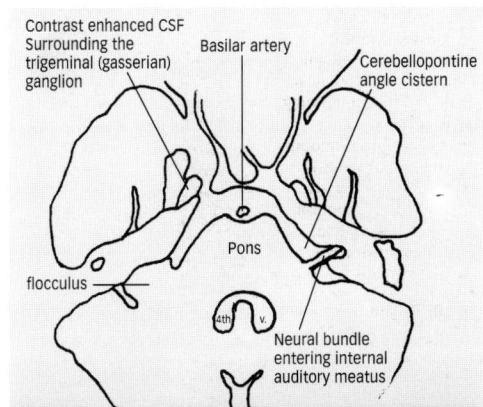

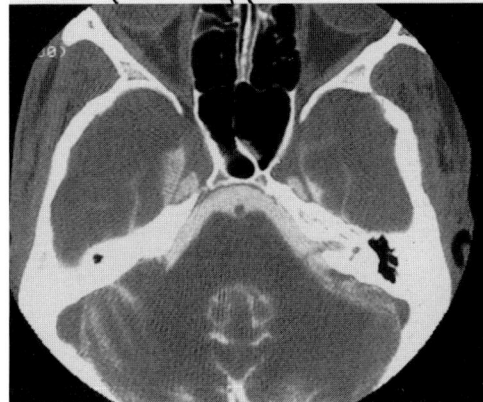

Fig 1.
Positive contrast CT cisternogram. Axial scan through the auditory meatus.

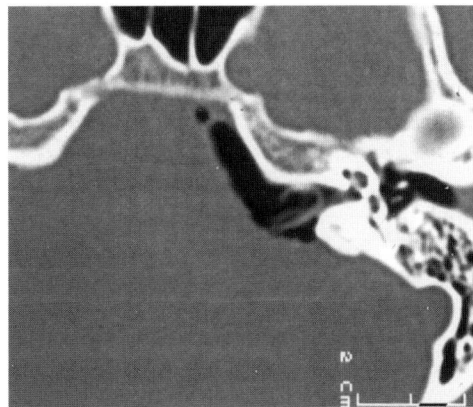

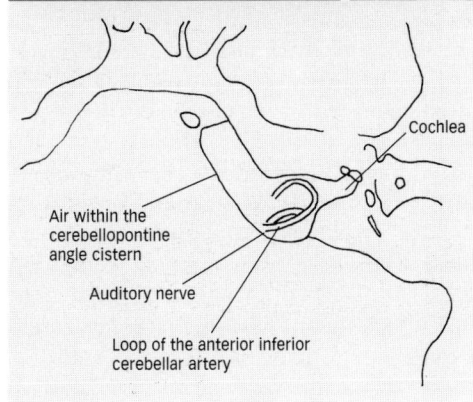

Fig 2(a).
Negative contrast CT cisternogram. Axial section showing the loop of the anterior inferior cerebellar artery entering the internal auditory meatus.

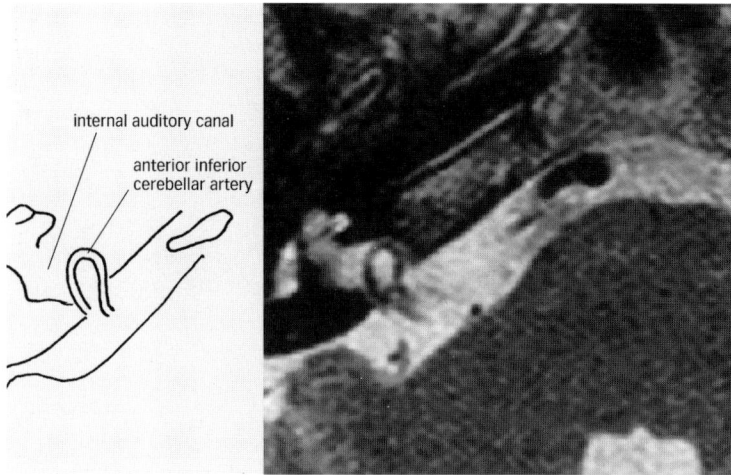

Fig 2(b).
Axial T2 weighted MRI showing a similar vascular loop.

Conventional radiography, including tomography, has largely been superseded by CT and MRI but is retained by some centres to assess the contour of the internal auditory canals.

Development

The inner ear develops early in gestation, with the formation of the otic capsule at about the third week. At birth, the inner ear is essentially of adult size and form, and the bony labyrinth is the only part of the cranium to have ossified fully.

The pinna, external auditory meatus and middle ear appear around the eighth week of gestation and arise separately from the inner ear, from the first and second branchial arches. It can thus be appreciated that whereas congenital anomalies of the external ear and middle ear are commonly associated, those of the inner ear are usually found in isolation.

Anatomy

External auditory meatus and tympanic membrane

The external auditory meatus is an S-shaped canal which leads to the tympanic membrane at its medial end. Its lateral one-third is cartilaginous and the medial two-thirds are osseous. The meatus is oval in cross-section and lined by closely adherent skin. It is narrowed slightly within its osseous portion at the isthmus (Fig. 3).

The tympanic membrane is also elliptical and is set at an angle to the floor of the meatus (Fig. 4). It is separated into the pars flaccida above and the larger pars tensa below. The pars tensa consists of an outer layer of thin, hairless skin, an intervening fibrous layer and an inner lining of mucosa continuous with that of tympanic (middle ear) cavity. The pars flaccida has no fibrous layer.

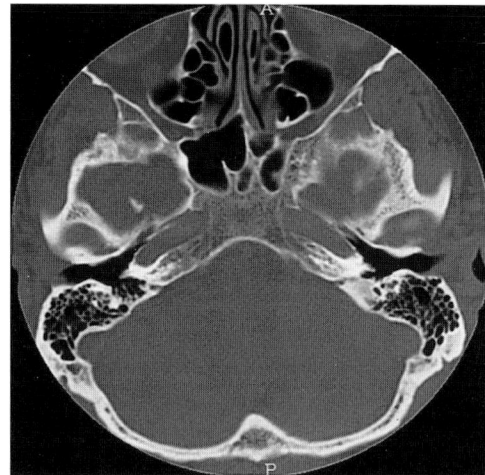

Fig 3.
Axial HRCT to show the Eustachian tube and isthmus of the external auditory meatus.

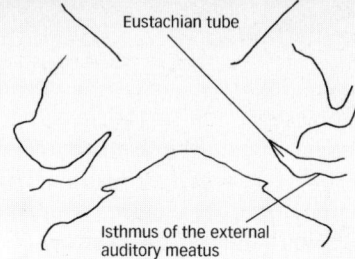

The tympanic membrane is embedded in the bone of the tympanic ring. The superior portion of this ring is known as the scutum and represents the lateral wall of the epitympanum. The scutum is a prominent feature on coronal HRCT and both superior and inferior parts of the tympanic ring are shown in Fig. 4.

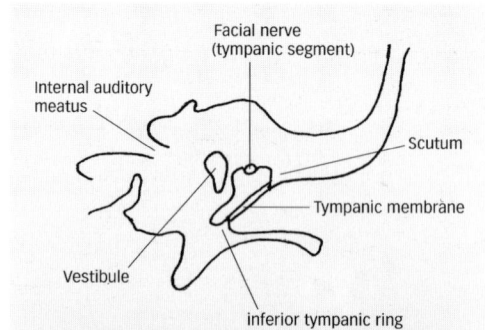

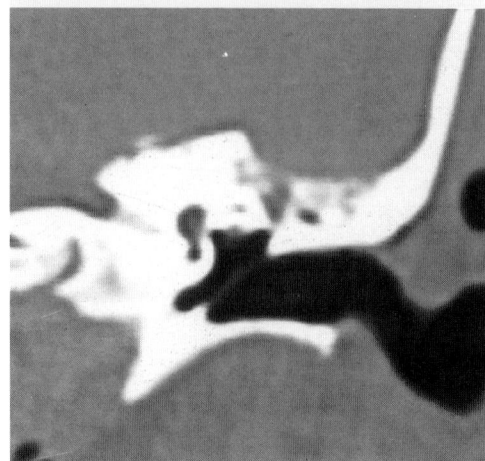

Fig 4.
Coronal HRCT to show the tympanic membrane and ring.

86

gram of the lateral wall
iddle ear. M, malleus;
cus; s, stapes.

gram of the medial wall
iddle ear.

gram of the auditory
cles. TM, tympanic
nbrane; M, malleus;
cus; s, stapes.

The middle ear and mastoid

In order to describe accurately the location of pathology within the middle ear, it is useful to divide the cavity in the coronal plane into epitympanum or attic, mesotympanum and hypotympanum by lines drawn along the superior and inferior margins of the external auditory meatus. In the axial plane, lines drawn through the anterior and posterior margins of the exterior auditory meatus separate the middle ear cavity into protympanum, mesotympanum and posterior tympanum (Figs. 5, 6 and 7).

The roof of the tympanic cavity is a thin plate of bone, called the tegmen tympani, which separates the tympanic cavity from the middle cranial fossa (Fig. 8). The floor also consists of a thin plate of bone beneath which is the bulb of the internal jugular vein. The tympanic membrane forms most of the lateral wall.

The medial wall of the middle ear cavity includes a number of important structures and landmarks. The promontory, which projects laterally, overlies the basal turn of the cochlea (Fig. 8). Above the promontory is the oval window or fenestra ovalis and below it the round window otherwise known as the fenestra cochlea or rotunda (Fig. 9). More posteriorly, the tympanic segment of the facial nerve passes beneath the lateral semicircular canal, itself a medial relation of the attic.

From the anterior tympanic wall in the hypotympanum, the Eustachian or pharyngotympanic tube passes anteromedially as a bony canal proximally which becomes fibrocartilaginous distally (Fig. 3). Just above the Eustachian tube is another bony canal for the tensor tympani muscle, which inserts into the malleus. Both tensor tympani, supplied by the trigeminal (Vth) cranial nerve, and stapedius muscle, supplied by the facial (VIIth) nerve, act together to dampen the effect of high intensity sound.

On the posterior wall of the tympanic cavity, the pyramidal eminence separates the sinus tympani medially from the facial recess laterally (Fig. 10). Stapedius muscle extends from the pyramidal eminence to insert into the neck of the stapes. From the posterior surface of the attic, a large aperture, the aditus, leads to the upper part of the mastoid antrum (Figs. 11, 14).

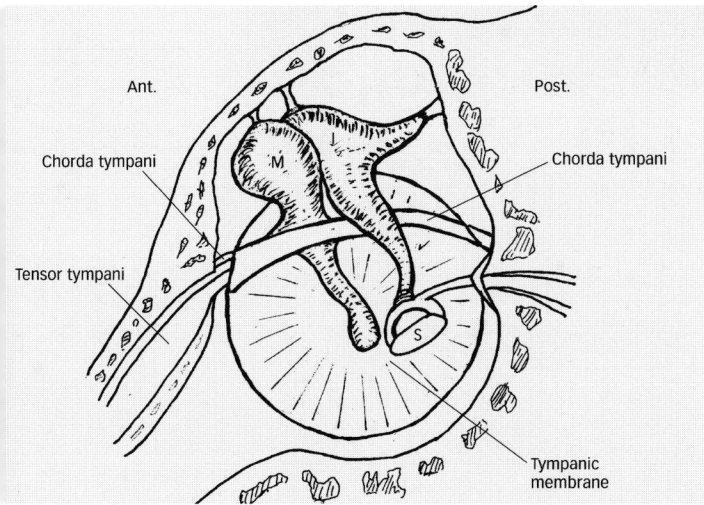

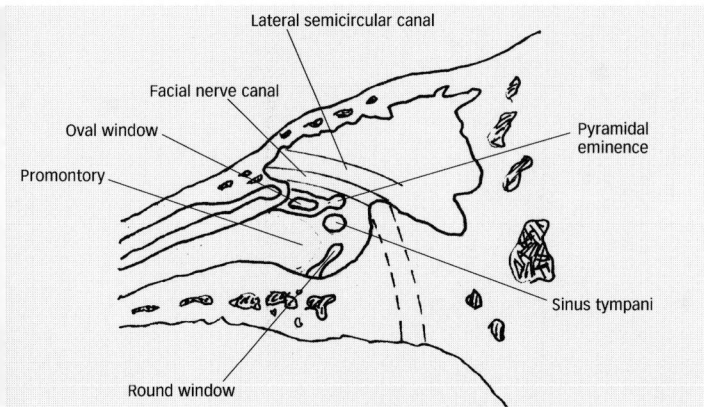

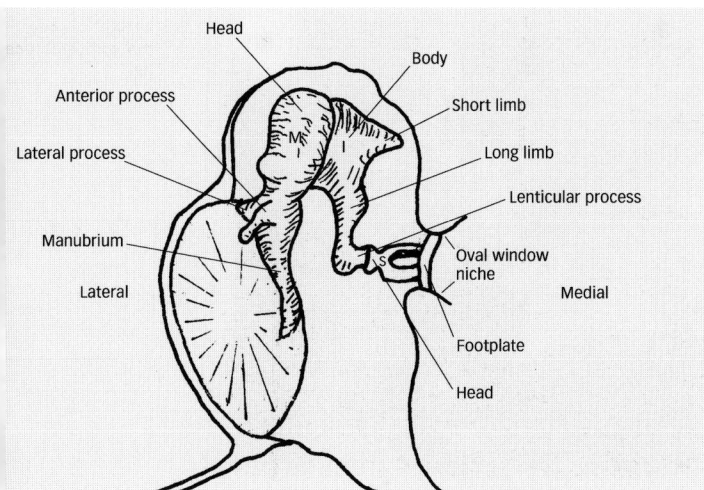

Fig 8.
Coronal HRCT through the vestibule

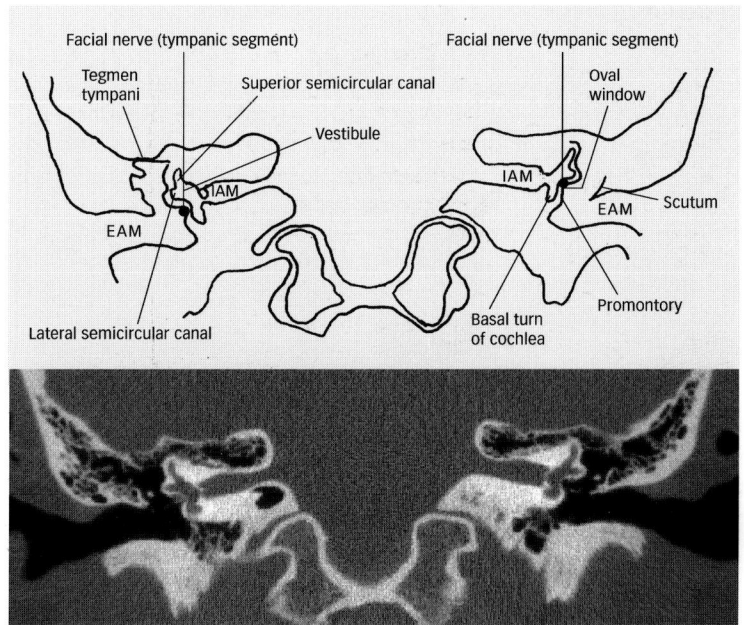

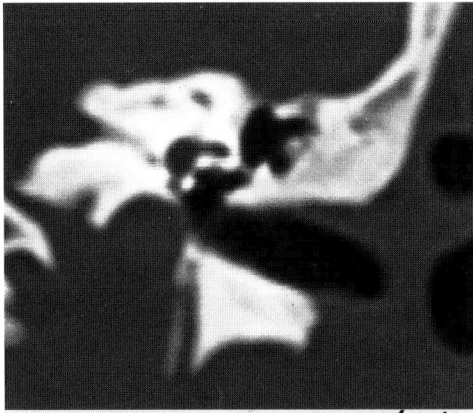

Fig 9.
Axial HRCT to show the oval and round windows.

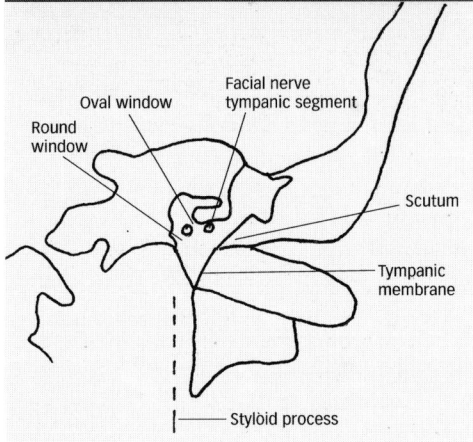

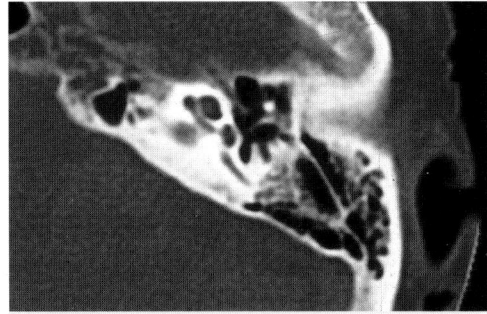

Oval window
Round window
Facial nerve tympanic segment
Scutum
Tympanic membrane
Styloid process

Fig 10.
Axial HRCT to show the posterior wall of the tympanic cavity.

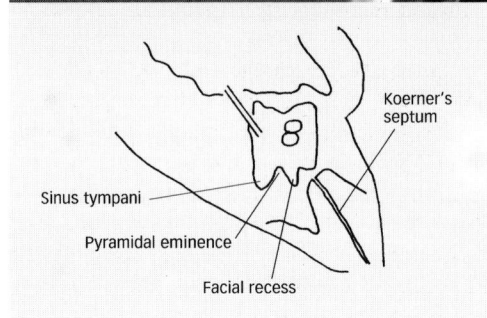

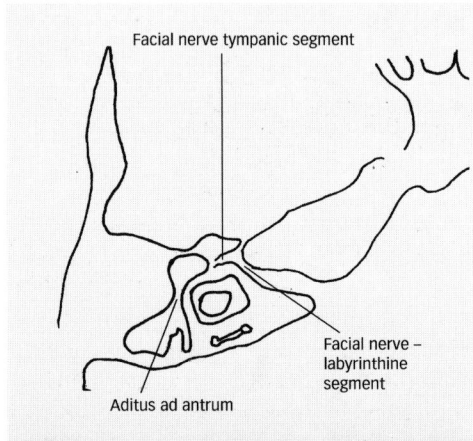

Koerner's septum
Sinus tympani
Pyramidal eminence
Facial recess

Fig 11.
Axial HRCT to show the aditus and the course of the facial nerve.

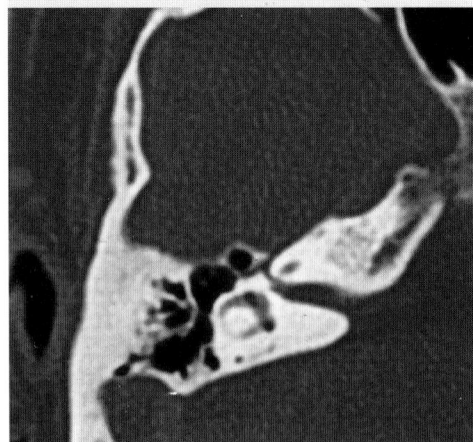

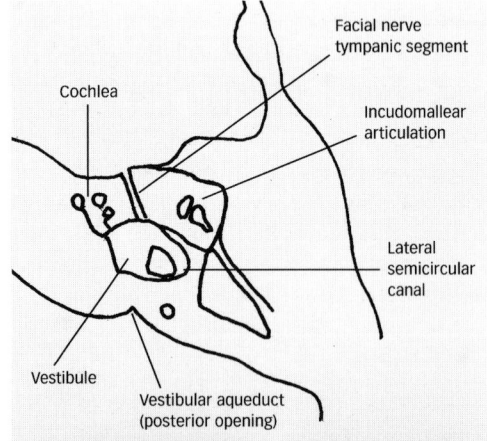

Facial nerve tympanic segment
Facial nerve – labyrinthine segment
Aditus ad antrum

Fig 12.
Axial HRCT to show the incudomallear articulation in the epitympanum and bony labyrinth.

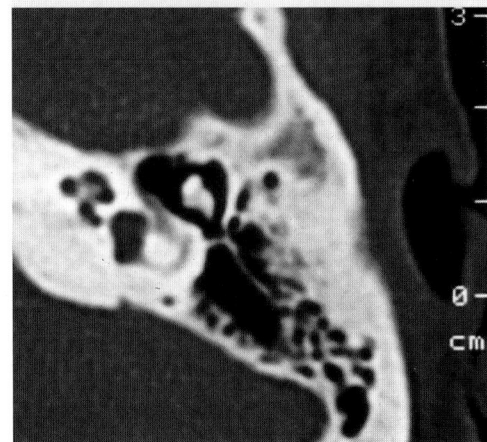

Cochlea
Facial nerve tympanic segment
Incudomallear articulation
Lateral semicircular canal
Vestibule
Vestibular aqueduct (posterior opening)

The degree of pneumatization of the mastoid and indeed of the temporal bone as a whole varies widely between individuals. There is, however, considerable symmetry between right and left sides.

The mastoid antrum is shaped like an inverted cone and in a proportion of patients is partitioned by Koerner's septum which, if well developed, can be mistaken for the medial limit of the antrum during exploratory surgery (Fig. 10).

The ossicular chain connects the tympanic membrane with the oval window within the middle ear and consists of the descriptively named malleus, incus and stapes. The orientation and anatomy of the ossicles are shown in Fig. 7.

The head of the malleus and the incudomallear articulation are situated in the epitympanic recess (Fig. 12). The manubrium and the lateral process of the malleus are attached to the tympanic membrane. Between the pars flaccida laterally and the neck of the malleus medially is the superior recess of the tympanic membrane or Prussak's space which is the site of origin of acquired cholesteatomas.

The incus lies posterior to the malleus. The short limb of the incus is attached via ligaments to the fossa incudis in the posterior epitympanum (Fig. 13). Its long limb is orientated vertically and lies posterior and parallel to the manubrium of the malleus (Fig. 14). It ends inferiorly in the rounded lenticular process with its facet for articulation with the head of the stapes. The footplate of the stapes is firmly embedded in the oval window (Fig. 15).

It is important to recognize that both the incudomallear and incudostapedial joints are synovial articulations and are thus prone to those diseases affecting synovial joints elsewhere in the body.

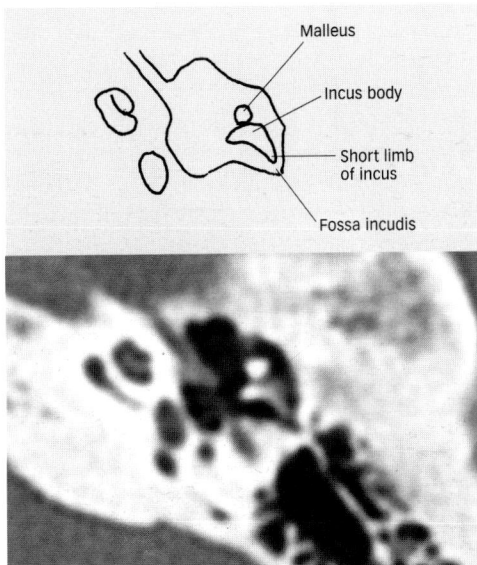

Fig 13.
Axial HRCT to show the fossa incudis.

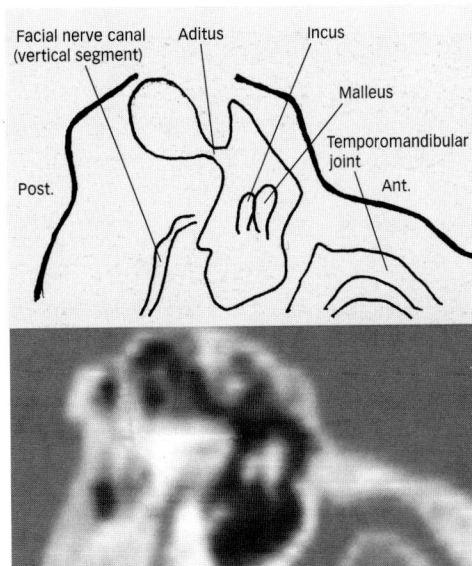

Fig 14.
HRCT reformatted in the sagittal plane to show normal incudomallear alignment, 'the molar tooth' sign.

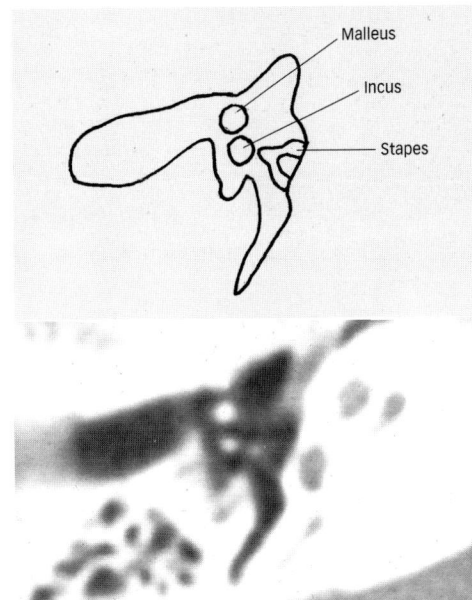

Fig 15.
Axial HRCT to show the ossicular chain.

The inner ear

The bony labyrinth of the inner ear is demonstrated by HRCT and surrounds the membranous labyrinth, whose component parts are shown by MRI (Fig. 16). The bony labyrinth comprises the vestibule, the cochlea, which lies anterior to it, and the semicircular canals, which lie posteriorly (Fig. 12).

The cochlea contains the Organ of Corti for the reception of sound transmitted through the ossicular chain. Its base is at the medial end of the internal auditory meatus; its apex or cupola points anterolaterally. A spiral lamina projects from a central modiolus, which can be identified with HRCT (Fig. 12).

There are three semicircular canals, the lateral (horizontal), the anterior (superior) and the posterior. They communicate with the

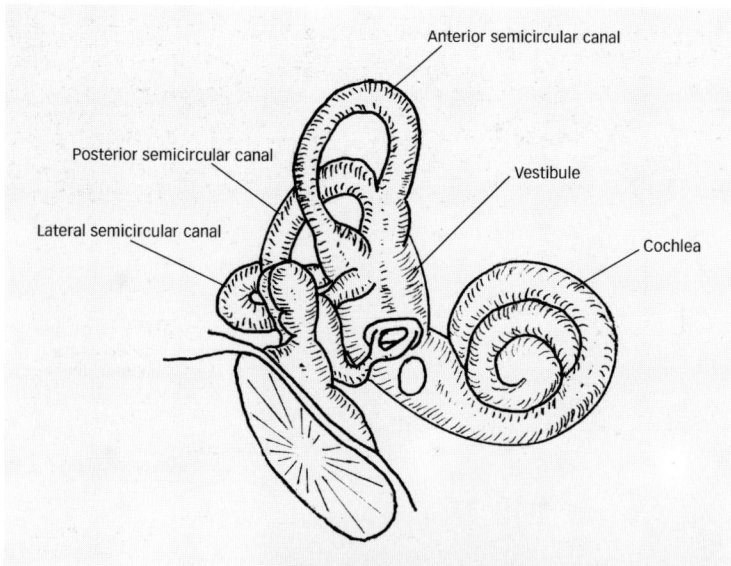

Fig 16(a).
**Diagram of
bony labyrinth.**

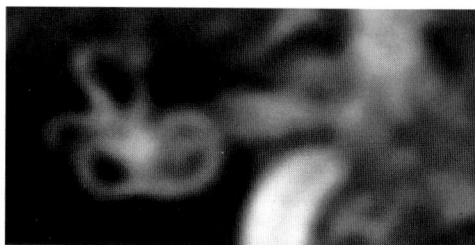

Fig 16(b).
**MRI 3D volume
acquisition to show the
membranous labyrinth.**

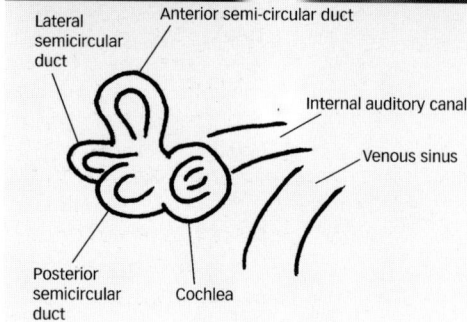

Fig 17.
**Axial HRCT to show the
semicircular canals.**

The membranous labyrinth consists of the saccule, utricle and semicircular ducts, which together are concerned with the maintenance of equilibrium. The saccule and utricle, situated anteriorly and posteriorly, respectively, within the vestibule, cannot as yet be resolved separately by MRI. The semicircular ducts occupy the semicircular canals and open into the utricle.

The fluid which surrounds the membranous labyrinth in the form of perilymph within and endolymph without determines its high signal intensity on T2-weighted MR images (Figs. 18, 19 and 20).

The cochlear duct, containing perilymph, extends from the cochlea and passes medially to open into the subarachnoid space inferior to the internal auditory meatus. Because of similarities in shape and course between the cochlear aqueduct and the internal auditory meatus, the two can be confused (Fig. 21).

The vestibular aqueduct arises from the posteromedial part of the vestibule near the common crus. It is directed posteriorly in an arched fashion, passing first superiorly and then inferiorly to reach the posterior surface of the petrous temporal bone. The posterior opening may be seen on axial CT (Fig. 12) but the aqueduct is best shown by the reformatting of axial sections in a sagittal plane taken through the vestibule (Fig. 22). The vestibular aqueduct contains the endolymphatic duct and sac and, in common with the cochlear aqueduct, is widest distally.

The internal auditory meatus

The internal auditory meatus (canal) is directed approximately horizontally in the coronal plane and can thus be seen on CT in both axial and coronal planes (Fig. 23). It can

vestibule by five openings including the common crus, which is shared by the anterior and posterior canals (Fig. 22). Each semicircular canal describes about two-thirds of a circle and is at right angles to the others, although the anterior and the posterior canals both lie in the vertical plane. The anterior semicircular canal is orientated perpendicular to the long axis of the petrous 'wedge' and can be identified on axial CT scans through the superior portion of the petrous bone (Fig. 17). On coronal scans it is seen beneath the rounded arcuate eminence (Fig. 25). This bony landmark can also be recognized on skull radiographs (see chapter 'Skull and brain'). The plane of the posterior semicircular canal is parallel to the long axis of the petrous 'wedge'.

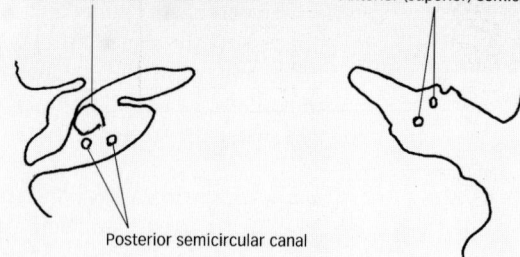

The lateral semicircular canal is the favoured site for a labyrinthine fistula complicating middle ear disease. From Fig. 8, the anatomical basis for this can be appreciated.

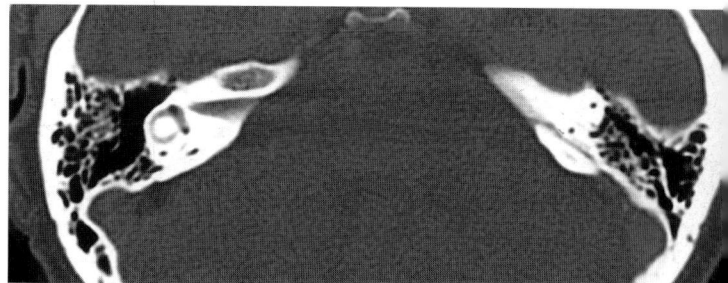

Fig 20.
Axial T2-weighted MRI to show the facial (VIIth) and vestibulocochlear (VIIIth) nerves within the internal auditory meatus.

(VIIIth) nerves, and the labyrinthine artery, which enter its medial opening into the posterior fossa, the porus acousticus. The facial and vestibulocochlear nerves may form a single bundle as they cross the cerebellopontine angle cistern but in the majority of cases studied with axial T2W MRI the facial nerve can be seen separately anterior to the vestibulocochlear nerve (Figs. 20, 24).

The internal auditory meatus is divided by the horizontal crista falciformis (Fig. 25) and vertical crests into four compartments. The facial nerve and the intermediate nerve occupy the anterosuperior quadrant, the cochlear branch of the vestibulocochlear nerve, the anteroinferior quadrant. The superior and inferior vestibular branches of the vestibulocochlear nerve are found in the posterior quadrants. At the lateral end of the internal auditory meatus is the lamina cribrosa through which the facial nerve passes to enter the facial canal and the vestibulocochlear nerve which gives branches to the cochlea and vestibule (Fig. 24).

The facial (VIIth) nerve
The facial nerve has a large motor root and a smaller sensory root (Fig. 23). The latter, known as the intermediate nerve, is too small to be identified either by CT cisternography or by MRI. The complex course of the facial nerve within the petrous temporal bone requires a combination of axial and coronal scans for a complete study. The first, or labyrinthine, segment of the facial nerve canal extends anterolaterally from the internal auditory meatus towards the geniculate fossa which contains the geniculate ganglion, in which the intermediate nerve terminates (Figs. 11, 26). The greater superficial petrosal nerve arises from the geniculate ganglion and carries secretomotor fibres to the lacrimal gland and taste

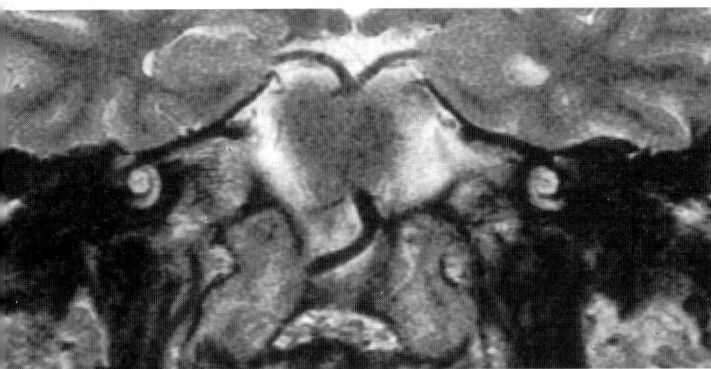

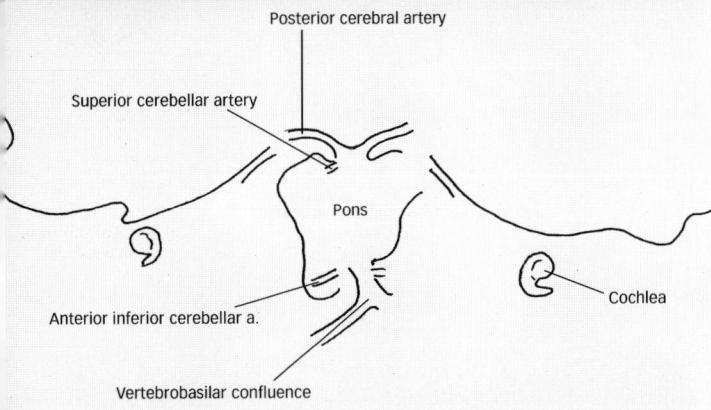

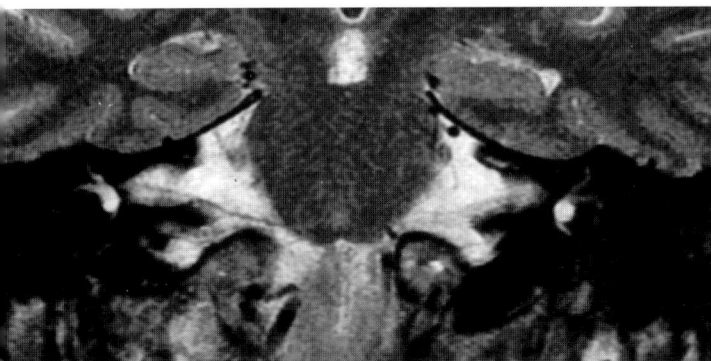

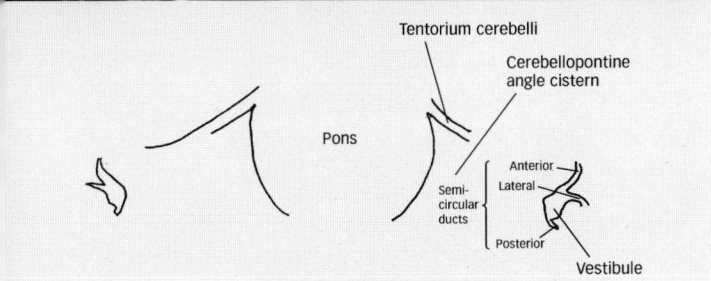

18. *(top)*
ronal T2-weighted MRI
ough the cochleae.

19.
ronal T2-weighted MRI
ough the vestibules
sterior to Fig. 18).

also be appreciated from Figs. 1 and 2 that the posterior wall of the internal auditory canal is shorter than the anterior.

There is some variation in the size and the shape of the normal canal between individuals but the two canals should be near mirror-images of one another. The meatus, which contains cerebrospinal fluid, is lined completely with dura and pia-arachnoid and transmits the facial (VIIth) and vestibulocochlear

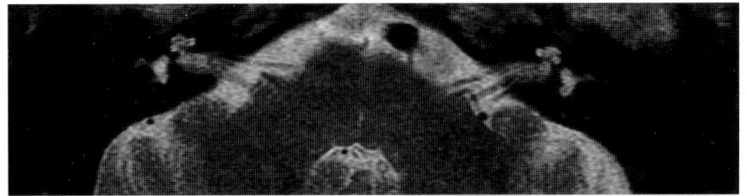

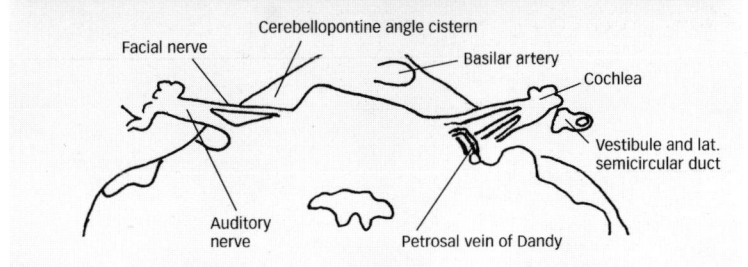

(a)

(b)

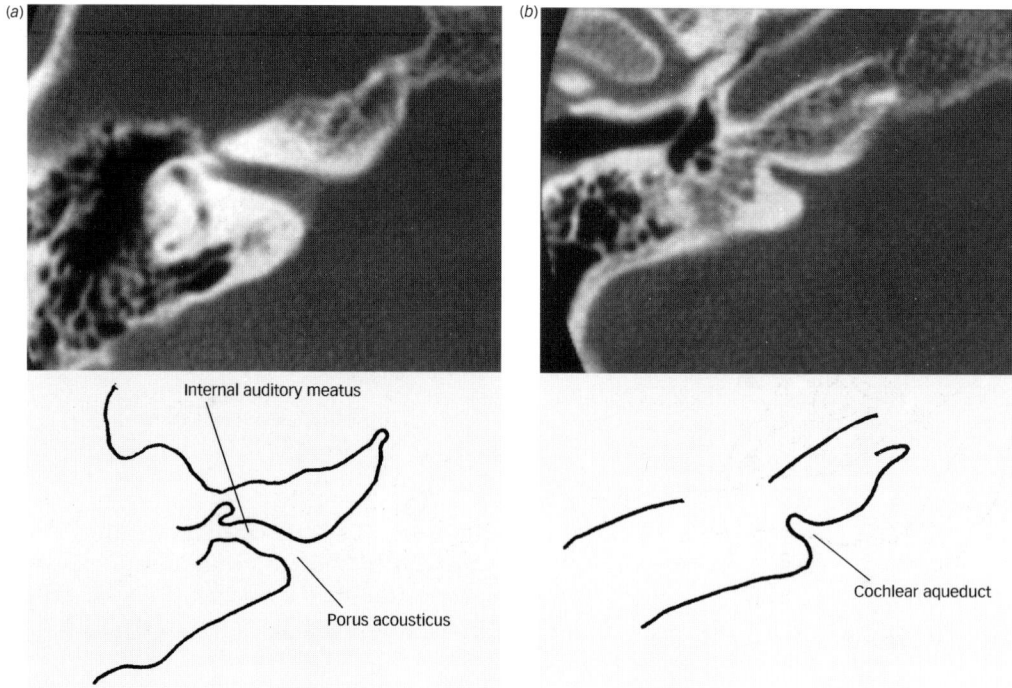

Fig 21.
Axial HRCT to show the similar orientation of the cochlear duct and internal auditory meatus; (a) is superior to (b).

Internal auditory meatus

Porus acousticus

Cochlear aqueduct

fibres to the palate. The labyrinthine segment of the facial nerve may be damaged by a transverse petrous fracture (at right angles to the long axis of the petrous bone). The facial nerve is directed posteriorly from the geniculate ganglion (the first genu) and continues as the tympanic segment within the tympanic cavity passing along the medial wall beneath the lateral semicircular canal (Figs. 8, 9). The bony canal here may be thin and is absent in some cases, but even when present may not be seen with HRCT. Predictably this second part of the facial nerve is vulnerable to inflammatory disease of the middle ear.

Coronal CT scans taken through the cochlea section the facial canal twice to produce the appearance known as 'snake's eyes' seen above the cochlea (Fig. 27). The medial 'eye' is the labyrinthine segment in cross-section, the lateral 'eye' represents the tympanic segment.

The second genu occurs at the fossa incudis and is therefore posterior to the first. From this point the canal is directed inferiorly as the mastoid segment (Fig. 14) and the nerve emerges from the skull base through the stylomastoid foramen. In the axial plane the mastoid segment may be difficult to identify but will be located lateral to the jugular foramen and posterior to the external auditory meatus.

The chorda tympani nerve arises from the mastoid segment of the facial nerve just proximal to the stylomastoid foramen. It travels superiorly and anteriorly in its own canal to reach the posterior part of the tympanic membrane passing forwards between its fibrous

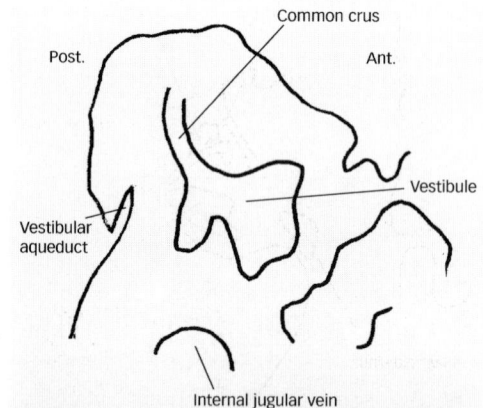

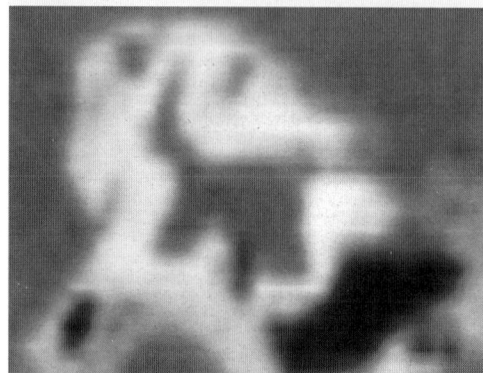

Post.

Common crus

Ant.

Vestibule

Vestibular aqueduct

Internal jugular vein

Fig 22.
HRCT reformatted in the sagittal plane to show the vestibular aqueduct.

and mucosal layers. In doing this, it also courses between the manubrium of the malleus and the incus. The nerve transmits taste fibres from the anterior two-thirds of the tongue to the lingual nerve and secretomotor fibres to the submandibular and sublingual glands.

z 23.
agram of the
anial nerves in
e internal
ditory meatus
ewed from above.

Facial nerve (labyrinthine segment)

Ant.

Foramen ovale

Lesser petrosal nerve

Greater superficial petrosal nerve

Cochlea

Cochlear nerve

Geniculate ganglion

Facial nerve (tympanic segment)

Vestibular nerve (superior and inferior divisions)

Malleus

Incus

Endolymphatic duct

Vestibule

Post.

Arcuate eminence

Crista falciformis

Scutum

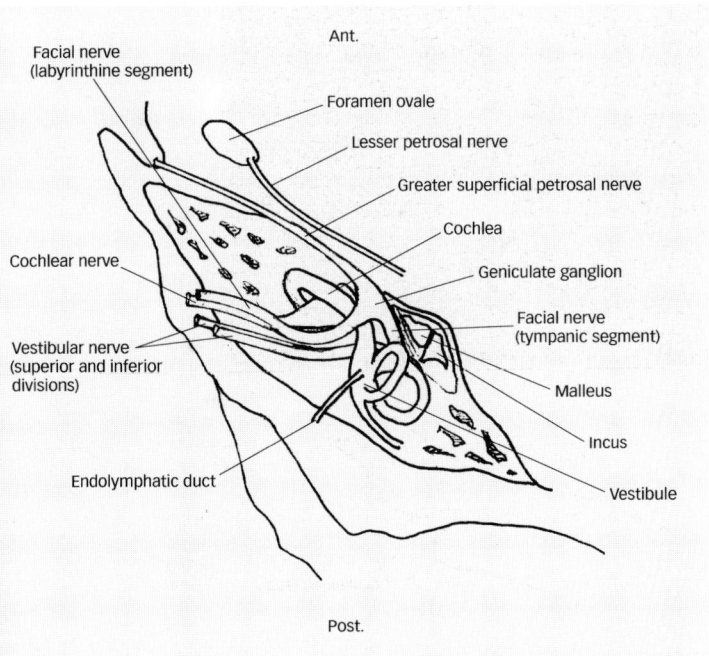

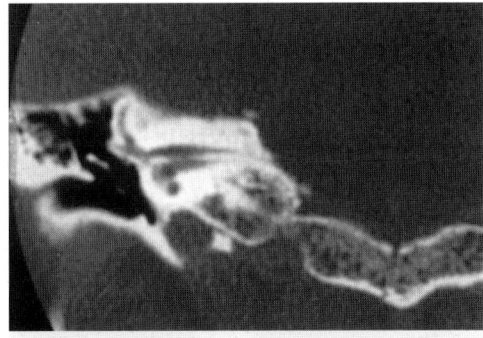

Fig 25.
Coronal HRCT to show the crista falciformis.

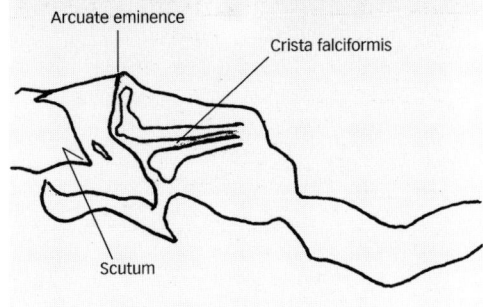

Vestibular nerve

Cochlear nerve

Facial nerve

Flocculus

Sigmoid sinus

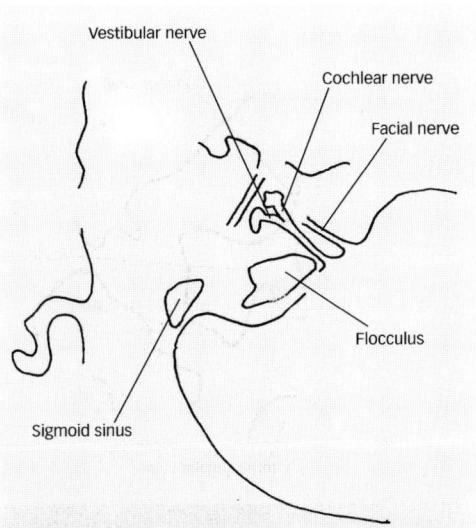

Fig 24.
Axial T1-weighted MRI to show the terminal division of the vestibulocochlear (VIIIth) nerve.

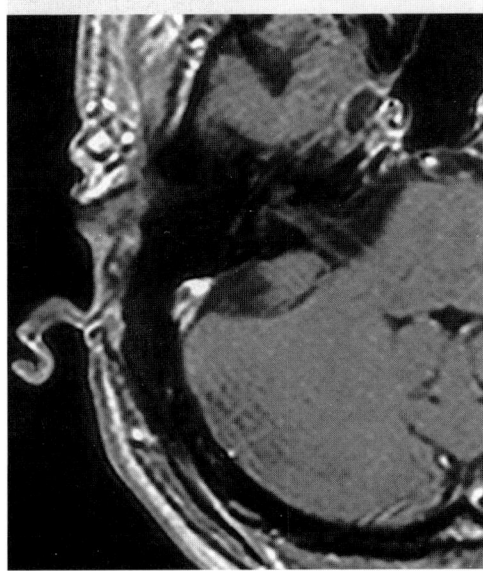

The cerebellopontine angle cistern

(see also Chapter 2 'The skull and brain')

The cerebellopontine angle cistern is one of a series of interconnecting subarachnoid spaces at the base of the brain. it is bounded by the posterior surface of the petrous bone laterally, the pons medially and the flocculus of the cerebellum posteriorly. The cistern is roughly triangular in shape in both the axial and the coronal planes (Figs. 1, 19 and 20).

The flocculus may appear to enhance with intravenous contrast medium, owing to the proximity of the anterior inferior cerebellar artery and may become hyperdense in comparison with the remainder of the cerebellum. This normal appearance should not be mistaken for an acoustic neurinoma.

The cerebellopontine angle cistern transmits the following structures: the facial (VIIth) and vestibulocochlear (VIIIth) nerves (the nerve 'bundle'), the anterior inferior cerebellar artery, and petrosal vein of Dandy and the trigeminal (Vth) nerve, which travels in the anterior part of the cistern.

The meatal loop of the anterior inferior cerebellar artery, from which the labyrinthine artery usually arises, lies very close to, and may even enter, the internal auditory meatus (Fig. 2). This can be responsible for enhancement seen within the internal auditory meatus on intravenous contrast enhanced CT and be misinterpreted as an acoustic neurinoma.

The jugular foramen

The jugular foramen transmits the jugular vein and the glossopharyngeal (IXth), vagus

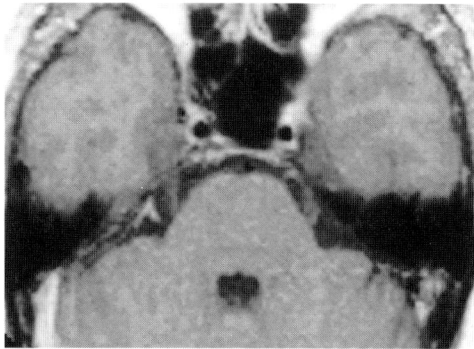

Fig 26.
Axial T1-weighted MRI to show the facial (VIIth) nerve. The nerve has enhanced after intravenous gadolinium DTPA. The patient has Bell's palsy and enhancement indicates that the nerve is inflamed. Normal nerves do not show contrast enhancement.

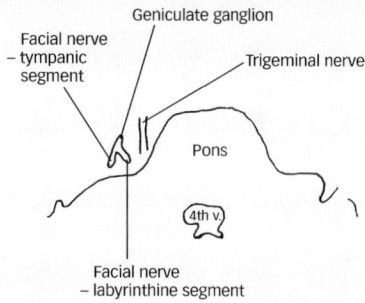

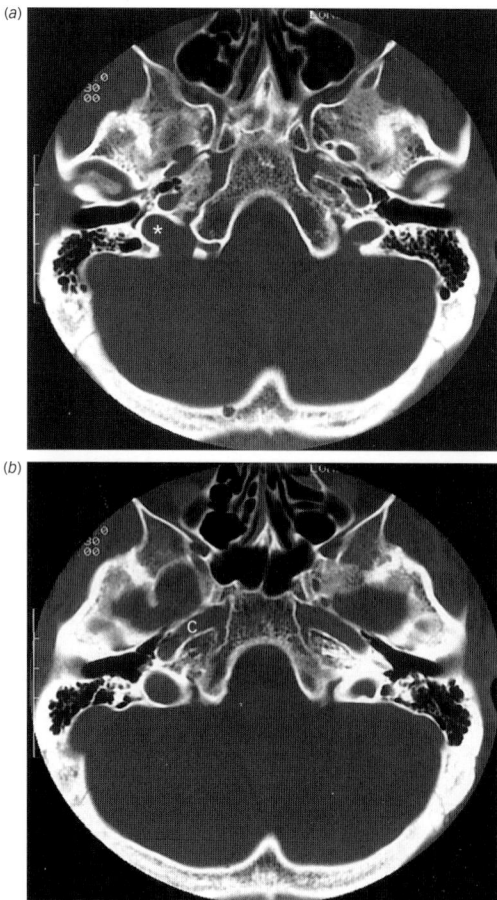

Fig 27.
Coronal HRCT through the cochleae to show the 'snake's eyes' appearance of the facial nerve.

Fig 28.
Axial HRCT to show the jugular foramina and carotid canals; (a) is inferior to (b). *jugular foramen; C, carotid canal.

(a)

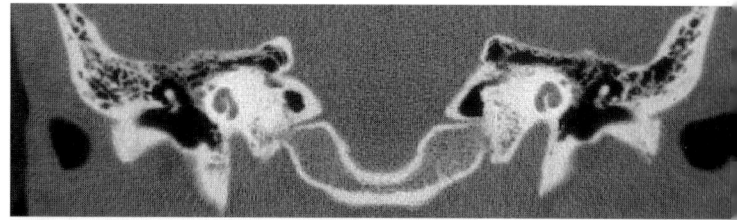

(b)

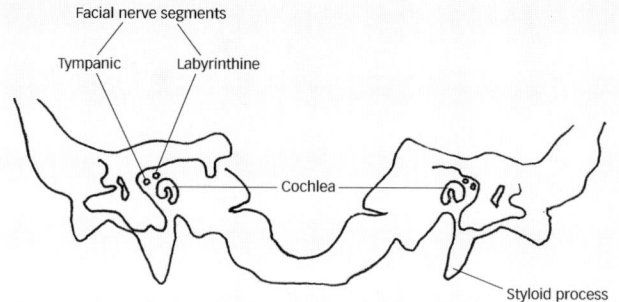

(Xth) and spinal accessory (XIth) cranial nerves. A fibrocartilaginous band separates the smaller, anteromedial pars nervosa from the pars vascularis. Despite the nomenclature, the pars nervosa contains the inferior petrosal sinus as well as the glossopharyngeal nerve. The pars vascularis contains the vagus and spinal accessory nerves as well as the jugular bulb.

Whereas the hallmark of the normal internal auditory canals is symmetry between right and left, the normal jugular foramina commonly differ in size. The right foramen is usually the larger, which reflects the difference in calibre of the right and left lateral dural venous sinuses.

The jugular foramen lies inferior to the hypotympanum and is separated anteriorly by a plate of bone from the carotid (Fig. 28). In rare instances, the jugular bulb may occupy an unusually high position and the bone separating it from the hypotympanum may be deficient or 'dehiscent'. In other cases, also rare, the petrous portion of the internal carotid artery may extend more laterally than is the norm.

These two congenital variants, the high jugular bulb and the aberrant carotid artery, result in the presence of a vascular 'mass' within the tympanic cavity which must be differentiated from a glomus tympanicum tumour.

5

Extracranial head and neck

J. BHATTACHARYA
and P. BUTLER

Development of the face, lips and palate (H. Ellis)

The basic morphology of the face is created between the fourth and tenth weeks by the development and fusion of five prominences around the primitive mouth, or stomodaeum. These are:

(a) The frontonasal process, which projects downwards from the cranium. Two olfactory pits develop in it and rupture into the pharynx to form the nostrils. Definitively, this process forms the nose, the nasal septum, nostril, the philtrum of the upper lip and the premaxilla, the V-shaped anterior portion of the upper jaw which usually bears the four incisor teeth.

(b) The maxillary processes, one on each side, which fuse with the frontonasal process and become the cheeks, upper lip (exclusive of the philtrum), upper jaw and palate (apart from the premaxilia).

(c) The mandibular process on each side which meet in the midline to form the lower jaw. The groove between the frontonasal process and the adjacent maxillary process is called the nasolacrimal groove. During the seventh week, the ectoderm at the floor of this groove invaginates to form a tube which becomes the nasolacrimal duct.

Abnormalities of this complex fusion process are numerous and constitute one of the commonest groups of congenital deformities. It is estimated that 1 child in 600 in the United Kingdom is born with some degree of either cleft lip or palate (Fig. 1). Frequently, these anomalies are associated with other congenital conditions.

The anomalies associated with defects of fusion of the face are macrostoma and micro-stoma, conditions where either too little or too great a closure of the stomodaeum occurs.

Cleft upper lip (or 'hare lip'). This is only very rarely like the upper lip of a hare, i.e. a medium cleft, although this may occur as a failure of development of the philtrum from the frontonasal process. Much more commonly, the cleft is on one or both sides of the philtrum, and results from failure of fusion of the maxillary and frontonasal processes. The cleft may be a small defect of the lip or may extend into the nostril, split the alveolus or even extend along the side of the nose as far as the orbit. There may be an associated cleft palate.

Cleft lower lip occurs very rarely but may be associated with a cleft tongue and cleft mandible. Cleft palate is a failure of fusion of the segments of the palate. The following stages may occur:

(a) a bifid uvula, which is of no clinical importance;

(b) partial cleft, which may involve the soft palate only or the posterior part of the hard palate also;
complete cleft, which may be (c) unilateral, running the full length of the maxilla and then alongside one face of the premaxilla; or (d) bilateral, in which the palate is cleft with an anterior V which separates the premaxilla completely.

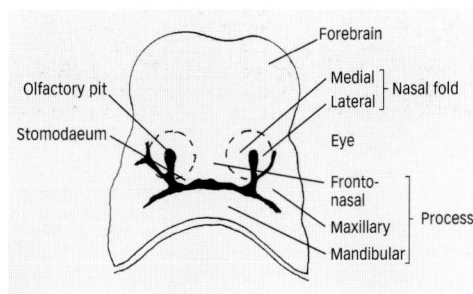

Fig. 1.
The ventral aspect of a fetal head showing the three processes, fronto-nasal, maxillary and mandibular, from which the face, nose and jaws are derived (Ellis, 1997).

Inclusion dermoids may form along the fines of fusion of the face. The most common of these is the external angular dermoid at the lateral extremity of the eyebrow. Occasionally, this dermoid extends through the skull to attach to the underlying dura.

The tongue

The tongue develops from the floor of the pharynx and derives from the first, third and fourth pharyngeal arches. At the end of the fourth week of embryonic life, the first pharyngeal arch forms a median swelling, the tuberculum impar. Early in the fifth week this is overgrown by the lateral lingual swellings, which develop on either side, also from the first arch. These swellings continue to grow and form the anterior two-thirds of the tongue (Fig. 2).

Later in the fourth week, a further midline swelling, the copula develops from the second arch. This is rapidly overgrown by a midline swelling, the hypobranchial eminence derived mainly from the third arch but also with a small contribution from the fourth arch to the most posterior aspect of the tongue. The line of circumvallate papillae demarcates the boundary between the first and third arch derivatives. A depression, the foramen caecum, is visible at the centre of this line and marks the site of origin of the thyroid gland.

The muscles of the tongue are derived from the myotomes of the occipital somites, innervated by the hypoglossal (XIIth) nerve. The only exception to this rule is the palatoglossus, which is innervated by the pharyngeal plexus of the vagus (Xth) nerve, and which can be considered to be a palatal rather than a tongue muscle.

This complex development reflects the multiple cranial nerve innervation of the tongue. The anterior two-thirds receives sensory supply from the mandibular branch of the trigeminal (Vth) nerve, which is the nerve of the first arch, and the taste buds in this region receive their supply from the chorda tympani branch of the facial (VIIth) nerve, the nerve of the second arch. The mucosa of the posterior one-third of the tongue receives both sensory and taste fibres, mainly from the glossopharyngeal (IXth) nerve, the nerve of the third arch, except for a small area of the most posterior aspect of the tongue which receives innervation from the superior laryngeal branch of the vagus (Xth) nerve, the nerve of the fourth arch.

The thyroid gland

The thyroid gland first appears late in the fourth week of embryonic life as a nodule of endoderm at the apex of the foramen caecum on the developing tongue. This nodule descends through the neck at the end of a slender thyroglossal duct, which breaks down by the end of the fifth week. The thyroid continues its descent to reach its definitive position by the seventh week (Fig. 3).

Normally, the only remnant of the thyroglossal duct is the foramen caecum itself. This is found in the midline of the tongue immediately behind the line of the circumvallate papillae. Rarely the whole or part of the gland remains as a swelling at the tongue base (lingual thyroid). More commonly is persistence of a thyroglossal cyst or sinus along the pathway of descent. Such a sinus can be dissected from the midline of the neck along the front of the hyoid (in such intimate contact with it that the centre of the hyoid must be excised during the dissection), then backwards through the muscles of the tongue to the foramen caecum. Descent of the thyroid may go beyond the normal position in the neck into the superior mediastinum (retrosternal goitre).

Fig. 2.
Development of the tongue
(Ellis, 1997).

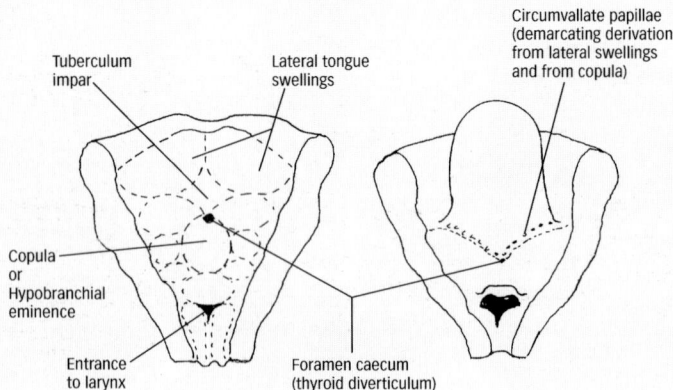

Tuberculum impar
Lateral tongue swellings
Circumvallate papillae (demarcating derivation from lateral swellings and from copula)
Copula or Hypobranchial eminence
Entrance to larynx
Foramen caecum (thyroid diverticulum)

Fig. 3.
The descent of the thyroid showing possible sites of ectopic thyroid tissue or thyroglossal cysts, and also the course of a thyroglossal fistula. (The arrow shows the further descent of the thyroid which may take place retrosternally into the superior mediastinum.)
(Ellis, 1997).

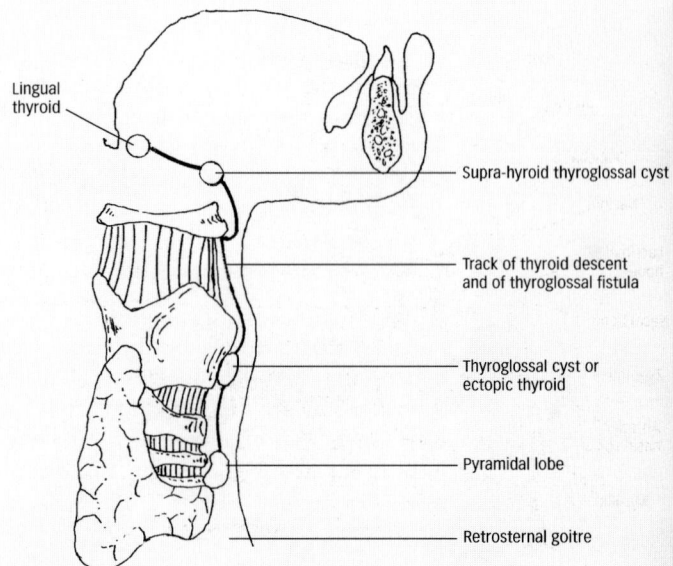

Lingual thyroid
Supra-hyoid thyroglossal cyst
Track of thyroid descent and of thyroglossal fistula
Thyroglossal cyst or ectopic thyroid
Pyramidal lobe
Retrosternal goitre

The commonest evidence of the embryologic thyroid descent is the small pyramidal lobe, which projects upwards from the isthmus of the thyroid gland, more commonly on the left than on the right side.

Osseous anatomy of the facial skeleton

With the exception of the mandible and the auditory ossicles, the bones of the skull and face are united by immobile sutures or synchondroses (see Chapter 2). The facial skeleton is joined to the skull base by the orbital walls, the zygomatic arches and the pterygoid plates, (Fig. 4). The halves of the face are joined inferiorly by the hard palate, and the face is supported centrally by the bony nasal septum which is formed from the perpendicular plate of the ethmoid bone and from the vomer (see p. 9). The facial skeleton can thus be represented as three groups of interconnected struts oriented in the coronal, sagittal and horizonal planes. The coronal struts include the frontal and nasal bones and the alveolar processes anteriorly and the posterior walls of the maxillary antra and pterygoid processes posteriorly. Sagittal struts include the medial and lateral walls of the maxillary antra and orbits and the nasal septum. Horizontal struts consist of the orbital floor and roof (and cribriform plate), the zygomatic processes and the hard palate. For descriptive purposes, the facial skeleton is often divided into the upper face, consisting of the supraorbital ridge and frontal bone; the midface extending from the supraorbital margin to the maxillary alveolus; and the lower face comprising the mandible.

Plain radiographs provide the first-line imaging in facial trauma. The occipito-mental (OM) or Water's view (Fig. 5), occipito-frontal, (OF), or Caldwell view (Fig. 6), and lateral views, (Fig. 7) are the usual projections. The symmetry of the facial anatomy on the frontal and basal views is important in diagnosis and, to facilitate interpretation, Dolan has described three lines of reference on the OM view which provide useful visual cues (Fig. 8).

Fig. 4.
Diagram of the skull and facial skeleton (a) frontal view, (b) lateral view.

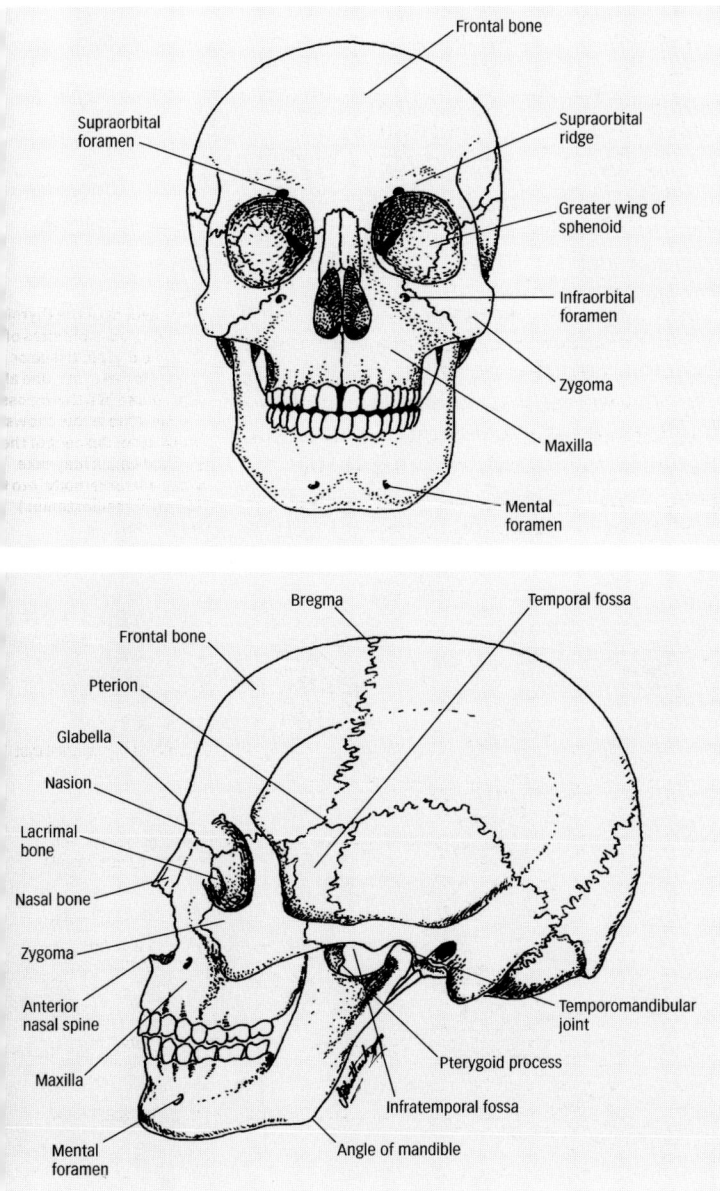

Fig. 5.
Occipitomental radiograph (Water's view). The petrous ridges should be projected just below the maxillary antra. This is the best single view for the antra. Note the lucency of the canal for the posterior superior alveolar nerve in the lateral antral wall*.

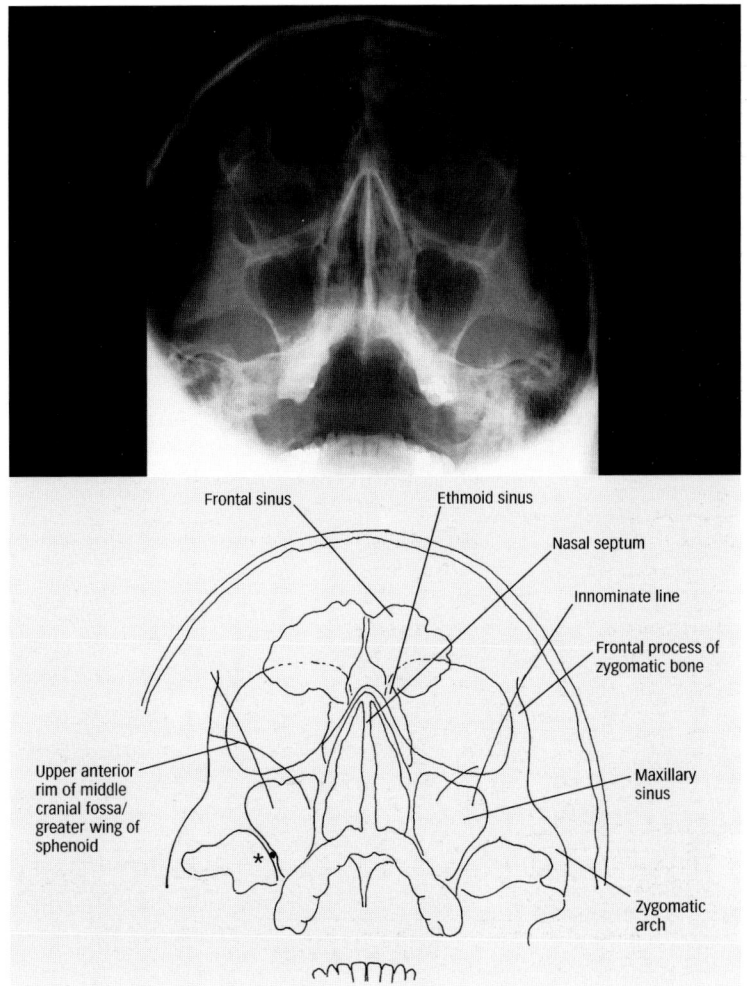

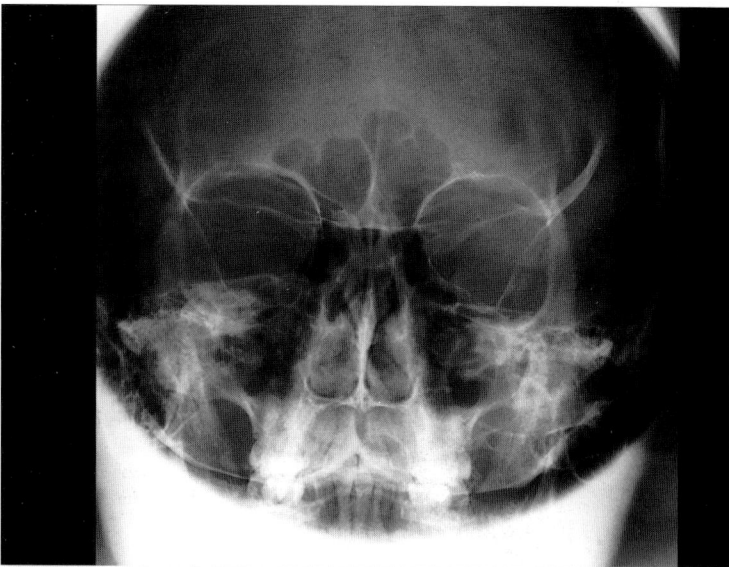

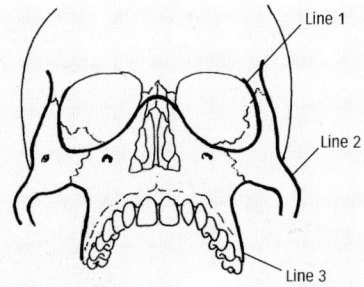

Fig. 8.
Diagram of Dolan's three lines of reference on the OM projection. Lines 2 an[d] form 'Dolan's elephant'. These lines are useful vis[ual] cues for facial symmetry i[n] excluding fractures.

The submentovertical (basal) projection is no longer part of the standard facial series but may be useful for assessing the zygomatic process and the anterior and posterior walls of the frontal sinus (see Chapter 2).

The facial musculature
The facial muscles, or muscles of expression, supplied by the facial nerve, function as sphincters or dilators of the orifices of the mouth, eye, nose and ear (Fig. 9). They are not normally readily separated by CT or MRI. The muscles of mastication, supplied by the trigeminal nerve, conversely are well demonstrated by both techniques. The masseter, pterygoid and temporalis muscles are well shown in the axial and coronal planes (Fig. 10). It can be seen from the coronal images that the bulk of the lateral pterygoid muscle lies craniad to the medial pterygoid. The two muscles occupy approximately similar positions on axial scans.

The infratemporal and pterygopalatine fossae
The infratemporal fossa is situated behind the maxilla and inferior to the greater wing of sphenoid. It communicates with the temporal fossa superiorly through the gap between the zygomatic arch and lateral wall of the skull

Fig. 6. (*left*)
Occipitofrontal radiograp[h] (Caldwell view). The petrous ridges should be projected over the lower third of the orbit. This is the best frontal view for t[he] ethmoid and frontal sinuses. Note the foramen[?] rotundum, which always lies immediately below th[e] superior orbital fissure.

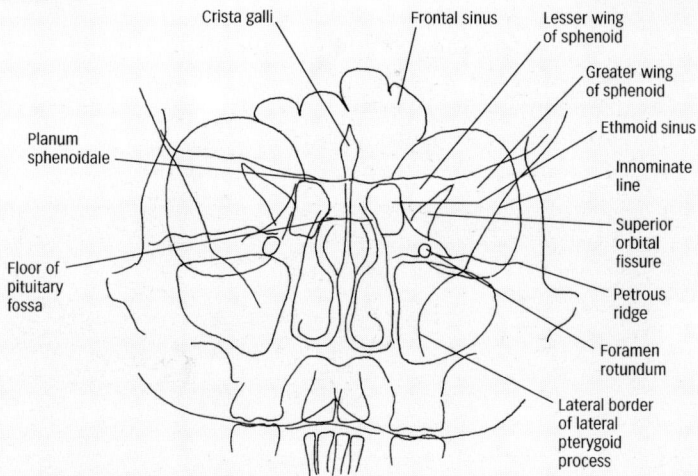

Fig. 7. (*below left*)
Lateral radiograph of the facial bones. Note the V-shaped shadows of the zygomatic recesses of the maxillary antra and the shadows of the middle and inferior conchae. The posterior walls of both antra are visible.

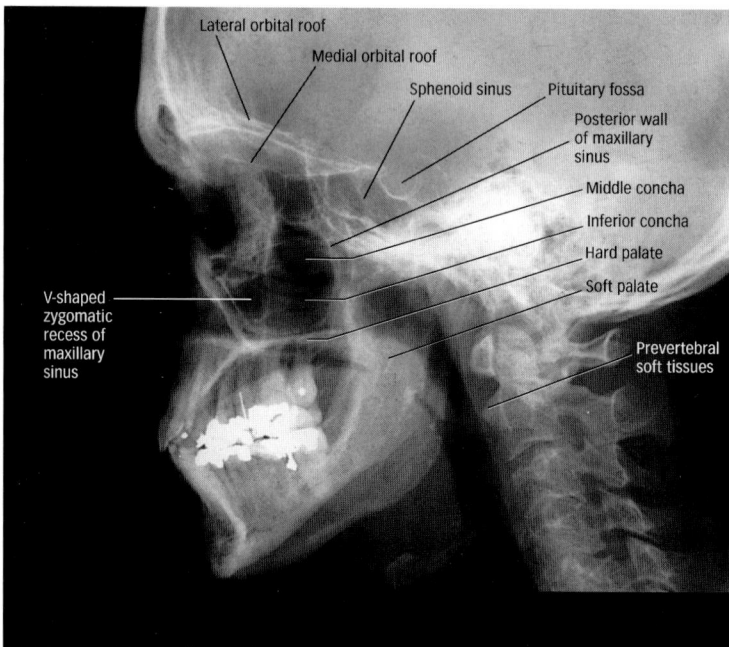

Fig. 9. (*below*)
The facial muscles. These are not normally readily distinguished by current imaging.

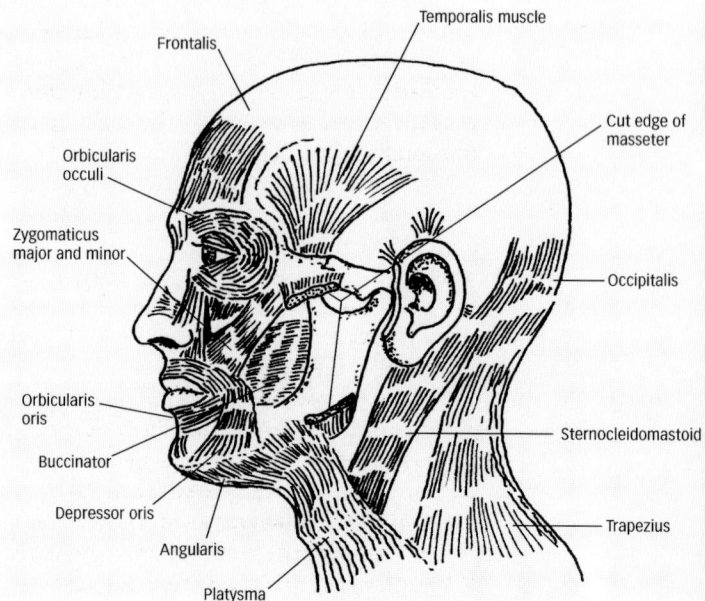

98

(b)

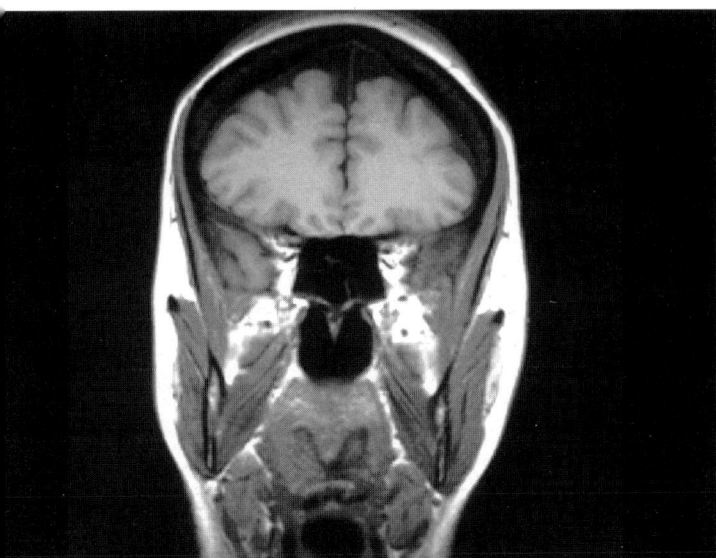

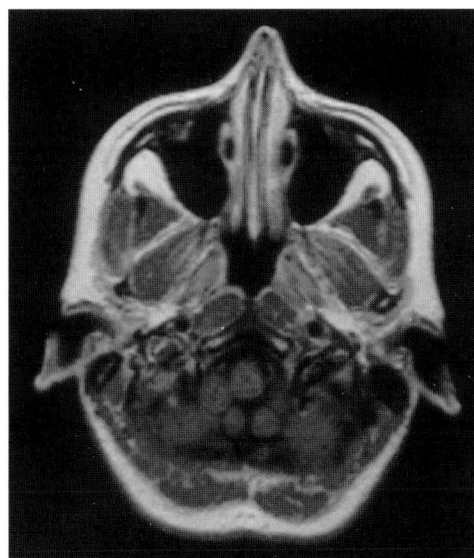

Fig. 10.
MRI demonstrating the muscles of mastication (*a*) **coronal and** (*b*) **axial T1W studies. The axial image following intravenous gadolinium DTPA demonstrates normal enhancement of the pharyngeal mucosa.**

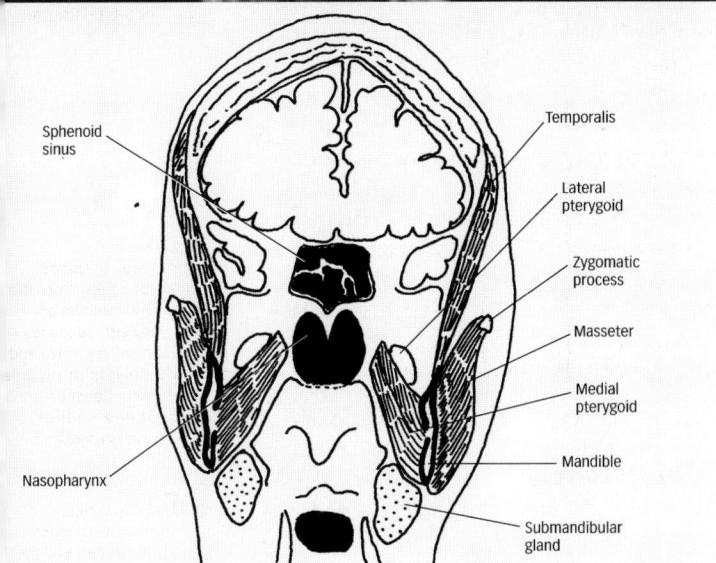

Sphenoid sinus

Temporalis

Lateral pterygoid

Zygomatic process

Masseter

Medial pterygoid

Mandible

Nasopharynx

Submandibular gland

Nasolacrimal duct

Maxillary sinus

Temporalis

Masseter

Lateral pterygoid

Levator veli palatini

Longus capitis

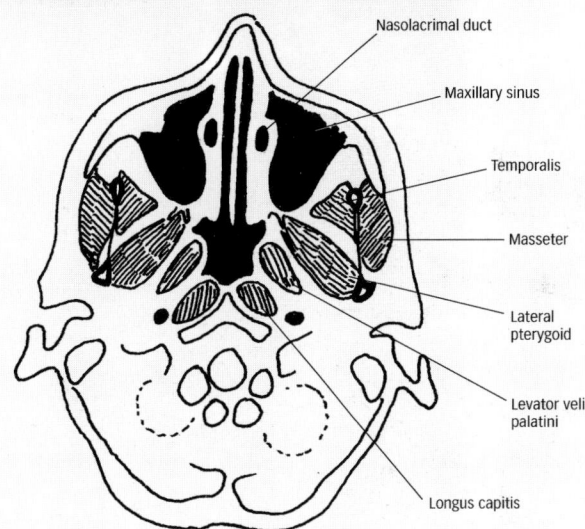

vault. The pterygomaxillary fissure connects the infratemporal and pterygopalatine fossae (Fig. 11), which both communicate with the orbit via the inferior orbital fissure. The pterygopalatine fossa additionally communicates with the nasal cavity through the sphenopalatine foramen (Fig. 20(*a*)).

The infratemporal fossa transmits the maxillary artery which runs deep to the temporalis muscle (see p. 117), and the mandibular nerve which emerges from the foramen ovale in the roof of the fossa, to send branches to the muscles of mastication. Its inferior alveolar branch enters the mandibular canal.

The pterygopalatine fossa contains the pterygopalatine ganglion and the terminal part of the maxillary artery, the sphenopalatine branch of which passes through the sphenopalatine foramen to supply the nasal cavity. The foramen rotundum opens onto the posterior wall of the fossa which thus also transmits the maxillary nerve.

The mandible and temporomandibular joint

The mandible (Fig. 12), is the strongest of the facial bones and is particularly well shown by dental panoramic radiography (or orthopantomography) (Fig. 13). Each half of the mandible consists of a vertical ramus and body which are fused anteriorly in the midline at the mental symphysis.

The teeth are borne by the inferior alveolar process and are apposed to those of the superior alveolar process of the maxilla. The mandibular foramen opens onto the inner surface of the ramus and admits the inferior alveolar branch of the trigeminal nerve into the mandibular canal, which in turn opens on the outer surface of the body of the mandible as the mental foramen.

The muscles of the tongue and floor of the mouth take their origins from the inner surface of the body of the mandible. The powerful muscles of mastication insert on the ramus, angle and neck.

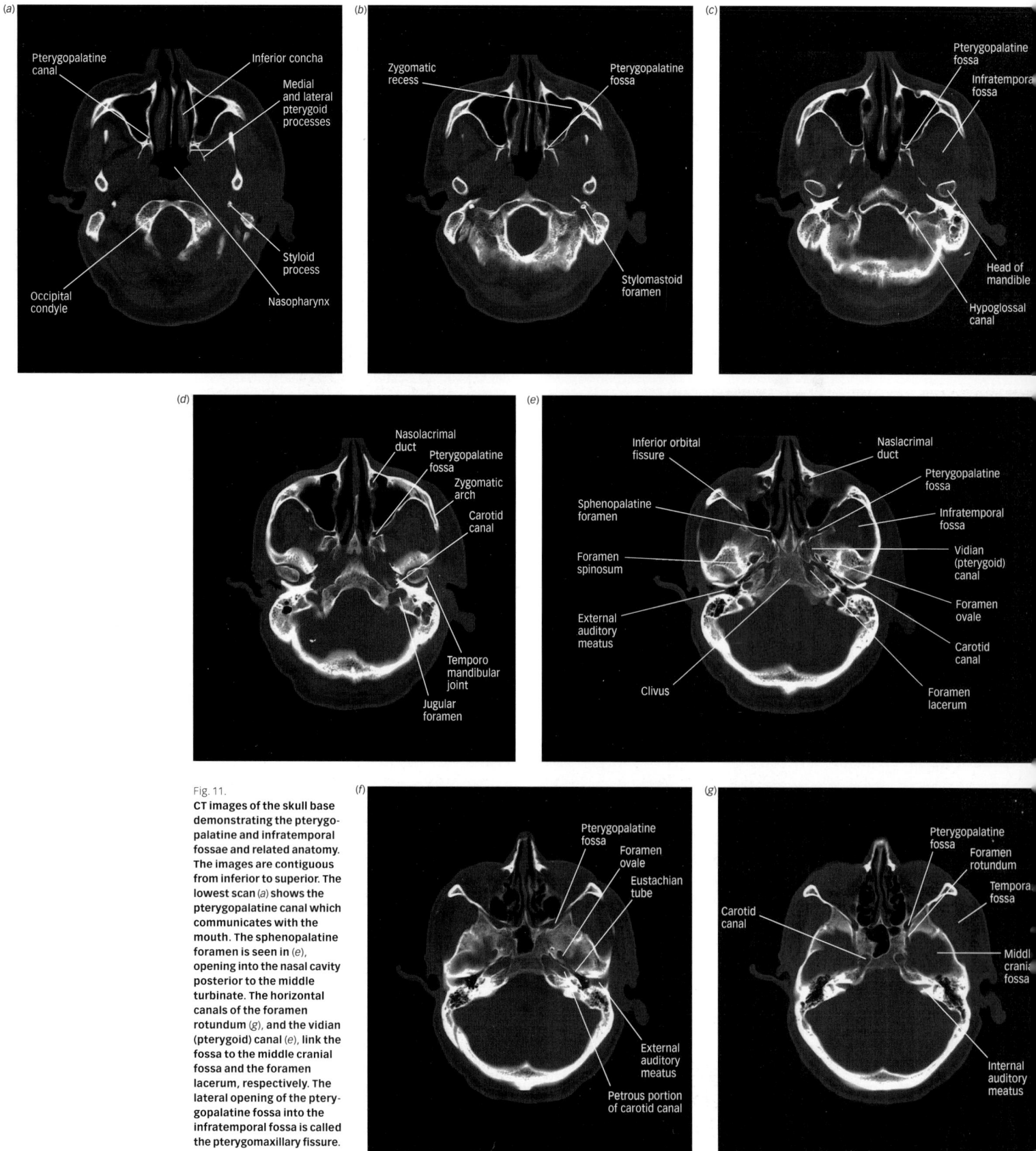

(a)

Pterygopalatine canal
Inferior concha
Medial and lateral pterygoid processes
Styloid process
Nasopharynx
Occipital condyle

(b)

Zygomatic recess
Pterygopalatine fossa
Stylomastoid foramen

(c)

Pterygopalatine fossa
Infratemporal fossa
Head of mandible
Hypoglossal canal

(d)

Nasolacrimal duct
Pterygopalatine fossa
Zygomatic arch
Carotid canal
Temporo mandibular joint
Jugular foramen

(e)

Inferior orbital fissure
Naslacrimal duct
Sphenopalatine foramen
Pterygopalatine fossa
Foramen spinosum
Infratemporal fossa
Vidian (pterygoid) canal
External auditory meatus
Foramen ovale
Carotid canal
Clivus
Foramen lacerum

Fig. 11.

CT images of the skull base demonstrating the pterygopalatine and infratemporal fossae and related anatomy. The images are contiguous from inferior to superior. The lowest scan (a) shows the pterygopalatine canal which communicates with the mouth. The sphenopalatine foramen is seen in (e), opening into the nasal cavity posterior to the middle turbinate. The horizontal canals of the foramen rotundum (g), and the vidian (pterygoid) canal (e), link the fossa to the middle cranial fossa and the foramen lacerum, respectively. The lateral opening of the pterygopalatine fossa into the infratemporal fossa is called the pterygomaxillary fissure.

(f)

Pterygopalatine fossa
Foramen ovale
Eustachian tube
External auditory meatus
Petrous portion of carotid canal

(g)

Pterygopalatine fossa
Foramen rotundum
Temporal fossa
Carotid canal
Middle cranial fossa
Internal auditory meatus

Fig. 12.
Diagram of the mandible. The masseter and medial pterygoid muscles insert on the outer and inner aspects of the angle, respectively. lateral pterygoid muscle inserts on the neck and the temporalis inserts on the coronoid process.

13. (*below*)
Dental panoramic radiograph (orthopantomogram) of the mandible and maxilla. This technique, in which the X-ray tube and film cassette rotate synchronously and reciprocally around the patient's head, gives a good survey of the upper and lower jaws.

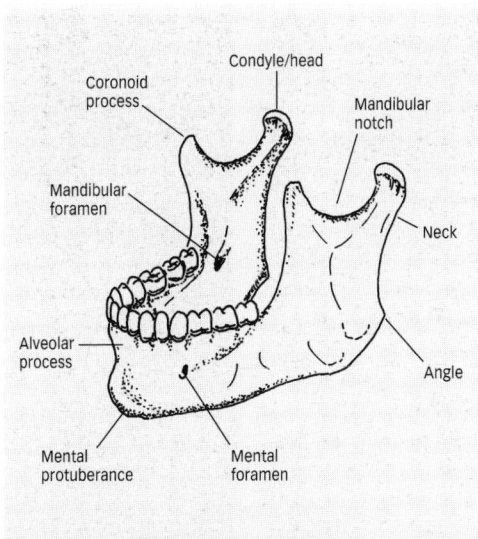

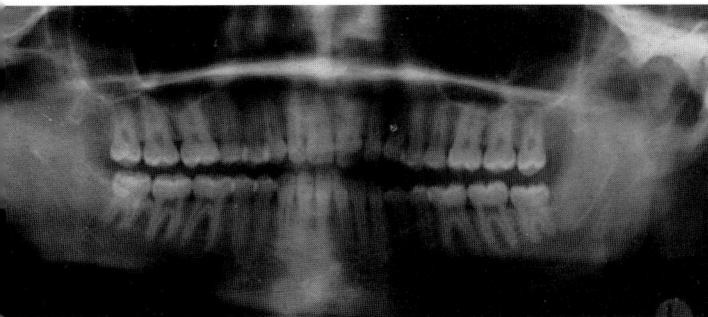

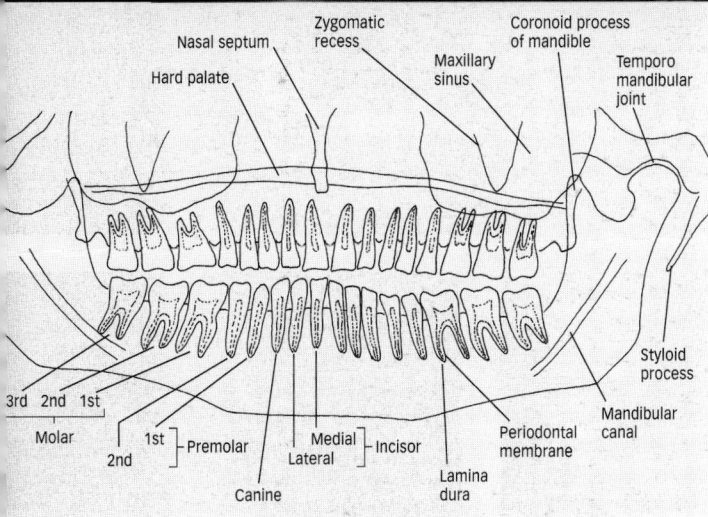

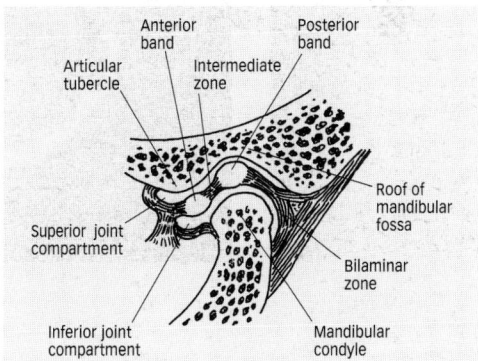

Fig. 14.
Schematic diagram of the temporomandibular joint.

The mandibular condyle articulates with the mandibular (or glenoid) fossa of the temporal bone at the temporomandibular joint (TMJ) (Fig. 14). The joint lies immediately anterior to the external auditory meatus (Fig. 11(*c*)–(*e*)). A fibrous articular disc separates the articular cartilage of the two bones which appears biconcave in the sagittal plane and crescentic in the coronal plane. The disc consists of anterior and posterior bands and a thinner mid-portion which normally lies between the mandibular condyle and articular eminence of the temporal fossa. It divides the joint cavity into a superior, and larger inferior compartments, which function as separate joints and which do not communicate. Anteriorly, medially and laterally the disc is attached to the joint capsule and mandibular condyle, and moves forward with the condyle when the mouth is opened. The posterior attachment to the condyle and temporal bone, called the bilaminar zone, consists of loose elastic and fibrous connective tissue and permits this forward translation. Rotational condylar movements take place mainly between the inferior aspect of the disc and the superior condylar surface, while translational movements occur between the glenoid fossa and the superior surface of the disc.

Arthrography, usually, only of the inferior compartment is still commonly used to study joint function, to diagnose perforation of the articular disc and identify anterior dislocation (Fig. 15). Although it is often technically difficult to obtain a good result, arthrography has the advantage of providing a true dynamic record of joint movement. MRI, however, has become the technique of choice for imaging the TMJ, providing more information on the morphology and position of the disc, in both the sagittal and coronal planes, along with the surrounding soft tissues.

Static scans may be performed in open and closed mouth positions (Fig. 16), or a pseudo-dynamic method employed, using a single slice, gradient-echo sequence in varying degrees of mouth-opening, with the resulting images displayed on a cine loop. Echo planar imaging offers the possibility of real-time dynamic MRI studies. The main use of CT is in the assessment of complex trauma.

The teeth

There are 20 deciduous teeth and the central incisors are the first to erupt at around 6 months. The first molar tooth is usually the first of the permanent dentition to erupt at about 6 years and for both deciduous and permanent teeth. The second permanent molar does not erupt until 12 years of age.

Fig. 15.
Arthrography of temporomandibular joint with the mouth closed (a), and open (b). Between 0.2 and 0.4 ml of contrast medium have been introduced into the lower joint compartment. Note the forward translation of the mandibular head and disc as the mouth opens and the posterior pooling of the contrast medium.

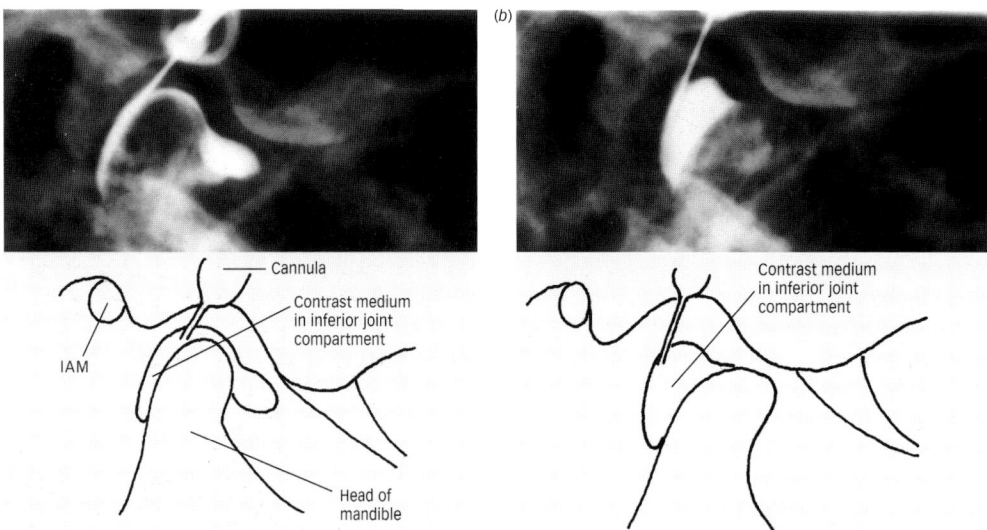

(a)

(b)

Cannula

Contrast medium in inferior joint compartment

IAM

Head of mandible

Contrast medium in inferior joint compartment

Fig. 16.
Sagittal proton density (PD) MRI of temporomandibular joint: (a) mouth closed, (b) mouth open. PD images are better than T1W images in distinguishing the disc from surrounding tissues. T2W images give an 'arthrographic effect' that may be useful for effusions and perforations.

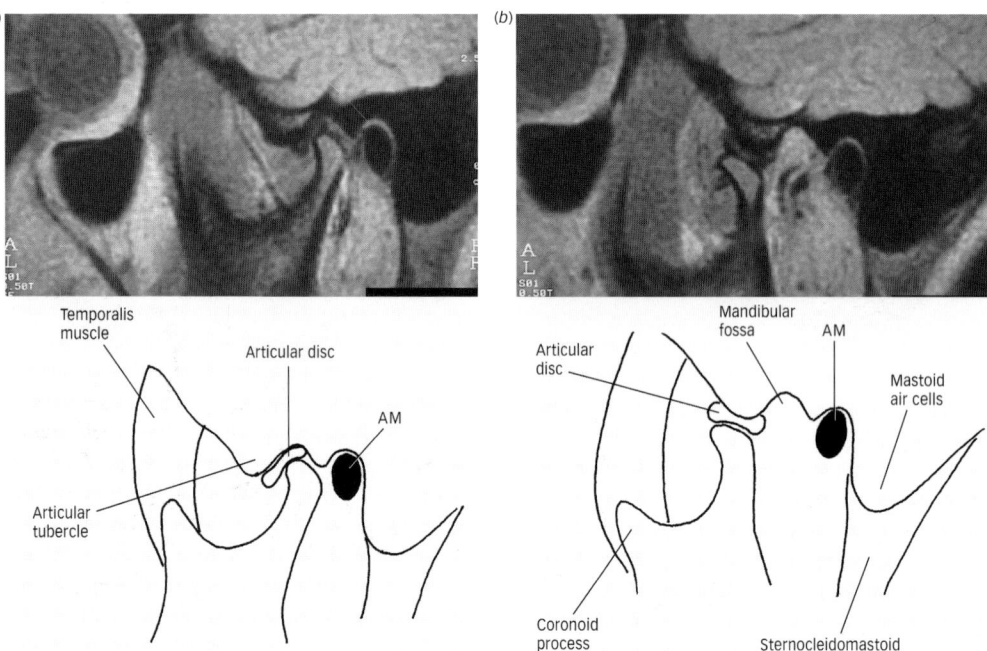

(a)

(b)

Temporalis muscle

Articular disc

AM

Articular tubercle

Articular disc

Mandibular fossa

AM

Mastoid air cells

Coronoid process

Sternocleidomastoid

Fig. 17.
Schematic diagram of a tooth.

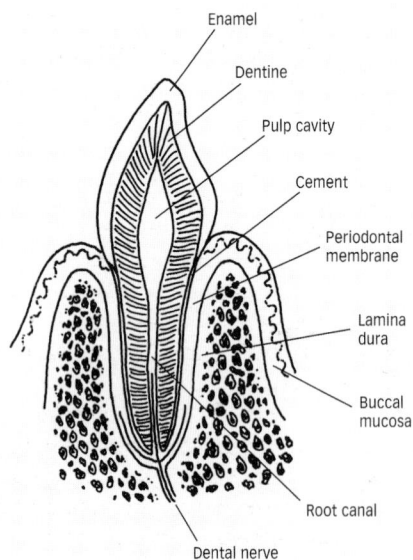

Enamel

Dentine

Pulp cavity

Cement

Periodontal membrane

Lamina dura

Buccal mucosa

Root canal

Dental nerve

In the intervening period the five deciduous teeth of each half-jaw are replaced. The order of replacement is the first incisors, central and lateral, then the milk molars, first and second, and, last of all, the long-rooted canine (Table 1).

There are 32 permanent teeth each of which occupies a bony socket, or alveolus, in the mandible and maxilla (Figs. 13, 17). The alveoli are lined by a dense rim of cortical bone known as the lamina dura, the loss of which is an important radiological sign of inflammation, or of metabolic disorders such as hyperpara-thyroidism. The periodontal membrane, the pulp cavity and root canals are radiolucent. For descriptive purposes the teeth are divided into quadrants. Thus on each side in the upper and lower jaw there are two incisors, one canine, two premolars and three molars.

TABLE 1
Permanent teeth

yrs	
6	First permanent mo
7	Central incisors
8	Lateral incisors
9	First premolars
10	Second premolars
11	Canines
12	Second molars
18	Wisdom teeth

Nasal cavity

The external nose consists of a bony component superiorly and a more substantial cartilaginous portion inferiorly. The nostrils, or nares, are braced by the U-shaped alar cartilages. The nasal cavity extends from the base of the skull to the roof of the mouth and is divided by the nasal septum into two approximately symmetrical nasal fossae. The nose communicates via the choanae with the nasopharynx posteriorly while apertures in the lateral wall of the nasal cavity communicate with the paranasal air sinuses. The complex anatomy of this region is best demonstrated by CT. Plain films have a limited role, mainly in trauma (Fig. 18).

Fig. 18.
Lateral radiograph of the nasal bones. The sutures and grooves for branches of the nasociliary nerves should not be mistaken for fractures. Note also the anterior nasal spine of the maxilla (arrow).

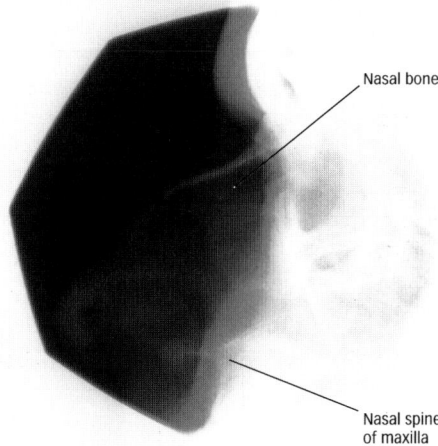

Nasal bone

Nasal spine of maxilla

The nasal cavity is roofed anteriorly by the nasal and frontal bones and posteriorly by the sphenoid bone. Its mid-portion is formed by the 3 mm wide cribriform plate of the ethnoid bone which is perforated by about 20 foramina transmitting fibres of the olfactory nerve, and the anterior ethmoidal vessels and nerve. The floor of the nasal cavity is formed by the hard palate, and the medial wall of each nasal fossa,

19.
gram of the nasal tum demonstrating cartilaginous and y components.

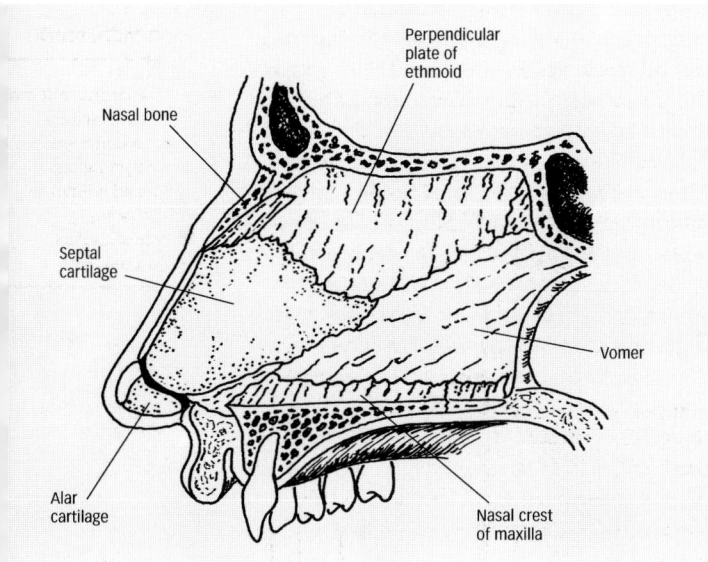

Perpendicular plate of ethmoid

Nasal bone

Septal cartilage

Vomer

Alar cartilage

Nasal crest of maxilla

by the nasal septum (Fig. 19). Deviation of the septum is commonly observed on radiographs and CT scans and is present in up to 25% of the population either developmentally or secondary to trauma.

The lateral wall of the nasal cavity has a complex structure (Fig. 20 (*a*), (*b*)), which is dominated by the three bony projections, the superior, middle and inferior conchae (turbinates). Beneath each cocha is a correspondingly named meatus (i.e. the superior meatus lies beneath the superior concha).

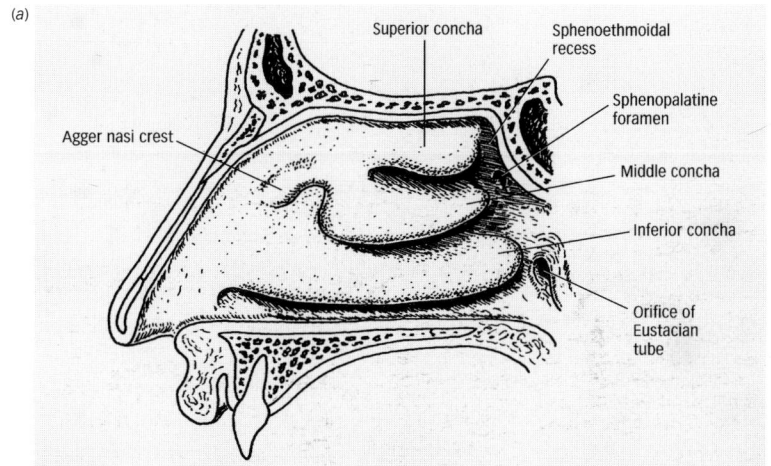

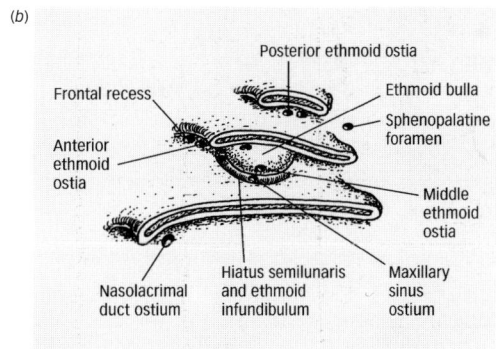

(*a*)

Superior concha

Sphenoethmoidal recess

Sphenopalatine foramen

Agger nasi crest

Middle concha

Inferior concha

Orifice of Eustacian tube

(*b*)

Posterior ethmoid ostia

Frontal recess

Ethmoid bulla

Sphenopalatine foramen

Anterior ethmoid ostia

Middle ethmoid ostia

Nasolacrimal duct ostium

Hiatus semilunaris and ethmoid infundibulum

Maxillary sinus ostium

Fig. 20.
Diagrams of the lateral wall of nasal fossa (*a*) before and (*b*) after removal of the turbinates to expose the underlying meati. Note that only the posterior ethmoid cells open into the superior meatus and only the nasolacrimal duct opens into the inferior meatus.

The inverted crescent of the hiatus semilunaris is situated beneath the bulging ethmoid bulla in the middle meatus (Fig. 20 (*b*)). The ethmoid, maxillary and frontal sinuses drain into the hiatus with the frontal recess opening into the anterior part.

Each of the paired sphenopalatine foramina lies immediately behind the superior meatus and transmits the nasopalatine nerve and vessels to the nasal cavity. They communicate with the pterygopalatine fossae and provide a conduit for infection or neoplasm to reach the orbit and cranial cavity.

The nasal mucosa is highly vascular and includes special areas of erectile cavernous tissue on the middle and inferior conchae and on the anterior nasal septum (the septal swell body). Periodic vascular engorgement of the mucosa of each nasal fossa results in the

Fig. 21.
Axial T2W MRI showing
congestion of the mucosa
of the left nasal fossa,
a normal finding.

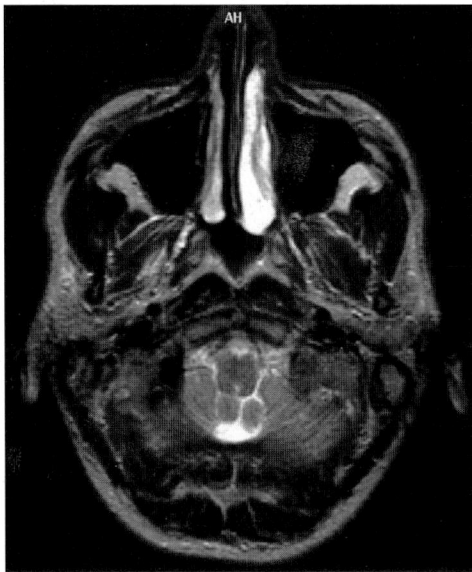

so-called nasal cycle causing the opening and closing of alternate sides of the nasal airway every 2 to 3 hours. This results in the commonly observed normal asymmetric congestion of nasal mucosa on MRI scans (Fig. 21).

The main blood supply to the nasal cavity is from the sphenopalatine branch of the maxillary artery but the rich blood supply derives from both internal and external carotid arterial branches. For example, the anterior ethmoidal branches of the ophthalmic artery penetrate the cribriform plate to join the anastomotic network, a portion of which, on the antero-inferior aspect of the nasal septum, is known as Little's area, the most common site of origin for epistaxis.

The paranasal sinuses and ostiomeatal complex
The paranasal sinuses (frontal, maxillary, ethmoid and sphenoid) arise as outgrowths of the nasal cavity and communicate with the cavity via ostia at the sites of their original evagination. There are traces of the maxillary and sphenoid sinuses in the neonate; the remainder become evident about the age of 7 or 8 years in association with the eruption of the permanent dentition. They only become fully developed in adolescence.

The frontal sinuses (Figs. 5–7, 22(*a*)), are asymmetrical, paired cavities between the tables of the frontal bone. Numerous incomplete bony septa frequently give a scalloped margin on plain radiographs and, because of differential growth, the dividing septum is often deviated to one side, usually returning to the midline inferiorly. The shape and size of the frontal sinus is highly variable and there may be hypoplasia or even aplasia. In the presence of a persisting metopic suture, the frontal sinuses develop separately on either side of the suture, which may be helpful in excluding frontal fractures. Drainage is via the frontal recess into the ostiomeatal complex (vide infra) and middle meatus.

The maxillary sinus, or antrum, lies within the body of the maxilla (Figs. 5, 6, 22). It is shaped like a tilted pyramid with its base forming the medial wall. Its apex points laterally into the zygoma forming a zygomatic recess which produces the V-shaped shadows projected over the antra on the lateral radiograph (Fig. 7). Hypoplasia of one maxillary sinus is present in up to 10% of the population and results in increased density of the sinus on plain films. This should not be confused with inflammation. The roof forms the floor of the orbit and is grooved by the infraorbital canal for the maxillary nerve. The floor of the sinus is formed by the alveolar recess. The roots of the molar and pre-molar teeth may project into the sinus but are usually covered by a thin layer of bone and mucosa.

The narrow posterior wall forms the anterior border of the pterygopalatine fossa. The bony medial wall of the sinus is deficient postero-superiorly at the maxillary hiatus. This large opening is partially closed by the inferior concha and the uncinate process of the ethmoid bone leaving, in addition to the ostium, anterior and posterior fontanelles which are covered only by periostium and mucosa. These accessory fontanelles may contain accessory ostia, which may be visible on axial CT scans. The main ostium is in the most superior part of the medial wall and opens into the ethmoid infundibulum, a narrow channel between the uncinate process, the lamina papyracea and the anterior surface of the ethmoid bulla. The ethmoid infundibulum opens into a curved groove in the middle meatus below the ethmoid bulla: the hiatus semilunaris (Fig. 20(*b*)). The frontal recess, with the aperture of the frontal sinus, opens into the anterior end of this groove. Drainage of mucus is thence into the middle meatus proper.

The term ostiomeatal complex or unit refers to the maxillary sinus ostium, ethmoid infundibulum, hiatus semilunaris and frontal recess. It is the final common pathway for drainage of secretions from the maxillary, frontal, and anterior and middle ethmoid sinuses into the middle meatus; obstruction here thus has a pivotal role in the development and persistence of sinusitis. Coronal high resolution CT (HRCT) reveals these structures in exquisite detail (Fig. 22), and is the imaging modality of choice.

Coordinated beating of the cilia of the sinus epithelium results in a continuous motion of

(a)

(b)

Anterior
ethmoid
air cells

Crista galli

Septal
swell
body

Lacrimal
fossa

22.
ronal CT series on bone
ndow settings
monstrating the anatomy
the paranasal sinuses and
tiomeatal complex from
terior, (a) to posterior (f).

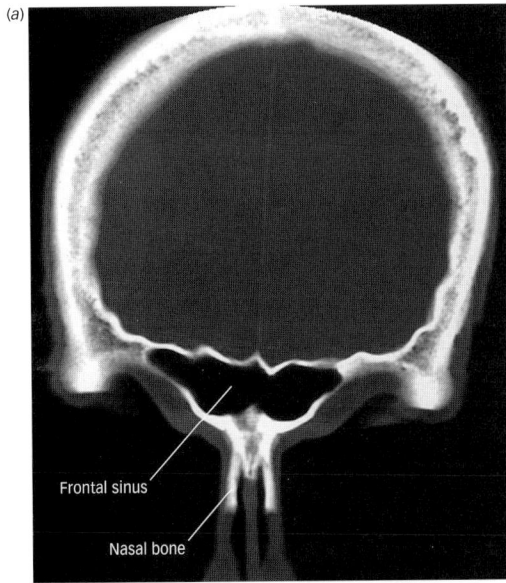

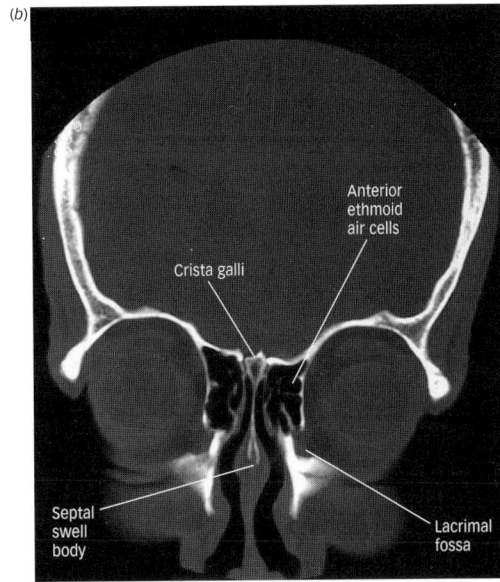

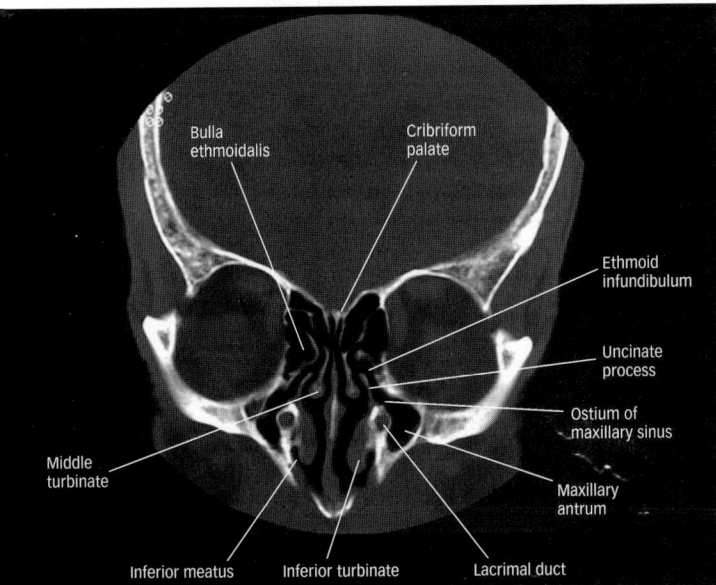

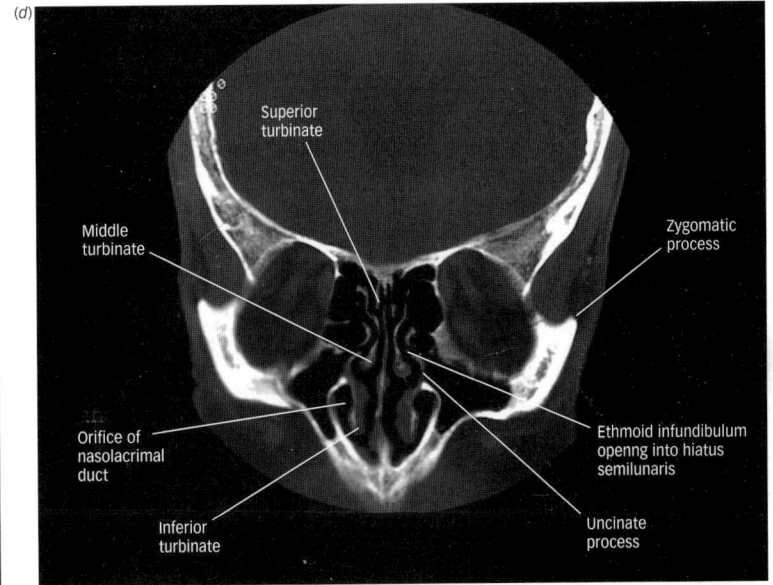

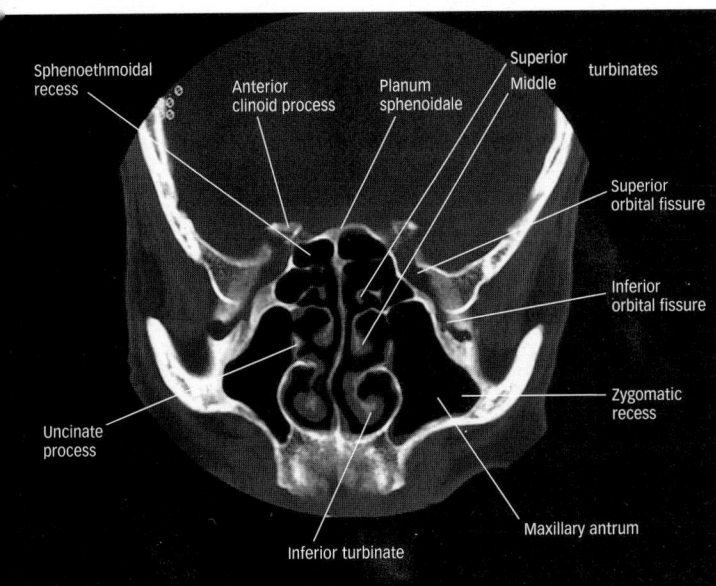

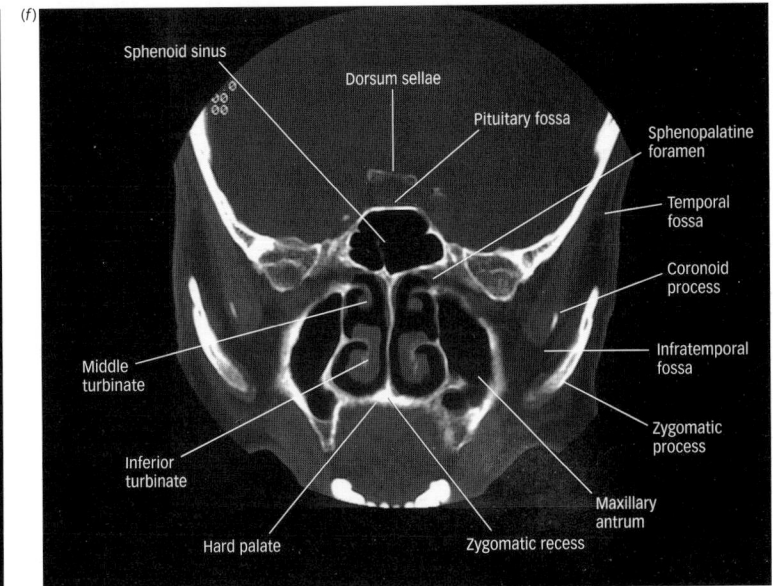

Frontal sinus

Nasal bone

(d)

Bulla
ethmoidalis

Cribriform
palate

Ethmoid
infundibulum

Uncinate
process

Ostium of
maxillary sinus

Middle
turbinate

Maxillary
antrum

Inferior meatus

Inferior turbinate

Lacrimal duct

Superior
turbinate

Middle
turbinate

Zygomatic
process

Orifice of
nasolacrimal
duct

Ethmoid infundibulum
openng into hiatus
semilunaris

Inferior
turbinate

Uncinate
process

Sphenoethmoidal
recess

Anterior
clinoid process

Planum
sphenoidale

Superior
Middle

turbinates

Superior
orbital fissure

Inferior
orbital fissure

Zygomatic
recess

Uncinate
process

Maxillary antrum

Inferior turbinate

(f)

Sphenoid sinus

Dorsum sellae

Pituitary fossa

Sphenopalatine
foramen

Temporal
fossa

Coronoid
process

Infratemporal
fossa

Zygomatic
process

Maxillary
antrum

Middle
turbinate

Inferior
turbinate

Hard palate

Zygomatic recess

mucus towards the ostia. This mucociliary escalator is the normal mechanism for clearance of the sinuses and maintenance of their aeration. The belief that ensuring a clear physiological outflow from the sinus would allow natural resolution of sinusitis forms the theoretical basis of functional endoscopic sinus surgery (FESS). This contrasts with the traditional treatment of creating additional unphysiological iatrogenic ostia low down on the medial wall.

The ethmoid sinuses comprise a group of thin-walled air cells within the ethmoid labyrinth which vary in size and in number from three to eighteen on each side. They are divided into three groups: anterior, middle and posterior, although some authors include the middle with the anterior group. The posterior group drains into the superior meatus, the remainder into the middle meatus as described above. The most anterior group, the agger nasi cells, invaginate beneath the ridge of the same name on the lateral wall of the nasal cavity anteriorly (Fig. 20 (a)), and are medial relations of the lacrimal sac and duct. Large anterior and middle cells may develop medially beneath the orbital floor and are known as Haller's cells. The ethmoid bulla contains the largest and most constant of the middle ethmoid cells.

Pneumatization may extend into the middle concha in 4–12% of individuals and into the body and wings of the sphenoid bone lateral to the sphenoid sinus.

The sphenoid sinuses develop within the body of the sphenoid bone (Figs. 7, 11, 22). The degree of pneumatization and thus the posterior extent of the sinus within the bone is highly variable. In nearly half of subjects, pneumatization extends into the greater or lesser wing or the pterygoid process. The anterior midline septum often becomes deviated to one side posteriorly and identification of this septation is important prior to trans-sphenoidal surgery. The sphenoid sinuses drain into the spheno-ethmoidal recesses, one on each side of the nasal septum. Located centrally within the skull base, the sphenoid sinuses are closely related to a number of important structures (see Chapter 2).

The oral cavity, tongue and salivary glands
The oral cavity consists of two parts: an external vestibule lying between the cheek externally and the teeth and gums internally and the buccal cavity proper. The buccal cavity is bounded by the teeth and alveolar processes and roofed by the hard and soft palates. From the soft palate the palatoglossal folds arch downwards on each side of the tongue demarcating the

posterior border of the cavity and marking the entrance to the pharynx. The floor of the buccal cavity is formed by the anterior two-thirds of the tongue, the mylohyoid muscle and the anterior 'bellies' of the digastric muscles. The mylohyoid muscles originate from the mylohyoid line of the mandible and insert on the hyoid bone. Together they are known as the 'diaphragma oris' which divides the floor of the mouth into a sublingual space superomedially and a submandibular space inferolaterally (Fig. 23).

The tongue contributes to the floor of the mouth anteriorly and the anterior wall of the pharynx posteriorly. The V-shaped sulcus terminalis marks this division on the surface. Taste buds are present in the anterior part, whereas the pharyngeal surface is covered in lymphoid tubercles giving an irregular appear-

Fig. 23.
T1W MRI of the head coronal (a), and sagittal (b), demonstrating the structures of the floor of the mouth and tongue.

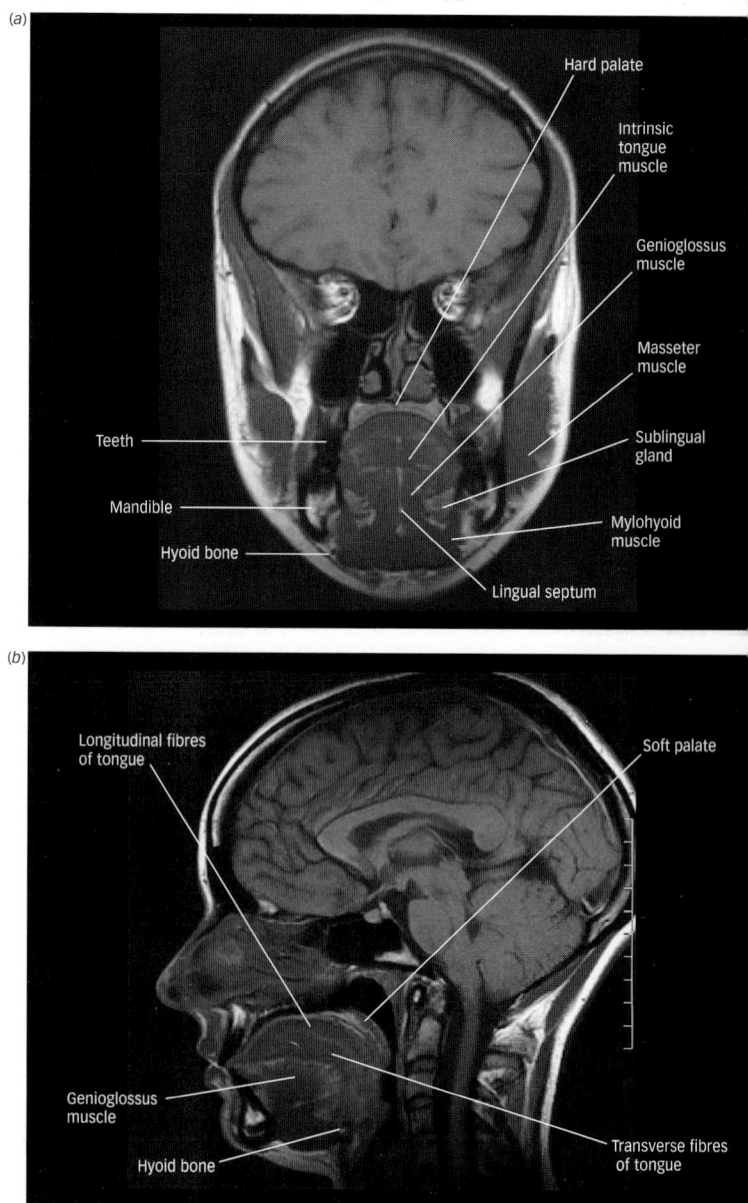

106

ance on axial images which should not be confused with superficial neoplasms. The tongue is made up of intrinsic muscles, which lie in transverse, vertical and longitudinal planes. The muscle groups are separated by fat planes which together with a midline fibro-fatty septum constitute important landmarks on CT and MRI (Fig. 24). They are reinforced by extrinsic muscles. These are: genioglossus (the largest) arising from the genial tubercle on the posterior aspect of the symphysis of the mandible; hyoglossus, arising from the hyoid body; styloglossus, arising from the styloid process; palatoglossus which lies deep to the palatoglossal fold and which arises from the soft palate. The first three of these are supplied by the hypoglossal (XIIth) nerve but palatoglossus (a palatal muscle), is supplied by the cranial part of the accessory (XIth) nerve via the vagus (Xth).

The parotid gland is the largest of the three and lies over the ramus of the mandible and masseter muscle (Fig. 25). A deep retro-mandibular portion curls around the posterior border of the mandible and forms part of the lateral margin of the parapharyngeal space (see section on parapharyngeal space). The gland is encapsulated and divided internally into lobules which vary in size. It is traversed by the facial nerve which follows the posterior belly of the digastric muscle from the skull base to enter the posterior border of the gland where it divides into its five terminal branches. The course of the nerve divides the gland by convention into superficial and deep 'lobes'. The facial nerve is not visible on CT, although its course can be traced (Fig. 25), but is sometimes visible on coronal T1W MRI as a linear low intensity structure.

Fig. 25.
Intravenous contrast-enhanced axial CT through the parotid gland. Note the typical attenuation of the adult parotid gland in (a), intermediate between fat and muscle density. In children and some adults the parotid can be nearly isodense with muscle (b) which can make identification of mass lesions difficult.

24.
V axial MRI of the floor of mouth.

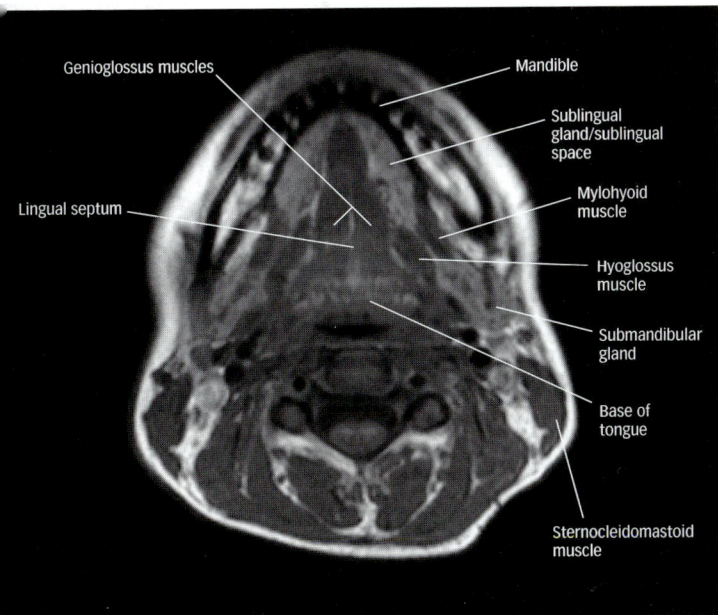

Genioglossus muscles
Lingual septum
Mandible
Sublingual gland/sublingual space
Mylohyoid muscle
Hyoglossus muscle
Submandibular gland
Base of tongue
Sternocleidomastoid muscle

(a)

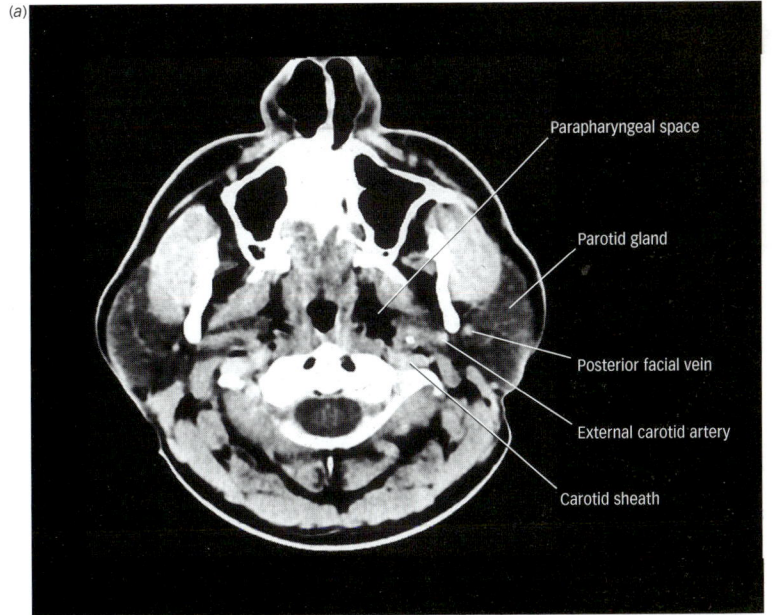

Parapharyngeal space
Parotid gland
Posterior facial vein
External carotid artery
Carotid sheath

Hypoglossus defines the lateral aspect of the tongue on axial imaging. The lingual artery courses medial to it. The hypoglossal (XIIth) nerve and lingual veins are lateral to it.

The salivary glands

The paired parotid, submandibular and sublingual glands are the major salivary glands, together with multiple minor salivary glands distributed throughout the oral and pharyngeal mucosa. Both CT and MRI are well suited for examining the morphology of the salivary glands and their relation to surrounding structures.

Sialography of the parotid and submandibular glands demonstrates their duct systems. This is normally undertaken with conventional radiography but CT sialography is occasionally performed.

(b)

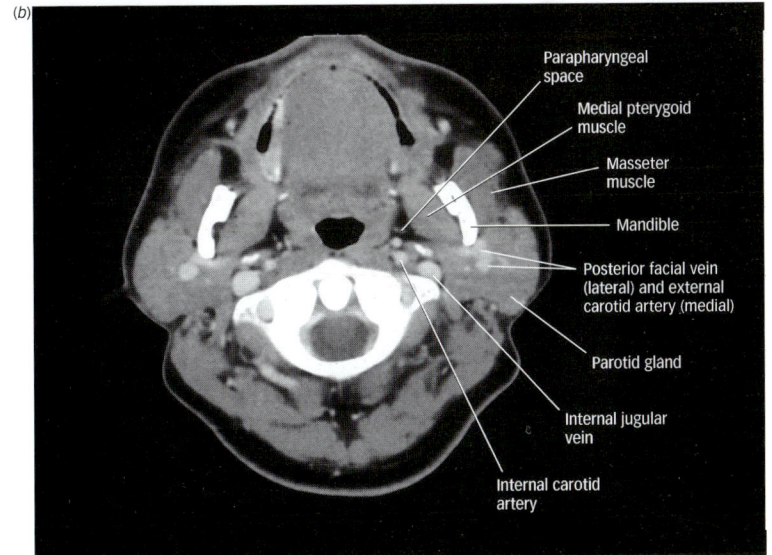

Parapharyngeal space
Medial pterygoid muscle
Masseter muscle
Mandible
Posterior facial vein (lateral) and external carotid artery (medial)
Parotid gland
Internal jugular vein
Internal carotid artery

The parotid gland produces serous secretion and has a fatty interstitial structure. The CT attenuation of the gland is between that of muscle and fat and it has a faintly inhomogeneous appearance. On MRI scans the gland is hyperintense to muscle. In children and occasionally in adults the normal gland approaches muscle attenuation or intensity. The parotid gland has lymph nodes within its substance as well as on its surface but these are not normally identified on CT or MRI.

The parotid duct (of Stenson), about 5 cm in length, emerges from the gland anteriorly. It runs forward superficial to the masseter and turns medially, piercing the buccinator to open at the vestibule opposite the second upper molar tooth. Sialography demonstrates the normal arborizing ductal pattern (Fig. 26), and the duct is also usually visible on thin-section axial CT. Accessory glandular tissue is seen along the course of the duct in 20% of subjects.

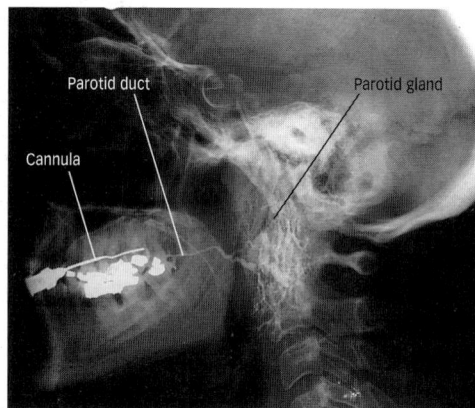

Fig. 26.
Parotid sialogram. Note the long branching ductal pattern. The tip of the cannula is adjacent to the second upper molar tooth.

Fig. 27.
Diagram of the submandibular and sublingual glands. The submandibular gland wraps around the posterior border of the mylohyoid muscle giving superficial and deep portions. Note the course of the digastric muscle which takes origin from the mastoid notch of the temporal bone, passes through a sling on the hyoid bone (which divides it into anterior and posterior bellies), to insert on the inner aspect of the mandible.

The submandibular gland is the principal structure in the submandibular space (Fig. 27). Because the gland wraps around the posterior border of the mylohyoid, its deep portion lies in the sublingual space accompanied by the submandibular duct, sublingual gland, lingual nerve and veins. Posteriorly the stylomandibular ligament separates it from the parotid

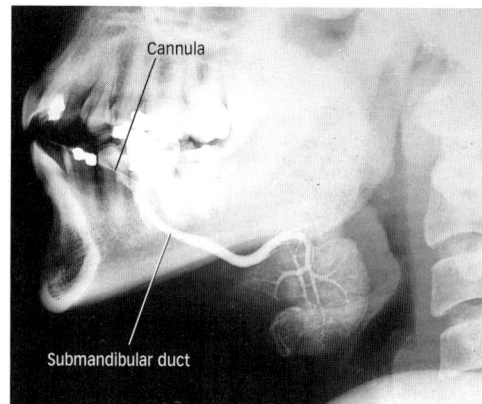

gland. The submandibular gland produces mixed serous and mucus secretions and its CT attenuation is approximately that of muscle and higher than that of the parotid gland. It actively secretes iodine and shows strong contrast enhancement.

The submandibular duct (of Wharton), like the parotid duct, is about 5 cm long and emerges anteriorly from the deep portion of the gland to run forward with the lingual nerve. It opens on the sublingual papilla on the floor of the buccal cavity (Fig. 28).

The sublingual gland is the smallest of the major salivary glands. It rests on the medial aspect of the mylohyoid muscle just anterior to the submandibular gland and just below the mucosa of the floor of the mouth. The sublingual gland produces mainly mucus secretions which drain via the ducts of Rivinius, about 20 in number, on to the sublingual papilla posterior to the orifice of the submandibular duct.

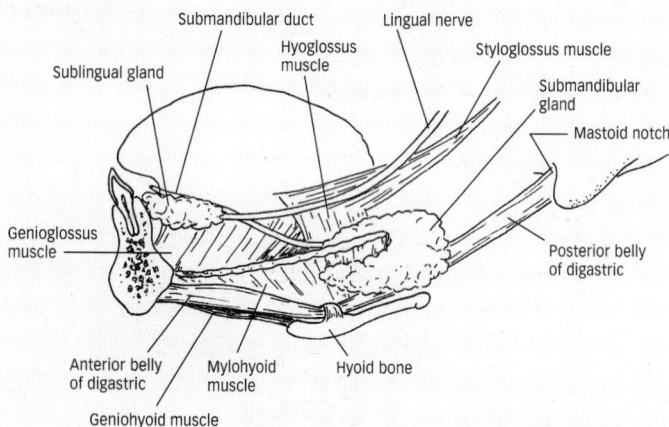

Fig. 28.
Submandibular sialogram
The duct branches are typically shorter than tho
within the parotid gland.

Some of the ducts may join to form Bartholin's duct to drain into the submandibular duct. The sublingual gland is not amenable to sialography.

The pharynx

The pharynx is a fibromuscular tube, about 14 cm long, which forms the upper part of the aerodigestive tract. It has the shape of an inverted J and extends from the base of the skull to the lower border of the cricoid cartilage at the level of the sixth cervical vertebra, where it becomes continuous with the oesophagus. It communicates with the nasal, oral and laryngeal cavities and is divided accordingly into the nasopharynx, oropharynx and laryngopharynx (Fig. 29). The prevertebral fascia and muscles are posterior to the pharynx. Its lateral relations, from above downwards are the pharyngotympanic (Eustachian) tube, the styloid process of the temporal bone and associated muscles, the carotid sheath and the thyroid gland.

The pharynx consists of mucosal, submucosal and muscular layers. The muscular layer consists of five paired muscles. The superior, middle

Fig. 29.
Diagram of the
subdivisions of
the pharynx.

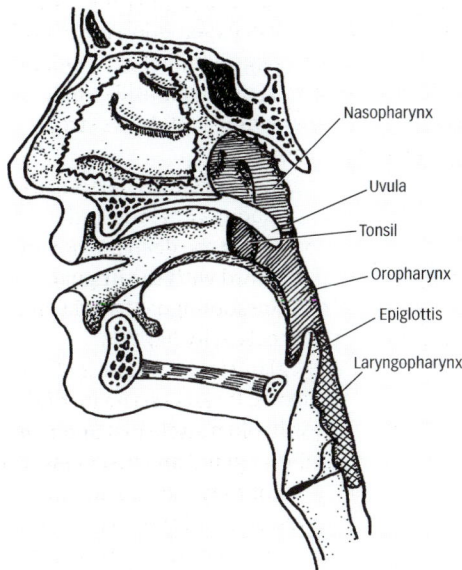

- Nasopharynx
- Uvula
- Tonsil
- Oropharynx
- Epiglottis
- Laryngopharynx

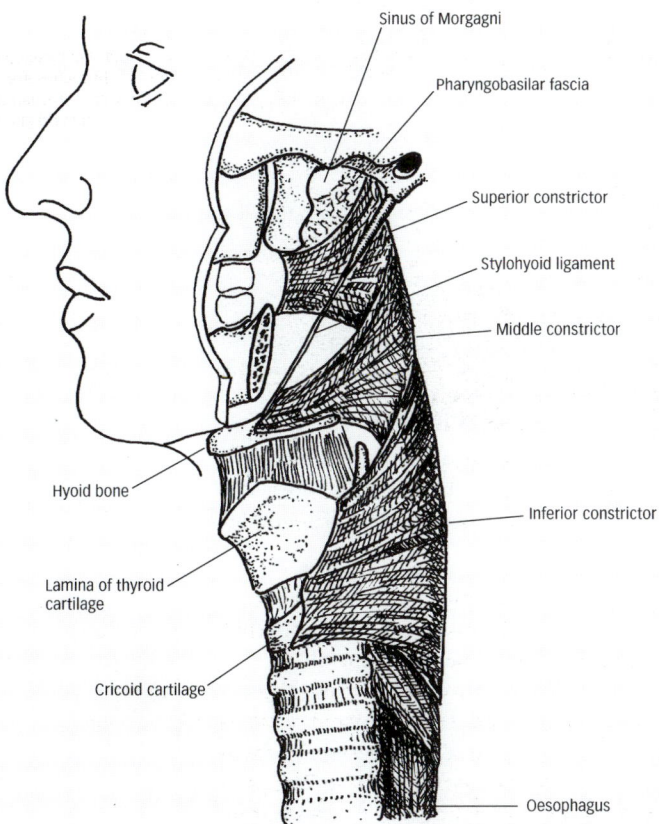

- Sinus of Morgagni
- Pharyngobasilar fascia
- Superior constrictor
- Stylohyoid ligament
- Middle constrictor
- Hyoid bone
- Inferior constrictor
- Lamina of thyroid cartilage
- Cricoid cartilage
- Oesophagus

30.
gram of the
aryngeal constrictors.
e longitudinal muscles
 not shown.

Pharyngeal morphology and adjacent structures are well shown by cross-sectional techniques while the mucosal surface is evaluated by barium studies. The major function of the pharynx is swallowing, the dynamics of which are best studied by videofluoroscopy.

The nasopharynx begins anteriorly at the nasal choanae and measures approximately 4 cm in width and 2 cm in height. Its roof slopes beneath the sphenoid bone and clivus and it is closely related to the foramina of the central skull base, accounting for the frequency of neurological involvement in invasive nasopharyngeal carcinomas (Fig. 31). The floor of the nasopharynx is formed by the hard and soft palates, the latter marking the transition to the oropharynx. The superior constrictor thins out superiorly to be replaced by pharyngobasilar fascia at the level of the nasopharynx. This fascia is deficient superiorly where the

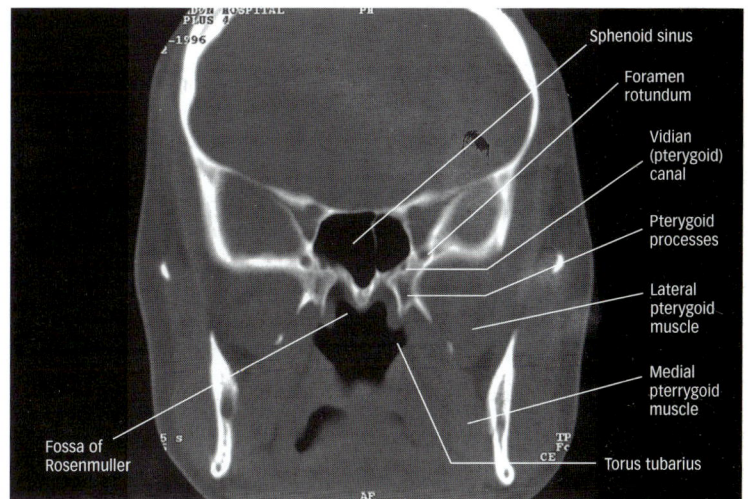

- Sphenoid sinus
- Foramen rotundum
- Vidian (pterygoid) canal
- Pterygoid processes
- Lateral pterygoid muscle
- Medial pterrygoid muscle
- Torus tubarius
- Fossa of Rosenmuller

Fig. 31.
Coronal CT through the nasopharynx showing the pharyngeal recesses. Also demonstrated are the foramen rotundum superolaterally, and the vidian canal linking the pterygopalatine fossa and the foramen lacerum, inferomedially.

and inferior constrictors form an outer circular coat, and the stylo- and palatopharyngeus contribute an inner longitudinal coat (Fig. 30).

The three pairs of constrictor muscles fan out from their anterior attachments to meet in the midline posteriorly in a fibrous raphe which is attached superiorly to the occipital bone and inferiorly to the oesophagus. The muscle coat is deficient superiorly and is replaced by the pharyngobasilar fascia, which extends from the superior constrictor to the base of the skull.

sinus of Morgagni serves as a potential conduit for neoplastic or inflammatory processes to reach the skull base.

The auditory tube anteriorly and levator palatini muscle posteriorly pass through the sinus of Morgagni, whilst more posteriorly still, the pharyngeal mucosa herniates outwards through the fascial defect to form the lateral recess, or fossa of Rosenmuller (the site of origin of up to 50% of nasopharyngeal carcinomas). These structures produce the characteristic appearance of the lateral nasopharyngeal wall on axial CT and MRI scans (Fig. 31), with bilateral paired recesses separated by the ridge of the levator palatini muscle. On coronal scans the fossa of Rosenmuller appears superior to the cartilaginous opening of the auditory tube, known as the torus tubarius (Fig. 32).

The adenoids, or pharyngeal tonsils, are collections of lymphatic tissue in the recesses of the nasopharynx. They atrophy progressively after puberty but small remnants may persist

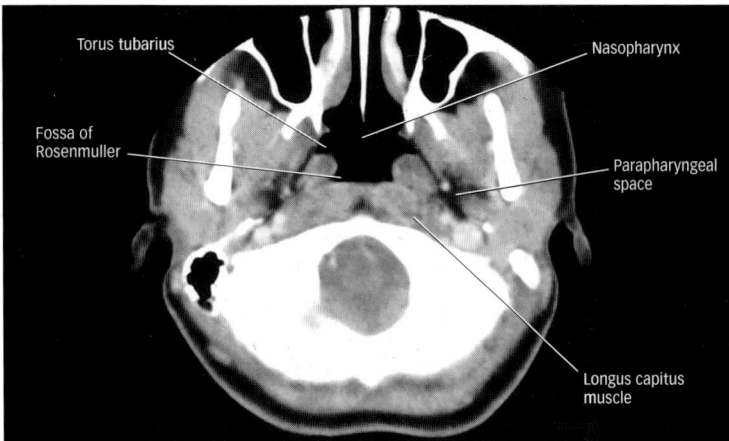

Fig. 32.
Axial CT of the nasopharynx showing the pharyngeal recesses. Note the fatty triangle of the parapharyngeal space.

into adulthood. In young patients normal adenoidal tissue may fill and obliterate the fossa of Rosenmuller, whilst in the elderly these recesses may normally appear shallow because of loss of muscle bulk.

The oropharynx extends from the nasopharynx to the upper border of the epiglottis inferiorly which, in turn, marks the upper limit of the laryngopharynx. The buccal cavity lies anteriorly, with the posterior third of the tongue forming the anterior wall of the oropharynx. Two folds of mucous membrane (the faucial pillars) arch downwards from the soft palate on each side. These are the palatoglossal fold anteriorly, which separates the oral cavity from the oropharynx, and the palatopharyngeal fold. Between the two folds are the palatine tonsils. The tonsils and faucial pillars together appear as symmetrical soft tissue densities on either side of the airway on CT. Both tonsils and adenoids appear slightly hyperintense to muscle on T1W MRI scans and markedly hyperintense on T2W images.

The laryngopharynx extends from the upper border of the epiglottis to the oesophagus at the level of the sixth cervical vertebra. The laryngeal opening or aditus lies anteriorly, roofed by the epiglottis. On each side of the laryngeal aditus the cavity extends forwards to form the piriform fossa which form the laryngopharynx. Each fossa is limited laterally by the thyroid cartilage. The inferior constrictor forms the posterior and lateral walls of the laryngopharynx and consists of two parts. The fibres of the upper portion or thyropharyngeus run obliquely and those of the lower portion or cricopharyngeus are oriented more horizontally. Between these two groups of fibres posteriorly is a potentially weak area known as Killian's dehiscence through which a pharyngeal pouch (Zenker's diverticulum), may protrude.

The pharyngeal lumen is narrowest at its junction with the oesophagus at the site of the cricopharyngeus, which forms the upper

oesophageal sphincter. Cricopharyngeal incoordination during swallowing is common in the elderly and may result in the smooth posterior indentation at the C 5/6 level commonly observed at barium swallow studies. A mucosal irregularity seen anteriorly, also at the level of the cricoid cartilage, is produced by the cricoid venous plexus.

The fascial layers of the neck and the parapharyngeal space
Traditional surgical anatomy recognizes a number of muscular triangles of the neck, (Fig. 33), but cross-sectional imaging, in contrast, emphasizes the importance of the deep, fascia-lined spaces of the head and neck. The potential spaces defined by the fascial layers are illustrated in Fig. 34 and their contents are summarized in Table 2.

Fig. 33.
Diagram of the muscular triangles of the neck.

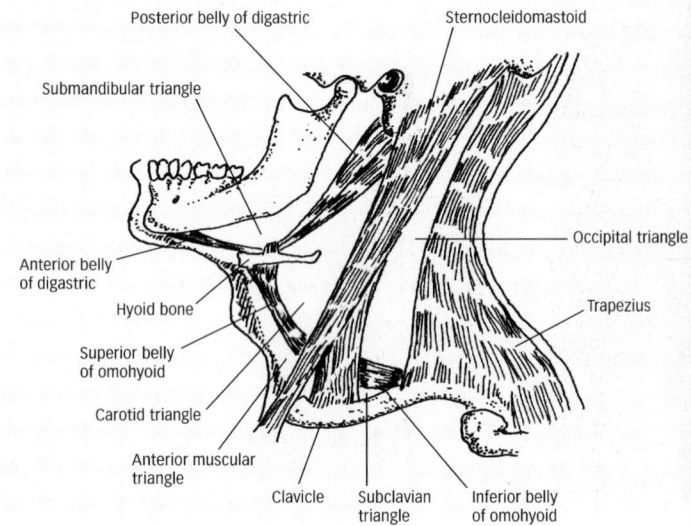

(a)

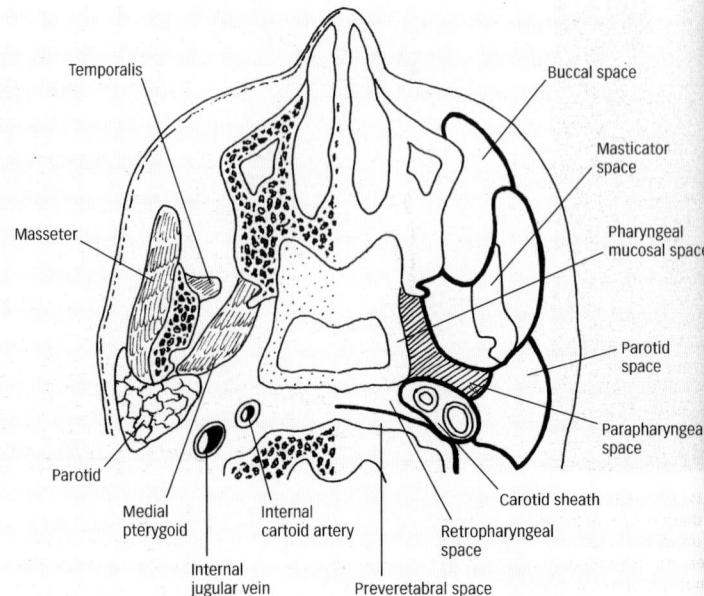

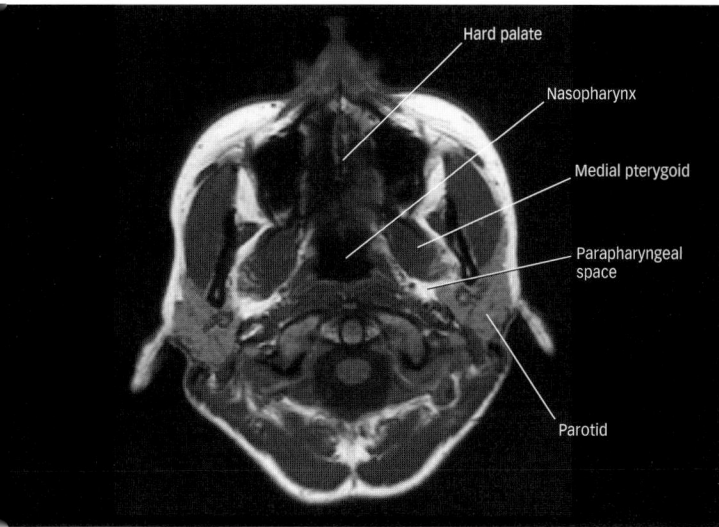

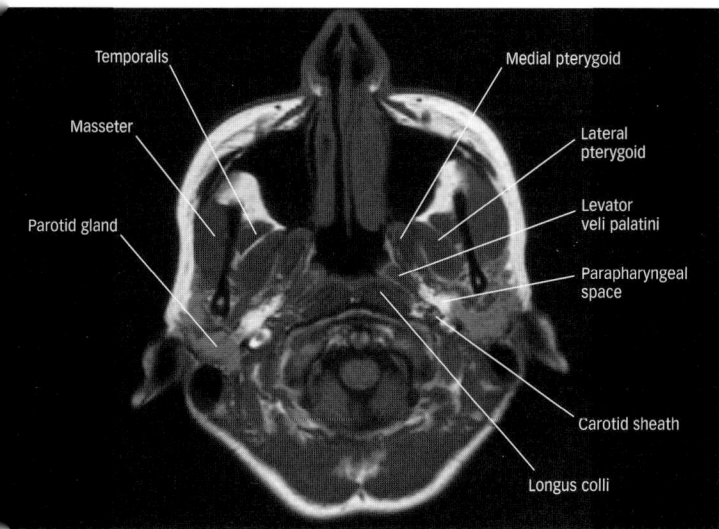

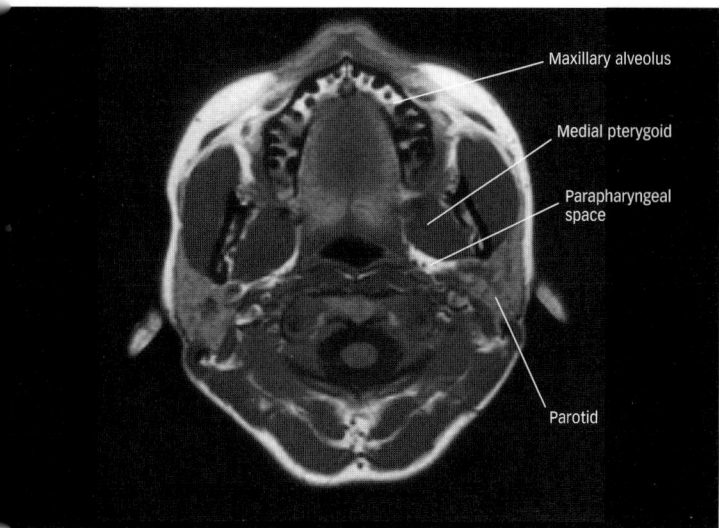

The fascial layers form a barrier against the spread of inflammatory or neoplastic disease which may thus be contained or localized within them.

The fascia of the neck are divided into superficial and deep layers. The superficial cervical fascia is a subcutaneous layer that completely encircles the head and neck and extends inferiorly to the thorax. The deep cervical fascia is further divided into three layers which, although they cannot be visualized directly by cross-sectional imaging, define the deep spaces of the head and neck. The superficial or investing layer of the deep cervical fascia encircles all the deep structures except the platysma and superficial lymph nodes. It envelops the parotid and submandibular salivary glands and extends inferiorly to the clavicles, sternum and scapulae. The middle or visceral layer lies deep to the anterior strap muscles (omohyoid, sternohyoid, sternothyroid and thyrohyoid). It surrounds the thyroid gland, contributes to the carotid sheath and invests the trachea and oesophagus. Its posterior portion forms the anterior border of the retropharyngeal space and inferiorly it fuses with the deep layer.

The deep or prevertebral layer surrounds the vertebrae, paraspinal muscles and brachial plexus. It extends from the skull base to the superior mediastinum, where it fuses with the middle layer and merges with the carotid sheath and aortic adventitia. The carotid sheath receives contributions from all three layers of the deep fascia.

The parapharyngeal space is easily recognized on both CT and MRI as a fatty triangle (Fig. 34). It is unusual for disease processes to arise in the parapharyngeal space itself and its main diagnostic importance is in the characteristic manner in which it is infiltrated, displaced or distorted by surrounding masses (Babbel & Harnsberger, 1990).

The larynx

The larynx forms the superior part of the lower respiratory tract and lies anterior to the laryngopharynx at the levels of the third and sixth cervical vertebrae. It consists of a cartilaginous skeleton (Fig. 35), within which lie the intrinsic muscles and the vocal folds covered by mucosa and submucosa. The laryngeal aditus projects into the pharynx, with its upper, anterior border formed by the epiglottis. The leaf-like epiglottis arises from the posterior surface of the thyroid cartilage and is separated from the back of the tongue by paired depressions, the valleculae, situated either side of the median glossoepiglottic fold. The piriform fossa of the laryngopharynx is interposed between the

TABLE 2

Main contents of the fascial spaces of the face and upper neck

Parapharyngeal space
Fat
Maxillary artery
Ascending pharyngeal artery
Pharyngeal venous plexus
Mandibular nerve branches

Masticator space
Medial pterygoid muscle
Lateral pterygoid muscle
Masseter muscle
Temporalis muscle
Inferior alveolar nerve
Mandible

Parotid space
Parotid gland
Facial nerve
External carotid artery
Maxillary artery
Lymph nodes

Carotid space
Internal carotid artery
Internal jugular vein
CNs IX, X, XI and XII
Sympathetic plexus
Lymph nodes

Buccal space
Buccal fat pad
Facial artery
Facial vein
Parotid duct (terminal portion)
Buccinator muscle

Pharyngeal mucosal space
Pharyngeal constrictors
Extrinsic muscles of pharynx
Pharyngobasilar fascia
Lymphoid tissue, adenoids, tonsils
Torus tubarius

Retropharyngeal space
Fat
Retropharygeal lymph nodes

Prevertebral space
Prevertebral muscles
Vertebral artery and veins
Phrenic nerve
Brachial plexus
Scalene muscles

34. (*left and above*) deep spaces of the face upper neck. (*a*) *left* ematic diagram through nasopharynx showing deep spaces of the face

on the right and some of their contents on the left. The central position of the parapharyngeal space (shaded) is emphasized.

(*b*)–(*d*) *above* contiguous axial T1W MRI from superior to inferior demonstrating the high-signal fatty triangle of the parapharyngeal space.

lateral border of the aditus (the aryepiglottic fold) and the thyroid cartilage on each side.

The lower border of the cricoid cartilage forms the inferior limit of the larynx. The cricoid cartilage is in the shape of a signet ring and bears articular facets on its posterosuperior surface for the paired arytenoid cartilages. Each arytenoid cartilage is pyramidal in shape with medial, posterior and anterolateral surfaces. Its base overlies the cricoid cartilage. The arytenoids are capable of rotational and gliding movements which alter the tension of the vocal cords and the shape of the glottis. Phonating a high pitched 'eee' will cause adduction of the cords.

The cricoid cartilage also articulates with the thyroid cartilage as well as with the arytenoid cartilages. These joints are synovial and are therefore susceptible to systemic arthropathies.

The posterior margins of the vocal cords are attached to the anterior vocal processes of the arytenoids, which are therefore useful landmarks on axial CT to identify the vocal folds. The interior of the larynx is marked by the parallel horizontal bands of the true vocal cords inferiorly, and the vestibular folds or false

Fig. 35. (a)
Diagram of the cartilaginous skeleton of the larynx
(a) **external view**
(b) **cutaway view.**

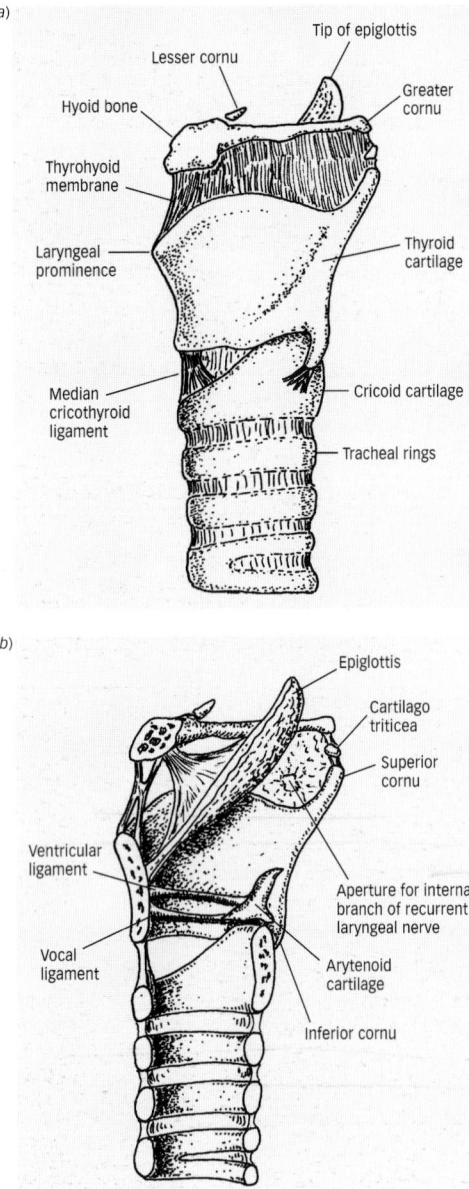

Fig. 36.
Axial CT of the larynx from superior to inferior. (a) CT a level of hyoid bone showin tip of epiglottis and the valleculae anteriorly. Note the piriform fossae are below the level of the valleculae and are

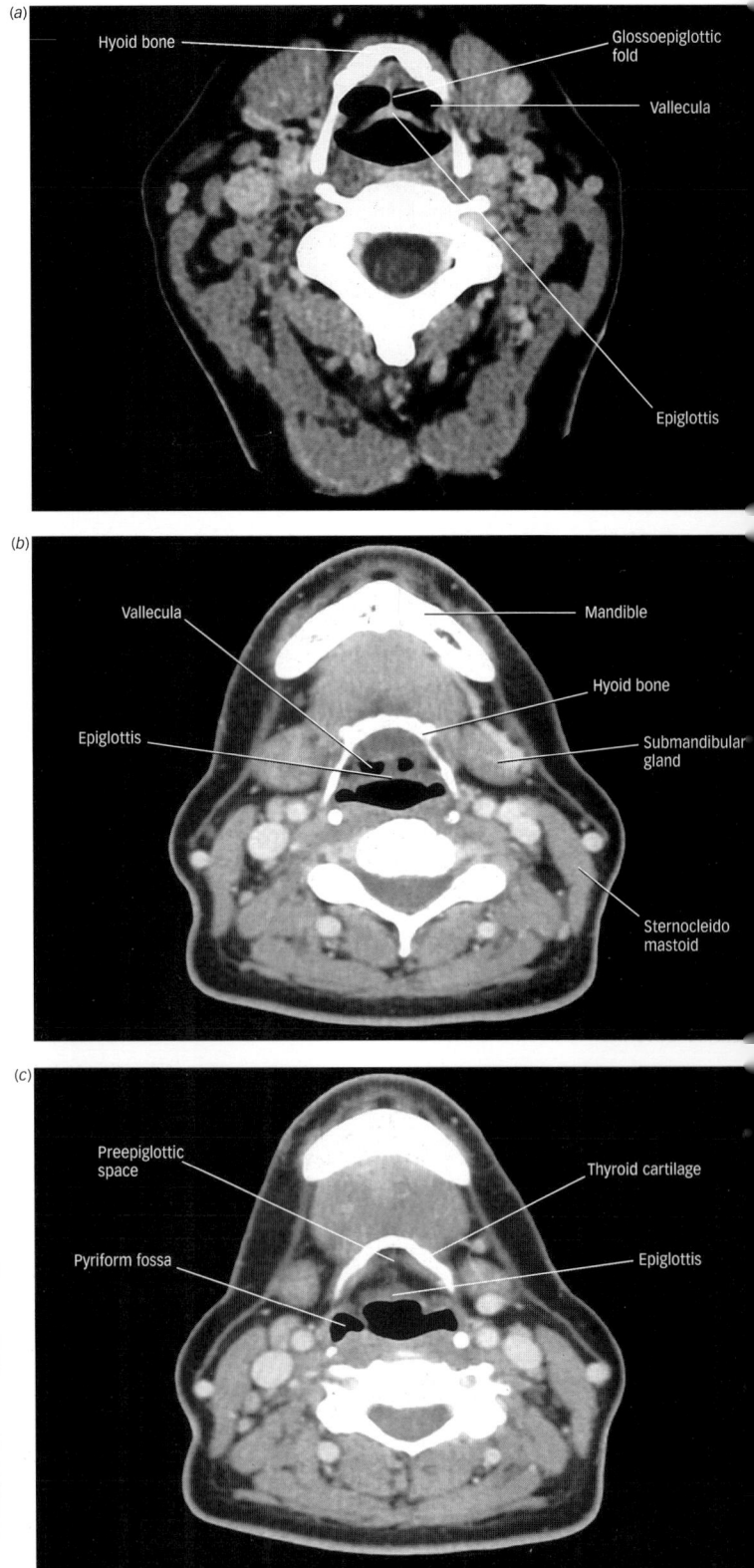

ominent laterally on
–(f). Note also the
rmally fatty pre-
iglottic and paraglottic
aces and that the fat is
placed by the glottic
uscles at the level of the
ottis.

cords superiorly. Between these is the slit like cavity of the laryngeal sinus (ventricle). Both CT and MRI demonstrate the fatty spaces of the larynx (Fig. 36). Of these, the paraglottic (or paralaryngeal) spaces lie deep to the false and true cords. It should be noted that the para-glottic space terminates at the upper border of the cricoid cartilage so that normally there is no soft tissue within the cricoid ring. The fat-containing pre-epiglottic space lies between the epiglottis and the hyoid bone. The relationships of the true and false cords are well seen in the coronal plane, on soft tissue radiographs and MRI scans (Fig. 37).

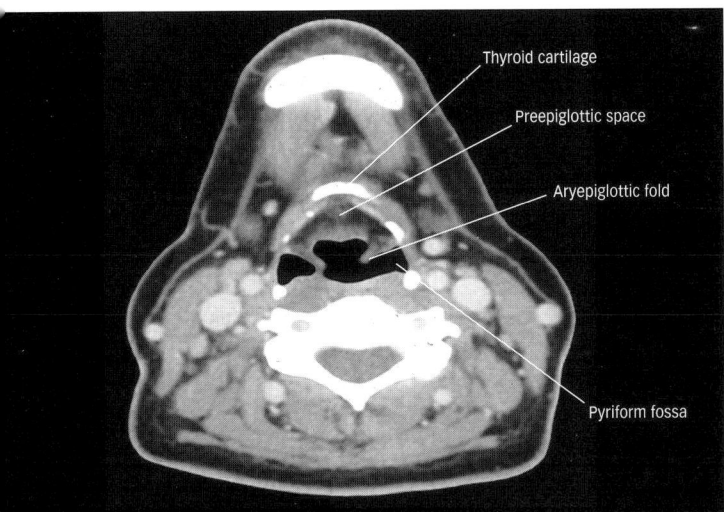

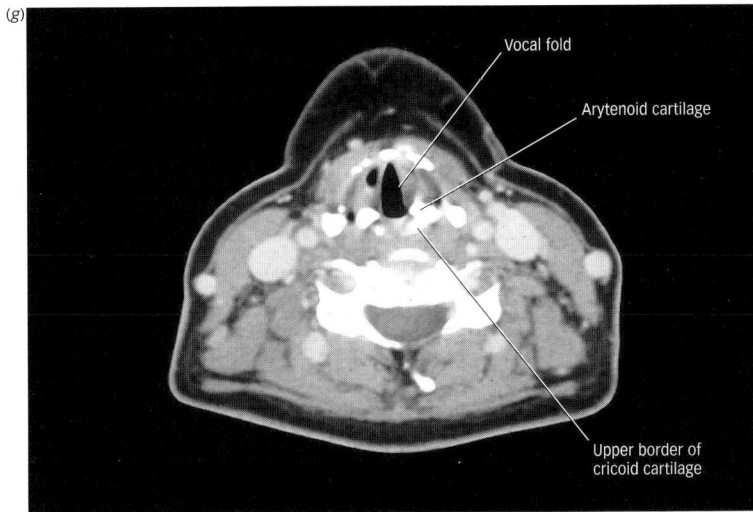

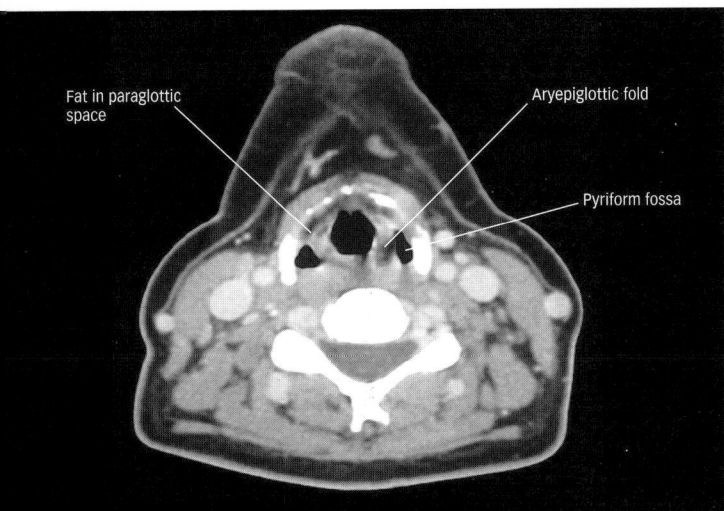

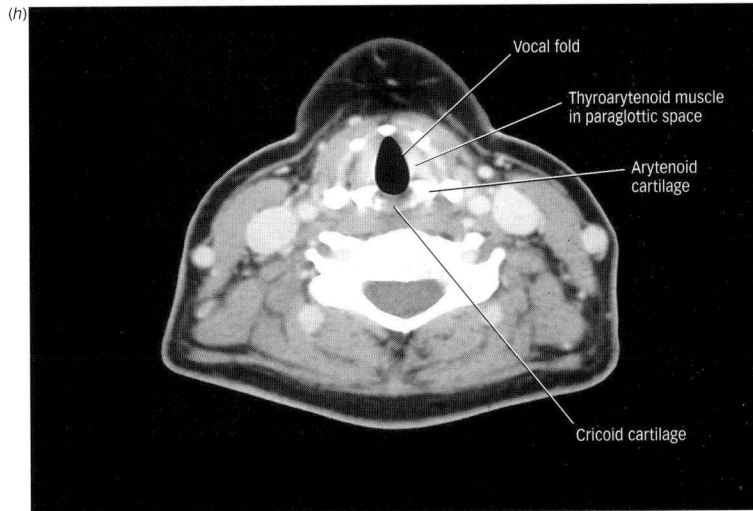

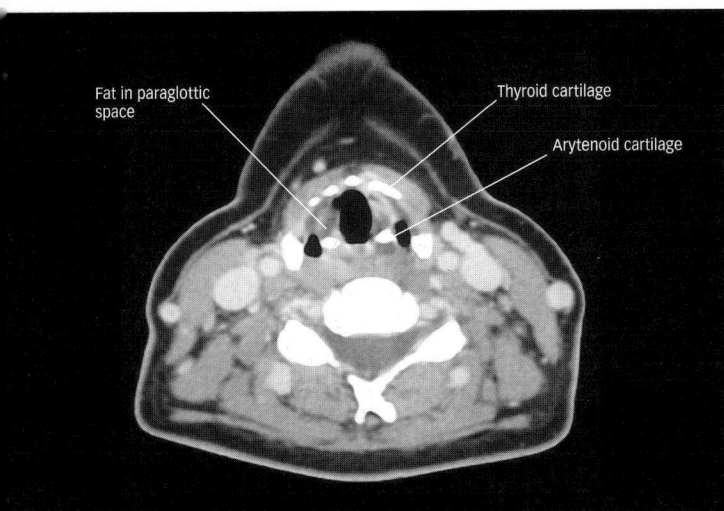

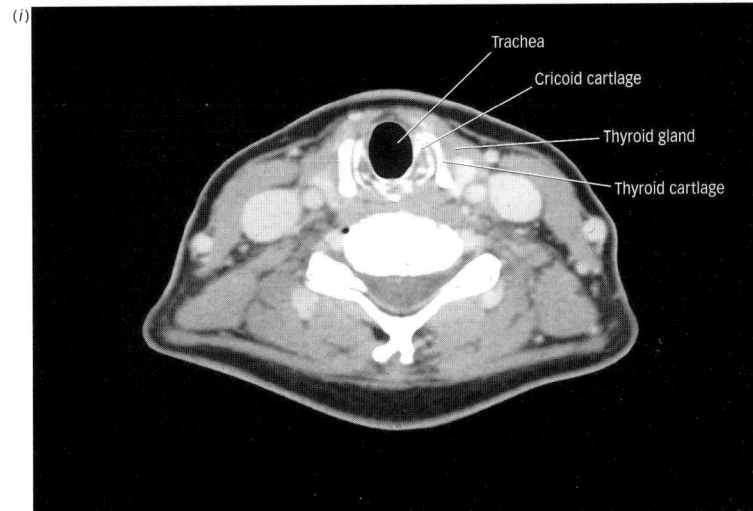

(g)

(h)

(i)

Fig. 37. (a)
**Coronal views of the larynx
(a) soft tissue radiograph
and (b) T1W MRI.**

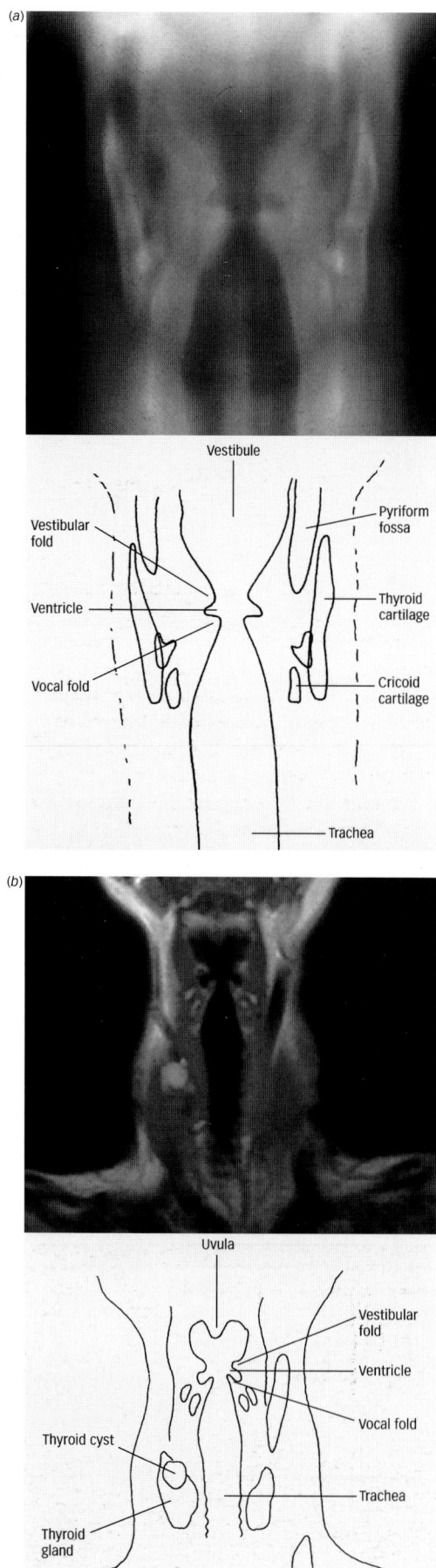

Vestibule

Vestibular
fold

Pyriform
fossa

Ventricle

Thyroid
cartilage

Vocal fold

Cricoid
cartilage

Trachea

(b)

Uvula

Vestibular
fold

Ventricle

Thyroid cyst

Vocal fold

Thyroid
gland

Trachea

Thyroid and parathyroid glands

The two lobes of the thyroid gland lie on either side of the trachea linked anteriorly by an isthmus from which a small midline pyramidal lobe may extend superiorly in 40% of subjects (Fig. 38). The gland is enclosed by the visceral layer of deep cervical fascia and covered anteriorly by the strap muscles. The gland shows great individual variation in size and is relatively larger in women and children. The right lobe is often slightly larger and more vascular than the left and tends to enlarge more in diffuse disorders. The follicular nature of the thyroid is not resolved by current imaging techniques and it thus presents a relatively homogeneous texture. Its superficial location makes the thyroid gland an ideal organ for sonographic examination (Fig. 39).

Radionuclide imaging may be performed with [Tc^{99m}] pertechnetate. This readily available radionuclide is trapped by the thyroid in the same way as iodine, but is not organified. It yields morphological information and will reveal the presence of ectopic thyroid tissue (Fig. 40). Functional data can be obtained with the use of ^{123}Iodine which is both trapped and organified.

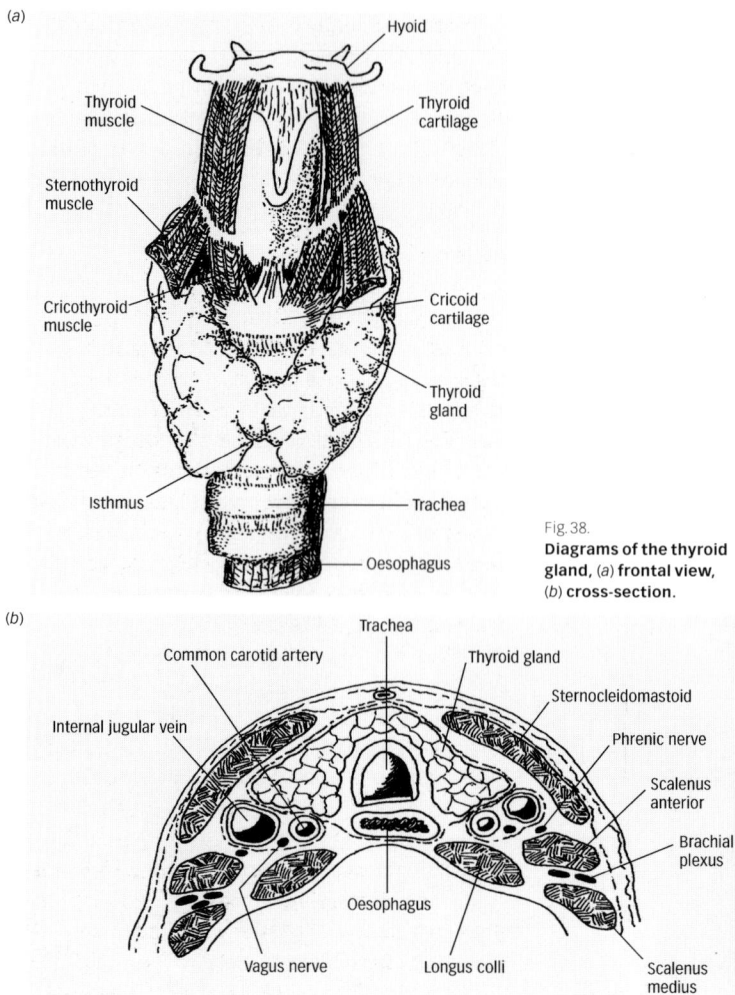

(a)

Hyoid

Thyroid
muscle

Thyroid
cartilage

Sternothyroid
muscle

Cricothyroid
muscle

Cricoid
cartilage

Thyroid
gland

Isthmus

Trachea

Oesophagus

Fig. 38.
**Diagrams of the thyroid
gland, (a) frontal view,
(b) cross-section.**

(b)

Trachea

Common carotid artery

Thyroid gland

Sternocleidomastoid

Internal jugular vein

Phrenic nerve

Scalenus
anterior

Brachial
plexus

Oesophagus

Vagus nerve

Longus colli

Scalenus
medius

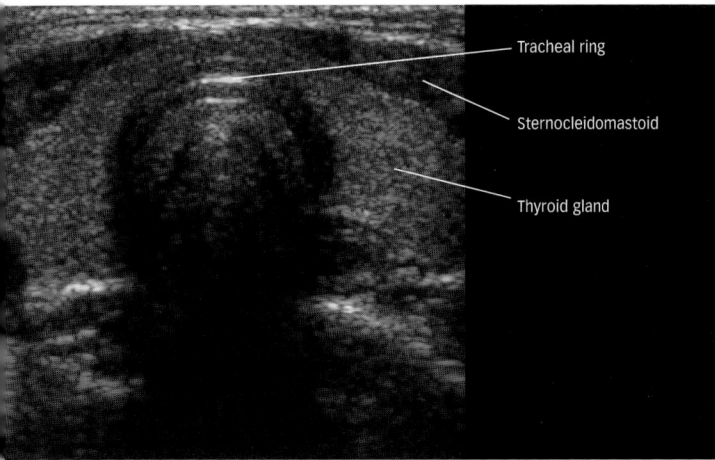

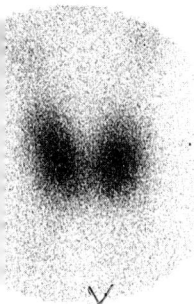

The thyroid gland is highly vascular and demonstrates intense contrast enhancement on CT and MRI (Fig. 42). Its blood supply derives from the external carotid and the thyrocervical trunk (a branch of the subclavian artery), via the paired superior and inferior thyroid arteries, respectively. Occasionally, a small branch may arise from the brachiocephalic artery (or the aortic arch) to supply the inferior portion of the right lower lobe (the thyroidea ima).

There are usually four parathyroid glands, embedded in the capsule of the thyroid gland. There are superior and inferior pairs. Each gland is ovoid and measures 5–6 mm across. The glands are very flattened in cross-section and are not normally visible by current imaging methods, including scintigraphy.

The craniocervical lymphatic system

Normal cervical lymph nodes are not readily identified by CT or MRI, but when seen, are of homogeneous soft tissue density or intensity respectively and are generally considered enlarged if greater than 1.5 cm in the sub-mandibular region, or in the jugulodigastric group of the internal jugular chain. Nodes elsewhere in the neck are considered abnormal if larger than 1 cm. With nearly 300 lymph nodes concentrated in a relatively small area, there is a complex relationship between the different nodal groups and a number of classifications exist. Broadly, however, there is a circular chain of nodes around the base of the skull, encompassing the occiptal, parotid, submandibular and submental regions (Fig. 41). Efferent vessels from these pass to the deep cervical chain around the internal jugular vein. The upper part of this chain extends medially to include the retropharyngeal nodes. Its lower part extends laterally to embrace the supra-clavicular nodes. Of the deep cervical chain, the jugulodigastric node, behind the angle of the mandible, is notable as it drains the tonsil

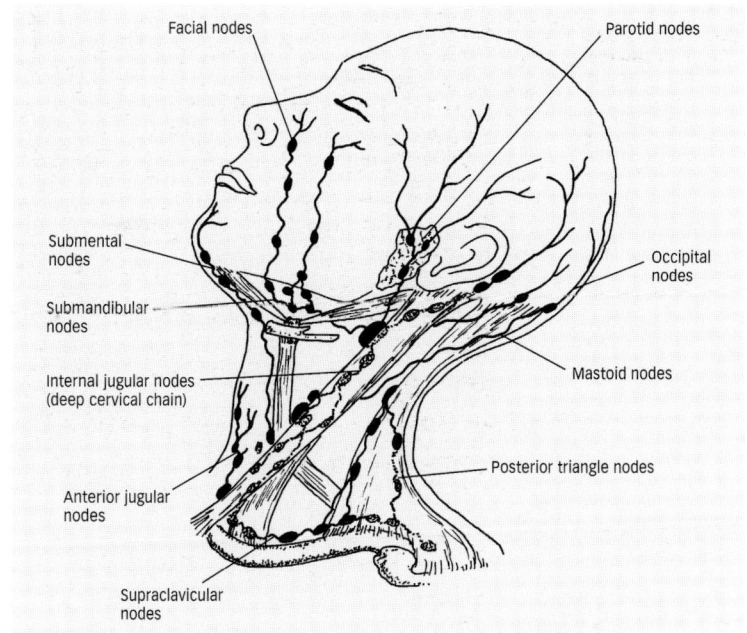

and the lymphatic drainage of the tongue converges on the jugulo-omohyoid node.

The deep cervical group serves as the common route for drainage of all the main structures from the nasopharynx above the thyroid below. There is also a chain of nodes around the spinal accessory nerve within the posterior triangle of the neck.

Lymph drainage is ultimately via the jugular trunks into the thoracic duct on the left and either into the right lymphatic duct or directly into the junction of the subclavian and internal jugular veins on the right.

The cervical arteries

The right common carotid artery arises from the brachiocephalic artery behind the right sternoclavicular joint. The left common carotid artery arises directly from the aortic arch and therefore, unlike the right, has thoracic as well as cervical portions. Both common carotid arteries are enclosed within the carotid sheath with the internal jugular vein laterally (Fig. 42) and the vagus nerve situated between artery and vein and lying posterior to both.

Fig. 41.
Diagram of the cervical lymph nodes.

Fig. 42.
Intravenous contrast-enhanced CT of the neck at the level of the C7 vertebra. The thyroid gland shows intense enhancement. Posterolaterally lie the carotid sheaths. The vertebral vessels have not yet entered the foramen transversarium.

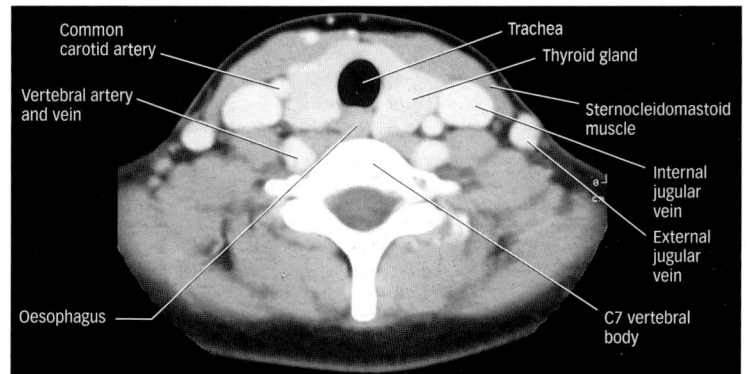

The common carotid artery divides into its internal and external branches at the level of the fourth cervical vertebra which also corresponds to the upper border of the thyroid cartilage (Fig. 43). The external carotid artery, the smaller of the two terminal branches lies initially anteromedial to the internal carotid artery.

The external carotid artery, about 7 to 8 cm in length and 8 mm in diameter ascends, coursing posterolaterally to divide into its two terminal branches, the superficial temporal and maxillary arteries within the parotid gland at the level of the neck of the mandible (Figs. 43, 44, Chapter 2, Fig. 19).

The external carotid artery supplies the upper cervical organs, facial structures, scalp and dura. With the development of therapeutic angiography, the detailed anatomy of the external carotid artery and its branches has assumed greater importance. Traditionally, eight branches are described, but individual variation is common and it is more accurate to state that there are between four and twelve branches. Many anastomoses exist between the branches of the external carotid artery; between those of the internal and external carotid arteries and between those of the external carotid artery and vertebral artery.

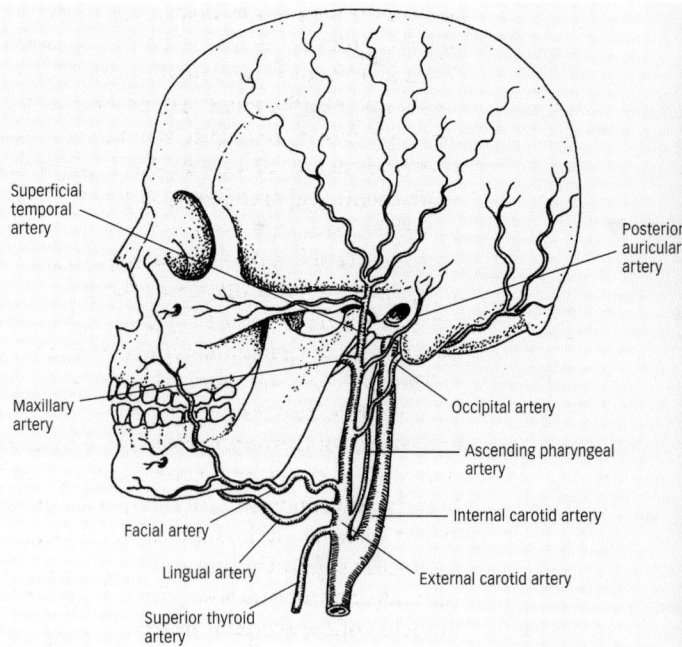

Fig. 44.
Diagram of the external carotid artery and its branches.

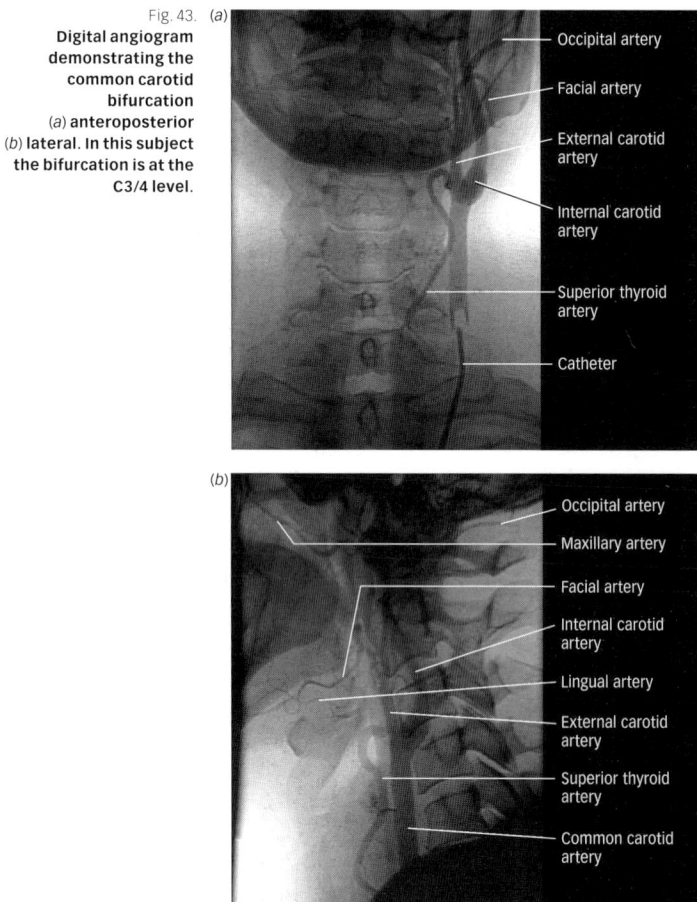

Fig. 43. (a)
Digital angiogram demonstrating the common carotid bifurcation (a) anteroposterior (b) lateral. In this subject the bifurcation is at the C3/4 level.

The main branches are described in the usual order in which they arise.

The superior thyroid artery arises anteriorly and descends to the superior pole of the thyroid. It supplies the thyroid and parathyroid glands, the pharynx, larynx and infrahyoid muscles.

The ascending pharyngeal artery, a small posterior branch, ascends between the internal and external carotid arteries on the posterolateral wall of the pharynx to supply the pharynx, tonsil, soft palate and auditory tube. It also sends branches to the meninges, middle ear and lower cranial nerves. It participates in extensive anastomoses with other branches of the external carotid artery and also with cavernous branches of the internal carotid artery and meningeal branches of the vertebral artery. It is commonly involved in craniofacial vascular lesions and, in spite of its small size, is of great importance in interventional radiology.

The lingual artery arises anteriorly and has a characteristic U-shaped upward curve. It passes forwards deep to the hyoglossus to supply the tongue. Branches also supply the submandibular gland and pharynx. In 20% of subjects, the lingual artery shares a common origin with the facial artery, forming a linguofacial trunk.

The facial artery arises just superior to the lingual. Following a tortuous course anteriorly, it crosses the inferior border of the mandible, then passes across the cheek to the nose, finally anastomosing with branches of the ophthalmic artery to form another important connection between the external and internal carotid arteries.

The occipital artery arises posteriorly. It travels backwards initially with the posterior belly of the digastric muscle and grooves the medial border of the mastoid process. It then follows a tortuous course to the occiput, supplying the upper part of the posterior neck, the skull and scalp. It may anastomose with branches of the vertebral artery, and also sends meningeal branches to the dura of the posterior fossa.

The posterior auricular artery, often not visible angiographically, arises above the occipital artery. This small vessel supplies the parotid gland, auricle and tympanic cavity.

The superficial temporal artery is the smaller of the two terminal branches of the external carotid artery. Crossing the posterior part of the zygomatic arch, its transverse facial branches anastomose with those of the facial artery. Branches of the superficial temporal artery also supply the anterior two-thirds of the scalp, and anastomose posteriorly with branches of the occipital artery.

The maxillary artery passes anteriorly from the parotid gland through the infra temporal fossa. It usually crosses the lateral surface of the lateral pterygoid muscle, passing deep to the temporalis muscle and enters the pterygopala-tine fossa to divide into its 15 terminal branches anterior to the pterygopalatine ganglion.

The maxillary artery is divided into three portions (Fig. 45). The largest branch of the first part, and of the whole vessel, is the middle meningeal artery which at first ascends almost vertically passing through the foramen spin-osum then turning horizontally as it enters the middle cranial fossa. Thereafter, it follows a wide upward curve, convex forwards and its relatively straight branches are easily dis-tinguished from the corkscrewing superficial temporal artery branches overlying it on the

45.
maxillary artery its branches.

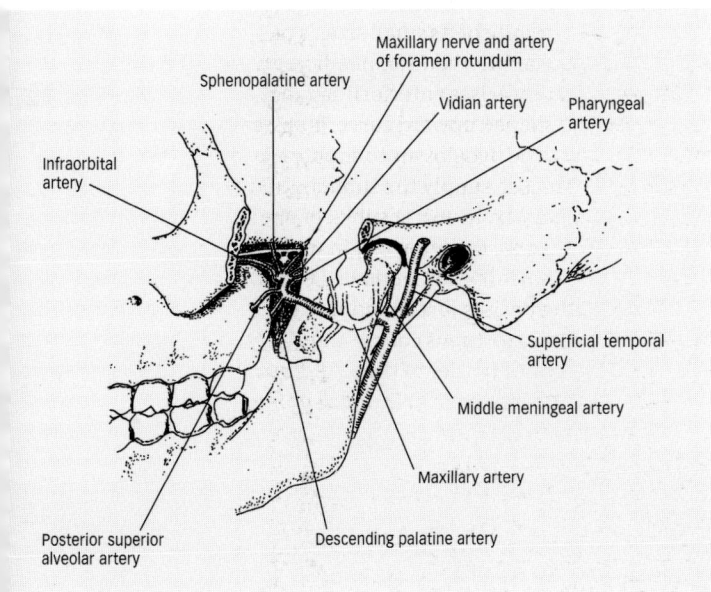

lateral angiogram. Its anterior division runs medial to the pterion and may be damaged by skull fractures to produce an extradural haematoma. The accessory meningeal artery, arising from either the maxillary or middle meningeal artery, traverses the foramen ovale and sends branches to the trigeminal ganglion. Small branches of the meningeal arteries may anastomose with cavernous branches of the internal carotid and with the ophthalmic arteries.

Branches arising from the second part of the maxillary artery supply the muscles of mastication. Of this group, the anterior deep temporal artery anastomoses with orbital vessels forming another potential external to internal carotid arterial connection.

The third part of the maxillary artery divides in the pterygopalatine fossa, its branches passing through the adjoining bony canals. The sphenopalatine artery, effectively the terminal part of the maxillary artery, passes through the foramen of the same name to supply the nasal cavity. Posterior branches traverse the foramen rotundum and the vidian (pterygoid) canals to enter the skull vault with other branches supplying the pharynx and adjacent structures. The anterior branches outline the maxillary sinus and supply adjacent structures including the maxilla, palate and orbit.

The vertebral artery is the first branch of the subclavian artery and travels through the foramina transversaria of the sixth to the third cervical vertebra. It then travels superolaterally to reach the foramen transversarium of the axis vertebra and then superiorly again through the foramen transversarium of the atlas. From the foramen transversarium the vertebral artery curves posteriorly around the atlanto-occipital joint and courses anteriorly, medially and superiorly to the vertebrobasilar junction, entering the skull through the foramen magnum (Fig. 46).

The vertebral artery sends branches to the cervical musculature and contributes to both the anterior and posterior spinal arteries.

Duplex sonography of the cervical arteries
Ultrasound examination of the carotid verte-bral arteries is a non-invasive procedure per-formed to identify, and to assess the severity of, cervical arterial narrowing in patients with suspected cerebral ischaemia.

The term 'duplex sonography' indicates that the examination has two components. The first of these, the B-mode study, provides images of the artery and is also used to study the morphology and extent of atheromatous deposits within the arterial lumen. The wall of

Fig. 46.
Vertebral angiography.
(a) Origin of the left
vertebral artery
(b), (c) anteroposterior and
(d), (e) lateral views of the
cervical portion of
the vertebral artery.
Note the muscular
branches, branches to
the anterior spinal artery
and the anastomoses
with the occipital artery.

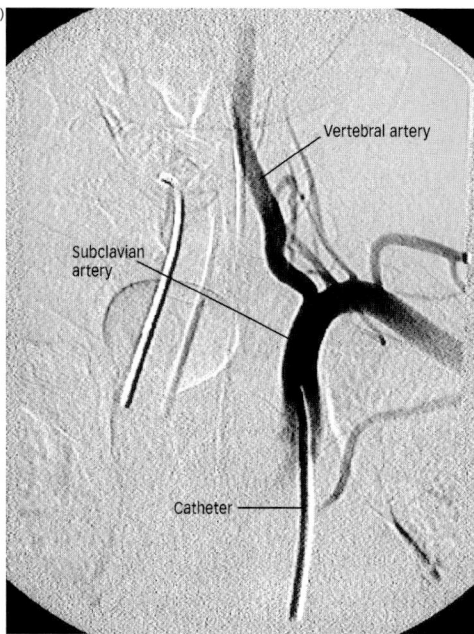

(a)

Vertebral artery

Subclavian artery

Catheter

the normal carotid artery produces two parallel echoes which correspond to the intima and adventitia with an intervening echolucent strip representing the media (Fig. 47).

The second element of duplex sonography is the Doppler flow study which is used to measure the velocity of blood flowing through the artery, its direction and flow characteristics. The results are displayed as a waveform (Fig. 48).

In the systemic arteries, flow is pulsatile and rapid, resulting in so-called 'plug flow' when velocity is uniform across the lumen. The frictional drag effect from the walls is negligible. This leads to a sharply defined waveform beneath which is the spectral window.

The internal carotid artery supplies a capacitance circulation with low total peripheral resistance. Blood flow is therefore seen to continue throughout the cardiac cycle and peak systolic velocity in the normal vessel should not exceed 110 cm per second.

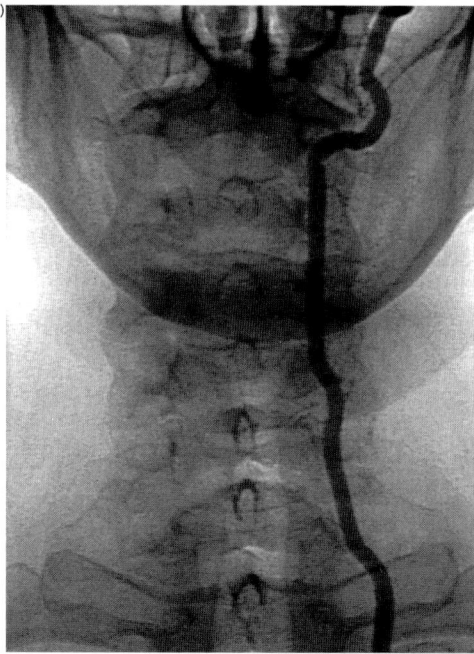

(b)

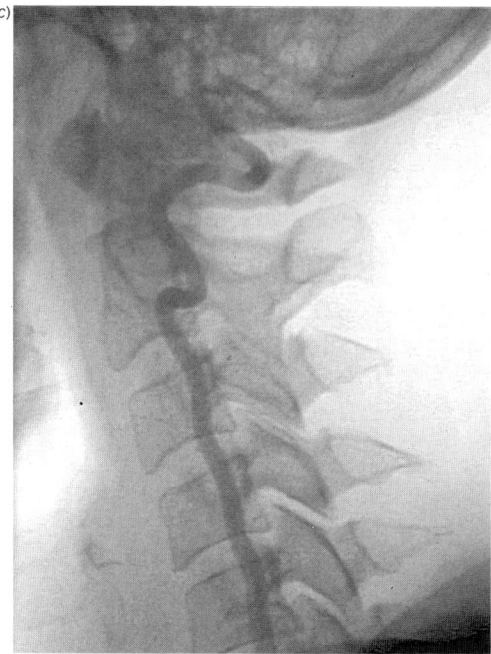

(c)

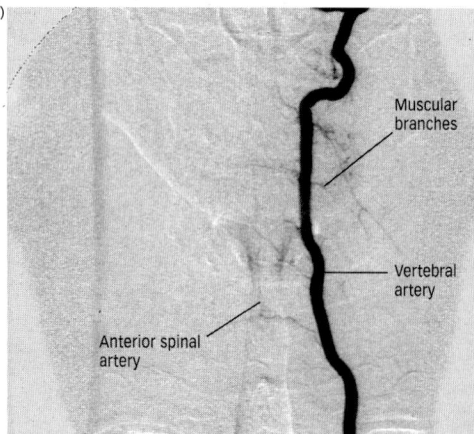

(d)

Muscular branches

Vertebral artery

Anterior spinal artery

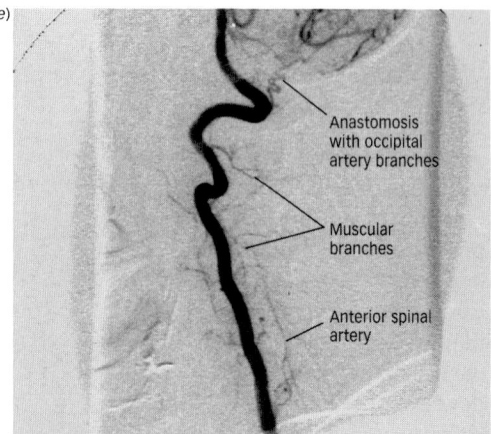

(e)

Anastomosis with occipital artery branches

Muscular branches

Anterior spinal artery

Fig. 47.
B-mode sonogram of the
common carotid bifurcation.

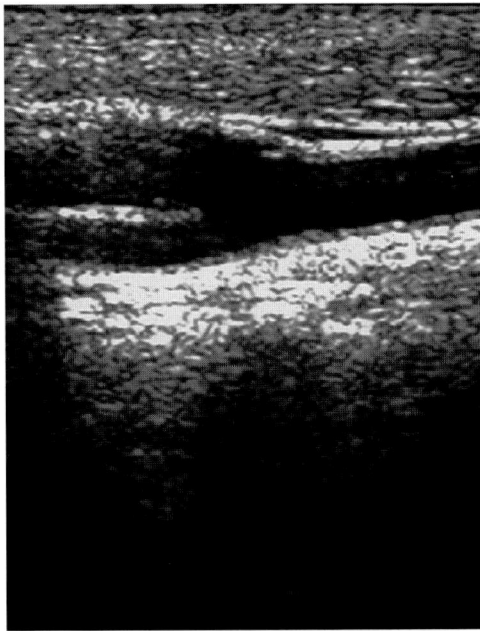

Fig. 48. (a)
Doppler waveforms
of the internal (a)
and external (b)
carotid arteries.

(b)

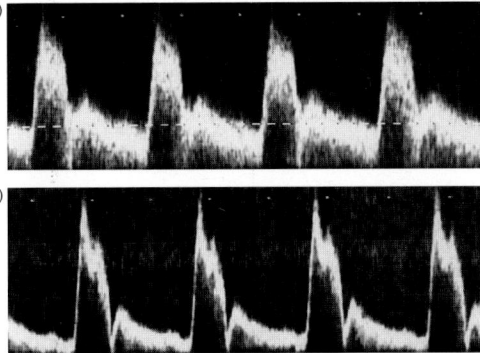

The external carotid artery circulation is one of high total peripheral resistance. It can be seen therefore that blood flow ceases or even reverses during diastole.

The common carotid arterial Doppler trace is a combination of the characteristics of both the internal and external carotid arteries. It resembles the internal carotid artery more closely since 70% of common carotid arterial blood flow is directed towards the brain.

The vertebral artery can also be studied using duplex sonography, but visualization of the vessel lumen is interrupted by acoustic shadows cast by the transverse processes of the cervical vertebrae.

Cervical carotid ultrasound can only be performed over a relatively short segment of the common carotid artery, the bifurcation and proximal external and internal carotid arteries. At the cervical bifurcation of the common carotid artery, a vortex occurs which may lead to flow reversal in the bulb. This is a normal feature particularly well demonstrated using 'colour-flow' Doppler ultrasound, where a variety of colours represents different directions of flow.

Venous drainage of the head and neck

The facial veins (Fig. 49), drain the anterior part of the scalp and face and communicate with the cavernous sinus through the ophthalmic veins. Externally, they drain via the pterygoid plexus to the retromandibular vein which is formed by the confluence of the superficial temporal and maxillary veins. The retromandibular vein is joined by the posterior auricular vein to form the external jugular vein. This descends superficially across the sternocleidomastoid, penetrates the cervical fascia immediately above the clavicle and enters the subclavian vein. Veins of the posterior scalp drain via the suboccipital plexus and vertebral veins into the brachiocephalic veins.

The anterior jugular veins, usually one on each side of the midline, enter the external jugular or subclavian vein near their confluence. Their junction, just above the sternum, is called the jugular arch. They may sometimes

Fig. 49.
Diagram of the craniofacial veins.

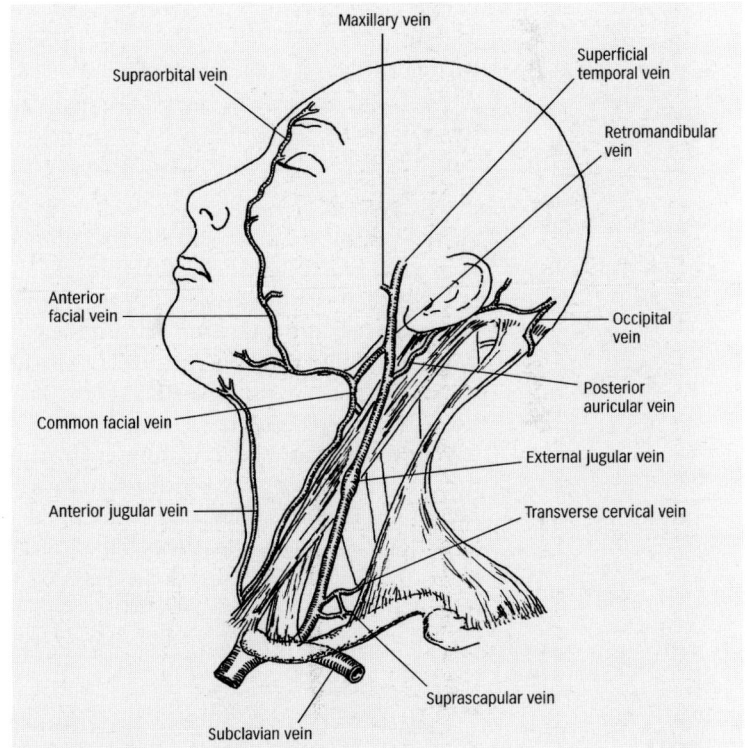

be replaced by a single midline vein.

The internal jugular vein emerges from the jugular foramen to enter the carotid sheath. Within the sheath, the internal and common carotid arteries lie medial to it with the vagus nerve posteriorly. The carotid sheath lies on the prevertebral fascia.

The internal jugular vein receives a number of tributaries as it descends (Fig. 50), and has a dilatation at each end, the superior and inferior jugular bulbs. Valves are usually present just above the inferior bulb beyond which the inter-

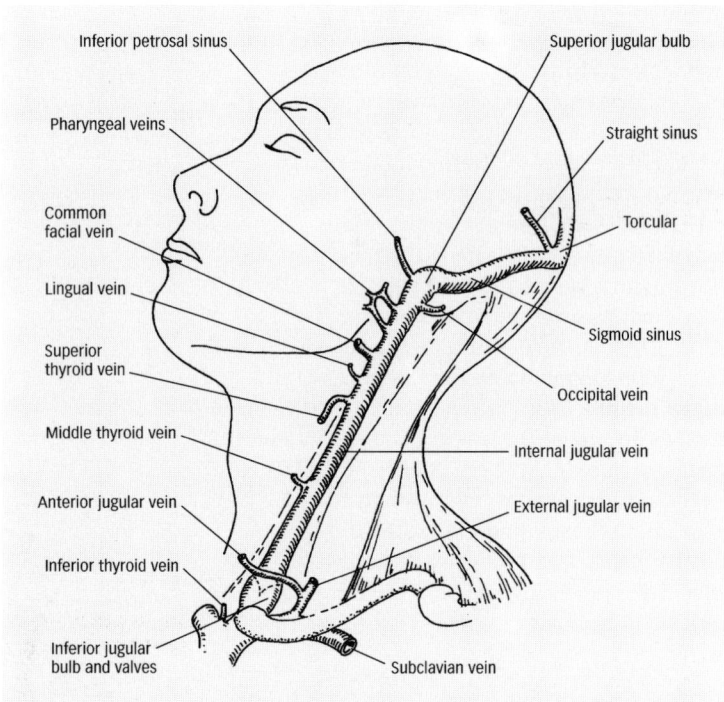

Fig. 50.
Diagram of the internal jugular vein and its tributaries.

The components of the brachial plexus bear constant relationships to landmarks identifiable on axial CT and MRI scans, in particular the subclavian vessels and scalene muscles. However, MRI scans in the coronal, sagittal and oblique planes are the most useful (Fig. 52).

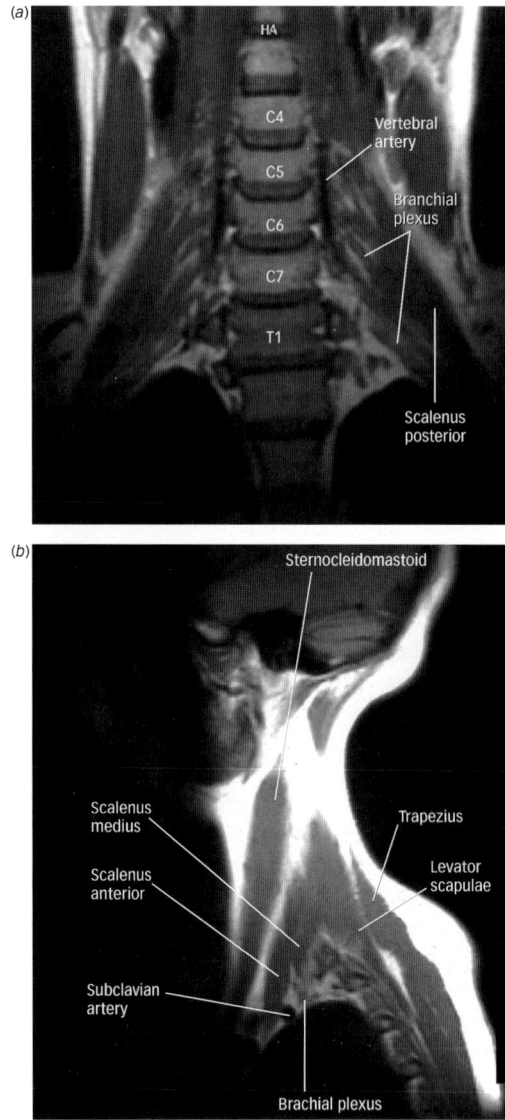

(a)

Fig. 52.
MRI of the brachial plexu T1W (a) coronal and (b) sagittal sections.

Reference
Dolan, D. D. & Jacoby, C. G. (19
Facial fractures. *Seminar Roentgenology*, **13**, 37–45

Further reading
Babbel, R. W. & Harnsberge
H. R. (1990). The paraphar
geal space: the key to
unlocking the suprahyoi
neck. *Seminars in Ultraso
CT and MR*, **11**; 444–59.
Ellis, A. H. (1997). *Clinical
Anatomy*, 9th edn. Oxfor
Basil Blackwell.
Gentry, L. R., Manor, W. F., Tu
P. A. & Strother, C. M. (198
High-resolution CT analy
of facial struts in trauma
1. Normal anatomy. *Amer
Journal of Roentgenology
140, 523–32.
Harnsberger, H. R. (1995).
Sinonasal imaging. In
*Handbook of Head and N
imaging*, 2nd edn. ed. R.
Harnsberger, pp. 357–61.
St Louis: Mosby.
Laine, F. J. & Smoker, W. R.
(1992). The ostiomeatal u
and endoscopic surgery:
anatomy, variations and
imaging findings in inflar
matory diseases. *Americ
Journal of Roentgenology
159, 849–57.
Lasjaunias, P. & Berenstein
(1987). *Surgical Neuroang
graphy*. vol. 1. *Functional
anatomy of craniofacial
arteries*. Heidelberg:
Springer-Verlag.
Payne, M. & Nakielny, R. A.
(1996). Review: temporo-
mandibular joint imaging
Clinical Radiology, **51**, 1–1
Sakai, F., Gamsu, F., Dillon, V
et al. (1990). MR imaging
the larynx at 1.5T. *Journa
Computer Assisted Tomo
raphy*, **14**, 60–72.
Zinriech, S. J., Kennedy, D. W
Kuman, M. et al. (1988). M
imaging of the normal na
cycle: comparison with s
pathology. *Journal of Com
puter Assisted Tomograp
12, 10–14.
Zwiebel, W. & Knighton, R.
(1990). Duplex examinat
of the carotid arteries.
*Seminars in Ultrasound,
CT and MR*, **11**, 97–135.

nal jugular joins the subclavian vein to form the brachiocephalic vein. These valves may sometimes prove difficult to pass with a guiding catheter during interventional procedures.

Brachial plexus

The brachial plexus is formed from the anterior rami of the fifth cervical to the first thoracic nerve roots. The fourth cervical and second thoracic roots may also contribute. The alternate division and union of these roots give rise to the complexity of the brachial plexus (Fig. 51). The five anterior nerve roots unite to form three trunks which divide into six divisions which in turn unite into three cords which again divide into six terminal branches. Since two of these branches immediately join to form the median nerve, the plexus commences as five anterior roots and ends distally as five nerves.

(b)

Fig. 51.
Diagram of the brachial plexus.

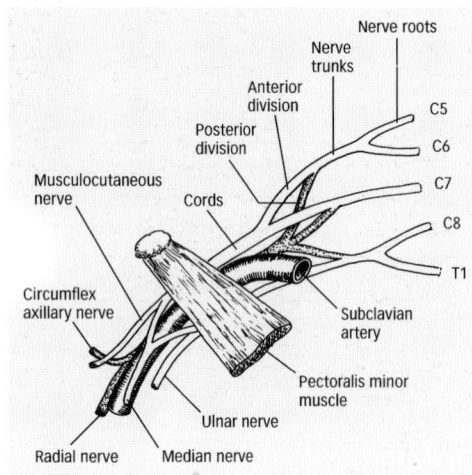

The roots and trunks of the brachial plexus lie in the neck. The fifth and sixth cervical roots descend anterolaterally from their exit foramina and are visible between the scalenus anterior and medius muscles, where they unite to form the upper trunk. Whereas the seventh cervical root continues alone as the middle trunk, the eighth cervical and first thoracic roots unite behind scalenus anterior forming the lower trunk. The divisions of the plexus lie behind the scalenus anterior or the clavicle. The cords form above and behind the pectoralis minor muscle and, surrounding the axillary artery, pass between the clavicle and first rib to enter the axilla. Within the axilla they divided into their terminal branches.

6 | # The chest

R. R. PHILLIPS
and P. ARMSTRONG

Imaging methods

Plain chest radiography (CXR) with frontal and lateral projections is the initial routine investigation. (Fig. 1(a), (b)).

Computed tomography (CT) allows assessment of the mediastinum, the lung parenchyma and the thoracic wall. The standard study uses contiguous axial 10 mm sections. Spiral (helical) acquisition, if available, ensures that no portions of the chest are missed due to variable inspiratory effort. Intravenous injection of iodinated contrast is helpful to opacify the vascular system. Spiral scan data can be reconstructed into coronal, sagittal or other planes and three-dimensional images to allow high quality images of the trachea and major airways (Fig. 2).

High resolution (thin-section) computed tomography (HRCT) uses a slice thickness of 1–2 mm and a high resolution algorithm to show fine detail of the lung parenchyma, pleura and tracheobronchial tree.

Fig. 1(a).
Normal PA chest X-ray (with accompanying diagram).

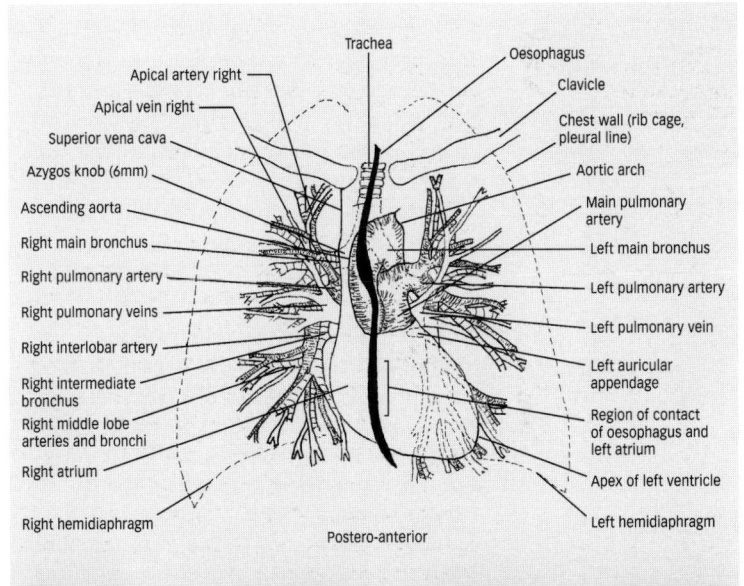

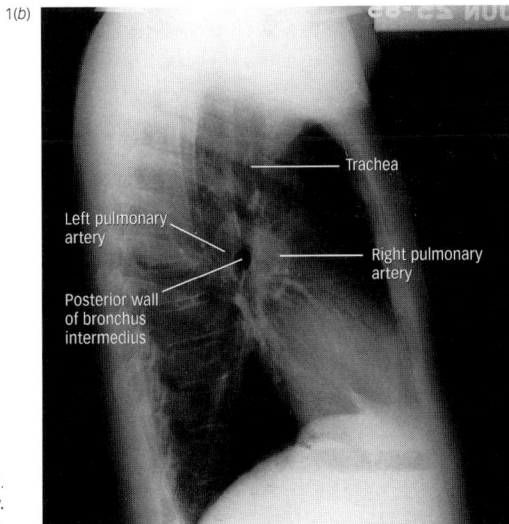

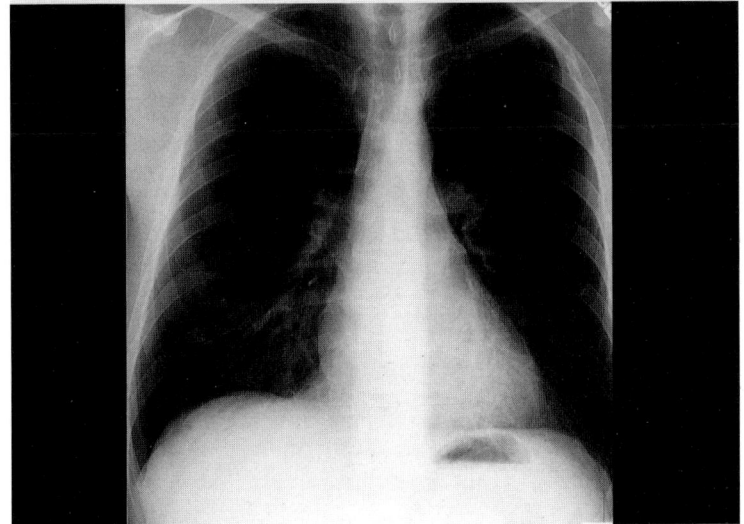

Trachea
Apical artery right
Apical vein right
Superior vena cava
Azygos knob (6mm)
Ascending aorta
Right main bronchus
Right pulmonary artery
Right pulmonary veins
Right interlobar artery
Right intermediate bronchus
Right middle lobe arteries and bronchi
Right atrium
Right hemidiaphragm

Oesophagus
Clavicle
Chest wall (rib cage, pleural line)
Aortic arch
Main pulmonary artery
Left main bronchus
Left pulmonary artery
Left pulmonary vein
Left auricular appendage
Region of contact of oesophagus and left atrium
Apex of left ventricle
Left hemidiaphragm

Postero-anterior

Trachea
Left pulmonary artery
Right pulmonary artery
Posterior wall of bronchus intermedius

Fig. 1(b).
**Normal lateral chest X-ray.
T, trachea.**

1(b)

1(a)

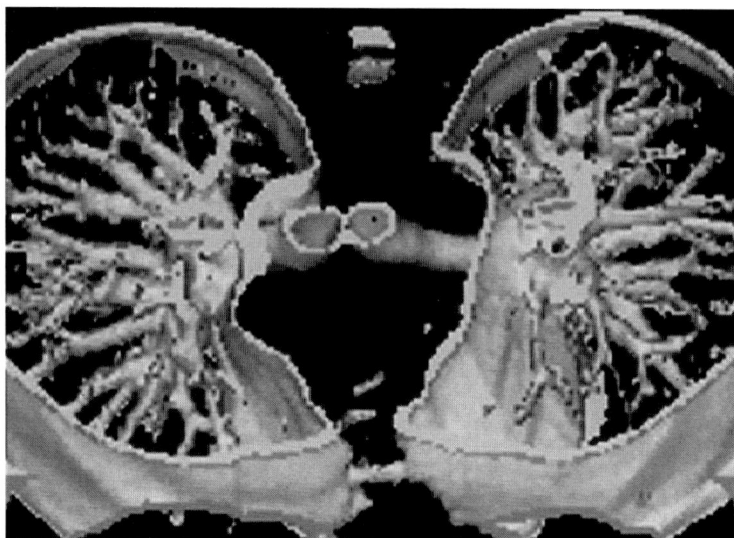

Fig. 2.
Three-dimensional CT image of bronchial tree.

Magnetic resonance (MRI) is a non-invasive modality that provides multiplanar imaging without the use of ionizing radiation and allows visualization of the chest wall, heart, mediastinal and hilar structures. The optimum technique for showing anatomical detail uses cardiac gating and respiratory compensation to overcome movement artefacts due to cardiac and respiratory movement. So-called T1-weighted sequences demonstrate the normal anatomy in superb detail. MRI is currently a poor technique for showing lung detail.

Angiography has a reduced role now that MRI and CT can be used to demonstrate the mediastinal vessels; it continues to be used to show the pulmonary vascular system. Arteriography of the systemic vessels is performed through catheters introduced via the femoral artery, or occasionally, a brachial artery; for pulmonary angiography, catheters are introduced via the venous system (Fig. 3(a), (b)).

Venography can be used to demonstrate the anatomy of the innominate veins, superior vena cava (SVC), and azygous and hemiazygous systems and is performed by injecting contrast into an indwelling line positioned in a central vein (Fig. 4(a), (b), (c)).

Lymphangiography is infrequently performed but allows depiction of the thoracic duct.

Bronchography, a procedure which involved passing a catheter or bronchoscope into the bronchial tree and injecting an appropriate contrast agent, has largely been superseded by CT (Fig. 5(a–d)).

Development of the respiratory tract

The development of the trachea and lungs

In the early fetus (the 3 mm embryo) a small slit appears on the ventral aspect of the caudal end of the pharynx. This slit is called the tra-

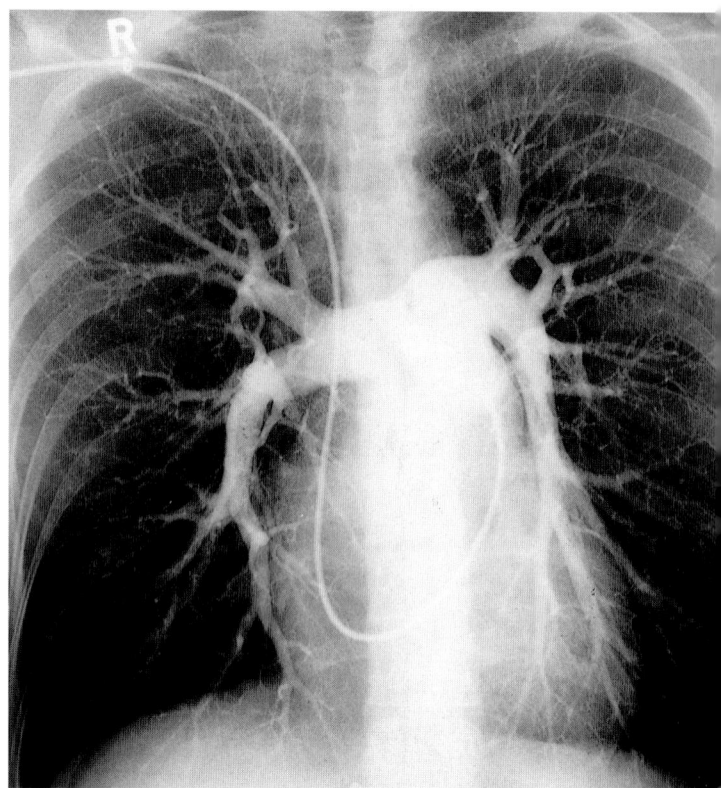

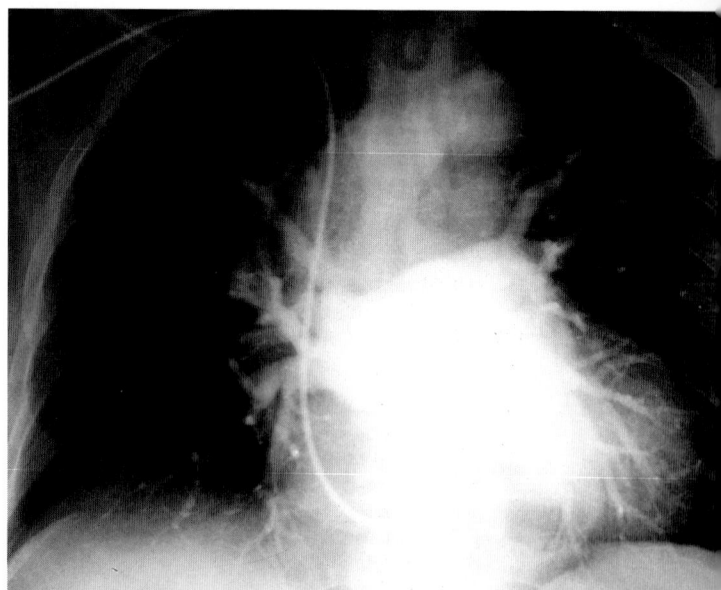

cheobronchial groove. This forms a diverticulum which grows downwards ventral to the pharynx as the tracheobronchial diverticulum. This bifurcates to form the primary broncial buds. These differentiate into the bronchi and their ramifications in each lung. Further branching produces the bronchioles, alveolar ducts and the alveoli. During embryonic life, the alveoli are lined by the same cuboidal epithelium that lines the rest of the respiratory tract. The transfer to the flattened pavement epithelium of the alveoli is accomplished when respiration commences at birth.

Fig. 3(a). *top*
Pulmonary angiogram showing right and left pulmonary arteries.
Fig. 3(b). *below*
Pulmonary angiogram during venous filling phase

(a)

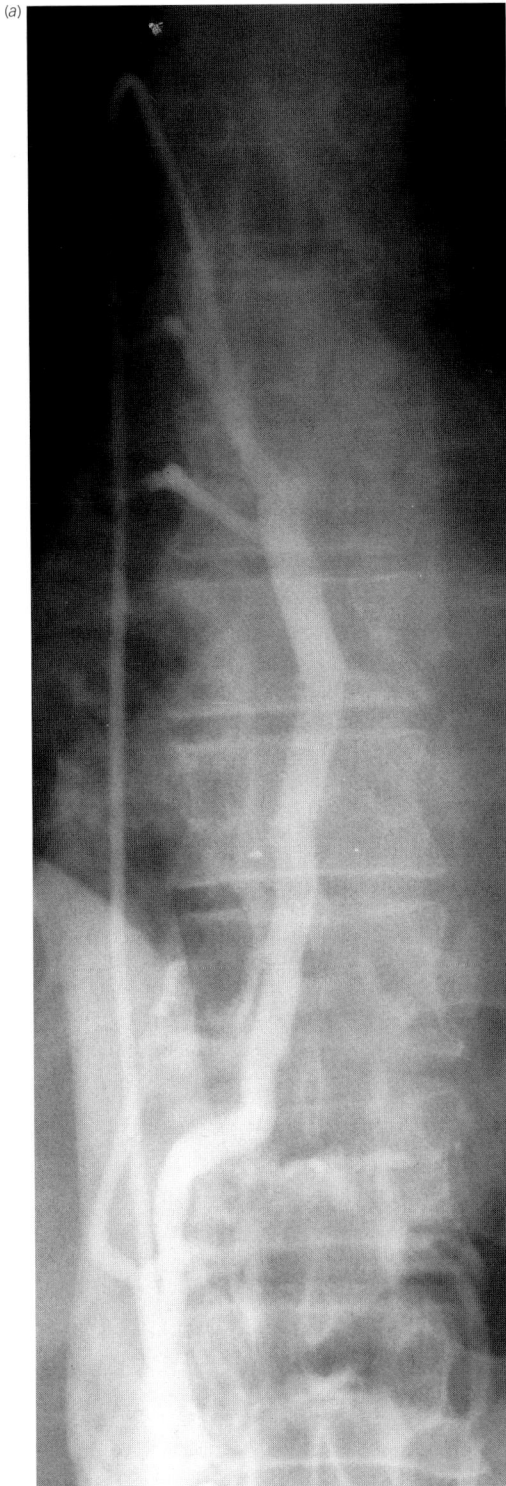

(b)

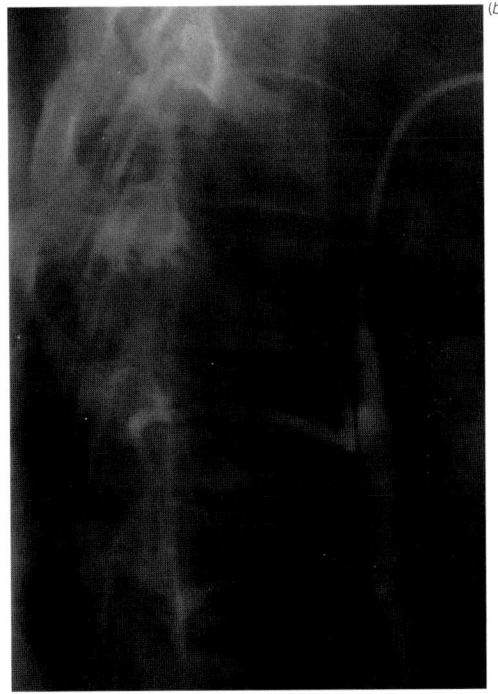

Fig. 4(b).
Azygos venogram: lateral
projection. (Courtesy of Dr
J.E. Dacie, London.)

(c)

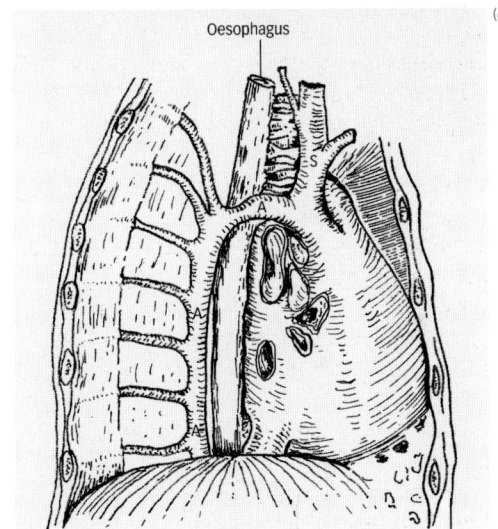

Oesophagus

Fig. 4(c).
Diagram shows the
relationship between the
azygos vein (a) and the right
posterior aspect of the
oesophagus (0). (S) denotes
the superior vena cava.

Fig. 4(a).
Azygos venogram: frontal
projection. (Courtesy of Dr
J.E. Dacie, London.)

A persistant tracheo-oesophageal fistula
may occur as an embryonic anomaly which
indicates the close developmental relationship between the foregut and the respiratory
passages. It is usually associated with a atresia
of the oesophagus, the fistula being situated
below the atretic segment.

At three weeks, the embryo develops a ventral outpouching of the endodermal foregut
termed the respiratory diverticulum, or lung
bud. This grows through the mesenchyme
which surrounds the foregut and, after a
week, bifurcates into the left and right primary bronchial buds, which are the primordia
of the lungs (Fig. 6). Progressive branching of
these buds produces the pulmonary respiratory tree, the stem proximal to the first
bifurcation becoming the definitive larynx
and trachea.

By the 36th week of fetal life, the terminal
sacs of the lung buds are surrounded by a
dense network of capillaries. These primitive
alveoli allow limited respiration but are few
and immature. Additional alveoli continue to
develop both before and after birth.

Congenital anomalies may result from failure of branching or differentiation of the respiratory tree. Errors in pulmonary branching

(a)

(b)

(c)

(d)

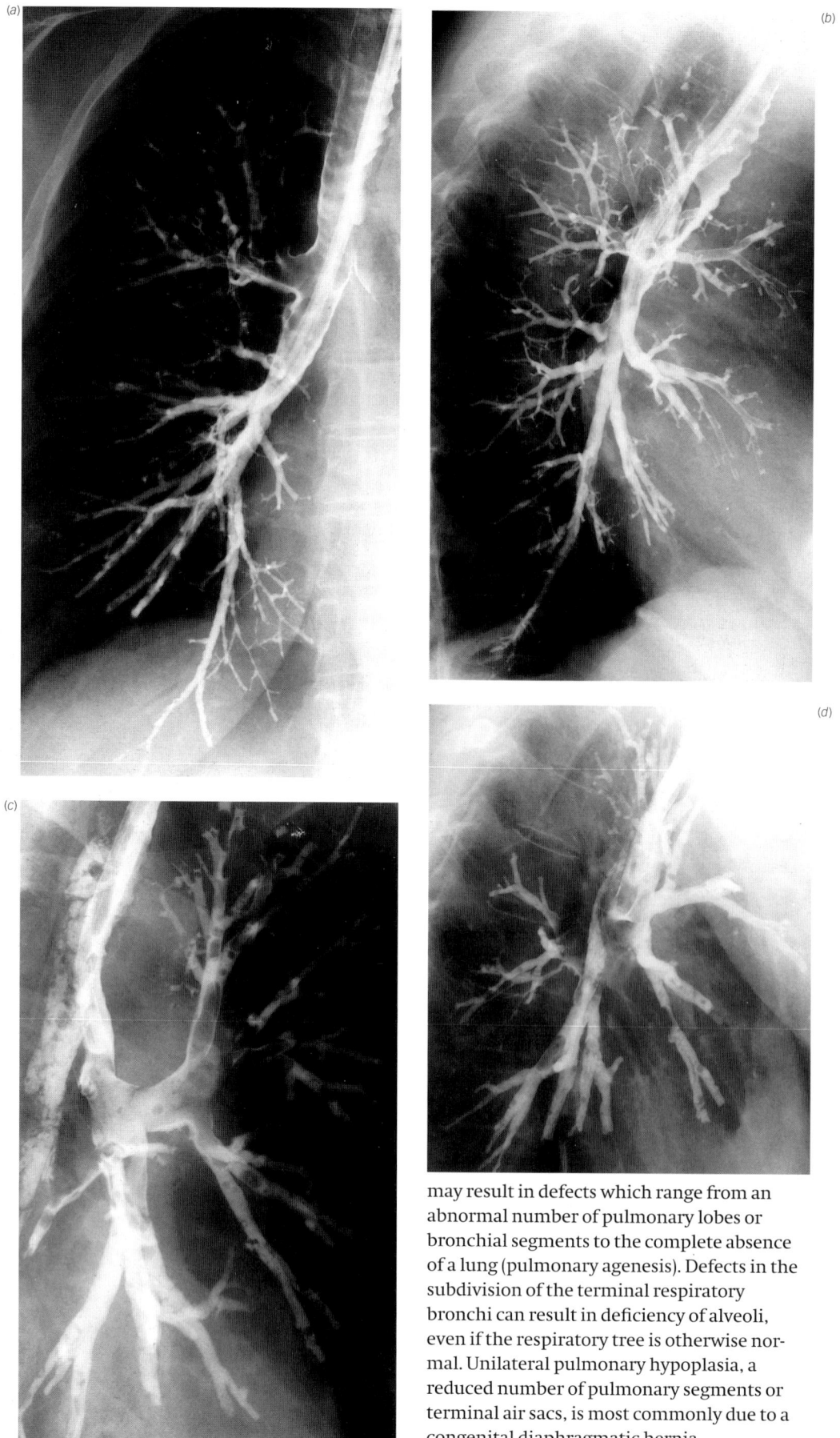

Fig. 5(a)–(d).
Bronchograms: (a) AP view
of the right bronchial tree,
(b) lateral view of right
bronchial tree, (c) oblique
view of left bronchial tree,
(d) lateral view of left
bronchial tree.

may result in defects which range from an abnormal number of pulmonary lobes or bronchial segments to the complete absence of a lung (pulmonary agenesis). Defects in the subdivision of the terminal respiratory bronchi can result in deficiency of alveoli, even if the respiratory tree is otherwise normal. Unilateral pulmonary hypoplasia, a reduced number of pulmonary segments or terminal air sacs, is most commonly due to a congenital diaphragmatic hernia.

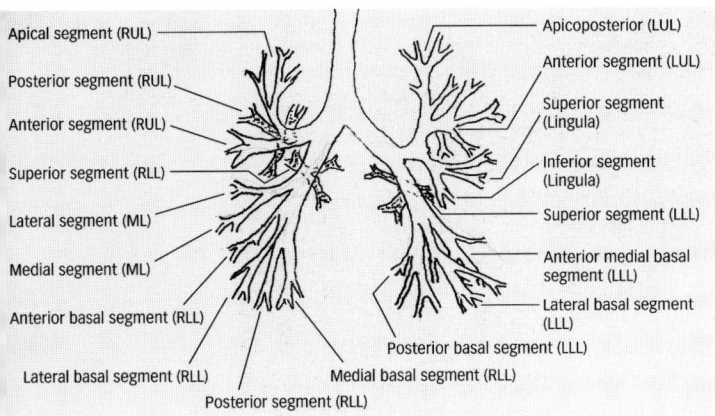

5(e)

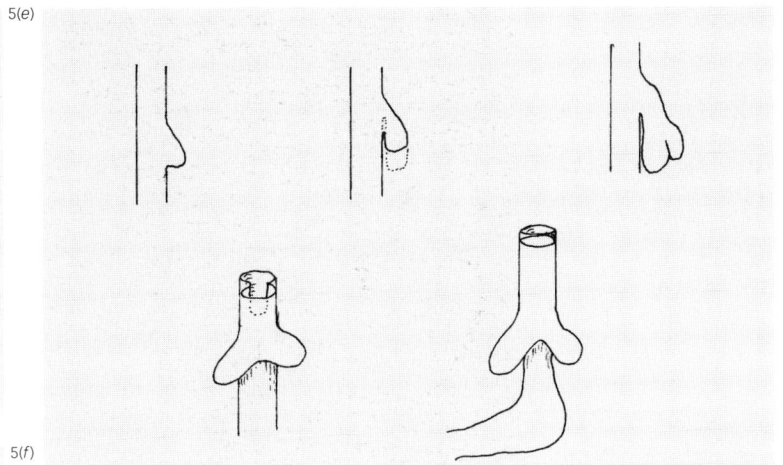

5(f)

Fig. 6.
Development of the lungs. A bifurcating diverticulum develops from the ventral pharynx.

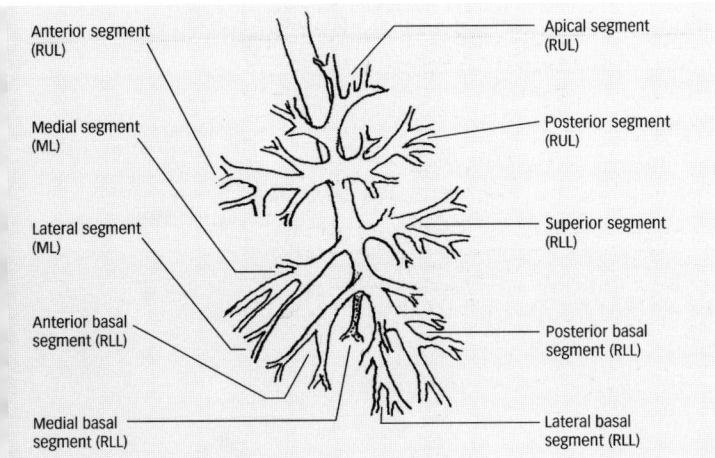

Fig. 7(a).
Axial CT section showing the muscles of the chest wall.

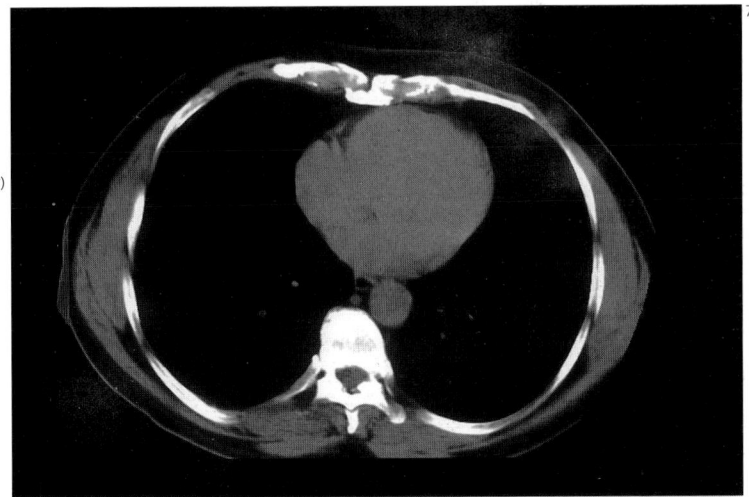

7(a)

5(g)

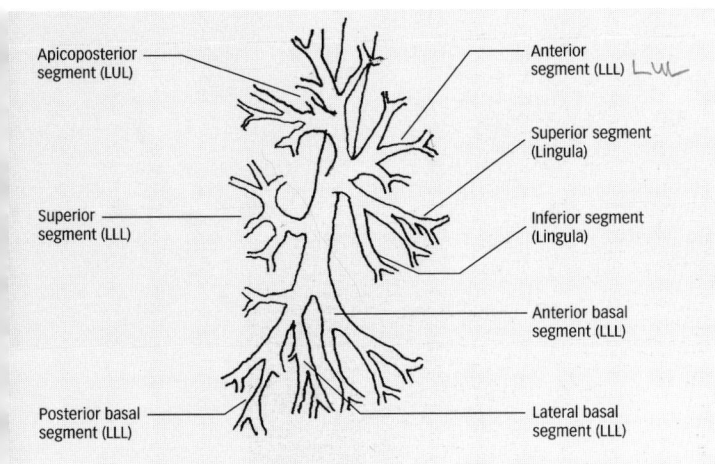

Fig. 5(e).
Diagram of AP view of bronchial anatomy.

Fig. 5(f).
Diagram of lateral view of right bronchial tree.

Fig. 5(g).
Diagram of lateral view of left bronchial tree.

Anatomy

The chest wall

The bony portion of the chest wall is formed by the 12 thoracic vertebrae posteriorly, the sternum anteriorly and the 12 pairs of ribs together with their costal cartilages. The thorax has a cylindrical configuration with a narrow inlet superiorly and a wide outlet inferiorly. The floor is formed by the diaphragm, which has three large openings which transmit the oesophagus, the aorta and the inferior vena cava (IVC). The muscular outer covering

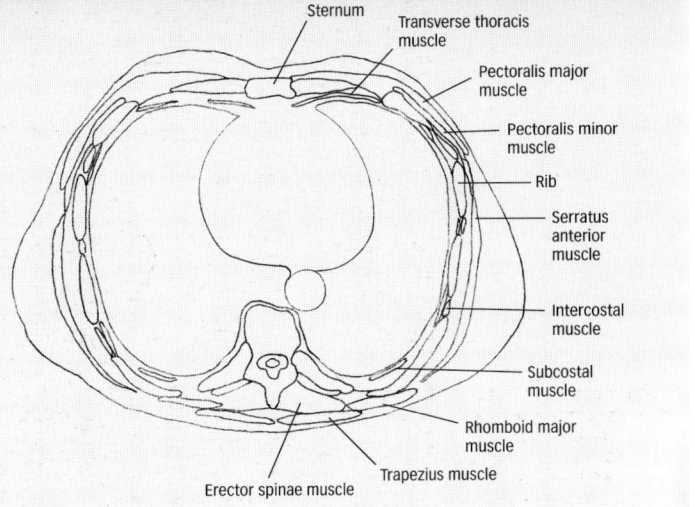

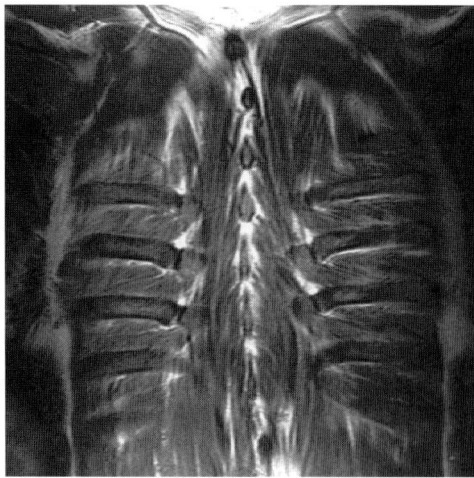

Fig. 7(*b*). Coronal MR section. The posterior chest wall muscles are well shown.

of the thoracic cage is formed anteriorly by the pectoralis major and minor, laterally by the serratus anterior, posterolaterally by the muscles of the shoulder girdle (teres major, subscapularis, rhomboids) and posteriorly by the erector spinae and trapezius. All of these muscles are seen on CT and MR images (Fig. 7(*a*),(*b*)). The deeper muscles of the chest wall consist of a group of muscles which connect adjoining ribs (the external, internal and innermost intercostal muscles), span several ribs between attachments (the subcostal muscles), connect the ribs to the sternum (the transverse thoracis) or the ribs to the vertebrae (the levatores costarum, serratus posterior, superior and inferior).

Blood supply to the chest wall

The intercostal vessels and nerves form a neurovascular bundle which passes forwards around the chest wall in the subcostal groove deep to the internal intercostal muscles. Most intercostal spaces are supplied by a single posterior and paired anterior intercostal arteries. The lower two spaces have only posterior

arteries. There are usually nine pairs of posterior intercostal arteries derived from the thoracic aorta. They arise from the posterolateral margin of the aorta and are distributed to the lower nine intercostal spaces, the first and second spaces being supplied by the superior intercostal artery derived from the subclavian artery via its costocervical trunk.

Each posterior intercostal artery gives off a spinal branch which is distributed to the vertebrae and spinal cord and has branches to the lateral chest wall and a collateral intercostal branch. The internal thoracic artery arises from the internal thoracic branch of the subclavian artery, is distributed to the upper six intercostal spaces (as the anterior intercostal artery) and ends in the sixth intercostal space dividing into musculophrenic and superior epigastric arteries.

The intercostal venous system

The intercostal spaces are drained by two anterior veins and a single posterior intercostal

Fig. 8(*a*). Enhanced axial CT study showing the azygos and hemiazygos veins in an infant with SVC obstruction.

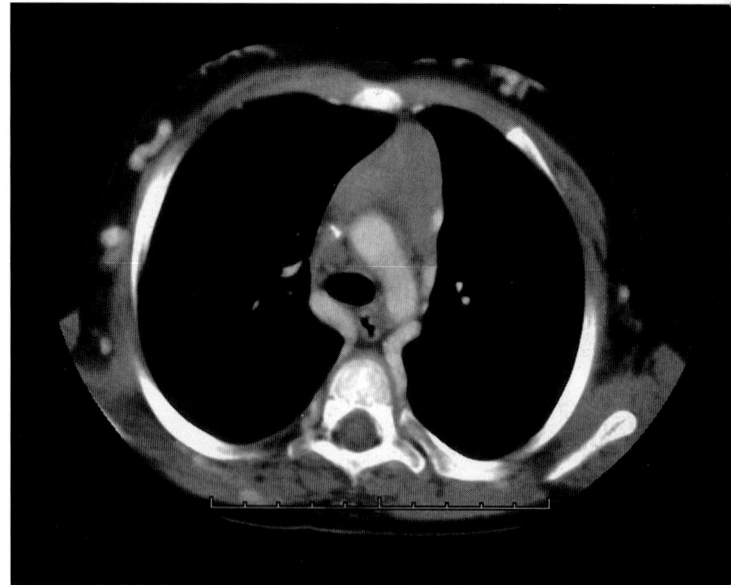

Fig. 8(*b*). Diagram illustrating mediastinal venous anatomy. (Redrawn from Godwin & Chen, 1986).

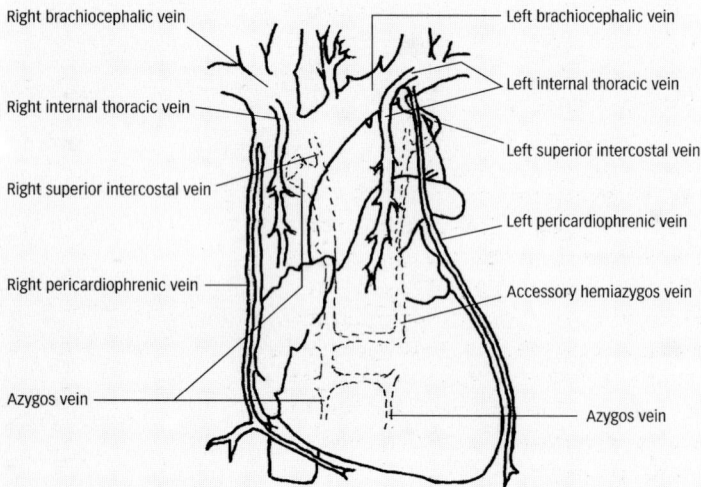

Right brachiocephalic vein
Right internal thoracic vein
Right superior intercostal vein
Right pericardiophrenic vein
Azygos vein
Left brachiocephalic vein
Left internal thoracic vein
Left superior intercostal vein
Left pericardiophrenic vein
Accessory hemiazygos vein
Azygos vein

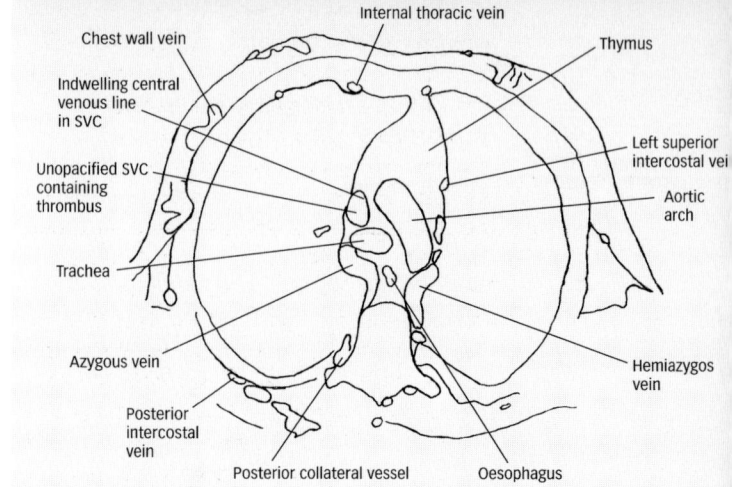

Chest wall vein
Indwelling central venous line in SVC
Unopacified SVC containing thrombus
Trachea
Azygous vein
Posterior intercostal vein
Posterior collateral vessel
Internal thoracic vein
Thymus
Left superior intercostal vei
Aortic arch
Hemiazygos vein
Oesophagus

vein (Fig. 8(*a*), (*b*)). The anterior veins drain into the musculophrenic and internal thoracic veins and the posterior veins drain into the brachiocephalic vein and azygos system.

The azygos vein ascends in the posterior mediastinum to the level of the fourth thoracic vertebra, where it arches forward above the root of the right lung and ends in the posterior aspect of the superior vena cava (SVC) just before it pierces the pericardium, approximately 1 cm below the junction of the left and right brachiocephalic veins (Fig. 4(*a*), (*c*)). Usually, the azygos vein remains within the mediastinum and occupies the right tracheobronchial angle. In the 1% of the population who have an azygos lobe, the azygos vein traverses the lung before entering the SVC, in which case the SVC may appear distorted, both on plain films and CT. The azygos vein lies anterior to the bodies of the lower eight thoracic vertebra, the anterior longitudinal ligament and the right posterior intercostal

Fig. 9.
Enhanced axial CT study showing the left superior intercostal vein (arrow).

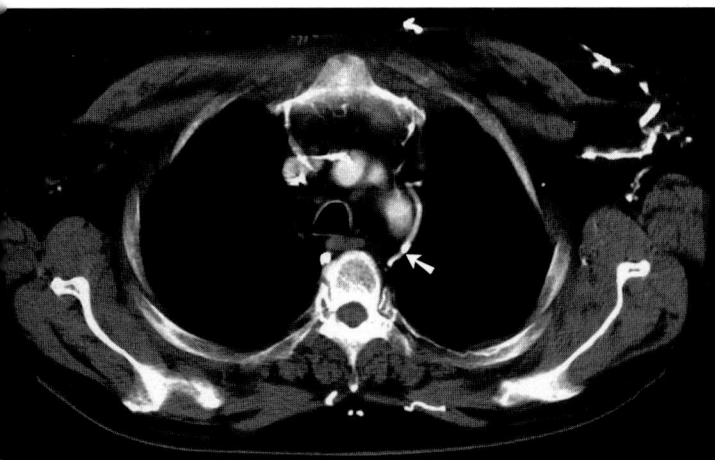

arteries just to the right of the midline. On its right are the greater splanchnic nerve, lung and pleura, on its left, throughout the greater part of its course, are the thoracic duct and aorta and higher up, where it arches forward above the root of the right lung, the oesophagus, trachea and right vagus. In the lower part of the thorax, it is covered anteriorly by a recess of the right pleural sac (the azygo-oesophageal recess), and by the oesophagus, but it emerges from behind the right edge of the oesophagus and ascends behind the root of the right lung. For a variable extent in the lower thorax, the azygos vein is quite closely applied to the right posterolateral aspect of the descending thoracic aorta and thus often reaches and sometimes crosses to the left of the midline. The azygos vein drains the posterior intercostal veins of the right side, with the exception of the first, the veins from the second, third and fourth intercostal spaces usu-

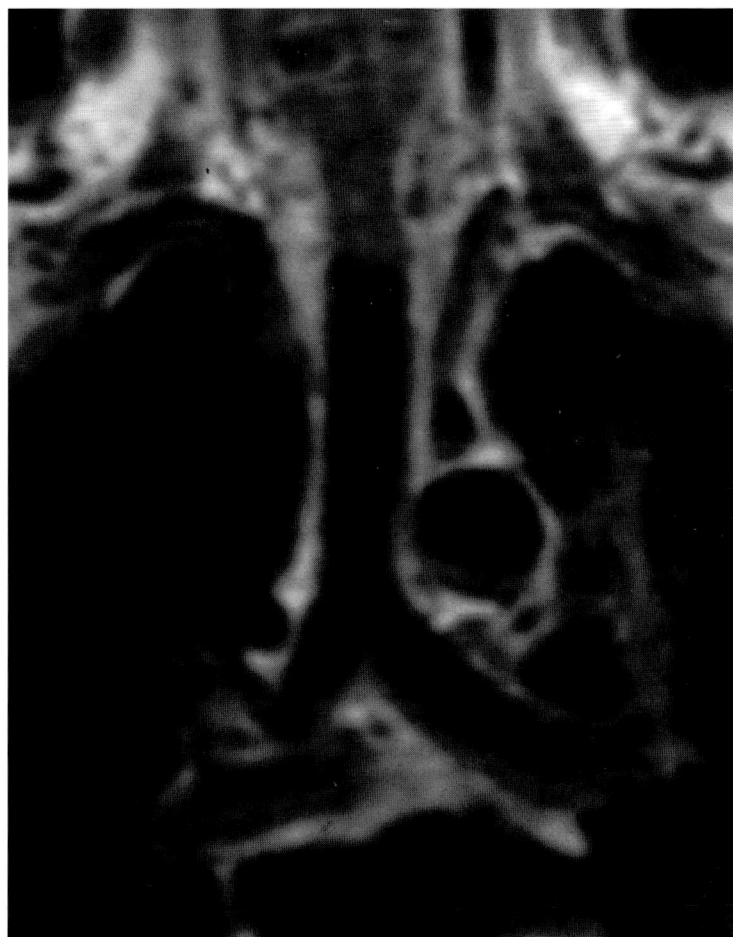

Fig. 10.
Coronal MR showing the trachea and carina.

ally drain via a common stem called the right superior intercostal vein. It also receives the hemiazygos and accessory hemiazygos veins, several oesophageal, mediastinal and pericardial veins, and near its termination, the right bronchial veins. Occasionally, the inferior vena cava (IVC) does not develop in the usual fashion, and the azygos vein then forms the venous conduit draining inferior vena caval blood back to the heart, an arrangement known as azygos continuation of the IVC. In this situation, the azygos vein is a large structure, but its anatomy is otherwise unaltered. Azygos continuation of the IVC may be confused for a mediastinal mass or lymphadenopathy on imaging studies.

The lower portion of the hemiazygos vein is similar to the azygos vein except that it lies to the left of the midline. It ascends anterior to the vertebra to the level of the eighth thoracic vertebra, then passes across the vertebral column, behind the aorta, oesophagus, and thoracic duct to drain into the azygos vein. Its tributaries are the lower three posterior intercostal veins and the common trunk formed by the union of the ascending lumbar and the subcostal veins of the left side, and some oesophageal and mediastinal veins.

The accessory hemiazygos vein also lies on the left side of the vertebral column. It receives the veins from the fourth (or fifth) to the eighth intercostal spaces of the left side, and sometimes the left bronchial veins. It may cross the body of the seventh thoracic vertebra to join the azygos vein and/or may drain into the left superior intercostal vein, which arches around the aorta more or less at the junction of the arch and the descending portion, to join the left brachiocephalic vein. The accessory hemiazygos vein sometimes joins the hemiazygos vein, and the resulting common trunk opens into the azygos vein. The azygos and hemiazygos veins are routinely identified on post-contrast CT studies.

The posterior intercostal veins number 11 on each side and accompany the posterior intercostal arteries. The first posterior intercostal vein ascends in front of the neck of the first rib and then arches forwards above the pleura to end in the corresponding brachiocephalic or vertebral vein. On the right side, the second, third and often the fourth posterior intercostal veins unite to form the right superior intercostal vein, which joins the terminal part of the azygos vein. The intercostal veins below the fourth drain individually into the azygos vein. On the left side, the second, third and sometimes the fourth posterior intercostal veins unite to form the left superior intercostal vein. The veins from the fourth (or fifth) to the eighth intercostal spaces inclusive drain into the accessory hemiazygos vein and the veins from the lower three spaces in to the hemiazygos vein.

The left superior intercostal vein is much smaller than the azygos vein and is only occasionally identified on plain films or CT scans (Fig. 9), though in 1–9.5% of normal patients, it is seen on plain chest radiography as a small nipple on the lateral margin of the aortic arch as it arches from back to front around the left side of the descending aorta to empty into the left brachiocephalic vein.

The anterior aspect of the chest is drained by the paired internal thoracic veins which drain into the brachiocephalic veins. In SVC obstruction, chest wall collateral vessels, including those from the lateral thoracic veins, can be observed draining to the IVC via musculophrenic branches.

The nerves to the chest wall

There are 12 thoracic nerves on each side. The upper 11 lie between the ribs (intercostal nerves) while the twelfth lies below the last rib (subcostal nerve). The intercostal nerves are the ventral rami of the upper 11 thoracic spinal nerves and have a collateral branch, muscular branches and the lateral cutaneous nerve, which divides into anterior and posterior branches. Each dorsal ramus supplies the extensor muscles of the back before ending in medial and lateral cutaneous branches which supply the skin of the back.

The sympathetic chain

The thoracic part of each sympathetic trunk contains a series of ganglia, which usually correspond approximately in number to the thoracic spinal nerves, but their number is variable. The first thoracic ganglion is usually fused with the inferior cervical to form the cervicothoracic (stellate) ganglion. The succeeding ganglia are numbered so that each corresponds numerically with the other segmental structures. With the exception of the last two or three, most of the thoracic ganglia rest against the heads of the ribs, and lie posterior to the costal pleura. Inferiorly, the thoracic sympathetic trunk passes posterior to the medial arcuate ligament (or through the crus of the diaphragm) to become continuous with the lumbar sympathetic trunk.

The medial branches from the upper five ganglia are very small, they supply filaments to the thoracic aorta and its branches. On the aorta, they form a delicate plexus (thoracic aortic plexus) together with filaments from the greater splanchnic nerve. Twigs from the second to fifth or sixth ganglia enter the posterior pulmonary plexus; others, from the second, third, fourth and fifth ganglia pass deep to the deep (dorsal) part of the cardiac plexus. Small branches from these pulmonary and cardiac nerves pass to the oesophagus and trachea. The medial branches from the lower seven ganglia are large. They distribute filaments to the aorta and unite to form the greater, the lesser, and the lowest splanchnic nerves, the last of which is not always identifiable. The greater splanchnic nerve consists mainly of myelinated, preganglionic and visceral afferent fibres. It is formed by branches from the fifth to the ninth or tenth thoracic ganglia, but the fibres in the higher branches may be traced upwards in the sympathetic trunk as far as the first or second thoracic ganglion. It descends obliquely, anterior to the vertebral bodies and supplies fine branches to the descending thoracic aorta. The lesser splanchnic nerve is formed by filaments from the ninth, tenth, and sometimes the eleventh, thoracic ganglia and from the trunk between the ganglia. The splanchnic nerves pierce the crus of the diaphragm to reach the abdominal ganglia.

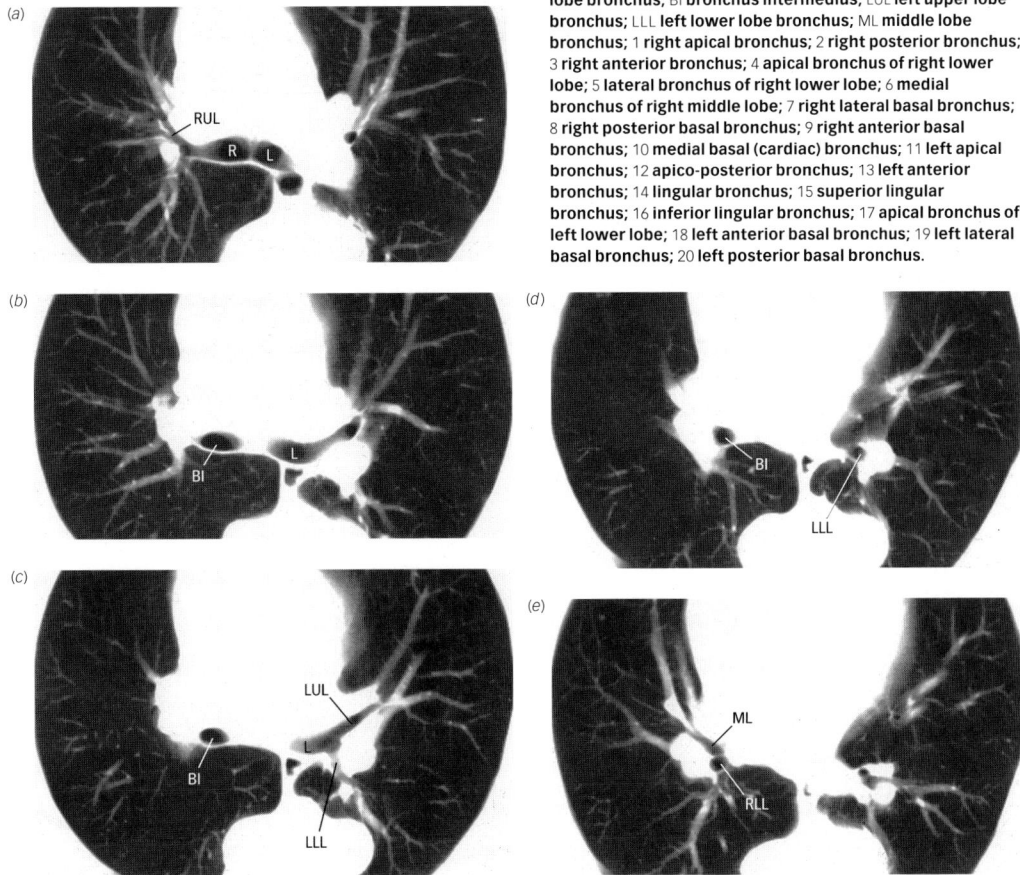

Fig. 11. (*a*)–(*e*).
Contiguous axial CT images showing bronchial tree. Key:
R **right main bronchus**; L **left main bronchus**; RUL **right upper lobe bronchus**; BI **bronchus intermedius**; LUL **left upper lobe bronchus**; LLL **left lower lobe bronchus**; ML **middle lobe bronchus**; 1 **right apical bronchus**; 2 **right posterior bronchus**; 3 **right anterior bronchus**; 4 **apical bronchus of right lower lobe**; 5 **lateral bronchus of right lower lobe**; 6 **medial bronchus of right middle lobe**; 7 **right lateral basal bronchus**; 8 **right posterior basal bronchus**; 9 **right anterior basal bronchus**; 10 **medial basal (cardiac) bronchus**; 11 **left apical bronchus**; 12 **apico-posterior bronchus**; 13 **left anterior bronchus**; 14 **lingular bronchus**; 15 **superior lingular bronchus**; 16 **inferior lingular bronchus**; 17 **apical bronchus of left lower lobe**; 18 **left anterior basal bronchus**; 19 **left lateral basal bronchus**; 20 **left posterior basal bronchus**.

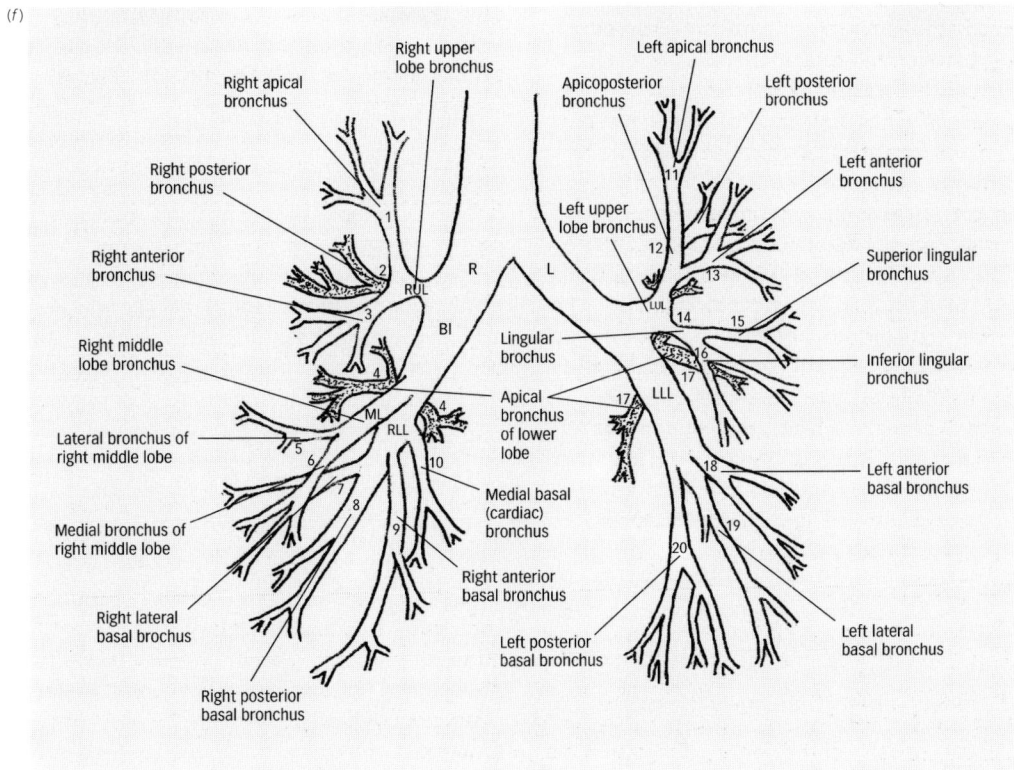

Fig. 11(*f*).
Diagram illustrating anteroposterior view of bronchial tree.

The lungs and airways

The trachea is a tube which travels inferiorly to lie just to the right of the midline at the level of the aortic arch. In cross-section it is usually round, oval or oval with a flattened posterior margin although it may occasionally show a square, inverted pear, or horseshoe configuration. At the carina it divides into the two main stem bronchi (Fig. 10). The angles of origin of these bronchi are symmetrical in children, but in adults the right main-stem bronchus has a steeper angle than the left. The left main bronchus is up to twice as long as the right main bronchus. The central, lobar and segmental bronchi can be identified routinely with CT sections (Fig. 11(*a*)–(*e*)). The lobar and segmental branching pattern is shown diagrammatically in Fig. 11(*f*) and demonstrated on the reformatted 3D CT study (Fig. 2).

The pulmonary hila (Naidich *et al.*, 1981; Webb *et al.*, 1981)

The normal hilar shadows on plain CXR and CT are composed of the major bronchi and hilar blood vessels. The normal lymph nodes, autonomic nerves and connective tissue do not contribute significantly to the bulk of the hila, and the small amount of fat between the vessels is usually visible only at MRI (Fig. 12(*a*)–(*e*)). The following points help to understand normal hilar anatomy on various imaging examinations:

(a) The right main-stem bronchus and its divisions into the right upper lobe bronchus and bronchus intermedius are outlined posteriorly by lung so that the posterior wall of these portions of the bronchial tree is seen as a thin stripe. On the left side, the lower lobe artery intervenes between the lung and the bronchial tree, and only a small tongue of lung can invaginate between the left lower lobe artery and the descending aorta to contact the posterior wall of the left main-stem bronchus.

(b) The right pulmonary artery passes anterior to the major bronchi to reach the lateral aspect of the bronchus intermedius and right lower lobe bronchus, whereas the left pulmonary artery arches over the left main bronchus and left upper lobe bronchus to descend posterolateral to the left lower lobe bronchus.

(c) The pulmonary veins are similar on the two sides. The superior pulmonary veins are the anterior structures in the upper and mid hilum on both sides, and the inferior pulmonary veins run obliquely forward beneath the divisions of each lower lobe artery to enter the left atrium (Fig. 13).

Because the central portions of the pulmonary arteries are so differently organized on the two sides, the relationship between the major veins and arteries differs. On the right, the superior pulmonary vein is separated from the central bronchi by the lower division of the right pulmonary artery, whereas on the left, the superior pulmonary vein is separated from the lower division of the left pulmonary artery by the bronchial tree.

(d) On plain chest radiographs, the transverse diameter of the lower lobe arteries prior to their segmental divisions should normally be 9 to 16 mm in diameter. The combination of the right pulmonary artery and the superior pulmonary vein may produce a large round shadow on lateral and oblique views of the right hilum.

(e) On lateral or oblique plain chest radiographs, there are normally no large vessels traversing the angle between the middle and lower lobe bronchi on the right or the angle between the upper and lower lobe bronchi on the left.

The lungs beyond the hila

The segmental bronchi divide into progressively smaller airways; after 6 to 20 divisions they no longer contain cartilage in their walls and become bronchioles. The last of the purely conducting airways is known as the terminal bronchiole. The walls of the segmental bronchi are invisible on a chest radiograph, except when seen end-on as ring shadows (Fig. 14), but are clearly seen on CT or bronchography. Beyond the terminal bronchioles lie the gas-exchange units of the lung, the acini (Fig. 15).

The bronchopulmonary segments (Lee *et al.*, 1991)

The bronchopulmonary segments are based on the divisions of the bronchi (Fig. 16). They can be identified with precision at bronchography and at CT. Segmental borders cannot be identified in normal lungs, but the boundaries of the broncho-pulmonary segments can be inferred from the course of the bronchi and the intersegmental arrangement of drainage veins. Segments vary considerably in shape and size, but in general, segments are wedge-shaped and radiate from each hilum. The boundaries between segments are complex in shape. With the rare exception of accessory fissures, they are not defined by septa.

Lobules of the lung (secondary pulmonary lobules)

A secondary pulmonary lobule is composed of up to ten acini. The acinus is the smallest functional unit of the lung. Acini are 8–20 mm

(a)

(b)

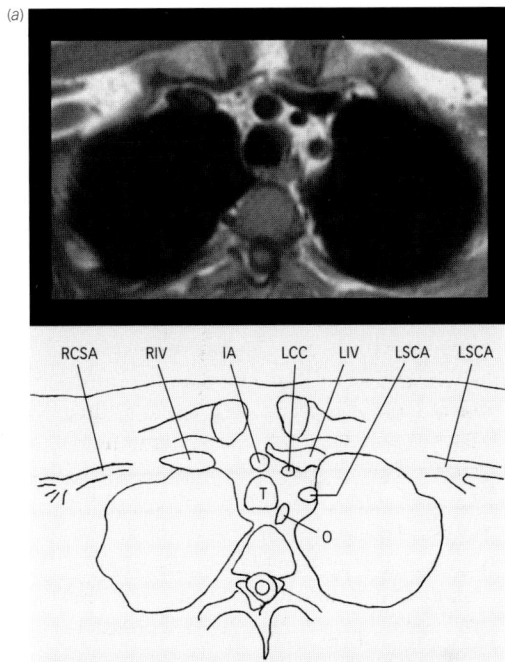

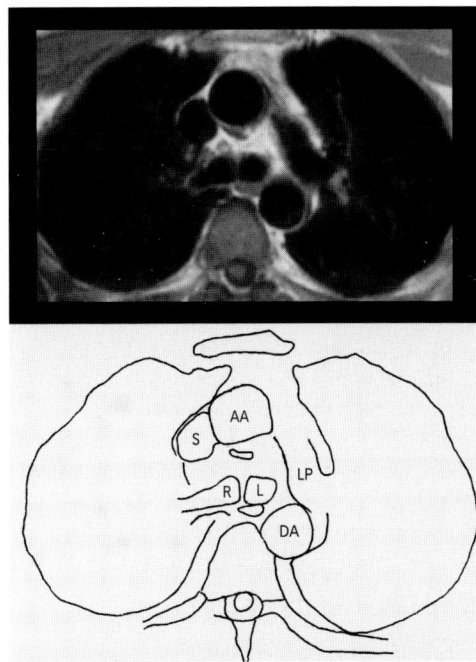

(c) Fig. 12(a)–(e).
Axial MR images showing mediastinal vessels. Key: A **aorta;** AA **ascending aorta;** Az **azygos vein;** BI **bronchus intermedius;** DA **descending aorta;** IA **internal thoracic vessels;** L **left main bronchus;** LA **left atrium;** LCC **left common carotid artery;** LIV **left brachiocephalic (innominate) vein;** LLLA **left lower lobe artery;** LSCA **left subclavian artery;** LP **left pulmonary artery;** LSPV **left superior pulmonary vein;** MLB **middle lobe bronchus;** MP **main pulmonary artery;** O **oesophagus;** R **right main bronchus;** RA **right atrium;** RIV **right brachiocephalic (innominate) vein;** RLLB **right lower lobe bronchus;** RP **right pulmonary artery;** RSCA **right subclavian artery;** RSPV **right superior pulmonary vein;** RV **right ventricle;** S **superior vena cava;** T **trachea.**

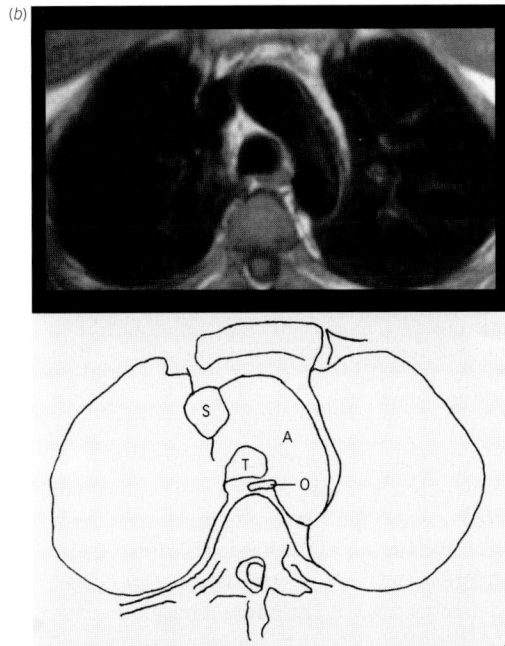

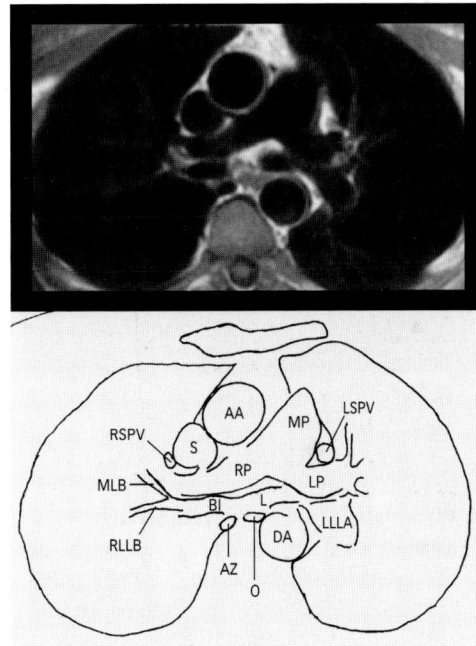

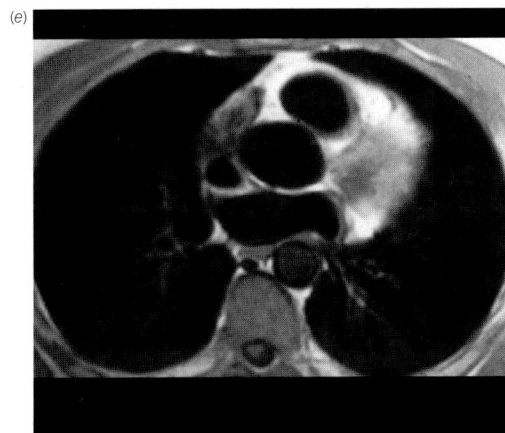

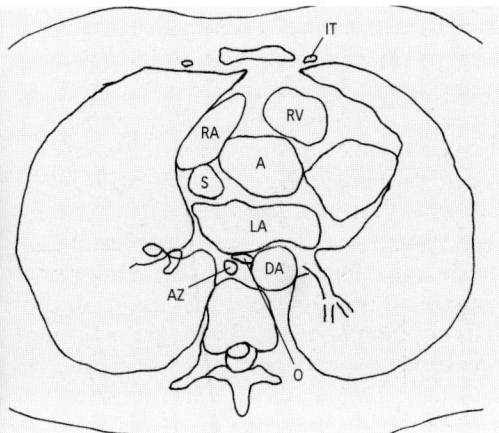

(d)

(e)

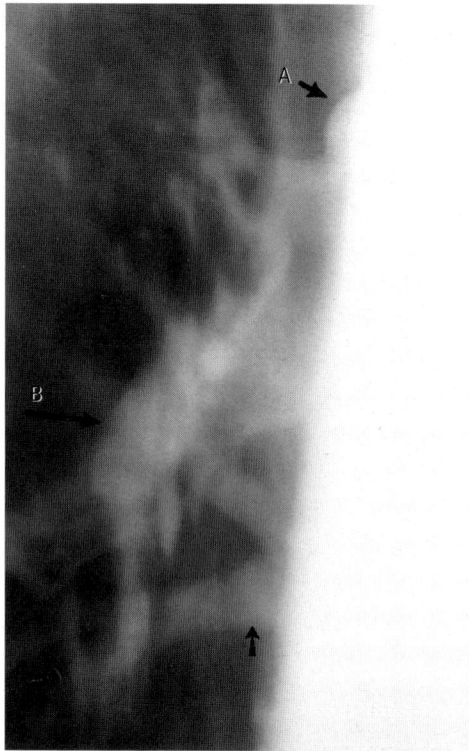

Fig. 13.
Representative plain tomogram of the hilum. **A** Azygos vein **B** Right lower lobe artery. Vertical arrow indicates tributary of inferior pulmonary vein.

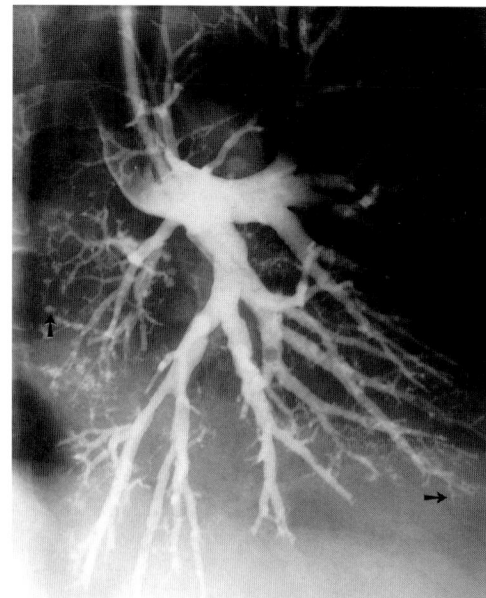

Fig. 14.
PA Chest X-ray showing bronchus 'end-on'. Horizontal arrows points to anterior segmental artery. Vertical arrow points to accompanying bronchus.

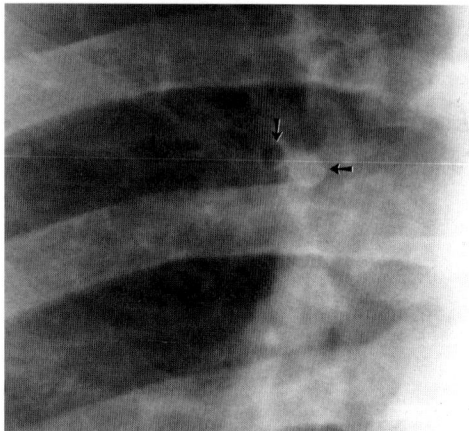

Fig. 15.
Bronchogram showing terminal bronchiolar filling in some segments. Horizontal arrow points to terminal bronchiole. Vertical arrow points to acinar filling.

septa, does not reach the pleural border.

The pulmonary blood vessels are responsible for the branching linear markings within the lungs, both on conventional films and at CT scanning. It is not possible to distinguish arteries from veins in the outer two-thirds of the lungs on plain radiography except by angiography or by sophisticated three-dimensional CT reconstruction. More centrally, the different orientation of the arteries and veins can be recognized even on plain PA radiography: the inferior pulmonary veins draining the lower lobes run more horizontally; the lower lobe arteries, more vertically. In the upper lobes, the arteries and veins show a similar gently curving vertical orientation, but the upper lobe veins (when not superimposed on the arteries), lie lateral to the arteries and can sometimes be traced to the main venous trunk – the superior pulmonary vein. The diameter of the blood vessels beyond the hilum varies according to the position of the patient. On plain chest radiographs taken with the patient in the upright position, there is a gradual increase in the diameter of both the arteries and the veins from apex to base: correlating with the physiological findings which show that, in an erect subject, there is a gradation of blood flow increasing from apex to base, a difference that is less marked when supine. It is usually not possible to distinguish artery from vein with certainty. Certain measurements have been suggested for upright chest films:

(a) The artery and bronchus of the anterior segment of either or both upper lobes are frequently seen end-on. The diameter of the artery is usually much the same as the diameter of the bronchus (4 to 5 mm) (Fig. 13).

in diameter and consist of respiratory bronchioles, alveolar ducts and alveoli. At the periphery of the lung, secondary pulmonary lobules are surrounded by connective tissue septa which contain veins and lymphatic vessels. Lobules are, therefore, best demonstrated in the periphery of the lung. On CT, they appear as polygonal structures in the subpleural region (Fig. 17(a)–(d)). The normal interlobular septa are not seen on conventional CT sections but can just be appreciated on some high resolution CT images. In the centre of the lobule is a branch of the pulmonary artery and an accompanying bronchiole. This bronchovascular bundle is demonstrated on axial CT sections as a rounded density approximately 1 cm away from the pleural border. The artery supplying the lobule appears as a finely branched structure, which, unlike the interlobular

Right lung : lateral view

Left lung : lateral view

Right lung : medial view

Left lung : medial view

Fig. 16.
Diagram demonstrating bronchopulmonary segments.

Key: right lung
upper lobe
1 apical segment
2 posterior segment
   upper lobe
3 anterior segment
middle lobe
4 lateral segment
5 medial segment
   middle lobe
lower lobe
6 superior segment
7 medial basal segment
8 anterior basal
   segment lower lobe
9 lateral basal segment
10 posterior basal segment

Key: left lung
upper lobe
1+2 apical posterior
   segment upper lobe
3 anterior segment superior
   division
4 superior segment
5 inferior segment lingula
   lower lobe
6 superior segment
8 anterior basal segment
9 lateral basal segment
   lower lobe
10 posterior basal segment

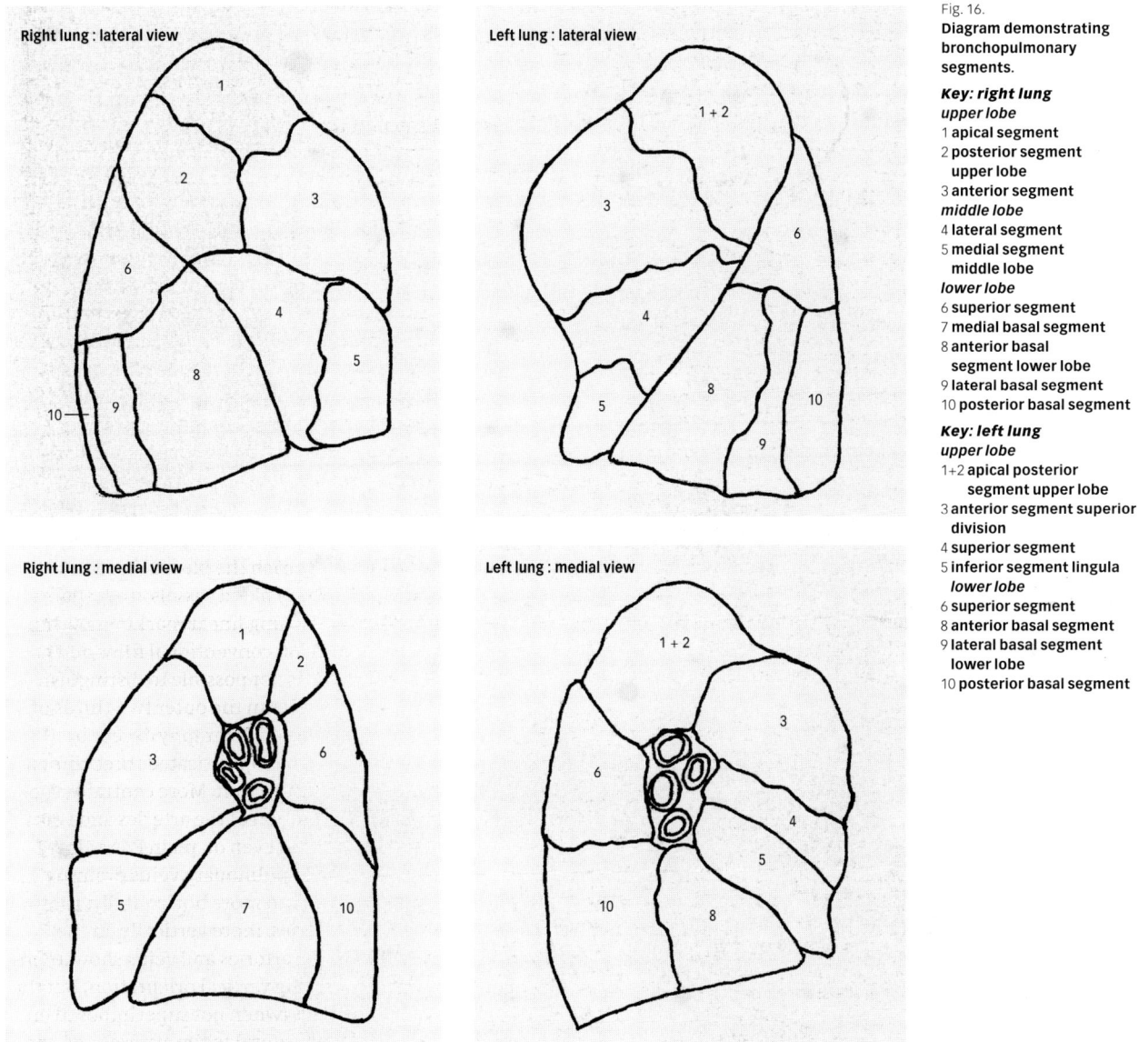

(b) In upright patients, the artery–bronchus ratio between the visible bronchi and immediately adjacent arteries is 0.85 (SD 0.15) for the upper zone and 1.34 (SD 0.25) for the lower zone.

(c) Vessels in the first anterior interspace should not exceed 3 mm in diameter.

The lymphatic network

A rich network of lymphatics drains the lung and pleura. The subpleural lymphatic vessels are found just beneath the pleura, at the junction of the interlobular septa and pleura, where they interconnect with each other as well as with the lymphatic vessels in the interlobular septa. The lymph then flows to the hilum by way of lymphatic channels that run peribronchially and in the deep septa. This normal lymphatic network is radiographically invisible.

The pleura

The visceral pleura (composed of a single layer of flat mesothelial cells) encloses the lobes of each lung. The parietal and visceral pleurae are continuous with each other at the hilum of the lung and along the inferior pulmonary ligament. Inferiorly, the parietal pleura tucks into the costophrenic sulcus. Together with the parietal pleura which lines the pleural cavity, a fine, soft-tissue interface is found, which in healthy individuals is recognizable on CT in the costoparietal and mediastinal regions. This intercostal stripe, a linear opacity of soft tissue density (1 to 2 mm thick), connects the inner aspects of the ribs at the lung–chest wall interface overlying an intercostal space and is produced by two layers of pleura, extrapleural fat, the endothoracic fascia, and the innermost intercostal muscle. The intercostal stripe disappears on the medial portion of the posterior ribs, since at this point it generally consists only of pleura, extrapleural fat and endo-thoracic fascia, which are too thin to resolve. Further peripherally a delicate layer of fat (extrapleural and subpleural fat), is located between the costoparietal pleura and endo-thoracic fascia. This layer of fat can be several millimetres thick in obese patients and can then be demonstrated on CT scans. On a plain chest radiograph, the pleura cannot be seen except where the visceral pleural invaginates into the lung to form the fissures and where the two lungs contact each other at junctional lines (Figs. 18, 19(*a*), (*b*)). The blood supply of the parietal pleura is from systemic vessels, while the visceral pleura is supplied by the pulmonary and bronchial circulations.

Standard fissures consist of a double layer of enfolded visceral pleura. They are normally very thin and are seen on plain radiographs only when tangential to the X-ray beam, appearing as a hairline of soft tissue density. Many fissures are incomplete. Where the fissures are incomplete there is parenchymal fusion between lobes and small bronchovascular structures, particularly veins, can be seen to cross fissural defects on HRCT (Berkmen *et al.*, 1989; Glazer *et al.*, 1991; Heitzman, 1984; Kent & Blades, 1942). The major fissure, also called the oblique or greater fissure, separates the upper lobe from the lower lobe on the left

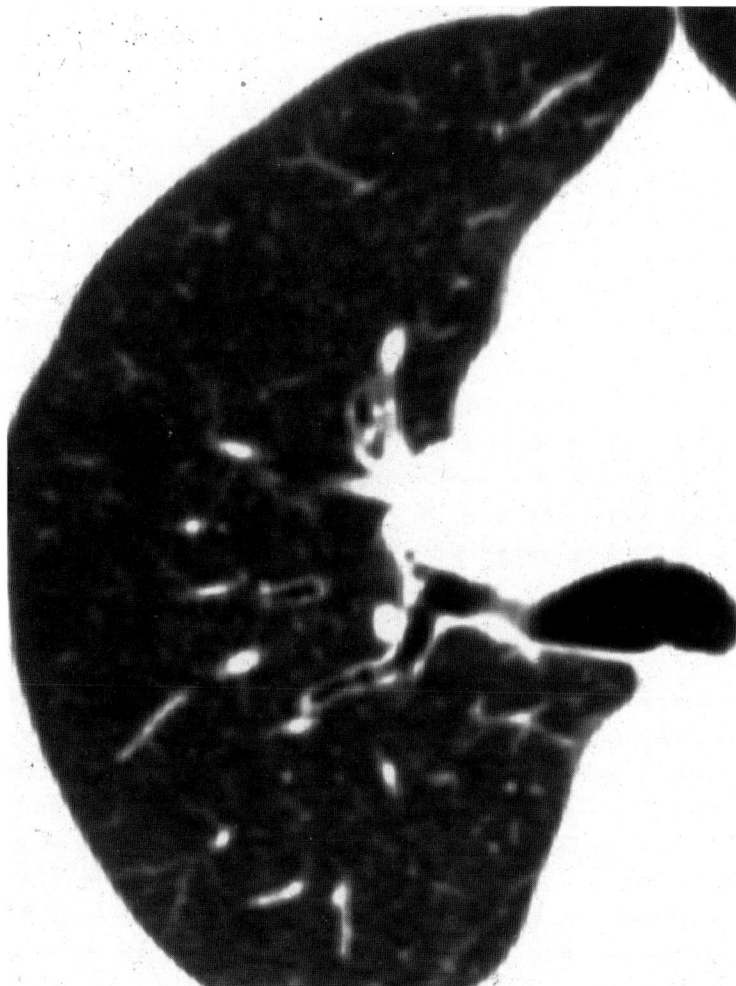

Fig. 17(*a*).
Normal HRCT. Note the bronchiolar lobules and the interlobular septa are not identified.

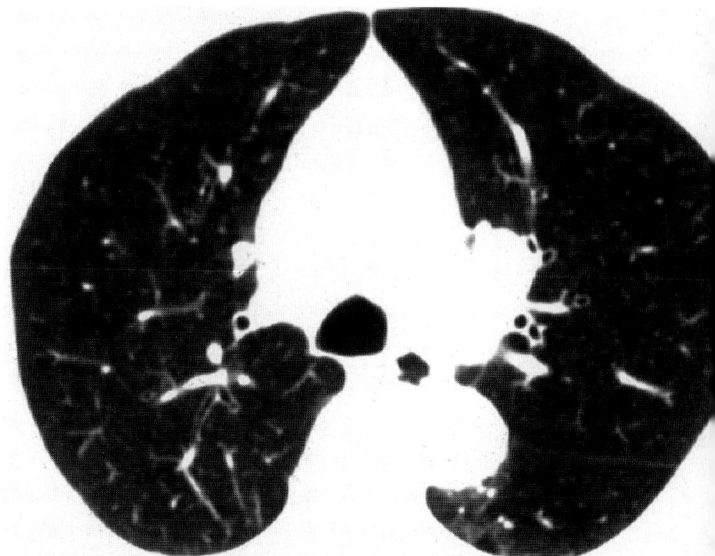

Fig. 17(*b*).
HRCT in lymphangitis carcinomatosa. The interlobular septa are irregularly thickened and easily defined.

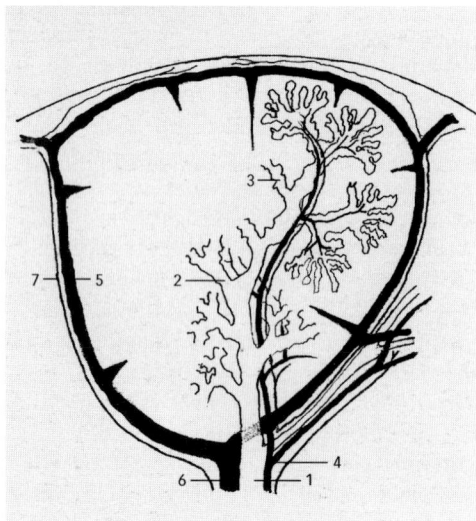

Fig. 17(*c*).
Diagram of secondary pulmonary lobule. In the central region, the bronchiole (1) merges with the lobule and branches via the terminal bronchiole (2) into the alveolar duct (3). The lobular artery (4) follows the branches of the bronchioles. Peripheral veins drain the lobule; the veins run along the interlobular septum (5), converging to form the interlobular vein (6). Lymph drainage is both interlobular (7) and central along the arteries. (Redrawn from Wegener, O.H., 1992.)

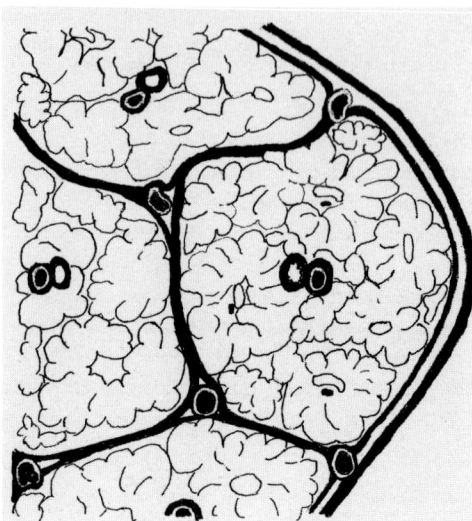

Fig. 17(*d*).
Diagram of secondary lobule on axial CT scan. In cross-section, the interlobular arteries app as punctate structures approximately 1 cm from the pleural boundary. So branching structures are also visible. The lobule ha a polygonal shape in cros section. (Redrawn from Wegener, O.H., 1992.)

and the upper and middle lobes from the lower lobe on the right. The major fissures face forward and pass obliquely downwards, parallel to the fifth rib, from about the body of the fifth thoracic vertebra, to meet the diaphragm several centimetres behind the sternum. They are most clearly seen on a lateral chest X-ray (Fig. 1(b)) (Felson, 1973; Proto & Ball, 1983; Proto & Speckman, 1979). Each major fissure follows a gently curving plane somewhat similar to that of a propeller blade, with the upper portion facing forward and laterally and the lower portion facing forward and medially. Below the hila, the lateral portions of the major fissures lie further forward than do the medial portions, whereas above the hila, this relationship reverses. Because of

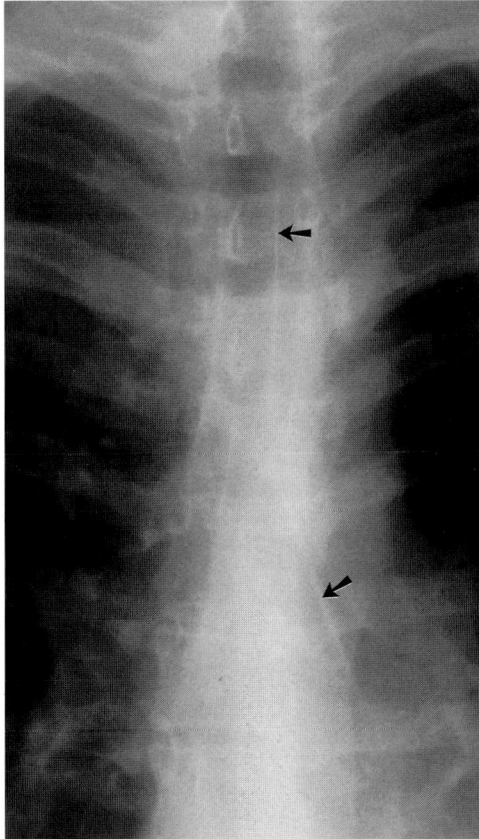

Fig. 18.
PA radiograph demonstrates anterior junction line (oblique arrow) and posterior junction line (horizontal arrow).

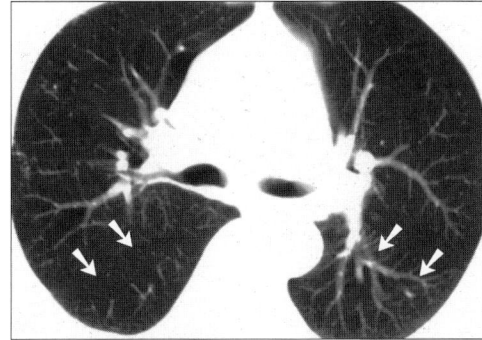

(a)

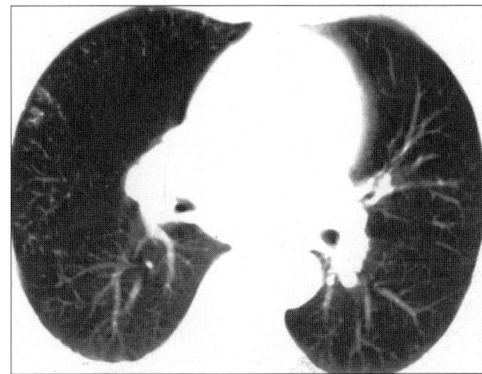

(b)

Fig. 20(a), (b).
Axial CT images demonstrating oblique fissures as a band of avascularity in upper zones (straight arrows). Note horizontal fissure seen as a lack of vessels in anterior two-thirds of right lung.

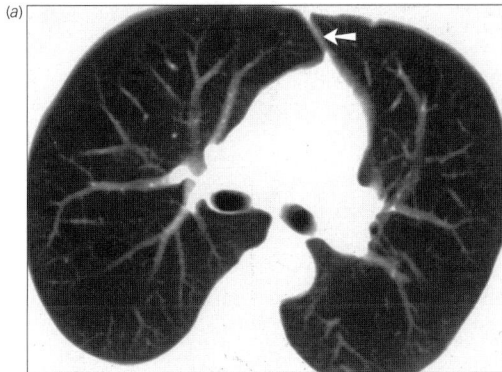

(a)

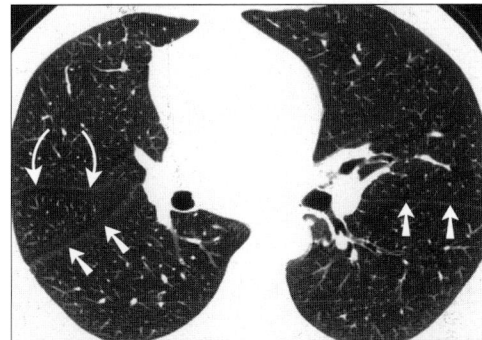

(c)

Fig. 19(a), (b).
Axial CT images demonstrate the anterior and posterior junction lines (arrow).

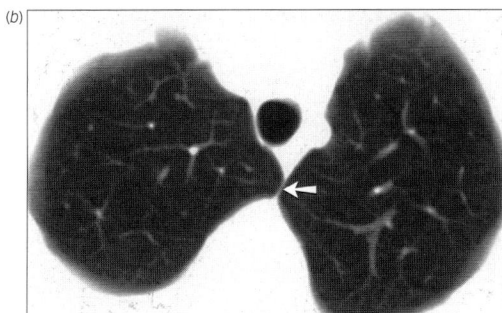

(b)

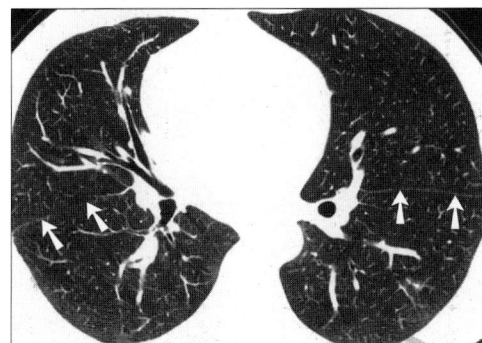

(d)

Fig. 20(c), (d).
Contiguous axial HRCT images demonstrating oblique fissures (straight arrows) and horizontal fissure (curved arrows).

these undulations, it is sometimes possible to identify the lateral aspect of the upper portion of either major fissure in the frontal view (Proto & Ball , 1983).

The position of the major fissures can be identified on standard 10 mm CT sections in the majority of patients (Fig. 20(a), (b)). The most common appearance is a curvilinear avascular band extending from the hilum to the chest wall, reflecting the lack of vessels in the subcortical zone of the lung (Frija *et al.*, 1982; Glazer *et al.*, 1991; Goodman *et al.*, 1982). Because of the obliquity of the major fissure, the fissure itself may be invisible or may be seen as a poorly defined curvilinear line or a band (Proto & Ball, 1983). On high resolution CT studies, the major fissure appears as a clearly defined line or, less commonly, as a band (Fig. 20(c), (d)).

Occasionally, the major fissure on HRCT appears as two parallel lines because of an artefact related to X-ray tube movement and breathing.

The minor fissure fans out forward and laterally in a horizontal direction from the right hilum and separates the anterior segment of the right upper lobe from the right middle lobe. It can be seen as a line shadow on both frontal and lateral chest radiographs. The fissure curves gently, the anterior and lateral portion usually curving downward. Because of the undulations of the major fissure, the minor fissure may be projected posterior to the right major fissure on a normal lateral view. On a standard upright frontal chest radiograph, the minor fissure contacts the lateral chest wall at, or close to, the axillary portion of the right sixth rib and ends medially at the interlobular pulmonary artery within about 1 cm of the point at which the superior venous trunk crosses (Felson, 1973). On frontal and lateral chest radiographs some or all of the fissure is seen in about 50% of patients (Proto & Speckman, 1979).

On conventional CT, the minor fissure is rarely seen as a line, but its position can usually be inferred by the large, triangular or oval-shaped deficiency of vessels extending from the major fissure to the chest wall on one or more sections at the level of the bronchus intermedius (Fig. 20(a), (b)). With thin-section CT, a variety of normal patterns (a line, an ill-defined band shadow or even as a rounded density) are encountered, depending on the precise shape of the minor fissure (Fig. 20(c),(d)).

Accessory fissures are clefts of varying depth in the outer surface of the lung.

The azygos fissure is the best-known accessory fissure and is so called because it contains the azygos vein within its lower margin. The fissure, which is almost invariably on the right side, results from failure of normal migration of the azygos vein from the chest wall through the upper lobe to its usual position in the tracheobronchial angle, so that the invaginated visceral and parietal pleurae persist to form a

Fig. 21.
Azygos fissure. (a) The azygos vein (curved arrow) is seen in the lower margin of the azygos fissure (horizontal arrow). Note the absence of the azygos vein in the right tracheobronchial angle (vertical arrow).

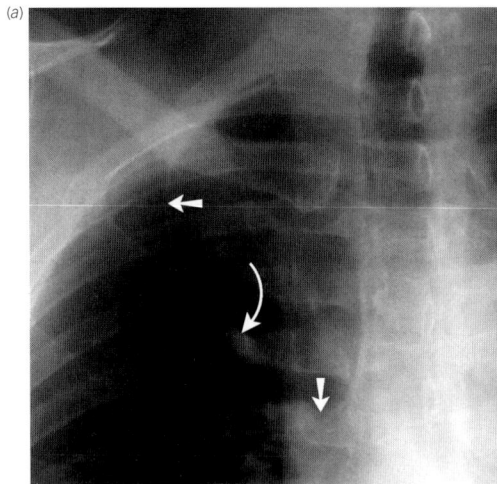

Fig. 21(b), (c).
Axial CT study demonstrates azygos vein (curved arrow) and azygos fissure (horizontal arrow).

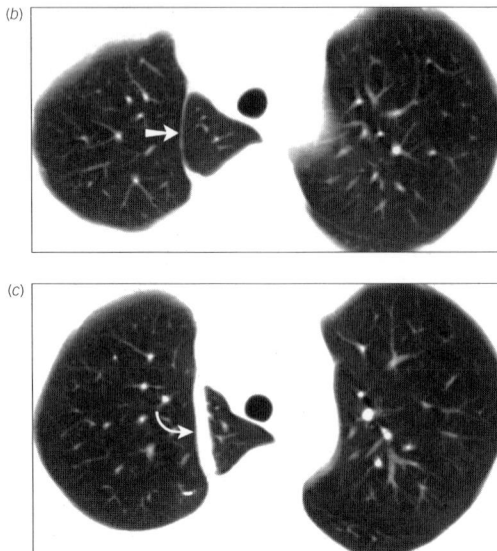

Fig. 22.
Inferior accessory fissur (arrows) separates the medial basal segment fr the anterior basal segme of the lower lobe. Consolidation in the anterior basal segment sharply demarcated by t inferior accessory fissur

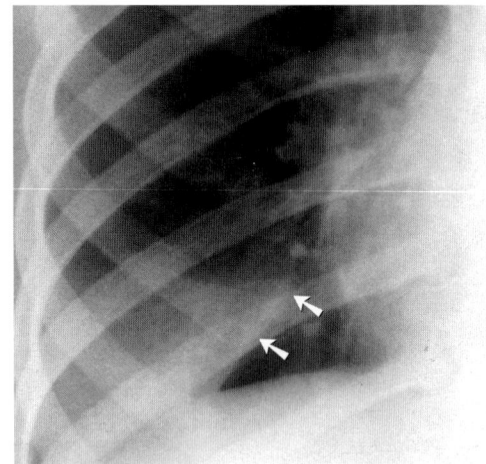

fissure. The azygos fissure produces a curvilinear opacity which extends from the chest wall to cross the right upper lobe obliquely, ending medially in the displaced azygos vein above and to the right of the normal position of the vein in the angle between trachea and right main stem bronchus (Fig. 21(*a*)). The segment of lung marginated by the fissure, though called the azygos lobe, is not a true segment or lobe because it does not have a specific bronchial supply; the airways to the 'azygos lobe' are derived from the apical or posterior segments of the right upper lobe. The altered course of the azygos vein together with the fissure is readily seen at CT and the azygos vein is demonstrated to lie 2 to 4 cm higher than usual, forming a curvilinear band coursing through the lung before entering the posterior aspect of the superior vena cava (Fig. 21(*b*), (*c*)). Above the azygos arch, the fissure is seen as a thin curvilinear line, its exact shape depending on the size of the 'lobe'. The lung invaginates against the mediastinum, coming to lie behind the superior vena cava outlining the posterior wall of the superior vena cava and sometimes even extends behind the trachea. A left 'azygos' fissure is rare and most commonly involves the hemiazygos and left superior intercostal veins in an analogous way to the azygos vein on the right. Fissures may, very rarely, be seen at the boundaries between bronchopulmonary segments. The inferior accessory fissure usually incompletely separates the medial basal segment from the rest of the right lower lobe. It runs obliquely upward and medially towards the hilum from the medial aspect of the diaphragm (Fig. 22). It is rarely seen on lateral radiographs. On CT the fissure appears on sections near the diaphragm as an arc, concave to the mediastinum, extending from the major fissure back to the mediastinum near the oesophagus. It is best demonstrated on high-resolution CT (Godwin & Tarver, 1985).

The superior accessory fissure separates the superior segment of one or other lower lobe from the basal segments and superficially resembles a minor fissure on a frontal radio-

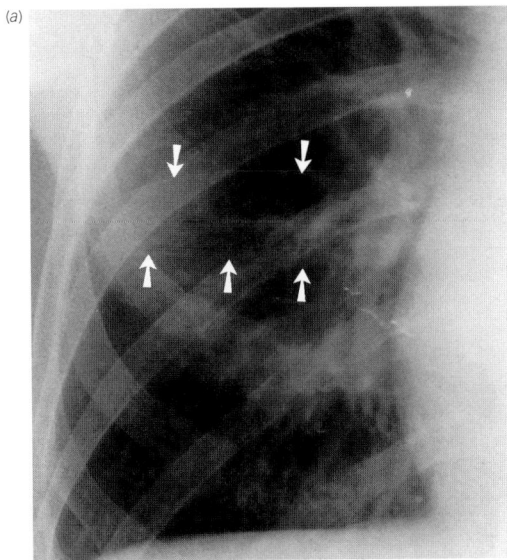

Fig. 23(*a*), (*b*). uperior accessory fissure. The downward pointing arrows indicate the horizontal fissure. The upward pointing arrows indicate the superior accessory fissure

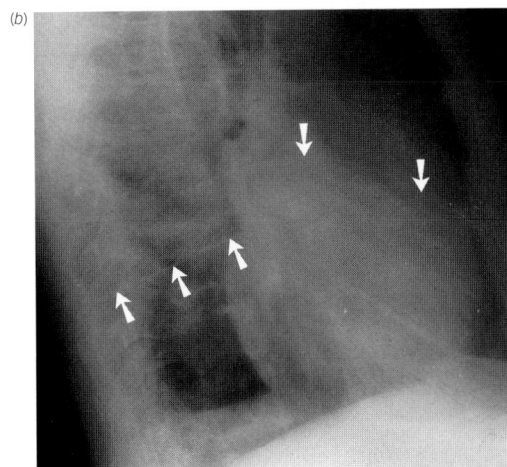

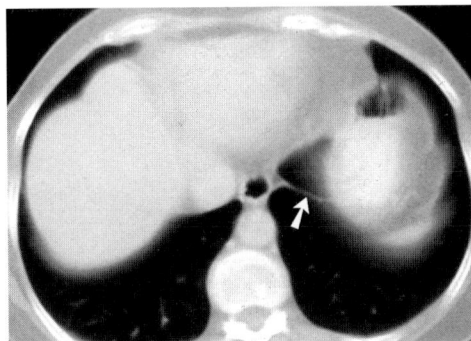

Fig. 24.
Inferior pulmonary ligament (arrow).

graph. However, the minor fissure lies above the middle lobe bronchus and the superior accessory fissure lies below the superior segmental bronchus. The superior accessory fissure is thus projected below the minor fissure on frontal radiographs (Fig. 23(*a*)). On the lateral view, unlike the minor fissure, the superior accessory fissure extends posteriorly across the vertebral bodies (Fig. 23(*b*)). On CT, like the minor fissure, it appears as an avascular area.

A left minor fissure is present in approximately 10% of people but is only rarely detected on posteroanterior and lateral radiographs. It separates the lingular segments from the rest of the left upper lobe and is analogous to the minor fissure.

The inferior pulmonary ligaments are pleural reflections that hang down from the hila like curtains and join the mediastinal surface of each lower lobe to the mediastinum and to the medial part of the diaphragm. The two layers of pleura contact each other below

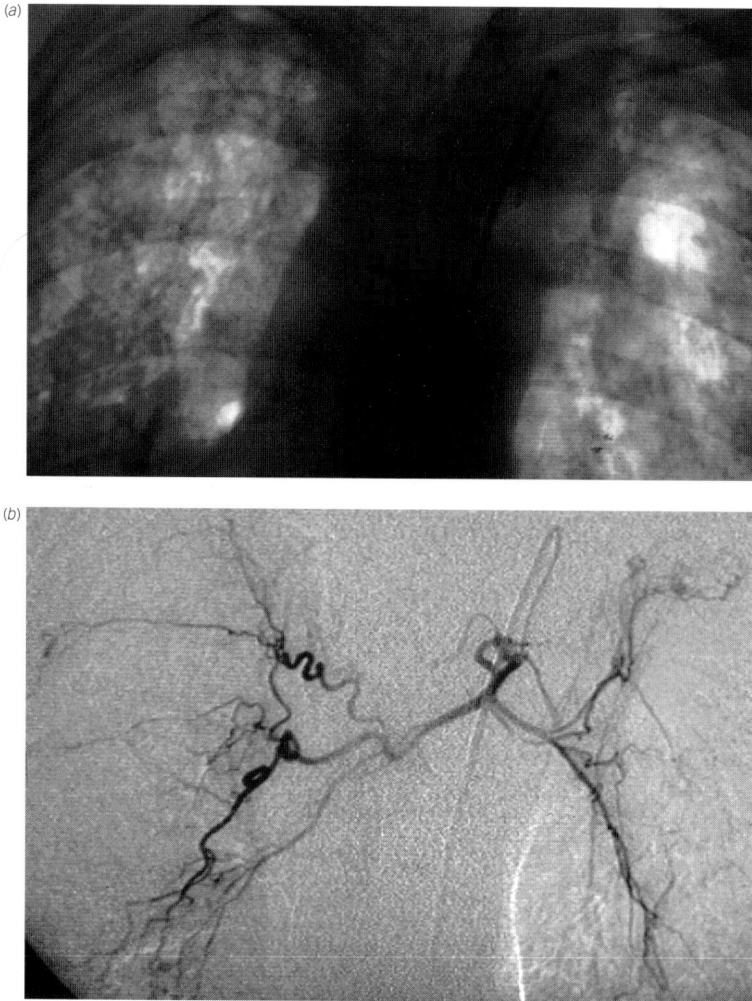

On CT the interlobular septum lying deep to the inferior pulmonary ligaments is visible in about 50% to 75% of patients (Fig. 24) (Berkmen et al., 1992) and is best detected just above the diaphragm as a thin curvilinear line passing into the lung laterally and slightly backward from the mediastinum at the level of the oesophagus.

Bronchial artery supply

The bronchial arteries vary in number, size and origin (Fig. 25(a), (b), (c)). As a rule, there is one right bronchial artery, which arises from the third posterior intercostal artery or from the upper left bronchial artery. It runs on the posterior surface of the right bronchus, dividing and subdividing along the bronchi, supplying them, the alveolar tissue of the lung and the bronchopulmonary lymph nodes and sends branches to the pericardium and the oesophagus. The left bronchial arteries, usually two in number, arise from the thoracic aorta, the upper one opposite the fifth thoracic vertebra and the lower one just below the left main bronchus. They run on the posterior surface of the left main bronchus and have a distribution similar to that of the right bronchial artery. The bronchial arteries supplying the bronchi form a capillary plexus which communicates with branches of the pulmonary artery in the walls of the smaller bronchi and in the visceral pleura and empties

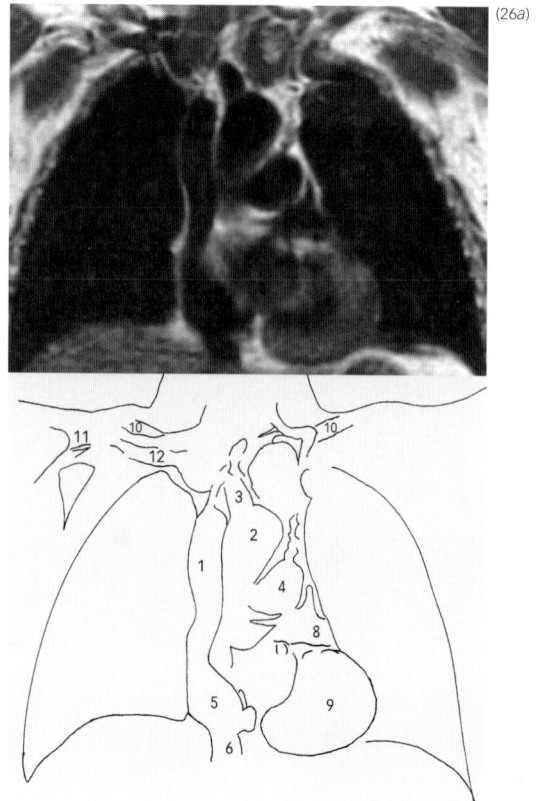

Fig. 25. Bronchial arteriogram (courtesy of Dr J.E. Jackson, London). (a) Image showing catheter positioned in thoracic aorta. (b) Image demonstrating moderately enlarged bronchial arteries. (c) Diagram of the bronchi and bronchial arteries. Note: the bronchial arteries normally run *behind* the bronchi and their branches. Key: 1 trachea, 2 left main bronchus; 3 right main bronchus; 4 aortic arch; 5 thoracic aorta; 6 origin of upper left bronchial artery; 7 origin of lower left bronchial artery; 8 origin of right bronchial artery; 9 left upper lobe bronchus; 10 left lower lobe bronchus; 11 right upper lobe bronchus; 12 bronchus intermedius; 13 right middle lobe bronchus; 14 right lower lobe bronchus.

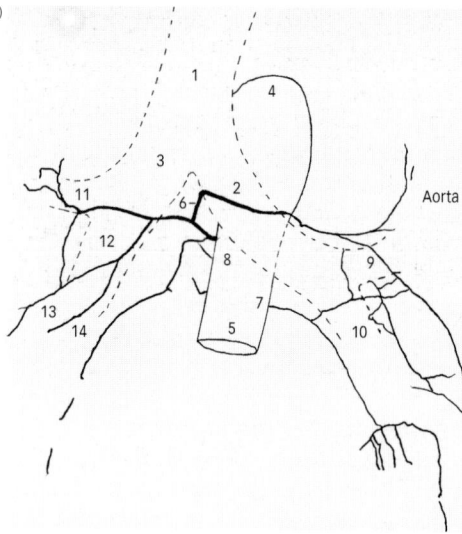

the inferior pulmonary vein and end in a free border that usually lies over the inner third of the hemidiaphragm, but is sometimes displaced towards the hilum. The bare area of the ligament contains connective tissue, bronchial veins, lymphatics and lymph nodes (Fraser et al., 1988). The inferior pulmonary ligaments are not visible on chest radiographs.

(b)

(d)

(c)

(e)

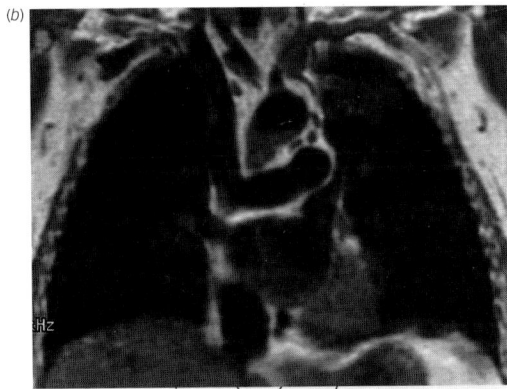

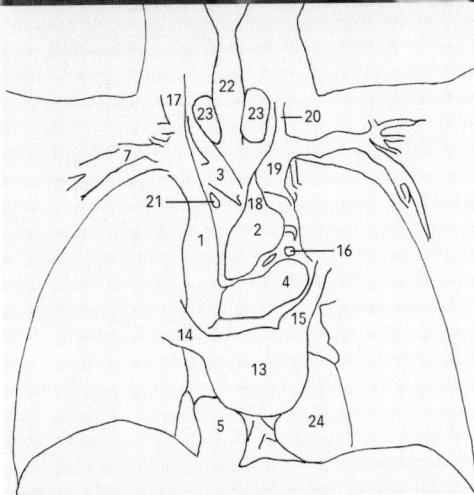

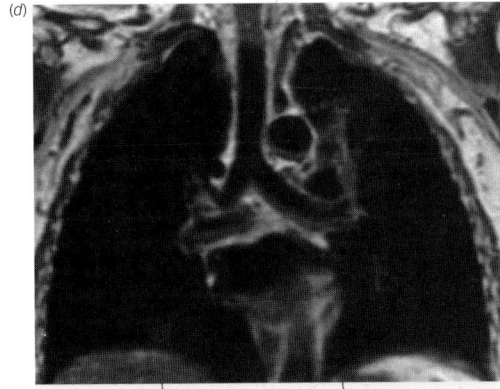

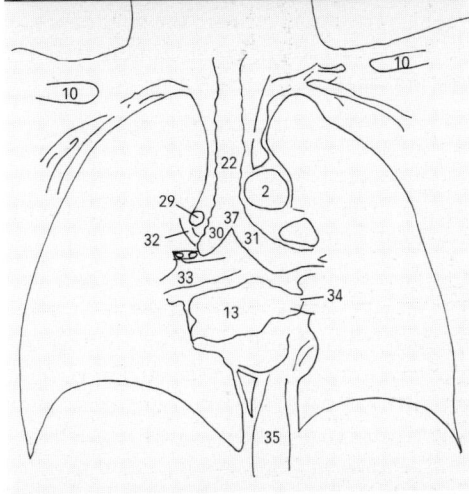

Fig. 26*(a)*–*(e)*.
Contiguous coronal MR images demonstrating mediastinal contents and borders. Key: 1 superior vena cava; 2 arch of aorta; 3 innominate artery; 4 pulmonary trunk; 5 right atrium; 6 inferior vena cava; 7 right subclavian vein; 8 left atrial appendage; 9 left ventricle; 10 clavicle; 11 brachial plexus; 12 right subclavian artery; 13 left atrium; 14 right superior pulmonary vein; 15 left superior pulmonary vein; 16 lymph node in aortopulmonary window; 17 right internal jugular vein; 18 left common carotid artery; 19 left subclavian artery; 20 left vertebral artery; 21 lymph node; 22 trachea; 23 thyroid gland; 24 left ventricular wall; 25 left pulmonary artery; 26 right pulmonary artery; 27 left axillary artery; 28 left axillary vein; 29 azygos vein; 30 right main bronchus; 31 left main bronchus; 32 right upper lobe pulmonary artery; 33 right lower lobe pulmonary artery; 34 left inferior pulmonary vein; 35 descending aorta; 36 vertebral body; 37 carina; 38 oesophagus

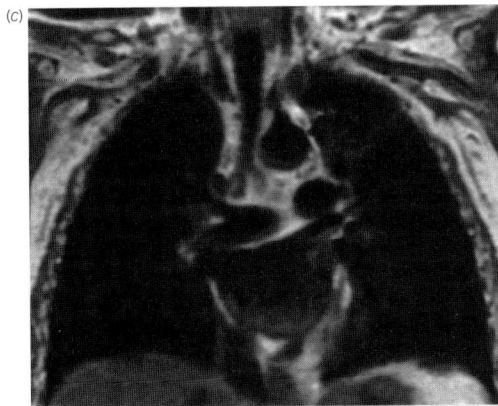

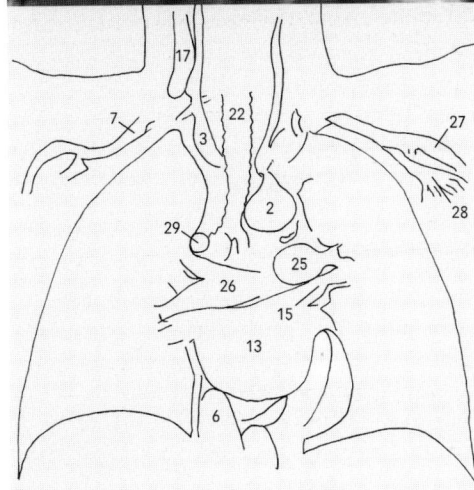

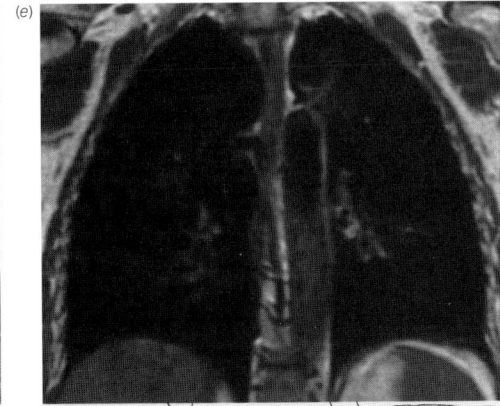

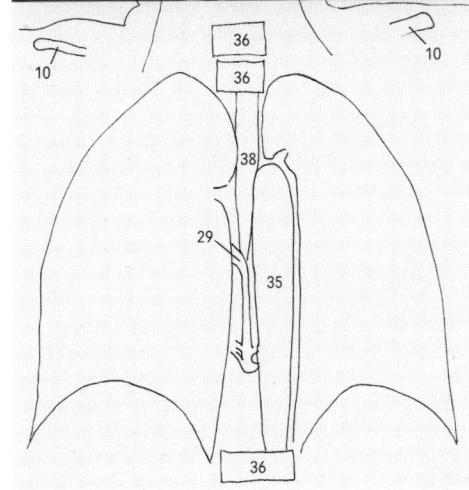

into the pulmonary veins. Others are distributed in the interlobular alveolar tissue and end in the deep or superficial bronchial veins. Lastly, some ramify upon the surface of the lung beneath the pleura, where they form a capillary network.

The bronchial veins form two distinct systems: (i) the deep bronchial veins, which communicate freely with the pulmonary veins and end in a main pulmonary vein or in the left atrium, (ii) the superficial bronchial veins which drain the extrapulmonary bronchi, the visceral pleura and the hilar lymph nodes; they also communicate with the pulmonary veins and end, on the right side in the azygos vein, and on the left in the left superior intercostal vein or the accessory hemiazygos vein. The bronchial veins do not receive all the blood conveyed to the lungs by the bronchial arteries, because some enters the pulmonary veins (Marchand *et al.*, 1950).

Pulmonary arteries and veins

The main pulmonary artery, together with the right and left pulmonary arteries, can be readily demonstrated on CT and MRI (Figs. 11, 26 (a)–(e)). The main pulmonary trunk runs obliquely backward and upward to the left of the ascending aorta before dividing into right and left branches. The right pulmonary artery travels more or less horizontally through the mediastinum, between the ascending aorta and the SVC anteriorly and the major bronchi posteriorly. The left pulmonary artery arches higher than the right pulmonary artery and passes over the left main bronchus to descend posterior to it. The left pulmonary artery is seen on a higher CT or MR section than the right pulmonary artery. The external diameter of the pulmonary trunk is slightly smaller than that of the ascending aorta, averaging 2.8 cm (Guthaner *et al.*, 1979). The right pulmonary artery is two-thirds the diameter of the main pulmonary trunk. The hilar vessels are more variable in position than the bronchi.

The right upper lobe pulmonary artery arises within the pericardium and is commonly seen just anterior to the right upper lobe bronchus. The right pulmonary artery crosses in front of the bronchus intermedius and then, at a more caudal level, lies alongside its lateral aspect as it becomes the right interlobar pulmonary artery, often causing a slightly nodular contour to the hilum at this level. More caudally, the right interlobar pulmonary artery assumes a vertical orientation and is positioned just lateral to the bifurcation of the middle and lower lobe bronchi. The

middle lobe pulmonary artery lies between the medial and lateral segmental bronchi of the right middle lobe. The segmental lower lobe pulmonary arteries generally lie more towards the periphery of the lung than their corresponding bronchi, and the segmental veins are positioned just central to the bronchi.

The veins of the upper lobe course in front of the arteries and bronchi towards the heart. The posterior branch of the right superior pulmonary vein usually lies within the angle formed by the bifurcation of the right upper lobe bronchus into the anterior and posterior segments: the anterior branch generally is located medial to the branches of the right upper lobe pulmonary artery. The right superior pulmonary vein lies anteromedial to the middle lobe bronchus as it enters the upper portion of the left atrium. Both inferior pulmonary veins travel medially and superiorly to enter the lower portion of the left atrium.

The left upper lobe pulmonary artery and the left superior pulmonary vein have much less constant anatomical relationships to the left upper lobe bronchus than their counterparts on the right side. The apicoposterior bronchus may lie medial or lateral to the branch of the left upper lobe pulmonary artery. The left pulmonary artery itself is first seen cephalad to the left main bronchus adjacent to the apicoposterior bronchus and generally lies posterior to the left superior pulmonary vein. The left superior pulmonary vein invariably lies in front of the left upper lobe bronchus as it courses to the left atrium; it frequently has a horizontal course at a slightly caudal level. The posterior wall of the left upper lobe bronchus is usually concave where it is indented superiorly and posteriorly by the left pulmonary artery.

The left pulmonary artery extends caudally posterior to the left upper lobe bronchus to become the left interlobar pulmonary artery. Just caudal to the left upper lobe bronchus, frequently at the level where the bronchus to the superior segment of the left lower lobe originates, the left interlobar pulmonary artery lies in the bifurcation behind the lingular bronchus and anterolateral to the lower lobe bronchus.

The mediastinum

The mediastinum is divided by anatomists into superior, anterior, middle and posterior divisions. The mediastinium is divided into superior and inferior compartments by an imaginary line from the lower border of the manubrium to the lower border of the fourth vertebra. The inferior compartment is further divided into anterior, middle and posterior compartments. The anterior mediastinum lies anterior to the pericardium and the root of the ascending aorta. The posterior mediastinum is bounded in front by the trachea, the pulmonary vessels and pericardium, and behind by the vertebral column. Its contents include the descending aorta, the oesophagus, the azygos and hemiazygos veins, and the thoracic duct. These divisions are not important to the radiologist because they do not provide a clearcut guide to disease, nor do they form barriers to the spread of disease. Moreover, different authors use different definitions (Felson, 1969; Fraser *et al.*, 1988; Heitzman, 1988; Zylak *et al.*, 1982).

The normal mediastinum
The normal mediastinal structures identified at CT and MRI (Figs. 12, 26) are the heart and blood vessels that make up the bulk of the mediastinum, the major airways, and the oesophagus. These structures are surrounded by a variable amount of connective tissue, largely fat, within which lie lymph nodes, the thymus, the thoracic duct and the phrenic and recurrent laryngeal nerves.

The oesophagus
The oesophagus is visible on all CT and MRI axial sections from the root of the neck down to the oesophageal hiatus through the diaphragm (Fig. 12). If there is sufficient mediastinal fat, the entire circumference of the oesophagus can be identified. In approximately 80% of normal individuals, the oesophagus contains a small amount of air. If air is present in the lumen, the uniform thickness of the wall can be appreciated. Without air, the collapsed oesophagus appears either circular or oval and is usually approximately 1 cm in its narrowest diameter. At MRI the signal intensity on T_1-weighted images is similar to that of muscle, but on T_2-weighted images the oesophagus often shows a much higher signal intensity than muscle.

The thoracic duct and its tributaries
The thoracic duct connects the cisterna chyli to the great veins in the root of the neck and transports all of the body lymph except that from most of the lungs and the right upper quadrant of the body. The thoracic duct is 2 to 8 mm in diameter (Nusbaum *et al.*, 1964) and, although thought of as a single structure, is commonly multiple in part of its course (Van Pernis, 1949). It may consist of up to eight separate channels. The duct or ducts pass up from the cisterna chyli behind the median

arcuate ligament and ascend between the azygos vein and aorta. At the level of T6, the thoracic duct crosses to the left of the spine and ascends along the lateral aspect of the oesophagus behind the aorta and left subclavian artery. It then arches forward across the subclavian artery and inserts into a large central vein within 1 cm of the junction of the left internal jugular and subclavian veins. Any, or all, of these vessels may end separately in the great veins. The thoracic duct cannot be visualised directly on plain chest radiographs or CT unless lymphangiographic contrast has been administered.

Mediastinal blood vessels
On transaxial images, the vertically oriented ascending and descending portions of the aorta appear round, whereas the arch is seen as a tapering oval that becomes more narrow as it gives rise to the arteries to the neck, head and upper limbs (Fig. 12). The average transverse diameter of the ascending aorta is 3.5 cm and that of the descending aorta is 2.5 cm. Sections above the aortic arch show the three major aortic branches arranged in a curve lying anterior and to the left of the trachea, the order from right to left being the brachiocephalic (innominate), left common carotid, and left subclavian arteries (Fig. 27(*a*), (*b*), (*c*)). The brachiocephalic artery is appreciably larger than the other two vessels and varies slightly in position. In about half the population, it is directly anterior to the trachea; in the remainder, while still anterior to the trachea, it is either slightly to the right or left of the midline (Gamsu, 1983). The left common carotid artery lies to the left of the trachea. The left subclavian artery also lies either to the left of the trachea or posterior to it. It is the most lateral vessel of the three and often contacts the left lung. In 0.5% of the population, the right subclavian artery arises distal to the left subclavian artery as a separate fourth major branch of the aorta, known as an aberrant right subclavian artery. Instead of arising from the brachiocephalic artery, it runs behind the oesophagus from left to right, at or just above the level of the aortic arch, to lie against the right side of the vertebral bodies before entering the root of the neck. In individuals with an aberrant right subclavian artery, the right common carotid artery is smaller than usual because the vessel does not give rise to a right subclavian artery and is, therefore, similar in diameter to the left common carotid artery.

As the descending aorta travels through the chest, it gradually moves from a position to

Fig. 27.
Aortic arch and branches.

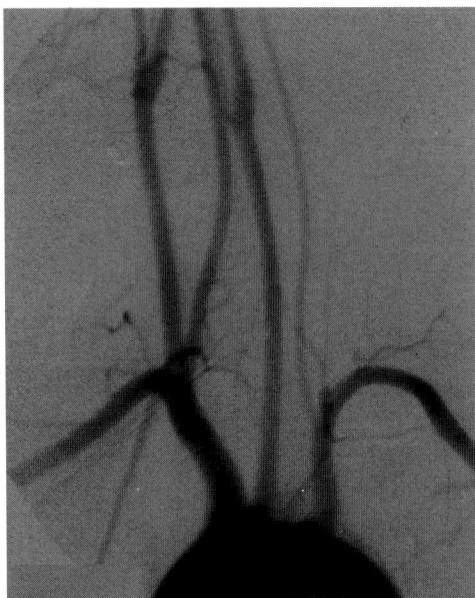

Fig. 27(*a*), (*b*).
Digital subtraction
angiogram demonstrating
vessels and background
structures. (Courtesy of Dr
J.E. Dacie, London.)

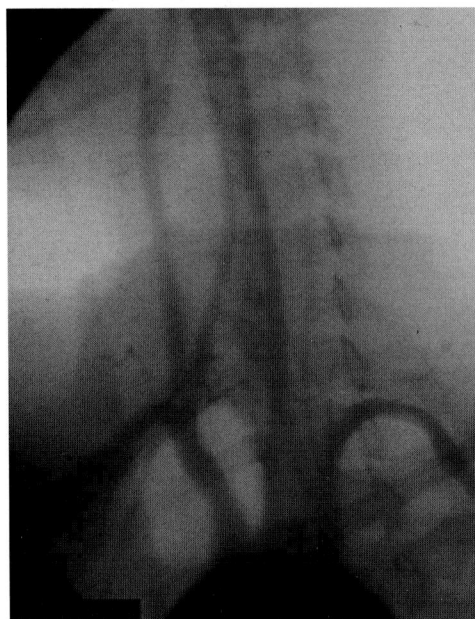

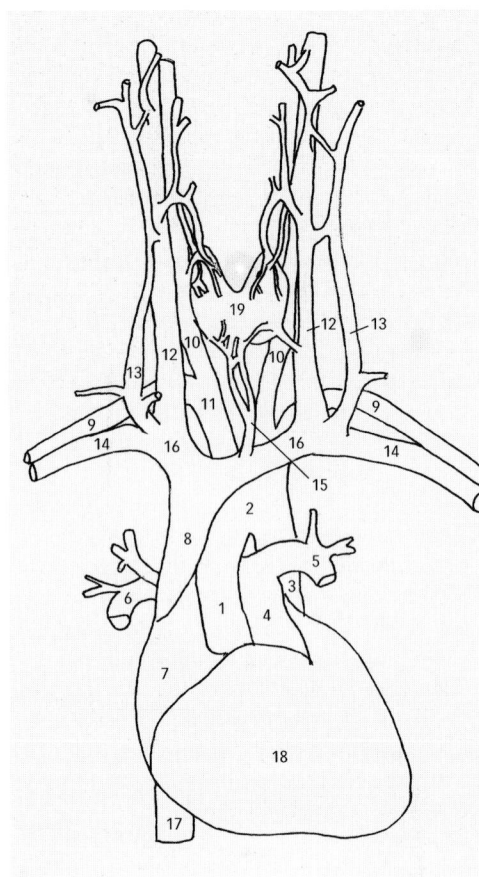

Fig. 27(*c*).
Diagram of mediastinal
vessels and branches to
the head and neck. Key: 1
ascending aorta; 2 arch of
the aorta; 3 descending
aorta; 4 pulmonary trunk;
5 left pulmonary artery;
6 right lower lobe
pulmonary artery;
7 right atrium; 8 superior
vena cava; 9 subclavian
artery; 10 common carotid
artery; 11 brachiocephalic
trunk; 12 internal jugular
vein; 13 external jugular
vein; 14 subclavian vein;
15 thyroid vein;
16 brachiocephalic vein;
17 inferior vena cava;
18 heart; 19 thyroid gland.

the left of the vertebral bodies to an almost midline position before exiting from the chest through the aortic hiatus in the diaphragm. With increasing age, the descending thoracic aorta becomes dilated and tortuous.

The brachiocephalic (innominate) veins are two large trunks in the root of the neck and the uppermost part of the thorax, and each is formed by the union of the ipsilateral internal jugular and subclavian veins.

The left brachiocephalic vein forms a curved band-like structure running obliquely downwards and to the right behind the upper part of the manubrium sterni to the sternal end of the first right costal cartilage, where it unites with the right brachiocephalic vein to form the superior vena cava. In its course, it crosses in front of the pleura over the left lung

apex, the left internal thoracic, subclavian and common carotid arteries, the left phrenic and the vagus nerves, the trachea and the brachiocephalic artery. It is formed by the junction of the left internal jugular and subclavian veins and it has tributaries from the left vertebral, internal thoracic, inferior thyroid and superior intercostal veins, and sometimes from the first left posterior intercostal vein and some thymic and pericardial veins. Since the left brachiocephalic vein takes an oblique, downward course to join the SVC, its image on axial sections is often oval rather than tubular in shape. On rare occasions it may descend vertically through the mediastinum before crossing the midline to join the right brachiocephalic vein and may mimic lymphadenopathy.

The right brachiocephalic vein begins behind the sternal end of the right clavicle and passes almost vertically downwards to join the left brachiocephalic vein and form the superior vena cava, behind the lower border of the first right costal cartilage, close to the right border of the sternum. It lies anterolateral to the brachiocephalic artery and the right vagus nerve. It is formed by the junction of the right internal jugular and subclavian veins and has tributaries from the right vertebral, internal thoracic and inferior thyroid veins and sometimes the first right posterior intercostal vein.

Fig. 28(a)–(d).
The mediastinal spaces.
PTS **pretracheal space;**
APW **aortopulmonary
window;** SCS **subcarinal
space;** RPS **right
paratracheal space;**
PPTS **posterior tracheal
space;** A **azygos vein;**
O **oesophagus.**

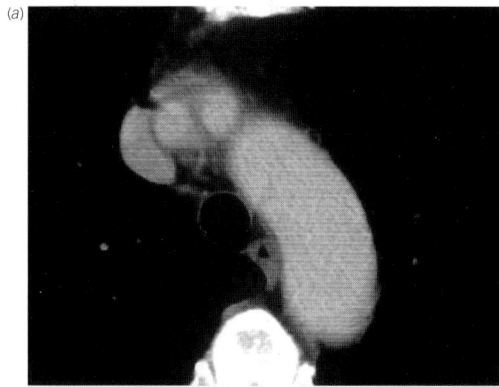

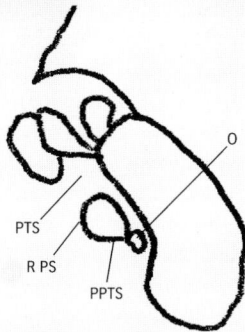

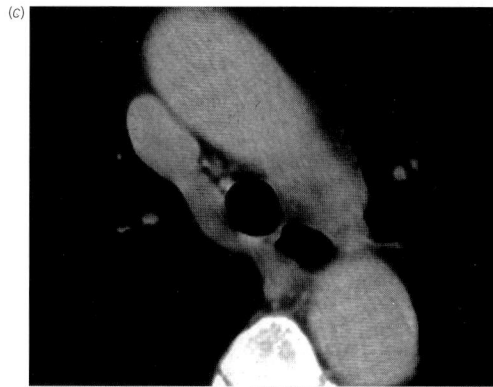

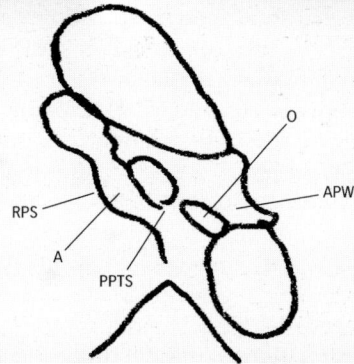

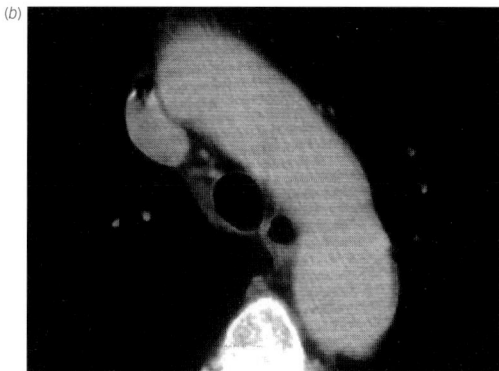

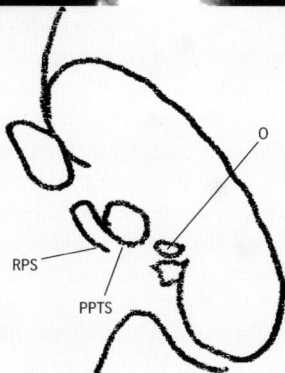

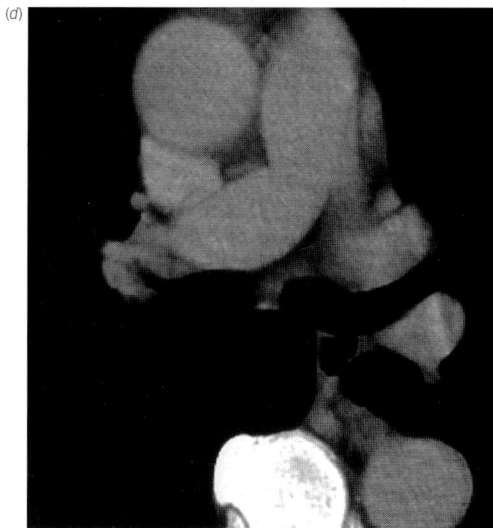

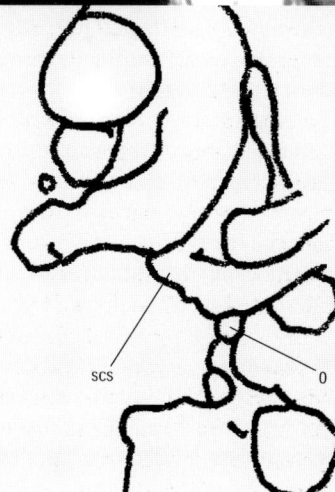

The right brachiocephalic vein travels vertically, anterolateral to the trachea in line with
the three major arteries. This vein is identifiable as the farthest right of the vessels. It is
larger than the arteries and is oval in shape.

The superior vena cava (SVC) collects blood
from the upper half of the body and is formed
by the junction of the two brachiocephalic
veins (Fig. 27(c)). The SVC begins behind the

143

lower border of the first right costal cartilage close to the sternum, descends vertically behind the first and second intercostal spaces and ends in the upper part of the right atrium opposite the third right costal cartilage. The lower half of the vessel is within the fibrous pericardium, which it pierces at the level of the second costal cartilage and here it is covered in front and on each side with serous pericardium. In front, the SVC is related to the anterior margins of the right lung and its pleura, with the pericardium intervening below. These structures separate it from the internal thoracic artery and the first and second intercostal spaces, and from the second and third costal cartilages. The trachea and the right vagus nerve lie posteromedially and the right lung lies posterolateral to its upper part, while the root of the right lung is a direct posterior relation below. On its right, it is related to the right phrenic nerve and right pleura; on its left, to the origin of the brachiocephalic artery and the ascending aorta. The tributaries of the SVC include the azygos vein and several small veins from the pericardium and other structures in the mediastinum.

The SVC has an oval or round configuration on transaxial section (Guthaner *et al.*, 1979). Its diameter is one-third to two-thirds the diameter of the ascending aorta. It can, however, be considerably smaller and may be much flattened in shape. Along an axial course, the SVC can be reliably traced posterolateral to the ascending aorta to the point where it enters the right atrium (Fig. 12). On occasion (in 0.3% to 0.5% of the healthy population, but in 4.4% to 12.9% of those with congenital heart disease) (Buirski *et al.*, 1986), there may be a persistent left SVC. This anomaly results from failure of obliteration of the left common cardinal vein during fetal development. A right SVC and an interconnecting brachiocephalic vein are also present in most cases. A left SVC arises from the junction of the left jugular and subclavian veins and travels vertically through the left mediastinum along the left side of the aortic arch passing anterior to the left main bronchus. In most instances, it drains into the coronary sinus on the posterior surface of the heart. The blood then flows through the coronary sinus into the right atrium, the coronary sinus being significantly larger than normal because of the increased blood flow.

The inferior vena cava

In most healthy subjects, the posterior wall of the inferior vena cava is visible just before it enters the right atrium (Fig. 26). Even patients with azygos continuation of the inferior vena cava may show a similar vessel formed by the continuation of the hepatic veins as they drain into the right atrium.

The 'mediastinal spaces' (Gamsu, 1983)

The nomenclature of the connective tissue spaces within the mediastinum is not standard, and there are no exact definitions for the boundaries between them. There are four named spaces surrounding the central airways (Fig. 28(*a*)–(*d*)): (i) the pretracheal space (ii) the aortopulmonary window (iii) the subcarinal space (iv) the right paratracheal space. All four contain lymph nodes that drain the lung and are therefore likely to be involved by bronchial carcinoma.

In addition to these central spaces, there are the so-called junction areas, where the two lungs approximate each other (Figs. 18, 19(*a*) (*b*)). The anterior junction line (or prevascular space), lies anterior to the aorta and pulmonary artery and the posterior junction line lies posterior to the trachea and oesophagus. In addition, there are the paraspinal lines on either side of the spine and the junctional area between the mediastinum and retroperitoneum known as the retrocrural space.

Pretracheal space

The pretracheal space has no boundary with the lung and is therefore not imaged on plain chest radiographs. It is well known to the surgeons, because it is the space explored by transcervical mediastinoscopy. The space is triangular in axial cross-section, the three boundaries being the trachea or carina posteriorly, either the superior vena cava or the right brachiocephalic vein anteriorly to the right, and the ascending aorta with its enveloping superior pericardial sinus anteriorly to the left.

The superior pericardial recess is a small pocket of pericardium investing the aorta. When distended, it is quite easy to recognize the pericardial configuration. In normal individuals, however, the small amount of pericardial fluid in the retroaortic extension of the superior pericardial recess may mimic lymphadenopathy on CT or MRI.

The pretracheal space is continuous with the right paratracheal space, the aorto-pulmonary window and the subcarinal space. Consequently, lymph nodes or other masses arising in any of these spaces may grow large enough to encroach on the pretracheal space and vice versa.

The aortopulmonary window

The aortopulmonary window is situated under the aortic arch above the pulmonary artery. It is bounded medially by the trachea and oesophagus and laterally by the lung. Its fatty density is not always appreciated at CT because the sections often include either the aortic arch or the left pulmonary artery, and volume averaging results in higher than fat density. The ligamentum arteriosum and the recurrent laryngeal nerve traverse this space. The ligamentum arteriosum may be calcified and may therefore, be identifiable on plain radiographs or CT.

The subcarinal space
The subcarinal space, lying beneath the tracheal carina, is bounded on either side by the major bronchi and the posterior boundary is partly formed by the oesophagus. The azygo-oesophageal recess of the right lung lies behind the subcarinal space.

The right paratracheal space and the posterior tracheal space
These two adjacent spaces (more properly called stripes), are best considered together. Normally, the right lung is separated from the trachea only by a thin layer of fat, the only exception being at the tracheobronchial angle where the azygos vein lies between the lung and the airway. The degree to which the lung envelopes the posterior wall of the trachea as it interposes between the spine and the trachea to contact the oesophagus is variable.

The anterior junction
The anterior junction (prevascular space) lies anterior to the pulmonary artery, the ascending aorta, and the three major branches of the aortic arch. It lies between the two lungs and is bounded anteriorly by the chest wall. If the two lungs approximate each other closely enough, the intervening mediastinum may consist of little more than four layers of pleura and is then known as the anterior junction line (Fig. 18). Coursing through this preaortic space superiorly is the left brachiocephalic vein. The internal thoracic vascular bundles are situated laterally and are only visible at CT if intravenous contrast material is administered. Embedded within the anterior junction fat are lymph nodes, the thymus, and the phrenic nerve.

The posterior junction and paraspinal areas
The term posterior junction describes the mediastinal region posterior to the trachea and the heart, where the two lungs lie close to each other (Fig. 18). The right lung always invaginates behind the right hilar structures and heart to contact the pleura overlying the azygos vein and oesophagus, forming the so-called azygo-oesophageal recess (Fig. 29). Above the level of the azygos arch, the lung contacts the oesophagus alone (the supraazygos recess). On the left, the lung interface is with the aortic arch and descending aorta rather than with the oesophagus, but in some individuals the lung below the aortic arch invaginates anterior to the descending aorta to almost reach the midline.

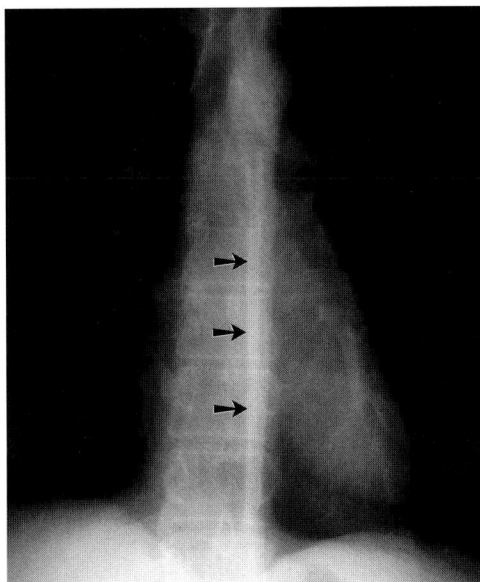

Fig. 29.
Azygo-oesophageal line (horizontal arrows).

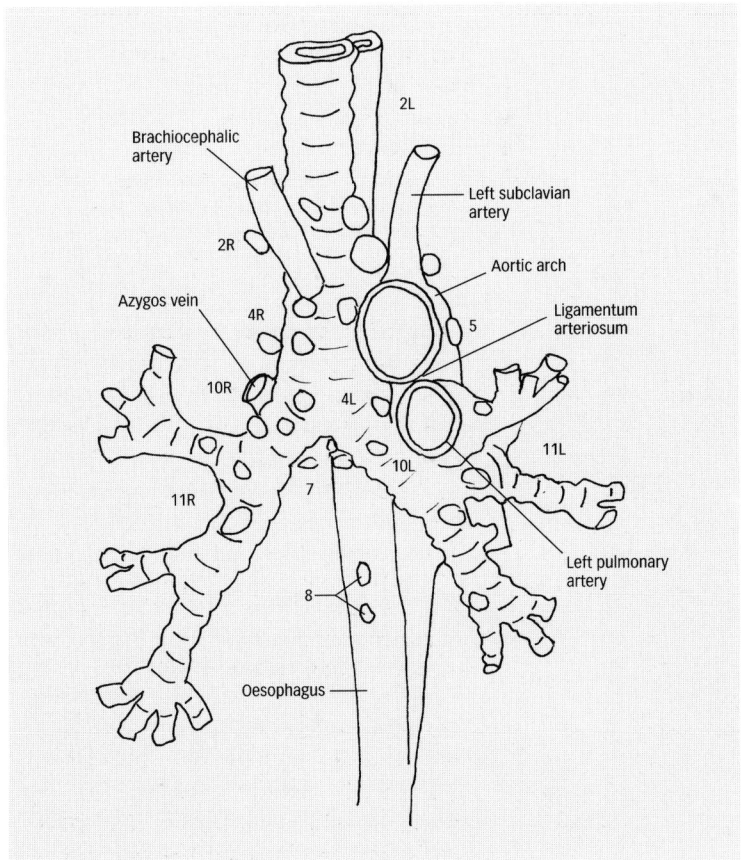

Fig. 30.
American Thoracic Society lymph node mapping scheme. (Redrawn from Glazer *et al*., 1986.)

American Thoracic Society definitions of regional nodal stations

X Supraclavicular nodes

2R Right upper paratracheal nodes: nodes to the right of the midline of the trachea, between the intersection of the caudal margin of the innominate artery with the trachea and the apex of the lung

2L Left upper paratracheal nodes: nodes to the left of the midline of the trachea, between the top of the aortic arch and the apex of the lung

4R Right lower paratracheal nodes: nodes to the right of the midline of the trachea, between the cephalic border of the azygos vein and the intersection of the caudal margin of the brachiocephalic artery with the right side of the trachea

4L Left lower paratracheal nodes: nodes to the left of the midline of the trachea, between the top of the aortic arch and the level of the carina, medial to the ligamentum arteriosum

5 Aortopulmonary nodes: subaortic and paraaortic nodes, lateral to the ligamentum arteriosum or the aorta or left pulmonary artery, proximal to the first branch of the left pulmonary artery

6 Anterior mediastinal nodes: nodes anterior to the ascending aorta or the innominate artery

7 Subcarinal nodes: nodes arising caudal to the carina of the trachea but not associated with the lower lobe bronchi or arteries within the lung

8 Paraesophageal nodes: nodes dorsal to the posterior wall of the trachea and to the right or left of the midline of the esophagus

9 Right or left pulmonary ligament nodes: nodes within the right or left pulmonary ligament

10R Right tracheobronchial nodes: nodes to the right of the midline of the trachea, from the level of the cephalic border of the azygos vein to the origin of the right upper lobe bronchus

10L Left tracheobronchial nodes: nodes to the left of the midline of the trachea, between the carina and the left upper lobe bronchus, medial to the ligamentum arteriosum

11 Intrapulmonary nodes: nodes removed in the right or left lung specimen, plus those distal to the main-stem bronchi or secondary carina

From Glazer *et al.* (1985).

The paraspinal areas are contiguous with the posterior junction. Normally, there is little or no discernible connective tissue between the lateral margins of the spine and the lungs. The only structures contained in these areas are intercostal vessels and small lymph nodes.

The retrocrural space

The aorta exits the chest passing through the aortic hiatus, which is bounded by the diaphgragmatic crura and the spine. The diaphragmatic crura are ligaments that blend with the anterior longitudinal ligament of the spine. Apart from the aorta, the structures that pass through the aortic hiatus are the azygos and hemiazygos veins and the commencement of the thoracic duct from the cisterna chyli.

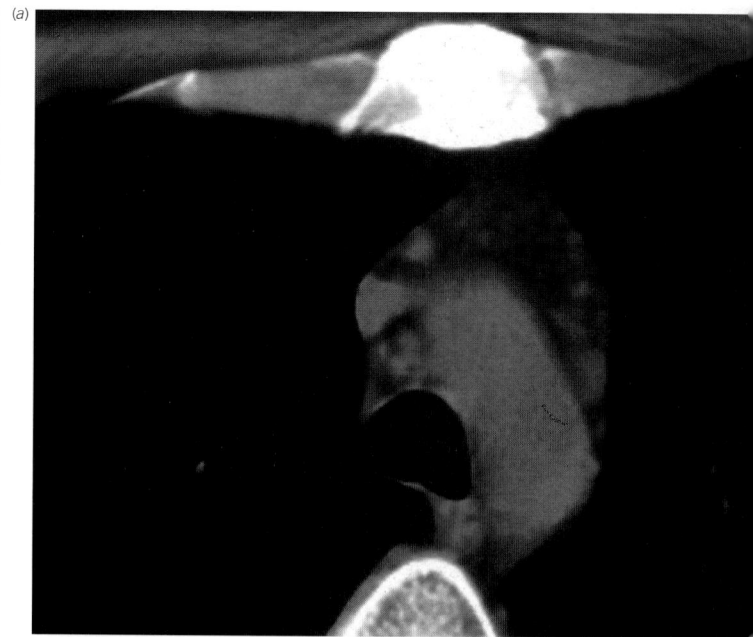

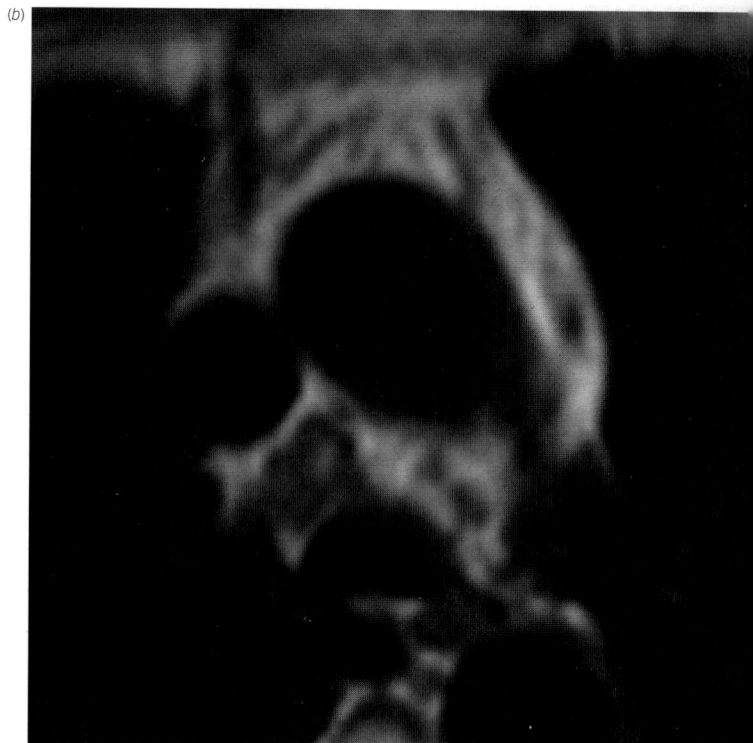

Mediastinal lymph nodes

Lymph nodes are widely distributed in the mediastinum. The nomenclature for these nodes is not standardised nor does it correspond exactly with the terms used for the mediastinal spaces. The following description uses terms in keeping with the nomenclature of the American Thoracic Society (ATS) designed for the staging of carcinoma of the bronchus (Table 1; Fig. 30; Glazer *et al.*, 1985, 1986).

Anterior mediastinal nodes lie anterior or anterolateral to the aorta and the brachiocephalic artery (station 6 in the ATS definitions).

Fig. 31.
Appearances of the norma thymus. (*a*) CT: Thymus almost entirely replaced b fat. (*b*) MRI: Residual thym parenchyma is visible as streaky densities within the anterior mediastinal fa (*c*) CT: Triangular-shaped thymus of soft tissue density fills the antero-superior mediastinum and closely moulds to the mediastinal vessels.

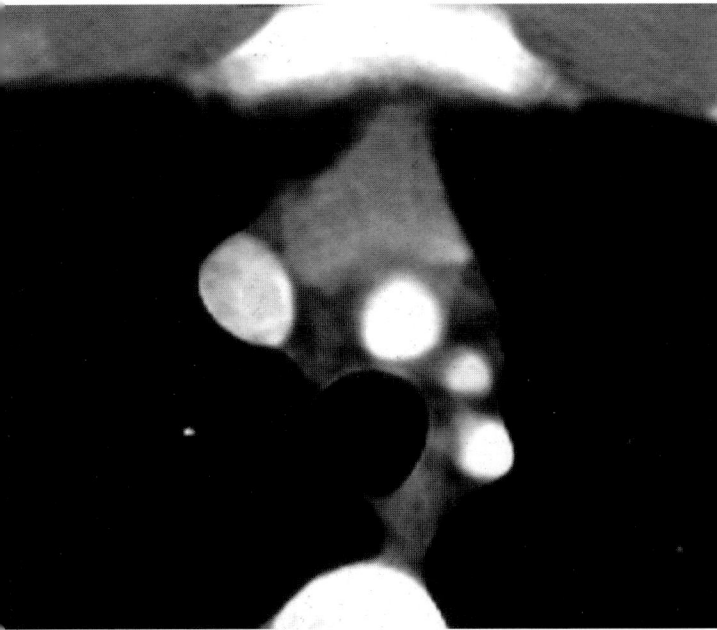

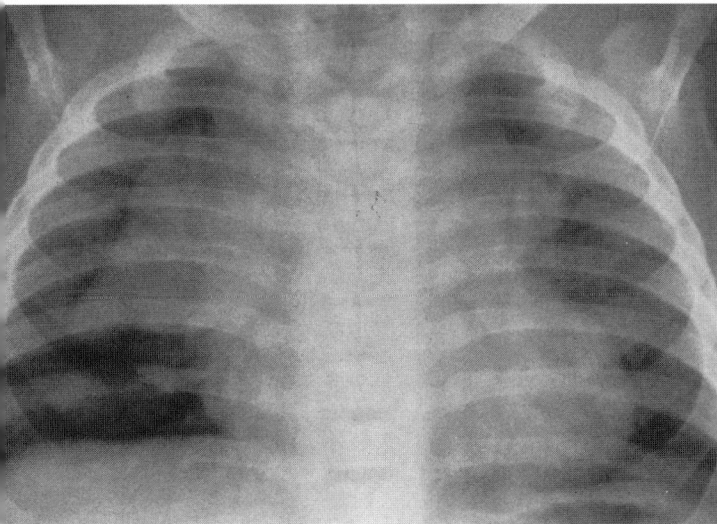

Fig. 32.
ɔrmal thymus in an infant.
Both lobes of the thymus
are prominent.

(c) Subcarinal nodes, a group that comprises all the nodes found beneath the carina and main bronchi (station 7).

(d) Tracheobronchial and hilar nodes. Tracheobronchial nodes (stations 10R and 10L) lie adjacent to right and left main stem bronchi and according to the ATS definition are mediastinal in location. The lower tracheobronchial nodes may, however, be removed at standard pneumonectomy. The hilar nodes (stations 11R and 11L) are defined as nodes distal to the main-stem bronchi, and these are always removed at pneumonectomy.

Posterior mediastinal nodes are divided into paraoesophageal (station 8) and pulmonary ligament nodes (station 9). Nodes are also present in the retrocrural areas and in the anterior cardiophrenic angles.

Normal lymph node size

There is a significant variation in the number and size of lymph nodes seen in different locations within the mediastinum. Of normal mediastinal lymph nodes, 95% are less than 10 mm in short-axis diameter, and the remainder, with very few exceptions, are less than 15 mm in diameter. Nodes in the region of the brachiocephalic veins are generally smaller, over 90% being 5 mm or less in short-axis diameter, whereas nodes in the aortopulmonary window, the pretracheal and lower paratracheal spaces, and the subcarinal compartment are often 6 to 10 mm in diameter. Nodes in the paracardiac areas are rarely visible in normal patients, measuring maximally 3.5 mm. Nodes in the retrocrural area do not normally exceed 6 mm in diameter (Genereux & Howie, 1984; Glazer *et al.*, 1985).

The thymus

The thymus is situated anterior to the aorta and the right ventricular outflow tract or pulmonary artery. At CT and MRI it is usually found inferior to the left brachiocephalic vein and superior to the level of the horizontal portion of the right pulmonary artery. It is often best appreciated on a section through the aortic arch (Fig. 31(a), (b), (c)). The thymus is soft, and fills in the spaces between the great vessels and the anterior chest wall as if moulded by these structures. The lateral margins may be concave, straight or bulged outward, and approximate symmetry is the rule. In childhood prior to puberty, the thymus occupies most of the mediastinum in front of the great vessels and may extend all the way into the posterior mediastinum (Francis *et al.*, 1985), as

Tracheobronchial nodes encircle the trachea and main bronchi except where the aorta, pulmonary artery, and oesophagus are in direct contact with the airway. There is no clear division between the various nodes in this group, but they can be divided according to site:

(a) Right and left paratracheal nodes, which can be further subdivided into upper and lower groups, depending on whether they lie above or below the level of the top of the aortic arch (stations 2R, 4R, 2L and 4L). In the ATS-approved nomenclature this group includes the pretracheal nodes.

(b) Aortopulmonary window nodes lateral to the ligamentum arteriosum, which include nodes along the lateral surfaces of the aorta and left or main pulmonary arteries (station 5).

147

well as projecting upwards in front of the trachea as far as the thyroid gland. In children under 5 years of age, the gland is usually quadrilateral in shape with convex lateral margins. A sharp angular border equivalent to the 'sail' sign on plain films (Fig. 32) is occasionally visible at CT. The gland remains fairly constant in weight, enlarging slightly until puberty, after which the thymic follicles atrophy and fatty replacement occurs until eventually it may no longer be possible to see any residual thymic tissue (Fig. 31(*a*)). In adults, the cross-sectional shape of any residual thymic tissue is triangular, or shaped like an arrowhead.

The thymus consists of two lobes, each enclosed in its own fibrous sheath. Up to 30% of the population have a fat cleft visible by CT at the junction of the two lobes. Of the two lobes, the left is usually larger and is situated slightly higher than the right (de Geer *et al.*, 1986). The maximum width and thickness of each lobe decrease with advancing age. Between ages 20 and 50, the average thickness measured by CT decreases from 8 or 9 mm to 5 or 6 mm, the maximum thickness of one lobe being up to 1.5 cm (Francis *et al.*, 1985). These diameters are greater at MRI, presumably because MRI demonstrates the thymic tissue even when it is partially replaced by fat. At MRI, sagittal images demonstrate that the gland is 5 to 7 cm in craniocaudad dimension (de Geer *et al.*, 1986). In younger patients, the CT density of the thymus is homogenous and close or slightly higher than muscle and often enhances following contrast. After puberty, the density gradually decreases owing to fatty replacement. In patients older than age 40, the thymus may have an attenutation value identical to that of fat and, in some patients, the whole gland shows fat density and is therefore indistinguishable from mediastinal fat. In others, residual thymic parenchyma is visible as a streaky or nodular density (Fig. 31). On T1-weighted MR images, the intensity of the normal thymic tissue is similar or slightly higher than that of muscle (Fig. 31). As fatty replacement progresses, the thymus shows higher signal intensity to eventually blend in with the surrounding fat. On T2-weighted images the signal intensity is similar or sometimes higher than fat and does not change with age. Proton density images show significantly less signal than the surrounding fat.

Normal mediastinal contours on plain chest radiographs

For descriptive convenience the frontal and lateral projections are treated separately, although in practice the information from these two views should be integrated (Proto & Speckman, 1979, 1980; Figs. 1(*a*), (*b*), 26(*a*)–(*e*)).

Frontal projection
The left mediastinal border

Above the aortic arch, the usual appearance is a gently curving border which fades out at the interface with the neck. This border is formed by the left subclavian artery or more usually by adjacent fat; occasionally the interface is with the left carotid artery. Below the aortic arch, the left mediastinal border is formed by the aortic–pulmonary pleural stripe, the main pulmonary artery and the heart (Keats, 1972). In children, the thymus may form the left mediastinal border in this region. The thymus in babies and young children may form a distinct bulge. A small 'nipple' may be seen projecting laterally from the aortic arch due to the left superior intercostal vein arching forward around the aorta just beyond the origin of the left subclavian artery. The left border of the descending aorta can be traced through the shadow of the main pulmonary artery and heart as a continuous border from the aortic arch down to the aortic hiatus in the diaphragm.

The right mediastinal border

The right mediastinal border is normally formed by the right brachiocephalic (innominate) vein, the SVC and the right atrium. In babies and young children, the thymus can be a prominent structure, and a sail shape is characteristic (Fig. 32). The right paratracheal stripe can be seen through the right brachiocephalic vein and SVC because the lung contacts the right tracheal wall from the clavicles down to the arch of the azygos vein. This stripe, which is of uniform thickness and up to 3 mm in width, is visible in approximately two-thirds of normal subjects. It consists of the wall of the trachea and adjacent mediastinal fat, and there are no focal bulges due to individual paratracheal lymph nodes. The azygos vein is outlined by air in the lung at the lower end of this stripe. The diameter of the azygos vein in the tracheobronchial angle is variable; the upper limit of normal on an upright PA chest radiograph is 8 mm. The nodes immediately beneath the azygos vein, which are sometimes known as azygos nodes, are not recognizable on normal chest radiographs.

The anterior junction line

When the two lungs anterior to the ascending aorta are separated only by pleura, an anterior junction line may be visible. The anterior junction line is usually straight and diverges to

Fig. 33.
Pleuro-oesphageal line (arrows)

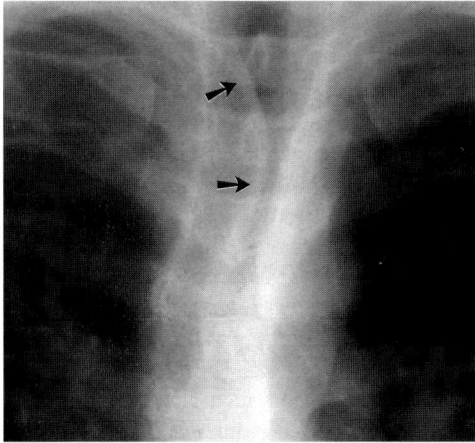

fade out superiorly as it reaches the clavicles (Fig. 18). It descends for a variable distance, usually deviating to the left. It cannot extend below the point where the two lungs separate to envelop the right ventricle.

The posterior junction and azygoesophageal recess

In some patients, the lungs almost touch each other behind the oesophagus to form the posterior junction line, a structure which can be thought of as an oesophageal 'mesentery' (Fig. 18). This line, unlike the anterior junction line, diverges to envelop the aortic and azygos arches. Above the aortic arch, the posterior junction line extends to the lung apices, where it diverges and disappears at the root of the neck, well above the level of the clavicles. The differences in the superior extent of the anterior and posterior junction lines are related to the sloping boundary between the thorax and neck. The width of the line depends on the amount of mediastinal fat. Whether both sides of the line are seen on plain chest radiograph depends on the tangent formed with the adjacent lung. If there is air in the oesophagus, the right wall of the oesophagus is seen as a stripe, usually 3 to 5 mm thick. This interface is known as the pleuroesophageal line or stripe (Fig. 33). Below the aortic arch, the right lower lobe makes contact with the right wall of the oesophagus and the azygos vein as it ascends next to the oesophagus. This portion of lung is known as the azygooesophageal recess, and the interface is known as the azygoesophageal line (Fig. 29). The shape of the azygos arch varies considerably in different subjects and, therefore, the shape of the upper portion of the azygooesophageal line varies accordingly. The upper few centimetres of the azygooesophageal line in adults are, however, always straight or concave toward the lung and a convex shape suggests a subcarinal mass. In children under 3, the azygooe-

sophageal line is usually convex and various configurations, including a high proportion showing a convex or straight border, are seen as the child gets older. The azygoesophageal line can be traced down into the posterior costophrenic angle in subjects with normal anatomy. Occasionally, the lung contacts the left wall of the oesophagus, and then the oesophagus will be outlined both from the right and the left.

The paraspinal lines

The term 'paraspinal line' refers to a stripe of soft tissue density parallel to the left and right margins of the thoracic spine. Although lymph nodes and intercostal veins share this space with mediastinal fat and pleura, these structures cannot normally be recognized individually. With little fat, the interface may closely follow the undulations of the lateral spinal ligaments, but with larger quantities of fat, these undulations are smoothed out. The thickness of the left paravertebral space is usually greater than that of the right. The paravertebral stripes are usually less than 1 cm in width, though they can be wider in obese subjects. Aortic unfolding contributes to the thickness of the left paraspinal line; as the aorta moves posteriorly, it strips the pleura from its otherwise close contact with the profiled portions of the spine.

Lateral view
The mediastinum above the aortic arch

A variable portion of the aortic arch and head and neck vessels are visible in the lateral view, depending on the degree of aortic unfolding. The brachiocephalic artery arises anterior to the tracheal air column and is the only artery recognised with any frequency. The origin is usually invisible, but, after a variable distance, the posterior wall can be seen as a gentle S-shaped interface crossing the tracheal air column. The left brachiocephalic vein often forms an extrapleural bulge behind the manubrium.

The trachea and retrotracheal area

The air column in the trachea can be seen throughout its length as it descends obliquely downward and posteriorly (Fig. 1(b)). The course of the trachea in the lateral view of adult subjects is straight, or bowed forward in individuals with aortic unfolding, with no visible indentation by adjacent vessels. The carina is not visible on the lateral view. The anterior wall of the trachea is visible only in a minority of patients, but its posterior wall is usually visible because lung often passes behind the trachea, thereby allowing one to see the 'posterior

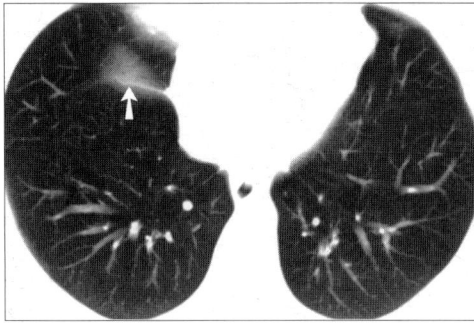

Fig. 34.
Phrenic nerve (arrow).

tracheal stripe or band'. It is uniform in width and measures up to 3 mm (rarely, 4 mm).

The restrosternal line

A band-like opacity may be seen along the lower half or third of the anterior chest wall on the lateral view. This density is due to the differing anterior extent of the left and right lungs. The left lung does not contact the most anterior portion of the left thoracic cavity at these levels because the heart and its epicardial fat occupies the space.

The diaphragm

The diaphragm consists of a large, dome-shaped central tendon with a sheet of striated muscles radiating from the central tendon to attach to ribs seven to twelve and to the xiphisternum (Panicek *et al.*, 1988). The two crura arise from the upper three lumbar vertebrae on the right and the upper two on the left, and arch upward and forward to form the margins of the aortic and oesophageal hiati. The median arcuate ligament connecting the two crura forms the anterior margin of the aortic hiatus, and the crura themselves form the lateral boundary. Accompanying the aorta through this opening are the azygos and hemiazygos veins and the thoracic duct. Anterior to the aortic hiatus lies the oesophageal hiatus,

through which run the oesophagus, the vagus nerves, and the oesophageal vessels. The most anterior of the three diaphragmatic hiati is the hiatus for the IVC, which is situated within the central tendon immediately beneath the right atrium. The diaphragm has a smooth dome shape in most individuals, but a scalloped outline is also common. At full inspiration, the normal right hemidiaphragm is found at about the level of the anterior sixth rib, being slightly higher in women and in individuals over 40 years of age (Lennon & Simon, 1965). The range covers approximately one interspace above or below this level. In most people, the right hemidiaphragm is 1.5 to 2.5 cm higher than the left, but the two hemidiaphragms are at the same level in some 9% of the population. In a few (3% in the series by Felson, 1973), the left hemidiaphragm is higher than the right, but by less than 1 cm. Partial incomplete muscularization, known as partial eventration, is so common that it could be regarded as a normal finding. An eventration is composed of a thin membranous sheet replacing what should be muscle. Usually it is partial, involving one-half to one-third of the hemidiaphragm, frequently the anteromedial portion of the right hemidiaphragm. The lack of muscle manifests itself radiographically as elevation of the affected portion of the diaphragm, and the usual pattern is a smooth hump on the contour of the diaphragm.

A linear density arising from the lateral wall of the IVC is often seen coursing over the superior surface of the right hemidiaphragm on CT. This line represents investing pleura and an envelope of fat surrounding either the phrenic nerve or the inferior phrenic artery and vein (Fig. 34).

References

Berkmen, Y.M., Auh, Y.H., Davis, S.D. *et al.* (1989). Anatomy of the minor fissure: evaluation with thin section CT. *Radiology*, **170**, 647–51.

Berkmen, Y.M., Drossman, S.R. & Marboe, C.C. (1992). Intersegmental (intersublobar) septum of the lower lobe in relation to the pulmonary ligament: anatomic, histologic and CT correlations. *Radiology*, **185**, 389–93.

Buirski, G., Jordan, S.C., Joffe, H.S. *et al.* (1986). Superior vena caval abnormalities: their occurrence rate, associated cardiac abnormalities and angiographic classification in a paediatric population with congenital heart disease. *Clinical Radiology*, **37**, 131–8.

de Geer, G., Webb, W.R. & Gamsu, G. (1986). Normal thymus: assessment with MR and CT. *Radiology*, **158**, 313–17.

Felson, B. (1969). The mediastinum. *Seminars in Roentgenology*, **4**, 41–58.

Felson, B. (1973). *Chest Roentgenology*. Philadelphia: W.B. Saunders.

Francis, I.R., Glazer, G.M., Bookstein, F.l. *et al.* (1985). The thymus re-examination of age-related changes in size and shape. *American Journal of Roentgenology*, **145**, 249–54.

Fraser, R.G., Pare, J.A.P., Pare, P.D. *et al.* (1988). *Diagnosis of Diseases of the Chest*, 3rd edn. Vol. 1. Philadelphia: W.B. Saunders.

Frija, J., Schmit, P., Katz, M., Vadrot, D. & Laval-Jeantet, M. (1982).

Computed tomography of the pulmonary fissures: normal anatomy. *Journal of Computer Assisted Tomography*, **6**, 1069–74.

Gamsu, G. (1983). Computed tomography of the mediastinum. In *Computed Tomography of the Body*, ed. A.A. Moss, G. Gamsu & H.K. Genant. Philadelphia: W.B. Saunders.

Genereux, G.P. & Howie, J.L. (1984). Normal mediastinal lymph node size and number: CT anatomic study. *American Journal of Roentgenology*, **142**, 1095–100.

Glazer, G.M., Gross, B.H., Quint, L.E., Francis, I.R., Bookstein, F.l. & Orrigen, M. (1985). Normal mediastinal lymph nodes: number and size according to American Thoracic Society mapping. *American Journal of Roentgenology*, **144**, 261–5.

Glazer, H.S., Aronberg, D.J., Sagel, S.S. & Friedman, P.J. (1986). CT demonstration of calicfied mediastinal lymph nodes: a guide to the new ATS classification. *American Journal of Roentgenology*, **147**, 17–25.

Glazer, H.S., Anderson, D.j, DiCroce, J.J., Solomon, S.L., Wilson, B.S., Molina, P.L. & Sagel, S.S. (1991). Anatomy of the major fissure: evaluation with standard and thin section CT. *Radiology*, **180**, 839–44.

Godwin, J.D. & Tarver, R.D. (1985). Accessory fissures of the lung. *American Journal of Roentgenology*, **144**, 39–47.

Godwin, J.D. & Chen, J.T.T. (1986). Thoracic venous anatomy. *American Journal of Roentgenology*, **147**, 674–84.

Goodman, L.R., Golkow, R.S., Steiner, R.M., Teplick, S.K., Haskin, M.E., Himmelstein, E. & Teplick, J.G. (1982). The right mid-lung window. *Radiology*, **143**, 135–8.

Guthaner, D.F., Wexler, L. & Harell, G. (1979). CT demonstration of cardiac structures. *American Journal of Roentgenology*, **133**, 75–81.

Heitzman, E.R. (1984). *The Lung: Radiologic–Pathologic Correlations*, 2nd edn. St Louis: CV Mosby Co.

Heitzman, E.R. (1988). *The Mediastinum: Radiologic Correlations With Anatomy and Pathology*, 2nd edn. Berlin: Springer-Verlag.

Jefferson, K. & Rees, S. (1973). *Clinical Cardiac Radiology*. London: Butterworths.

Keats, T.E. (1972). The aortic–pulmonary mediastinal stripe. *American Journal of Roentgenology*, **116**, 107–9.

Kent, E.M. & Blades, B. (1942). Surgical anatomy of pulmonary lobes. *Journal of Thoracic Surgery*, **12**, 18–30.

Lee, K.S., Bae, W.K., Lee, B.H., Kim, I.Y., Choi, E.W. & Lee, B.H. (1991). Bronchovascular anatomy of the upper lobes: evaluation with thin section CT. *Radiology*, **181**, 765–72.

Lennon, E.A. & Simon, G. (1965). The height of the diaphragm in the chest radiograph of normal adults. *British Journal of Radiology*, **38**, 937–43.

Marchand, P., Gilroy, J.C. & Wilson, H. (1950). Anatomical study of bronchial vascular system and its variations in disease. *Thorax*, **5**, 207–21.

Naidich, D.P., Jhouri, N.F., Scott, W.W.Jr, Wang, K.P. & Siegelmann, S.S. (1981). Computed tomography of the pulmonary hila: normal anatomy. *Journal of Computer Assisted Tomography*, **5**, 459–67.

Nusbaum, M., Baum, S., Hedges, R.C. *et al.* (1964). Roentgenographic and direct visualization of the thoracic duct. *Archives of Surgery*, **88**, 105–13.

Panicek, D.M., Benson, C.B., Gottlieb, R.H. & Heitzman, E.R. (1988). The diaphragm: anatomic, pathologic and radiologic considerations. *Radiographics*, **8**, 385–425.

Proto, A.V. & Ball, J.B. Jr. (1983). Computed tomography of the major and minor fissures. *American Journal of Roentgenology*, **140**, 439–48.

Proto, A.V. & Speckman, J.M. (1979). The left lateral radiograph of the chest. Part one. *Medical Radiography and Photography*, **55**, 29–74.

Proto, A.V. & Speckman, J.M. (1980). The left lateral radiograph of the chest. Part two. *Medical Radiography and Photography*, **56**, 38–64.

Van Pernis, P.A. (1949). Variations of thoracic duct. *Surgery*, **26**, 806–9.

Webb, W.R., Glazer, G. & Gamsu, G. (1981). Computed tomography of the normal pulmonary hilum. *Journal of Computer Assisted Tomography*, **5**, 476–84.

Wegener, O.H. (1992). *Whole Body Computed Tomography*. Oxford: Blackwell Scientific Publications.

Williams, P.L., Warwick, R., Dyson, M., *et al.* (eds) (1989) *Gray's Anatomy*, 37th edn. Edinburgh: Churchill Livingstone.

Wilson, A.G. (1995). Pleura and pleural disorders, *In Imaging of Diseases of the Chest*, 2nd edn. St Louis: Mosby.

Woodring, J.H. (1991). Pulmonary artery–bronchus ratios in patients with normal lungs, pulmonary vascular plethora, and congestive heart failure. *Radiology*, **179**, 115–22.

Zylak, C.J., Pallie, W. & Jackson, R. (1982). Correlative anatomy and computed tomography: a module on the mediastinum. *Radiographics*, **2**, 555–92.

7

The heart and great vessels

B. J. KENNY
and P. WILDE

Introduction

Imaging methods

The plain chest radiograph is widely used for initial assessment of the heart and great vessels. Despite its relative lack of sophistication in the face of the latest technology, there remains much to be gleaned from the humble 'chest X-ray'. Reliable assessment of the heart size, thoracic aorta and pulmonary vasculature can be made; and calcification of the cardiac vessels and valves can be easily seen. In the past, fluoroscopy of calcified cardiac valves was an important method of assessment of the valves; similarly, a lateral barium swallow was a frequently used method of assessing left atrial size.

Cardiac ultrasound (syn. echocardiography) has become the workhorse of cardiac imaging. All chambers and valves of the heart can be directly visualized in real time, allowing both structural and functional assessment. While it

is an examination requiring considerable expertise, the technology is both widely available and affordable.

By convention, the probe is positioned at the left parasternal, apical and subcostal windows (Fig. 1); and images are obtained in the long axis plane, short axis plane and four chamber plane (Fig. 2). These planes refer to the axis of the heart. The aorta and major vessels can be viewed through the suprasternal window. The exact probe position and angulation will vary according to the multitude of shapes and sizes of the human thorax. In addition, the morphology of the atria, cardiac valves and descending aorta are often better

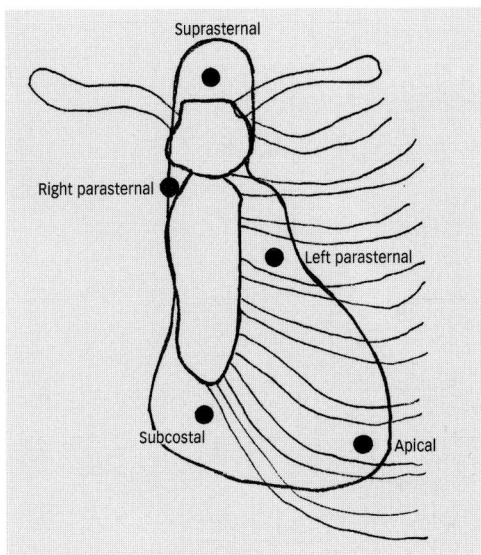

Fig. 1.
The probe positioning for echocardiography. (From Meire *et al.*, 1993.)

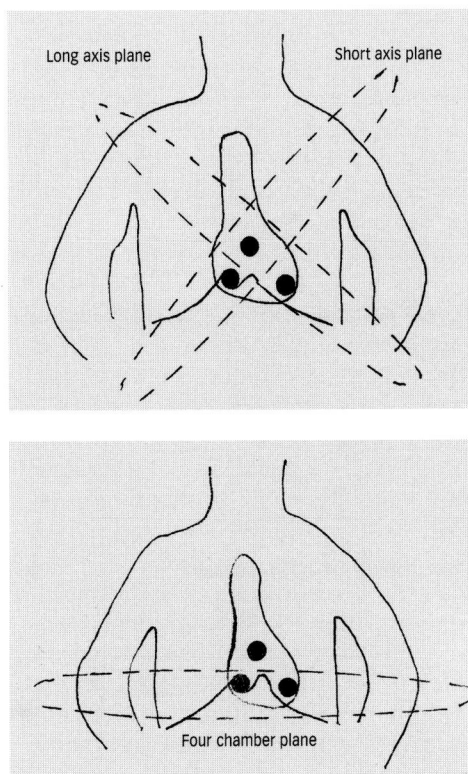

Fig. 2.
The axes and imaging planes of the heart. (From Meire *et al.*, 1993.)

seen on trans-oesophageal ultrasound. Trans-oesophageal echocardiography is widely used in emergency situations to view the arch and descending aorta, e.g. acute aortic dissection.

By attempting to obtain ultrasonic images in consistent reproducible planes, a variety of functional calculations can be made. Innumerable measurements have been devised; however, the parameters commonly observed include ventricular contractility, ejection fraction, blood velocity across valves and pressure gradients.

Conventional angiography is the best available means of imaging the coronary circulation and is widely practised; and also has the advantage of allowing a therapeutic procedure to be performed at the same time. The main disadvantage is that it is invasive and has a significant mortality and morbidity. Standard projections in coronary angiography include 30 and 60 degree left anterior oblique views, PA and cranio-caudal views; however, exact positioning varies from centre to centre. Magnetic resonance imaging and computed tomography are as yet unproven methods of coronary arterial imaging, but offer promising non-invasive possibilities for the future.

The aortic arch and great vessels are elegantly demonstrated by conventional angiography, which has long been regarded as the gold standard. In many centres, CT is the initial modality used to image the aortic arch for trauma, although MRI has been shown to be an effective and safe non-invasive alternative. Magnetic resonance imaging has allowed more detailed anatomic visualization of the heart; in particular, it has an important role to play in the structural assessment of congenital anomalies. However, the requirement for specialized monitoring equipment compatible with magnetic field restricts the use of MRI in the acute situation.

For many years, nuclear medicine has had a variety of cardiac applications in the assessment of both cardiac anatomy and function. The development of the multi-planar capability of SPECT, improved software and technetium-labelled perfusion agents have led to a greater role for nuclear medicine as a non-invasive imaging method of cardiac disease.

Development of the heart

The heart is the earliest organ to function since, even in the primitive embryo, it must not only contain the blood but also propel it. The primitive heart is formed by the fusion of two parallel tubes. Fusion commences at the anterior and extends to the caudal extremity to produce a single pulsating tube. This soon shows grooves which demarcate the sinus venosus, atrium, ventricle and bulbus cordis from behind forward (Fig. 3(a)). Venous blood drains into the sinus venosus from the umbilical and vitelline (yolk sac) radicles on each side which are joined by the common cardinal vein.

At the beginning of the fourth week the tube grows rapidly and kinks to form a U-shaped loop so that its caudal end, receiving venous blood, comes to lie behind its cephalic end with its emerging artery, the truncus arteriosus (Fig. 3(b)). The sinus venosus is later absorbed to form the main bulk of each definitive atrium and the bulbus becomes incorporated into the ventricle. Thus, in the fully developed heart, the atria and great veins come to lie posterior to the ventricles and to the roots of the great arteries.

Separation of the single atrial cavity from the single ventricle occurs by the development of a dorsal and ventral endocardial cushion which meet in the midline. These divide the common atrio-ventricular opening into a right (tricuspid) and left (mitral) orifice.

The single primitive atrium is divided into two by a complicated process which is of importance in the understanding of congenital septal defects. The septum primum grows downwards as a partition from the posterior and superior walls of the atrium to fuse with the endocardial cushions. However, before this fusion is completed, a defect appears in the upper part of this septum, which is termed the foramen secundum. A second membrane, the septum secundum, now grows to the right of the septum primum but this is never complete. It has a free lower edge which, however, extends low enough for this septum to overlap the foramen secundum in the septum primum and hence to close it (Fig. 4).

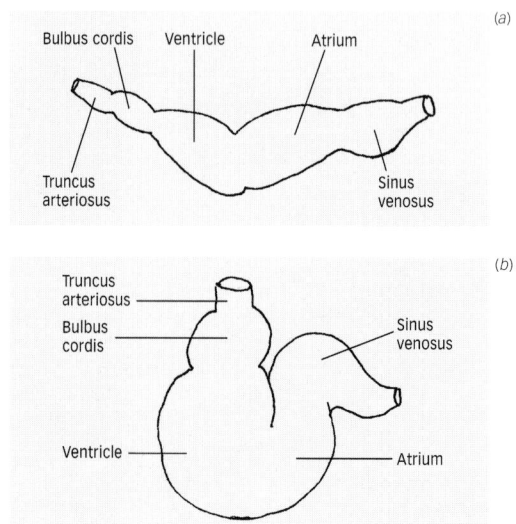

Fig. 3.
Diagram of the coiling of the heart tube into its definitive form (Ellis, 1997).

These two overlapping defects in the septa form the valve-like foramen ovale, which shunts blood from the right to the left side of the heart in the fetus. After birth, this foramen usually becomes completely fused, leaving only the fossa ovalis on the septal wall as its memorial. However, in about 10% of subjects, a probe can still be passed through an anatomically patent, although functionally sealed, foramen.

Division of the primitive single ventricle commences by the upgrowth of a fleshy septum from the apex of the heart towards the endocardial cushions. However, this stops short of completely dividing the ventricle and thus it has an upper free border which forms a temporary interventricular foramen. At the same time, the single truncus arteriosus is divided into the aorta and the pulmonary trunk by the spiral septum, which grows downwards to the ventricle and fuses accurately with the upper free border of the ventricular septum. This contributes the small pars membranacea septi, which completes the separation of the ventricle.

The primitive sinus venosus absorbs into the right atrium so that the venae cavae which drain into the sinus come to open separately into the right atrium. The smooth-walled part of the adult atrium represents the contribution of the sinus venosus, whereas the trabeculated portion represents the part derived from the fetal atrium, the adult right auricular appendage. In a similar manner, the adult left atrium has a double origin. The original single pulmonary venous trunk which enters the left atrium becomes absorbed into it and donates the smooth-walled part of this chamber with the pulmonary veins entering as four separate openings. The trabeculated part of the definitive left atrium is the remains of the original atrial wall and forms the definitive left auricular appendage.

The development of the aortic arches and their derivatives

A common arterial trunk, the *truncus arteriosus*, emerges from the bulbus cordis (Fig. 5). From the truncus arises six pairs of aortic arches. These are equivalent to the arteries which supply the gill clefts of the fish. These arteries curve dorsally around the pharynx on either side then join to form two longitudinally placed dorsal aortae. These fuse distally into the descending aorta. In man, the first, second and fifth arches disappear. On each side, the third arch becomes the carotid artery. On the right side, the fourth arch develops into the brachiocephalic artery and right subclavian artery, while on the left it differentiates into the aortic arch, gives off the left subclavian artery and links distally with the descending aorta. When the truncus arteriosus splits longitudinally by its spiral septum to form the ascending aorta and pulmonary trunk, the sixth arch (unlike the others), remains linked with the latter to form the right and left pulmonary arteries. On the left side, this sixth arch retains its connection with the dorsal aorta to form the ductus arteriosus, which becomes the ligamentum arteriosum of adult anatomy.

This asymmetrical development of the aortic arches accounts for the different course which is taken by the recurrent laryngeal nerve on each side. In the early fetus, the vagus nerve lies lateral to the primitive pharynx, separated from it by the aortic arches. What are to become the recurrent laryngeal nerves

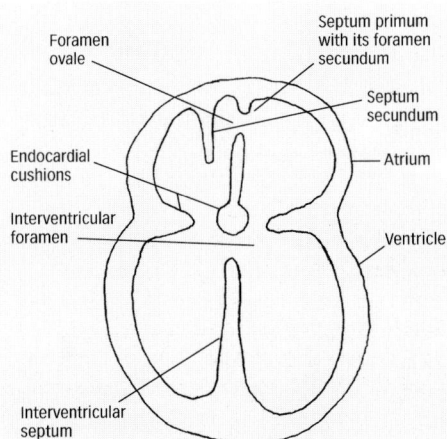

Fig. 4.
The development of the chambers of the heart. Note the septum primum and septum secundum which form the interatrial septum and which leave the foramen ovale as a valvular opening between them (Ellis, 1997).

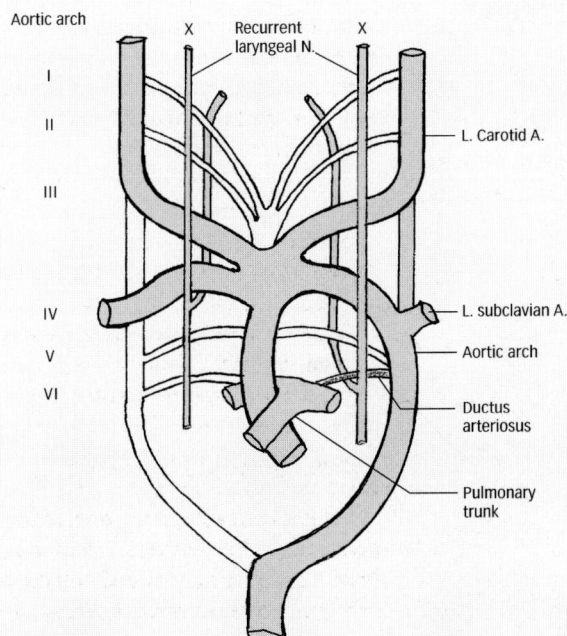

Fig. 5.
The primitive aortic arches and their adult derivatives. The parts of the arches which disappear are shown in white (Ellis, 1997).

155

pass medially and caudal to the aortic arches to supply the developing larynx. With elongation of the neck and caudal migration of the developing heart, the recurrent laryngeal nerves are caught up and dragged down by the descending aortic arches. On the right side, the fifth arch does not develop and the distal part of the sixth arch absorbs, thus leaving the nerve to hook around the fourth arch (that is to say, the right subclavian artery). On the left side, however, the nerve remains looped around the persistent distal part of the sixth arch (the ligamentum arteriosum), which is overlapped and dwarfed by the arch of the aorta.

Abnormal development of the primitive aortic arches may result in the aortic arch being on the right or actually being double. An abnormal right subclavian artery may arise from the dorsal aorta and pass behind the oesophagus, a rare cause of dysphagia.

Aortic coarctation is thought to be due to an abnormality of the obliterative process which normally occludes the ductus arteriosus. There may be an extensive obstruction of the aorta from the left subclavian artery to the ductus, which remains widely patent and maintains the circulation to the lower part of the body. This is often associated with multiple other defects. More commonly, there is a short segment involved in the region of the ligamentum arteriosum or the still-patent ductus. In these cases the circulation of the lower limb is maintained via collateral arteries around the scapula which anastomose with the intercostal arteries, and via the link-up between the internal thoracic and inferior epigastric arteries. Clinically, this circulation may be manifest by enlarged vessels which may be palpable around the margins of the scapula. Radiologically, enlargement of the engorged intercostal arteries results in notching of the inferior borders of the ribs.

Pericardium

The heart is contained within the pericardium, which has a visceral and parietal layer. These layers enclose the pericardial sac, a potential space containing only a few millilitres of lubricating pericardial fluid. Normally, the pericardial layers are not easily distinguished by conventional imaging methods. The pericardial reflections are the boundaries of the pericardial space and lie posteriorly between the inferior vena cava and pulmonary veins (i.e. the oblique sinus); and anterosuperiorly between the aorta and pulmonary trunk in front, and the atria and great veins behind (i.e. the transverse sinus).

The inner visceral pericardium (serous pericardium, epicardium) is adherent to the myocardium, though with age there may be a thin layer of fat between the two. Most of the myocardium is covered by the visceral pericardium except its reflection around the pulmonary veins where there is no pericardial space directly behind the left atrium.

The outer parietal pericardium blends with the adventitial fibrous covering of the aortic root and pulmonary trunk, to the extent that the aortic root and pulmonary trunk as far as the bifurcation are invested in the pericardium. Inferiorly it is in continuity with the diaphragmatic central tendon. Apart from inconstant slips to the sternum it is otherwise free and serves to limit distension of the heart. Areas of fat-filled spaces between the parietal pericardium and the mediastinal pleura are common in the anterior and lateral cardiophrenic angles, and are referred to as pericardial fat pads.

Heart chambers

Right atrium

The right atrium (Fig. 6) lies to the right of the midline forming most of the right heart border on the frontal chest radiograph, and is slightly above and to the right of the right ventricle (Figs. 7 and 8). It is anterior and to the right of the left atrium and its auricular appendage projects anteromedially to overlap the aortic root, from the right side. The interatrial septum lies in the left anterior oblique plane, to form the posteromedial wall of the chamber; while the aortic root lies anteromedial to the right atrium.

The inner wall of this globular-shaped chamber is smooth except anteriorly, where the auricular appendage is ridged by the musculi pectinati. A vertical ridge, the crista terminalis demarcates the smooth from the ridged portions of the inner wall. The appendage has a characteristic appearance, protruding upwards, forwards and to the left over the anterolateral surface of the aortic root and superior vena cava. The interatrial septum makes up the posteroinferior portion of the medial atrial wall. In the middle of the septum lies the depression of the fossa ovalis partially surrounded by a raised limbus of tissue. Anterosuperiorly the medial wall of the right atrium is in close proximity to the aortic root; where the non-coronary and anterior right coronary artery cusps form a slight bulge, the torus aorticus. A small portion of the membranous ventricular septum separates the right atrium from the subaortic region of the left

ventricle, due to offsetting of the atrioventricular valves where the hingepoint of the tricuspid valve is attached more apically than
that of the mitral valve (Figs. 9 and 10).

Entering the right atrium are the superior
and inferior venae cavae at the superior and
inferior extremities of the posterior wall. The
coronary sinus also enters on the posterior
wall (Fig. 11), between the inferior vena cava
and the tricuspid valve. The inferior vena cava
has a rudimentary valvular structure
(Eustachian valve), its function being the
direction of oxygenated blood flow to the foramen ovale in fetal life. A similar structure is
located at the coronary sinus opening (Thebesian valve). The anterior cardiac veins have
numerous small openings directly into the
atrium.

The tricuspid valve opens to the left and
anteriorly into the right ventricle.

The morphological right atrium is
characterized anatomically by:

- limbus of the fossa ovalis on the septal
  aspect;
- the crista terminalis;
- the characteristically shaped and positioned appendage.

Right ventricle

The right ventricle (Fig. 12) lies to the left of
the right atrium. It is a rhomboid-shaped cavity
with the bulkier left ventricle bulging into it
(Figs. 9, 10 and 13). The smaller top of the
rhomboid is formed by the pulmonary valve
which is anterior and to the left of the aortic
root. The interventricular septum lies in the
left anterior oblique plane, like the interatrial
septum. The right ventricle forms the front
of the heart. It does not usually contribute
significantly to the cardiac outline on the
frontal chest radiograph but forms the anterior
border on the lateral view, partially in contact
with the lower half of the sternum (Fig. 8).

The inner wall of the right ventricle is
coarsely trabeculated by thick muscular bundles the trabeculae carneae, except for the
smooth muscular conus (infundibulum) of the
outflow tract. The crista supraventricularis
demarcates the smooth conus from the trabeculated wall on the septal aspect of the conus.
A muscular bundle, the moderator band,
traverses the cavity carrying the right bundle
branch fibres of the conducting system. It
crosses from the lower ventricular septum to
the anterior wall joining the anterior papillary
muscle (Fig. 12). There are usually three papillary muscles in the right ventricle: a large
anterior papillary muscle arising from the
moderator band and the anterolateral ventricular wall (i.e. the free wall), the posterior papillary muscle from the inferior wall and a small
septal muscle originating from the infundibulum tethering the septal and posterior leaflets.

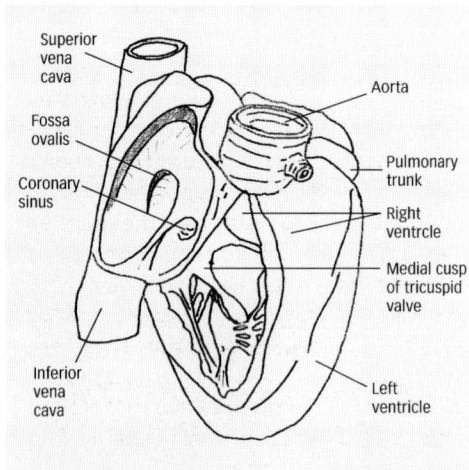

Fig. 6.
Right atrium.

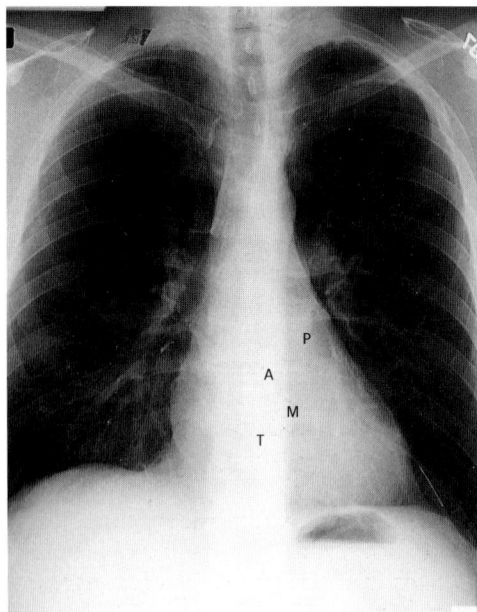

Fig. 7.
A frontal PA chest
radiograph showing the
cardiac outlines and
position of the heart valves.

P Pulmonary valve
A Aortic valve
T Tricuspid valve
M Mitral valve

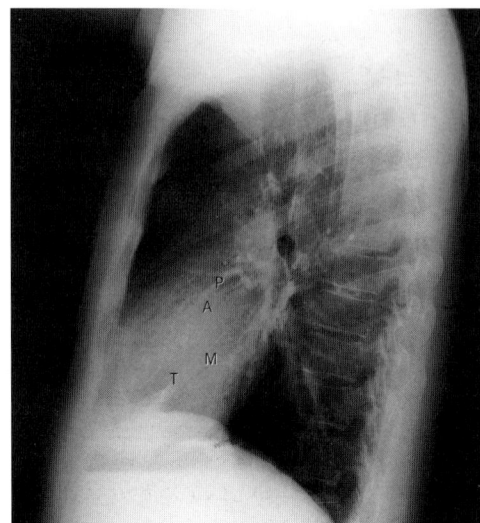

Fig. 8.
A lateral chest radiograph.

P Pulmonary valve
A Aortic valve
T Tricuspid valve
M Mitral valve

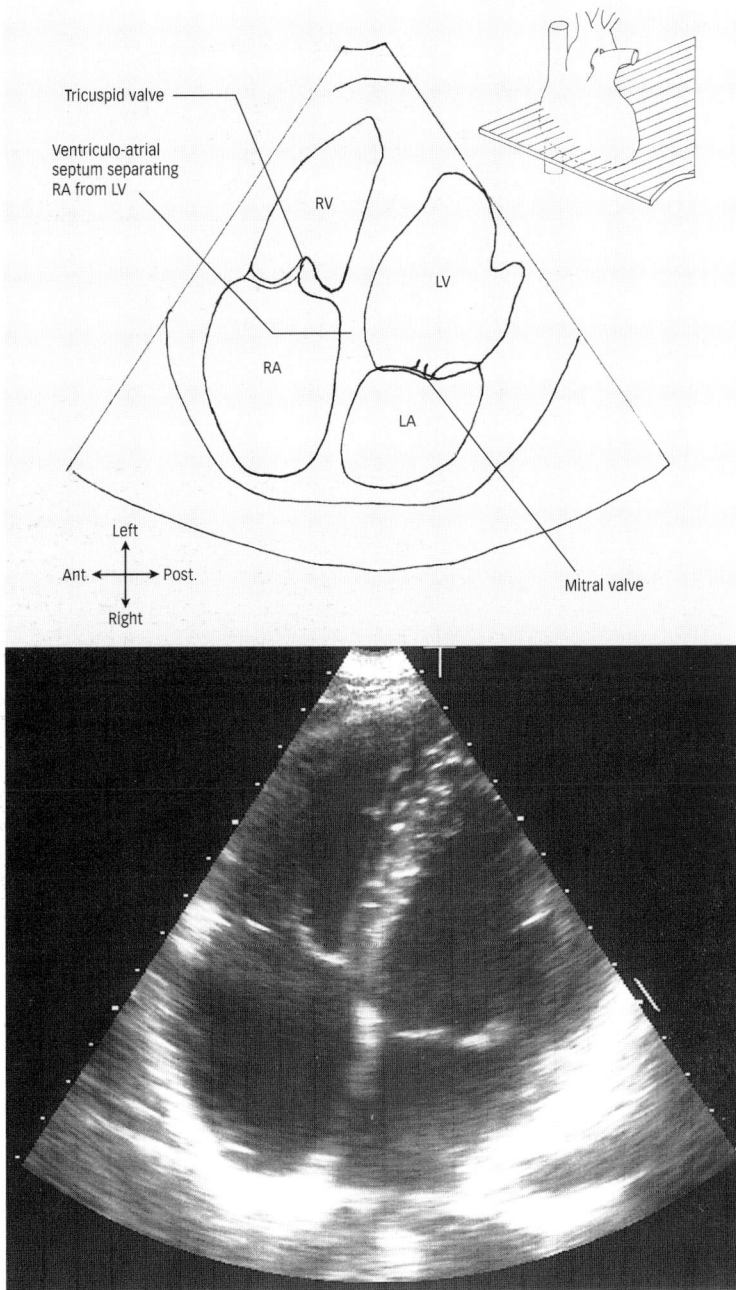

Fig. 9.
Transthoracic
echocardiogram. Apical
four-chamber view. Note
the position of the tricuspid
valve inferior to the mitral
valve, and hence the
portion of membranous
interventricular septum
separating the right atrium
from subaortic portion of
the left ventricle.

Fig. 9.
Transthoracic echocardiogram. Apical four-chamber view. Note the position of the tricuspid valve inferior to the mitral valve, and hence the portion of membranous interventricular septum separating the right atrium from subaortic portion of the left ventricle.

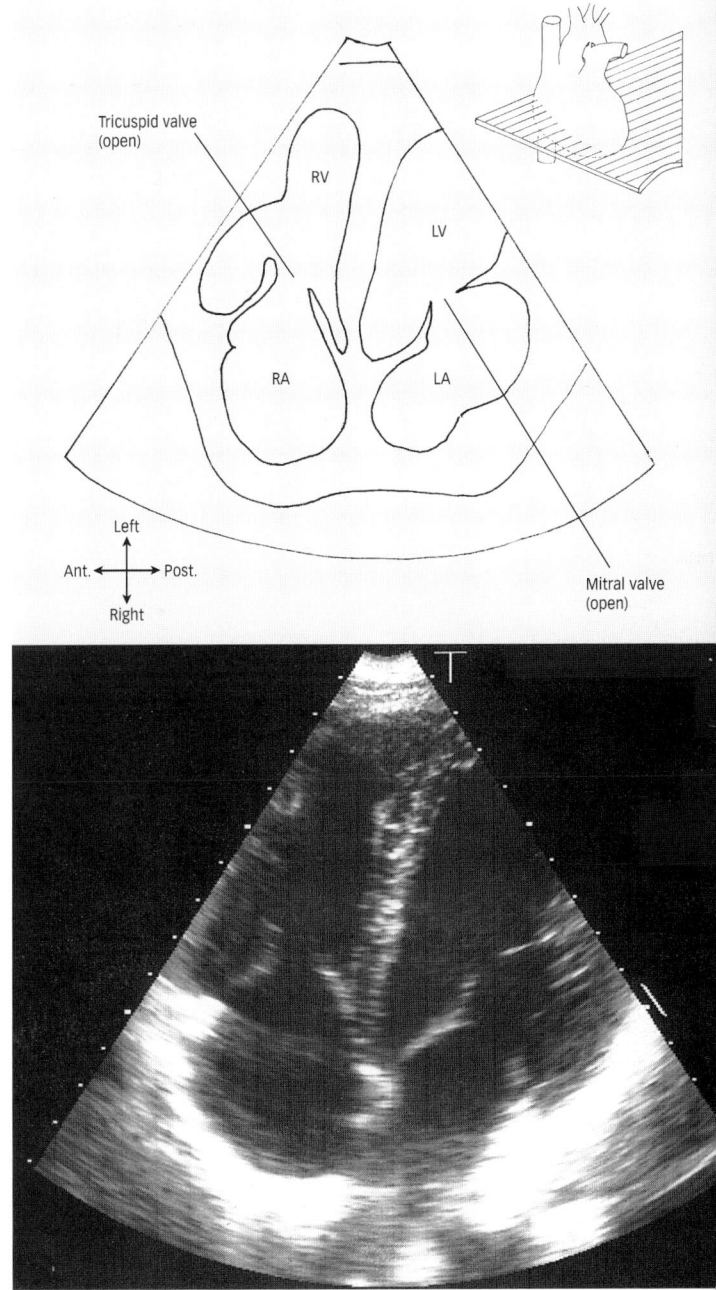

Fig. 10.
Transthoracic echocardiogram. Apical four-chamber view, valve open.

They are attached to the edges of the tricuspid valve leaflets by the chordae tendinae.

In the right ventricle, the atrioventricular valve is tricuspid, having septal (medial), anterior and posterior leaflets. The valve is attached to the fibrous atrioventricular ring and lies in right anterior oblique plane. This orientation of the atrioventricular orifices perpendicular to the interatrial and inter-ventricular septa can be easily seen on four-chamber views. The septal leaflet is attached at its base to the interventricular septum, while the larger anterior leaflet lies between the atri-oventricular opening and the infundibulum. The smaller posterior leaflet is attached to the posteroinferior portion of the fibrous ring.

Above the tricuspid valve the infundibulum curves over the left ventricular outflow tract to reach the pulmonary valve, which is the most anterior and superior of the cardiac valves (Figs. 12 and 14). There are three semilunar cusps: a right anterior, left anterior and posterior.

The morphological right ventricle is characterised anatomically by:

- a smooth muscular conus separating the inflow from the outflow tracts;
- trabeculated anterior and septal wall;
- a tricuspid atrioventricular valve.

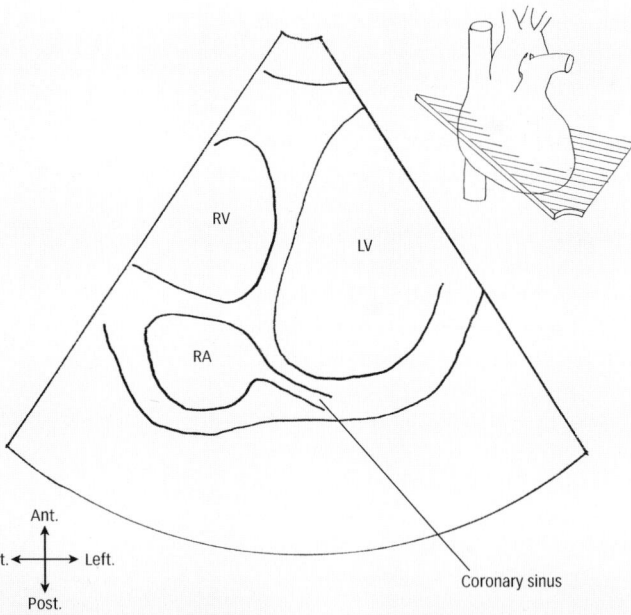

Ant.

Right. ←→ Left.

Post.

Coronary sinus

RV

LV

RA

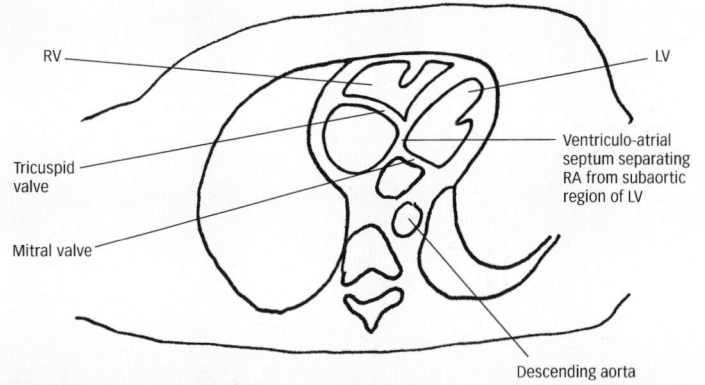

RV

LV

Tricuspid
valve

Ventriculo-atrial
septum separating
RA from subaortic
region of LV

Mitral valve

Descending aorta

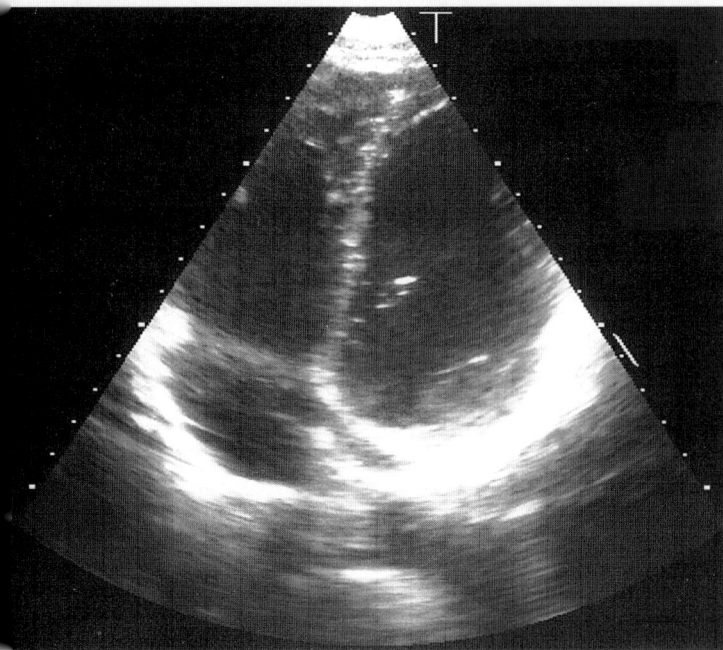

RH

SP 3
SL 5
FoV 400*4
128 *256c

Fig. 13.
**T$_1$-weighted axial oblique
MRI, giving a four-chamber
view. Note the membranous
interventricular septum
separating the right atrium
from subaortic portion of
the left ventricle.**

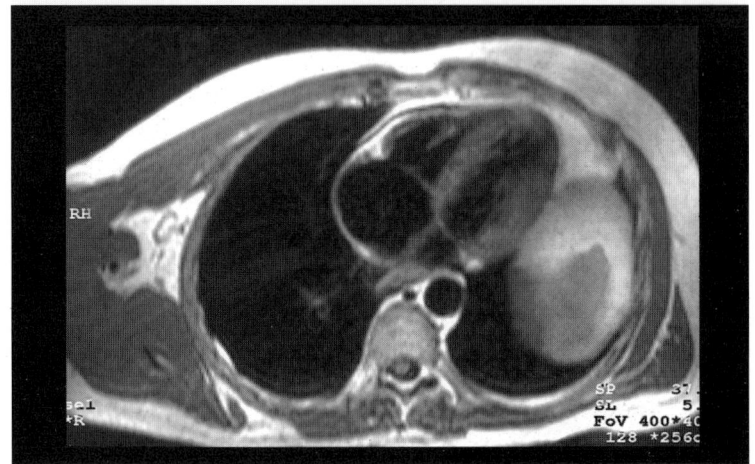

Fig. 11. above
**Transthoracic
echocardiogram. Apical
oblique view. Note the
coronary sinus entering the
right atrium.**

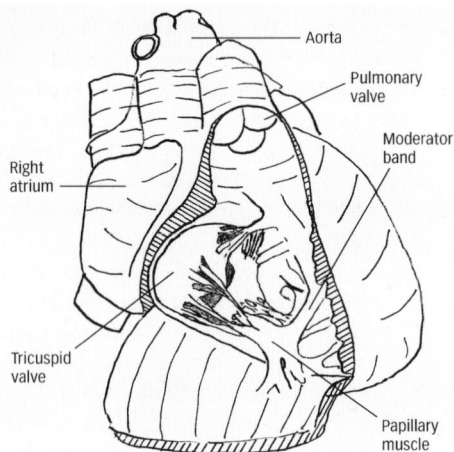

Aorta

Pulmonary
valve

Moderator
band

Right
atrium

Tricuspid
valve

Papillary
muscle

Fig. 12. right
**Right ventricle opened
(anterior view).**

Left atrium

The left atrium is a smooth-walled chamber
lying at the upper posterior aspect of the heart
shadow. It does not contribute to the normal
cardiac outline on the frontal radiograph,
even the normal auricular appendage is
obscured by epicardial fat as it curves around
the left heart border. Posteriorly the left
atrium is intimately related to the left lower
lobe bronchus and the oesophagus. On the
lateral radiograph it does not normally have
a clearly definable outline since there is no
direct lung interface. Thus when pathologically enlarged it elevates the left bronchus,
indents the oesophagus and overlaps the
right heart border giving a 'double outline'
appearance on the frontal radiograph.

Inflow from the lungs into the left atrium is
through four pulmonary veins, located at the
upper and lower posterolateral margins on
either side. Blood exits the left atrium via the
mitral valve, which is placed in the left lower
anterior aspect.

Morphologically the only reliable distinguishing feature is the long, curved and
trabeculated appearance of the appendage,
best seen at angiography.

159

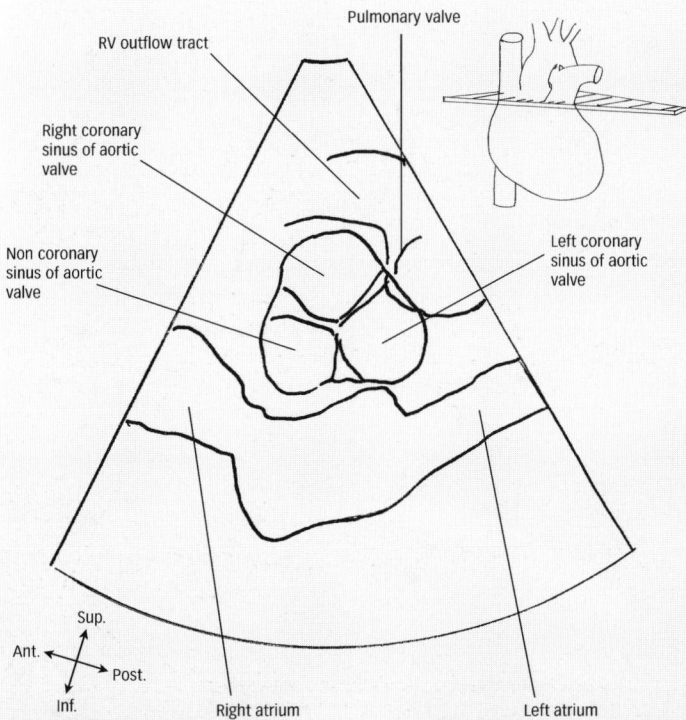

RV outflow tract

Pulmonary valve

Right coronary sinus of aortic valve

Non coronary sinus of aortic valve

Left coronary sinus of aortic valve

Sup.
Ant.
Post.
Inf.

Right atrium

Left atrium

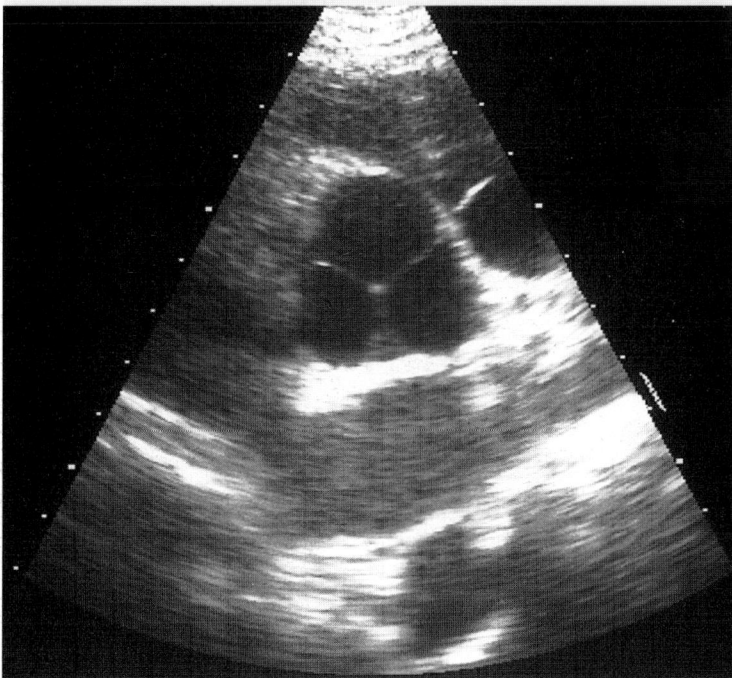

Fig. 14.
Transthoracic echocardiogram. Parasternal short axis at the level of the closed aortic valve. Note position of the pulmonary valve and outflow tract anterior to the aortic valve.

Left ventricle

The left ventricle (Fig. 15) is approximately a cone-shaped chamber with the long axis in the left anterior oblique plane. The circular base forms the fibrous ring of the mitral and aortic valves, while the muscular apex, pointing down and to left, forms the cardiac apex. On the frontal radiograph (Fig. 7) the left ventricle forms most of the left heart border, though the major portion of its external surface is posterolateral. The left ventricle is posterior and

to the left of the right ventricle; and anteroinferior and to the left of the left atrium (Figs. 9, 10 and 13).

Apart from the upper part of the septum, the inner wall of the left ventricle is finely trabeculated. Unlike the right side there is no infundibulum, the mitral and aortic valve having a continuous fibrous ring, and the anterior mitral leaflet separates the inflow from outflow tracts (Figs. 16 and 17). The interventricular septum lies in the left anterior oblique plane. It describes an arch over the chamber so that the thin proximal membranous portion faces to the right under the non-coronary and anterior coronary sinus, while the muscular septum faces to the left under the anterior and left posterior coronary sinuses.

Left ventricular inflow is from the left atrium through the bicuspid mitral valve (Figs. 15, 16 and 17), which lies on the lower posterior aspect of the chamber pointing towards the apex. The mitral valve arises from the infolded atrioventricular junction, but is closely related to the non-coronary and left posterior coronary sinuses and lies in the same right anterior

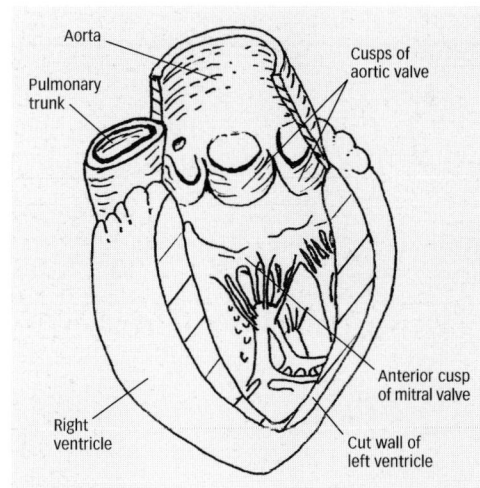

Aorta

Pulmonary trunk

Cusps of aortic valve

Anterior cusp of mitral valve

Right ventricle

Cut wall of left ventricle

Fig. 15.
Left ventricle.

oblique plane as the tricuspid valve. It has an anterior and posterior leaflet; each attached to a papillary muscle by chordae tendinae, but unlike the tricuspid valve there is no direct septal attachment. The anterior leaflet is convex, while the posterior leaflet has a slightly longer circumference (Figs. 18 and 19). The papillary muscles arise from the junction of the apical and middle third of the ventricular wall (Fig. 20).

The outflow is just above the mitral valve (Figs. 16 and 17), via the aortic valve (Fig. 21). This has three semilunar cusps: anterior, right posterior and left posterior cusps (i.e. a symmetrical arrangement to the pulmonary valve). Just above the valve in the aortic root are three focal dilatations, the sinuses of Valsalva.

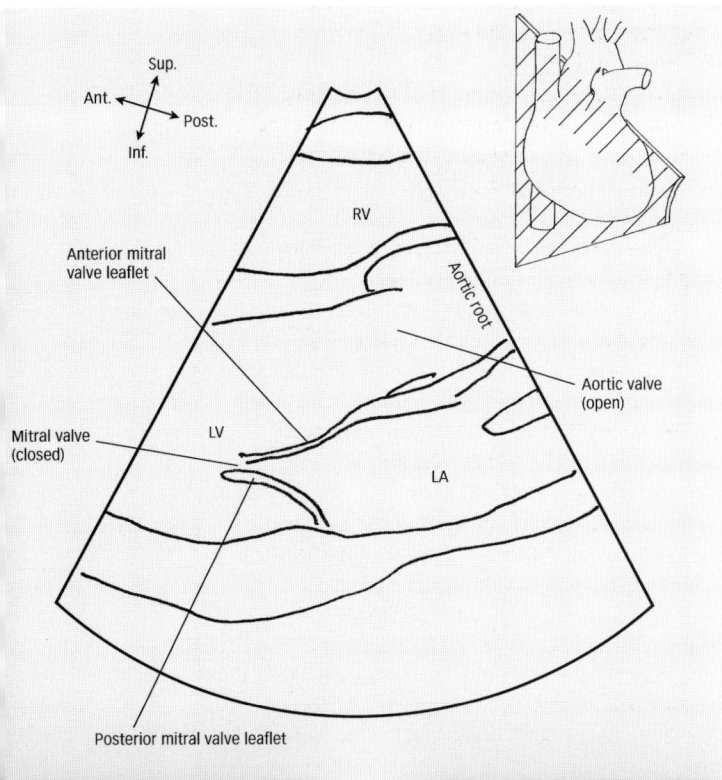

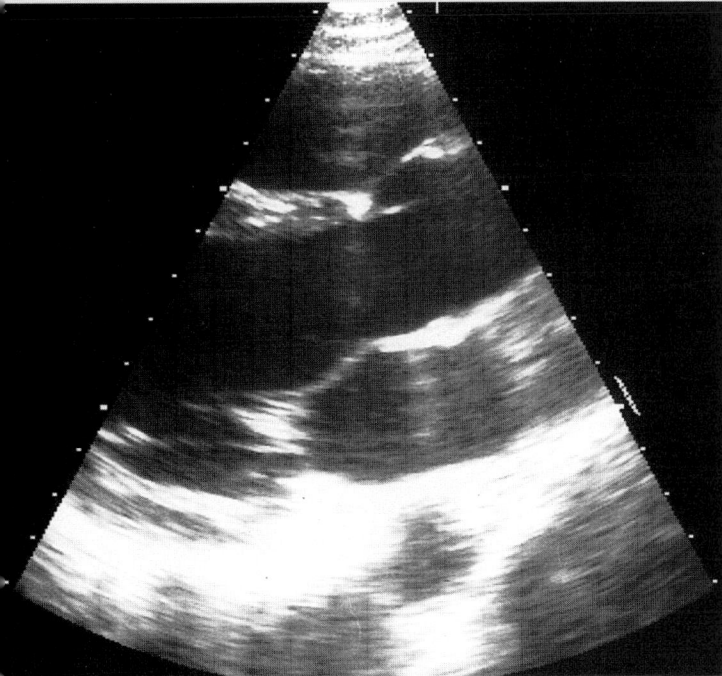

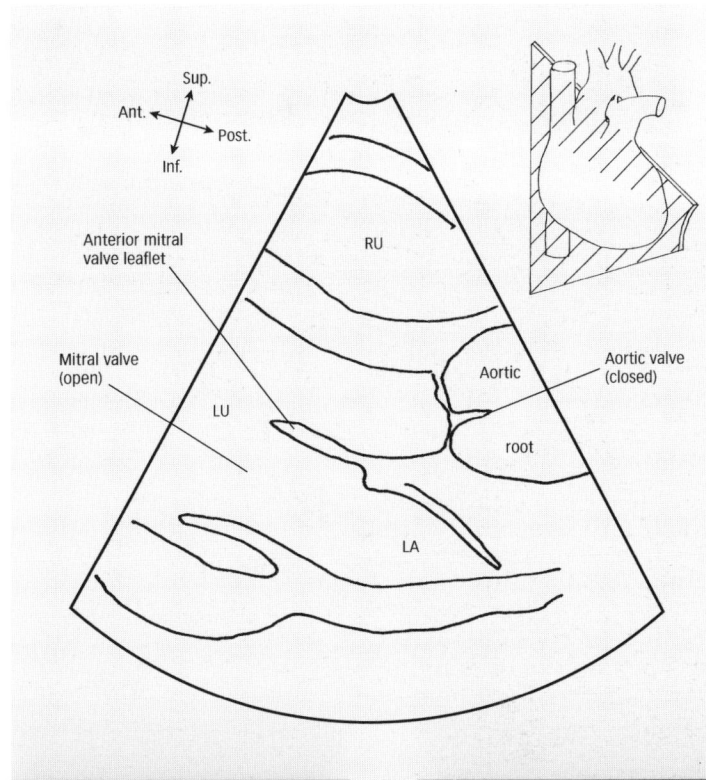

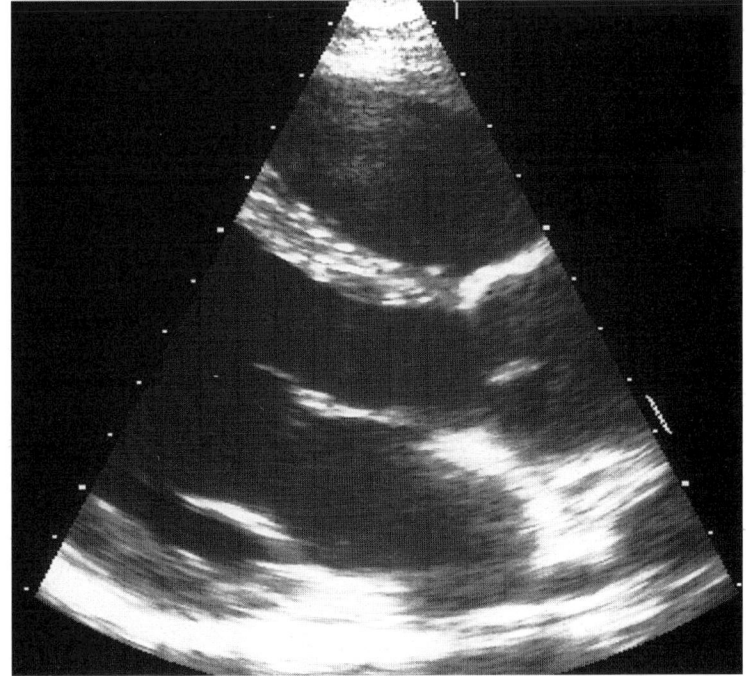

Fig. 16.
Transthoracic
echocardiogram.
Parasternal long axis
view showing the relative
positions of the closed
mitral valve and open
aortic valve.

The left coronary artery arises from the left posterior sinus, while the right coronary artery arises from the anterior sinus. The right posterior sinus is also known as the non-coronary sinus (Fig. 14).

The morphological left ventricle characterized by:

- a bicuspid atrioventricular valve without any septal attachments;
- absence of an infundibulum due fibrous continuity of the entry and exit orifices;

- finer trabeculation pattern than in the right ventricle.

Conducting system

The conducting system cannot be imaged by any current method; arterial supply to the sinus node is from the right coronary artery in 60% of people. The supply to the atrioventricular node is from the right coronary artery in 90% of people, and from the left coronary artery in 10%.

Fig. 17.
Transthoracic
echocardiogram.
Parasternal long axis with
the mitral valve open and
the aortic valve closed.
Note how the anterior
mitral valve leaflet
separates the left
ventricular inflow from
outflow.

Anterior mitral
valve leaflet

Commissure

Posterior mitral valve leaflet

Anterior mitral
valve leaflet

Valve
orifice

Posterior mitral
valve leaflet

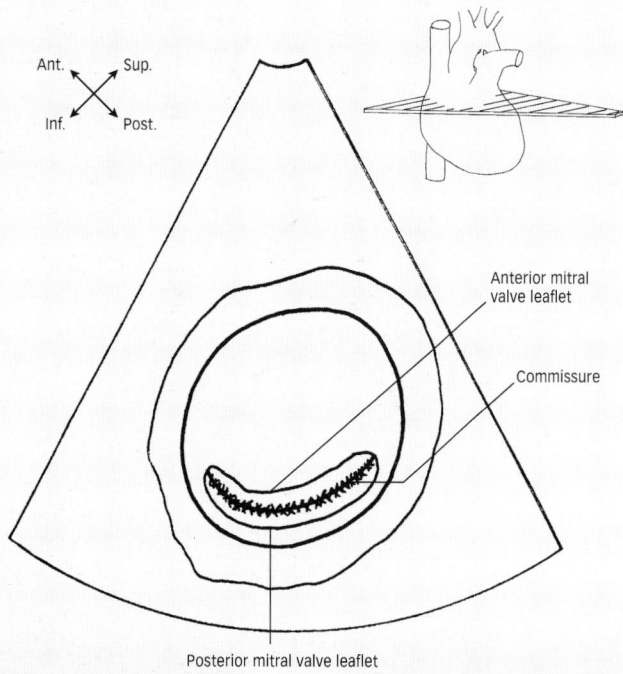

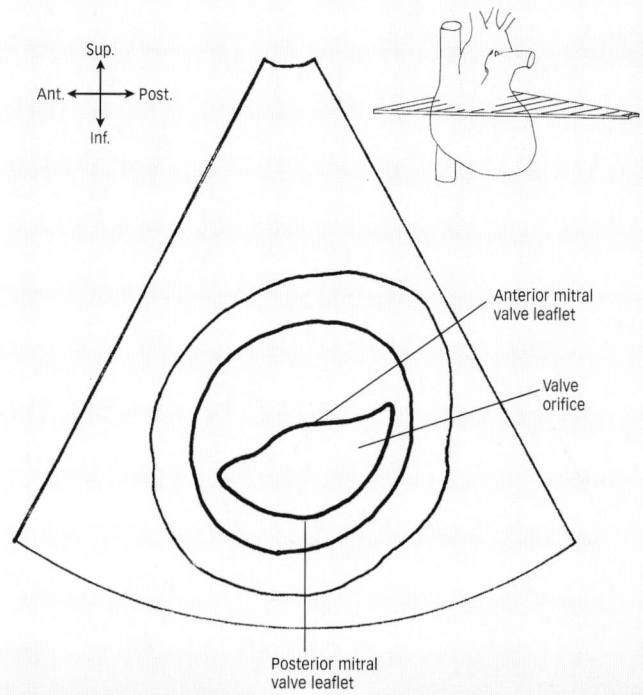

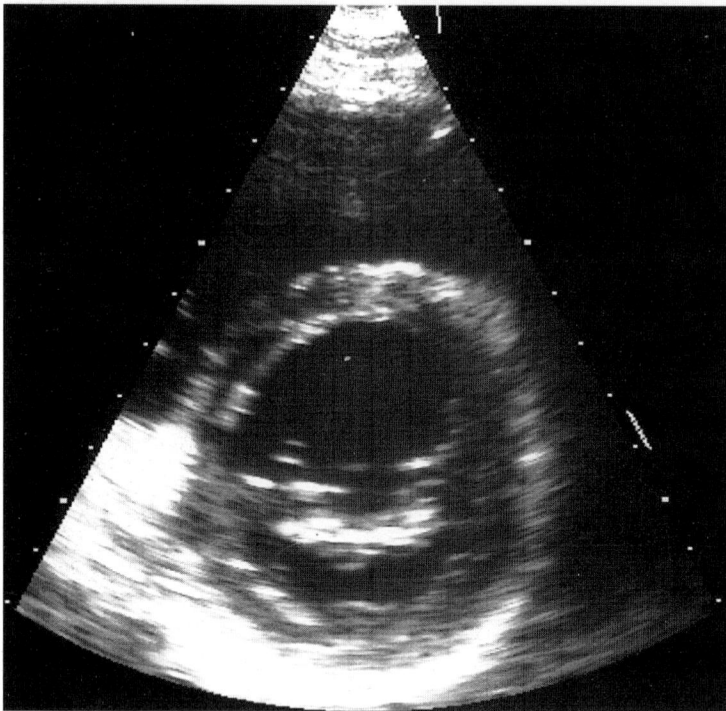

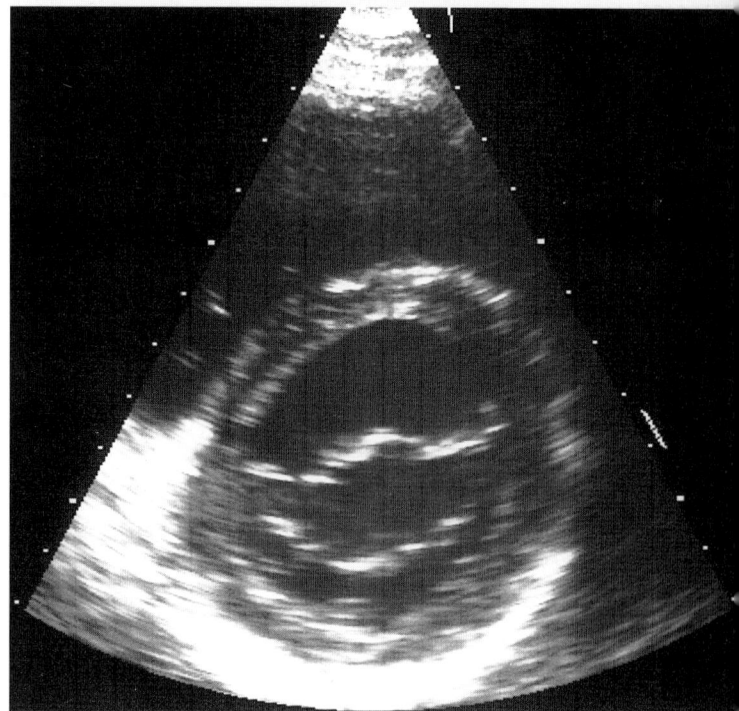

Fig. 18.
Transthoracic
echocardiogram.
Parasternal short axis view,
at the level of the mitral
valve. Note the asymmetry
of the cusps of the closed
valve. The anterior leaflet is
convex, while the posterior
leaflet is wider.

Sinus node

The sinus node is located posterosuperiorly within the sulcus terminalis to the right of the superior vena cava, at its junction with the right atrial appendage and the lateral wall of the right atrium. It is an oval-shaped structure measuring approximately 15 mm by 3 mm in size. From the sinus node there are anterior, middle, and posterior internodal tracts transmitting the impulse to the atrioventricular node. The anterior internodal tract passes

around the front of the superior vena cava and down the interatrial septum giving off fibres to the left atrium, to reach the atrioventricular node. The middle internodal tract passes around behind the superior vena cava and then runs down the interatrial septum to the atrioventricular node. The posterior internodal tract passes through the crista terminalis and posterior atrial septum towards the atrioventricular node.

Fig. 19.
Transthoracic
echocardiogram.
Parasternal short axis, at
the level of the partially
open mitral valve.

Atrioventricular node

The atrioventricular node is situated in the medial floor of the right atrium between the tricuspid septal leaflet and the opening of the coronary sinus. The bundle of His is an anterior continuation of the node and passes down underneath the membranous portion of the interventricular septum into the muscular septum between the non-coronary and the right aortic cusps. Numerous fibres are given off to the left ventricle over a variable distance, but the His bundle divides into two principle subdivisions within the muscular interventricular septum just after the membranous septum. These right and left bundle branches ramify within the ventricular myocardium, with the right bundle branch passing through the moderator band anterior papillary muscle of the right ventricle.

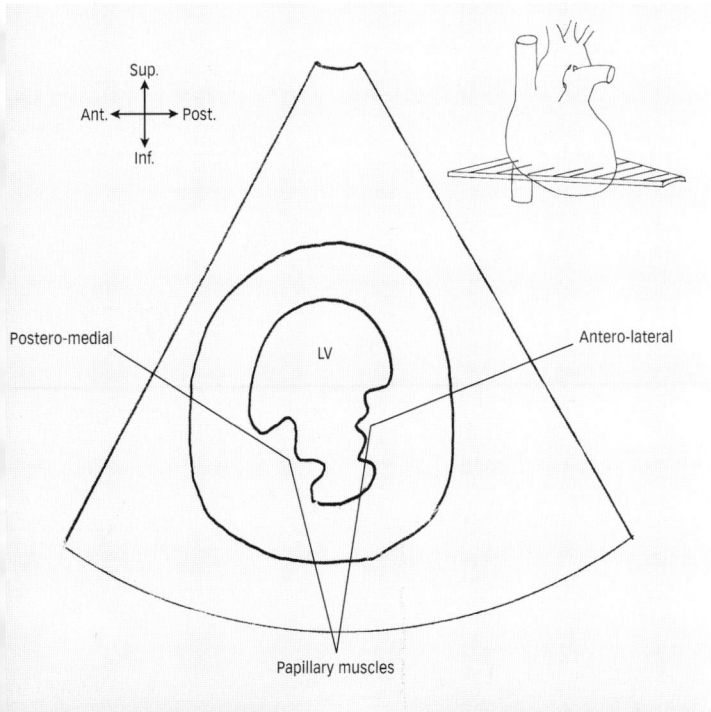

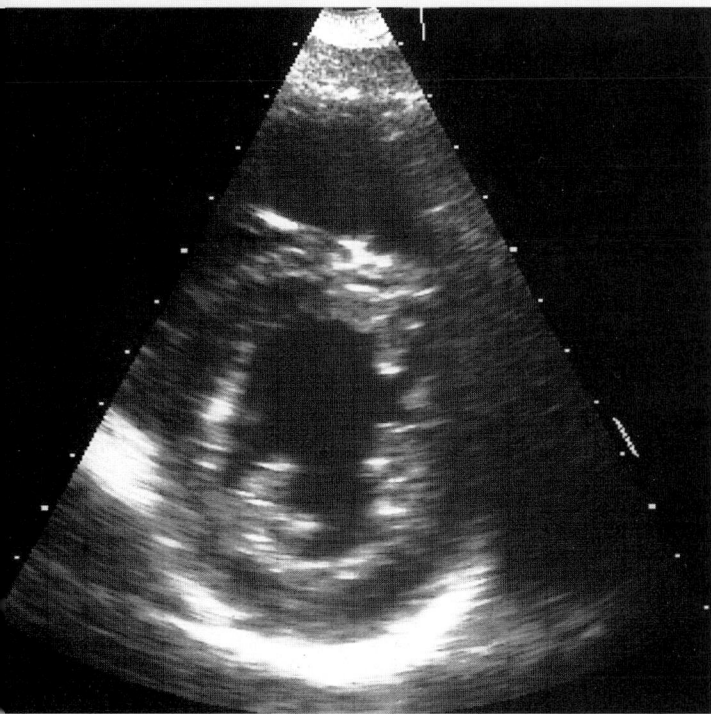

Fig. 20. Transthoracic echocardiogram. Parasternal short axis, at the level of the left ventricular papillary muscles.

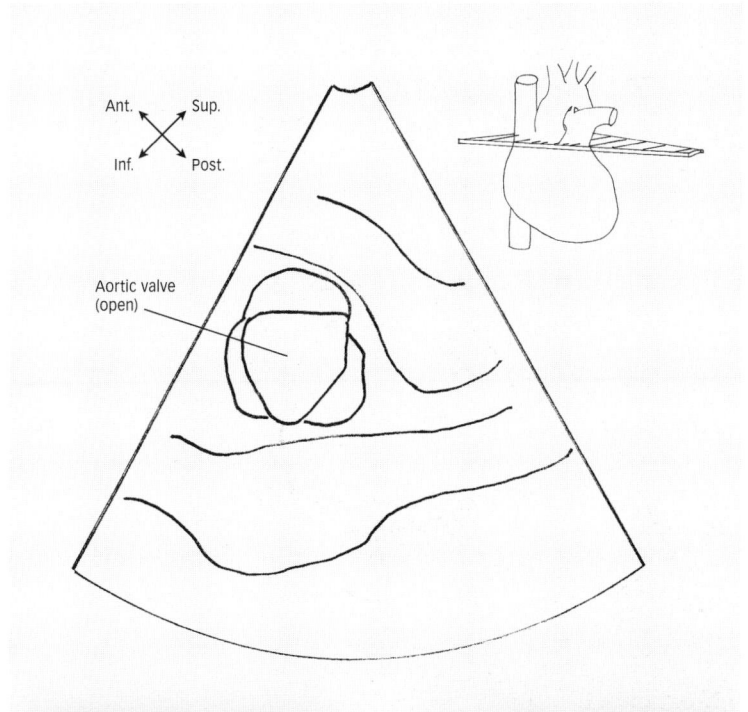

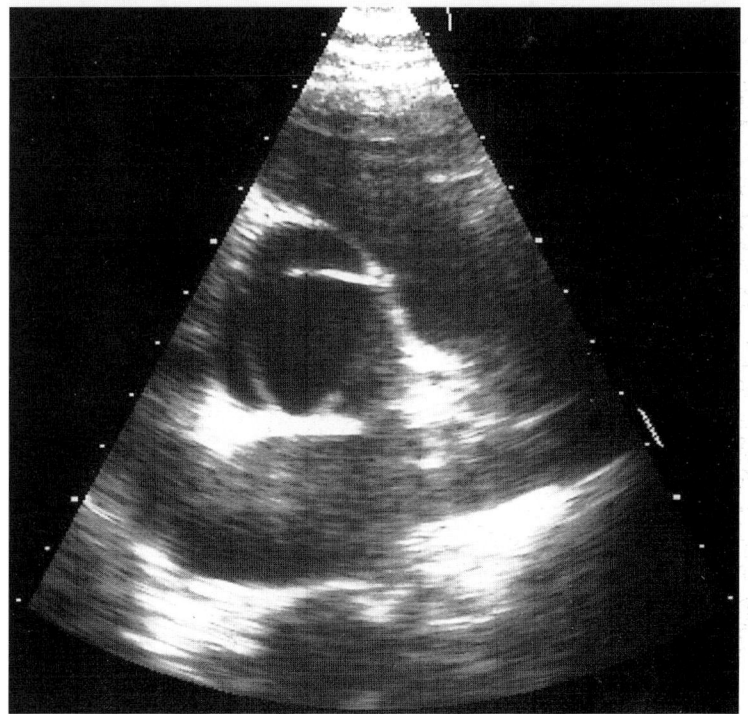

Fig. 21. Transthoracic echocardiogram. Parasternal short axis, at the level of the open aortic valve.

(a)

- Arch of aorta
- Pulmonary trunk
- Left coronary artery
- Circumflex branch
- Anterior descending (interventricular) artery
- Left marginal artery
- Atrioventricular nodal artery
- Diagonal artery
- Posterior descending (interventricular) artery

Sinus artery
Right coronary artery
Marginal artery

Anterior view

(b)

- Arch of aorta
- Superior vena cava
- Sinus artery
- Right pulmonary veins
- Right coronary artery
- Atrioventricular nodal artery
- Posterior descending (interventricular) artery
- Marginal artery

Left pulmonary artery
Left coronary artery
Circumflex branch
Anterior descending (interventricular) artery

Posterior view

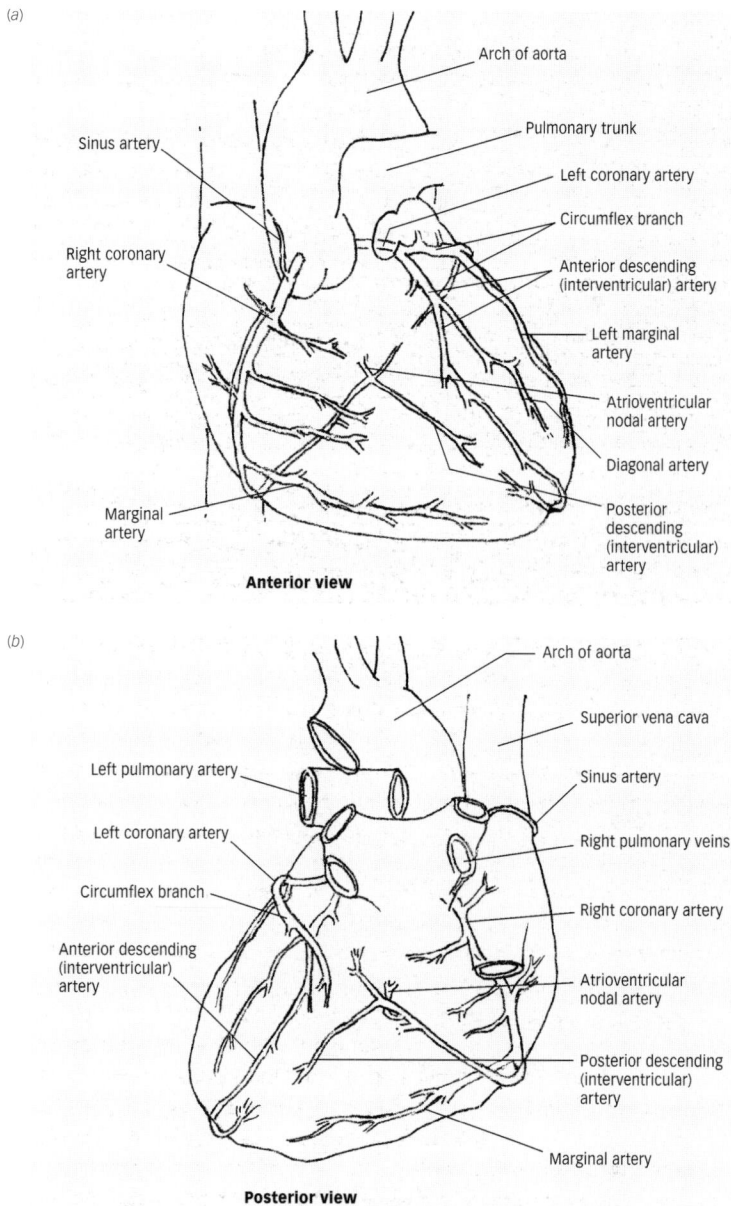

Fig. 22.
Coronary arteries.

(a)

- Aortic valve
- Left coronary artery
- Circumflex artery
- Anterior interventricular artery

Right coronary artery
Posterior interventricular artery
Right marginal artery

(b)

Fig. 23.
(*a*) Variants of coronary dominance. 85% of people have right dominance. (*b*) Less than 15% have left dominance.

Coronary circulation

Anatomically, the coronary circulation is right or left dominant, 'coronary dominance' referring to whether the left or right vessels supply the posterior diaphragmatic portion of the interventricular septum and the diaphragmatic surface of the left ventricle. In 85% of people there is right dominance. It should be noted that there is considerable anatomical variation of the coronary circulation, and in practice the nomenclature of the vessels is regarded as a guideline rather than a definitive description (Figs. 22 and 23).

Right coronary artery
Arises from the anterior sinus of Valsalva and passes to the right between the pulmonary trunk and the right atrium to the atrioventric-

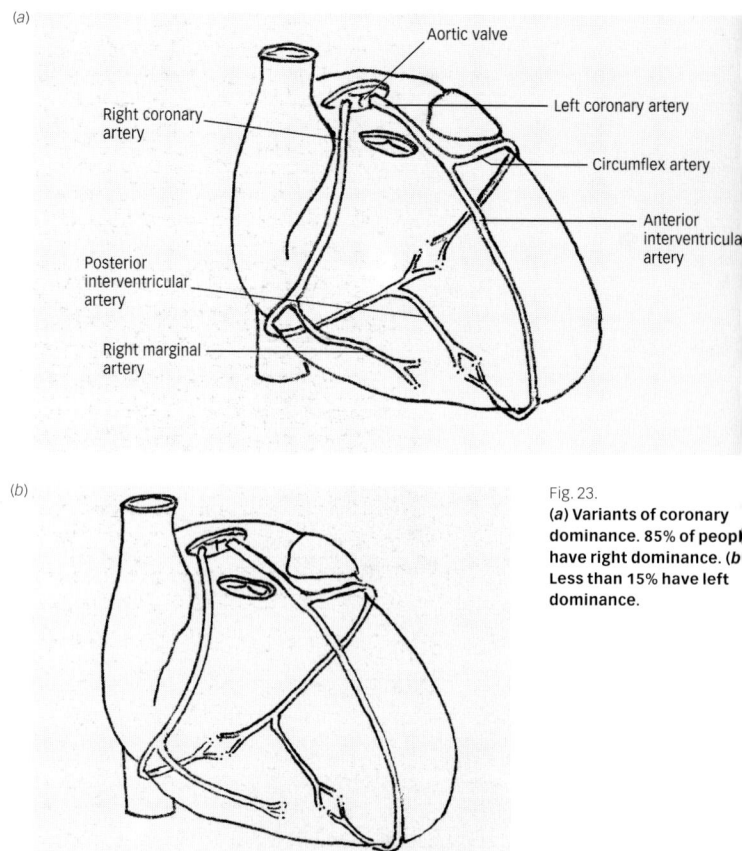

ular groove as the marginal artery. Ultimately, the right coronary artery anastomoses with the left circumflex artery on the inferior atrioventricular groove. It has the following branches (Figs. 22, 24 and 25):

(a) Conus artery: arises at the ostium, or within a few millimetres of it, to supply the pulmonary outflow tract. It may arise directly from the coronary sinus itself.
(b) Sinus artery: a branch of the right coronary artery in 60%, or alternatively from the left circumflex. Supplies the sino-atrial node.
(c) Atrial branches.
(d) Marginal branches: pass anteriorly to supply the right ventricle.
(e) Posterior descending artery (posterior interventricular artery): in 85% there is right dominance where the posterior descending artery arises at the junction of the atrioventricular groove and the interventricular septum (i.e. the crux) to run forward in the interventricular septum to supply the inferior surface of the left ventricle and the posterior two-thirds of the interventricular septum.
(f) Common variants: partial supply of the posterior descending artery territory by marginal branches, double posterior descending artery, early origin of the posterior descending artery proximal to the crux.

164

Fig. 24.
...onary arteriogram. Right
coronary artery, LAO 60
degrees.

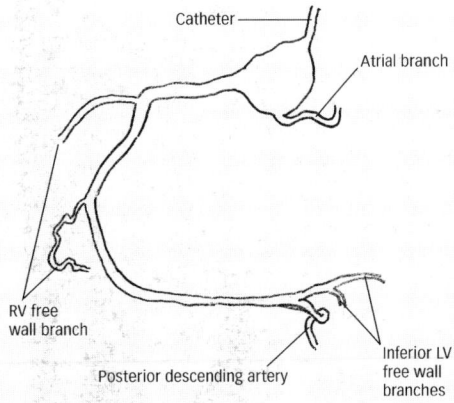

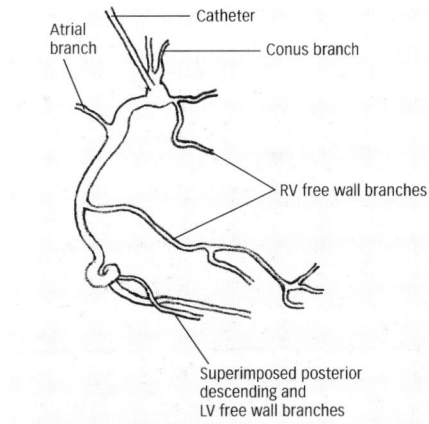

Fig. 25.
Coronary arteriogram.
Right coronary artery,
RAO 30 degrees.

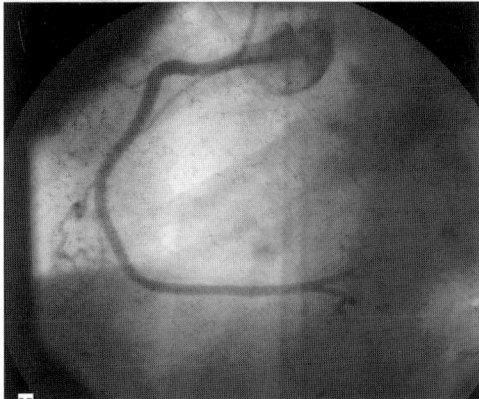

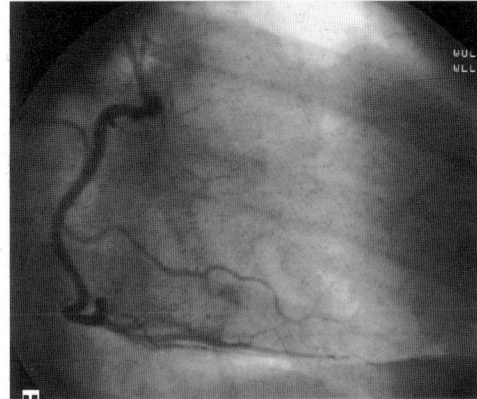

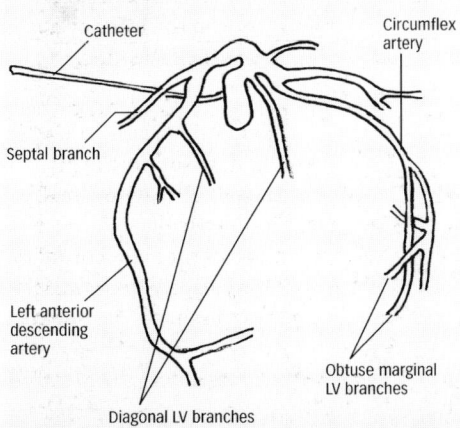

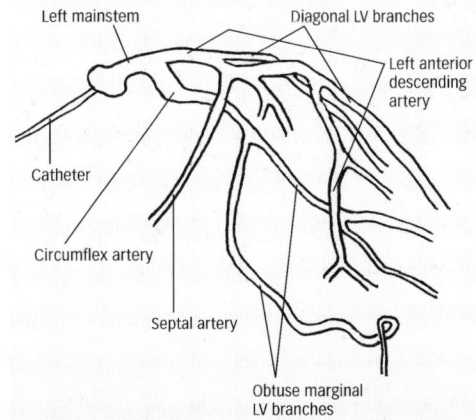

Fig. 26.
...ronary arteriogram. Left
coronary artery, LAO 60
degrees.

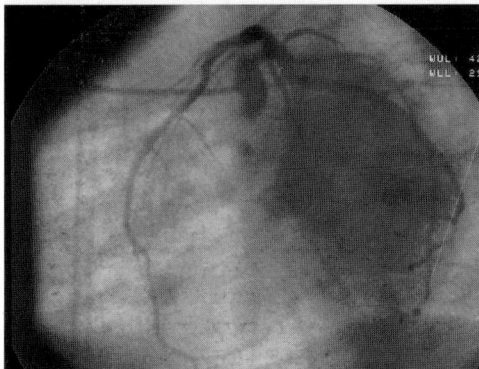

Fig. 27.
Coronary arteriogram.
Left coronary artery, PA

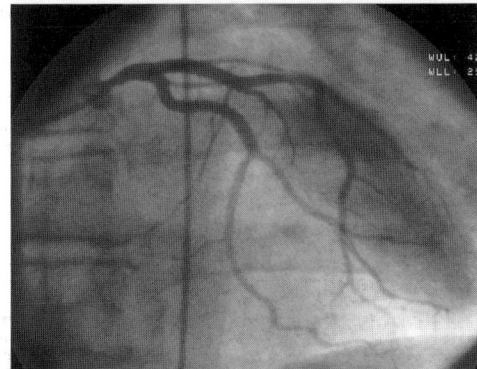

165

Left coronary artery

This arises from the left posterior sinus of Valsalva as the left main coronary artery. It passes to the left and behind the pulmonary trunk on to the left atrioventricular groove, where it bifurcates within 1 cm of its origin, into the left circumflex artery and anterior descending artery (Figs. 22, 26 and 27).

Left anterior descending artery

This descends in the anterior interventricular groove towards the apex, where in 80% it rounds the apex. It has the following branches:

(a) Septal branches: a variable number pass down into the septum, the first being the most prominent. Supplies the anterior one-third of the interventricular septum.
(b) Diagonal branches: a variable number run anterolaterally towards the apex, supplying the anterior wall of the left ventricle.

Common variants In a third of people, the main left coronary artery trifurcates to give a 'ramus medianus' (or intermediate artery) between the left anterior descending and left circumflex arteries, which supplies the anterior left ventricular wall. In 20%, the left anterior descending artery tapers out before reaching the apex. A single, large, septal branch may run deep and parallel to the left anterior descending artery. There may be separate left main and left circumflex ostia.

Left circumflex artery

This runs laterally around the atrioventricular groove to anastomose with the terminal branches of the right coronary artery; though such anastomosis is only considered to occur pathologically. In 10 to 15% of people, there is left dominance, where the right coronary artery is short and the left circumflex supplies the posterolateral wall of the left ventricle giving off the posterior descending artery. Within this group of subjects there is a spectrum in the degree to which the left ventricular myocardium is supplied by the left or right coronary arteries. The left circumflex has the following branches:

(a) Obtuse marginal branches: supplying the free lateral wall of the left ventricle.
(b) Inferior surface left ventricular branches: depending on dominance of right or left coronary arteries.
(c) Atrial branches: supplying the posterior and lateral aspects of the left atrium.

Coronary veins

The coronary sinus is the main conduit of venous drainage. The coronary sinus lies in the posterior atrioventricular groove and opens into the posterior wall of the right atrium (Fig. 11) to the left of the inferior vena cava. Veins that run alongside the arteries are its tributaries. It receives the following (Fig. 28):

(a) Great cardiac vein: runs up the anterior interventricular groove to become the coronary sinus.
(b) Middle cardiac vein: ascends in the posterior interventricular groove.
(c) Small cardiac vein: runs with the marginal branches of the right of the right coronary artery.
(d) Left posterior ventricular vein: accompanies the obtuse marginal branches of the left coronary artery.

A small portion of the venous drainage does not flow into the coronary sinus. The anterior cardiac veins are three or four veins draining the anterior surface of the right ventricle, and open directly into the right atrium. The venae cordis minimae are minute vessels within the myocardium which also drain directly into the heart chambers, mostly the atria.

Fig. 28.
Coronary veins.

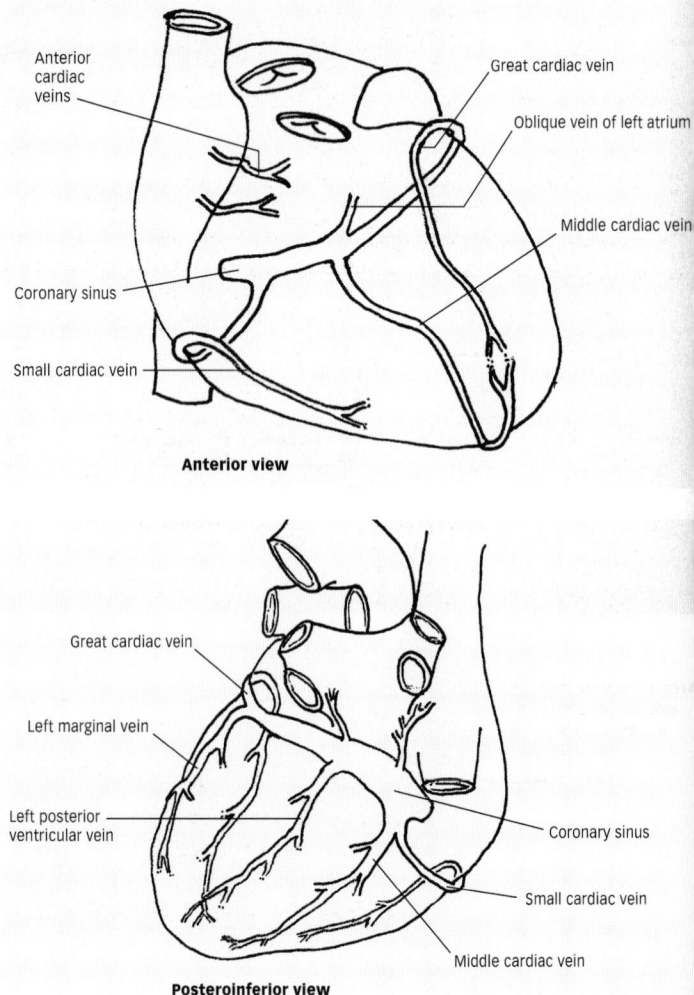

Anterior view

Posteroinferior view

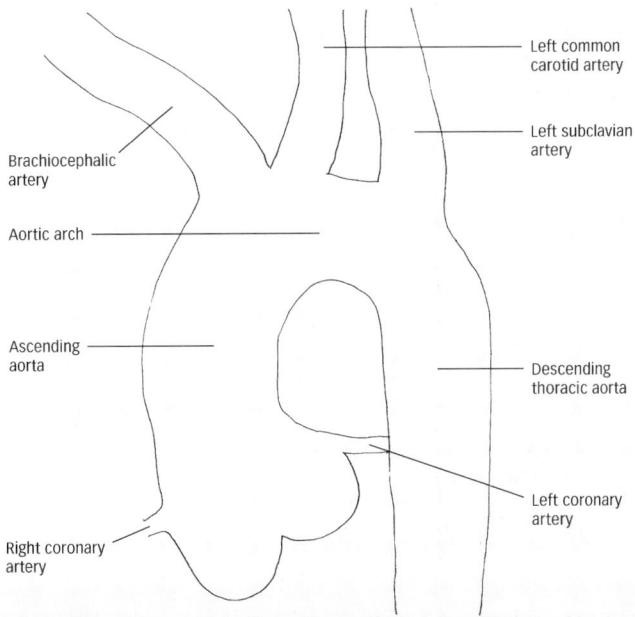

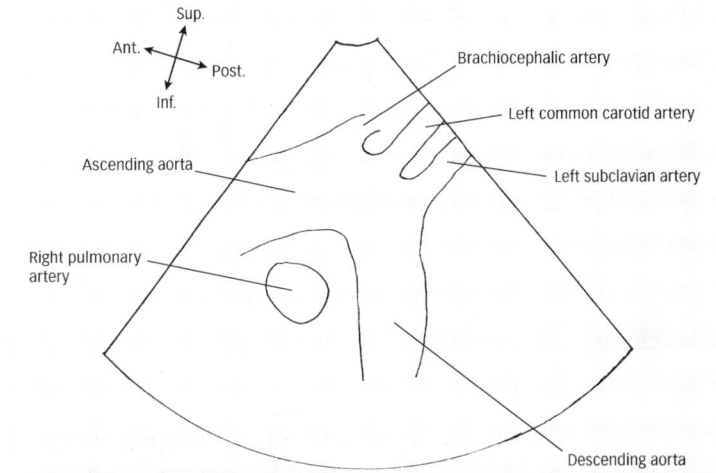

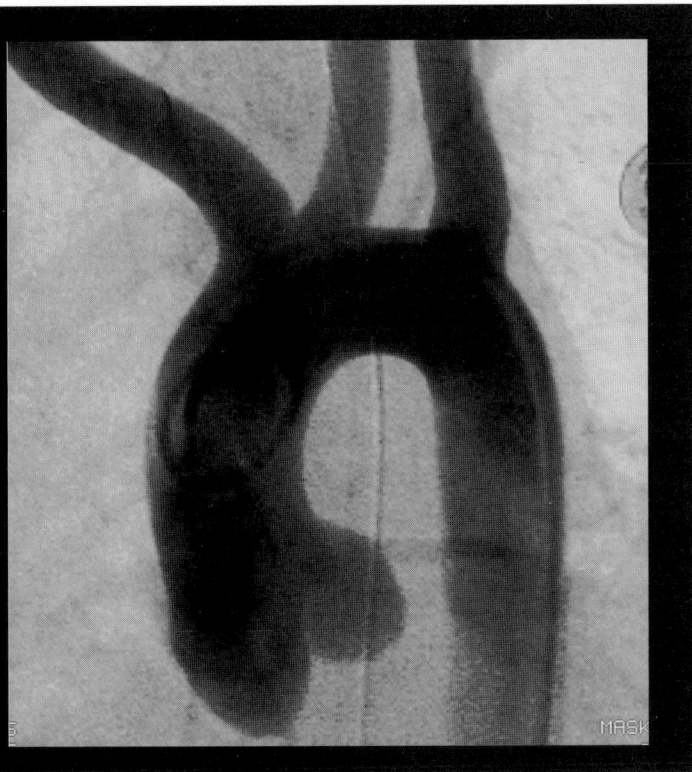

Fig. 30.
Transthoracic
echocardiogram.
**Suprasternal view, showing
the aorta and its main
branches.**

Fig. 29.
Arch aortogram. Note the
sinuses of Valsalva and
origin of the coronary
arteries.

Great vessels

Aorta

In the thorax the aorta can be divided into aortic root, ascending aorta, aortic arch and descending aorta (Figs. 29 and 30).

The aortic root is the first few centimetres of aorta from its valve to just above the coronary sinuses and is invested within the pericardium. It lies at the level of the right third costal cartilage anteriorly and the 5th thoracic vertebrae posteriorly, at a 15–30° angle to the long axis of the body. In the wall of the root there are three focal dilatations (an anterior, right posterior and left posterior) corresponding to the three semilunar cusps of the aortic valve. The left coronary artery arises from the left posterior sinus, while the right coronary artery arises from the anterior sinus. The right posterior sinus is also called the non-coronary sinus. The aortic root is related anteromedially to the right atrium, the non-coronary and anterior coronary sinuses forming a slight bulge, the torus aorticus, on the antero-superior part of the right atrial wall. The anterior sinus is also related anteriorly to the pulmonary outflow tract above, and the interventricular septum below.

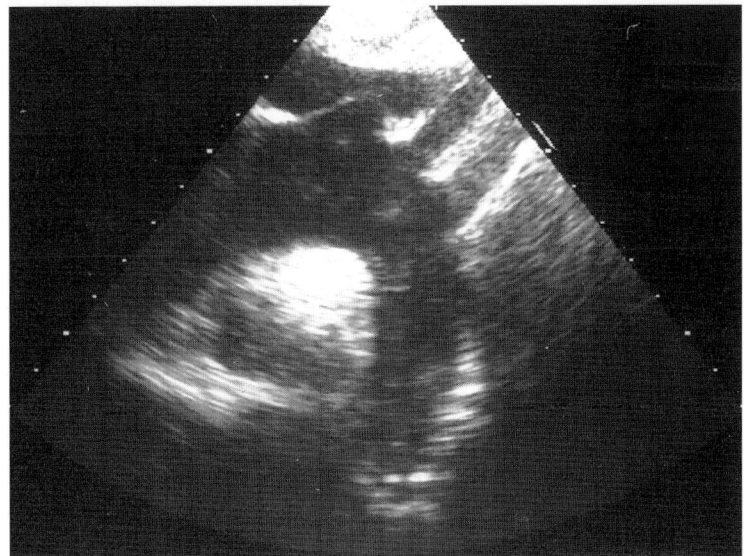

The ascending aorta continues upwards, anteriorly and to the right for a distance of approximately 5 cm, where it becomes the aortic arch at the level of the manubrial angle. The right ventricle is anterior and to the left, the pulmonary trunk is to the left, and the right atrium and superior vena cava are to the right of the ascending aorta.

167

The aortic arch runs upwards and posteriorly from right to left, at first anterior to the trachea and oesophagus, then over the pulmonary trunk and left main bronchus to a position left of the fourth dorsal vertebral body. Beneath the arch the pulmonary trunk bifurcates and the right pulmonary artery passes to the right under the arch. The left pulmonary artery is attached to the junction of the arch and descending aorta (i.e. the isthmus) by the ligamentum arteriosum. Anteriorly and to the left the arch is related to the medial aspect of the left lung and pleura; while posteriorly and to the right are the trachea, oesophagus, thoracic duct and vertebral column. In the majority of people (65%) the major vessels arise from the arch in the following order (Fig. 31(*a*)):

- brachiocephalic artery, which subsequently divides into right common carotid and right suclavian arteries,
- left common carotid artery,
- left subclavian artery.

Variation is common (Fig. 31), in the most frequent of which (27%) the left common carotid artery arises from the brachiocephalic artery (Figs. 31(*b*) and 31 (*c*)) rather than directly from the arch. In 2.5%, the left vertebral arises directly from the arch (Fig. 31(*d*)), between the left common carotid and left subclavian arteries. An aberrant right subclavian artery is seen in 0.5%, and arises distal to the left subclavian and crosses the mediastinum posterior to the oesophagus (Fig. 31(*g*)).

The descending aorta passes down the posterior mediastinum from its junction with the arch (the isthmus), to the aortic hiatus of the diaphragm at the 12th dorsal vertebral body. Laterally lies the right lung and pleura, while posteriorly and medially is the vertebral column. The oesophagus is an anterio-medial relation to the descending aorta, except in its upper portion where it lies to the right. The descending aorta passes behind the left main-stem bronchus, pulmonary artery and left atrium. The descending aorta gives off the following branches:

- nine pairs of intercostal arteries.
- bronchial arteries, the number and location of which are variable. Any systemic artery in the mediastinum may be a potential source of bronchial circulation. A frequent appearance is of three vessels with a right bronchial artery from the 3rd intercostal artery at the level of T5 and two left bronchial arteries directly from the aorta, somewhat more inferior.
- oesophageal branches; up to five arteries to the oesophagus which form an anastomotic plexus with branches of the inferior thyroid and phrenic and left gastric arteries.
- spinal arteries, two or three branches.
- mediastinal branches.
- a pair of superior phrenic arteries.
- a pair of subcostal arteries.

At certain anatomical points the aorta is fixed within the thorax: at the aortic isthmus (by the ligamentum arteriosum), aortic valve, the main aortic branches, the intercostal vessels, the diaphragm.

Great veins

The superior vena cava (Fig. 32) is formed by the union of right and left brachiocephalic veins, behind the junction of the manubrium and the first costal cartilage, and enters the right atrium at the level of the right third costal cartilage (Fig. 33). The lower half is enclosed

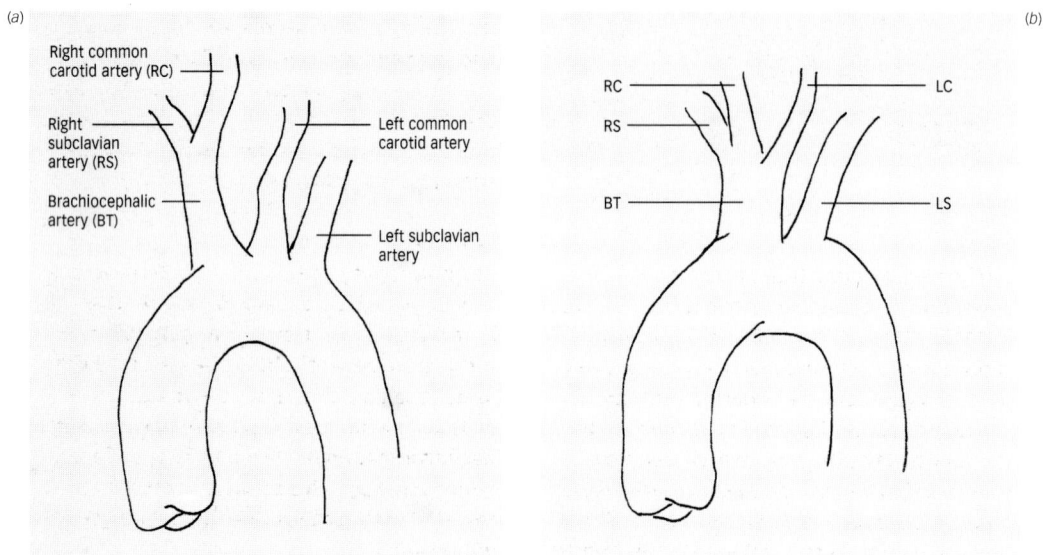

(a)

(b)

(c)

(d)

(e)

(f)

(g)

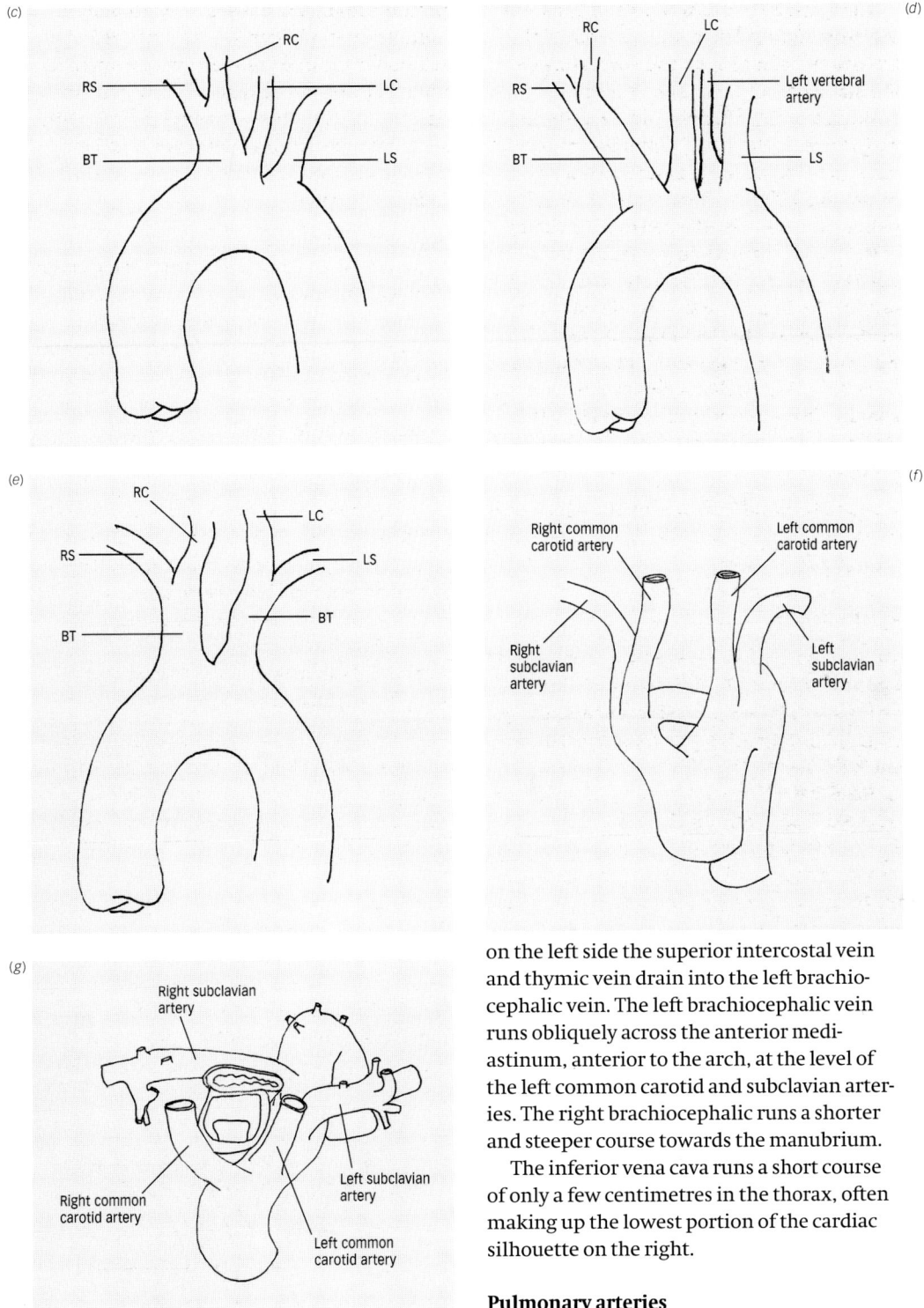

Fig. 31.
The normal arch (a) and its anomalies (b)–(e), (f) double aortic arch, (g) anomalous right subclavian; note how it passes posterior to the oesophagus.

by the pericardium. It lies to the right of the aortic arch and anterior to the right mainstem bronchus. The azygos vein arches over the right mainstem bronchus to drain into the posterior aspect of the superior vena cava.

The brachiocephalic veins are formed by the union of the internal jugular and subclavian veins behind the medial end of either clavicle. Both receive the internal thoracic (mammary) and inferior thyroid veins, while on the left side the superior intercostal vein and thymic vein drain into the left brachiocephalic vein. The left brachiocephalic vein runs obliquely across the anterior mediastinum, anterior to the arch, at the level of the left common carotid and subclavian arteries. The right brachiocephalic runs a shorter and steeper course towards the manubrium.

The inferior vena cava runs a short course of only a few centimetres in the thorax, often making up the lowest portion of the cardiac silhouette on the right.

Pulmonary arteries

The pulmonary trunk curves postero-superiorly to the left from the pulmonary valve, anterior to the aortic root, for 5 cm to its bifurcation beneath the aortic arch into right and left main pulmonary arteries. It is surrounded by the commencements of the coronary arteries and the two atrial appendages, which together with the aortic root are invested within the pericardium (Figs. 34, 35 and 36).

The right main pulmonary artery exits the pericardium and passes under the arch in front of the right main bronchus, and behind the ascending aorta and superior vena cava. It is crossed anteriorly by the right superior pulmonary vein, which is recognizable on the frontal radiograph as the right hilar point. Before entering the hilum of the lung the right main pulmonary artery divides into an upper and lower branch.

The left main pulmonary artery passes to the left, initially in front of the left main bronchus but then curves superior to the bronchus as the latter gives off its upper lobe bronchus. The ligamentum arteriosum, the fibrous remnant of the fetal ductus arteriosus, runs posteriorly from the left main pulmonary artery through the pericardium to its attach-ment at the aortic isthmus. In addition to being shorter than its fellow on the right, the left main pulmonary artery lies in a higher position. The superior pulmonary vein crosses anterior to the left main pulmonary artery, thus marking the left hilar point which is approximately 1 cm higher than the right hilar point.

Pulmonary veins

The pulmonary veins enter the left atrium, two from each lung, at the posterolateral margins (Fig. 37). They converge on the left atrium beneath the level of the pulmonary arteries and run horizontally as they approach the heart. However, on one or both sides, they may become confluent before entering the left atrium.

Fig. 32.
T$_1$-weighted coronal MRI, showing relationship of SVC to ascending aorta and pulmonary trunk.

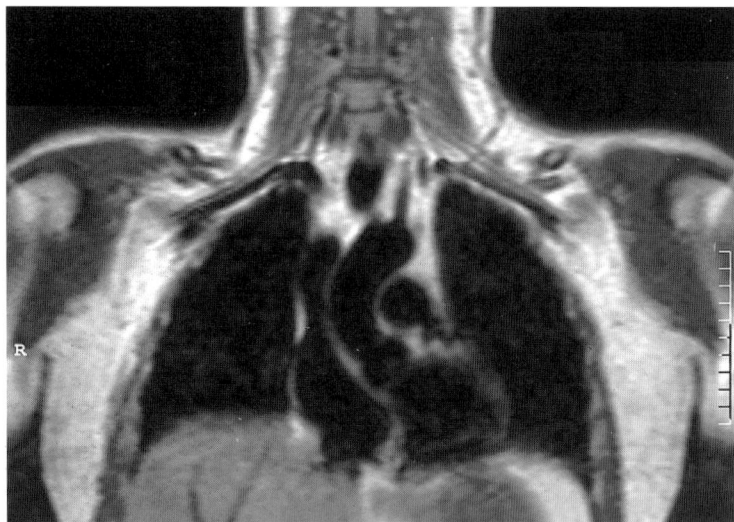

Fig. 33.
Axial CT with IV contrast, at level of SVC entering right atrium.

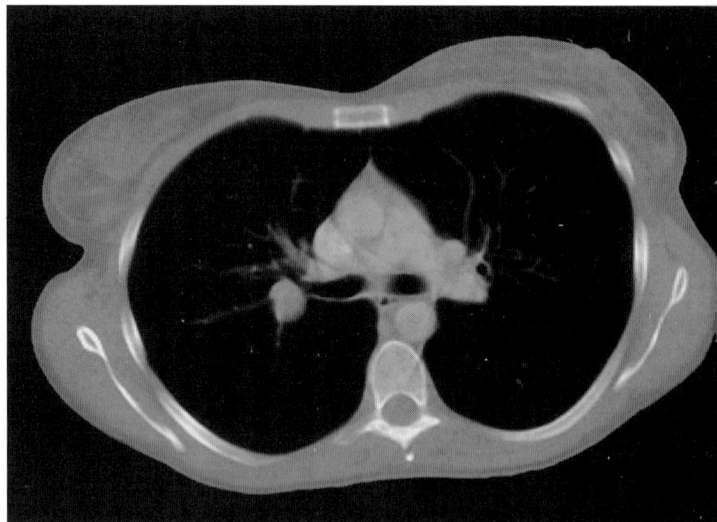

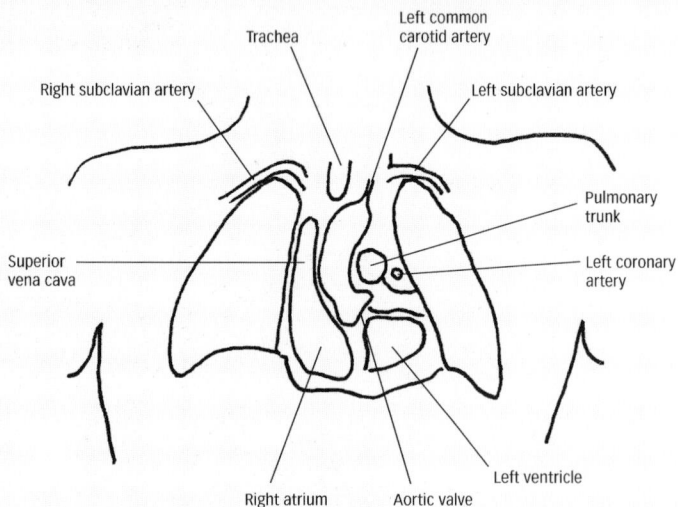

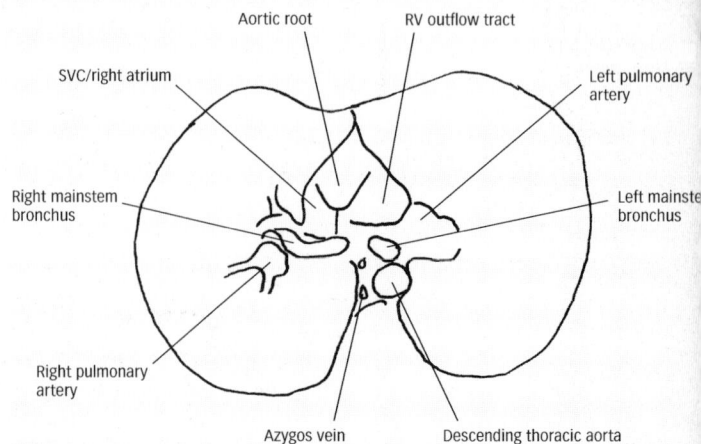

Ascending aorta   Pulmonary trunk

Left pulmonary
artery

SVC/RA
junction

Left bronchus

Left pulmonary
artery (distal)

Right main
pulmonary artery   Right bronchus

Descending aorta

Aortic root

SVC/right atrium

Pulmonary
trunk

Right pulmonary
artery

Left pulmonary
artery

Right mainstem
bronchus

Left mainstem
bronchus

Oesophagus   Azygos vein   Descending aorta

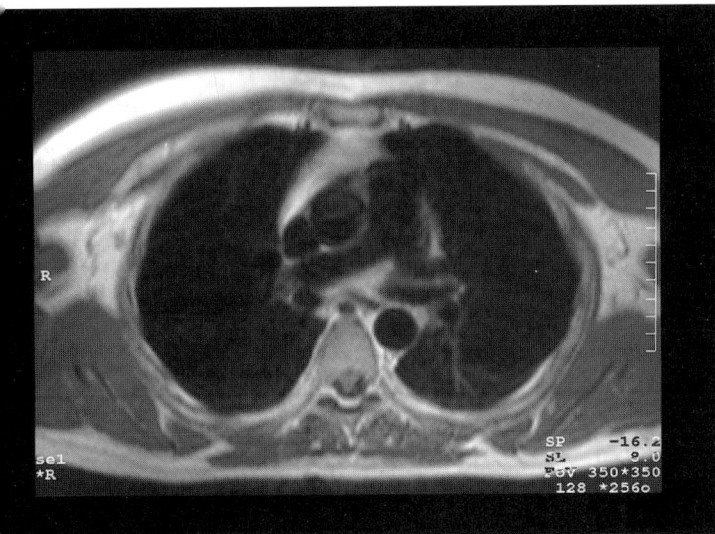

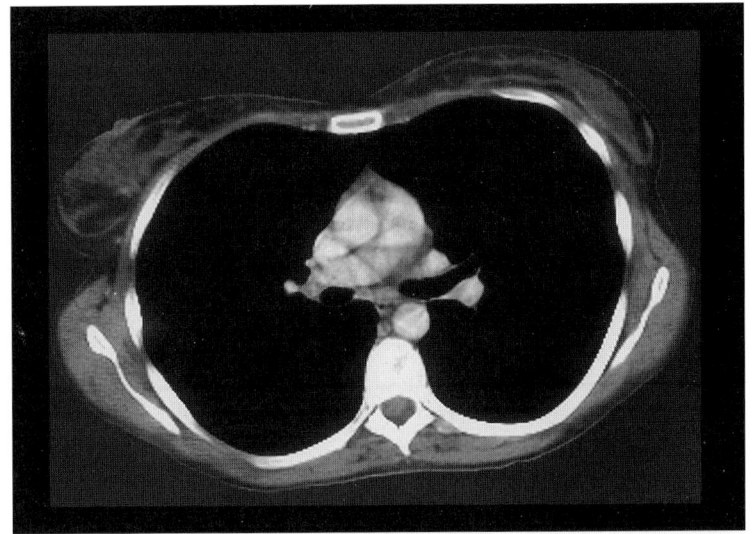

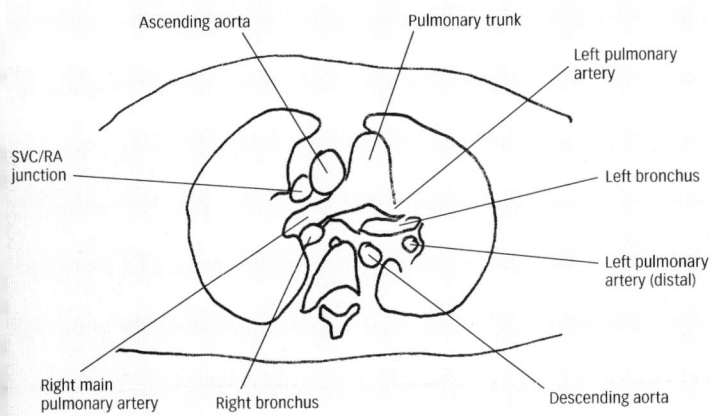

Fig. 34.
T_1-weighted axial oblique
MRI, showing the
relationships of the
pulmonary trunk.

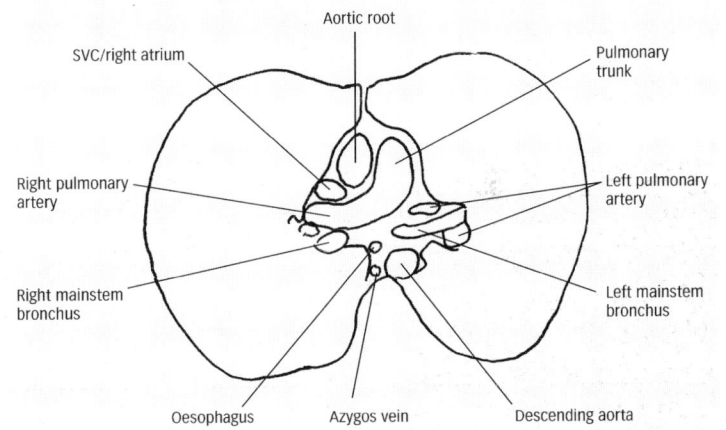

Fig. 35.
Axial CT with IV contrast,
showing pulmonary trunk.

Fig. 36.
Pulmonary angiogram, arterial
phase. Note position of the
pulmonary trunk to the left of the
midline and the unequal lengths
of the main pulmonary arteries.

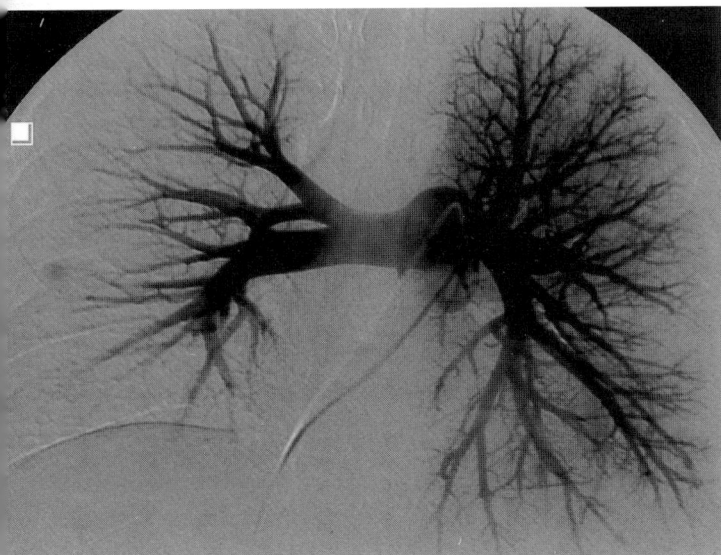

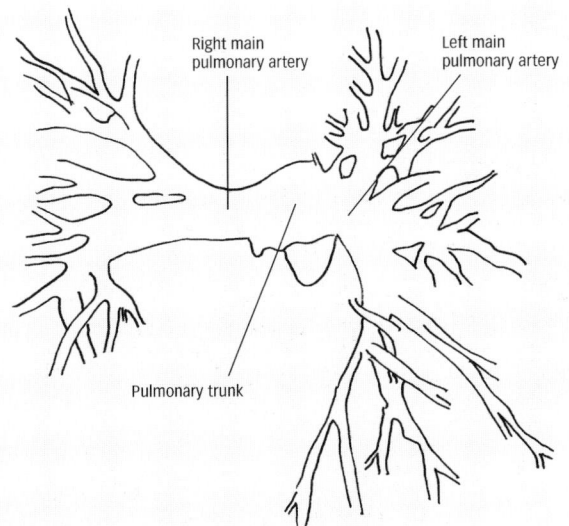

Right main
pulmonary artery

Left main
pulmonary artery

Pulmonary trunk

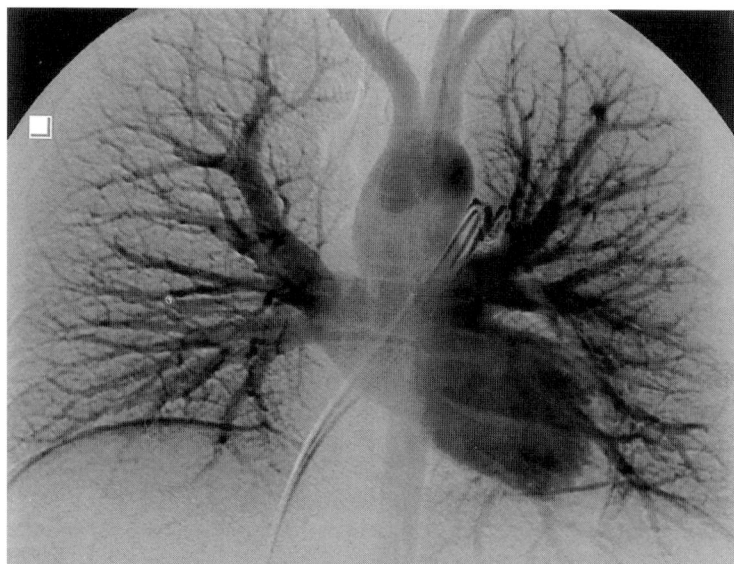

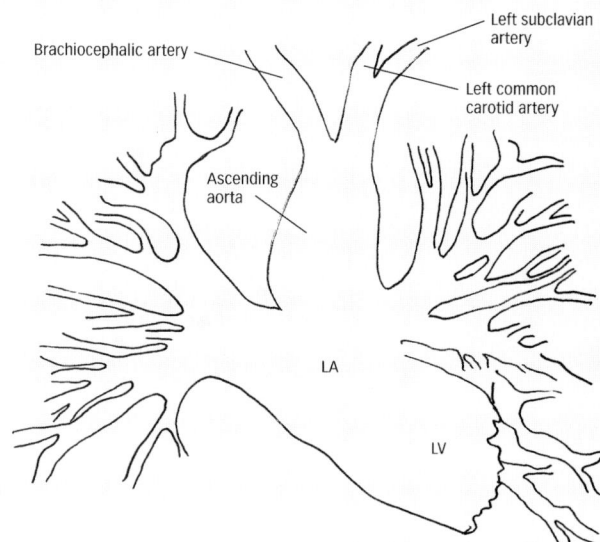

Fig. 37.
Pulmonary angiogram, venous phase.

References

Ellis, H. (1997). *Clinical Anatomy*, 9th edn., Oxford: Blackwell.

Meire, H., Cosgrove, D., Dewbury, K. & Wilde, P. (1993). *Clinical Ultrasound, A Comprehensive Text: Cardiac Ultrasound*. London: Churchill Livingstone.

Runge, V.M. (1990). *Clinical Magnetic Resonance Imaging*. Philadelphia: J.B. Lippincott Co.

Further reading

Hurst, J.W., Logue, R.B., Rackley, C.E., Schlant, R.C., Sonnenblick, E.H. & Wallace, A.G. & Wenger, N.K. (1986). *The Heart*. New York: McGraw-Hill Book Co.

Roelandt, J.R.T.C., Sutherland, G.R., Iliceto, S. & Linker, D.T. (1993). *Cardiac Ultrasound*. London: Churchill Livingstone.

Schiller, N.B., Shah, P.M., Crawford, M. *et al*. (1989). Recommendation for quantitation of the left ventricle by two dimensional echocardiography. *Journal of the American Society of Echocardiography*, **2**, 358–67.

8

The breast

J. A. HANSON
and N. M. PERRY

The introduction of population screening for breast cancer using mammography, combined with increasing attention to symptomatic breast care, has resulted in rapid expansion of breast imaging and the need for skilled radiological interpretation. An average department taking part in the United Kingdom National Breast Screening Programme might expect to perform 10 000–15 000 screening and up to 5000 symptomatic examinations per year. The need for correct understanding of the typical radiological appearances of the breast, its anatomy and normal variations has never been greater.

Development

The breast is a tubulo-acinar type of modified apocrine sweat gland. A primitive embryonic ectodermal milk line runs from the base of the forelimb to the region of the hindlimb (Fig. 1). During the fifth–seventh week of intrauterine fetal development, the thoracic section will specialize and thicken to form the mammary ridge. A number of epithelial cords penetrate the underlying mesenchyme, giving rise to 15–20 solid outbuddings. At term these have canalized to form a branching system of ducts, representing the future lobes of the breast. The ducts open on to a surface pit, which undergoes mesenchymal proliferation and eversion at about the time of birth to become the nipple (Fig. 2).

The breast retains a rudimentary glandular structure until puberty, when the female gland enlarges under the influence of pituitary, ovarian and other hormones. The lactiferous ducts proliferate to form ductules, acinar ducts and simple acini. These are lined by a single layer of cuboidal epithelial cells and a

Fig. 1.
The milk line. Mammary glands normally develop in humans from the pectoral portion of the line. (Adapted from Skandalakis, Gray & Rowe, 1983, with permission.)

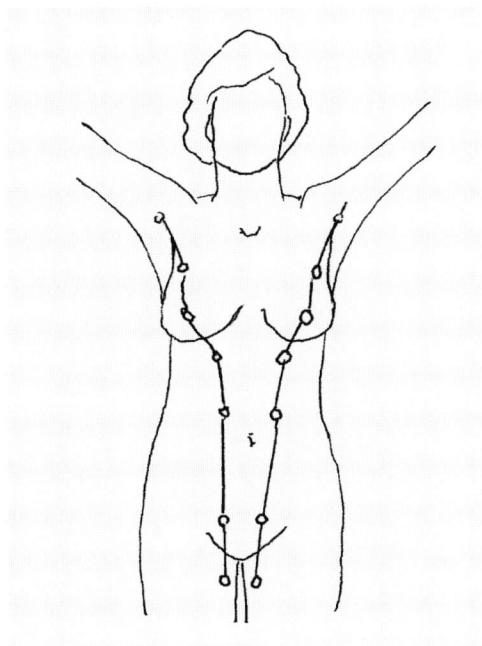

Fig. 2.
Development of the breast. (*a*)–(*d*). Stages in the development of the duct system and potential glandular tissue from the epidermis. Connective tissue septa form from the epidermis. (*e*) Eversion of the nipple near the time of birth. (Adapted from Skandalakis, Gray & Rowe, 1983, with permission.)

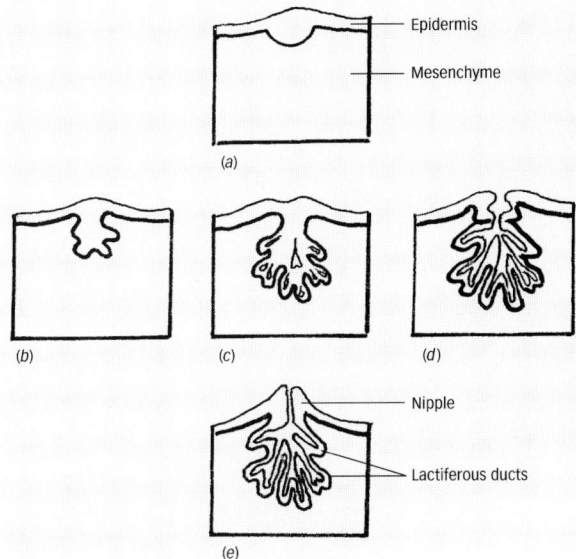

flattened layer of myoepithelial cells, the ducts being lined by columnar cells. The male breast maintains a simple ductal system, although temporary gynaecomastia may occur in response to pubertal hormonal stimuli.

In the mature female breast, some 15–20 lobes drain by lactiferous ducts onto the nipple. Each lactiferous duct shows a small dilatation, or sinus, just proximal to its termination. The lobes are further subdivided into lobules surrounded by a fibrous and fatty interlobular stroma. A lobule consists of a group of acini supplied by one terminal duct and supported by loose connective tissue. Parks (1959) and subsequently Wellings and Wolfe (1978) developed the concept of the basic functional unit of the breast being the terminal duct lobular unit (TDLU). Most pathological entities can be referred to this microstructure (Fig. 3).

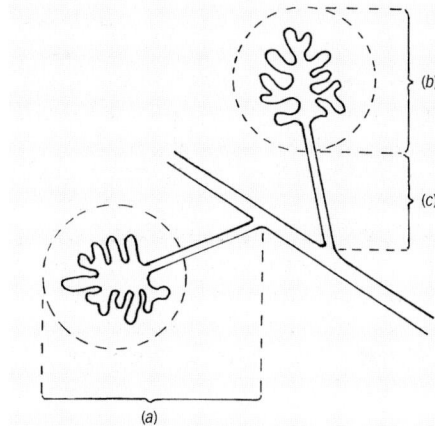

Fig. 3.
The terminal duct lobular unit (TDLU). (*a*) Terminal duct lobular unit, (*b*) margin of lobule, (*c*) extralobular terminal duct.

Topographic anatomy

The breast lies entirely within the superficial fascia of the chest wall, separated from the deep fascia by the potential retromammary space. It extends from the second rib superiorly to the sixth or seventh costal cartilage inferiorly, and medially from the sternal edge as far laterally as the mid-axillary line. The breast is divided arbitrarily into quadrants extending peripherally from the nipple. The upper outer quadrant contains the greatest proportion of fibroglandular tissue and gives rise to the axillary tail of Spence, which passes superolaterally towards the axilla, and may reach as far as the posterior axillary line. The medial two-thirds of the breast overlie the pectoralis major muscle with pectoralis minor lying deep to this, whereas the lateral aspect of the gland overlies the serratus anterior and external oblique muscles. Fibrous strands or extensions of the superficial fascia pass through the breast towards the skin and nipple, and are known as the suspensory ligaments of Cooper.

The nipple arises centrally as a conical elevation of skin on to which the lactiferous ducts drain separately. Bands of smooth muscle run parallel to the ducts and circularly at the base, and contract to produce nipple erection. The nipple is surrounded by a circular zone of pigmented skin, the areola, which contains numerous small elevations due to specialized sebaceous glands, known as Montgomery's tubercles. The secretion of these glands helps protect the nipple during suckling.

The major vascular supply to the breast arises from the internal thoracic and lateral thoracic arteries, with additional supply from the thoracoacromial and intercostal arteries. Venous drainage occurs via the internal thoracic, axillary, subclavian and azygos veins. Anastomoses occur between the azygos system and the vertebral venous plexus, which are important in the spread of metastatic disease to the spinal column.

Lymphatic drainage of the breast deserves careful attention because of its importance in the spread and staging of malignant disease. The majority of lymph drains towards the axillary nodes but some passes to the intercostal and internal thoracic chains, with nodes arranged in groups. Some lymphatic flow also occurs to the opposite breast. Three surgical levels of nodes are recognized in the axilla according to their relationship to the pectoralis minor muscle. Level I nodes are inferolateral, level II nodes deep and level III nodes superomedial to this muscle. Excision of level III nodes requires more radical surgery, often with division of the pectoralis minor muscle (Scanlon & Caprini, 1975; Fig. 4).

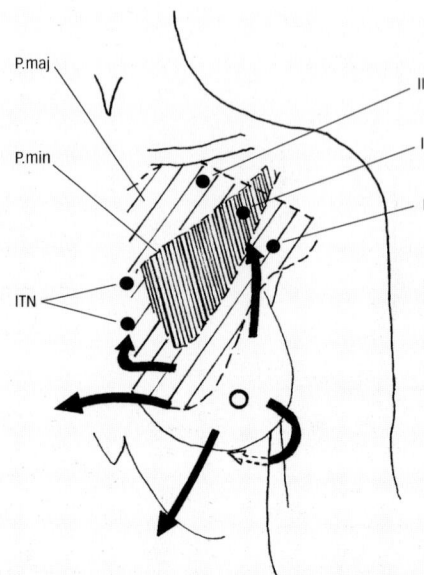

Fig. 4.
Lymphatic drainage of the breast. Relationship of three levels of axillary nodes (I, II, III) to pectoralis minor muscle (P. min) is shown. Additional lymphatic flow occurs to internal thoracic nodes (ITN), intercostal, contralateral chest wall and upper abdominal nodes.

Pathophysiological changes

In the non-pregnant state, cyclical changes occur. Rising oestrogens in the proliferative phase cause epithelial proliferation followed by duct dilatation and differentiation under the influence of progestogens in the secretory phase. During pregnancy, marked epithelial proliferation occurs within the TDLU with relative decrease in the surrounding fat and connective tissue. Prolactin, insulin and growth hormone induce the ductules to form secretory acini. Lactation produces further dilatation of the acini and ducts. The process of regression of the fibroglandular tissue with fatty replacement commences following pregnancy and lactation. More rapid involution occurs with reduction in hormonal levels with the menopause. The effect of hormone replacement therapy is to arrest or reverse these changes, either focally or diffusely. It is quite possible to observe many of these changes mammographically, manifested by overall density, nodularity and ductal prominence proportional to the amount of fat content visible.

Mammographic anatomy

Contrast between fat and soft tissue is optimized by the use of low energy X-ray spectra from dedicated units, 17.4 and 19.6 keV being the characteristic peaks from a molybdenum anode. A small focal spot, compression and a sensitive film screen combination are employed to maximize resolution, reduce scatter and minimize the dose of ionizing radiation to the breast. Provided that the positioning and technical aspects of a mammogram are adequate, various landmarks should be easily identified, but will vary according to the projection used. Mammography is now performed exclusively using a film-screen technique. This has replaced the xeroradiographic technique which reached a height of popularity 20 years ago. This latter technique required a higher dose of ionizing radiation but had certain advantages, which included a wide latitude capable of demonstrating lungs, ribs and breast tissue on a single image (Fig. 18).

The standard mammographic projection is the 45° mediolateral oblique view (Fig. 5). This projection demonstrates the maximum breast tissue on a single film and is particularly chosen in single view screening programmes as it demonstrates the upper outer quadrant to best effect. The pectoralis major muscle should be well seen posteriorly, ideally as far down as the nipple level. The nipple itself should be in profile and the inframammary fold should also be visible. The skin is shown peripherally and tangentially and will be focally thickened in the areolar region. The skin thickness varies in the normal breast,

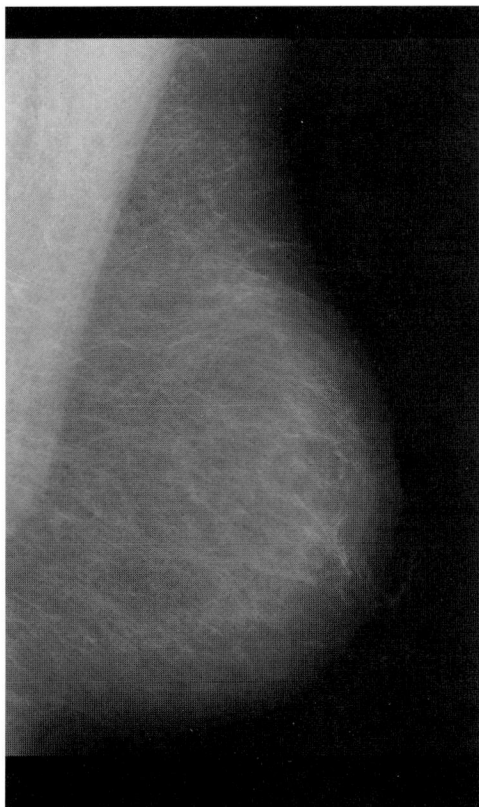

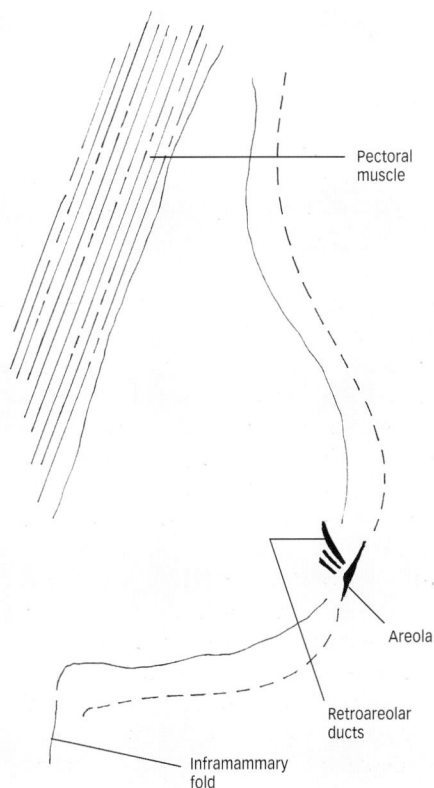

Fig. 5.
Normal mammogram. The background pattern is involuted. The majority of fibroglandular tissue has been replaced by fat, which appears lucent. The pectoral muscles come well down to the level of the nipple and the inframammary fold is demonstrated. The areola is represented as focal skin thickening with fine linear ductal structures running up to it (Wolfe N1).

Pectoral muscle

Areola

Retroareolar ducts

Inframammary fold

being thinnest medially and thickest over the upper outer quadrant. Demonstration of abnormal thickening indicates possible underlying inflammatory or neoplastic conditions.

It is no longer regarded as a priority for the skin to be clearly visible on mammograms. Modern mammographic image quality places great emphasis on contrast and penetration of fibroglandular tissue in order to detect small tumours, and the optical density of a high-quality mammogram has been increased significantly over recent years. Consequently, it may be necessary to use a bright light to visualize the skin and subcutaneous region to best effect.

Ducts may be identified in the retroareolar region as tubular densities, which pass back from the nipple and fan out in the breast, particularly the upper outer quadrant. However, entirely normal and non-thickened ducts are thread-like and extremely difficult to visualize unless completely surrounded by fat. Vascular structures may be clearly seen. Arteries are smaller and may be best visualized in the upper outer quadrant, whereas superficial veins can be very prominent wherever they occur. Other linear structures identified in the breast include the suspensory ligaments of Cooper, seen as fine shallow curvilinear densities.

Intramammary lymph nodes are often seen in the normal breast, and appear as rounded, ovoid or reniform masses of low soft tissue density, classically sited towards the upper outer quadrant and close to a vascular bundle. The presence of a small fatty hilum confirms their origin (Fig. 6).

The mammographic appearance of the normal breast otherwise varies according to the age of the woman and the proportion of fibroglandular tissue to fat present. Mammography is rarely if ever performed in adolescence, largely because of the radiation risk, but also because of the lack of detail obtained. The breast tissue at this age is extremely dense and homogeneous and the subcutaneous fat layer relatively sparse. With increasing age, the subcutaneous layer becomes thicker and mammographically more visible. Also, the fibroglandular tissue becomes better differentiated, with fatty interlobular deposits and septa breaking up the homogeneous density into a more recognizable structure. The progressive decrease of dense fibroglandular tissue with fatty replacement has obvious diagnostic advantages.

Parenchymal or fibroglandular thickening within a breast may still be regarded as within normal range even if it is particularly florid. When marked, it is commonly described as benign breast change; however, this is in itself an aberration of normal development and involution. Ductal prominence and thickening is an important component of this condition and may create a very nodular appearance on the mammograms. The amount and distribution of fibroglandular tissue within a breast was described and graded by Wolfe (1976) into four categories:

Nl. Normal largely adipose tissue (Fig. 5).
Pl. The breasts are still adipose but there is parenchymal thickening with ductal prominence anteriorly, usually in the

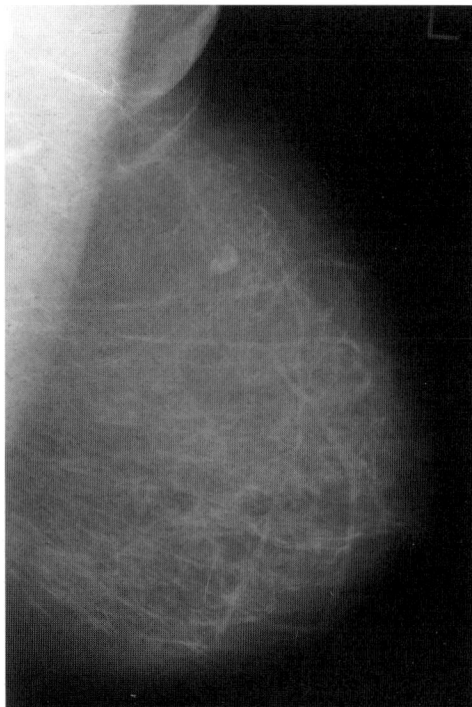

Fig. 6
Normal intramammary lymph node. A well-defined ovoid mass of soft tissue density lies in the upper part of the breast adjacent to the vascular bundle. A lucent fatty hilum is clearly seen within this. Normal branching vascular structures can be identified inferiorly.

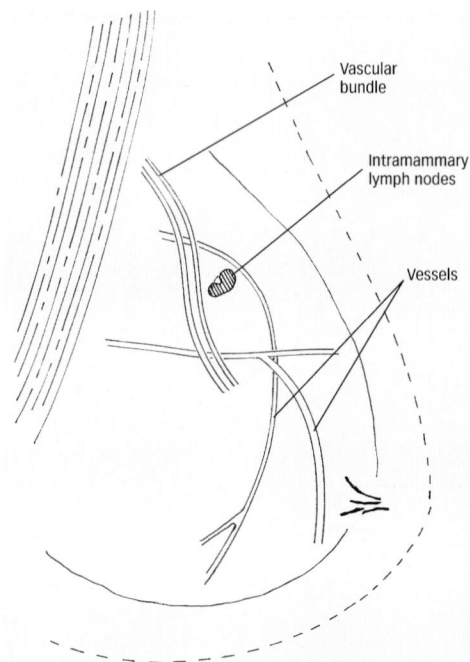

Vascular bundle

Intramammary lymph nodes

Vessels

retroareolar region but occupying less than one quarter of the breast volume (Fig. 13).

P2. A much more prominent ductal and fibroglandular pattern involving greater than one-quarter of the breast volume (Fig. 14).

DY. Generalized increased density of the fibroglandular pattern, without a recognizable ductal or nodular appearance (Fig. 15).

It is generally accepted that there is an increased risk of malignancy with the P2 and DY patterns, largely related to the amount of fibroglandular tissue and epithelial components present. The Wolfe classification is not used in everyday reporting, but remains of value for descriptive and comparative purposes, especially when collating data.

The most commonly used second projection, used routinely for symptomatic examinations in addition to the oblique view, is the cranio-caudal examination (Fig. 7). This does not demonstrate as much breast tissue as the oblique view. However, it has advantages of a second near orthogonal projection for diagnostic purposes and technically is a better quality image than the oblique owing to more complete compression. It demonstrates the anterior portion of the breast well but usually the pectoralis major muscle is not visualized posteriorly, unless it is caught as a shallow curved feature on the back edge of the image. Other projections are usually reserved for specialized assessment views. These include the true lateral projection (taken mediolaterally). This resembles the oblique view except that the pectoral muscle is less well shown. The other projections are more concerned with radiographic positioning and are outside the scope of this chapter.

The male breast may be demonstrated mammographically usually in attempting a differential diagnosis of gynaecomastia from male carcinoma of the breast. The normal male mammogram appears small and fatty with vascular and rudimentary duct structures barely visible (Fig. 8). In general terms, the appearance is very different to that of a small female breast, where almost always there is a moderate amount of fibroglandular tissue visible.

Fig. 7.
A standard cranio-caudal projection showing a small amount of pectoral muscle posteriorly. Also demonstrated are vessels, fibrous septa and some slightly prominent retroareolar ducts.

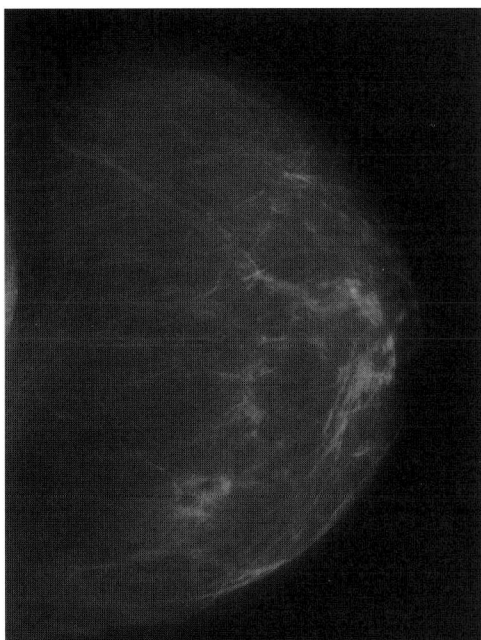

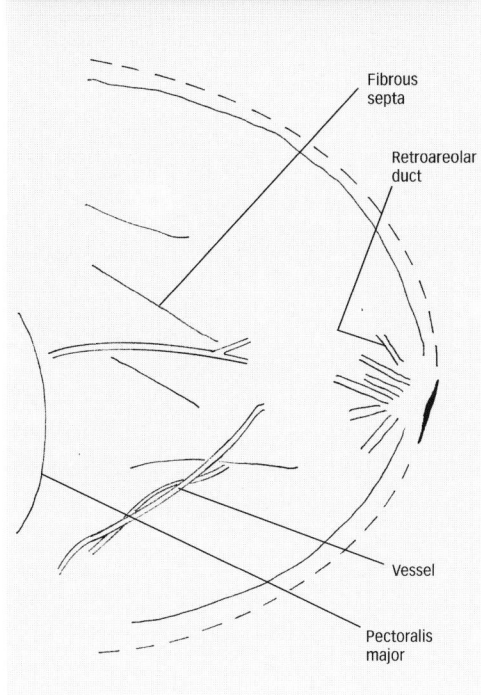

Fig. 8.
A normal male breast with no discernable fibroglandular structure. The breast is small and fatty with tiny vessels just visible.

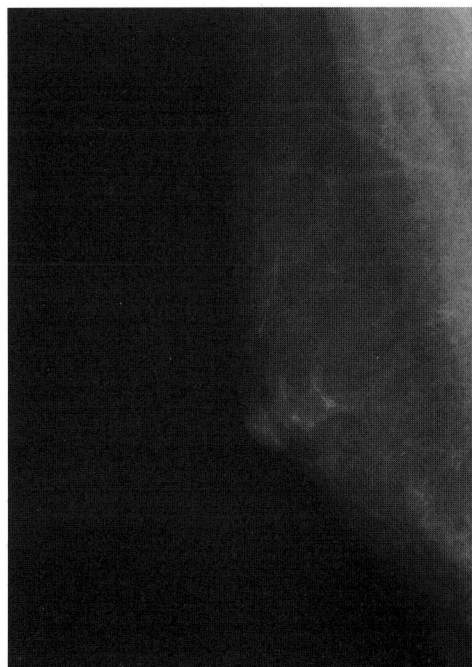

Fig. 9.
A double areolar nipple. An ovoid 1.5 cm well-defined soft tissue mass is projected directly posterior to the normal nipple. On clinical examination there were two normal size nipples on the areola.

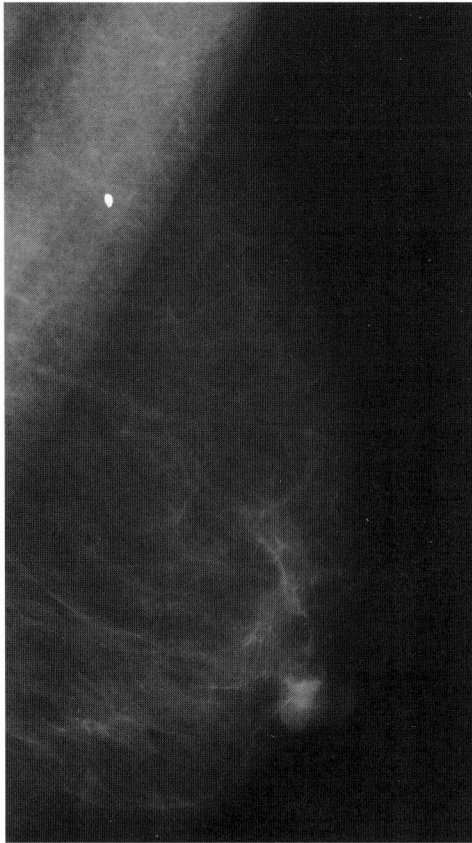

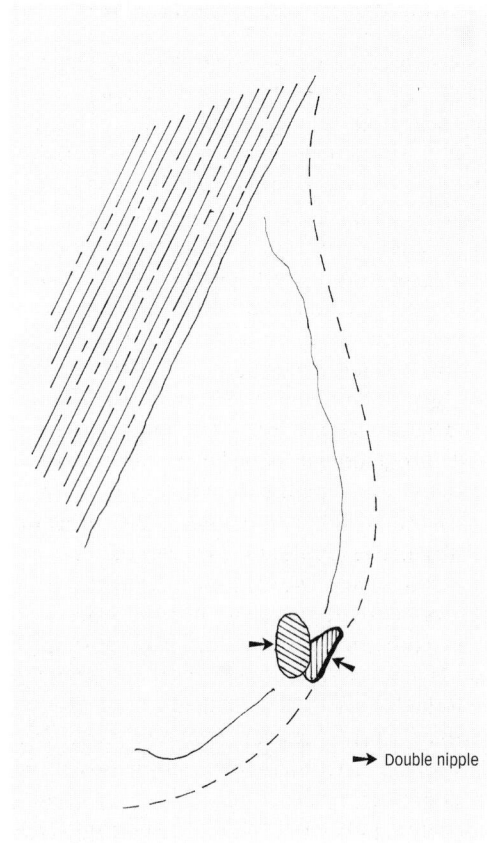

→ Double nipple

Fig. 10.
An axillary breast. An axillary nipple was also present clinically. The outline of the axillary breast can be made out with central thickening from fibroglandular tissue. The prominent branching vascular structure identified in the breast represents a normal vein.

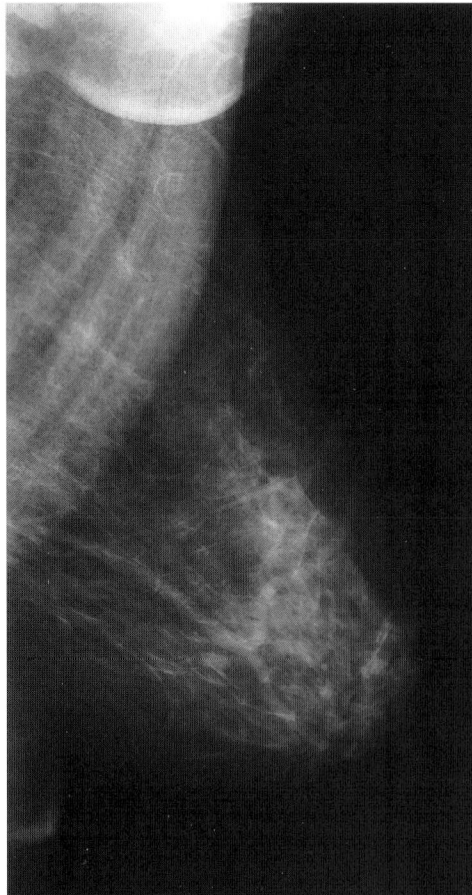

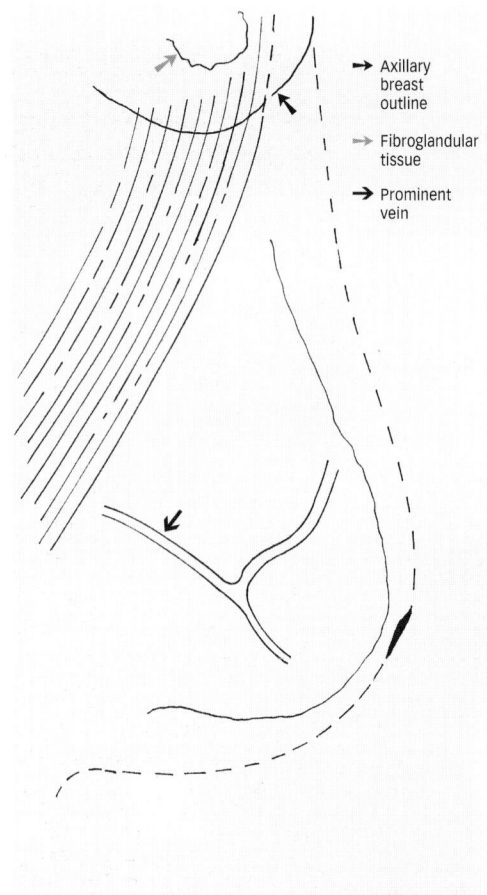

→ Axillary breast outline

→ Fibroglandular tissue

→ Prominent vein

Developmental and normal variants

Incomplete regression of the milk line occurs in 2%–6% of women. This may result in an accessory nipple (polythelia), commonly just inferior to the normal breast, but occasionally anywhere along the milk line. This is usually a clinical as opposed to radiological finding but duplication of the nipple on the areola may occur (Fig. 9). Accessory breasts (polymastia) may also occur and mammographically may be visualized when present in the axilla (Fig. 10). However, it is more common to find accessory glandular tissue in a similar position (Fig. 11). This can be recognized as identical to normal fibroglandular tissue but higher towards the axilla and separate from the main breast tissue (Adler, Rebner & Pennes, 1987). Congenital absence of nipple and all breast tissue (amastia) is rare. The condition of amazia occurs when a nipple is present, but when there is absence of any underlying breast tissue. Hypoplasia of the breast may occasionally be linked to under-development of the structures of the chest wall or forelimb (Poland's Syndrome). Asymmetry of breast tissue occurs in 3% of women, although it may be seen temporarily at puberty. It is rarely associated with any significant pathology (Kopans *et al.*, 1989). Congenital nipple inversion is easily distin-guished from acquired retraction, since the former is present from birth.

Certain normal structures may simulate breast pathology. Calcification of sebaceous glands may be clearly identified as such, and should not be confused with pathological intramammary calcification. The appearance is usually fine, dense and punctate, often with very tiny central lucencies. Tangential projection on to the skin surface is diagnostic (Fig. 12). A skin papilloma or wart may appear to be an intramammary mass but can be readily distinguished by its appearance. Most commonly, these lesions appear as low density, extremely well-circumscribed masses, their clear definition being often enhanced by a thin lucent rim representing a halo caused by air trapped between the skin and the compression plate (Fig. 13).

Calcification in arterial walls is a normal finding and shows typical tubular and occasionally segmented morphology (Fig. 14). Increased vascular calcification is also found in various pathological conditions.

Ultrasound

Ultrasound of the breast is performed either in the investigation of younger women unsuitable for mammography, for further assessment of a

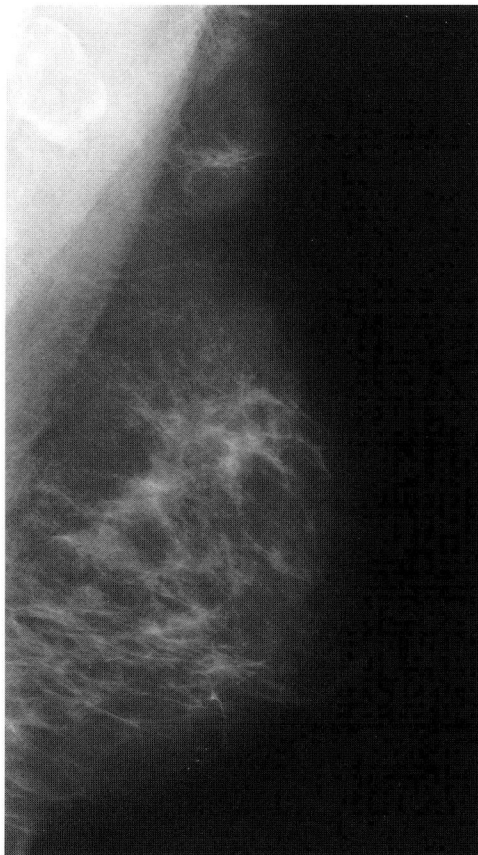

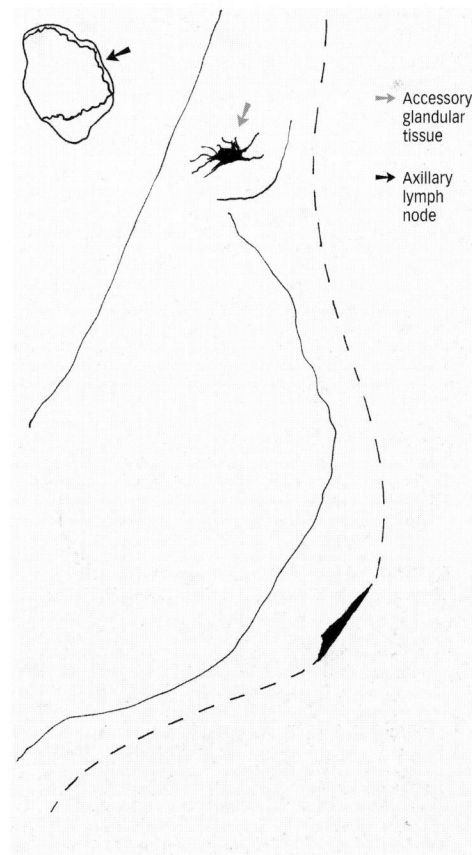

Fig. 11.
Accessory glandular tissue. A small amount of fibroglandular tissue can be seen lying high in the breast towards the axilla. This normal variant may be sufficient to cause pain and discomfort and occasionally a lump. Incidental note is made of a large, but still normal, fat-replaced axillary lymph node.

Accessory glandular tissue

Axillary lymph node

mammographically detected abnormality, or in the investigation of a clinical mass where the breast tissue is dense and no discrete mammographic lesion can be identified (Fig. 15). A 7.5 MHz frequency transducer typically is used, but higher frequences such as 10 MHz or 12.5 MHz are becoming increasingly popular in dedicated breast units. The skin, subcutaneous and interlobular fat deposits, fibroglandular tissue, fascial layers and fibrous septa are clearly demonstrated (Figs. 16 and 17). Structural adipose tissue appears hypoechoic, compared to the increased echogenicity of organic fat. Ducts may be seen clearly in the retroareolar region and have a tubular appearance, with a typical distribution running up towards the nipple (Fig. 18).

Fibrous tissue has an echogenic appearance, and fibroglandular tissue therefore is relatively

Fig. 12.
Multiple sebaceous gland calcifications. These are rounded, dense and are either punctate or have a very fine lucent centre. They can be seen as skin associated if tangentially projected.

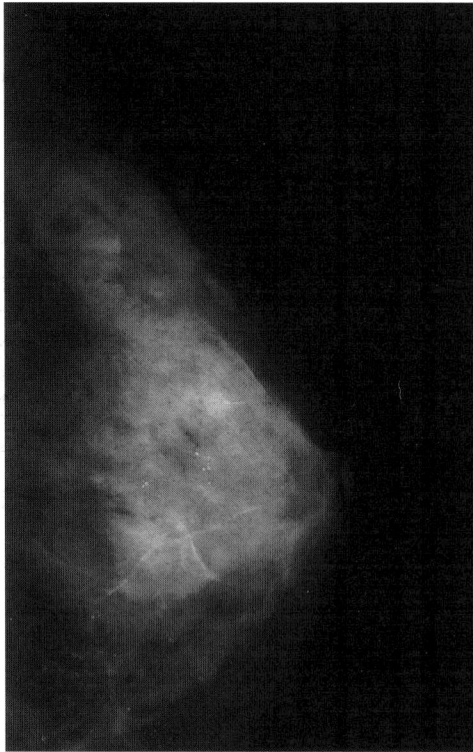

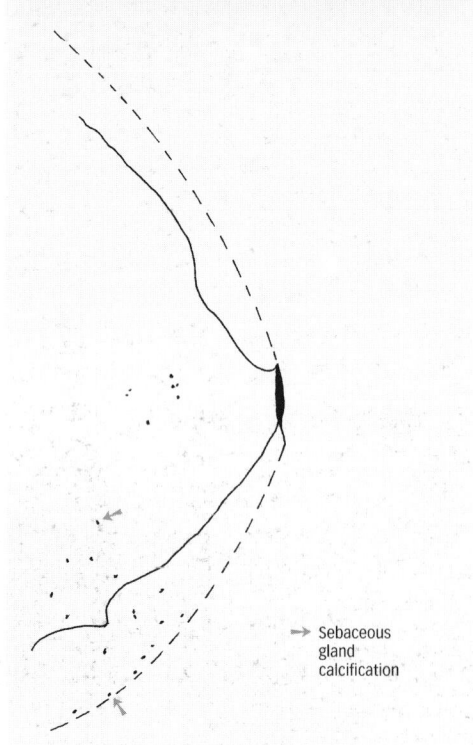

→ Sebaceous gland calcification

Fig. 13.
A large skin naevus appearing as an ovoid soft tissue mass with fine lobulations. On most borders this mass is exceptionally well defined and anteriorly and inferiorly can be seen to be outlined by an air halo (Wolfe P1).

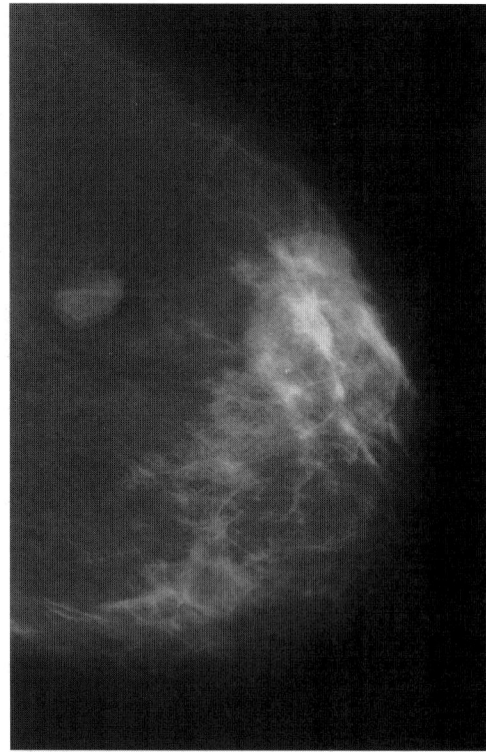

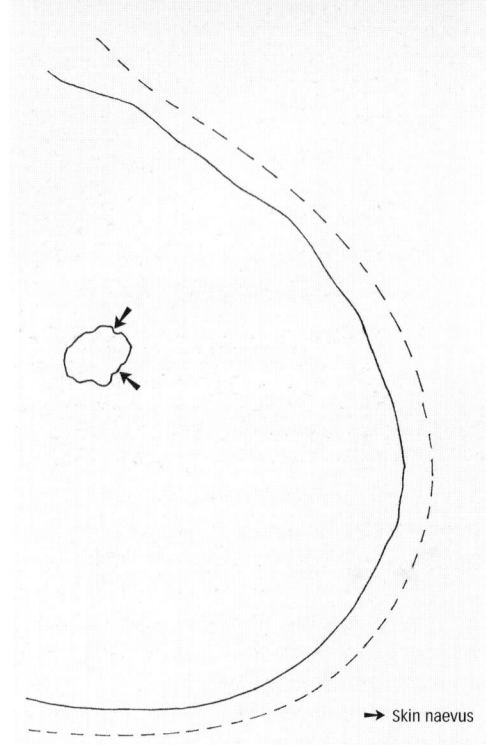

→ Skin naevus

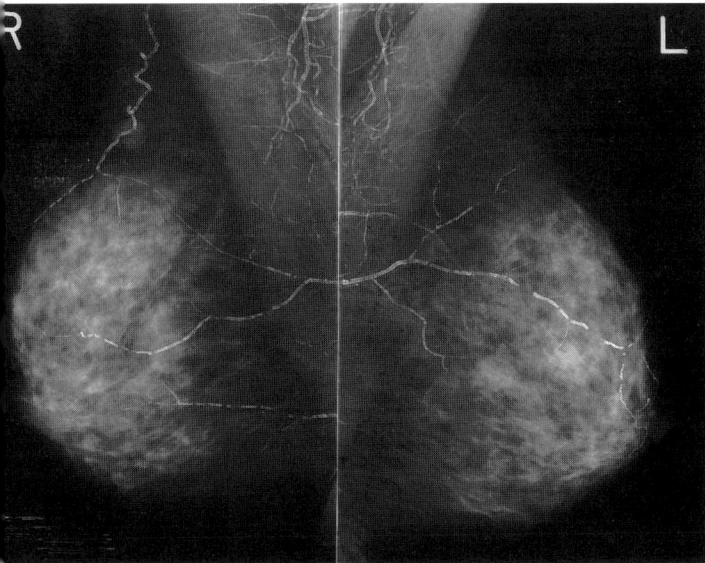

Fig. 14.
...cular calcification.
...tiple calcified arteries
...be seen running into the
...ast from posteriorly and
...eriorly having a typical
...lar and branching
...cture. In some vessels
...calcification is
...tinuous, and in others it
...egmented (Wolfe P2).

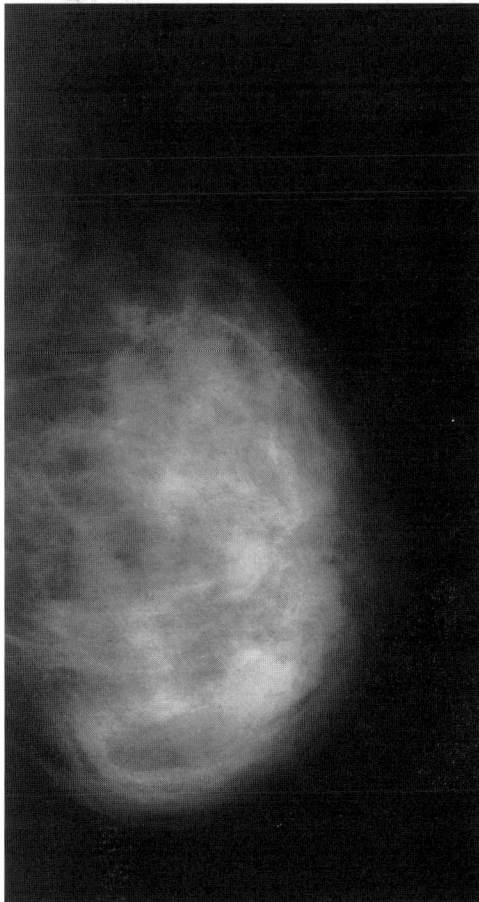

Fig. 15.
An extremely dense
fibroglandular pattern.
Such dense tissue may
...scure small masses and,
if a discrete clinical
...normality is present, an
...asound examination will
be required (Wolfe DY).

the ribs, which cast dense acoustic shadowing. The pleura can usually be identified. Intra-mammary or axillary lymph nodes can be detected and have an ovoid configuration of low echogenicity with an echogenic fatty hilum (Fig. 19).

Acoustic shadowing is a sonographic finding associated with malignancy, but it must be remembered that small zones of shadowing are common in the normal breast and may be caused by fibroglandular tissue or the bright curvilinear bands of Cooper's ligaments.

Other imaging techniques

Ductography
Cannulation of a duct orifice on the nipple surface followed by injection of contrast into that system produces an image known as a

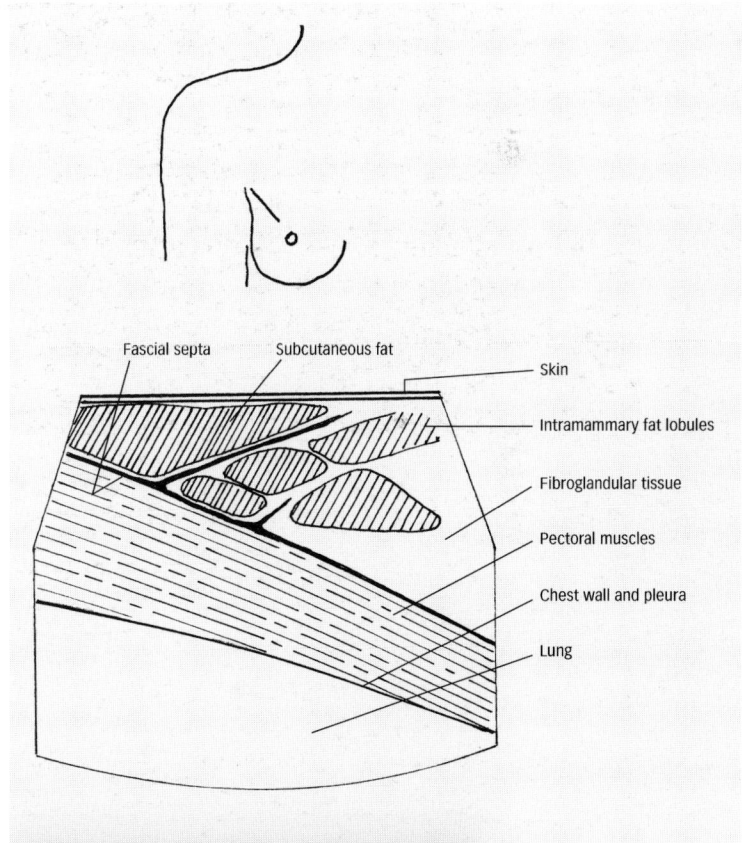

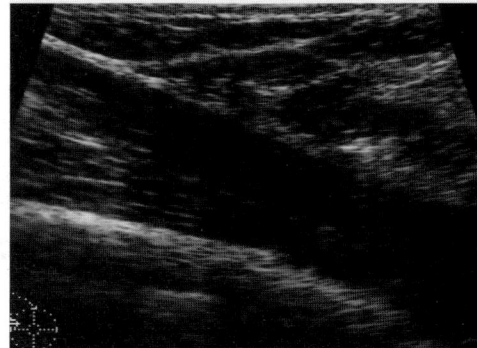

Fig. 16.
Normal breast ultrasound. In the region of the axillary tail the fascia divides to enclose the breast tissue between its layers. Skin and subcutaneous fatty lobules lie anteriorly. A mixture of intramammary fat lobules and fibroglandular tissue can be seen in the breast. The deeper fibres of pectoralis major muscle are well demonstrated.

hyperechoic compared to the anterior subcutaneous fatty lobules. Fibroglandular tissue in the breast is often interspersed with small fatty lobules. These, and the smaller ducts, break up what would otherwise be a uniformly bright appearance. The skin is displayed as two echogenic layers separated by a thin hypoechoic layer. Deep to the breast the pectoral muscle fibres are seen draped over

Fig. 17.
Normal breast ultrasound. There is little fibroglandular tissue remaining in this involuted breast. Echogenic septa surround fatty lobules.

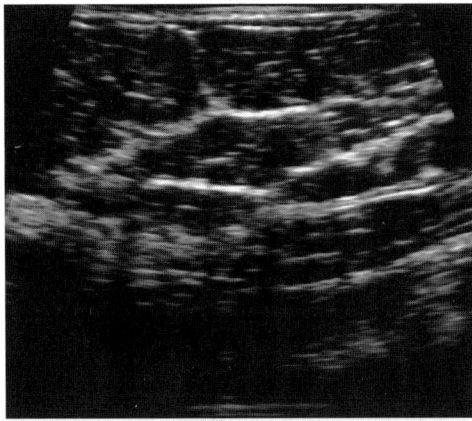

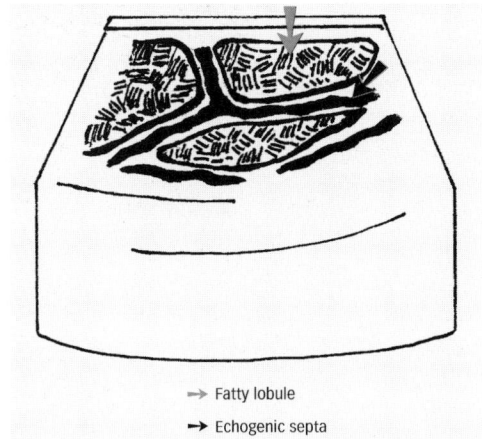

→ Fatty lobule

→ Echogenic septa

Fig. 18.
Normal retroareolar ducts. Two ducts converge to form a single duct running up towards the nipple.

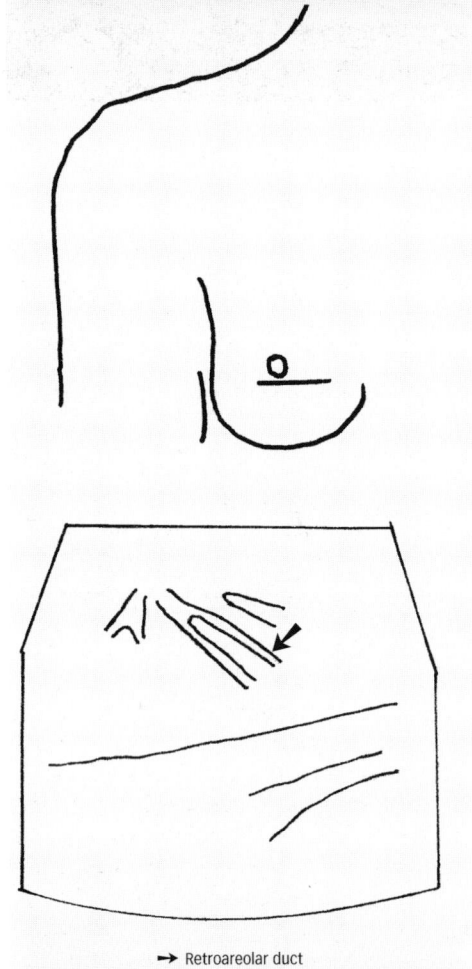

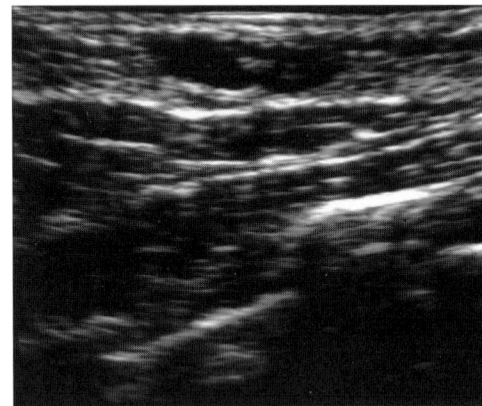

→ Retroareolar duct

Fig. 19.
Normal lymph node. Typ features are seen of an ovoid hypoechoic struct without increased throu transmission of sound a with a central echogenic focus representing hilar

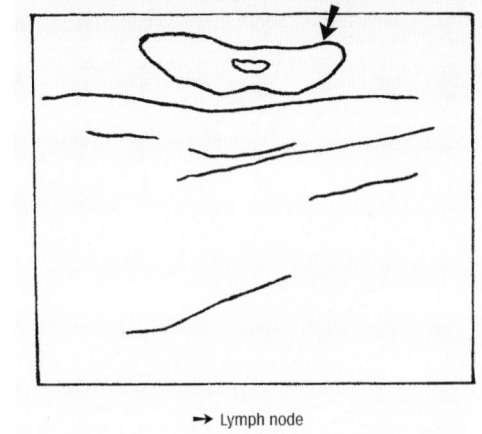

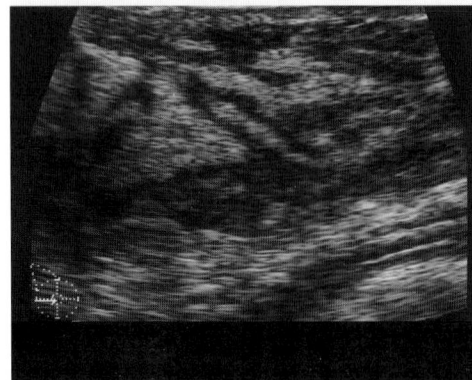

→ Lymph node

ductogram or galactogram but currently this is used infrequently. Previously, its prime role was the investigation of a bloody uniduct nipple discharge in order to demonstrate an intraluminal abnormality such as a papilloma. The use of high frequency ultrasound and alternative management approaches to nipple discharge including cytology, now allow relatively few indications for a ductogram. An adequate examination will demonstrate the major duct system down to at least three or four branching subdivisions (Fig. 20).

Fig. 20.
Normal ductogram. A xeroradiograhic technique was used for this examination. Normal branching ductal structures are present. This particular technique demonstrates multiple anatomical features including ribs and lung tissue.

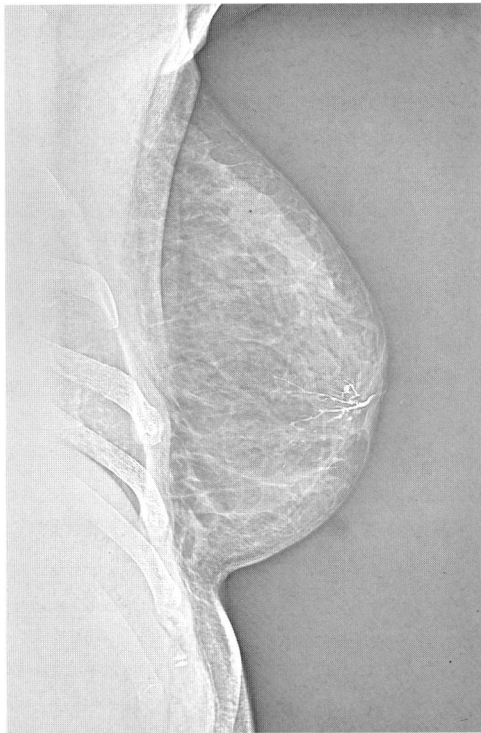

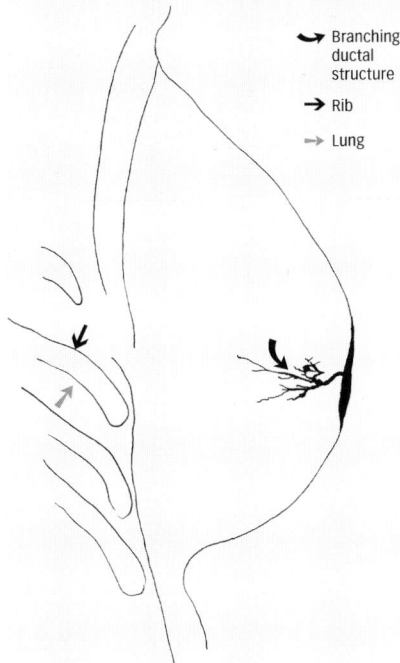

→ Branching ductal structure
→ Rib
→ Lung

→ Fibroglandular tissue
→ Fatty tissue
→ Branching vessel

Magnetic resonance mammography

The present role of magnetic resonance imaging (MRI) in breast investigation is limited, partly by technical factors. Images may be compromised by motion artefact, noise and suboptimal resolution. However, considerable effort is being spent on further evaluation and refinement of the technique. Surface coils and specialist imaging techniques with fat suppression, and the use of contrast material improve image quality and diagnostic factors substantially. Excellent contrast is provided between fat and fibroglandular tissue (Fig. 21). MRI is not suitable as a screening investigation, but may have a place in imaging of implants, attempting to differentiate scarring from recurrent malignancy following conservative surgery, establishing the extent of tumour, and other selected problem cases.

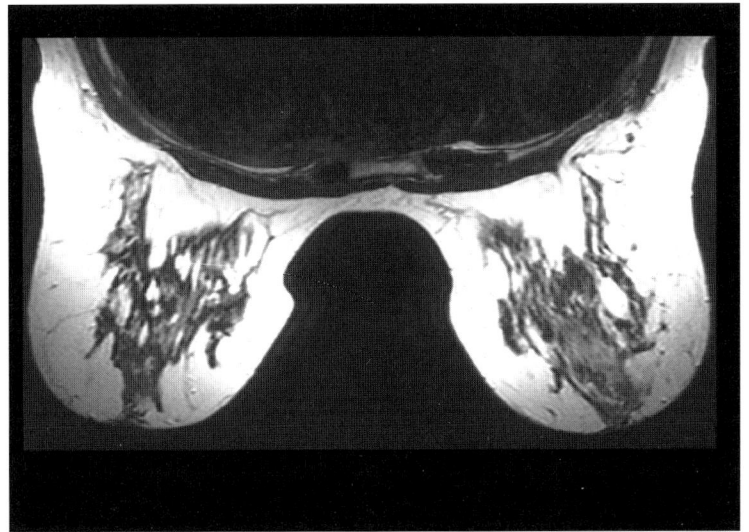

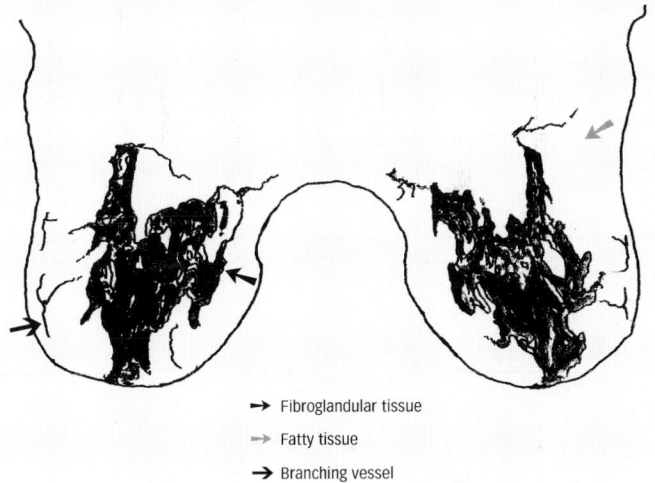

Fig. 21.
Magnetic resonance mammogram. Fibroglandular tissue is easily identified compared to the higher signal fat. Small branching vessels are demonstrated in the subcutaneous region.

References

Adler, D.D., Rebner, M. & Pennes, D.R. (1987). Accessory breast tissue in the axilla: mammographic appearance. *Radiology*, **163**, 709–11.

Kopans, D.B., Swann, C.A. *et al.* (1989). Asymmetric breast tissue. *Radiology*, **171**, 639–43.

Parks, A.G. (1959). The micro-anatomy of the breast. *Annals of the Royal College of Surgeons*, **25**, 235–51.

Scanlon, E.F. & Caprini, J.A. (1975). Modified radical mastectomy. *Cancer*, **35**, 710–13.

Skandalakis, J.E., Gray, S.W. & Rowe, J.S. Jr (1983). *Anatomical Complications in General Surgery*, p. 38. New York: McGraw-Hill Book Co.

Wellings, S.R. & Wolfe, J.N. (1978). Correlative studies of the histological and radiographic appearance of the breast parenchyma. *Radiology*, **129**, 299–306.

Wolfe, J.N. (1976). Breast parenchymal patterns and their changes with age. *Radiology*, **121**, 545–52.

9

Embryology of the gastrointestinal tract and its adnexae

H. ELLIS

The primary endodermal gut tube comprises the blind-ending foregut, closed by the buccopharyngeal membrane; the blind-ending hindgut, closed by the cloacal membrane; and the midgut, which communicates ventrally with the yolk sac. Conventionally, the limits of these three segments are defined by their blood supply, so that the coeliac axis supplies the foregut (and its adnexae), down to the superior half of the duodenum; the superior mesenteric artery supplies the midgut, down to the splenic flexure; and the inferior mesenteric artery supplies the hindgut, which extends to the upper part of the anal canal.

Foregut development

By the beginning of the fifth week of fetal life, the gut tube within the peritoneal cavity is suspended by the dorsal mesentery into the coelomic cavity (Fig. 1). In addition, in the region of the primitive stomach, the gut tube is connected to the ventral body wall by the ventral mesentery derived from the septum transversum. The stomach expands into first a fusiform swelling and then, by differential growth, bulges dorsally to form its greater

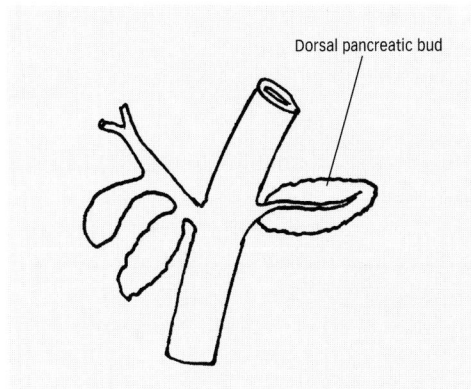

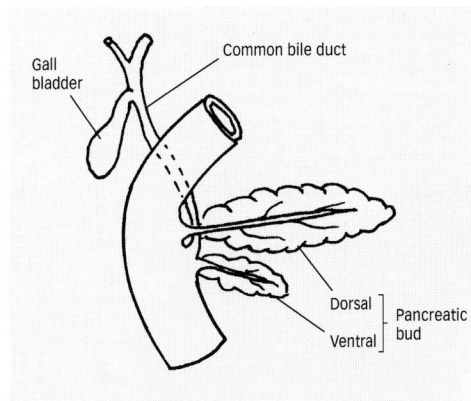

Fig. 1.
Development of the intestinal adnexae
(Ellis, 1997).

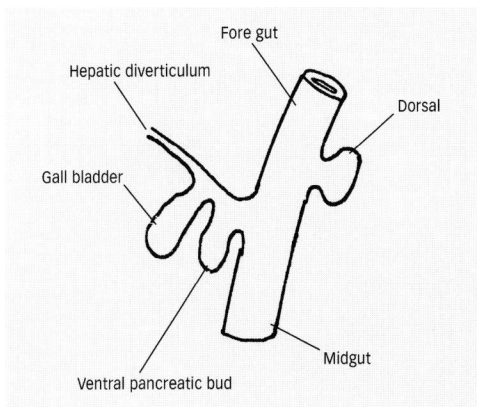

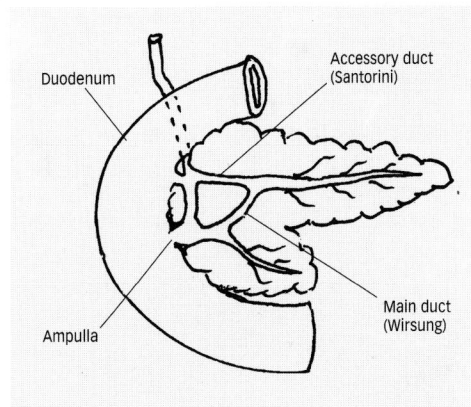

185

curvature and fundus. During the seventh and eighth week, the stomach rotates through 90° around a cranio-caudal axis, so that its lesser curvature now lies to the left and its greater curvature to the right. At the same time, the duodenum curves into a C-shape, displaces to the right and adheres to the dorsal body wall.

Rotation and expansion of the dorsal mesogastrium produces the lesser sac. This diverticulum of peritoneum bulges downwards from beyond the greater curvature of the stomach to produce the greater omentum.

The spleen develops as a condensation of mesenchyme in the dorsal mesogastrium of the lesser sac during the fifth week. It is a mesodermal derivative and not a product of the gut tube endoderm. The rotation of the stomach displaces the spleen to the left side to take up its definitive position at the left extremity of the lesser sac.

The liver develops in the third week of fetal life from a hepatic diverticulum which buds from the duodenum. This grows into the inferior aspect of the septum transversum and gives rise to ramifying cords of liver cells, the hepatic ducts and the bile canaliculi. A further budding from the hepatic diverticulum produces the gall bladder and cystic duct.

The pancreas develops from a larger dorsal and smaller ventral pancreatic bud. The dorsal bud forms as a second diverticulum from the duodenum opposite the hepatic diverticulum and projects into the dorsal mesentery, while the ventral bud sprouts from the hepatic diverticulum into the ventral mesentery proximal to the gall bladder diverticulum.

In the fifth week, the opening of the common bile duct and ventral pancreatic bud migrates behind the duodenum to the dorsal mesentery and fuses with the larger dorsal bud. The dorsal bud gives rise to the head, body and tail of the pancreas, while the ventral bud produces the uncinate process, with the superior mesenteric vessels trapped between the two buds. As with the duodenum, the pancreas then fuses to the dorsal body wall to become retroperitoneal.

An occasional anomaly is for the pancreas to form a complete ring around the duodenum (annular pancreas). This probably results from the ventral pancreatic bud being bilobed and the two lobes migrating in opposite directions around the duodenum to fuse with the dorsal bud.

Fusion of the ventral and dorsal pancreatic buds is accompanied by the interconnection of their ductal systems. The ventral pancreatic duct becomes the main pancreatic duct, which is united with the termination of the common bile duct as a short ampulla, which opens on to the second part of the duodenum as the duodenal papilla. The dorsal pancreatic duct usually persists as an accessory pancreatic duct, which empties about 2 cm above the duodenal papilla as the minor duodenal papilla.

Development of the midgut

The midgut enlarges rapidly in the five-week fetus and is thrown into a hairpin fold termed the primary intestinal loop (Fig. 2). The cranial limb of this loop gives rise to most of the ileum, while the caudal limb develops into the ascending and transverse colons. At its apex, the primary intestinal loop is attached to the umbilicus by the vitelline duct. The superior mesenteric vessels run in the dorsal mesentery down the long axis of the loop. By the beginning of the sixth week, the continued growth of the midgut, combined with the intra-abdominal pressure due to the rapid growth of the other abdominal organs, in

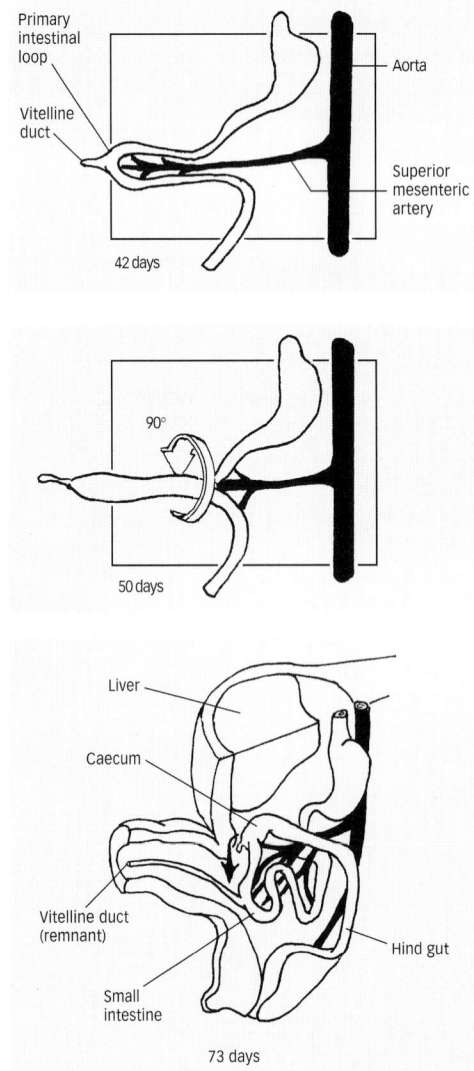

Fig. 2.
Development of the midg
(Ellis, 1997).

particular the liver, forces the intestinal loop to herniate into the umbilical cord. Even at this early stage of fetal life, the vitelline duct is reduced to a fibrous strand. A bud, which develops on the caudal segment of the primary intestinal loop, indicates the site of subsequent formation of the caecum. It may well be that this bud delays the return of the caudal limb in favour of the cephalic gut during the subsequent reduction of the herniated bowel. The appendix develops as a sprout from the enlarging caecum.

As the primary intestinal loop herniates into the umbilicus, it rotates around the axis of the superior mesenteric vessels by 90° in a counter-clockwise direction, so that the cephalic limb now lies to the right, and the caudal limb to the left.

During the tenth week, the midgut retracts into the abdomen. The mechanism for this is not known, but may be due to an increase in the size of the peritoneal cavity. As the loop re-enters the abdomen, it rotates counter-clockwise through an additional 180°. The cephalic limb returns first, passing upwards and to the left into the space left available by the bulky liver. In doing so, this mid-gut loop passes behind the superior mesenteric vessels (which thus come to cross the third part of the duodenum), and also to push the hindgut (the definitive distal colon), over to the left. When the caudal limb of the primary intestinal loop returns, it comes to lie in the only space remaining to it, superficial to, and above, the small intestine, with the caecum lying immediately below the liver. The caecum then descends into its definitive position in the right iliac fossa, dragging the ascending colon down with it. The transverse colon thus comes to lie in front of the superior messenteric vessels and the small intestine.

Finally, the mesenteries of the ascending and descending parts of the colon blend with the posterior peritoneal wall by a process termed zygosis. This forms an avascular plane which the surgeon employs in mobilization of the right and left colon.

During the sixth week of fetal life, a remarkable proliferation of the endodermal lining of the gut takes place, which completely occludes its lumen. Recanalization then takes place and is completed by the ninth week. Incomplete or abnormal recanalization may result in duplication of the lumen or stenosis of the gut.

Hindgut development

The distal hindgut terminates in the cloaca. Between the fourth and sixth weeks, the cloaca is divided into an anterior urogenital sinus and a posterior rectum. The superior part of the anal canal is formed from the distal part of the hindgut. Its lower part is derived from an ectodermal invagination termed the proctodeum. The anal membrane, which separates the endodermal and ectodermal portions of the anorectal canal, breaks down during the eighth week. This junction is marked in the adult anal canal by the pectinate line.

Developmental anomalies

Numerous anomalies may occur in the highly complex developmental process of the alimentary canal:

(a) Atresia or stenosis of the bowel may result from failure of recanalization of the lumen. Another cause of this may damage to the blood supply of the bowel within the fetal umbilical hernia with consequent ischaemic changes.

(b) Meckel's diverticulum represents the remains of the embryonic vitello-intestinal duct.

(c) The caecum may fail to descend. The peritoneal fold, which normally seals it in the right iliac fossa, passes instead across the duodenum and causes a neonatal intestinal obstruction (Ladd's band). The mesentery of the small intestine in such a case is left as a narrow pedicle which allows volvulus of the whole small intestine to occur (Volvulus neonatorum).

(d) Occasionally reversed rotation occurs, in which the transverse colon comes to lie behind the superior mesenteric vessels with the duodenum in front of them. This may again be accompanied by extrinsic duodenal obstruction due to a peritoneal fold.

Reference
Ellis, H. (1997). *Clinical Anatomy*, 9th edn. Oxford: Blackwell Scientific.

10

The anterior abdominal wall and peritoneum

J.C. HEALY
and R. H. REZNEK

Imaging methods

Peritoneum

Computed tomography is the method of choice in evaluating the peritoneal spaces and their associated peritoneal reflections. Careful opacification of the bowel with dilute gastrograffin will allow evaluation of peritoneal collections of fluid or masses, and intravenous contrast enhancement will allow identification of blood vessels in the peritoneal reflections. There is little need for positive contrast CT peritonography in evaluating suspected peritoneal disease. MRI provides good visualization of the peritoneal spaces and reflections; however, as the scans take longer to acquire than CT, bowel peristalsis and respiratory movement can degrade the images. Ultrasound is an inexpensive and effective method of seeking peritoneal collections, but as bowel gas reflects sound, this modality cannot survey the entire peritoneum. Conventional radiography, including barium examinations, only display peritoneal pathology indirectly and thus it has been superseded by CT.

Anterior abdominal wall

Computed tomography (CT) and magnetic resonance imaging (MRI) provide excellent anatomical detail of the anterior abdominal wall in the axial plane. MRI has superior soft-tissue contrast resolution than CT and can interrogate the patient in other planes, but the images are often degraded by movement associated with respiration. Ultrasound is useful in evaluating focal masses in the anterior abdominal wall, but does not demonstrate the anatomy as elegantly as CT or MRI. Conventional plain film radiography has no place in the evaluation of the anterior abdominal wall.

Anatomy of the peritoneum

The peritoneum is the largest and most complexly arranged serous membrane in the body, which in the male forms a closed sac, and in the female is penetrated by the lateral ends of the Fallopian tubes. The peritoneal cavity is a potential space between the parietal peritoneum lining the abdominal wall and the visceral peritoneum enveloping the abdominal organs. It consits of a main region, termed the greater sac, and a diverticulum, the omental bursa or lesser sac, situated behind the stomach. These two areas communicate via the epiploic foramen (foramen of Winslow). The free surface of the peritoneum has a layer of flattened mesothelial cells kept moist and smooth by a thin film of serous fluid. The potential peritoneal spaces, the peritoneal reflections forming peritoneal ligaments, mesenteries, omenta, and the natural flow of peritoneal fluid determine the route of spread of intraperitoneal fluid and disease processes within the abdominal cavity. The flow of intraperitoneal fluid is directed by gravity to its most dependent sites. It is also directed in a cephalad direction by the negative intra-abdominal pressure generated in the upper abdomen by respiration. Peritoneal ligaments, mesenteries, and omenta serve as boundaries for disease processes and also as conduits for disease spread.

The anatomy of the peritoneum will be described in detail, dealing first with the peritoneal spaces, and then with the peritoneal reflections including the peritoneal ligaments, the mesenteries, and the omenta. This anatomy will be illustrated on axial CT in a patient with chronic renal failure on continuous ambulatory peritoneal dialysis (CAPD). The peritoneal space has been opacified using positive contrast medium in this patient in an attempt to visualize inflammatory adhesions.

Peritoneal spaces

The peritoneal cavity is divided into two main compartments, supramesocolic and inframesocolic, by the transverse colon and its mesentery connecting it to the posterior abdominal wall (Fig. 1(a), (b)). The root of the transverse mesocolon extends across the infraampullary segment of the descending duodenum, the head of the pancreas, and continues along the lower edge of the body and tail of the pancreas (Fig. 1(b)).

The supramesocolic compartment

can be divided arbitrarily into right and left supramesocolic peritoneal spaces. These regions can also be divided into a number of subspaces, which are normally in communication, but often become separated by inflammatory membranes in disease.

Right supramesocolic space The right supramesocolic space has three subspaces; (a) the right subphrenic space, (b) the right subhepatic space, which can be further arbitrarily divided into anterior and posterior areas and (c) the lesser sac. (Figs. 1(a), 2(a), (b), c)).

The right subphrenic space This extends over the diaphragmatic surface of the right lobe of the liver to the right coronary ligament postero-inferiorly and the falciform ligament medially, which separates it from the left subphrenic space (Figs. 1(a), 2(a), (b), 3(a), (b)). In the presence of infected fluid, pyogenic membranes may divide the right subphrenic space into anterior and posterior compartments.

The right subhepatic space This can be divided arbitrarily into anterior and posterior spaces (Figs. 1(a), 2(b), 5(a), (b)). The anterior right subhepatic space is limited inferiorly by the transverse colon and its mesentery. The posterior right subhepatic space, also known as the hepatorenal fossa or Morison's pouch, extends posteriorly to the peritoneum overlying the right kidney.

Superiorly, the right subhepatic space is bounded by the inferior surface of the right lobe of the liver. It communicates freely with the right subphrenic space and the right paracolic gutter (Figs. 1(a), 6(a), (b)). In the supine patient, the posterior right subhepatic space (the hepatorenal fossa or Morison's pouch) is more dependent than the right paracolic gutter, and thus under the force of gravity, fluid collections are common in this location.

The lesser sac This extends to the left behind the stomach, anterior to the pancreas (Figs. 1(a), 2(a), (c), (d)). It is considered part of the right supramesocolic space as embryologically the growth of the liver into the right peritoneal space, stretching the dorsal mesentery,

Fig. 1(a).
Coronal view of posterior peritoneal spaces.

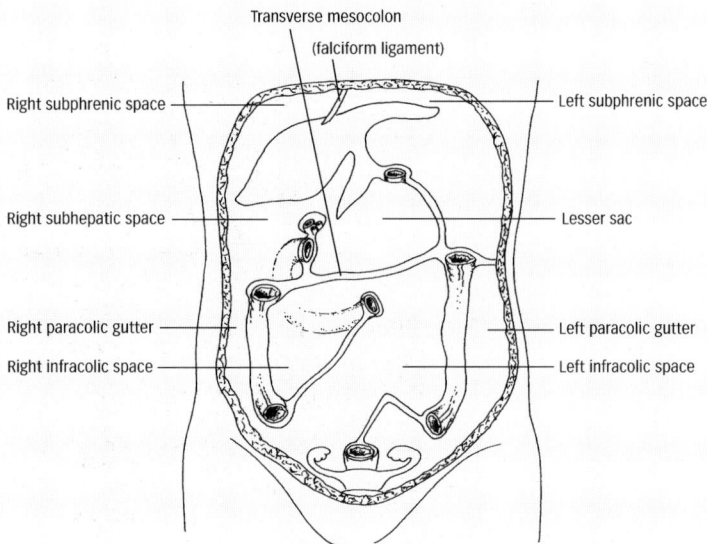

1(a)

Fig. 1(b). below left
Coronal view of peritoneal attachments to the abdominal wall.

Fig. 1(c). below
Sagittal view of pelvic peritoneal spaces.

1(b)

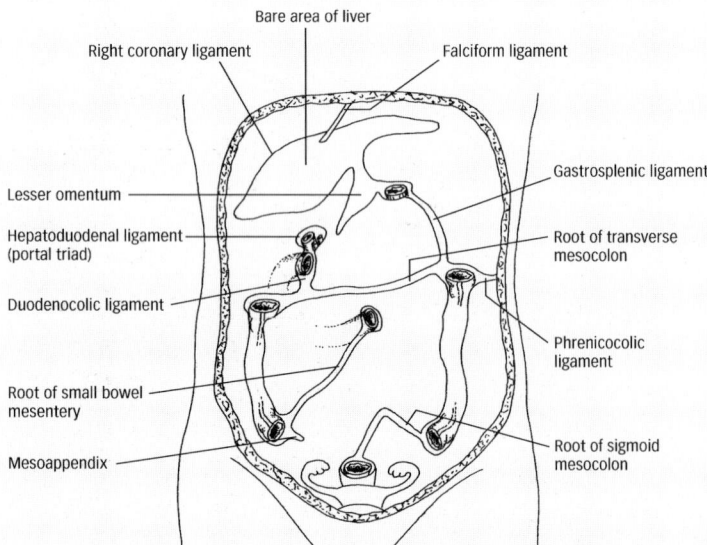

1(c)

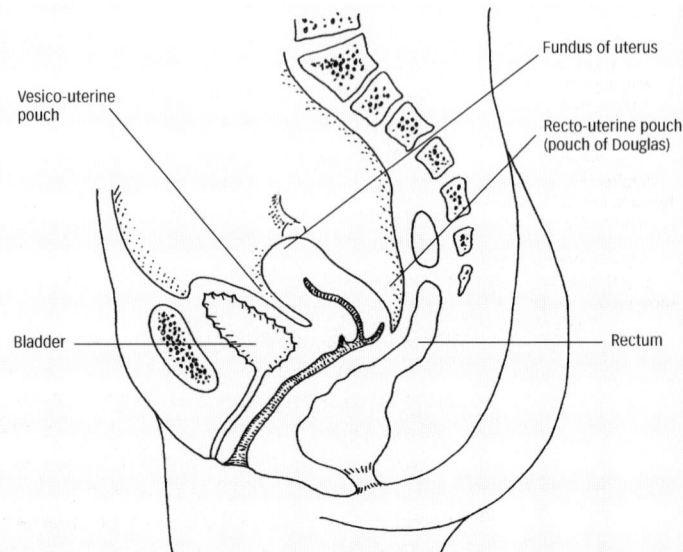

2(a)

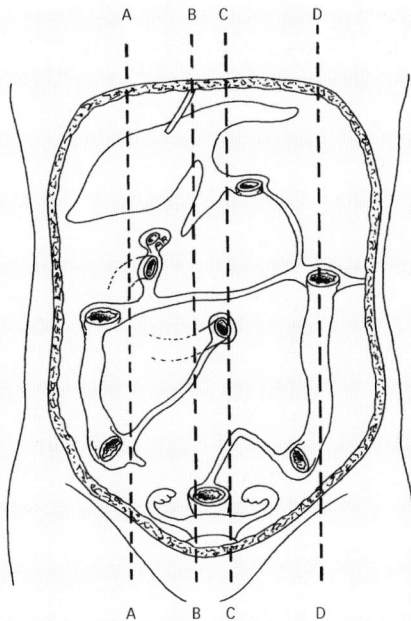

Fig. 2(a). top left
**sition of sagittal sections
through upper abdomen.**

Fig. 2(b). top right
**Sagittal section A–A
through the right lobe of
liver and right kidney.**

2(b)

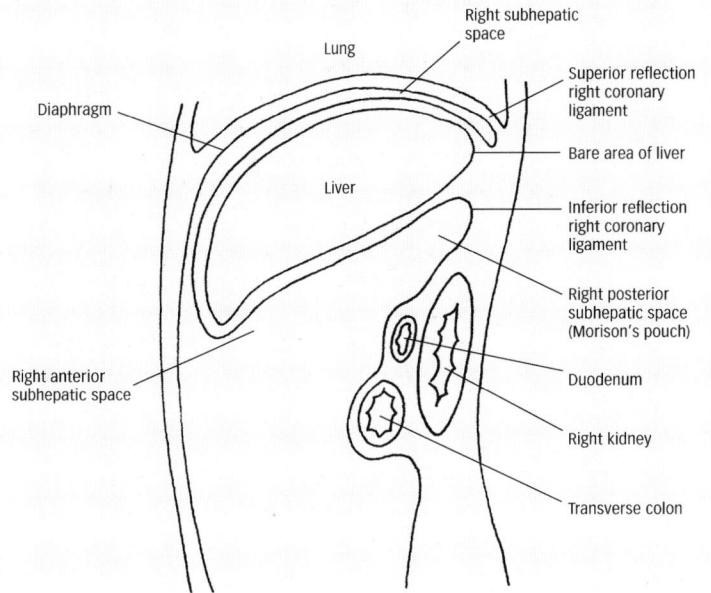

2(c)

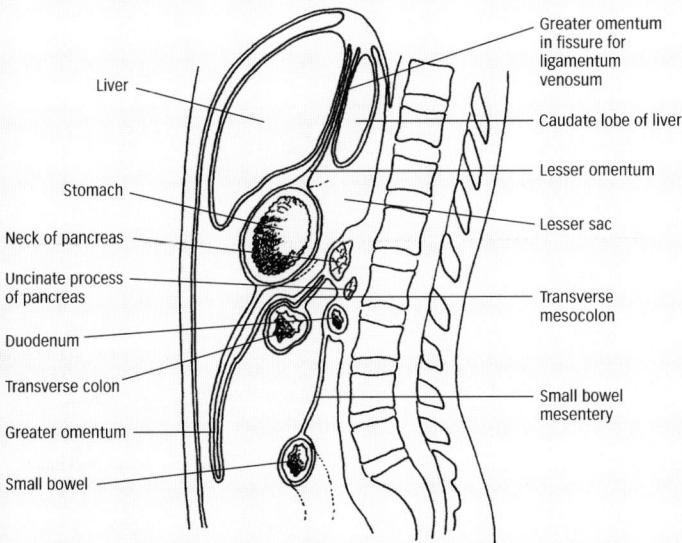

Fig. 2(c). middle left
**Mid-sagittal section
through the upper
abdomen B–B.**

Fig. 2(d). middle right
**Sagittal section C–C
through the left lobe of
liver and lesser sac.**

Fig. 2(e). bottom right
**Sagittal section D–D
through the spleen and
left kidney.**

2(d)

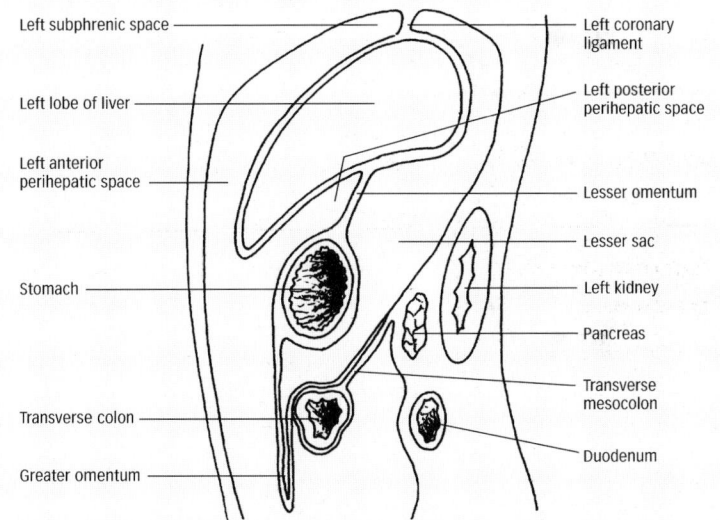

2(e)

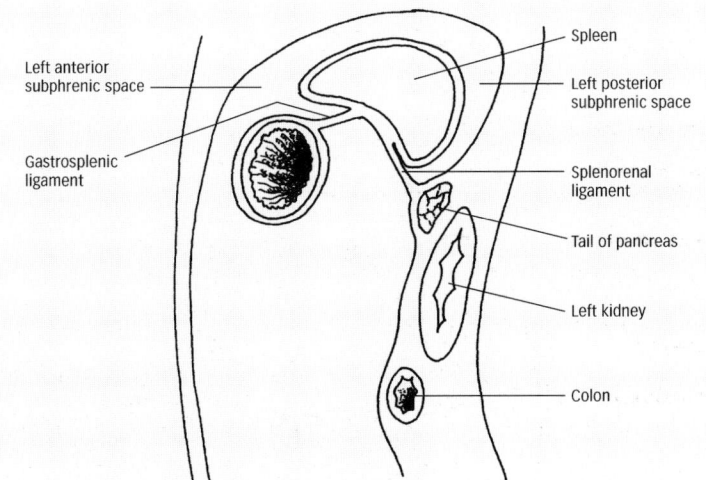

forms the future lesser sac posterior to the stomach. It communicates with the rest of the peritoneal cavity through a narrow inlet, the epiploic foramen (foramen of Winslow), between the inferior vena cava and the free margin of the hepatoduodenal ligament. The lesser sac lies posterior to the lesser omentum, stomach, duodenal bulb, and gastrocolic ligament. A prominent oblique fold of peritoneum is raised on the posterior wall of the lesser sac by the left gastric artery, dividing it into two major recesses. The smaller superior recess completely encloses the caudate lobe of the liver. At the porta hepatis this recess lies posterior to the portal vein. Superiorly, it extends deep into the fissure for the ligamentum venosum and posteriorly lies adjacent to

3(a)

4(a)

3(b)

Falciform ligament

Right subphrenic space

Left anterior subphrenic space

Liver

Left posterior (perisplenic) space

Superior recess of lesser sac

Spleen

4(b)

Falciform ligament

Portal vein

Left anterior perihepatic space

Left Posterior perihepatic space

Caudate lobe of liver

Stomach

Superior recess of lesser sac

Left posterior subphrenic space

Right diaphragmatic crus

Spleen

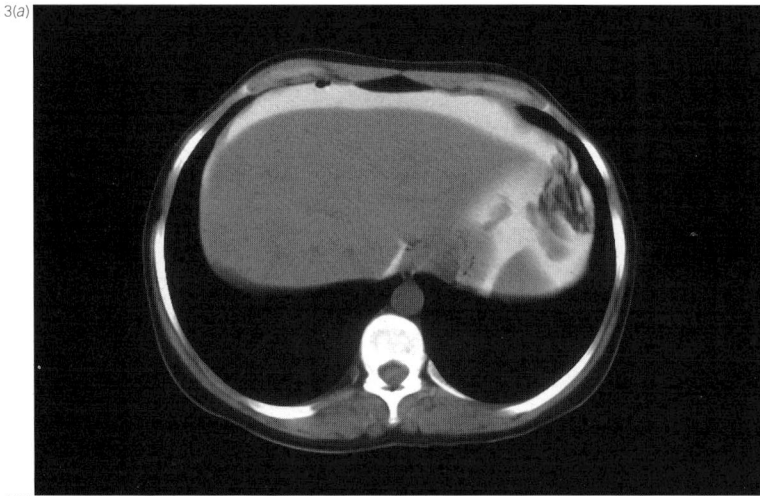

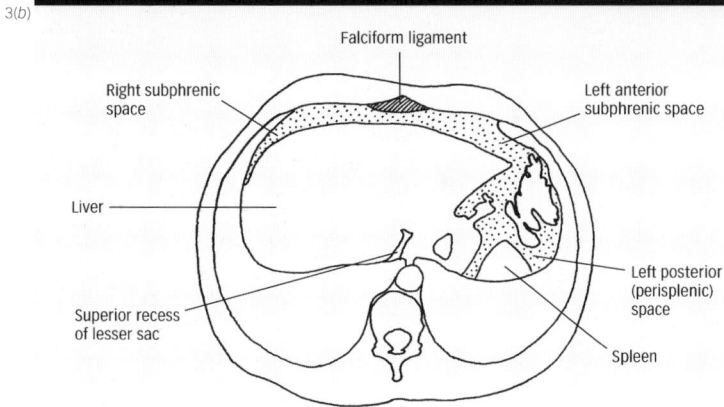

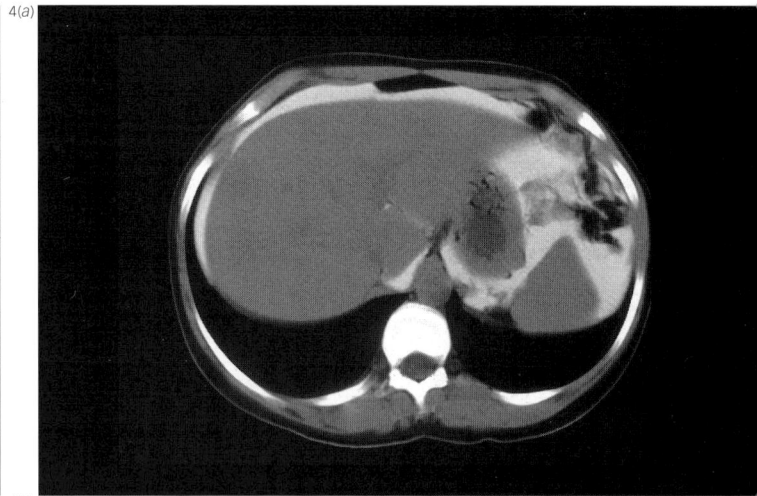

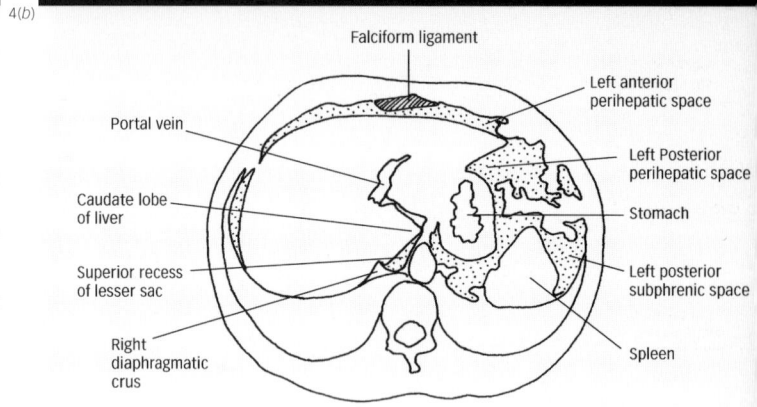

Fig. 3(a). top
Axial CT with contrast in peritoneal cavity to show the subphrenic spaces

Fig. 3(b).
Diagram to show the subphrenic spaces.

the right diaphragmatic crus (Fig. 4(a), (b)). The larger inferior recess lies between the stomach and the pancreas (Fig. 5(a), (b)). It is bounded inferiorly by the transverse colon and its mesentery, but can extend for a variable distance between the leaves of the greater omentum. To the left it is bounded by the gastrosplenic and splenorenal ligaments (Fig. 1(a), (b)), which meet at the splenic hilum. Clinically, fluid collections in the pelvis spreading to the left supramesocolic space, for example, the left subphrenic space, do not generally involve the lesser sac.

Left supramesocolic space The left supramesocolic space has four arbitrary subspaces which are in communication in normals (Fig. 1(a)); (a) the anterior left perihepatic space, (b) the posterior left perihepatic space, surrounding the lateral segment of the left hepatic lobe, (c) the anterior left subphrenic spaces, and (d) the posterior left subphrenic (perisplenic) space, superior to gastric fundus and spleen (Fig. 2(d), (e)).

The left anterior perihepatic space This is bounded medially by the falciform ligament, posteriorly by the liver surface and left coronary ligament, and anteriorly by the diaphragm (Figs. 2(d), 4(a), (b)). It communi-

cates superiorly and to the left with the left anterior subphrenic space, and inferiorly with the greater peritoneal cavity over the surface of the transverse mesocolon.

The left posterior perihepatic space This is also called the gastrohepatic recess and follows the inferior surface of the lateral segment of the left hepatic lobe, extending into the fissure for the ligamentum venosum on the right anterior to the main portal vein (Figs. 2(d), 4(a), (b)). Posteriorly, the lesser omentum separates this space from the superior recess of the lesser sac. On the left this space is bounded by the lesser curve of the stomach (Fig. 2(d)). It communicates with the the left anterior perihepatic space anteroinferiorly.

The left anterior subphrenic space This lies between the stomach posteriorly and the left hemidiaphragm (Figs. 2(d), (e), 3(a), (b)). It communicates on the right with the left anterior perihepatic space, and posteriorly with the posterior subphrenic (perisplenic) space.

The left posterior subphrenic (perisplenic) space This covers the superior and inferolateral surfaces of the spleen (Figs. 2(d), (e), 4(a), (b), 5(a), (b)). It is limited inferiorly by the splenorenal and phrenicocolic ligaments, and more superiorly by the gastrosplenic ligaments.

Fig. 4(a). top
Axial CT with contrast in peritoneal cavity to show the left perihepatic space and superior recess of the lesser sac.

Fig. 4(b).
Diagram to show the left perihepatic spaces and superior recess of the lesser sac.

6(a)

6(b)

Fig. 5(a) diagram labels:
- Right anterior subhepatic space
- Stomach
- Lesser sac – inferior recess
- Head of pancreas
- Liver
- Left posterior subhepatic (perisplenic) space
- Right posterior subhepatic space (Morison's pouch)
- Spleen
- Kidneys

Fig. 6(b) diagram labels:
- Transverse mesocolon
- Right paracolic gutter
- Right inframesocolic space
- Liver
- Right subphrenic space
- Left paracolic gutter
- Right posterior subphrenic space (Morison''s pouch)
- Small bowel mesentery

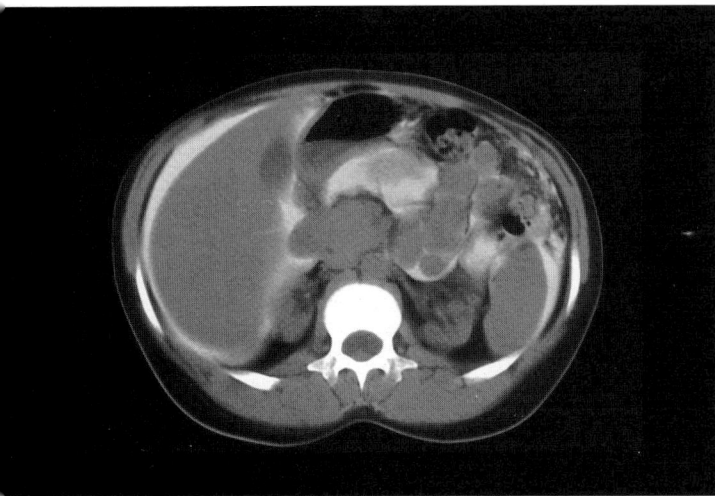

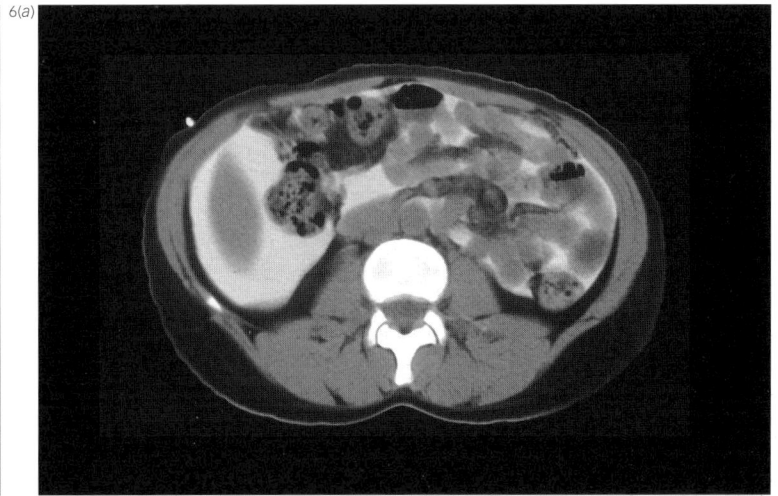

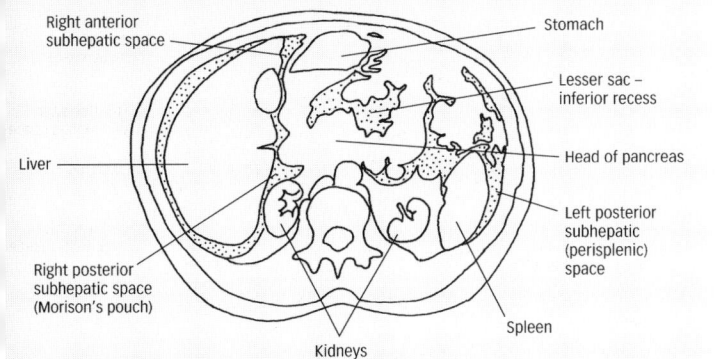

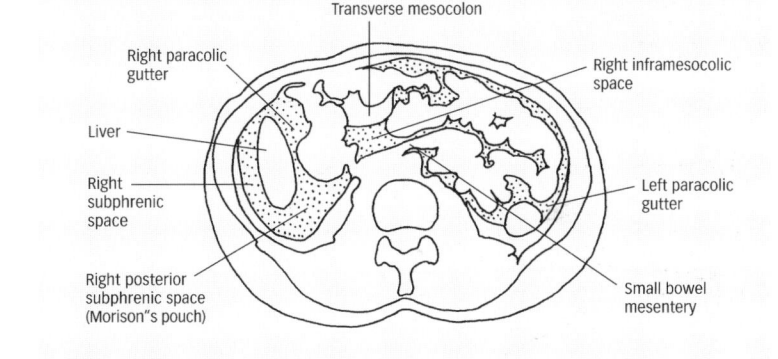

Fig. 5(a). top
Axial CT with contrast in peritoneal cavity to show the anterior right subhepatic space, the posterior right subhepatic space (Morison's pouch), and the inferior recess of the lesser sac.

Fig. 5(b).
Diagram to show the right subhepatic space (Morison's pouch) and the inferior recess of the lesser sac.

The phrenicocolic ligament, extending from the splenic flexure of the colon to the diaphragm, partially separates the left posterior subphrenic (perisplenic) space from the rest of the peritoneal cavity (Figs. 1(a), (b), 10(a), (b), 12(a), (b)). It forms a partial barrier to the spread of fluid from the left paracolic gutter into the left subphrenic space, explaining why left subphrenic collections are less common than right-sided collections.

The inframesocolic compartment

is divided into two unequal spaces posteriorly by the root of the small bowel mesentery, as this runs from the duodenojejunal flexure in the left upper quadrant to the ileocaecal valve in the right lower quadrant. It also contains the right and left paracolic gutters lateral to the ascending and descending colon (Figs. 1(a), (b)).

The right inframesocolic space This triangular space is smaller than its counterpart on the left. It is bounded by the transverse colon superiorly and to the right, and by the root of the small bowel mesentery, as this runs from the duodenojejunal flexure to the ileocaecal junction, inferiorly and to the left (Figs. 1(a), 6(a), (b)).

The left inframesocolic space This space is larger than its counterpart on the right and is in free communication with the pelvis on the right of the midline. The sigmoid colon and its associated mesentery forms a partial barrier on the left of the midline (Figs. 1(a), (b), 7(a), (b)).

The paracolic gutters These are the peritoneal recesses on the posterior abdominal wall lateral to the ascending and descending colon (Fig. 1(a)). The right paracolic gutter is continuous superiorly with the right subhepatic and subphrenic spaces (Fig. 6(a), (b)). It is larger than the left paracolic gutter, which is partially separated from the left subphrenic spaces by the phrenicocolic ligament (Figs. 1(a), (b), 10(a), (b), 12(a), (b)). Both paracolic spaces are in continuity with the pelvic peritoneal spaces.

The pelvic peritoneal spaces
Inferiorly, the peritoneum is reflected over the fundus of the bladder, the anterior and posterior surface of the uterus and upper posterior vagina in females, and on to the front of the rectum at the junction of its middle and lower thirds (Fig. 1(c)). The urinary bladder subdivides the pelvis into right and left paravesical spaces (Fig. 8(a), (b)). In men, there is only one potential space for fluid collection posterior to

Fig. 6(a). top
Axial CT with contrast in peritoneal cavity to show the confluence of the right subphrenic space, the right subhepatic space, and right paracolic gutter. Also shown is the right inframesocolic space.

Fig. 6(b).
Diagram to show the confluence of the right subphrenic space, the right subhepatic space, and right paracolic gutter. Also shown is the right inframesocolic space.

7(a)

8(a)

7(b)

Small bowel mesentery

Anterior abdominal wall hernia

Right inframesocolic space

Left inframesocolic space

Right paracolic gutter

Left paracolic gutter

8(b)

Right paravesical space

Bladder

Uterus

Peritoneal dialysis catheter

Uterovesical pouch

Rectouterine pouch (pouch of Douglas)

Rectum

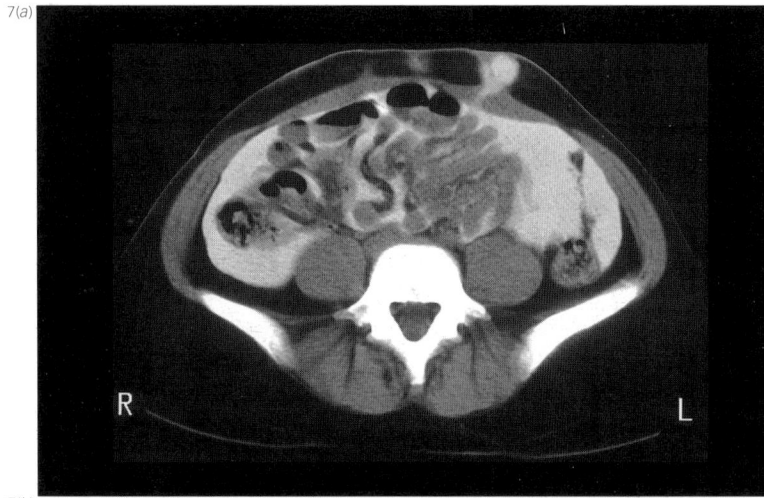

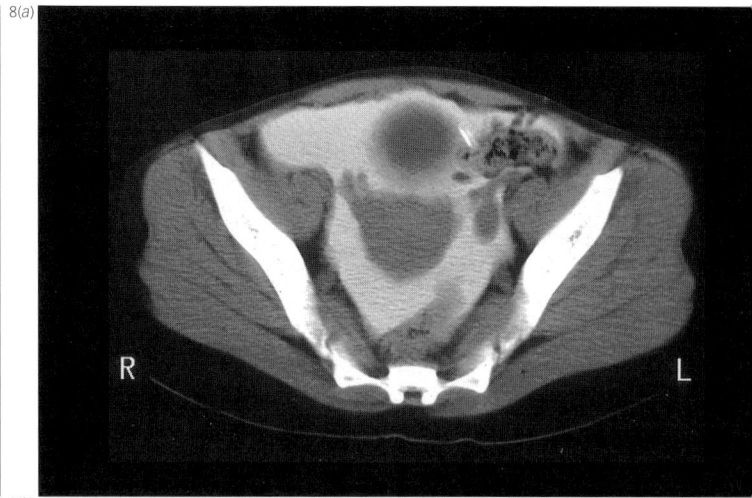

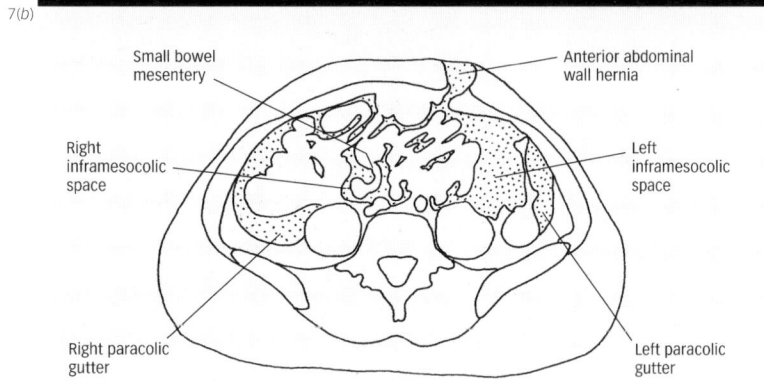

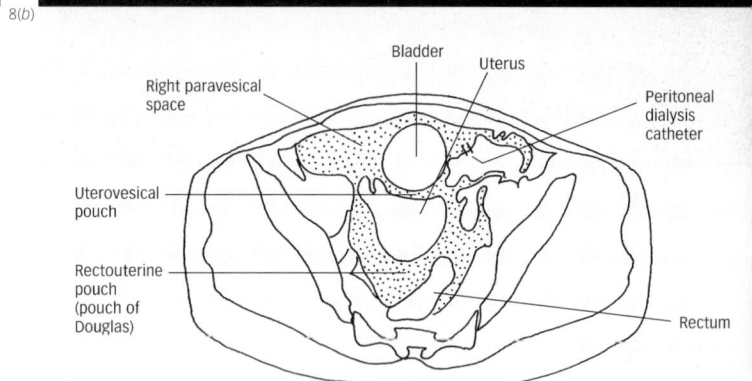

Fig. 7(a). top
Axial CT with contrast in peritoneal cavity to show the left inframesocolic space and the paracolic gutters.

Fig. 7(b).
Diagram to show the left inframesocolic space and the paracolic gutters.

the bladder, the recto-vesical pouch. In women, there are two potential spaces posterior to the bladder, the utero-vesical pouch, and posterior to the uterus, the deeper rectouterine pouch (pouch of Douglas) (Figs. 1(c), 8(a), (b), 9(a), (b)). The layers of peritoneum on the anterior and posterior surfaces of the uterus are reflected laterally to the pelvic side walls as the broad ligaments, containing the uterine (Fallopian) tubes.

Peritoneal reflections

In early fetal life, as the abdominal cavity divides into two major compartments (the retroperitoneum and the peritoneum), the parietal peritoneum is reflected over the peritoneal organs to form a series of supporting ligaments, mesenteries and omenta. These peritoneal reflections carry with them areolar tissue, vessels, nerves, and lymphatics from the retroperitoneum to the peritoneal organs. Consequently, a natural connection is formed between the retroperitoneum and peritoneum, which has been termed the subperitoneal space, providing pathways for the extension of intra-abdominal disease.

The peritoneal reflections in the upper abdomen comprise:

(a) eight ligaments; the right and left coronary, falciform, hepatoduodenal, duodenocolic, gastrosplenic, splenorenal, and phrenicocolic ligaments;

(b) four mesenteries; the small bowel mesentery, the transverse mesocolon, the sigmoid mesocolon, and the mesoappendix;

(c) two omenta; the lesser and greater omentum.

These reflections are generally recognizable as fat-containing structures on computed tomography scans, either by their typical location and organ relationships or by the landmarks provided by their major constituent vessels.

Peritoneal ligaments

The right coronary ligament This ligament on the right is formed by the reflection of the peritoneum from the diaphragm to the posterior surfaces of the right lobe of the liver (Fig. 1(b)). Between the two layers of this ligament, there is a large, triangular area of the liver devoid of peritoneal covering; the bare area of the liver (Fig. 10(a), (b)). Here the liver is attached to the diaphragm by areolar tissue and this bare area is continuous with the anterior pararenal space. The peritoneal reflections continue to the left, becoming closely applied to form the left coronary ligament (left trian-

Fig. 8(a). top
Axial CT with contrast in peritoneal cavity to show the paravesical spaces, the uterovesical pouch, and the rectouterine pouch (pouch of Douglas).

Fig. 8(b).
Diagram to show the paravesical spaces, the uterovesical pouch, and the rectouterine pouch (pouch of Douglas).

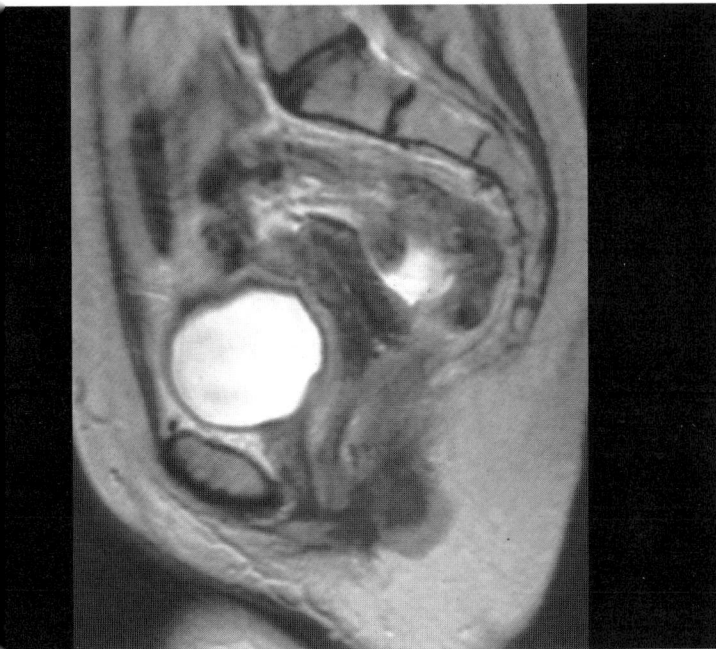

10(a)

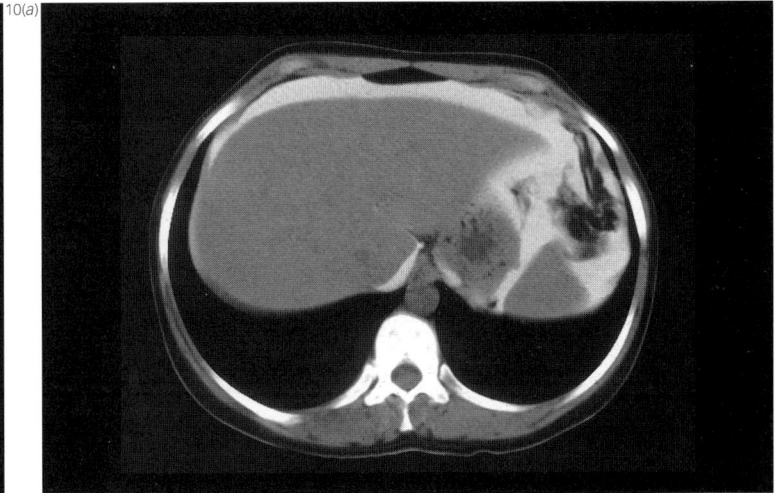

10(b)

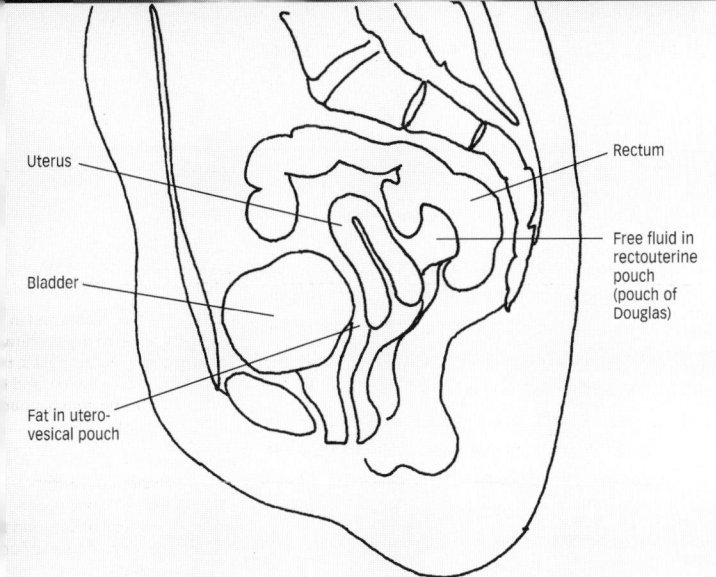

Fig. 9(a). top
Sagittal MRI which shows free fluid in the rectouterine pouch (pouch of Douglas).

Fig. 9(b).
Diagram to show the rectouterine pouch (pouch of Douglas)

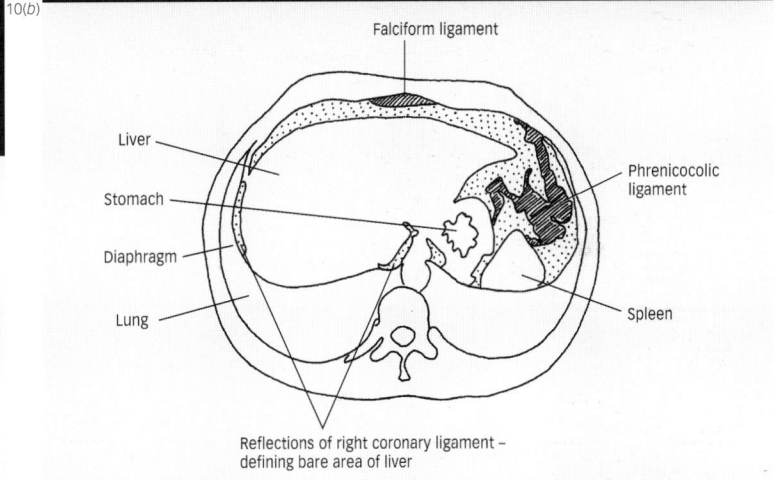

Fig. 10(a). top
Axial CT with contrast in peritoneal cavity to show the bare area of the liver and phrenicocolic ligament.

Fig. 10(b).
Diagram to show the bare area of the liver and phrenicocolic ligament.

gular ligament), a flimsy structure of little anatomical or pathological consequence (Fig. 1(b)).

The gastrosplenic ligament This is a short ligament continuous with the greater omentum extending from the greater curve of the stomach to the spleen (Fig. 1(b)). It contains the left gastroepiploic vessels and short gastric vessels. It can be identified on CT scans by its fat and vascular content at the site between the stomach and spleen (Fig. 11(a), (b)).

The falciform ligament This extends from the anterosuperior surface of the liver to the diaphragm and anterior abdominal wall, carrying the ligamentum teres (the obliterated left umbilical vein) in its free edge (Fig. 1(b)). It is in continuity with the fissure for the liga-

mentum venosum. It may be identified on CT by its predominantly fatty attenuation (Fig. 12(a), (b)).

The phrenicocolic ligament This extends from the splenic flexure of the colon to the diaphragm at the level of the eleventh rib. It is continuous with the transverse mesocolon and splenorenal ligament and thus provides support for the spleen (Fig. 1(b)). It can be identified on CT by its fat content (Fig. 12(a), (b)). It forms a potential barrier to the spread of infected fluid from the pelvis and left paracolic gutter to the left subphrenic space.

The splenorenal ligament This sweeps from the extremity of the pancreatic tail and inserts into the splenic hilus, transmitting the splenic vessels. It can be identified on CT by its fat content and the presence of the distal splenic artery. Together with the gastrosplenic ligament, with which it is in continuity, it forms the boundary of the lesser sac on the left side of the abdomen (Figs. 1(a), (b), 13(a), (b)).

The hepatoduodenal ligament This extends from the flexure between the first and second

11(a)

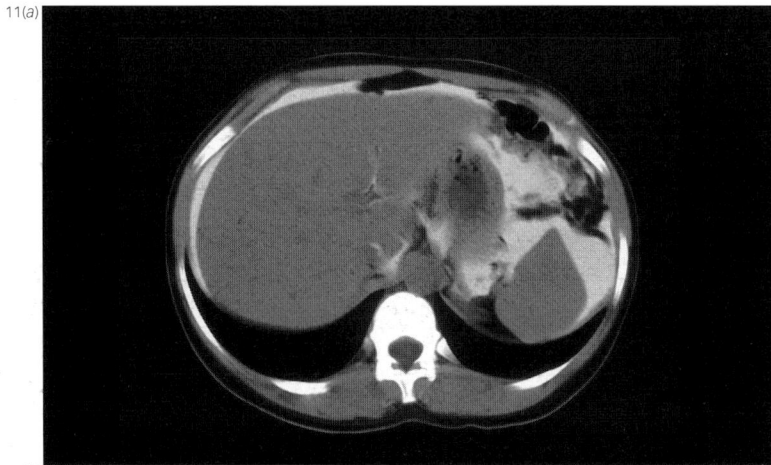

11(b)

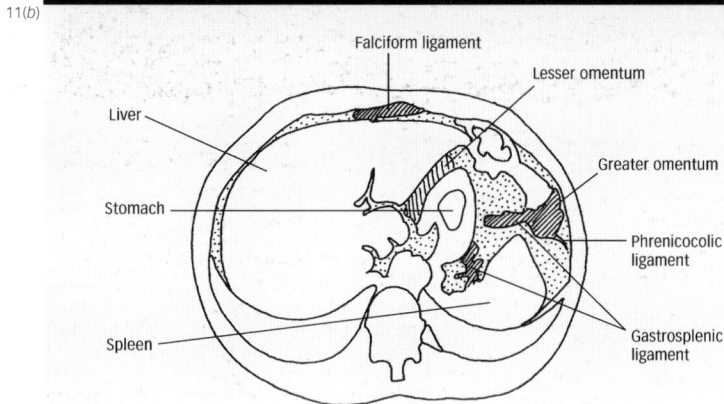

12(a)

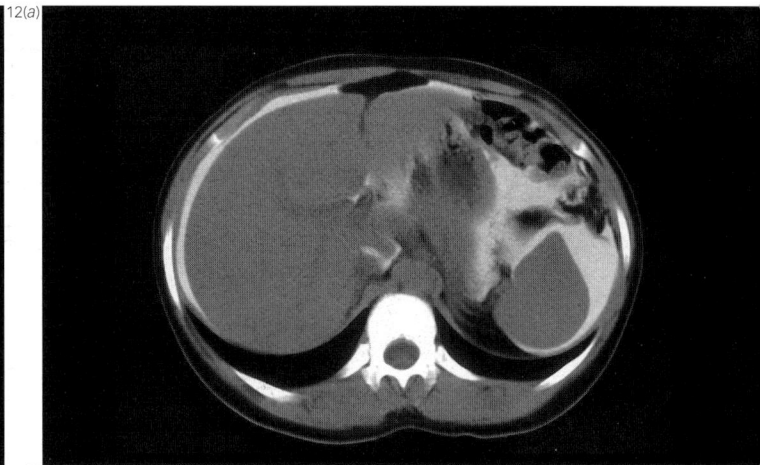

12(b)

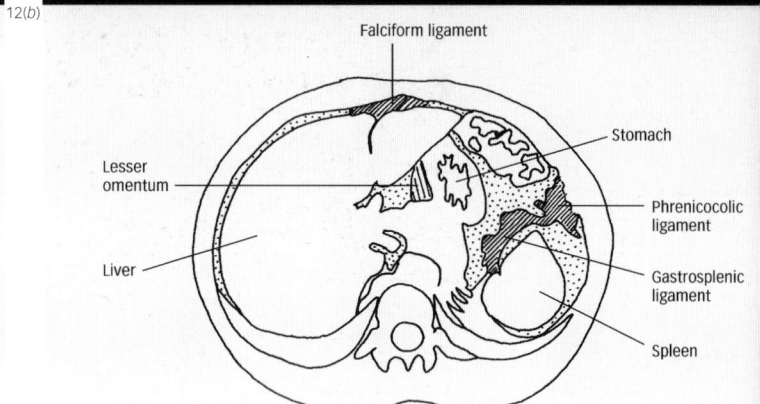

Fig. 11(a). top
Axial CT with contrast in peritoneal cavity to show the lesser and greater omentum, and the gastrosplenic ligament.

Fig. 11(b).
Diagram to show the lesser and greater omentum, and the gastrosplenic ligament.

parts of the duodenum to the porta hepatis and transports the portal triad, that is the hepatic artery, the portal vein and the common bile duct (Fig. 1(b)). It represents the thickened right edge of the lesser omentum. Immediately behind it is the epiploic foramen leading into the lesser sac. Identification of the hepatic artery, portal vein, and common duct on CT allow its precise location (Fig. 14(a), (b)).

The duodenocolic ligament This extends from the right colic flexure to the descending duodenum and is continuous with the transverse mesocolon (Fig. 1(b)). The lymphatic drainage of the right-sided colon is via this ligament to the central superior mesenteric nodes, in common with the transverse duodenum (Fig. 15(a)(b)).

Mesenteries
The small bowel mesentery This is a broad fan-shaped fold of peritoneum connecting the loops of jejunum and ileum to the posterior abdominal wall. Its connection with the posterior abdominal wall, its root, measures about 15 cm and extends obliquely from the duodenojejunal flexure, on the left of the second lumbar vertebra, to the right lower quadrant, anterior to the upper part of the right sacroiliac joint (Fig. 1(b)). The root is a bare area continuous with the left anterior pararenal space superiorly, and the right anterior pararenal space inferiorly. In its course it passes from left to right, successively in front of the horizontal part of the duodenum (where the superior mesenteric vessels enter the mesentery), the abdominal aorta, the inferior vena cava, the right ureter, and right psoas muscle. It suspends 20–25 feet of small bowel. The intestinal border of the mesentery is characteristically thrown into a number of pleats or frills. The mesentery consists of two layers of peritoneum between which lie the jejunal and ileal branches of the superior mesenteric arteries, and their accompanying veins, nerves, and lymphatics. The normal small bowel mesentery can be seen axially on CT (Figs. 16(a), (b)), and sagittally and coronally on MRI (Figs. 17(a), (b), 18(a), (b)), containing fat and vessels.

The transverse mesocolon This is a broad peritoneal fold which connects the transverse colon to the posterior abdominal wall (Fig. 1(b)). Its two layers pass from the anterior surface of the head and the anterior border of the body of the pancreas to the posterior surface of the transverse colon where they separate to surround the gut. The upper layer is adherent to, but separable from, the greater omentum.

Fig. 12(a).
Axial CT with contrast in peritoneal cavity to show the falciform, gastrosplen and phrenicocolic ligaments.

Fig. 12(b).
Diagram to show the falciform, gastrosplenic a phrenicocolic ligaments.

14(a)

14(b)

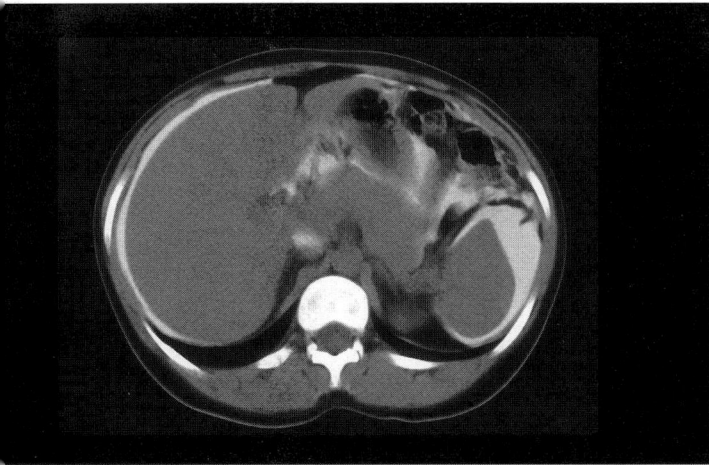

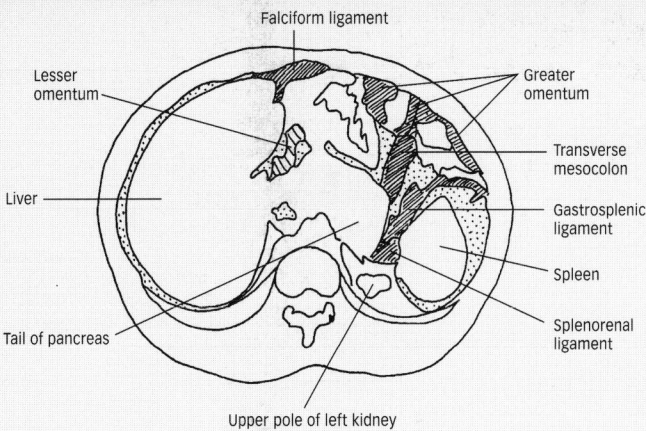

Between the layers run the middle colic vessels, autonomic nerves, and lymphatics, which supply the transverse colon. Near the uncinate process of the pancreas its root becomes confluent with the root of the small bowel mesentery. On CT scans the transverse mesocolon can be identified as a fatty plane extending from the pancreas to the ventrally situated transverse colon, with the middle colic vessels coursing through it (Figs. 15(a), (b)).

The sigmoid mesocolon This is a fold of peritoneum which attaches the sigmoid colon to the pelvic wall. Its line of attachment is an inverted V, the apex of which is near to the division of the left common iliac artery (Fig. 1(b)). The left limb descends medially to the left psoas muscle, the right limb descends into the pelvis and ends in the midline anterior to the third sacral segment. The sigmoid and superior rectal vessels run between the layers of the sigmoid mesocolon and the left ureter descends into the pelvis behind its apex. It can be identified on CT by its fat content and vessels coursing within it (Fig. 19(a), (b)).

The mesoappendix This is a fold of peritoneum around the vermiform appendix, which is attached to the lower end of the small

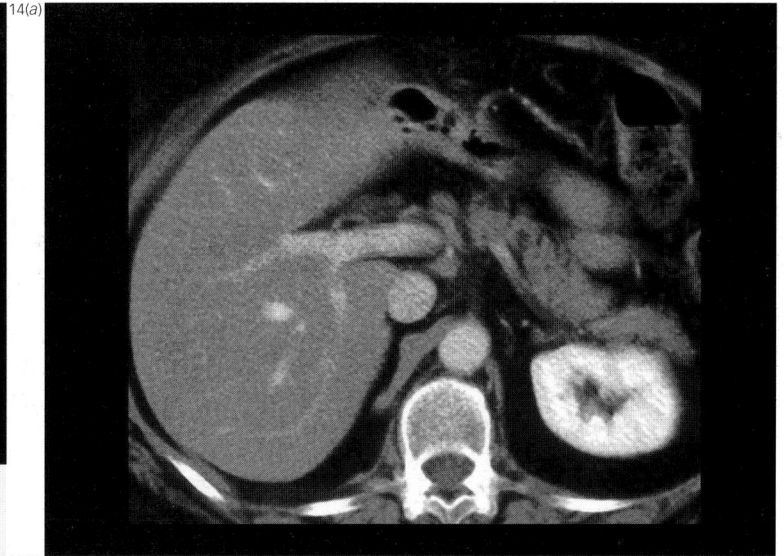

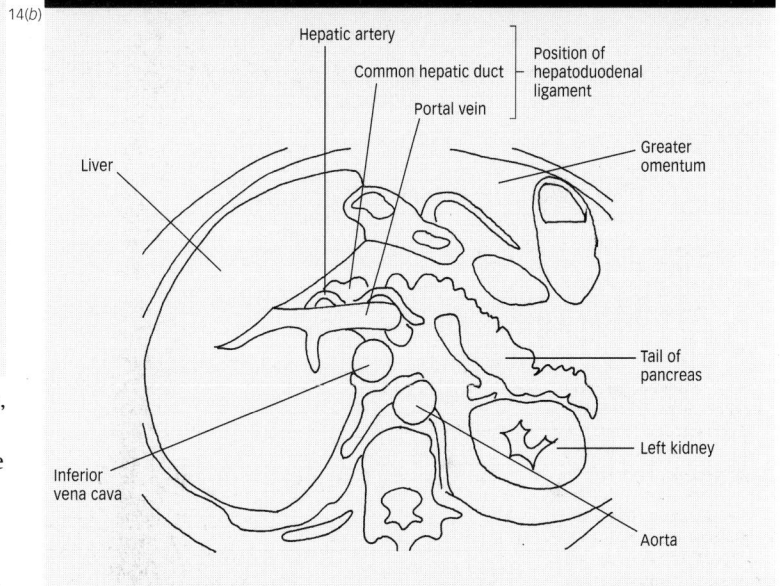

bowel mesentery, close to the ileocaecal junction (Fig. 1(b)). It usually extends to the tip of the appendix and sometimes suspends the caecum. On CT, it is identified by its fat content and contained vessels (Fig. 16(a), (b)).

Omenta

The greater omentum This is the largest peritoneal fold consisting of a double sheet, folded upon itself and thus made up of four layers. The two layers of peritoneum descend from the greater curve of the stomach and proximal duodenum passing inferiorly, anterior to the small bowel for a variable distance, and then turn superiorly again to insert into the anterosuperior aspect of the transverse colon. The left border is continuous with the gastrosplenic ligament; the right extends as far as the origin of the dodenum. The greater omentum always contains some adipose tissue, which in fat people can be considerable; this is easily

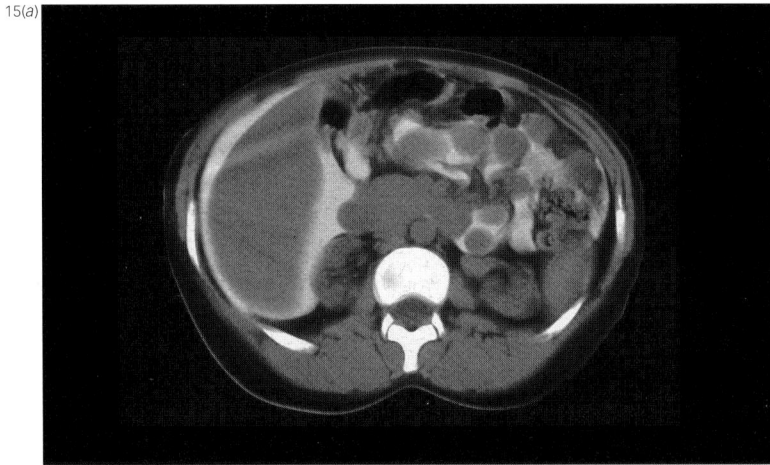

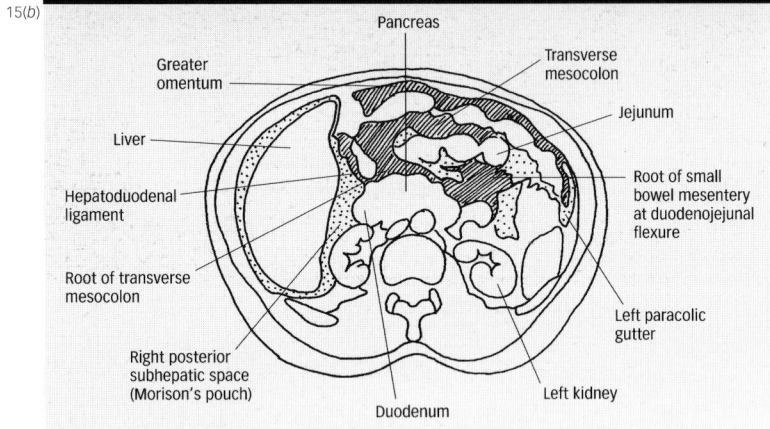

15(a)

16(a)

15(b)

Pancreas

Greater omentum

Transverse mesocolon

Liver

Jejunum

Hepatoduodenal ligament

Root of small bowel mesentery at duodenojejunal flexure

Root of transverse mesocolon

Left paracolic gutter

Right posterior subhepatic space (Morison's pouch)

Duodenum

Left kidney

16(b)

Root of small bowel mesentery in right lower quadrant

Caecum

Small bowel mesentery

Mesentery of caecum and appendix

Small bowel

Inferior vena cava

Fig. 15(a).
Axial CT with contrast in peritoneal cavity to show the root of the transverse mesocolon, the root of the small bowel mesentery, the greater omentum, and the duodenocolic ligament.

Fig. 15(b).
Diagram to show the root of the transverse mesocolon, the root of the small bowel mesentery, the greater omentum, and the duodenocolic ligament.

identified on CT anterior to the transverse colon superiorly, and loops of small bowel inferiorly (Figs. 15(a), (b)).

The lesser omentum (gastrohepatic ligament)

This is the fold of peritoneum extending from the lesser curvature of the stomach and proximal 2 cm of the duodenum to the liver. It forms the anterior surface of the lesser sac. At its free edge, which extends to the porta hepatis, it forms the hepatoduodenal ligament. It is attached in its superior extent to the fissures for the porta hepatis and ligamentum venosum. The lesser omentum is generally wedge-shaped and contains considerable adipose tissue, through which course the gastric artery, the coronary vein, and the left gastric nodal chain. The presence of the fissure for the ligamentum venosum immediately inferior to the oesophagogastric junction on CT scans can be used to identify this reflection (Figs. 11(a), (b), 13(a), (b)).

Anatomy of the anterior abdominal wall

The anterior abdominal wall extends from the xiphoid and lower six costal cartilages to the anterior aspect of the pelvic bones. It is composed of several layers, including skin, superficial fascia, subcutaneous fat, anterolat-

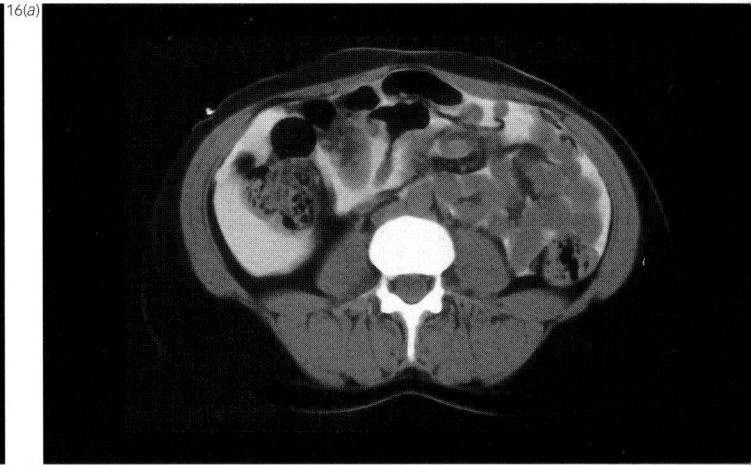

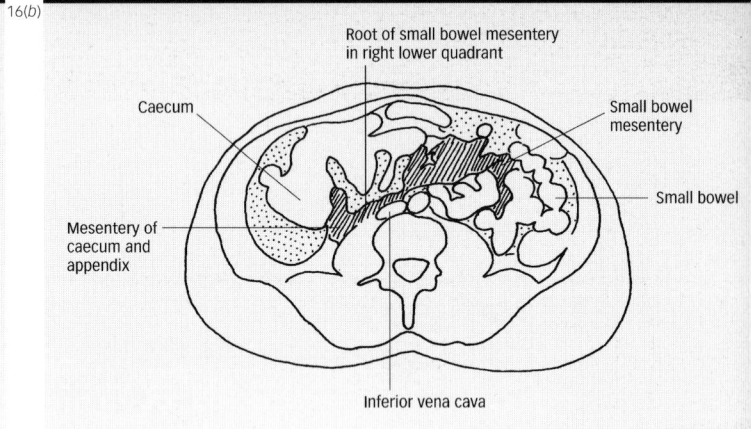

eral and midline muscle groups, tranversalis fascia, extraperitoneal fat and peritoneum.

The superficial fascia

The superficial fascia of the superior and central abdominal wall is a single layer containing a variable amount of fat. Inferiorly it divides into two layers, superficial and deep, between which run vessels, nerves and lymphatics. The superficial layer is thick and contains areolar tissue and variable amounts of fat. It passes over the inguinal ligament and is continuous with the superficial fascia of the thigh. The deep layer is more membranous and contains elastic fibres. This fascia is connected to the aponeurosis of the external oblique muscle laterally and to the linea alba and symphysis pubis medially. Superiorly, it is continuous with the superficial fascia over the trunk. Inferolaterally, it passes over the inguinal ligament to fuse with the underlying fascia of the thigh. Inferomedially, it forms the superficial perineal fascia by passing over the penis and scrotum, in males, and into the labia majora in females.

Muscles

Four muscles are found in the anterior and lateral abdominal wall. Anteriorly there are

Fig. 16(a).
Axial CT with contrast in peritoneal cavity to show the confluence of the ro of the small bowel mesentery and the mesentery around the caecum and appendix.

Fig. 16(b).
Diagram to show the confluence of the root o the small bowel mesent and the mesentery arou the caecum and append

18(a)

Liver

Superior
mesentery
artery

Vessels in
small bowel
mesentery

18(b)

Fat in small
bowel
mesentery

Small bowel

Small bowel
mesentery
containing
blood
vessels

Small
bowel

Sigmoid
colon

Uterus

Bladder

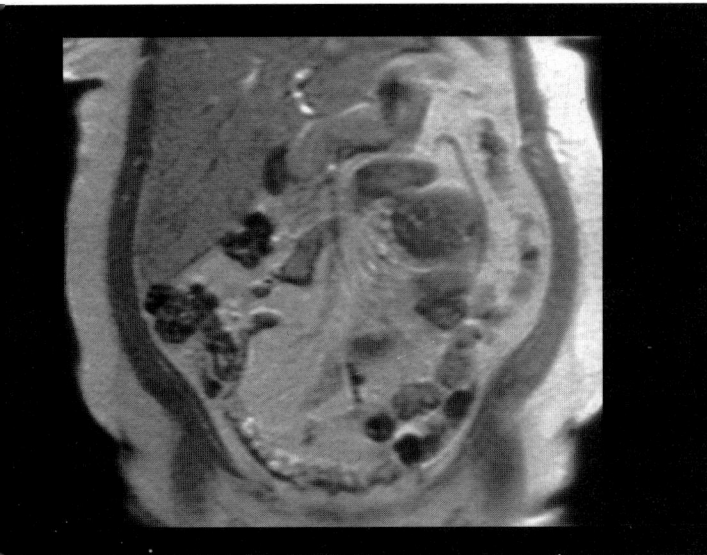

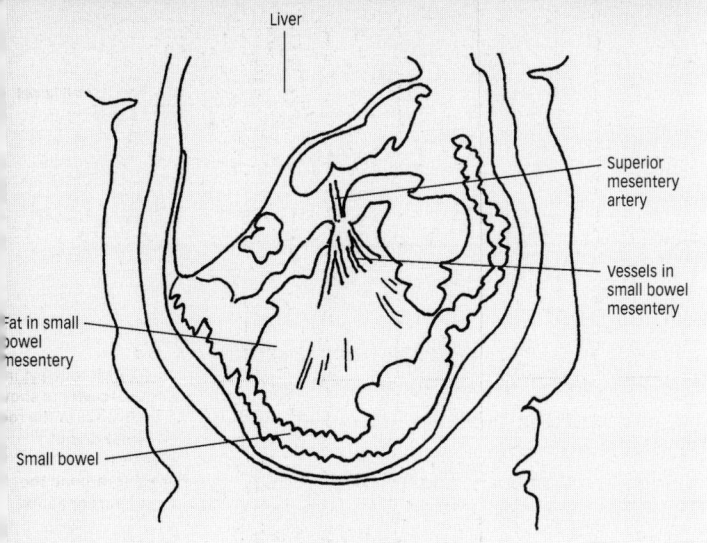

Fig. 17(a).
**Coronal MRI to show the
small bowel mesentery.**

Fig. 17(b).
**agram to show the small
bowel mesentery**

the paired paramedian rectus abdominis muscles. Three muscles make up the anterolateral
surface. Superficial to deep, these are: external
olique, internal oblique, and the transversus
abdominis. These muscles are separated by a
variable amount of areolar tissue that allows
them to move over one another. The presence
of fat in the intermuscular connective tissue
allows the individual muscle layers to be
identified on CT and MRI (Figs. 20, 21(a), (b),
22(a), (b), 23(a), (b)). In patients with poorly
developed fat planes, these muscles are seen
as a single mass on imaging. Two smaller muscles, not usually seen on axial imaging, cre-
master and pyramidalis, which are concerned
with suspension of the testis and tensing the
midline tendinous raphe of the abdominal
wall, respectively, are also present.

Rectus abdomini
These are paired paramedian strap muscles
that extend from the ventral lower thorax to

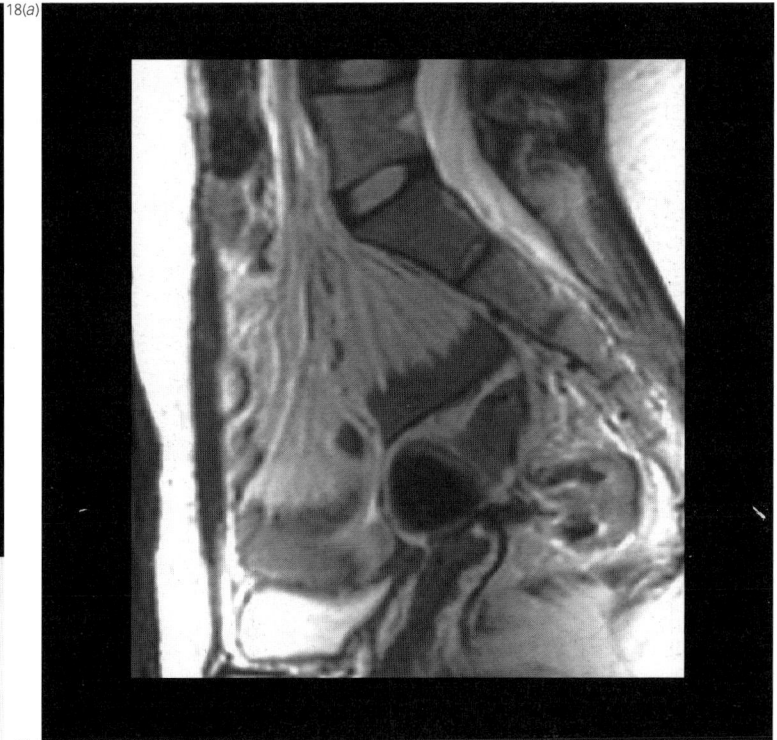

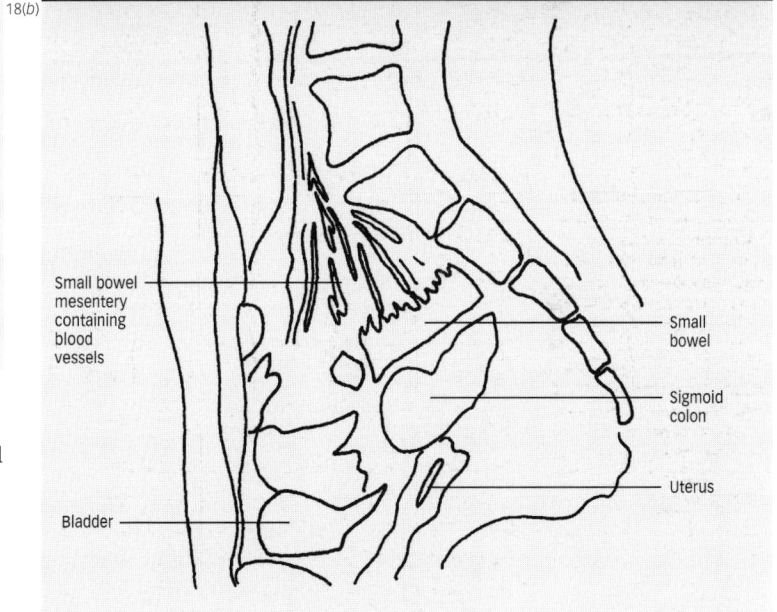

the pubis, separated from each other by the
linea alba. These muscles are narrow and thick
inferiorly, becoming broader and thinner
superiorly (Figs. 24(a), (b), 25(a), (b)). They arise
from two tendons inferiorly, the larger lateral
tendon originates on the crest of the pubis and
may extend beyond the pubic tubercle to the
pecten pubis, the medial tendon interlaces
with the contralateral tendon and is continuous with the ligamentous fibres covering the
front of the symphysis pubis. Superiorly, the
muscle is attached by three slips to the 5, 6,
7th costal cartilages and occasionally to the
costoxiphoid ligaments and xiphoid process

Fig. 18(a).
**Sagittal MRI to show the
small bowel mesentery.**

Fig. 18(b).
**Diagram to show the small
bowel mesentery**

19(a)

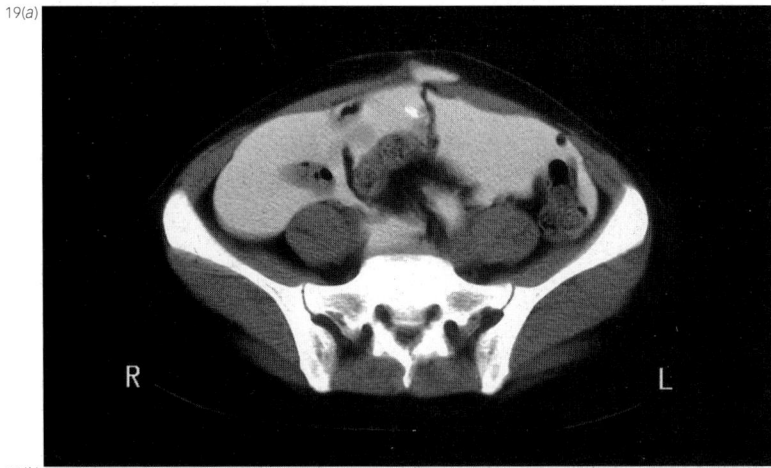

21(a)

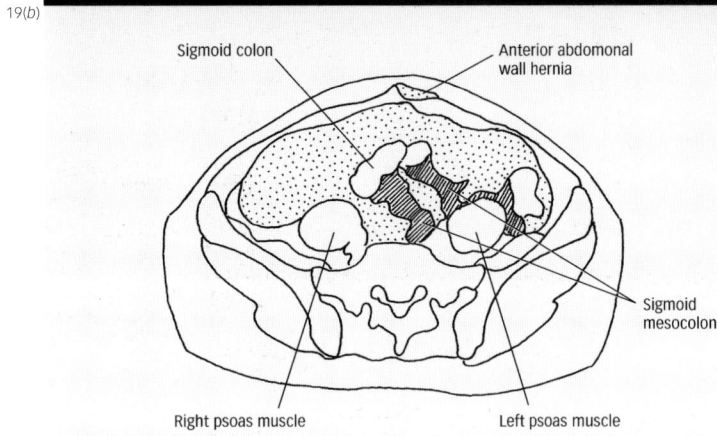

19(b)

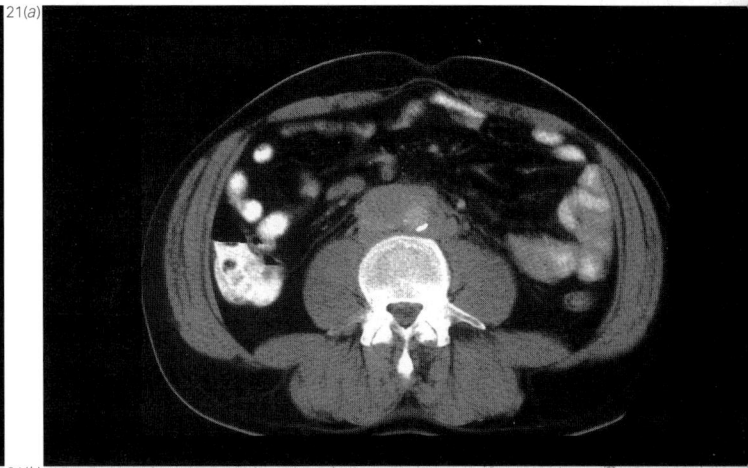

Sigmoid colon

Anterior abdomonal wall hernia

Sigmoid mesocolon

Right psoas muscle

Left psoas muscle

21(b)

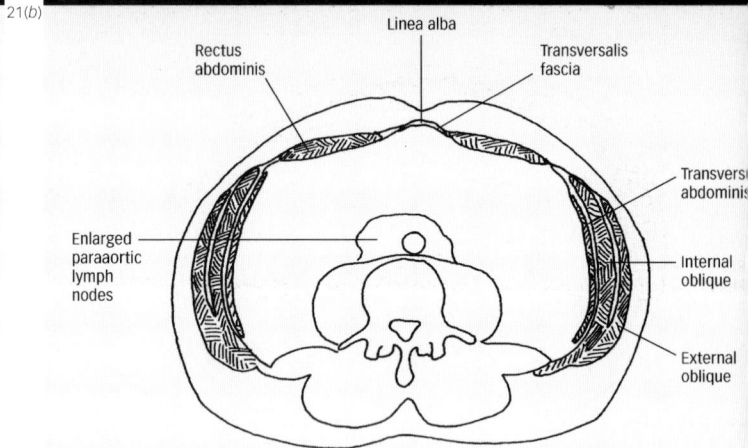

Linea alba

Rectus abdominis

Transversalis fascia

Transversi abdominis

Enlarged paraaortic lymph nodes

Internal oblique

External oblique

20

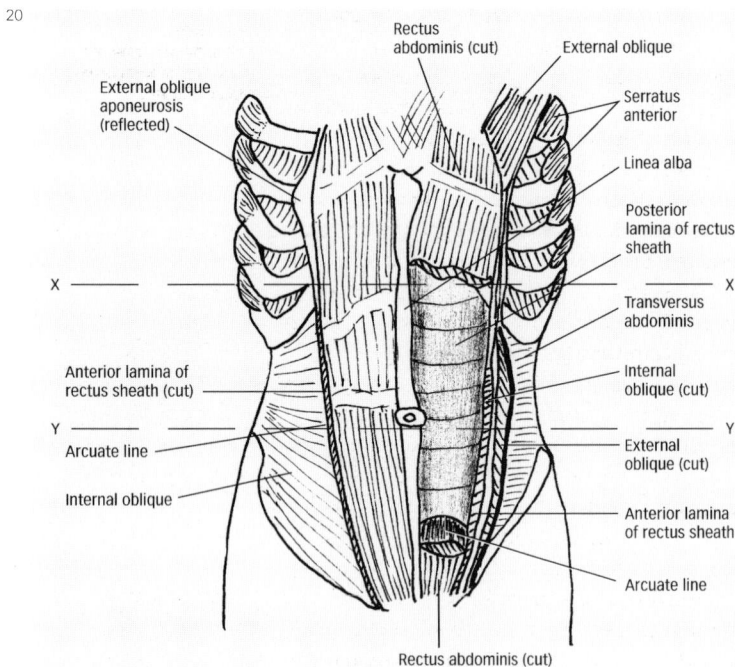

External oblique aponeurosis (reflected)

Rectus abdominis (cut)

External oblique

Serratus anterior

Linea alba

Posterior lamina of rectus sheath

X   X

Transversus abdominis

Anterior lamina of rectus sheath (cut)

Internal oblique (cut)

Y   Y

External oblique (cut)

Arcuate line

Anterior lamina of rectus sheath

Internal oblique

Arcuate line

Rectus abdominis (cut)

Fig. 19(a). top left
Axial CT with contrast in peritoneal cavity to show the root of the sigmoid mesocolon.

Fig. 19(b). middle left
Diagram to show the root of the sigmoid mesocolon.

Fig. 20. above
Coronal diagram of the muscles of the anterior abdominal wall. On the right, external oblique and the anterior lamina of the rectus sheath have been removed. On the left, most of the external and internal obliques and most of rectus abdominis have been removed.

(Fig. 26(a), (b)). The muscle fibres of the recti are interrupted by three fibrous bands named tendinous intersections, one opposite the umbilicus, one opposite the free edge of the xiphoid process, and one midway between these points.

The muscles are enclosed by the aponeuroses of the oblique and transverse muscles, which form the rectus sheath. From the costoxiphoid margin to the level of the umbilicus the anterior layer of the rectus sheath is formed by the aponeurosis of the external oblique and the superficial layer of the internal oblique aponeurosis (Fig. 27(a), (b)). The posterior layer is formed by the aponeurosis of the transversus abdominis and deep layer of the internal oblique aponeurosis. Below the umbilicus, the aponeurosis of all three flat anterolateral muscles pass in front of the rectus abdominis (Fig. 28(a), (b)). Medially, the sheaths are bound by the linea alba, a complex tendinous raphe between the recti, extending from the xiphoid process to the symphysis pubis and public crest. It is composed of aponeurotic fibres from both sets of the oblique and transversus muscles. Above the umbilicus, where the recti diverge, the linea alba has a transverse diameter of 4–6 mm and

Fig. 21(a).
Axial CT to show the anterolateral abdomina wall musculature above the umbilicus.

Fig. 21(b).
Diagram to show the anterolateral abdomina wall musculature above the umbilicus.

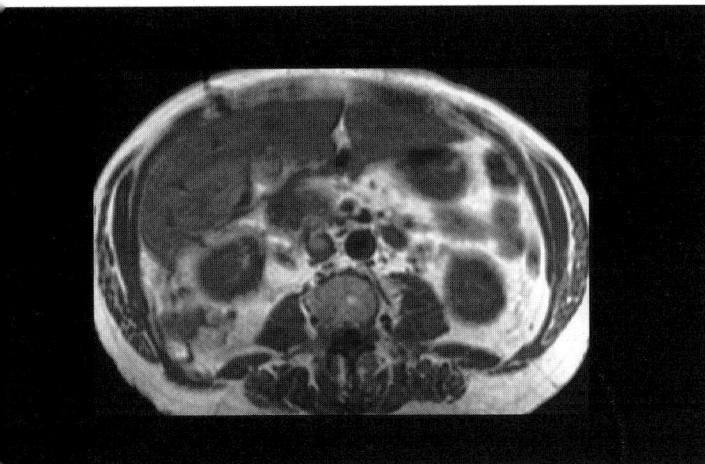

23(a)

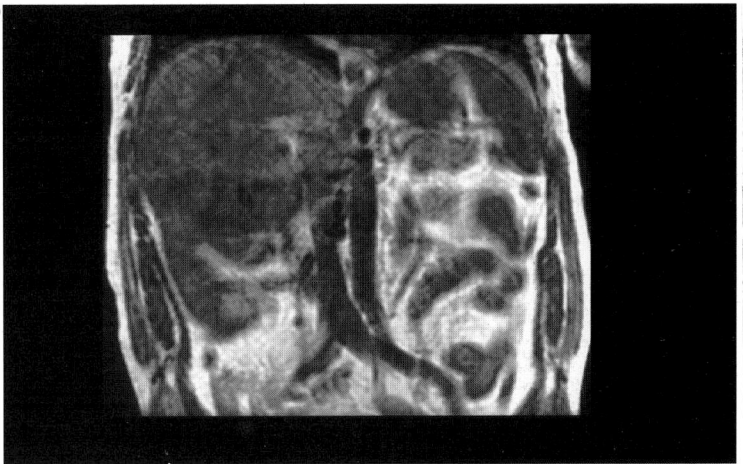

23(b)

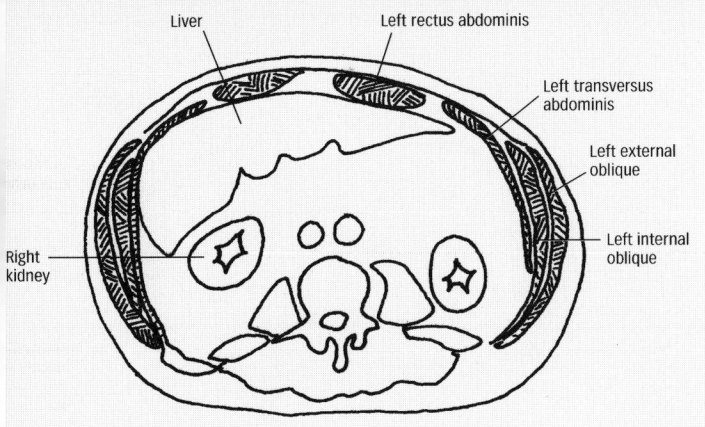

Fig. 22(a).
Axial MRI to show the anterolateral abdominal wall musculature above the umbilicus.

Fig. 22(b).
Diagram to show the anterolateral abdominal wall musculature above the umbilicus.

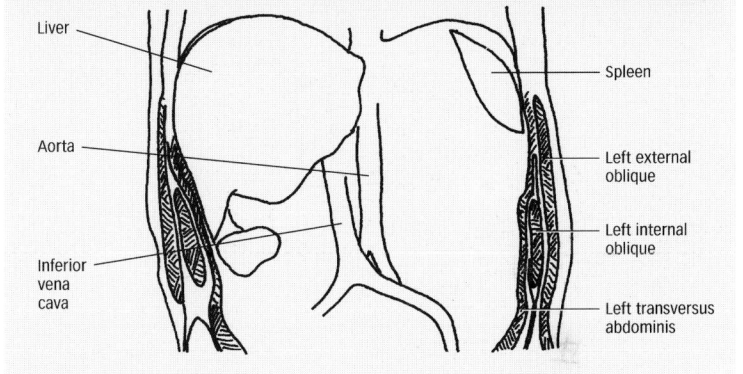

Fig. 23(a).
Coronal MRI to show the abdominal wall musculature laterally.

Fig. 23(b).
Diagram to show the lateral abdominal wall musculature.

is thin in its anteroposterior depth, below the umbilicus its transverse diameter narrows but its anteroposterior dimension deepens (Figs. 29(a), (b), 30(a), (b)). Inferiorly, its superficial fibres pass anterior to the medial tendons of the recti to reach the pubis. Its deeper fibres pass behind the recti to insert on the pubic crest as the adminiculum lineae albae. The rectus sheath is bound laterally by the linea semilunaris, the fused aponeuroses of the lateral muscles, passing from the tip of the ninth costal cartilage to the pubic tubercle.

Pyramidalis is a triangular muscle anterior to the lower part of the rectus abdominis and in its sheath. It originates from the front of the pubic body and the anterior ligaments of the pubic symphysis, ascending and diminishing in size, to become embedded in the linea alba itself, half-way between the pubis and umbilicus. The posterior rectus sheath contains the superior and inferior epigastric vessels and terminal parts of the lower intercostal nerves.

The external oblique
This is the largest and most superficial of the three flat anterolateral muscles curving around the lateral and anterior part of the abdominal wall (Figs. 20, 21(a), (b), 22(a), (b),

23(a), (b)). It arises from eight slips from the external and inferior borders of the lower eight ribs, interdigitating with the origins of the serratus anterior and latissimus dorsi, extending downwards and backwards. Its fibres diverge inferomedially. The posterior fibres, from the lower ribs, pass vertically to insert into the anterior half of the iliac crest. The middle and upper fibres pass anteriorly and forwards to end in the muscle's aponeurosis. The muscles fibres rarely descend beyond a line from the anterior superior iliac spine to the umbilicus. The aponeurosis of the external oblique forms a strong tendinous sheet, which medially contributes to the rectus sheath and linea alba (Fig. 31(a), (b)). Inferiorly, the aponeurosis is attached to the pubic symphysis as far laterally as the pubic tubercle. The free margin of the aponeurosis between the anterior superior iliac spine and pubic tubercle forms a thick band, the inguinal ligament. Its length is convex towards the thigh and is continuous with the fascia lata. In adults, the inguinal ligament is 12–14 cm in length, inclined 40–35 degrees to the horizontal, its medial half gradually widens towards its attachment to the pubis. The medial (pectineal part) of the inguinal ligament is known as the lacunar ligament, which forms the medial margin of the femoral ring. The superficial inguinal ring is a

24(a)

24(b)

Rectus abdominis

Linea alba

linea semilunaris

Small bowel

Iliopsoas

26(a)

26(b)

Right rectus abdominis

Right 6th rib

Xiphisternum

Left rectus abdominis

Hepatic metastasis

Liver

Stomach

25(a)

25(b)

Right rectus abdominis

Linea alba

Small bowel

Left rectus abdominis

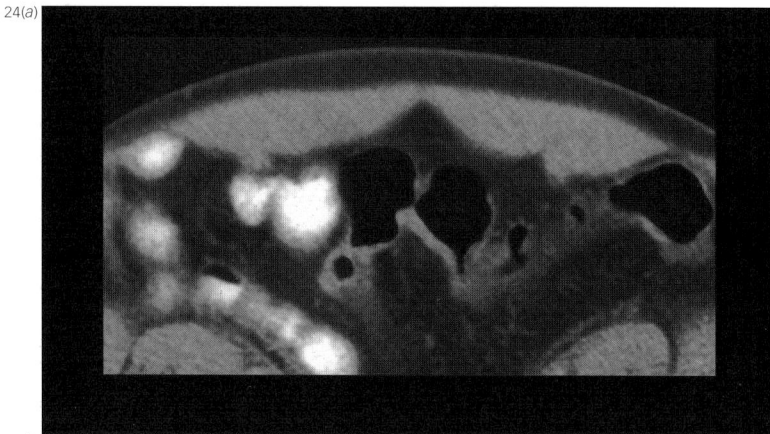

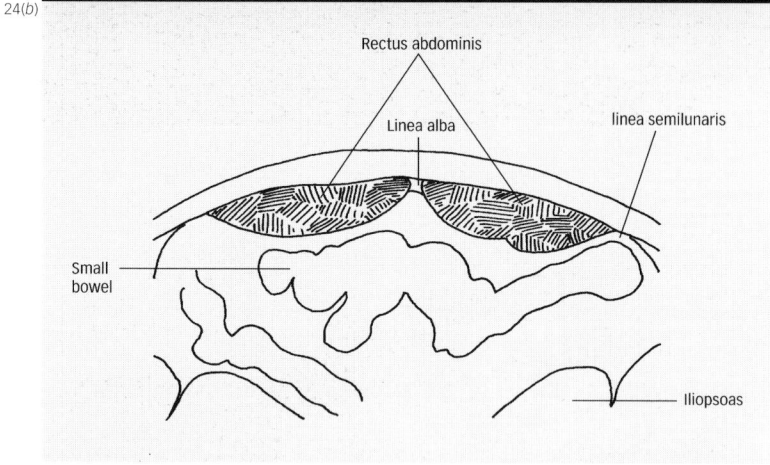

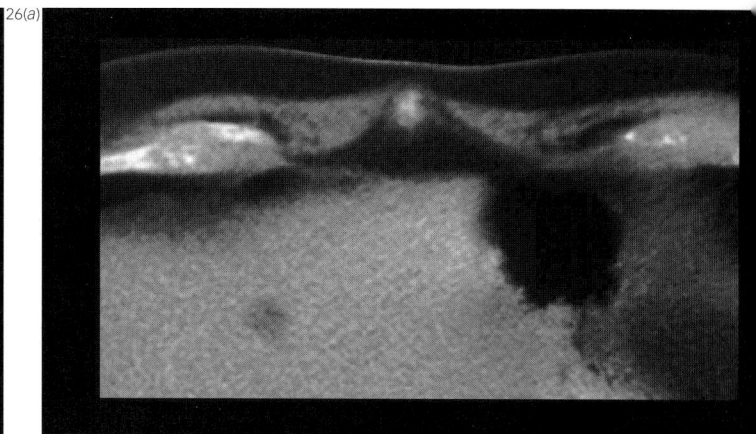

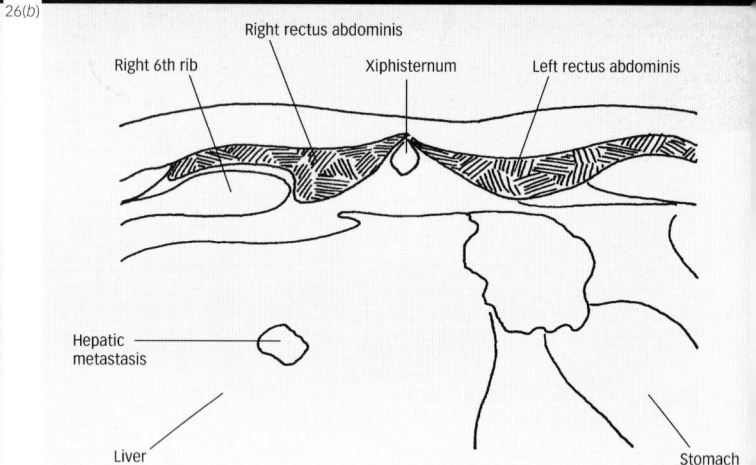

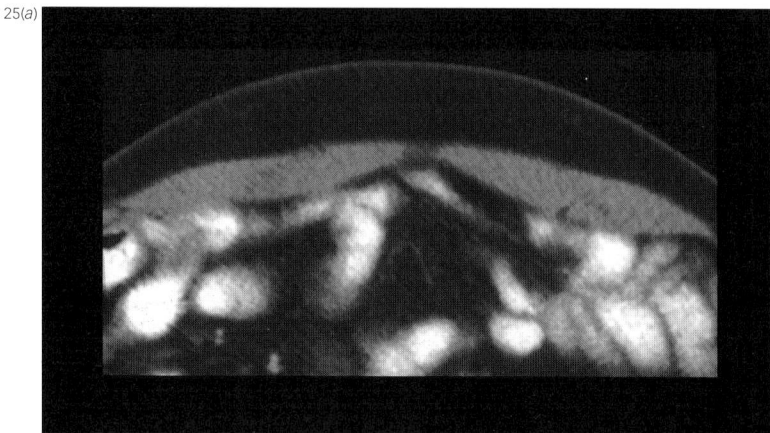

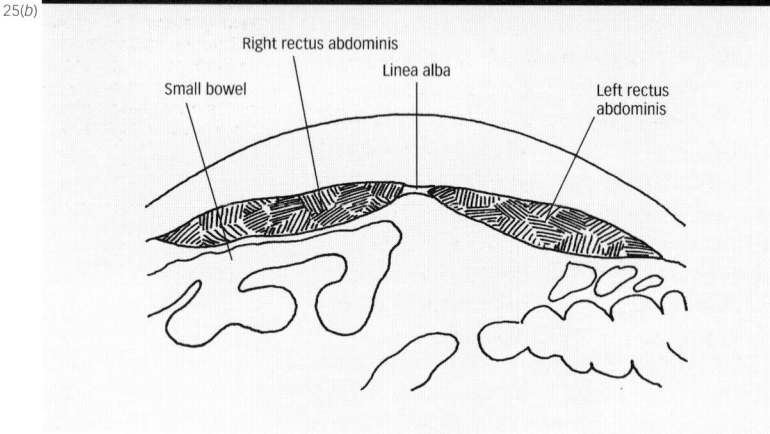

hiatus in the external oblique aponeurosis lying superolaterally to the pubic crest. It transmits the spermatic cord in males, the round ligament of the uterus in females, and the ilioinguinal nerve is both.

The internal oblique

This lies internal to the external oblique and is generally thinner and less bulky (Figs. 20, 21(a), (b), 22 (a), (b), 23(a), (b)). It arises from the lateral two-thirds of the inguinal ligament, from the anterior two-thirds of the iliac crest, and from the thoracolumbar fascia. The posterior fibres pass upwards and laterally to the inferior borders of the lower three or four ribs, where they are continuous with the intercostal muscles. The rest of the fibres diverge and end in an aponeurosis which gradually broadens from below upwards. In its upper two-thirds this aponeurosis splits to form part of the anterior and posterior layers of the rectus sheath (Fig. 27(a), (b)). Superiorly, the aponeurosis is attached to the cartilages of the seventh, eighth and ninth ribs. In the lower part of the abdominal wall the whole aponeurosis passes with that of the transversus abdominis aponeurosis, to lie anterior to the recti muscles to help form the linea alba medially (Fig. 28(a), (b)).

Fig. 24(a). top left
Axial CT through the pelvis to show the rectus abdomini.

Fig. 24(b).
Diagram to show the rectus abdomini muscles

Fig. 25(a).
Axial CT through the mid abdomen to show the rectus abdomini.

Fig. 25(b). bottom left
Diagram to show the rect abdomini in the mid-abdomen.

Fig. 26(a). top right
Magnified axial CT throug the upper abdomen to sh the attachment of the rectus abdomini into the xiphisternum.

Fig. 26(b).
Diagram to show the attachment of the rectus abdomini into the xiphisternum.

28(a)

28(b)

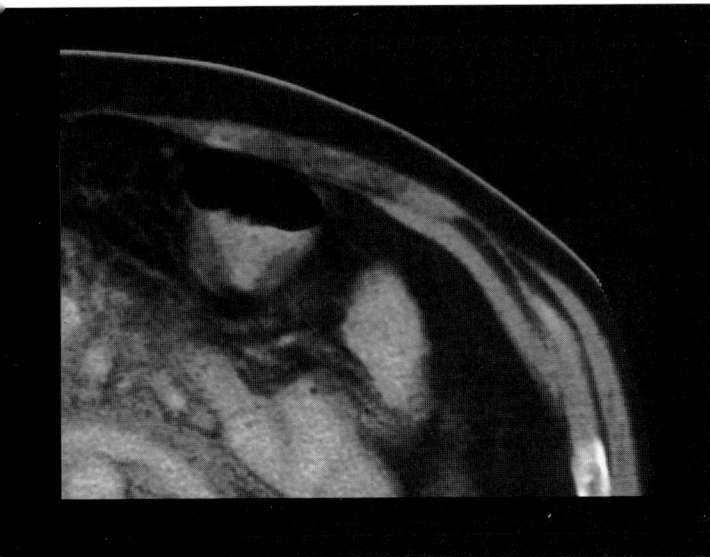

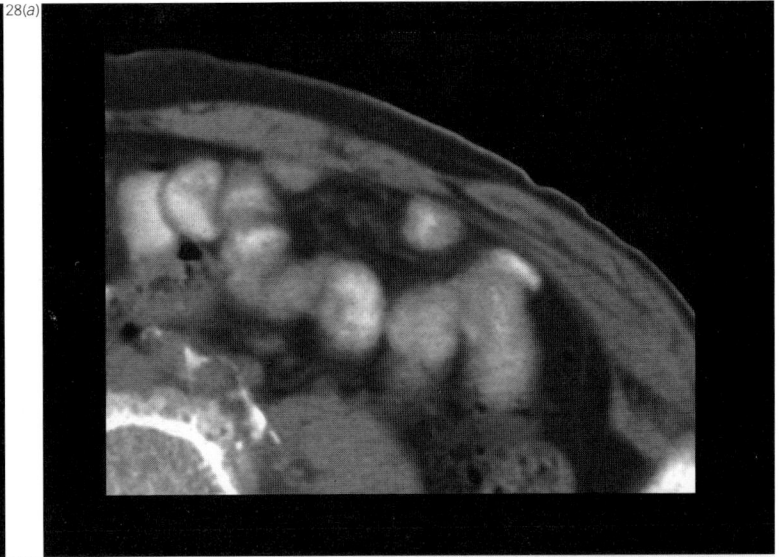

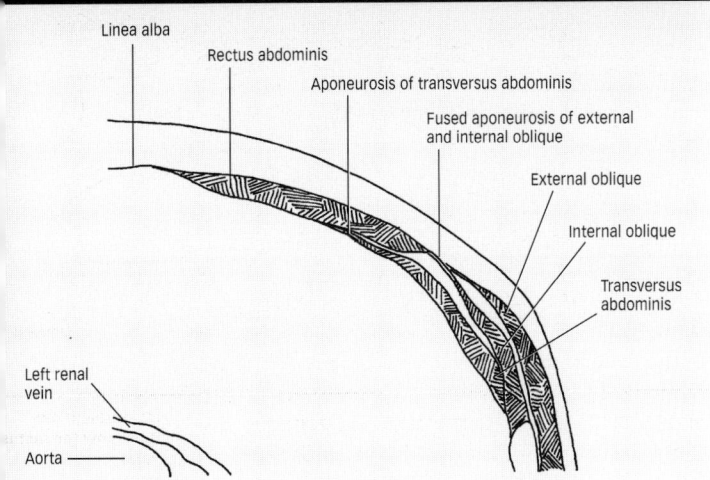

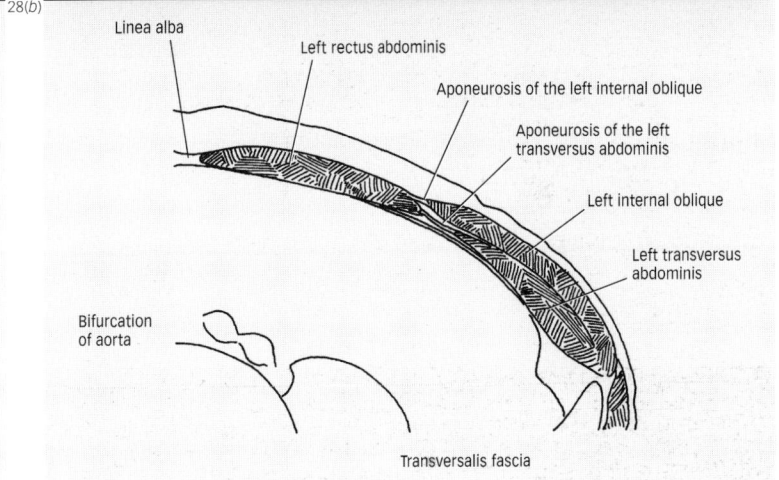

Fig. 27(a).
Magnified axial CT through the abdomen at level X–X (Fig. 20), above the umbilicus, to show the aponeuroses of the external and internal oblique passing anterior to the left rectus to form the rectus sheath. The aponeurosis of the transversus abdominis passes behind the rectus sheath.

Fig. 27(b).
Diagram to show the aponeuroses of the external and internal oblique passing anterior to the left rectus and that of the transversus abdominis passing posteriorly to form the rectus sheath.

The transversus abdominis

This is the innermost of the flat muscles of the abdominal wall (Figs. 21(a), (b), 22(a), (b), 23(a), (b)). It arises from the lateral third of the inguinal ligament, the inner two-thirds of the iliac crest, the thoracolumbar fascia between the iliac crest and the 12th rib, and the internal aspects of the lower six costal cartilages, where it interdigitates with the insertions of the diaphragm. The muscle ends in an aponeurosis of variable extent inferomedially. The lower fibres of the aponeurosis curve inferomedially with the fibres of the internal oblique aponeurosis to insert in to the crest and pecten of the pubis, forming the cojoint tendon or falx inguinalis, a tendon attached to the pubic crest and pecten. The rest of the aponeurosis passes medially to the rectus and helps form the linea alba medially. Above the umbilicus it passes behind the rectus abdominis and below it passes in front of the muscle (Figs. 27(a), (b), 28(a), (b)).

The transversalis fascia

This is a thin areolar membrane lying between the transversus abdominis and the extraperitoneal fat (Fig. 28(a), (b)). Superiorly, it is continuous with the inferior diaphragmatic fascia and inferiorly with the iliac and pelvic fascia. Posteriorly, it fuses with the thoracolumbar fascia. The spermatic cord in the male, or round ligament in the female, passes through the transversalis fascia at the deep inguinal ring.

The extraperitoneal connective tissue

This lies between the peritoneum and inner surface of the transversalis fascia which lines the interior of the abdominal and pelvic cavities. It contains a considerable amount of areolar connective tissue. This tissue is particularly abundant around the posterior wall of the abdomen, especially around the kidneys, where it contains fat. It is scanty on the anterior abdominal wall, except in the pubic region and above the iliac crest.

Fig. 28(a).
Magnified axial CT through the pelvis, at level Y–Y (Fig. 20), below the umbilicus, to show the internal oblique and transversus abdominis and their aponeuroses passing anterior to the left rectus to form the rectus sheath. Also shown is the transversalis fascia.

Fig. 28(b).
Diagram to show the aponeuroses of the internal oblique and transversus abdominis passing anterior to the left rectus to form the rectus sheath. Also shown is the transversalis fascia.

29(a)

30(a)

29(b)

Aponeurosis of the right transversus abdominis

Linea alba

Left rectus abdominis

Duodenum

Inferior vena cava

Aorta

30(b)

Transversalis fascia

Linea alba

Left rectus abdominis

Aortic bifurcation

Left psoas

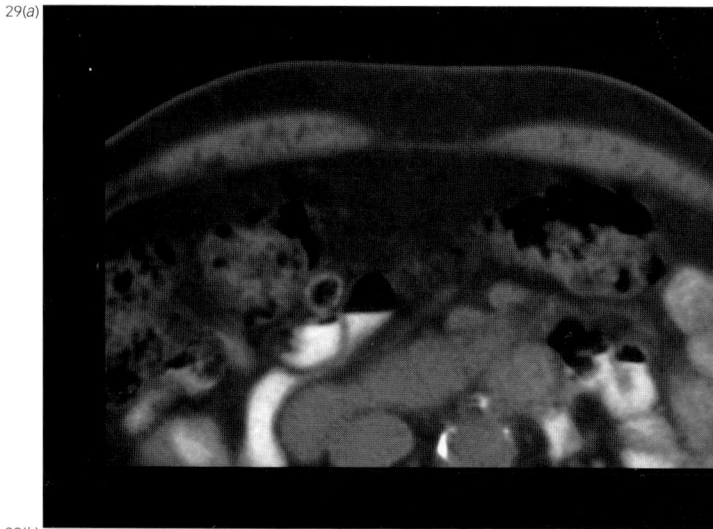

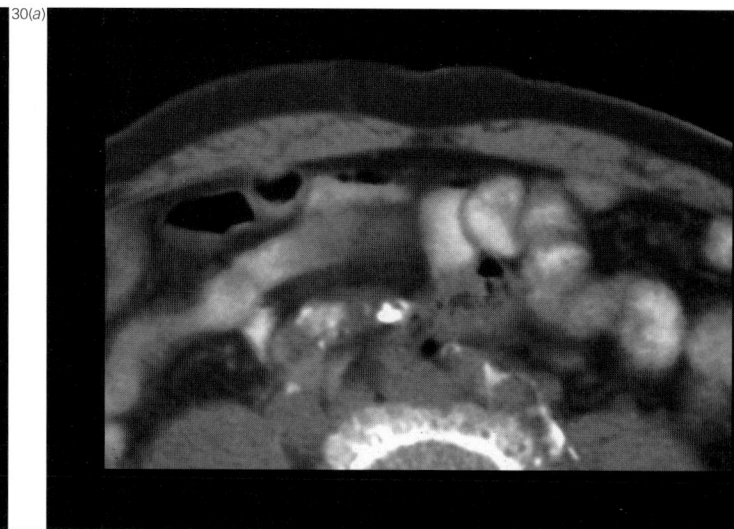

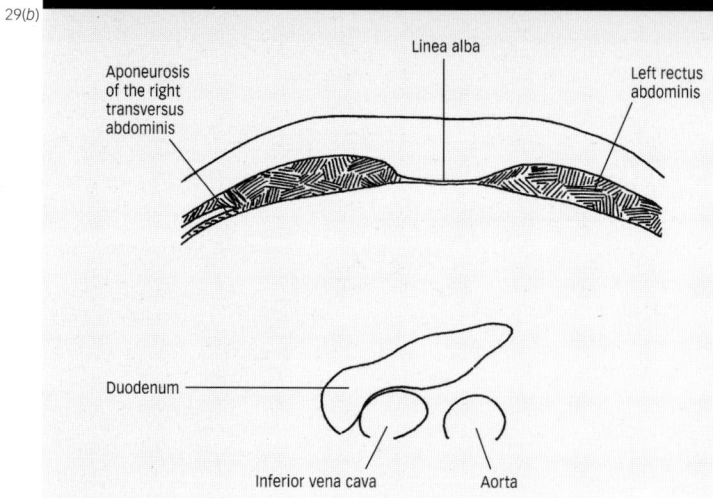

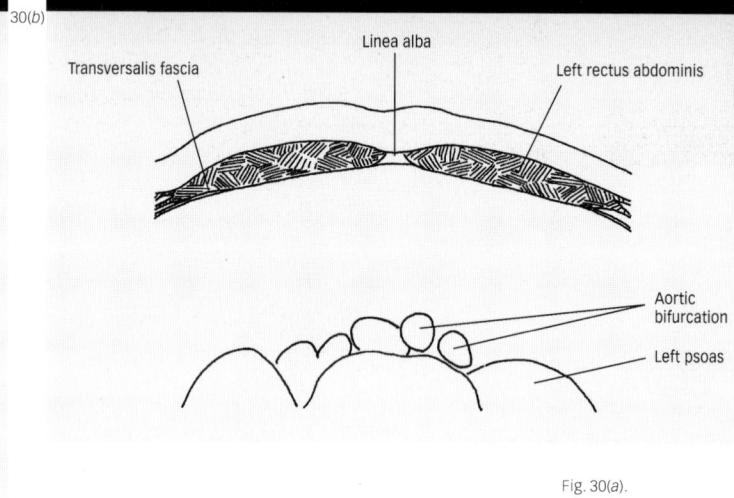

Fig. 29(a).
Magnified axial CT at the level X–X (Fig. 20) to show the linea alba in the upper abdomen.

Fig. 29(b).
Diagram to show the linea alba in the upper abdomen

The superior epigastric artery, which runs in the sheath of the rectus abdominis, is a branch of the internal thoracic (mammary) artery. Initially it lies behind the muscle, and then perforates and supplies it. Inferiorly, it anastomoses with the inferior epigastric artery, which is a branch of the external iliac artery. The inferior epigastric artery leaves the external iliac artery immediately above the inguinal ligament, piercing the transversalis fascia, and runs in the rectus sheath behind the muscle. It demarcates the medial margin of the deep inguinal ring. It also perforates and supplies the rectus abdominis.

Fig. 30(a).
Magnified axial CT at level Y–Y (Fig. 20) to show the linea alba in the lower abdomen.

Fig. 30(b).
Diagram to show the linea alba in the lower abdomen

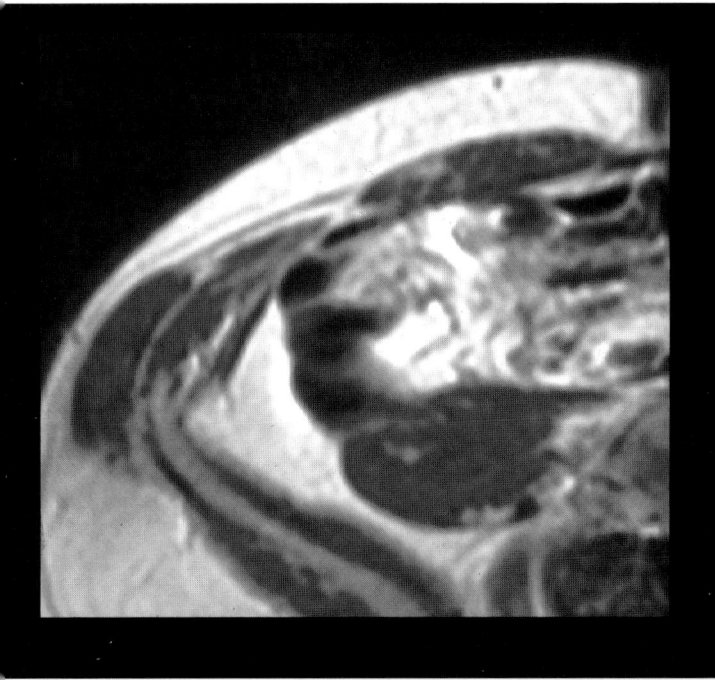

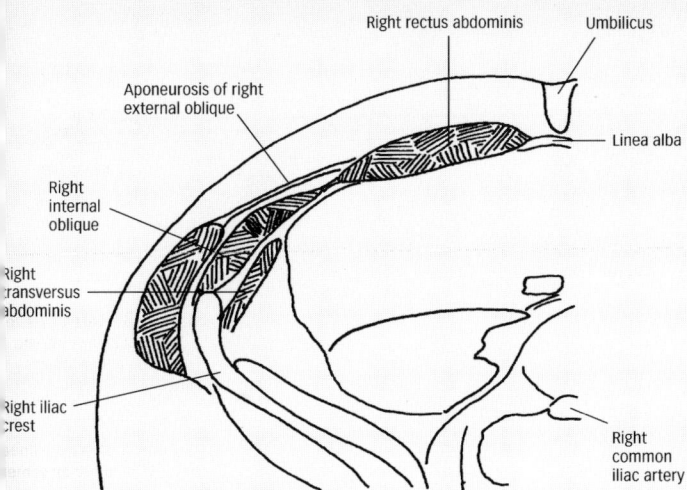

Fig. 31(*a*).
Magnified axial MRI to show the aponeurosis of the external oblique.

Fig. 31(*b*).
Diagram to show the aponeurosis of the external oblique.

References

Auh, Y.H., Rubenstein, W.A., Markisz, J.A., Zirinsky, K., Whalen, J.P. & Kazam, E. (1986). Intraperitoneal paravesical spaces: CT delineation with US correlation. *Radiology*, **159**, 311–17.

Brooke-Jeffrey, R., Federle, M.P. & Goodman, P.C. (1981). Computed tomography of the lesser peritoneal sac. *Radiology*, **141**, 117–22.

Dodds, W.J., Foley, W.D., Lawson, T.L., Stewart, E.T. & Taylor, A. (1985). Anatomy and imaging of the lesser peritoneal sac. *American Journal of Radiology*, **144**, 567–75.

Fisch, A.E. & Brodey, P.A. (1981). Computed tomography of the anterior abdominal wall. Normal anatomy and pathology. *Journal of Computer Aided Tomography*, **5**, 728–33.

Goodman, P. & Raval, B. (1990). CT of the abdominal wall. *American Journal of Radiology*, **154**, 1207–11.

Heiken, J.P. (1989). Abdominal wall and peritoneal cavity. In *Computed Body Tomography with MRI Correlation*, 2nd edn, ed. J.K.T. Lee, S.S. Sagel & R.J. Stanley, pp. 661–706. New York: Raven Press.

Meyers, M.A. (1994). *Dynamic Radiology of the Abdomen and Pathological Anatomy*. 4th edn. New York, Berlin, Heidelberg: Springer-Verlag.

Meyers, M.A., Oliphant, M., Berne, A.S. & Feldberg, M.A.M. (1987). Annual oration. The peritoneal ligaments and mesenteries: pathways of intraabdominal spread of disease. *Radiology*, **163**, 593–604.

Oliphant, M. & Berne, A.S. (1982). Computer tomography of the subperitoneal space: demonstration of direct spread of intraabdominal disease. *Journal of Computer Aided Tomography*, **6**, 1127–37.

Rubenstein, W.A., Auh, Y.H., Whalen, J.P. & Kazam, E. (1983). The perihepatic spaces: computer tomography and ultrasound. *Radiology*, **149**, 231–9.

Silverman, P.M., Kelvin, F.M., Korobkin, M. & Dunnick, N.R. (1984). Computed tomography of the normal mesentery. *American Journal of Radiology*, **143**, 953–7.

Williams, P.L., Warwick, R., Dyson, M. & Bannister, L.H. (1989). *Gray's Anatomy*. 37th edn. Edinburgh, London, Melbourne, New York: Churchill Livingstone.

The gastrointestinal tract

S. E. ROBBINS
and J. VIRJEE

Imaging methods

The choice of imaging modality for optimal demonstration of gastrointestinal anatomy is highly dependent on the clinical symptoms and signs. With the advent of newer technology, the role of plain abdominal radiography has diminished, although characteristic gas and soft tissue patterns can be of great importance in the diagnosis of the 'acute abdomen'.

Double contrast barium examinations are the most sensitive way of examining the gastrointestinal tract, providing information on distribution of the gut, mucosal and muscular detail, and, using dynamic investigations as in the case of the barium swallow, functional information. The diagnostic information gained from the barium examination is dependent on adequate preparation of the patient and attention to technique. The use of short-acting muscle relaxants, such as hyoscine or glucagon, reduces peristalsis, and improves visualization of the mucosa.

Transabdominal ultrasound scanning has a limited application in the gastrointestinal tract due to bowel gas, but is used to identify intra-abdominal collections. It is particularly useful in children, in the diagnosis of pyloric stenosis, appendicitis, and intussusception. Endoscopic ultrasound is a technique which is being increasingly used in the staging of gastrointestinal tumours. It has been used chiefly in the oesophagus, stomach, colon and rectum. It is performed with high frequency (7.5–20 MHz) probes (either radial or linear array in type). The use of such high frequency probes provides information about the bowel wall which cannot be obtained with other techniques. It can also be used to examine and perhaps biopsy those structures in close proximity to the bowel wall such as the pancreas, biliary tract and lymph nodes. Endoscopic linear array probes, with colour Doppler, can also be used to assess blood flow in the mesenteric and portal vessels.

Nuclear medicine can be an invaluable adjunct to other forms of imaging. Poor spatial resolution limits the amount of morphological information but radio isotope scans are used to study function, as in gastric emptying, to assess the activity of inflammatory bowel disease and to investigate gastrointestinal bleeding.

The chief use of mesenteric arteriography is in the diagnosis of unexplained gastrointestinal bleeding or ischaemia (see the next section).

Computed tomography has a limited role in investigation of the gastrointestinal tract, although it is used in combination with oral or rectal contrast agents to demonstrate masses in or around the bowel wall.

Magnetic resonance imaging has become the investigation of choice for anorectal fistulae. Elsewhere in the gastrointestinal tract its use has been limited. However, this may change with the introduction of superparamagnetic oral and rectal contrast agents.

The digestive system

The gastrointestinal tract is subdivided on topographical, histological and functional grounds into several different regions: the mouth, the pharynx, the oesophagus, the stomach, and the small and large intestine. The small intestine is divided further into the duodenum, jejunum, and ileum. The large intestine is subdivided into the caecum and appendix, the ascending, transverse, and descending colon, the rectum and anal canal. Embryologically the gut is divided into the foregut (from the pharynx to the second part of the duodenum), the midgut (from the second part of duodenum to the junction of the proximal two-thirds and distal third of transverse colon), and the hindgut (from the distal third of the transverse colon to the rectum).

The vascular supply of the bowel is determined by these embryological divisions. The upper third of the oesophagus is supplied by the inferior thyroid artery; the middle portion by oesophageal branches from the aorta, and the lower part and the remainder of the foregut are supplied by branches of the coeliac axis.

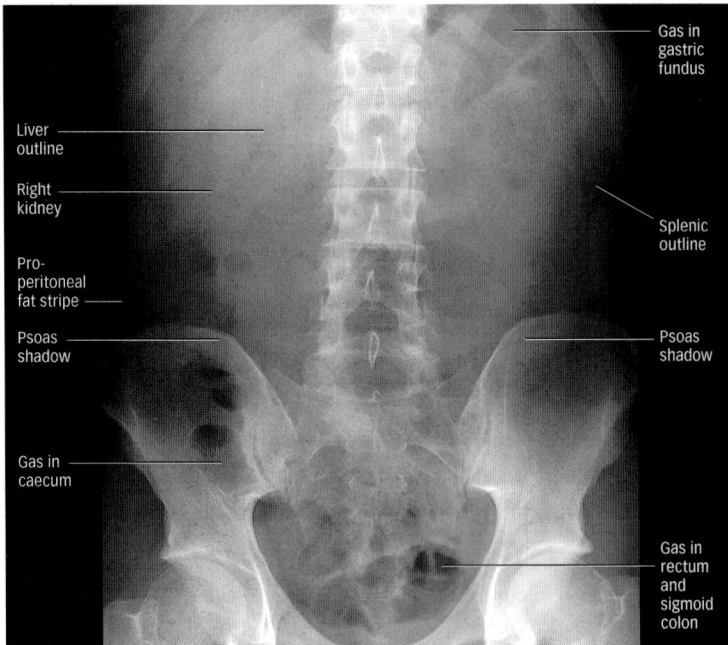

Fig. 1.
Plain abdominal radiograph.

The midgut is supplied by the superior mesenteric artery and its branches and the hindgut by the inferior mesenteric artery and its branches.

The plain abdominal radiograph

Relatively large amounts of gas are normally present in the stomach and colon of adults, with only a small amount in the small bowel (Fig. 1). In children who have been crying there is often considerably more gas in the stomach and small bowel. The gastric rugae may be seen on a supine radiograph, and on an erect film a fluid level is present in the stomach. The presence of fluid in the fundus of the stomach on a supine radiograph can give the appearance of a gastric 'pseudotumour', which may be mistaken for a soft tissue mass. Occasionally, short segments of the small bowel are seen, but the thin bands of the valvulae conniventes are not normally identified. Fluid levels may be present in the small bowel, although more than five is abnormal. The transverse diameter of the small intestine on a plain radiograph should not exceed 2.5 cm.

The caecum is seen as a speckled area on plain

supine film, and 20% of the normal population have a fluid level in the caecum on an erect film. The amount of gas present in the normal colon is very variable and the colonic haustra are usually seen. There may be several fluid levels in the normal colon, the calibre of which is variable.

The borders of the kidneys, psoas muscles, bladder, the posterior borders of the liver and spleen are often seen outlined by fat. However, it is not unusual for these fat lines to be obscured. For example, the spleen is not outlined in 42% of normal individuals; the outlines of the psoas muscles are only seen in 48% of normal radiographs, and the bladder in 60%. The properitoneal fat lines are seen in each flank, particularly in the obese, and represent the borders of the peritoneum.

Deglutition

Swallowing consists of a complex series of voluntary and involuntary muscle actions. Video radiography can be employed as part of the barium swallow examination and both structure and function can be assessed using solids and liquids.

Swallowing is initiated by the tongue, which forces the bolus of food backwards and downwards. The larynx rises and the pharyngeal space is closed for a fraction of a second. The bolus then passes the epiglottis, fills the pyriform recesses and enters the oesophagus. Air then enters the nasopharynx and the soft palate, larynx and epiglottis return to their normal positions. From the upper third of the oesophagus, the food is carried to the stomach by peristalsis.

The oesophagus

The oesophagus is a muscular tube which extends from the pharynx at the level of the cricoid cartilage at the sixth cervical vertebra to the cardiac orifice of the stomach at the level of the tenth thoracic vertebra. It is approximately 25 cm long, and most of its course is within the posterior mediastinum. The cervical portion of the oesophagus lies to the left of the midline. It enters the thorax in the midline, deviating to the left to lie behind the trachea and left main bronchus. It is separated from the left atrium by the pericardium, but remains in contact with the thoracic vertebrae throughout its course. The oesophagus inclines forward to pierce the diaphragm 2.5 cm to the left of the midline at the level of the tenth thoracic vertebra. The oesophageal opening of the diaphragm is bounded by a sling of muscle fibres derived from the right crus of the diaphragm. It also transmits the right and left vagus (Xth cranial), nerves, the oesophageal branches of the left gastric vessels and the lymphatics draining the lower third of the oesophagus. The abdominal portion of the oesophagus measures between 1 cm and 3 cm in length and runs in the oesophageal groove on the posterior surface of the liver.

Anatomy of the oesophagus
The wall of the oesophagus is composed of four layers: fibrous, muscular, submucous and mucous. The muscular layer, in turn, consists of superficial longitudinal and inner circular layers. The circular layer at the lower end of the oesophagus and adjacent part of the stomach acts as a functional sphincter. In the upper third of the oesophagus the muscle fibres are striated, in the middle third both striated and smooth fibres are found, and in the lower third the muscular layer consists only of smooth muscle fibres. The oesophageal mucosa is thrown into longitudinal folds, which can be seen in a normal barium swallow.

Anatomical relations of the oesophagus
In the neck
Posteriorly lie the prevertebral muscles. Anteriorly is the trachea. The recurrent laryngeal nerve lies between the oesophagus and trachea. Laterally are the lateral lobes of the thyroid and the carotid sheath (containing the common carotid artery, internal jugular vein and vagus nerve).

In the thorax
Posteriorly lie the prevertebral muscles, the thoracic duct, the azygos veins and the right posterior intercostal arteries. The thoracic aorta passes obliquely to run posterior to the oesophagus at and below the level of the seventh thoracic vertebra (Fig. 2). Anteriorly, from above downwards, are the trachea, the left main bronchus at the level of the fifth thoracic vertebra, the right pulmonary artery and the left atrium and pericardium. The vagal plexus lies just below the carina. In the lower part of the thorax the anterior and posterior vagal trunks form predominantly from the left and right vagus nerves, respectively. Laterally are the pleural cavities. On the right, the azygos vein lies between the pleura and the oesophagus. The thoracic duct lies to the right of, and posterior to, the lower part of the thoracic oesophagus. The duct crosses posterior to the oesophagus at the level of the fifth thoracic vertebra to lie behind the left border of the upper thoracic and cervical vertebrae. On the left, from superior to inferior, lie the left subclavian artery, the aortic arch, and the upper part of the descending aorta.

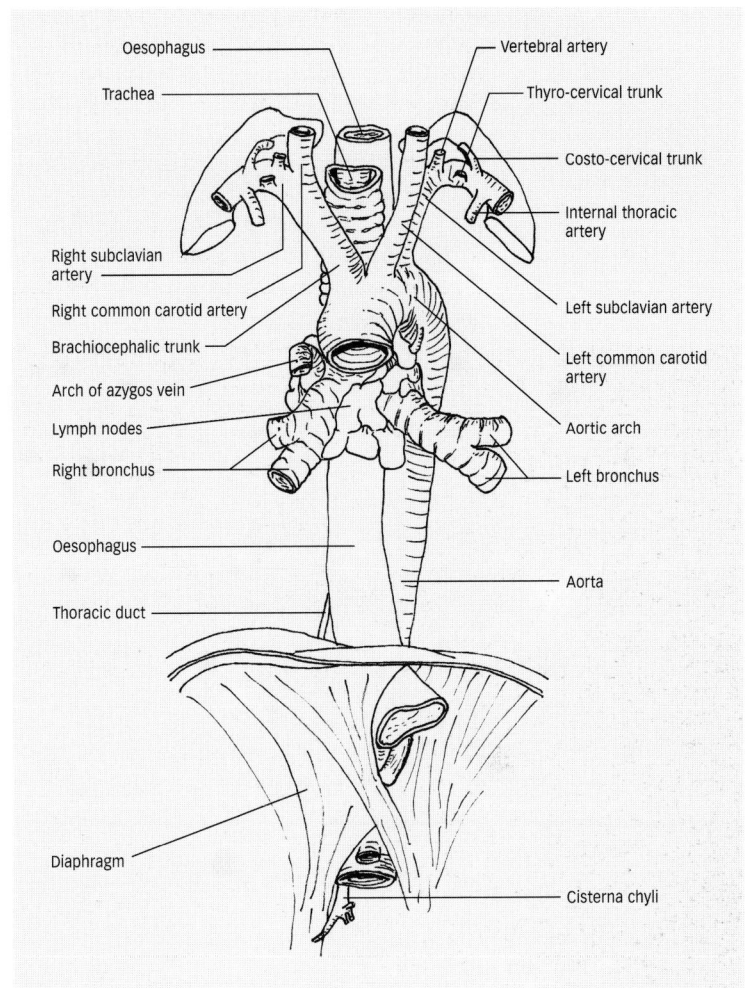

Fig. 2.
Anatomical relations of the oesophagus in the thorax – anterior view.

In the abdomen
Posteriorly lies the left crus of the diaphragm. Anteriorly is the left lobe of the liver.

Vascular supply of the oesophagus
The arterial supply of the upper third of the oesophagus is derived from the inferior thyroid branch of the subclavian artery. The oesophageal branches of the aorta supply the middle third. Oesophageal branches from the left gastric artery, a branch of the coeliac trunk, supply the lower third.

Veins run adjacent to the arteries. The upper third of the oesophagus drains to the brachiocephalic veins, the middle third to the azygos veins, and the left gastric vein drains the lowest portion into the portal vein. Thus there is an important anastomosis between the azygos system and the portal system via the left gastric vein.

Lymphatic drainage of the oesophagus
Lymphatic drainage is predominantly along the length of the oesophagus. Lymphatics follow the arteries to the deep cervical nodes,

from the upper oesophagus, to the posterior mediastinal nodes, from the mid portion of the oesophagus, and to the pre-aortic nodes of the coeliac group from the lower oesophagus.

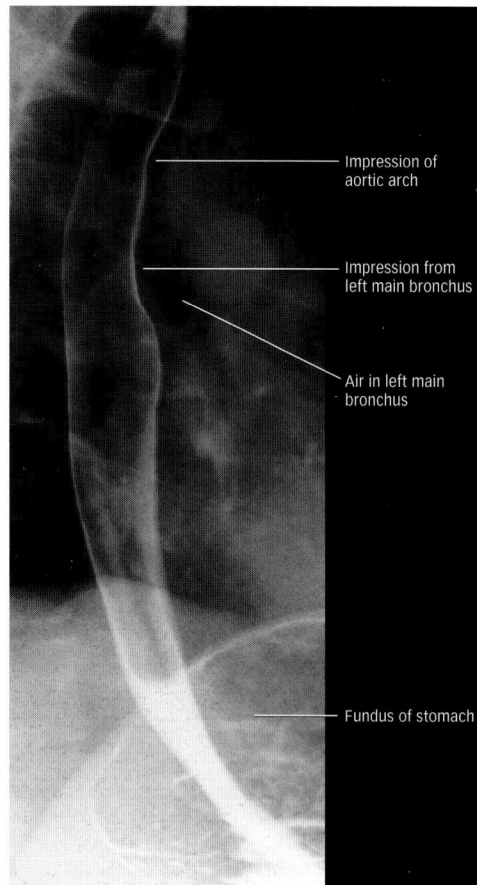

Fig. 3.
Barium swallow: right anterior oblique view.

first is where the pharynx joins the upper end of the oesophagus; the second is where the aortic arch and left main bronchus cross the anterior surface of the oesophagus; the third occurs where the oesophagus passes through the diaphragm.

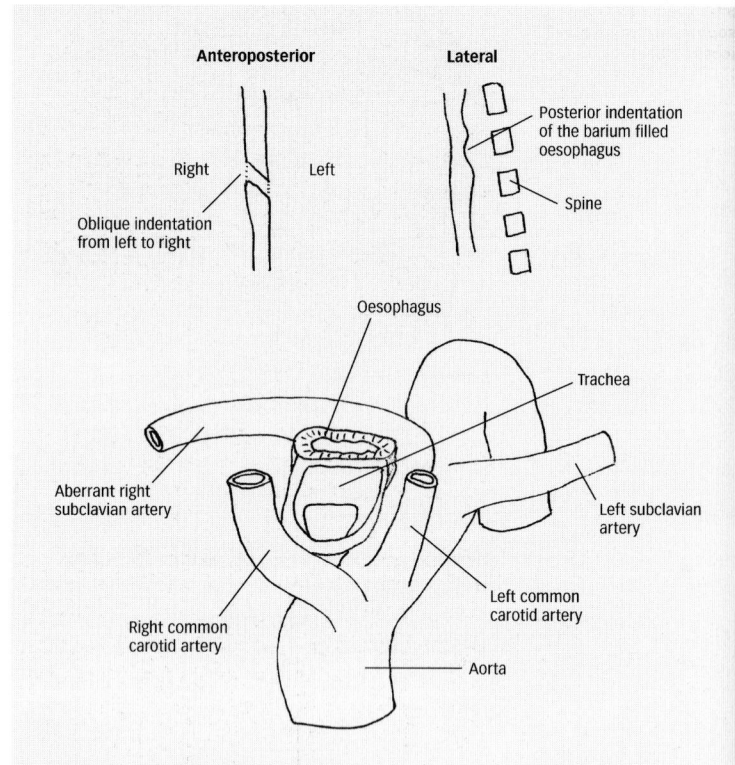

Fig. 4.
The anatomy of the aberrant right subclavian artery

Radiological examination of the oesophagus

The chest radiograph, particularly if performed at a high kV, may demonstrate the right wall of the oesophagus and azygos vein as they are outlined by lung. This appearance produces the azygo-oesophageal line. Above the arch of the azygos vein (at the level of the fourth thoracic vertebra), the pleura abuts the right oesophageal wall to form the pleuro-oesophageal line. If it contains air, the oesophagus can be identified on a lateral chest radiograph posterior to the trachea. The oesophagus can be examined by the oral administration of barium sulphate suspension. The examination is usually performed with the patient upright. Oesophageal motility is assessed with the patient prone. The pharynx and oesophagus are examined in sequence, in two planes at right angles to each other. Swallowing results in a long column of barium with a rounded or tapering end which descends rapidly to the cardia and then passes into the stomach by instalments. There are three anatomical and physiological constrictions in the oesophagus, which are seen anteriorly and to the left on a barium swallow (Fig. 3). The

At the level of the left atrium there is a long shallow anterior concavity. Occasionally, additional indentations can be seen in the barium column due to anomalous origins of the great vessels and it is important that these are not misinterpreted. The commonest is an aberrant right subclavian artery from a left-sided aortic arch (Fig. 4). In this anomaly, the right subclavian artery is the last brachiocephalic branch of the aorta. It passes cephalad obliquely from left to right, posterior to the oesophagus and can be recognized by a posterior indentation

Fig. 5.
The anatomy of the anomalous left main pulmonary artery.

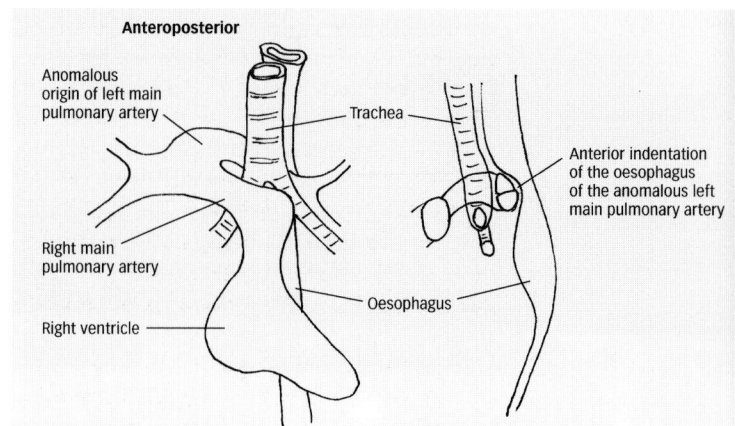

of the barium column. An important, but rare, anomaly is an aberrant left main pulmonary artery which produces an anterior indentation of the oesophagus (Fig. 5).

6.
uble contrast barium
allow demonstrating the
ction between
ophageal and gastric
cosa ('Z'line).

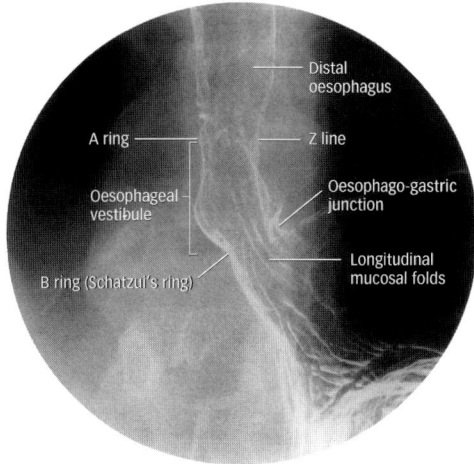

The lower end of the oesophagus (Fig. 6), is slightly dilated to form the vestibule, just above the oesophagogastric junction. The upper limit of this is referred to as 'A'ring, and the lower limit as the 'B' ring or 'Schatzki ring', which is usually below the diaphragm and not identified radiologically unless there is a small hiatus hernia.

The longitudinal folds of the mucous membrane can be outlined with barium, particularly at the lower end of the oesophagus, but these are readily distended by the passage of a bolus of barium. The mucosal junction between the oesophagus and stomach is sometimes seen as a fine line (or 'Z'line) on a double contrast barium swallow.

The stomach

The stomach is the widest part of the alimentary tract. It is a muscular cavity which is fixed at both ends but otherwise mobile. It has a maximum capacity of approximately 1500 ml. It is situated in the upper abdomen, extending from the left upper quadrant downwards, forwards, and to the right. It has two surfaces, anterosuperior and posteroinferior, which are bounded by two borders, the lesser and greater curvatures.

There are great variations in the size and shape of the stomach depending on the volume of its contents and also on the subject's body habitus. In short obese people, the stomach is arranged transversely in a 'steer horn' shape. In tall thin people it is more longitudinal and 'J-shaped'.

The stomach is divided for descriptive purposes into the fundus, body, pyloric antrum, and pylorus. The fundus is dome-shaped and

projects above and to the left of the cardiac orifice to lie in contact with the left dome of the diaphragm. The body extends from the fundus to the incisura angularis, which is a constant notch at the lower end of the lesser curvature. The pyloric antrum extends from the incisura angularis to the proximal part of the pylorus, where it narrows to become the pyloric canal. The pyloric orifice is formed by the pyloric canal. The muscular layer of the stomach wall is much thicker at this point and forms an anatomical and physiological sphincter. The pylorus lies approximately at the level of the first lumbar vertebra in the transpyloric plane, about 2.5 cm to the right of the midline. The stomach is completely covered by peritoneum. This passes as a double layer from the lesser curve as the lesser omentum and from the greater curve as the greater omentum.

The structure of the stomach

As with most of the gastrointestinal tract, the stomach is composed of four layers: an outer fibrous layer, a muscular layer, submucosa and mucosa. The muscular coat consists of inner

Fig. 7.
Axial CT section through the abdomen at the level of the first lumbar vertebra (oral and rapid intravenous contrast). Note the relations of the stomach and the second part of the duodenum.

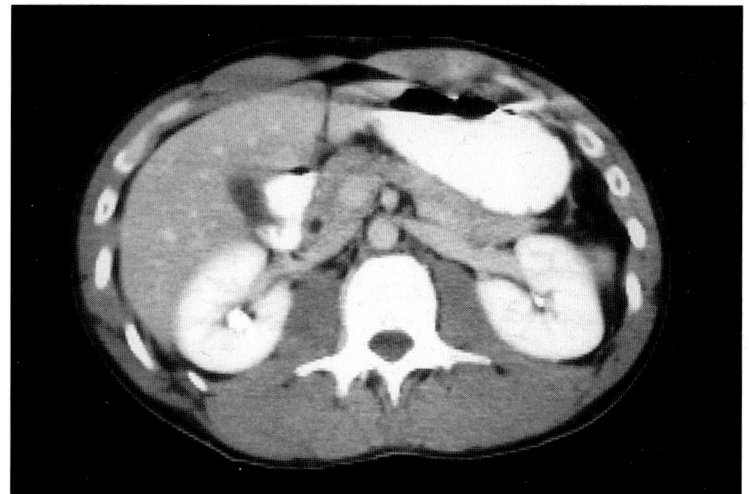

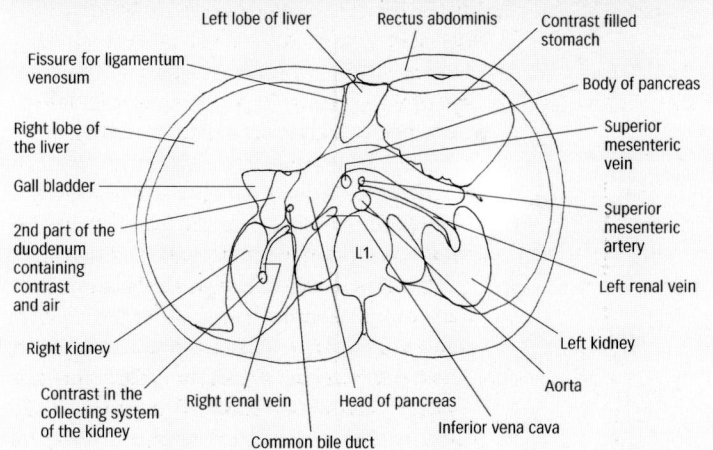

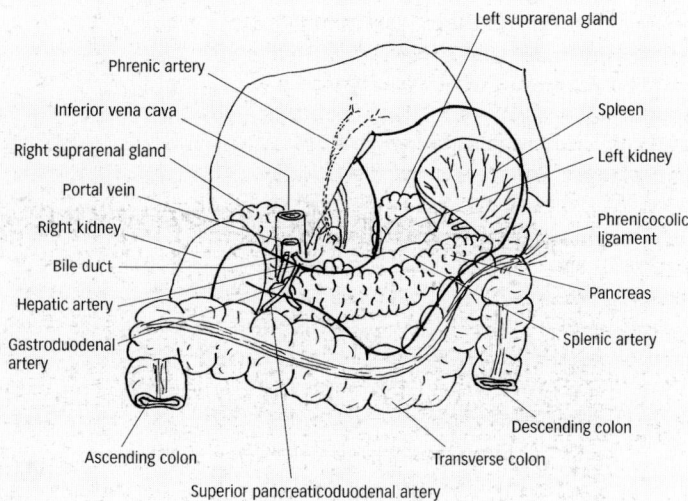

Fig. 8.
Structures of the stomach bed.

oblique, middle circular and outer longitudinal layers. The oblique layer runs parallel to the lesser curve, looping over the fundus. Its contraction raises the greater curvature. The circular layer surrounds the body of the stomach and forms the pyloric sphincter. The longitudinal fibres are concentrated around the greater and lesser curvatures.

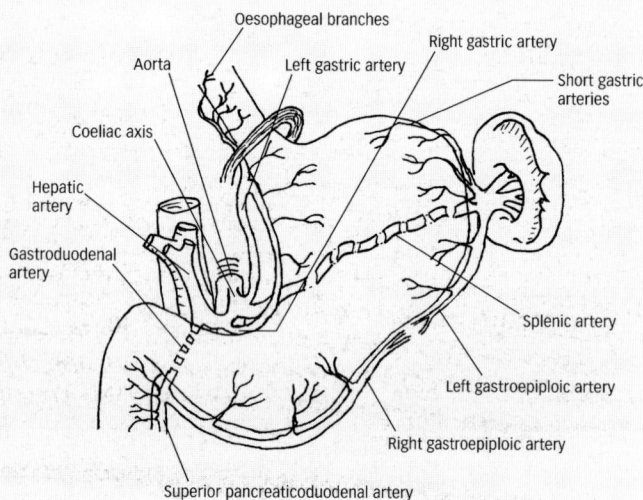

Fig. 9.
Diagram of the branches of the coeliac axis demonstrating the arterial supply of the stomach.

Anatomical relations of the stomach

Anteriorly lie the anterior abdominal wall and diaphragm. The sharp inferior border of the left lobe of the liver overlaps the lesser curvature (Fig. 7). Posteriorly the stomach is covered by the peritoneum of the lesser sac. Posteroinferior to the stomach is the stomach bed (Fig. 8). This is composed of a small part of the diaphragm, the left suprarenal gland, the gastric surfaces of the spleen and left kidney, the anterosuperior surface of the pancreas, the mesocolon and the transverse colon.

Vascular supply of the stomach

The arterial supply of the stomach is derived from all three branches of the coeliac trunk (Fig. 9).

Lymphatic drainage of the stomach

Lymphatic drainage of the stomach follows the arterial supply. All the gastric lymph vessels drain eventually into the coeliac lymph nodes, which surround the origin of the coeliac artery.

Radiological investigation of the stomach

The double contrast barium meal is the principal radiological investigation of the stomach. It provides anatomical information, and fine mucosal detail. A complete barium meal examination should also include imaging of the duodenum and oesophagus. When the stomach is empty, the mucosa is thrown into numerous folds or rugae (Fig. 10). In the lesser curve these are longitudinally arranged but in the remainder of the stomach they are less regular, having a mosaic appearance in the

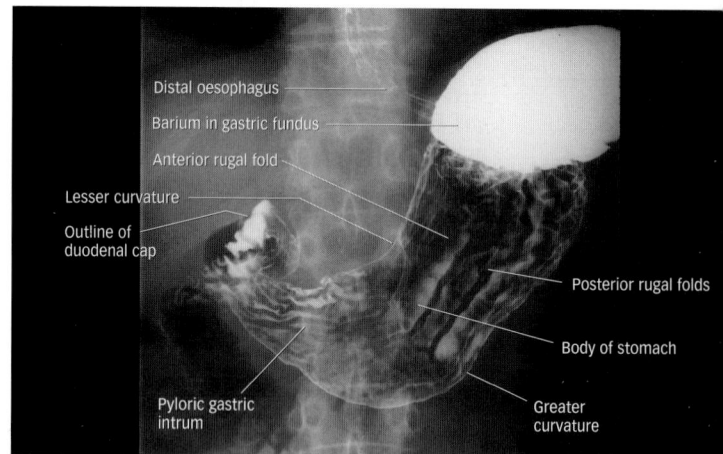

Fig. 10.
Supine barium meal examination demonstrati rugal folds. The anterior surface of the stomach ca be differentiated from the posterior in the supine position due to pooling of barium around the posterior folds.

region of the greater curvature. The rugae are arranged in fine parallel lines in the pyloric canal. The areae gastricae (Fig. 11), are small nodular elevations of the mucosal surface which measure 2–3 mm in diameter. These are readily seen on double contrast barium meal, particularly in the gastric antrum.

Because the stomach is a gas filled structure, ultrasound scanning is usually inappropriate, an exception being its use in the diagnosis of infantile pyloric stenosis. Cross-sectional imaging of the stomach by MRI or CT scanning does not show the stomach wall adequately and its chief application is to assess the local spread of stomach tumours. Isotope scanning is sometimes used in the assessment of gastric motility, particularly in patients who have had previous ulcer surgery.[111m] Indium DTPA in either a solid or liquid meal is used to

11.
ble contrast barium
al examination
nonstrating prominent
ae gastricae in the
rum.

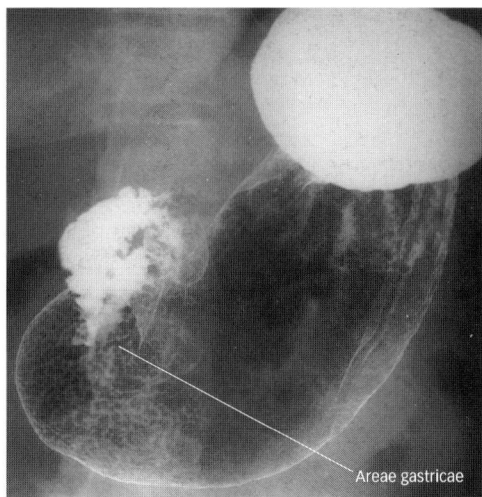

Areae gastricae

assess gastric emptying. Arteriography of the coeliac trunk is used in the investigation of gastrointestinal bleeding.

The duodenum

The duodenum is a 'C'-shaped tube which measures 25 cm long and runs from the pylorus to the proximal jejunum (Fig. 12). The bile and pancreatic ducts open into its second part. The duodenum curves around the head of the pancreas, and arches over the aorta and inferior vena cava. The first inch (2.5 cm) of the duodenum is intraperitoneal, the remainder is retroperitoneal, being covered only anteriorly by peritoneum. It is best demonstrated with a double contrast barium meal. It is described in four parts.

12.
ble contrast barium
al examination: right
erior oblique position,
nonstrating the
denal loop.

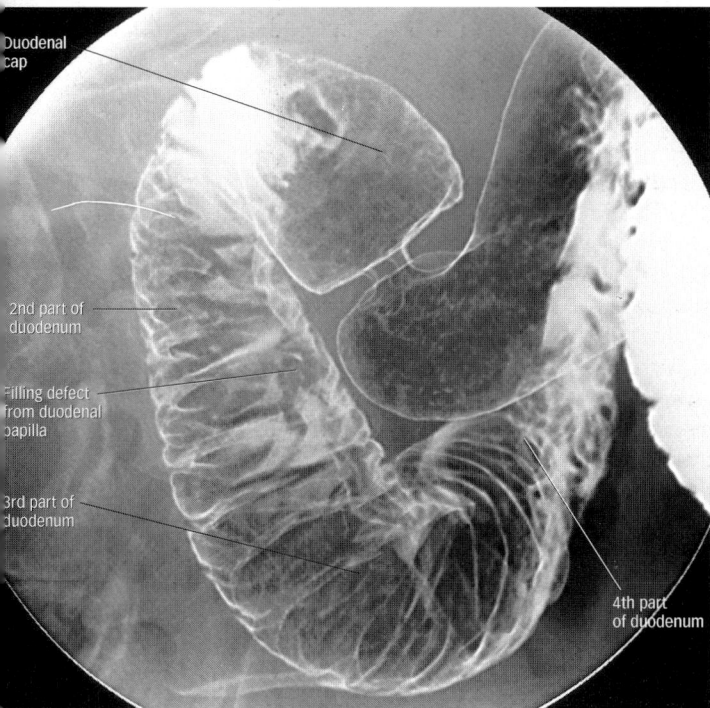

Duodenal
cap

2nd part of
duodenum

Filling defect
from duodenal
papilla

3rd part of
duodenum

4th part
of duodenum

The first part of the duodenum

This is continuous with the pylorus and is in the transpyloric plane at the level of the first lumbar vertebra. It is 5 cm long and runs from the pylorus upwards, backwards and to the right. The first 2 cm of the duodenum is known as the duodenal cap (duodenal bulb), which is slightly conical in shape. The duodenal cap resembles the pylorus in that it has the same rugal pattern and is intraperitoneal, lying between the folds of the greater and lesser omentum.

Anatomical relations of the first part

Anteriorly lie the quadrate lobe of the liver and the gall bladder (Fig. 13). Posteriorly, the lesser sac is related to the cap only. The gastro-duodenal artery runs inferiorly behind the first part. The bile duct runs posteriorly towards its opening in the second part. The portal vein is formed from the splenic vein and superior mesenteric vein and runs superiorly. The inferior vena cava lies behind this. Superiorly is the epiploic foramen (the opening of the lesser sac). Inferiorly lies the head of the pancreas.

Fig. 13.
Anatomical relations of the duodenum.

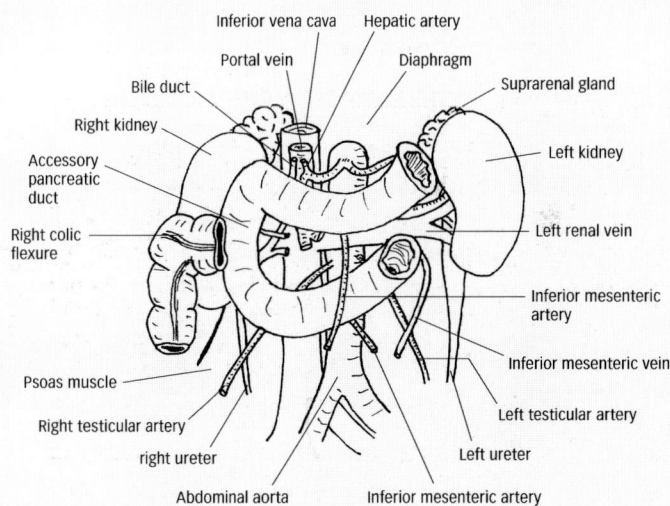

Inferior vena cava   Hepatic artery

Portal vein   Diaphragm

Bile duct

Right kidney   Suprarenal gland

Accessory   Left kidney
pancreatic
duct

Right colic   Left renal vein
flexure

                                          Inferior mesenteric
                                          artery

                                          Inferior mesenteric vein

Psoas muscle

Right testicular artery   Left testicular artery

right ureter   Left ureter

Abdominal aorta   Inferior mesenteric artery

The second part of the duodenum

This is 8 cm long. It runs inferiorly over the hilus of the right kidney and to the right of the second and third lumbar vertebrae. Postero-medially, at the junction of the upper two-thirds and lower one-third of the second part, is the duodenal papilla or ampulla of Vater. This is the opening of the bile and pancreatic ducts into the gut. The ducts usually have a common opening, but may be separate. There may also be an additional accessory duct from the pancreas which opens more proximally.

Anatomical relations of the second part

Anteriorly lie the fundus of the gallbladder and the right lobe of the liver (Fig. 7). The attachment of the transverse mesocolon crosses the midpoint of the second part. Loops of small intestine also lie anteriorly. Posteriorly is the hilus of the right kidney and the right ureter. Laterally are the ascending colon, the hepatic flexure and the right lobe of the liver. Medially is the head of the pancreas. The bile duct and pancreatic duct enter the duodenal papilla posteromedially.

The third part of the duodenum

This is 8 cm long. It crosses from right to left curving forward over the right psoas muscle, inferior vena cava and aorta, following the lower margin of the head of the pancreas.

Anatomical relations of the third part

Anteriorly, the superior mesenteric vessels exit from behind the neck of the pancreas to run over the duodenum. The third part is crossed by the root of the mesentery of the small bowel sloping down from the duodeno-jejunal flexure and loops of jejunum. Posteriorly, from right to left, are the right ureter and right psoas muscle, the inferior vena cava and aorta. Superiorly, the upper border of the third part hugs the lower border of the pancreas. Inferiorly are loops of jejunum.

The fourth part of the duodenum

This is 4 cm long. It runs upwards and to the left lying on the left psoas muscle. It ends by turning forward at the duodenojejunal junction, at the level of the second lumbar vertebra, where it is held in place by the ligament of Treitz, a peritoneal fold which ascends to the right crus of the diaphragm. This is an important landmark particularly when examining children as an abnormal position of the ligament of Treitz indicates malrotation.

Anatomical relations of the fourth part

Anteriorly, it is covered by coils of jejunum and the beginning of the root of the mesentery of the small bowel. Posteriorly, it runs along the left border of the aorta and the left psoas muscle.

Structure of the duodenum

The structure of the small intestine is generally similar throughout but there are certain regional differences. The mucous membrane of the first part of the duodenum is smooth but that of the rest of the small bowel is broken up into 'plicae circulares' or 'valvulae conniventes' which are circular folds which encircle two thirds of the inner mucosal wall. The plicae circulares become more prominent towards the distal duodenum.

The vascular supply of the duodenum

The duodenal cap is supplied by numerous small branches from the hepatic and gastroduodenal arteries. Venous blood drains into the prepyloric vein and thence the portal vein. The remainder of the duodenum is supplied by the superior and inferior pancreaticoduodenal arteries.

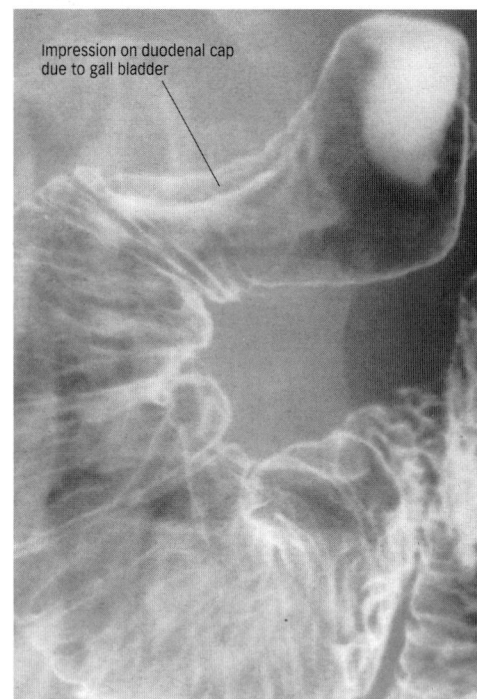

Impression on duodenal cap due to gall bladder

Fig. 14.
Double contrast barium meal examination: right anterior oblique position demonstrating impression of gall bladder on the duodenal cap.

Lymphatic drainage of the duodenum

This follows the arterial supply. The proximal duodenum is drained via the pancreatico-duodenal nodes to the gastroduodenal nodes and thus to the coeliac nodes. Distally, drainage is via the pancreatico-duodenal nodes to the superior mesenteric nodes around the origin of the superior mesenteric artery.

Radiological investigation of the duodenum

The duodenum is examined as part of the barium meal investigation. The appearance of the duodenal cap varies with body habitus of the patient. The gallbladder is often seen compressing the duodenal cap (Fig. 14). In about two-thirds of patients, the duodenal ampulla will either fill with barium or produce a filling defect, which can be quite prominent. Less frequently an accessory pancreatic duct opening is seen. The aorta can also impress the third part of the duodenum, particularly in thin patients. In children, the position of the ligament of Treitz is of the utmost importance in the diagnosis of malrotation. It should be demonstrated to the left of, and at the same level, or above, the first part of the duodenum.

The small intestine

The jejunum and ileum together are approximately 6.5 metres in length, the jejunum comprising the proximal two-fifths (Fig. 15). There are distinctive features to each, but there is a gradual transition from one to the other.

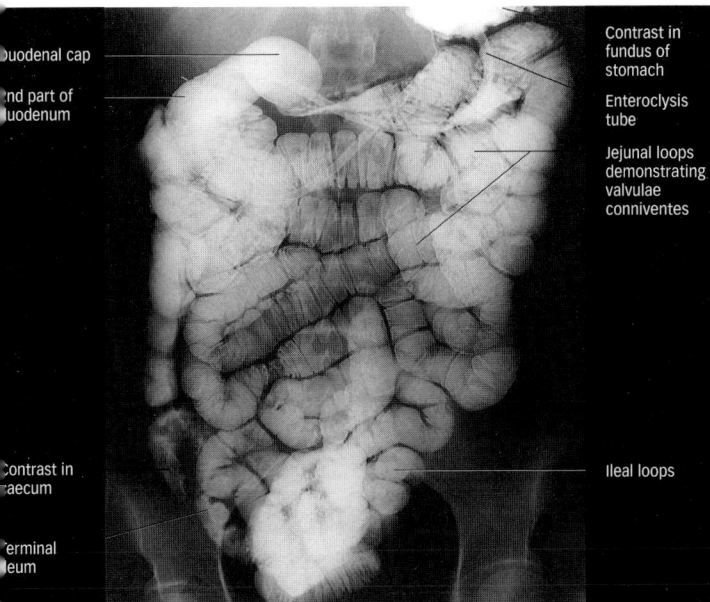

Duodenal cap

2nd part of duodenum

Contrast in fundus of stomach

Enteroclysis tube

Jejunal loops demonstrating valvulae conniventes

Contrast in caecum

Terminal ileum

Ileal loops

15.
Small bowel enema (enteroclysis) examination.

The small bowel begins at the duodeno-jejunal junction, and ends at the ileocaecal junction. A Meckel's diverticulum, a remnant of the embryological vitellointestinal duct, is present in 2% of the population. It is found in the ileum, 60 cm (two feet), from the caecum, and can vary in length from a small outpouching of the intestinal wall to 15 cm (six inches), long. Its blind end may contain gastric mucosa and occasionally liver or pancreatic tissue, (Fig. 16).

The small intestine is attached to the posterior abdominal wall by its own fan-shaped mesentery. The root of that mesentery is continuous with the parietal peritoneum of the posterior abdominal wall along a line running from the left of the second lumbar vertebra, to the region of the right sacroiliac joint. It measures approximately 15 cm. The root of the small bowel mesentery allows the passage of vessels, lymphatics and nerves between the two layers of peritoneum to supply the bowel. The long, free edge of the mesentery encloses the intestine.

Anatomical relations of the small bowel mesentery

Posteriorly, from left to right, lie the fourth part of the duodenum, the aorta, the inferior vena cava, the right gonadal vessels, the right ureter and psoas muscle.

The structure of the jejunum and ileum

As in the duodenum, the plicae circulares encompass two-thirds of the inner surface of the small bowel. They become less prominent and less numerous in the ileum until, at the terminal ileum, the folds are almost entirely absent.

Radiological differences between the jejunum and ileum

(a) The jejunum is situated principally in the upper abdomen, to the left of the midline, whereas the ileum is in the lower part of the abdomen and pelvis.

(b) The jejunum (2.5 cm in diameter) is wider than the ileum (2 cm).

(c) The plicae circulares are more numerous and deeper set in the jejunum than the ileum.

(d) The jejunal mesenteric vessels form only one or two arcades, with long and less frequent branches into the bowel wall. The ileum receives numerous short vessels arising from a series of three or four arcades.

Vascular supply of the small intestine

The small intestine is supplied by branches of the superior mesenteric artery – the jejunal, ileal and ileocolic arteries. Venous drainage of the small intestine follows the arterial supply to drain into the superior mesenteric vein.

Lymphatic drainage of the small intestine

Lymphatics drain to the superior mesenteric group of preaortic lymph nodes.

Radiological examination of the small bowel

The small bowel can be examined by the small bowel follow through or enema. These will

Fig. 16.
Meckel's scan after 60 minutes: anterior view, demonstrating uptake of 99 m technetium by the gastric mucosa of the stomach and Meckel's diverticulum. Activity is also seen in the bladder following excretion by the kidneys.

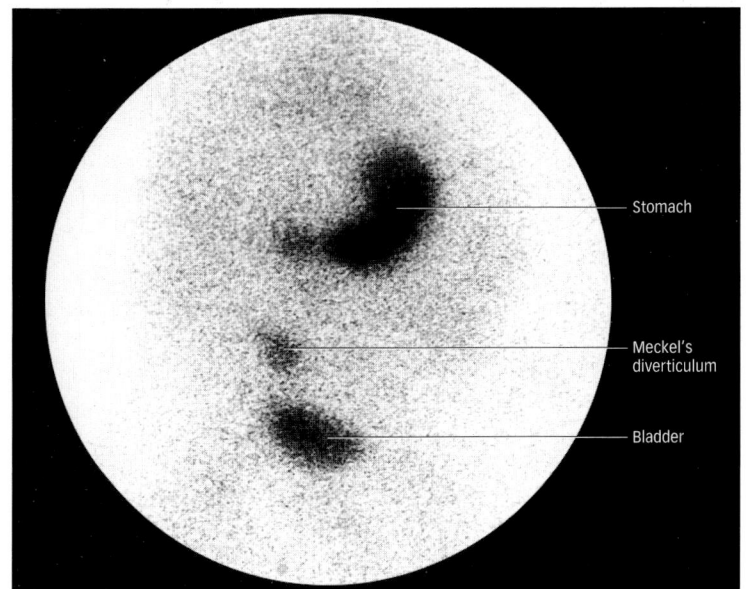

Stomach

Meckel's diverticulum

Bladder

provide information about small bowel calibre, its disposition, the wall thickness, and the distribution of the valvulae conniventes. The small bowel enema involves rapid infusion of a large continuous column of dilute contrast medium via a feeding tube placed in the first part of the jejunum. It gives better visualization of the bowel but is more time-consuming and can be more unpleasant for the patient than a follow-through. The small bowel enema distends the bowel and the calibre is increased to 4 cm in the jejunum, and 3 cm in the ileum. The differences between the jejunum and ileum as outlined above are well demonstrated.

Radionuclide investigation of the small bowel is used to detect occult bleeding (with [99m] Technetium-labelled colloid or red cells); to detect Meckel's diverticulum containing gastric mucosa ([99m] Technetium pertechnetate); or in the assessment of inflammatory bowel disease ([111] Indium or [99m] Technetium-labelled white blood cells).

Selective visceral angiography of the small bowel is used in the investigation of bleeding, where other examinations have failed to locate a cause. To detect small intestinal haemorrhage, angiography should be performed whilst the patient is actively bleeding at a rate of greater than 0.5 ml per minute. Angiography may also be of use in detecting a vascular malformation and in the investigation of mesenteric ischaemia.

The large intestine

The caecum

The caecum is a blind pouch of large intestine in the right iliac fossa, lying below the ileocaecal valve and thus proximal to the ascending colon. It is 6 cm long, mobile and easily distensible and is covered anteriorly and on both sides by peritoneum. The peritoneum is reflected upwards behind the caecum and is then downwards to the floor of the right iliac fossa. The presence of peritoneal folds around the caecum creates the superior ileocaecal, the inferior ileocaecal, and the retrocaecal fossae.

The appendix arises from the caecum medially, below the ileocaecal valve.

The ileocaecal valve (Fig. 17), marks the opening of the terminal ileum into the large bowel at the junction of the caecum and ascending colon. It consists of an upper and a lower fold which project into the large bowel. The valve plays a little part in the prevention of reflux from the caecum to the ileum, which is controlled by thickening of the distal part of the terminal ileum which acts as a physiological sphincter. The ileocaecal valve may be seen as a filling defect on a barium enema, which should not be mistaken for pathology.

Anatomical relations of the caecum

Anteriorly lie coils of small intestine, sometimes a part of the greater omentum and the anterior abdominal wall. Posteriorly are the psoas and iliacus muscles, the femoral nerve, and the lateral cutaneous nerve of the thigh (Fig. 18). The appendix is commonly retrocaecal. Medially the appendix arises from the caecum.

Vascular supply of the caecum

The arterial supply of the caecum consists of the anterior and posterior caecal arteries and

Fig. 17.
Double contrast barium enema: supine view, with reflux of barium suspension into the terminal ileum.

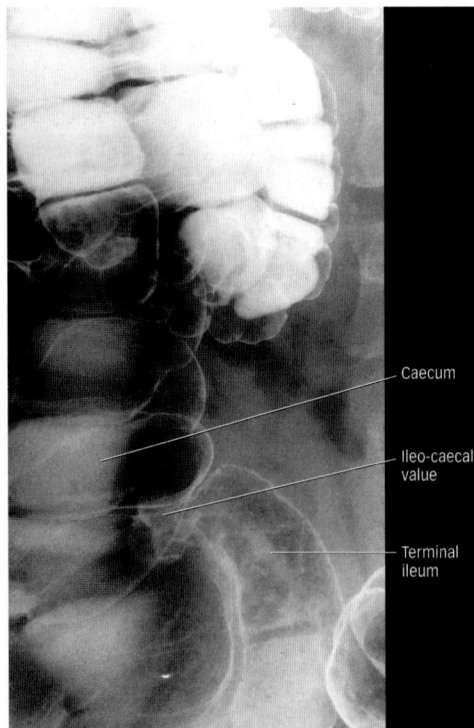

Fig. 18.
Posterior relations of the colon.

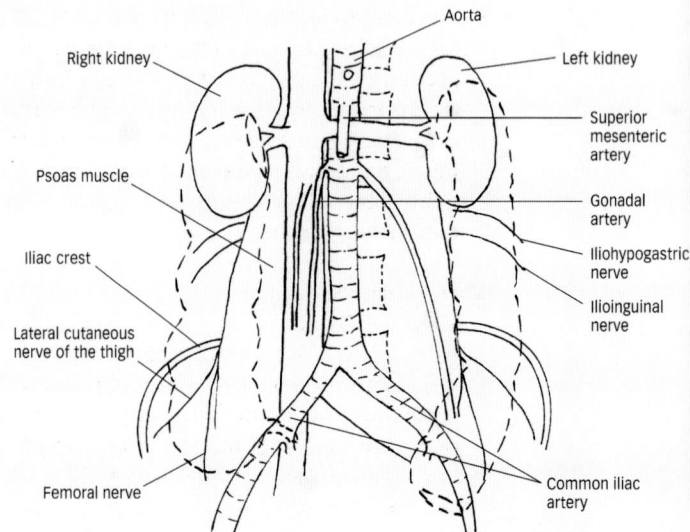

the terminal branches of the colic artery, which arises from the ileocolic artery. Veins corresponding to the arteries drain into the superior mesenteric vein.

Lymph drainage of the caecum
Lymph from caecum drains to the epicolic nodes, lying along the left side of the gut. These drain, in turn, to the paracolic nodes lying along the ileocolic and right colic arteries and thus to the superior mesenteric group of para-aortic nodes.

The appendix
The appendix is a long thin organ which contains lymphoid tissue. It is attached by its base to the posteromedial surface of the caecum, 2.5 cm below the ileocaecal junction. It is variable in length, but is usually about 5 cm long. It is attached to the meso-appendix, which is a peritoneal fold enclosing the appendicular vessels. The tip of the appendix lies in the region of the pelvic brim, but its position is variable. The appendix is most commonly encountered directed inferiorly into the pelvis against the right pelvic wall, or coiled in the retrocaecal fossa.

Vascular supply of the appendix
The appendicular artery is a branch of the posterior caecal artery and passes to the appendix in the mesoappendix. The appendicular vein joins the posterior caecal vein.

Lymphatic drainage of the appendix
Lymph nodes in the meso-appendix drain into the paracolic nodes lying along the ileocolic artery and thus to the superior mesenteric group.

Radiological examination of the appendix
Appendicoliths may be visible on the plain film in 7–15% of the normal population. In those patients with acute abdominal pain, their presence indicates a 90% chance of appendicitis. On ultrasound examination the appendix can be seen as a blindly ending tube arising from the posterior aspect of the caecum. The appendix will fill with barium during a barium enema if the lumen is patent but failure of the lumen to fill does not necessarily indicate disease.

The ascending colon
The ascending colon extends from the ileocaecal valve to the inferior surface of the liver where it turns to the left to become the hepatic flexure of the colon. It is about 15 cm long and is covered anteriorly and on both sides by peritoneum, which binds it to the posterior abdominal wall.

Anatomical relations of the ascending colon
Anteriorly lie the coils of small intestine, the greater omentum and the anterior abdominal wall (Fig. 18). Posteriorly are the iliac crest and the iliacus and quadratus lumborum muscles, and the origin of the transversus abdominis. The iliohypogastric and ilioinguinal nerves lie posteriorly as they cross quadratus lumborum. Laterally the peritoneum forms the paracolic gutter. Medially is the right infracolic gutter.

Arterial supply of the ascending colon
The arterial supply to the ascending colon arises from the ileocolic, right colic and middle colic branches of the superior mesenteric artery. Venous drainage is via corresponding veins which drain into the superior mesenteric vein.

Lymphatic drainage of the ascending colon
Drainage of lymph, of both the ascending colon and caecum, is into the epicolic nodes and to the superior mesenteric group of nodes.

The transverse colon
The transverse colon is approximately 45 cm long. It extends from the hepatic flexure just below the right lobe of the liver, passing upwards to the splenic flexure inferior towards the spleen. The splenic flexure is attached to the diaphragm by the phrenicocolic ligament. The transverse colon is completely invested in peritoneum. It is suspended by the transverse mesocolon and hangs down between the flexures to a variable extent, sometimes reaching the pelvis.

The greater curve of the stomach is attached to the transverse colon by the gastrocolic ligament. The greater omentum is a continuation of the gastrocolic ligament extending inferiorly from the lower convexity of the transverse colon.

Anatomical relations of the transverse colon
Anteriorly are the greater omentum and the anterior abdominal wall. Posteriorly lie the second part of the duodenum, the head of the pancreas, and the coils of small bowel (Fig. 18). The transverse mesocolon is attached from the inferior part of the right kidney, across the second part of the duodenum and pancreas to the inferior pole of the left kidney.

Vascular supply of the transverse colon
The proximal two-thirds of the transverse colon are supplied by the middle colic artery, a branch of the superior mesenteric artery. The distal third of the transverse colon is supplied by the ascending branch of the left colic artery, a branch of the inferior mesenteric artery. The veins draining the transverse colon follow the arterial supply and enter the superior and inferior mesenteric veins.

Lymphatic drainage of the transverse colon

Lymph drains into nodes lying along the course of the colic blood vessels and thence into the superior and inferior mesenteric nodes.

The descending colon

The descending colon is approximately 30 cm long. It extends from the splenic flexure to the pelvic brim where it continues as the sigmoid colon. It is covered on its front and sides by peritoneum, which binds it to the posterior abdominal wall.

Anatomical relations of the descending colon

Anteriorly lie the coils of small intestine, the greater omentum and the anterior abdominal wall. Posteriorly, from above down, the descending colon, which passes over the lateral border of the left kidney, the origin of the transversus abdominis muscle, the quadratus lumborum, the iliac crest and iliacus muscle and the left psoas muscle. The iliohypogastric and the ilioinguinal nerves, the lateral cutaneous nerve of the thigh and the femoral nerve also lie posteriorly.

Vascular supply of the descending colon

The descending colon is supplied by branches of the inferior mesenteric artery. The veins correspond to the arterial supply and drain into the inferior mesenteric vein.

Lymphatic drainage of the descending colon

Lymph drains into lymph nodes lying along the course of the colic blood vessels, and ultimately to the inferior mesenteric nodes at the origin of the inferior mesenteric artery at the level of the third lumbar vertebra.

The sigmoid colon

The sigmoid colon is that part of the colon which lies within the pelvis. It commences at the pelvic brim, and ends at the rectum where its peritoneal attachment also ends. It is subject to great variations in length, but is usually less than 45 cm.

The sigmoid colon is completely invested in peritoneum and is attached to the posterior pelvic wall by the fan-shaped sigmoid mesocolon. The root of the mesocolon is shaped like an inverted V. The left limb of the inverted V is medial to the left iliac vessels, and the right limb runs down in front of the sacrum to the level of the third sacral vertebra. The sigmoid vessels run between the layers of the sigmoid mesocolon.

Anatomical relations of the sigmoid mesocolon

Anteriorly, in the male, is the urinary bladder. In the female, the posterior surface of the uterus and upper part of the vagina lie anteriorly.

Posteriorly lie the rectum and sacrum, and lower coils of the terminal ileum.

Vascular supply of the sigmoid colon

The three or four sigmoid branches of the inferior mesenteric artery supply the sigmoid colon. The veins run alongside the arteries and drain into the inferior mesenteric vein. The marginal artery of Drummond is a single arterial trunk formed by the anastomosis of arteries around the 'inner' border of the colon.

Lymphatic drainage of the sigmoid colon

Lymph vessels drain to nodes along the course of the sigmoid arteries, and these drain to the inferior mesenteric nodes.

The structure of the colon

The large intestine, with the exception of the appendix and rectum, has three narrow bands, the taeniae coli, on its outer wall, which are formed by thickenings of the longitudinal muscle layer. The three taeniae lie anteriorly, posteromedially and posterolaterally, and converge on the appendix proximally and the rectum distally. The taeniae are shorter than the colon, and thus the wall of the colon is thrown into sacculations which give the appearance on radiographs of folds, or haustra.

The mucous membrane of the large intestine is thrown into irregular folds, which become smooth when the bowel is distended.

Small pieces of fat, known as the appendices epiploicae, are attached to the free surface of

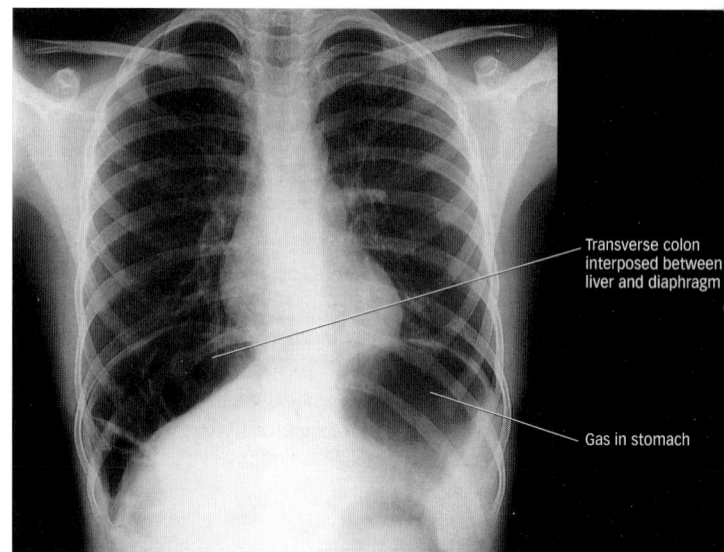

Transverse colon interposed between liver and diaphragm

Gas in stomach

the colon. Their function is unknown. They are sparse over the caecum and rectum, and most numerous over the sigmoid colon. They are supplied by arteries which perforate the muscle wall. Herniation of mucous membrane through the appendices epiploicae leads to formation of diverticula.

Fig. 19.
Erect chest radiograph in 8-year-old girl demonstrating Chilaiditi syndrome.

218

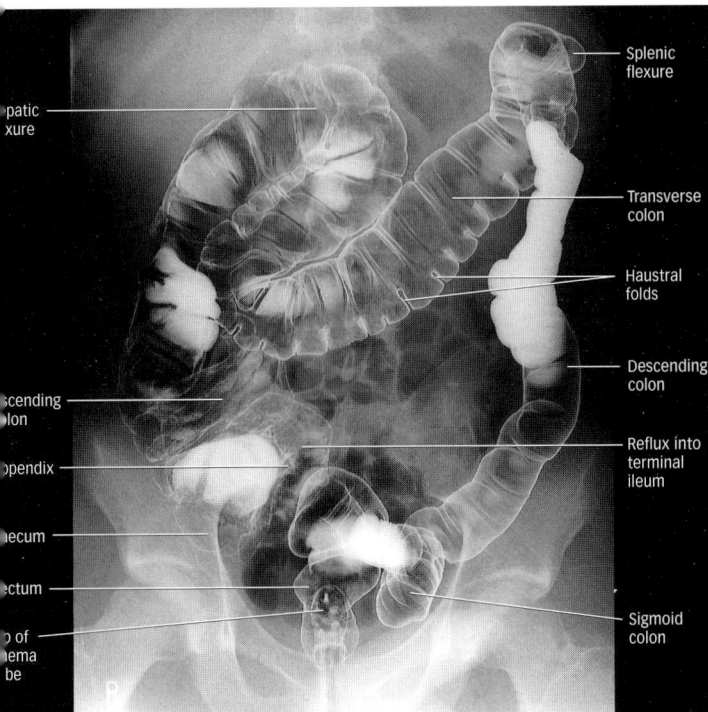

Splenic flexure

Transverse colon

Haustral folds

Descending colon

Reflux into terminal ileum

Sigmoid colon

patic xure

scending lon

ppendix

ecum

ctum

o of ema be

20.
ble contrast barium ma: supine film.

Radiological examination of the large intestine
Plain radiographs of the gas-filled large bowel demonstrate the haustral pattern of incomplete septations arising from the bowel wall (as compared with the valvulae conniventes of the small bowel, which are complete). The long mesentery of the transverse colon allows for considerable mobility in this region, and in some individuals this can lead to the interposition of the transverse colon between the liver and the diaphragm. Chilaiditi syndrome (Fig. 19), is generally an asymptomatic condition in which there is hepatodiaphragmatic interposition of intestine. It is regarded as a normal variant, but can mimic the appearance of free intraperitoneal gas and potentially lead to unnecessary laparotomy. The double contrast barium enema (Fig. 20), is the routine method of examination of the large bowel. When performed in an adequately prepared colon, with the use of a hypotonic agent such as hyoscine, it is an extremely sensitive method for the examination of anatomical and fine mucosal detail. Techniques for the performance of the barium enema vary, and the patient is moved in such a way as to demonstrate the various anatomical regions in double contrast. The rectum and sigmoid colon are well shown in the right anterior oblique, prone, left posterior oblique, and lateral positions. The splenic and hepatic flexures are best demonstrated upright in the left anterior oblique and right anterior oblique positions, respectively. The caecal pole can be shown in the left anterior oblique view, with the patient tilted slightly head down. A

varying number of overcouch films can also be taken, at the end of the examination, with the patient lying down to demonstrate all of the large bowel. The innominate grooves are seen as numerous thin parallel lines with short intercommunicating branches, and are a normal appearance which can be very pronounced in some patients (Fig. 21).

Ultrasound of the large bowel is used to identify appendicitis or pericolic abscesses. Some centres also use ultrasound in the investigation of bowel wall thickness, e.g. in patients with cystic fibrosis on pancreatic enzyme supplements. Angiography of the superior and inferior mesenteric vessels is used chiefly in the evaluation of acute bleeding. Radionuclide scanning is used in the investigation of bleeding or for the localization of inflammation as described for the small bowel.

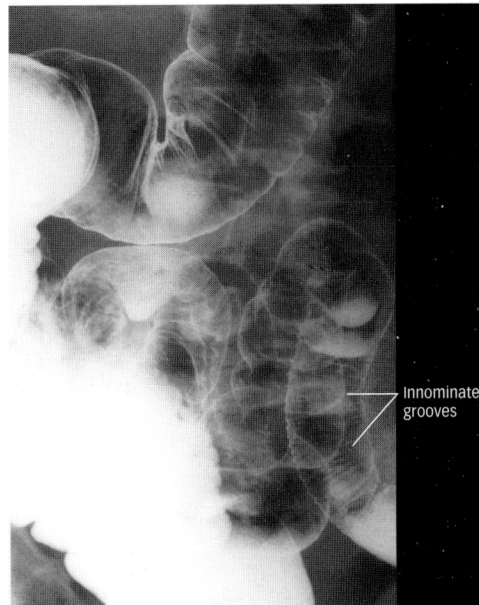

Innominate grooves

Fig. 21.
Double contrast barium enema examination showing prominent innominate grooves in the sigmoid colon (normal variant).

The rectum
The rectum is about 13 cm long, commencing at the level of the third sacral vertebra, and ending at the upper end of the anal canal (Fig. 22). The taeniae coli of the sigmoid colon join together over the rectum to invest it in a complete muscle coat. Thus, there are no haustra in the rectum.

There is no change in structure at the rectosigmoid junction, but the rectum, unlike the sigmoid, has no mesentery. The pelvic peritoneum of the posterior wall of the pouch of Douglas is draped over the upper part of the rectum. Thus the upper third of the rectum is covered in front and on both sides by peritoneum, the middle third in front only, and the lower third is uncovered. The lower part of the rectum, which lies on the pelvic diaphragm, is dilated to form the rectal ampulla. The upper

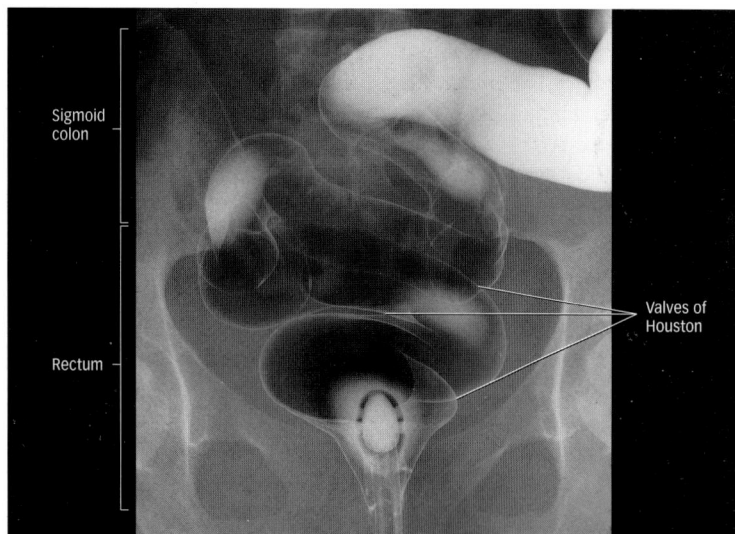

Fig. 22.
Double contrast barium enema: prone view of the rectum and sigmoid colon.

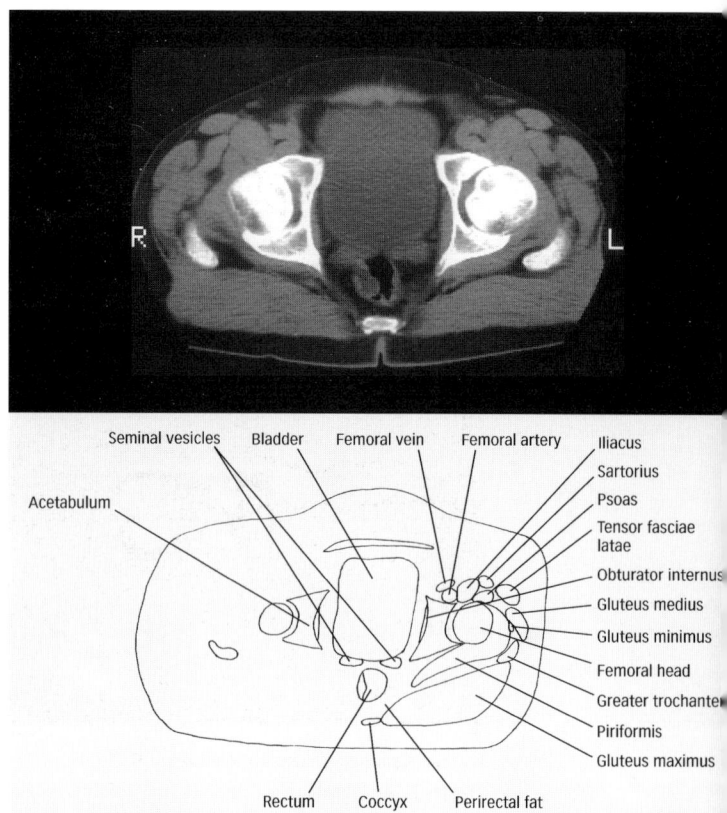

Fig. 23.
Axial CT through the male pelvis, demonstrating the relations of the rectum.

and lower parts of the rectum are in the midline, but the ampulla is convex to the left. This produces three lateral curves which are marked by horizontal shelves or valves (the valves of Houston). There are two valves to the left and one to the right between them. In the normal population, on the lateral view of the rectum, the postrectal space, between the levels of the third to the fifth sacral vertebrae, should measure less than 1.5 cm. However, this is subject to variation, and can be wider in large or obese individuals.

Anatomical relations of the rectum
Posteriorly, the rectum is in contact with the sacrum and coccyx, the piriformis, coccygeus, and levatores ani muscles, the sacral plexus and sympathetic trunks. Anteriorly, in the male (Fig. 23), the upper two-thirds of rectum are related to the sigmoid colon and coils of ileum. The lower third lies behind the posterior surface of the bladder, the termination of the vas deferens, the seminal vesicles on each side, and the prostate gland. These structures are invested in visceral pelvic fascia. In the female (Fig. 24), anteriorly is the rectouterine pouch (the pouch of Douglas), which contains the sigmoid colon, coils of ileum and often the ovaries, separating the rectum from the posterior aspect of the uterus. The lower third of the rectum is related to the vagina.

The vascular supply of the rectum
The superior rectal artery is the continuation of the inferior mesenteric artery. The middle rectal artery is a branch of the internal iliac artery and provides a further supply to the muscle wall of the rectum. The inferior rectal artery is a branch of the internal pudendal artery which anastomoses with the middle rectal artery at the anorectal junction. The median sacral artery, which is the attenuated

continuation of the abdominal aorta, supplies some small branches to the back of the rectum.

The veins of the rectum follow the arterial supply. The superior rectal vein is a tributary of the inferior mesenteric vein, which drains into the portal vein. The middle and inferior rectal veins drain into the internal iliac and internal pudendal veins, respectively, which drain to the systemic venous system. Thus, there is an important portosystemic anastomosis in this region.

Fig. 24.
Sagittal T1 weighted MRI female, demonstrating the relations of the rectum.

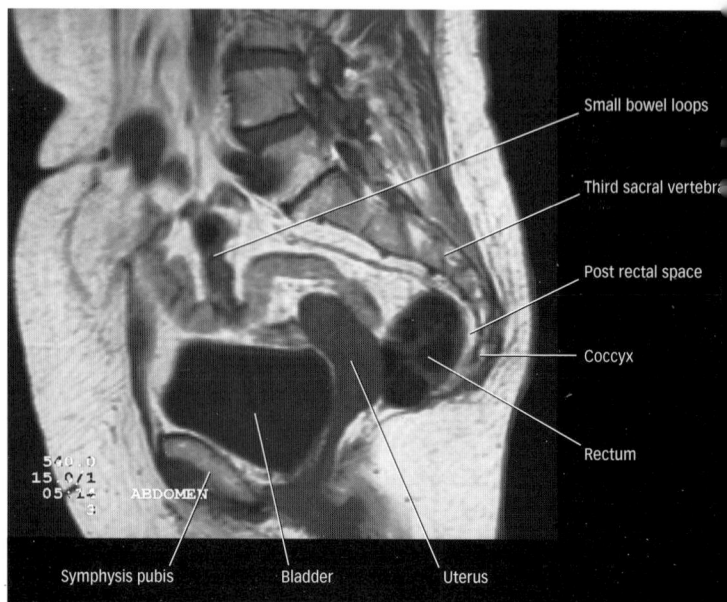

25.
Diagrammatic
presentation of the anal
canal and sphincters, (b)
coronal MRI of the anal
sphincters.

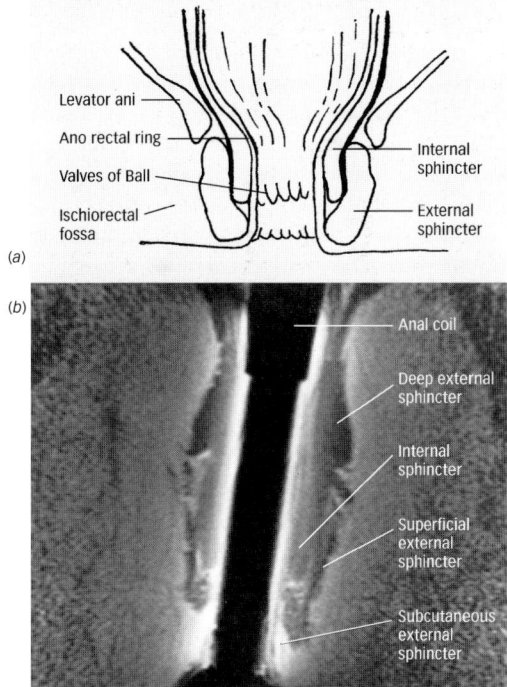

(a)

(b)

junction (Hilton's white line) is a watershed dividing upper and lower zones of arterial supply, venous and lymphatic drainage. The lining membrane of the anal canal has between six and ten vertical folds, which are the anal columns. These are flattened out when the canal is distended. The lower ends of the columns are joined together by folds which are known as the anal valves (the valves of Ball).

The anal sphincters consist of the internal (smooth muscle) and external (striated muscle) sphincters, which are always closed except during the passage of faeces or flatus. Each sphincter occupies two-thirds of the canal, so that they overlap in the middle third. The internal sphincter is under involuntary control, but is relatively weak and is not competent when acting alone. The internal sphincter is a thickening of the circular muscle of the gut wall which surrounds the submucosa in the upper two-thirds of the anal canal. It is usually elliptical in cross-section and is thicker anteriorly. At the lower border of the internal sphincter, the longitudinal muscle coat of the rectum passes inferiorly, medially and then superiorly as a fascial extension which inserts at Hilton's white line. This can be identified on MRI and is sometimes referred to as the musculus submucosa ani.

The lymphatic drainage of the rectum

Lymph drainage of the rectum is to the pararectal nodes, which are embedded in the perirectal connective tissue. Drainage follows the vascular supply, the upper two-thirds of the rectum draining to the inferior mesenteric nodes, and the lower two-thirds draining to the internal iliac nodes.

The anal canal

The anal canal is about 3 cm long, and is directed posteriorly at right angles to the rectum. It is a muscular tube which comprises the internal and external sphincters. The junction of rectum and anus is at the pelvic floor where the puborectal sling angles the anal canal forwards. From this point, the anal canal passes downward and backwards to the skin surface.

Anatomical relations of the anal canal

Posteriorly lies the anococcygeal body, which is a mass of fibrous tissue lying between the anal canal and the coccyx. Laterally are the fat-filled ischiorectal fossae. Anteriorly, in the male, are the perineal body, the urogenital diaphragm, the membranous part of the urethra, and the bulb of the penis.

In the female anteriorly, are the perineal body, the urogenital diaphragm, and the lower part of the vagina.

Structure of the anal canal

The anal canal is lined with mucous membrane in its upper two-thirds and skin in its lower one-third (Figs. 25 and 26). The mucocutaneous

Fig. 26.
T1W, axial MRI of the anal sphincters.

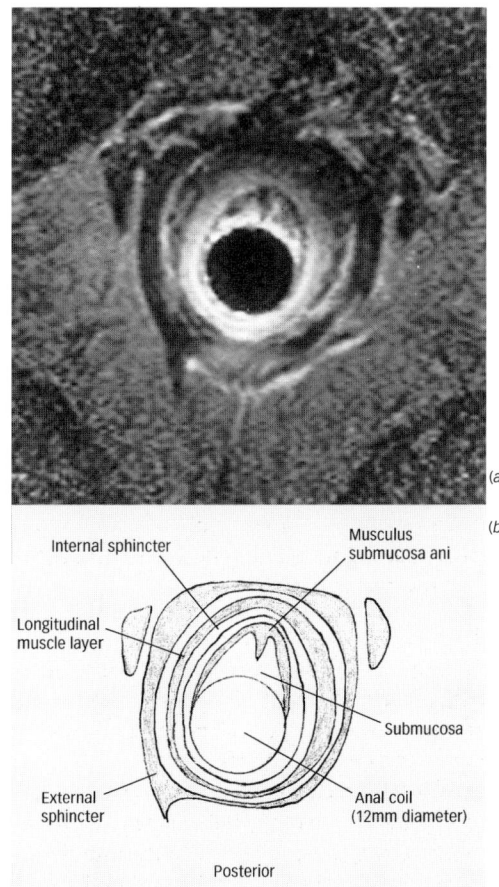

(a)

(b)

The external sphincter is under voluntary control and consists of striated muscle surrounding the lower two-thirds of the anal canal. It is composed of three parts: the subcutaneous, superficial and deep rings, which, however, are not clearly distinct and which are variable in appearance.

The subcutaneous external sphincter is a thick ring of muscle lying immediately beneath the skin. It is separated from the superficial external sphincter by fascia. The superficial external sphincter is the middle sphincter which attaches to the hip of the coccyx posteriorly and to the perineal body anteriorly.

The deep external sphincter is annular, encircling the lower part of the internal sphincter and blending posteriorly with the puborectalis muscle.

Vascular supply of the anal canal

The superior rectal artery supplies the upper part of the anal canal, and the inferior artery the lower half. The junction between these two halves (the mucocutaneous junction) marks the end of the hind gut.

The venous drainage follows the arterial supply, the superior rectal vein draining into the portal venous system, and the inferior rectal vein into the systemic venous system.

Lymphatic drainage of the anal canal

The lymph vessels from the upper half of the anal canal follow the superior rectal artery to drain into the inferior mesenteric nodes. The vessels from the lower half of the anal canal join the medial group of superficial inguinal nodes.

Radiological investigation of the rectum and anal canal

The rectum is examined as part of the double-contrast barium enema examination, but the anal canal is not well seen due to the position of the enema tube. Defaecation proctography studies the dynamics of rectal evacuation. Thick barium paste is injected into the rectum and a video recording is made of the voluntary evacuation of the paste. This provides information as to how rapidly the patient can evacuate and whether the sphincters relax completely. The position of the anorectal junction at rest, during evacuation and in recovery is also important. At rest, the junction is just above the level of the ischial tuberosities. During evacuation the pelvic floor descends about 30 mm and the anorectal angle widens from 90 to 115 degrees.

Magnetic resonance imaging is used increasingly in the investigation of the anal sphincters (Figs. 25, 26). MRI acquires images with superior soft tissue resolution to that gained with either ultrasound or CT. MRI is particularly useful in the investigation of patients with anal fistulae, the multiplanar capability giving valuable information to the surgeon with respect to the path of the fistulous track.

The structure of the anal canal can be demonstrated using MRI because of the different signal characteristics of the components.

The musculus submucosa ani has a low signal intensity and is readily discriminated from the high signal fat and submucosa. The internal sphincter has a high signal relative to the sphincter, on all sequences but particularly the T2W and STIR sequences. The subcutaneous fibres of the external sphincter have high signal components due to its proximity to the coil. The superficial and deep external sphincters are of low signal.

Vascular anatomy of the gastrointestinal tract

J. E. JACKSON

The vascular anatomy of the gastrointestinal tract is best demonstrated by direct catheterization of the coeliac axis and mesenteric arteries using a percutaneously placed catheter which is usually inserted via a transfemoral approach. While other less invasive imaging modalities such as ultrasound, computed tomography and, increasingly, magnetic resonance imaging are often used in order to demonstrate the abdominal vasculature, this section is devoted to the anatomy of the gastrointestinal tract as seen during catheter angiography.

Arteriographic techniques

Arteriographic images may be obtained using either cut film or digital subtraction techniques. Whilst cut film produces images of improved spatial resolution when compared with those obtained using digital subtraction equipment, this is generally offset by the advantages of the latter modality including improved contrast resolution (less contrast medium required, improved conspicuity of small vascular abnormalities) and the ability to review images immediately after their acquisition. The main disadvantage of DSA is the marked image degradation which occurs owing to movement, and this can be a particular problem in the abdomen because of bowel peristalsis and patient respiration. Bowel

Fig. 1.
Selective coeliac axis angiogram.

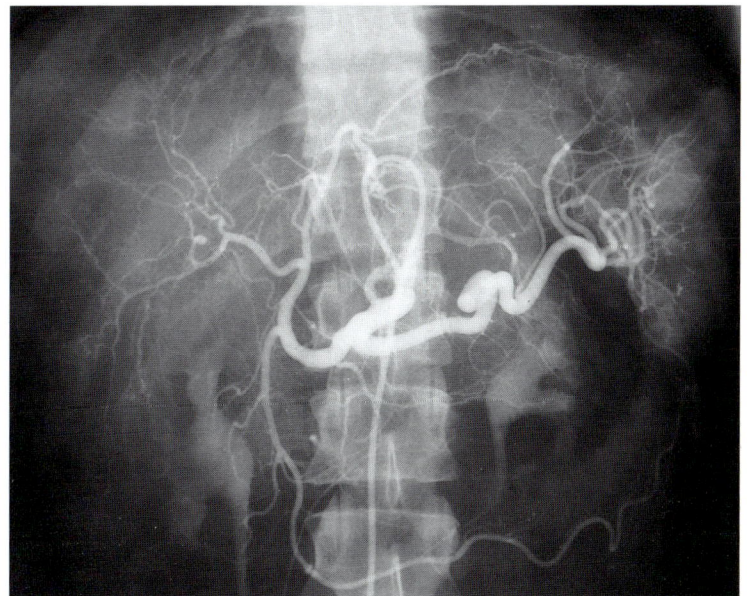

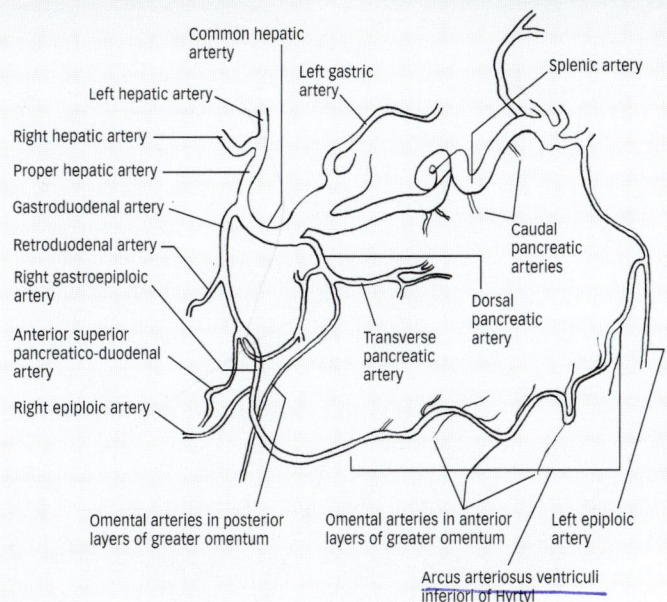

Common hepatic artery
Left gastric artery
Splenic artery
Left hepatic artery
Right hepatic artery
Proper hepatic artery
Gastroduodenal artery
Retroduodenal artery
Right gastroepiploic artery
Anterior superior pancreatico-duodenal artery
Right epiploic artery
Caudal pancreatic arteries
Dorsal pancreatic artery
Transverse pancreatic artery
Omental arteries in posterior layers of greater omentum
Omental arteries in anterior layers of greater omentum
Left epiploic artery
Arcus arteriosus ventriculi inferiori of Hyrtyl

223

(a)

Left gastric artery
Splenic artery
Common hepatic artery
Left hepatic artery
Gastroduodenal artery
Retroduodenal artery
Omental arteries
Left epiploic artery
Right epiploic artery
Right gastro-epiploic artery
Anterior superior pancreatico-duodenal artery
Arcus epiploicus magnus of Barkow

Cystic artery
Replaced right hepatic artery
Superior mesenteric artery
Dorsal pancreatic artery
First jejunal artery
Middle colic artery
Inferior pancreatico-duodenal arteries
Right colic/middle colic trunk
Right colic artery
Ileocolic artery

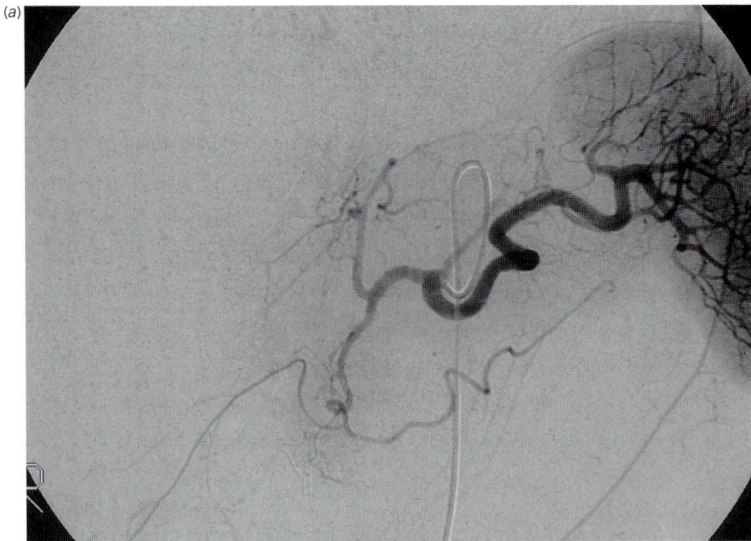

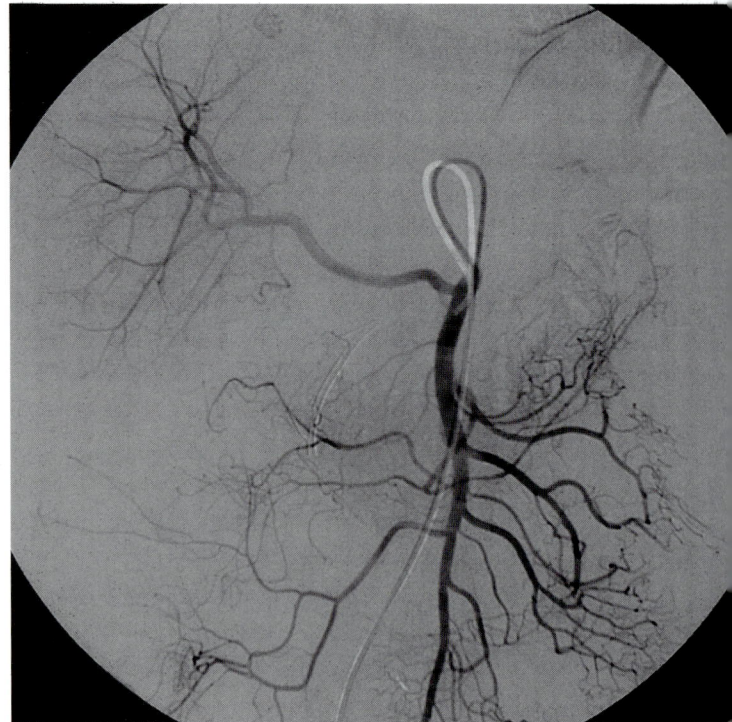

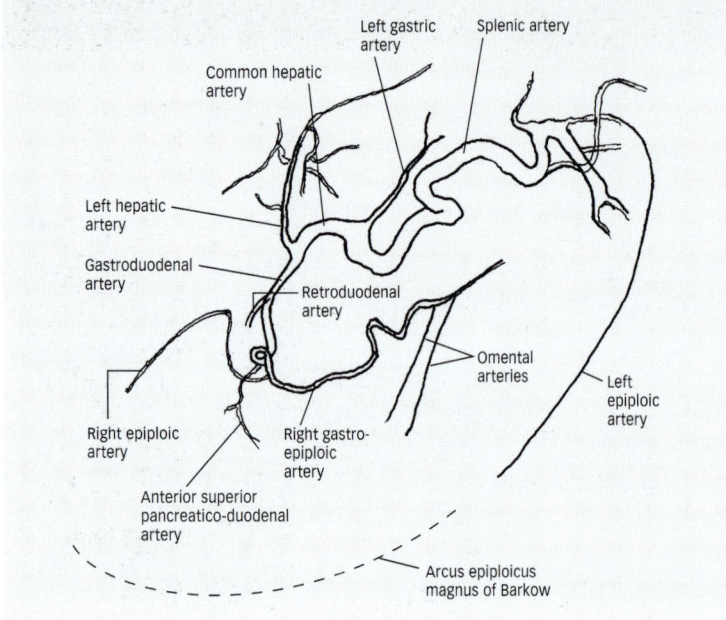

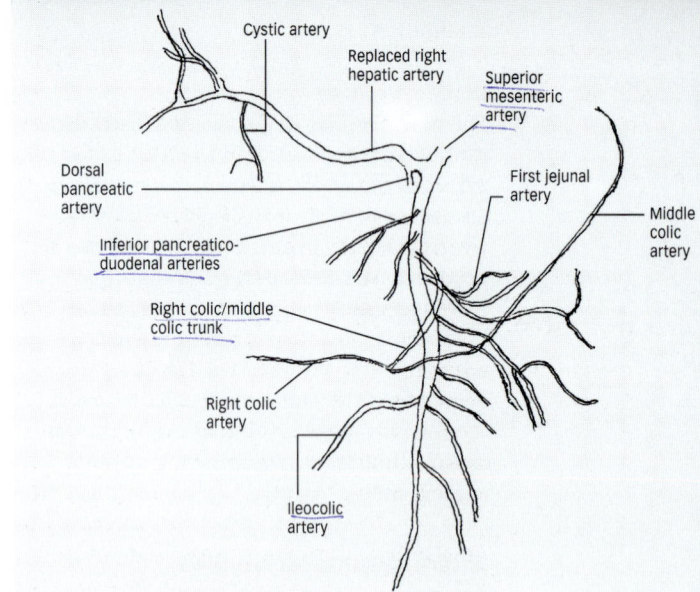

Fig. 2.
Variants of normal anatomy (a) coeliac axis angiogram; (b) Superior mesenteric angiogram demonstrating a replaced right hepatic artery.

movement can usually be obliterated, however, by the use of anti-peristaltic agents and patient movement, even in the most unco-operative individuals, can usually be overcome using a variety of techniques. These include continuous breathing during the angiographic 'run' with acquisition of multiple 'masks' before contrast medium injection so that a suitable mask exists for most of the subsequent images.

Arterial anatomy

Origins of coeliac and superior mesenteric arteries

The conventional anatomy of the coeliac axis is that of a single trunk which gives rise to the left gastric, splenic and common hepatic arteries (Fig. 1). The most common variant of normal anatomy, occurring in approximately 20% of individuals, is that in which a variable

amount of the liver is supplied by a branch arising from the proximal superior mesenteric artery (Fig. 2). A coeliacomesenteric trunk, in which the coeliac axis and superior mesenteric arteries arise from a common origin, is rare and is reported as occurring in 0.5% of individuals (Fig. 3). A lienohepatomesenteric trunk (common origin of the splenic, hepatic and superior mesenteric artery with the left gastric artery arising separately) is even less common, being seen in only 0.25% of persons.

The arc of Bühler is a large anastomotic channel between the proximal coeliac, common hepatic or splenic arteries and the proximal superior mesenteric artery and is

Fig. 3.
coeliacomesenteric trunk.

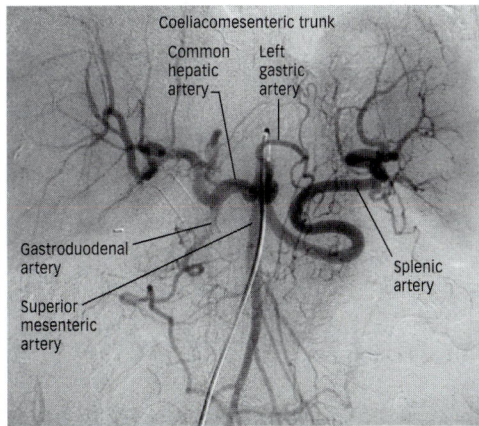

Coeliacomesenteric trunk

Common hepatic artery

Left gastric artery

Gastroduodenal artery

Superior mesenteric artery

Splenic artery

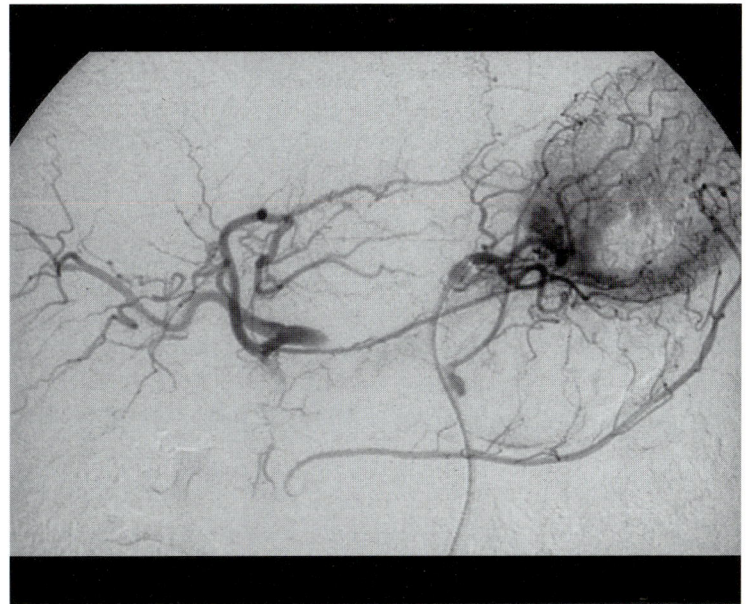

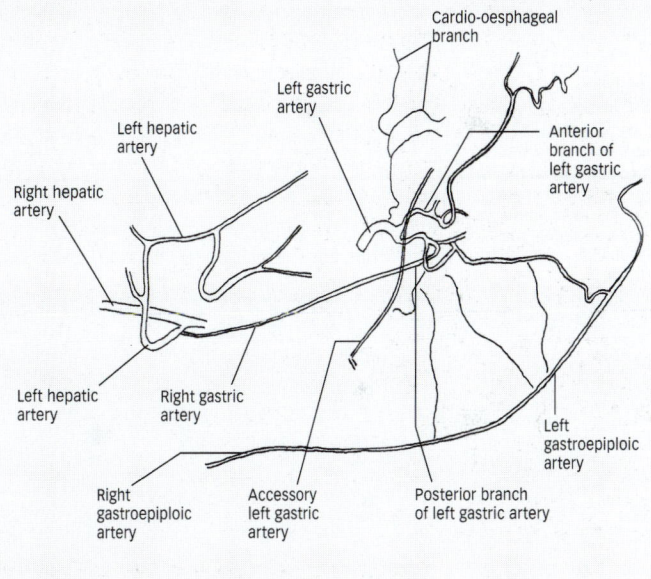

Cardio-oesophageal branch

Left gastric artery

Left hepatic artery

Anterior branch of left gastric artery

Right hepatic artery

Left hepatic artery

Right gastric artery

Right gastroepiploic artery

Accessory left gastric artery

Posterior branch of left gastric artery

Left gastroepiploic artery

reported as being present in 2% of individuals. It represents persistence of the embryonal ventral longitudinal anastomosis and may be difficult to differentiate on angiography from an hypertrophied dorsal pancreatic artery, a vessel which may form a similar anastomotic communication between the same vessels (see below).

Coeliac trunk

The coeliac axis arises from the anterior aspect of the aorta at a level between T12 and L1 (Figs. 1, 2, 3, 7 and 8). Its initial course is usually caudad, although it may pass directly horizontally or superiorly. It lies above the pancreas and splenic vein and below the left lobe of the liver. On its left is the cardia of the stomach and in front is the lesser omentum.

In a significant minority of individuals, it is compressed to a variable extent in its proximal portion by the median arcuate ligament of the diaphragm. This may be of sufficient severity to reduce, or even obstruct, antegrade flow with the subsequent enlargement of collateral vessels arising from the superior (Fig. 6), and occasionally inferior, mesenteric arteries. The vessels most commonly involved in this collateral circulation are those making up the pancreatico-duodenal arcade (see below) although the dorsal pancreatic, transverse pancreatic and middle colic vessels will often contribute (and may constitute the principal supply), in some individuals (Fig. 6).

The coeliac trunk conventionally divides after 1–2 cm into the left gastric (usually the first branch), splenic and common hepatic arteries (Fig. 1) and this pattern is seen in 65–75% of individuals. In the remainder, one or more of these vessels has a variant origin (see below).

Left gastric artery

This is usually the first and smallest branch of the coeliac axis and arises from its superior

aspect; in 3% it arises directly from the aorta (Figs. 1, 2, 3, 4 and 8). It courses upwards and to the left towards the gastric cardia, running close to the inferior phrenic artery and medial and anterior to the left suprarenal gland. At the cardia it divides into several branches, which supply the anterior and posterior gastric surfaces. One of these turns sharply downwards to follow the lesser curvature towards the pylorus and usually anastomoses with the terminal branches of the right gastric artery (Figs. 4 and 8). One to three small cardio-oesophageal arteries may arise from the main trunk (Fig. 4) or its divisions. Peripheral branches of the left gastric artery anastomose with branches of the short gastric arteries arising from the splenic artery, with branches of the gastroepiploic arteries (see Fig. 4) and with

Fig. 4.
A selective left gastric arteriogram.

cardio-oesophageal branches arising from the inferior phrenic artery.

In 25% of individuals, part or all of the left lobe of the liver is supplied by an aberrant left hepatic artery arising from the left gastric artery (Fig. 8).

Splenic artery

This is the largest branch of the coeliac axis (Figs. 1, 2, 3, 5, 6, 7 and 8). It is often very tortuous, measuring between 13 and 32 cm in length, and courses along the superior aspect of the pancreas above the splenic vein to supply the spleen. At first, it lies retroperitoneally behind the omental bursa, but it enters the lienorenal ligament before entering the spleen.

The dorsal pancreatic artery (Figs, 1, 2(*b*), 5, 7 and 11) most commonly arises from the proximal part of the splenic artery, although it may originate from the hepatic, superior mesenteric or coeliac arteries. It lies behind the junction of the splenic and superior mesenteric veins and supplies branches to the posterior surface of the pancreas. It gives off a single branch to the left, the transverse pancreatic artery (Figs. 1, 5, 6 and 11), which supplies the pancreatic body and tail and from which posterior epiploic arteries arise, which descend in the posterior layers of the greater omentum (Fig. 1). Two branches arise from the right side of the dorsal

pancreatic artery to supply the pancreatic head, one of which communicates with branches of the anterior superior pancreatico-duodenal, gastroduodenal or the right gastroepiploic artery, and the other of which supplies the uncinate process of the pancreas. A fourth branch of the dorsal pancreatic artery will often descend and communicate with the superior mesenteric, middle colic or accessory middle colic artery (Fig. 5). Rarely, a proximal jejunal artery will arise from the dorsal pancreatic artery.

The arteria pancreatica magna (Figs. 6 and 8) is usually the largest branch to the body of the pancreas. It arises from the mid-portion of the splenic artery and passes through the substance of the pancreas behind the pancreatic duct, where it divides into several branches which usually, but not invariably, anastomose with the transverse pancreatic and caudal pancreatic arteries (Fig. 6). *[greater pancreatic artery.]*

The caudal pancreatic arteries (Figs. 1 and 6), which are often multiple, arise from the distal portion of the main splenic artery or from its terminal branches, and supply the pancreatic tail, where they anastomose with branches of the arteria pancreatica magna and transverse pancreatic arteries (Fig. 6). In addition, the splenic artery provides several short pancreatic arteries to the body and tail along its course.

Fig. 5.
Selective dorsal pancreatic artery angiogram, demonstrating anastomoses between the superior mesenteric and middle colic arteries. ASPD, anterior superior pancreatico-duodenal artery.

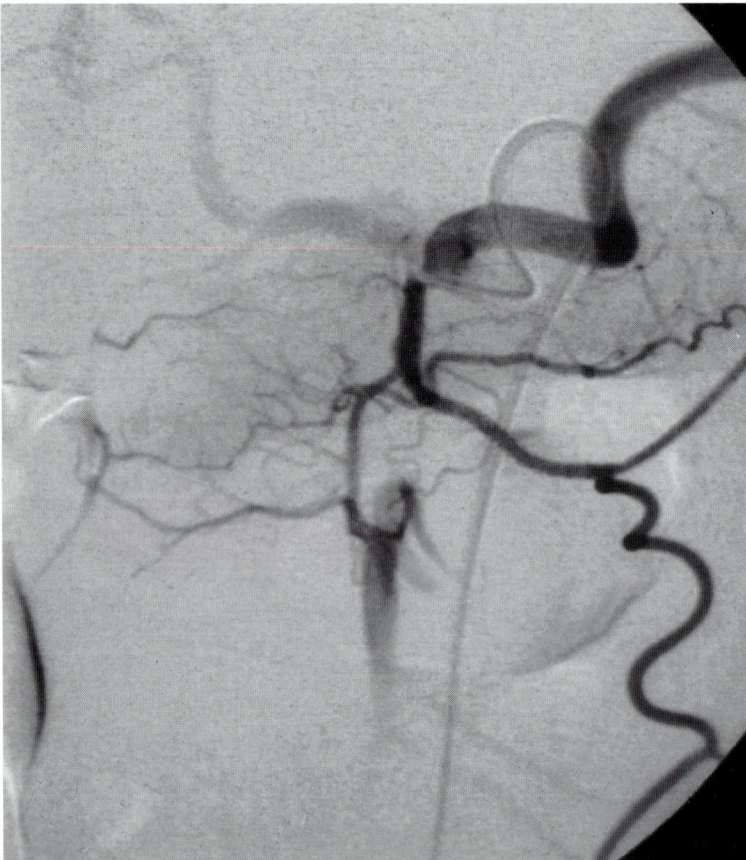

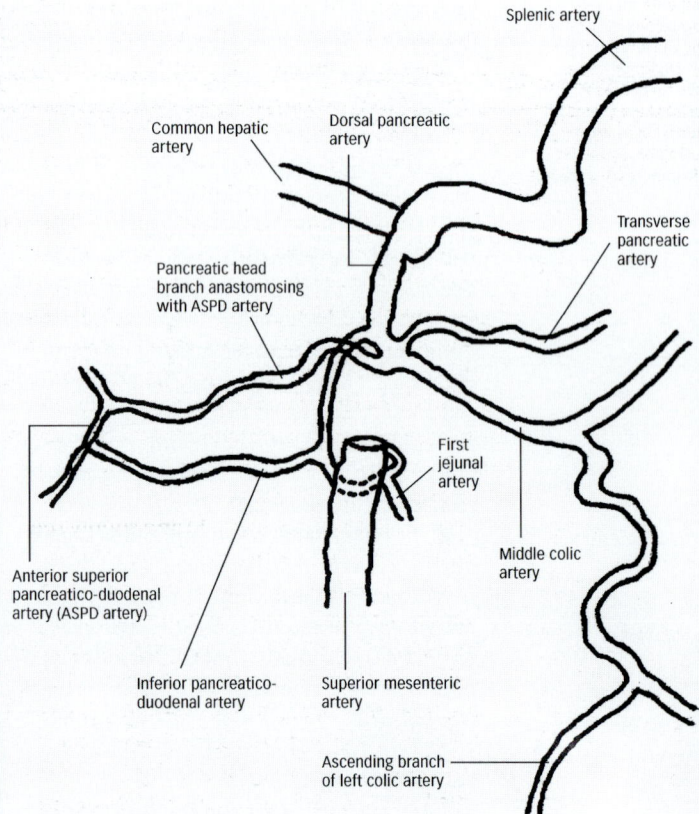

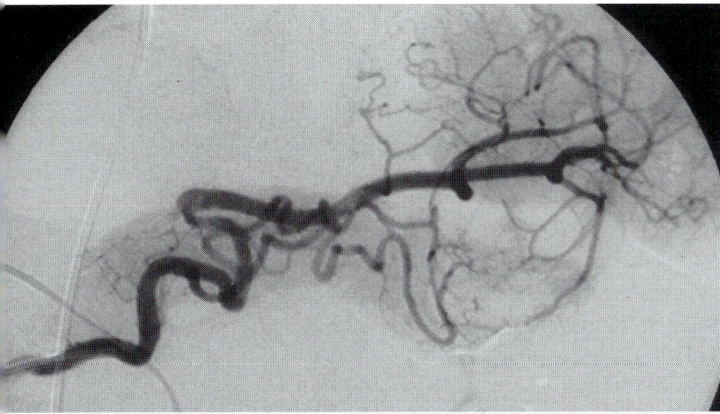

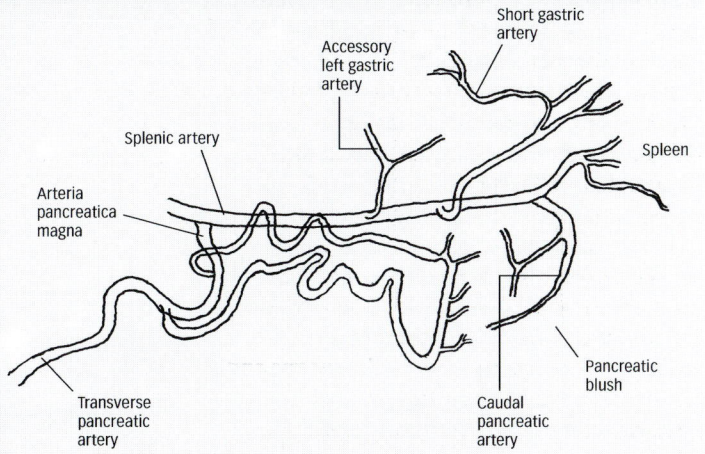

Fig. 6.
Selective transverse pancreatic arteriogram in a patient with marked compression of the coeliac axis by the left median arcuate ligament. The transverse pancreatic artery has hypertrophied to provide a collateral supply to the splenic artery via the arteria pancreatica magna.

main splenic artery, and this branch will often be of larger calibre than the short gastric arteries.

The splenic artery divides at the splenic hilum into superior and inferior, and occasionally middle, terminal arteries, each of which then subdivides into between four and six intrasplenic arteries. The superior terminal arteries are usually longer and tend to supply a greater proportion of the spleen. Not infrequently, superior and inferior polar arteries are present; a superior polar artery is seen in 65% of individuals and usually arises from the distal splenic artery and less frequently from the superior terminal artery. Occasionally, it will arise from the proximal splenic artery. An inferior polar artery is present in 82% and usually arises from the left gastroepiploic artery or from the distal splenic or inferior terminal artery.

The left gastroepiploic artery (Figs. 1, 4 and 7) also arises from the terminal portion of the main splenic artery or from one of its terminal branches. It descends in the anterior divisions of the greater omentum along the greater curvature of the stomach, where it usually anastomoses with the right gastroepiploic artery to form the arcus arteriosus ventriculi inferiori of Hyrtl (Fig. 1). The left epiploic artery (Figs. 1, 2(a) and 8) is a branch of the left gastroepiploic artery which anastomoses with the right epiploic artery to form the arcus epiploicus magnus of Barkow (see Fig. 2(a)), which is located in the posterior layers of the greater omentum below the transverse colon. The left epiploic artery is commonly larger and hence more visible on arteriography than the left gastroepiploic artery.

Between four and ten short gastric arteries originate from the distal splenic artery or from its terminal branches (Fig. 6) and supply the cardia and fundus of the stomach. These are often difficult to appreciate on splenic arteriograms because of the overlying intrasplenic branches and the splenic parenchymal blush. They may, however, become obvious in the presence of a hiatus hernia, when they are seen to be pulled up with the herniated stomach through the oesophageal opening.

An accessory left gastric artery (Figs. 4 and 6), may arise from the mid or distal portion of the

Fig. 7.
Coeliac axis angiogram. Separate origins of the right and left hepatic arteries from the coeliac axis. The gastroduodenal artery arises from the left hepatic artery.

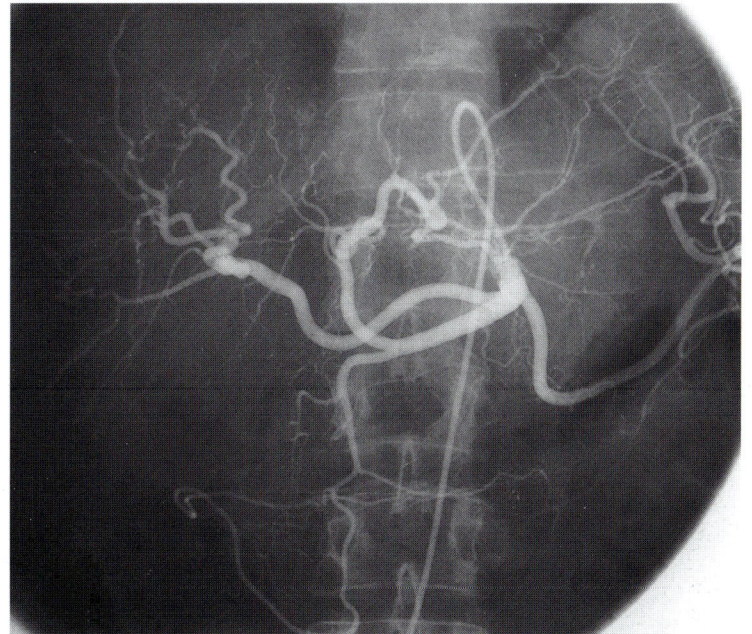

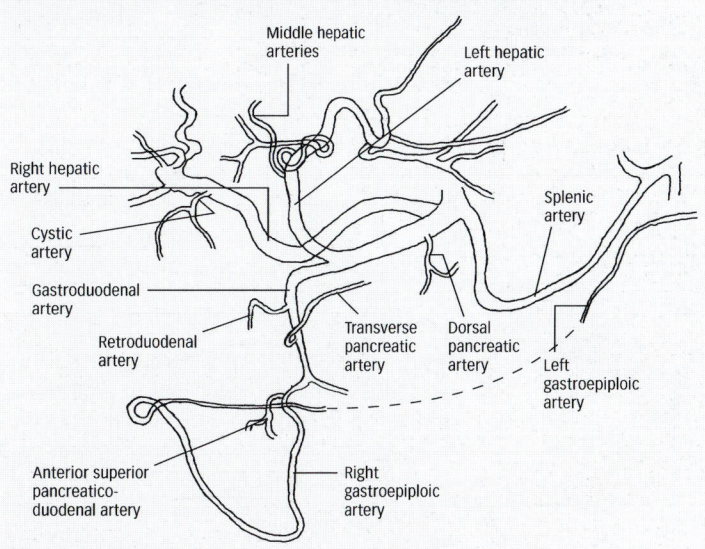

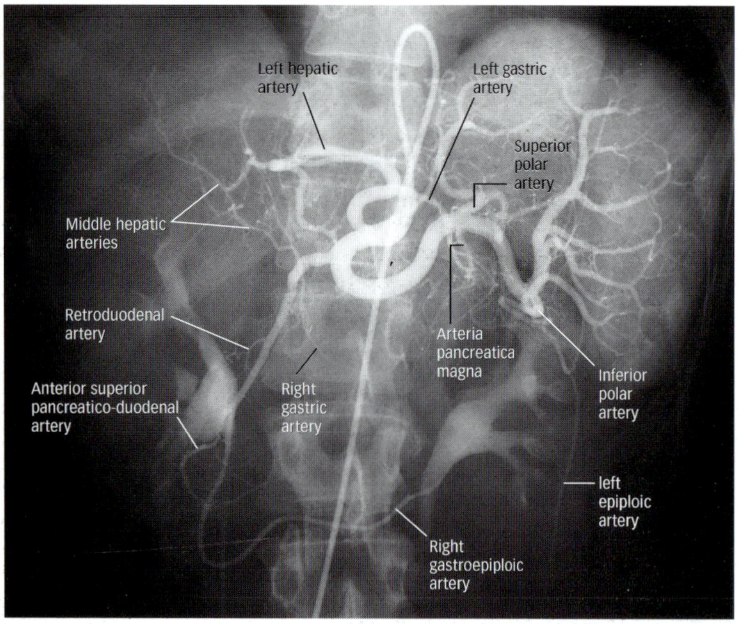

Fig. 8.
Coeliac axis angiogram. The left hepatic artery arises from the left gastric artery. Note the typical hairpin configuration of the anomalous left hepatic artery. Note the middle hepatic artery arising from the gastroduodenal artery.

Labels in figure:
Left hepatic artery
Left gastric artery
Superior polar artery
Middle hepatic arteries
Retroduodenal artery
Arteria pancreatica magna
Inferior polar artery
Anterior superior pancreatico-duodenal artery
Right gastric artery
left epiploic artery
Right gastroepiploic artery

Hepatic arteries

In conventional anatomy the common hepatic artery arises from the coeliac axis (Fig. 4). It initially runs along the upper border of the pancreatic head behind the posterior layer of the peritoneum of the omental bursa. At the upper margin of the duodenum, it passes anteriorly in the right hepatopancreatic fold and then ascends in the hepatoduodenal ligament at the right border of the lesser omentum towards the liver hilum immediately to the left of the common bile and common hepatic ducts and anterior to the portal vein. Its first major branch is usually the gastroduodenal artery, after which it continues as the proper hepatic artery before dividing into right, middle and left hepatic arteries.

The right hepatic artery crosses the common hepatic duct posteriorly in most individuals although it may rarely pass anteriorly; compression of the common duct by this vessel may sometimes be seen on cholangiography. It characteristically loops inferiorly in the cystohepatic angle, sometimes to such an extent that it reaches the cystic duct, where it may be injured during surgery. It then divides within the liver substance into an anterior segmental artery supplying segments V and VIII, and a posterior segmental artery, which supplies segments VI and VII. The anterior segmental artery often has a typical caterpillar loop configuration. The posterior segmental branch lies superior to the anterior branch and frequently provides a branch to the caudate lobe and the gallbladder.

The middle hepatic artery arises from the right and left hepatic arteries in equal proportions (45%), or from the proper hepatic, gastro-

duodenal or coeliac arteries (10%) (Fig. 8), and supplies the medial segment of the left lobe of the liver (segment IV or quadrate lobe). It may occasionally contribute a supply to the caudate lobe.

The left hepatic artery supplies the lateral segments of the left lobe of the liver and may contribute a supply to segment IV. It enters the left lobe of the liver inferior to the left portal vein and then courses upwards in the fossa for the ligamentum venosum, where it divides to supply the left lobe segments.

The 'conventional' hepatic arterial supply as described above occurs in just over half of all individuals; in the remainder, one of a number of variants exists (Figs. 2, 7, and 8). In approximately 20% of persons all, or part, of the hepatic arterial supply will arise from the superior mesenteric artery (Fig. 2). Of these, 10–12% will be replaced by right hepatic arteries (no right hepatic arterial supply arising from the coeliac axis), and 4–6% will be accessory (additional right hepatic arterial supply from coeliac axis). In 2.5%, the entire hepatic arterial supply will arise from the superior mesenteric artery. A replaced or accessory hepatic artery courses upwards to the right either behind or through the head of the pancreas before passing between the layers of the lesser omentum in the hepatoduodenal ligament, where it lies posterior to the portal vein.

In approximately 25% of persons, all or part of the left hepatic arterial supply arises in equal proportions from the left gastric artery (Fig. 8). A typical 'hairpin' configuration of the left hepatic artery is seen in this situation. Very rarely, the entire hepatic arterial supply arises from the left gastric artery. In 2%, the common hepatic artery has a separate origin from the aorta.

Cystic artery

This vessel typically (45%) arises from the right hepatic artery to the right of, and posterior to, the common hepatic duct (Figs. 2(b) and 7). In 20%, it originates from the common hepatic, left hepatic, middle hepatic, gastroduodenal or retroduodenal artery. Upon reaching the gall bladder the cystic artery divides into superficial and deep branches, the former distributed to the peritoneal and the latter to the non-peritoneal surface of the gallbladder. In 20%, there are two cystic arteries, which may arise from the same or different vessels.

Right gastric artery

This is usually a small vessel arising from the proper or left hepatic arteries in about equal proportions (40%) (Figs. 4 and 8). It may occasionally arise from the gastroduodenal or middle or right hepatic arteries. It descends to the pylorus, which it supplies, and courses along the lesser curvature of the stomach where it anastomoses with the left gastric artery. It frequently gives origin to the supraduodenal artery of Wilkie (which may alternatively arise from the retroduodenal or gastroduodenal arteries), which supplies the first inch of the duodenum.

Gastroduodenal artery (GDA)

The GDA most commonly arises from the common hepatic artery (75%) almost always before the division of the hepatic artery into right and left branches (Figs. 1, 3 and 9). The proper hepatic artery beyond the origin of the GDA is of variable length and may be absent altogether when the GDA and right and left hepatic arteries form a trifurcation. Other sites of origin include the left hepatic artery (4–11%), (Figs. 2 and 7), right hepatic artery (7%), or superior mesenteric artery via a replaced hepatic trunk (4–11%). When there are separate origins of the left and right hepatic arteries, the GDA will usually arise from that branch supplying the left lobe of the liver (Figs. 2 and 7) but this is not invariable.

The proximal GDA descends behind the first portion of the duodenum, anterior to the pancreas and to the left of the common bile duct. Erosion of the posterior wall of the duodenum, by an ulcer, can produce torrential and life-threatening haemorrhage if the GDA is involved. It then courses to the left, and at the lower bor-

der of the pancreas divides into its terminal branches, the right gastroepiploic and anterior superior pancreatico-duodenal arteries.

The first branch of the GDA is the retroduodenal artery (posterior superior pancreatico-duodenal artery) which arises 1–2 cm from its origin above the duodenum and pancreatic head (Figs. 1, 2, 7, 8 and 9). Here, it gives rise to the blood supply to the common duct. It then descends along the left side of the common duct, crosses its supraduodenal portion anteriorly (occasionally posteriorly), and then runs along its right side. At about the middle portion of the posterior surface of the pancreatic head, it anastomoses with the posterior inferior pancreatico-duodenal artery. Branches of the resulting arcade supply the posterior surface of the entire duodenum and part of the pancreatic head. A frequent branch of the retroduodenal artery (50%) or the proximal GDA (25%) is the supraduodenal artery of Wilkie (Fig. 9), which supplies both the anterior and posterior surfaces of the first part of the duodenum. The supraduodenal artery may also arise from the common hepatic, proper hepatic, right hepatic or the right gastric arteries. It is a small vessel, which is often difficult to appreciate on angiography.

The anterior superior pancreatico-duodenal artery arises as one of the terminal branches of the GDA behind the first part of the duodenum (Figs. 1, 2, 8 and 9). It supplies the gastric pylorus and then courses between the second part of the duodenum and the pancreatic head. Its distal portion enters the pancreas and, on emerging from the pancreatic head,

...tomy of pancreatico-
...denal arcade. Note the
...mon trunk of the
...rior pancreatico-
...denal arcade arising
...n the main trunk of the
...erior mesenteric artery.
...hermore, there is a
...ll anastomotic arcade
...ween the anterior
...rior pancreatico-
...denal artery and the
...jejunal artery. This is
...of the potential 'weak
...its' in the marginal
...ry of the small bowel
...en such an anastomosis
...osent. Note the
...sence of three
...creatico-duodenal
...des. AIPD, anterior
...rior pancreatico-
...denal artery.

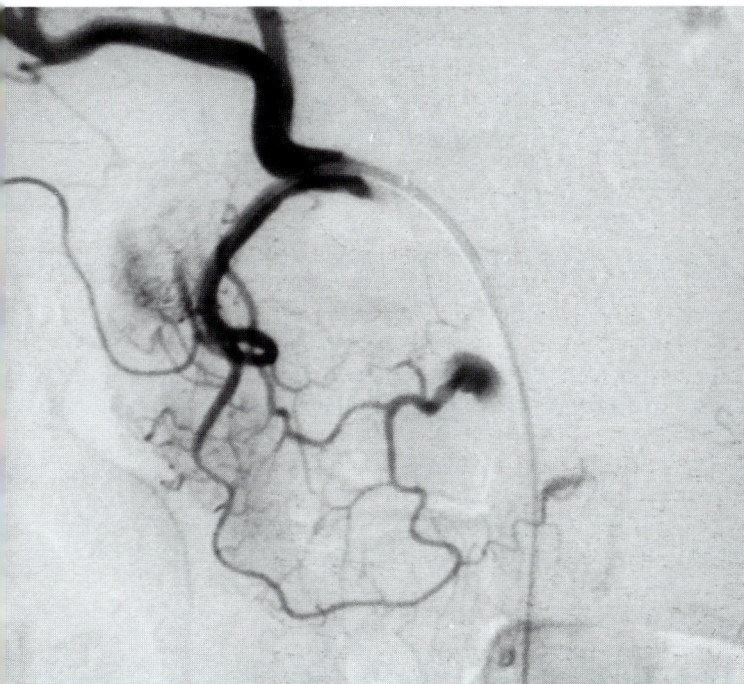

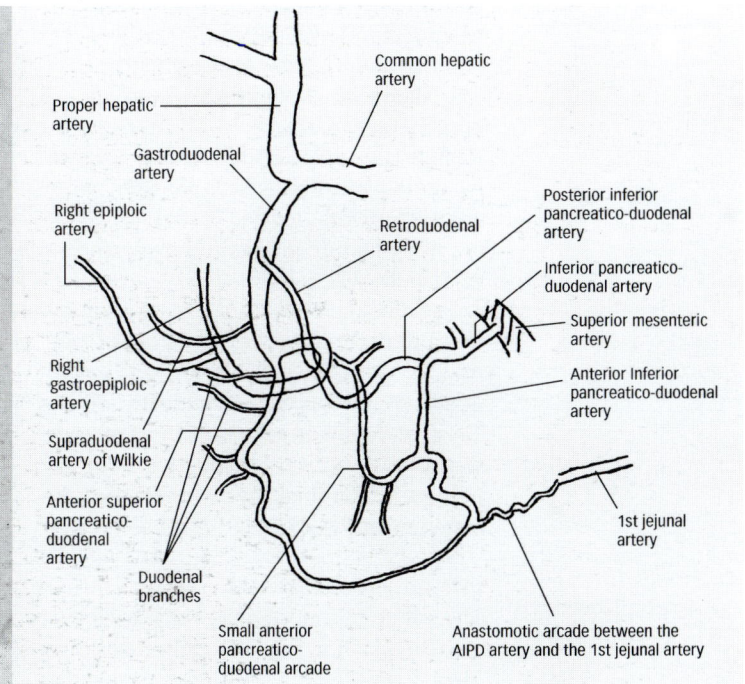

posteriorly anastomoses with the anterior inferior pancreatico-duodenal artery; the resulting anterior pancreatico-duodenal arcade lies inferior to the posterior arcade.

Both the anterior and posterior pancreatico-duodenal arcades may vary between one and four in number and, as well as communicating with one another, have numerous branches which anastomose with those of the dorsal and transverse pancreatic arteries. The anatomy of these arcades is very variable. The inferior pancreatico-duodenal arteries most commonly arise from the superior mesenteric trunk or a proximal jejunal artery but may originate from a right hepatic artery arising from the superior mesenteric artery.

The transverse pancreatic artery may arise from the anterior superior pancreatico-duodenal artery, an anomaly present in approximately 10% of individuals. As mentioned above, this vessel is more commonly (75%) a branch of the dorsal pancreatic artery.

The right gastroepiploic artery (Figs 1, 2(a), 3, 4, 7, 8 and 9) initially supplies one or two branches to the pylorus before passing to the left along the greater curvature of the stomach in the anterior layers of the greater omentum to anastomose with the left gastroepiploic artery. Both gastroepiploic arteries send branches superiorly to supply the greater curvature of the stomach and these anastomose with descending branches of the right and left gastric arteries (see Fig. 4).

The right epiploic artery (Figs. 1, 2(a) and 9) arises from the proximal portion of the right gastroepiploic artery. The anterior epiploic arteries (Figs. 1 and 2) arise from both gastroepiploic arteries and descend within the anterior layers of the greater omentum, at the free edge of which they turn upward to become the posterior epiploic arteries, which join the large epiploic arc of Barkow (formed by the anastomosis between the right and left epiploic arteries), located in the posterior layers of the greater omentum beneath the transverse colon (Fig. 2(a)).

The omental vessels are usually of small calibre and anastomose with branches of the middle colic, left colic, inferior pancreatico-duodenal and transverse pancreatic arteries. They commonly hypertrophy in pathological states, however, and are not infrequently a pointer to inflammatory disease in the abdomen on visceral angiography.

Inferior phrenic arteries

The inferior phrenic arteries have a very variable origin but in approximately one-third of individuals they will arise as a common trunk from the anterior aspect of the aorta (usually at a level between the twelfth thoracic and first lumbar vertebrae) or from the origin of the coeliac axis (Fig. 10). In the remainder the right and left inferior phrenic arteries will arise independently and these may originate from the aorta, coeliac axis origin, left gastric artery or renal artery. They pass superolaterally and anterior to the crus of the hemidiaphragm on each side close to the medial border of the suprarenal gland. The left inferior phrenic artery passes behind the oesophagus and then passes anteriorly around the left side of the oesophageal opening. The right inferior phrenic artery passes behind the inferior vena cava and to the right of the caval hiatus. Close to the central tendon of the diaphragm, each vessel divides into medial and lateral branches with the medial division curving forwards to anastomose with the musculophrenic (a terminal branch of the internal thoracic artery) and pericardiophrenic arteries in front of the central tendon. The lateral branch approaches the thoracic wall and anastomoses with the lower posterior intercostal and musculophrenic arteries.

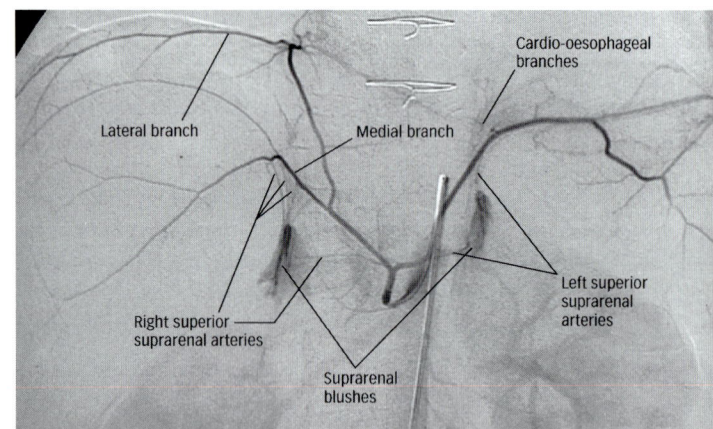

Two or three superior suprarenal arteries (Fig. 10) arise from the main trunk of the inferior phrenic artery or one of its divisions and these vessels supply part, or all, of the ipsilateral gland. In addition, the lateral branch of the right inferior phrenic artery supplies the inferior vena cava, while the left sends small branches to the oesophagus and stomach and renal capsular branches may be present on either side. Small vessels are also present bilaterally which supply the liver and spleen and the former may hypertrohy considerably and provide an important collateral supply to the liver in the presence of main hepatic artery occlusion.

Superior mesenteric artery (SMA)

The superior mesenteric artery arises from the anterior surface of the aorta at about the level

Fig. 10.
Common trunk of the inferior phrenic arteries

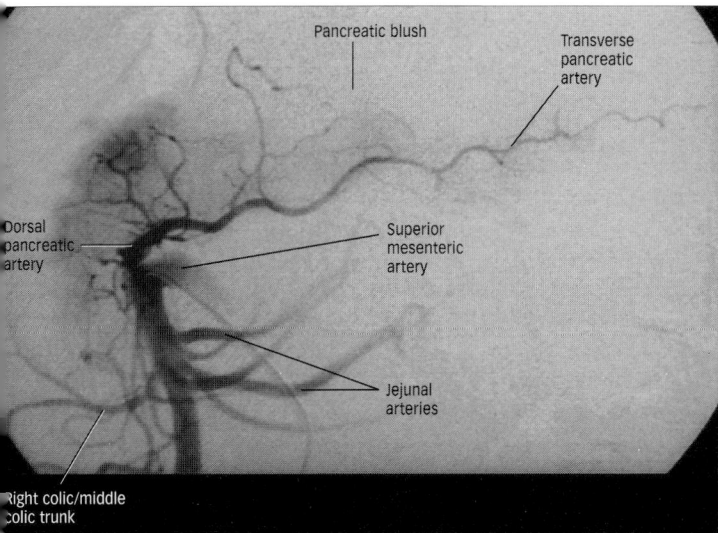

Pancreatic blush

Transverse pancreatic artery

Dorsal pancreatic artery

Superior mesenteric artery

Jejunal arteries

Right colic/middle colic trunk

11.
Superior mesenteric arteriogram. The dorsal pancreatic artery arises from the proximal superior mesenteric artery.

12.
Superior mesenteric arteriogram demonstrating the jejunal and ileal branches.

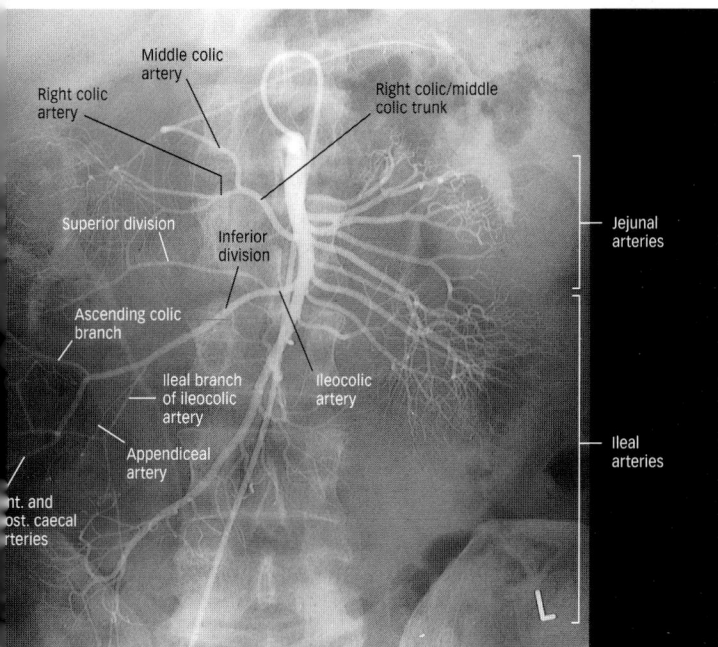

Middle colic artery

Right colic artery

Right colic/middle colic trunk

Superior division

Inferior division

Jejunal arteries

Ascending colic branch

Ileal branch of ileocolic artery

Ileocolic artery

Appendiceal artery

Ileal arteries

Ant. and post. caecal arteries

of the first lumbar vertebra and lies posterior to the body of the pancreas and the splenic vein (Figs. 2(*b*), 3, 5, 9, 11, 12, 13 and 17). It passes anteriorly, and occasionally superiorly, and descends in front of the uncinate process of the pancreas, the left renal vein and third part of the duodenum. The superior mesenteric vein lies on its right side.

A branch of the dorsal pancreatic artery arising from a branch of the coeliac axis (Fig. 5), or the main trunk of the dorsal pancreatic artery itself may arise from the proximal portion of the superior mesenteric artery (Fig. 11) or its first jejunal branch (Fig. 5).

The middle colic artery (Figs. 2(*b*), 5, 11, 12, 13, 14, 15 and 17) arises just inferior to the uncinate process of the pancreas and enters the transverse mesocolon. It most commonly arises from the right anterolateral aspect of

the SMA as a common trunk with the right colic artery (53%) (Fig. 12) but may arise separately (44%) (Fig. 13). It, or an accessory artery, may arise from the dorsal pancreatic artery, which itself may take origin from the splenic, coeliac or common hepatic arteries, and rarely it may originate from an accessory or replaced hepatic artery arising from the SMA. After a variable distance, it divides into right and left branches, the former of which anastomoses with the right colic artery and the latter with the ascending branch of the left colic artery arising from the inferior mesenteric artery. A large branch may be present, which runs parallel and posterior to the middle colic artery in the transverse mesocolon and which provides a direct communication between the superior and inferior mesenteric arteries; this is termed the arc of Riolan (Fig. 13).

The right colic artery (Figs. 2(*b*), 11, 12, 13, 15 and 17) most frequently arises with the middle colic artery as a common trunk. In 38% it arises separately from the right side of SMA and in 2% it is absent. When arising from the ileocolic artery (8%), it is called an accessory right colic artery. It passes behind the parietal peritoneum and supplies the ascending colon. An ascending branch anastomoses with the middle colic artery around the hepatic flexure, and a descending branch anastomoses with the marginal artery arising from the ileocolic or accessory right colic arteries.

The inferior pancreatico-duodenal artery (IPDA) (Figs. 2(*b*), 5, and 9) is a single branch in 40% of individuals which divides into anterior and posterior branches. In 60% these branches have separate origins. In at least half of all individuals the common trunk or one of the divisions arises from the first (or less commonly the second) jejunal artery. Selective catheterization of the IPDA will often be unsuccessful unless this anatomical variant is appreciated, as on a selective superior mesenteric arteriogram it will often appear as if the IPDA is arising from the right side of the SMA when its actual origin is the first jejunal artery. The IPD arteries cross behind the superior mesenteric vein (and artery when arising from a proximal jejunal branch) and course upwards and to the right to the dorsal aspect of the pancreatic head, where they anastomose with the corresponding superior pancreatico-duodenal arteries.

Four to six jejunal arteries (in 83%) (Figs. 2(*b*), 3, 9, 11, 12 and 13) arise from the superior mesenteric artery proximal to the origin of the ileocolic artery. These vessels usually arise from the left side of the SMA; the first jejunal artery commonly arises from its left postero-

to the jejunal arteries. The last ileal artery anastomoses with the ileocolic artery.

A persistent vitellointestinal artery, which supplies a Meckel's diverticulum (Fig. 14), arises from an ileal artery (often the sixth or seventh) at the embryological end-point of the superior mesenteric artery. This is defined as a point approximately 5 cm proximal to the anatomical end-point which is taken to be the anastomosis between the most distal ileal artery and the ileal branch of the ileocolic

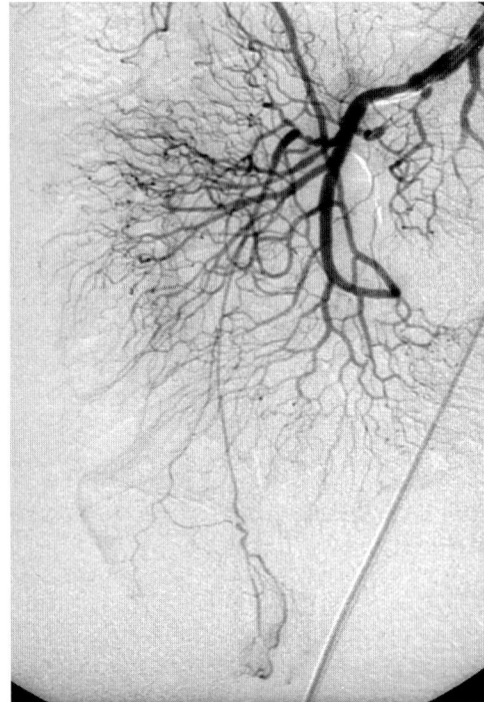

Fig. 14.
Distal superior mesenter[ic] angiogram. The catheter in the distal superior mesenteric artery just proximal to the seventh ileal artery. The anatomy [of] the vitellointestinal arter[y] is more easily appreciate[d]

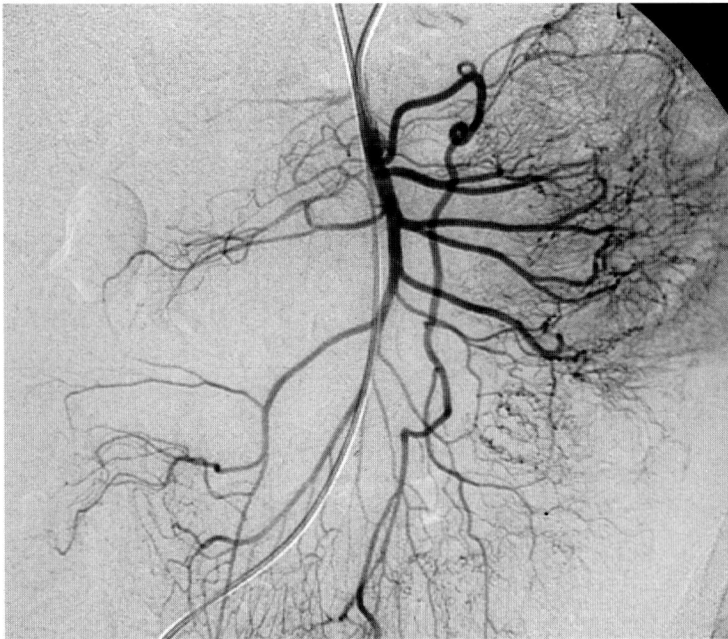

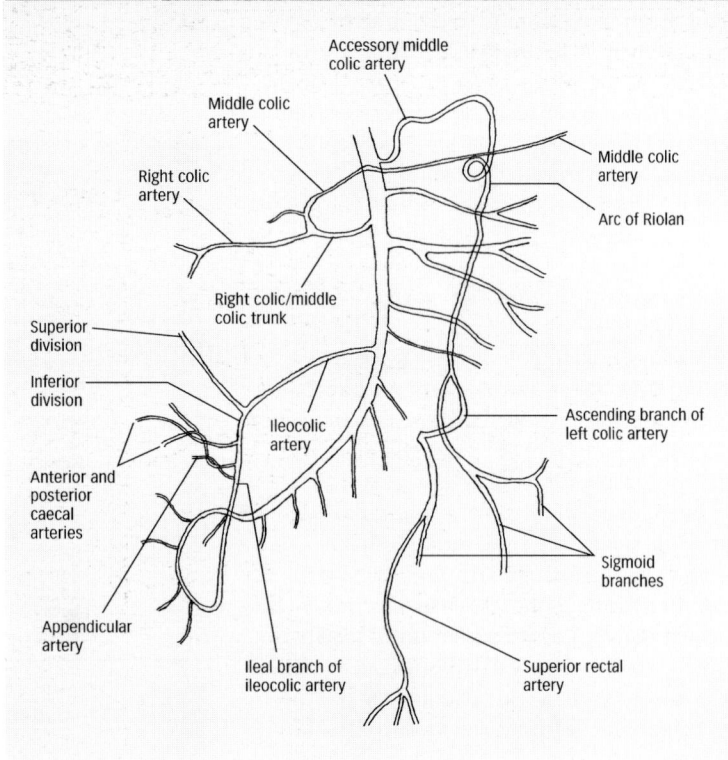

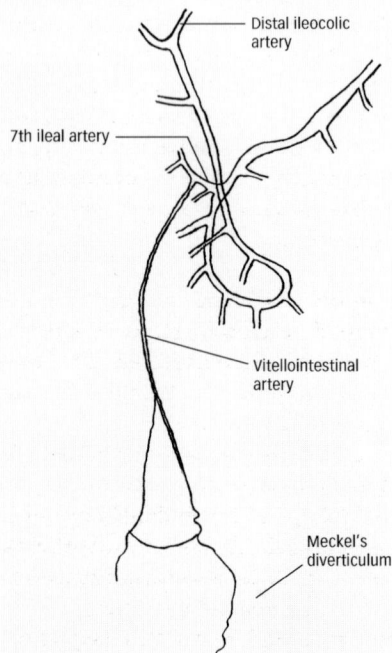

Fig. 13.
Superior mesenteric arteriogram demonstrating the arc of Riolan.

lateral aspect. Each jejunal artery divides into two vessels which communicate with the adjacent jejunal arteries to form a series of arcades which parallel the intestine. Between three and six further arcades are formed; the last of them sends out vasa rectae which divide to supply the anterior and posterior surfaces of the small bowel.

Beyond the origin of the ileocolic artery, nine to thirteen ileal arteries (in 83%) (Figs. 2(b), 12, 13 and 15) arise to supply the distal small bowel. These divide in a similar pattern artery. Although usually described as a long, non-branching vessel, a vitellointestinal artery is of variable length and is usually seen to have multiple branches when selectively catheterized.

The marginal artery of the small bowel (the marginal artery of Dwight) is defined as the artery which runs closest to, and parallel with, the wall of the intestine and from which the vasa rectae arise. This is made up of the arcades described above and usually consists of a continuous channel. Breaks in this anastomotic arcade in the small bowel may, however, be present at the junction between the inferior pancreatico-duodenal artery and first jejunal artery (Fig. 9) and the junction between the terminal ileal artery and the ileocolic artery.

The ileocolic artery crosses anterior to the right ureter, the right gonadal vessels and psoas major and distributes branches to the terminal ileum, the caecum and the ascending colon. Although it has many variations in its terminal distribution, it usually divides into a superior branch, which anastomoses with the right colic artery, and an inferior branch, which anastomoses with the distal superior mesenteric artery. The inferior division gives rise to several branches; a colic branch which supplies the proximal ascending colon; anterior and posterior caecal arteries; an appendicular artery; and an ileal artery which anastomoses with a terminal branch of the superior mesenteric artery. A variant of normal anatomy is shown in Fig. 15.

The appendicular artery (Figs. 12 and 13) descends behind the terminal ileum and enters the mesoappendix, where it gives off a recurrent artery which anastomoses with a branch of the posterior caecal artery. It then runs towards the tip of the appendix.

The anastomosis between the ileal branch of the ileocolic artery and the distal superior mesenteric artery is usually small and the terminal ileum often appears relatively avascular on angiography.

Inferior mesenteric artery (IMA)
The inferior mesenteric artery arises from the anterior or left antero-lateral aspect of the aorta at about the level of the third lumbar vertebra (Figs. 13, 16 and 17).

The left colic artery (Figs. 5, 13, 16 and 17) is its first branch which divides soon after its origin into ascending and descending branches. The ascending branch anastomoses with the middle colic artery while the descending branch anastomoses with the first sigmoid artery.

There are usually two or three sigmoid arteries, which communicate with the descending branch of the left colic artery

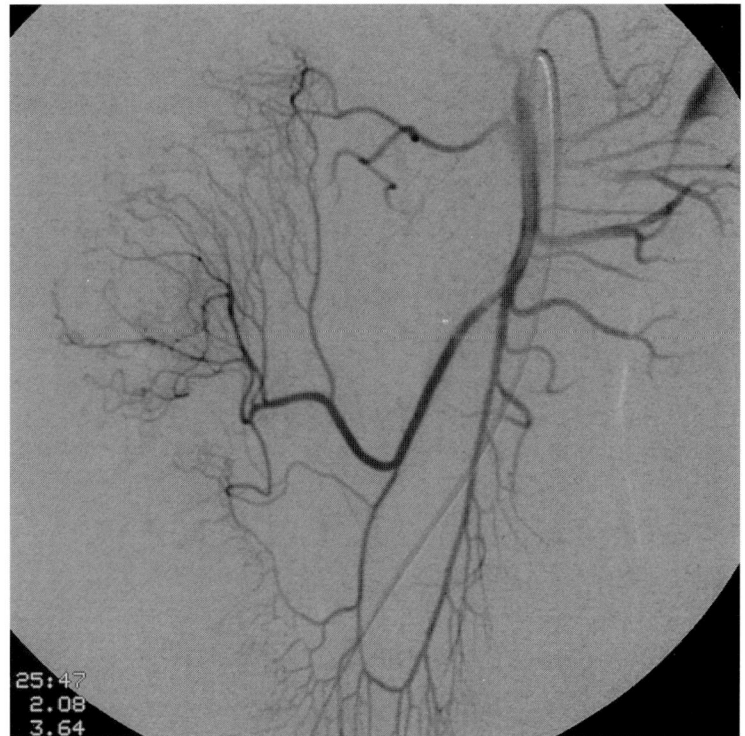

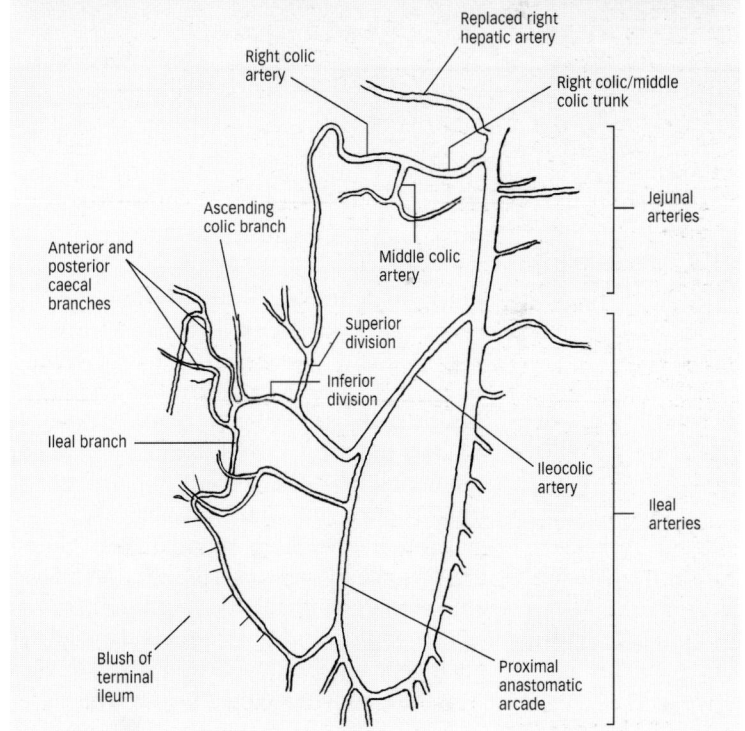

above and with the superior rectal (haemorrhoidal) artery below.

The superior rectal (haemorrhoidal) artery is the terminal artery of the IMA which supplies the proximal rectum. It divides into left and right branches, which intercommunicate with one another and with branches of the middle and inferior rectal arteries arising from the internal iliac arteries.

Fig. 15.
Superior mesenteric angiogram to demonstrate ileocolic anatomy. Note the presence of the two anastomotic arcades between the ileocolic artery and the distal superior mesenteric artery.

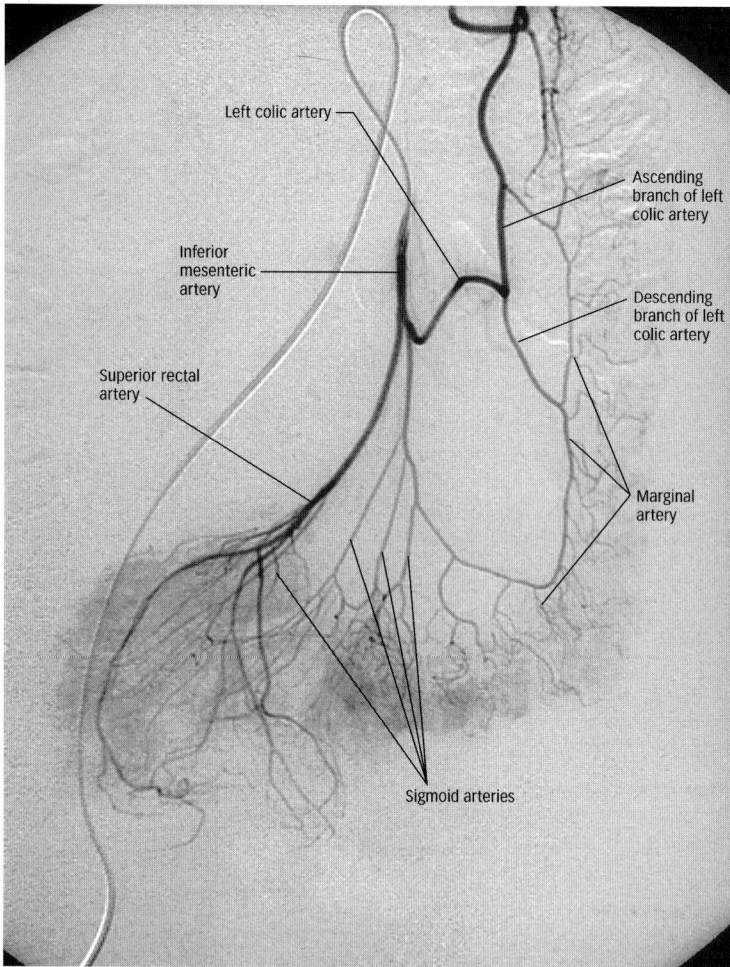

Fig. 16.
Inferior mesenteric arteriogram.

The marginal artery of the large bowel (marginal artery of Drummond) is that vessel which is closest to and which parallels the bowel wall from which the vasa rectae arise (Figs. 16 and 17). The marginal artery of Drummond is formed by the main trunks, and the arcades arising from, the ileocolic and right, middle and left colic arteries. It may be absent or tenuous at the splenic flexure. It may also hypertrophy significantly when one of the main visceral arteries is compromised. This is most commonly seen when the inferior mesenteric artery is stenosed or occluded and the main supply to the descending and sigmoid colon persists via the middle colic artery arising from the superior mesenteric artery (Fig. 13).

Venous anatomy

The portal venous system is most commonly demonstrated during the venous phase of coeliac, splenic and superior mesenteric arteriograms, a technique termed indirect portography. Direct portography involves a direct puncture of the spleen or catheterization of the portal vein via a percutaneous, or transjugular transhepatic approach or through the

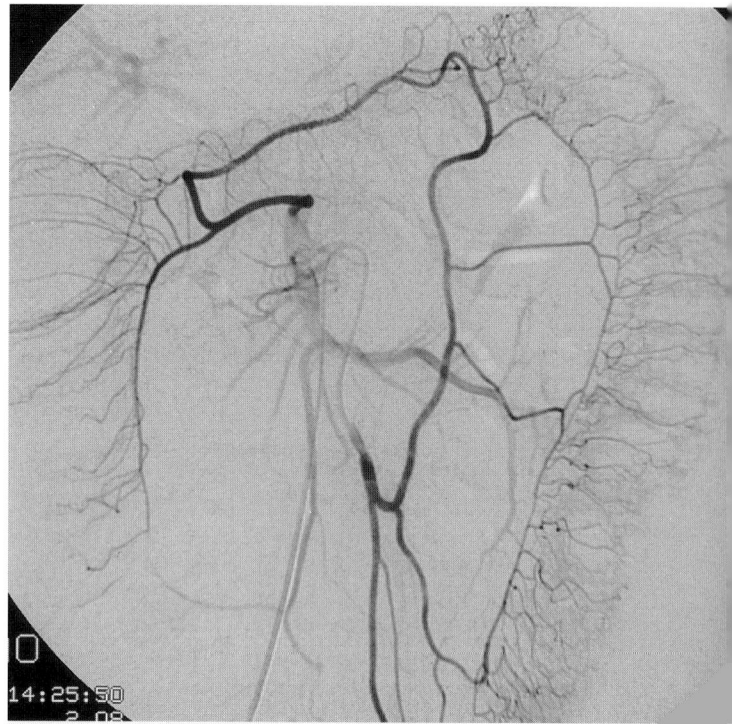

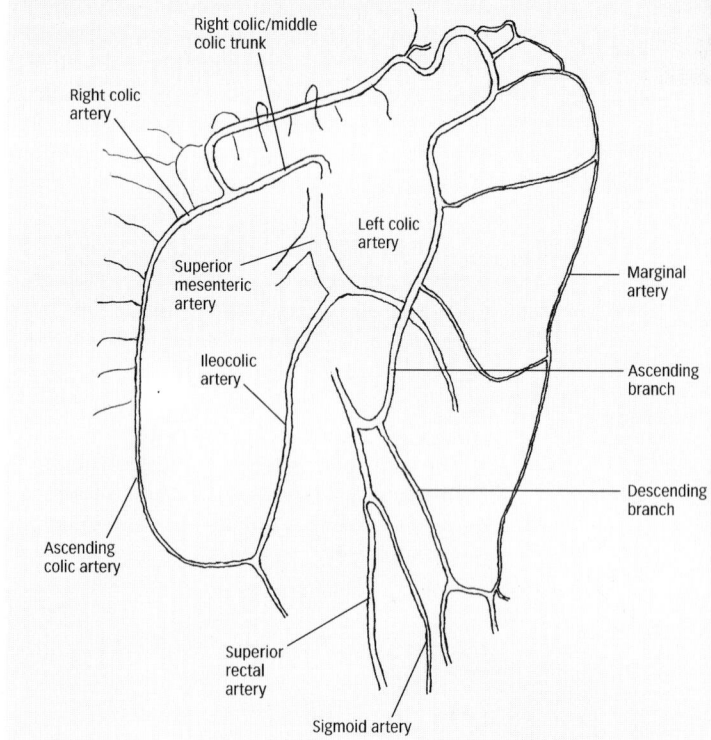

Fig. 17.
An inferior mesenteric arteriogram demonstrating the marginal artery of Drummond.

umbilical vein. Portal venous opacification may also be achieved in some individuals by performing a wedged hepatic venogram.

Portal vein

The splenic and superior mesenteric veins join to form the main portal vein at about the level of the first or second lumbar vertebrae, behind the pancreatic neck and slightly to the right of

The right portal vein is 2–3 cm in length and divides into anterior and posterior branches, which accompany the segmental hepatic arterial branches.

The left portal vein is 2–4 cm in length; its proximal (transverse) portion extends from the porta hepatis and supplies branches to the caudate (segment I) and quadrate (segment IV) lobes. Its distal (umbilical) portion divides into superior and inferior branches to supply the lateral segments (II and III) and the inferior portion of segment IV. The obliterated umbilical vein, which is normally only patent when it provides collateral shunting in the presence of portal hypertension, courses vertically from the umbilical portion of the left portal vein in the falciform ligament to the anterior abdominal wall.

Superior mesenteric vein

Drainage from the gut wall occurs into mesenteric arcades and subsequently segmental veins, which accompany their respective arteries. These unite to form the main superior mesenteric vein, which lies to the right side of the superior mesenteric artery. The right gastroepiploic, middle colic and anterior superior pancreatico-duodenal veins combine to form the gastrocolic trunk, which enters the right side of the superior mesenteric vein just anterior to the pancreatic head at the level of the uncinate process.

The posterior superior pancreatico-duodenal vein is smaller than its anterior counterpart and usually lies on the posterolateral surface of the pancreatic head adjacent and parallel to the common bile duct, before it drains into the undersurface of the main portal vein just superior to the head of the pancreas.

Splenic vein

The splenic vein lies postero-inferior to the splenic artery and the pancreatic body and tail. It receives tributaries from the inferior mesenteric (Fig. 19), left gastric, short gastric, pancreatic and gastroepiploic veins.

Inferior mesenteric vein

The inferior mesenteric vein is formed by superior rectal (haemorrhoidal), sigmoidal and left colic veins and lies to the right side of the inferior mesenteric artery (Fig. 19). It drains into the splenic vein in 40%, into the confluence of the splenic and superior mesenteric veins in 30% and into the superior mesenteric vein in 30%. The left colic vein anastomoses with the middle colic vein.

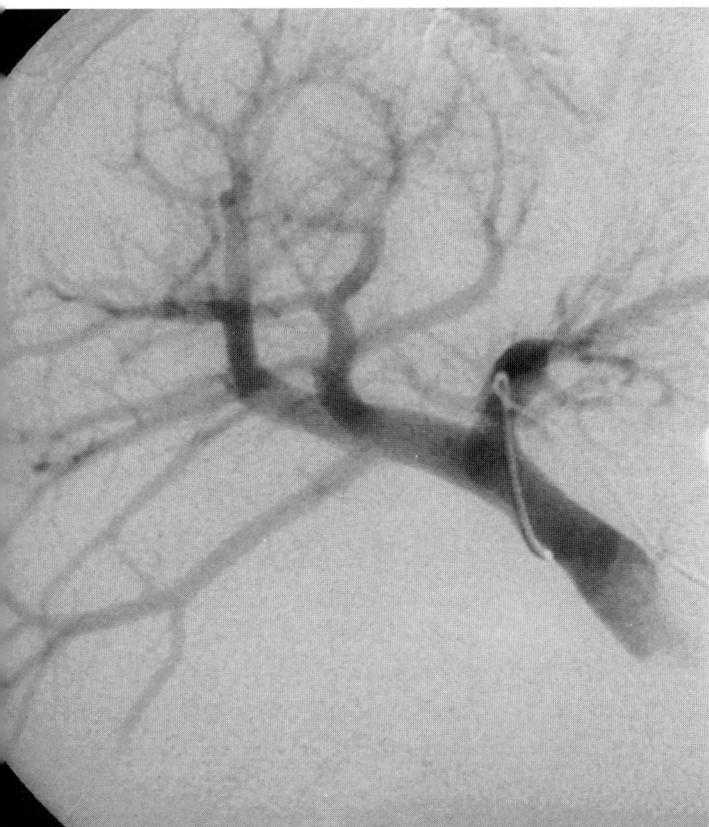

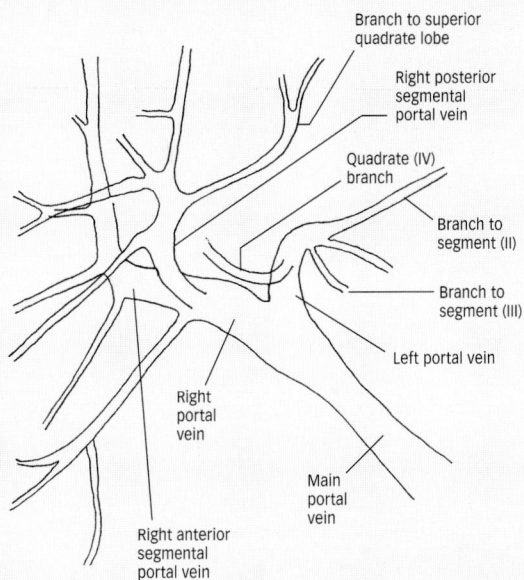

Fig. 18.
Main portal vein anatomy

the midline (Fig. 18). The extrahepatic portal vein is about 8 cm long. It lies between the common duct on the right and hepatic artery on the left and is posterior to both in the hepatoduodenal ligament except in the presence of a replaced or accessory hepatic artery arising from the superior mesenteric artery, when it lies anterior to this vessel. It crosses the inferior vena cava anteriorly and divides into right and left branches at the porta hepatis.

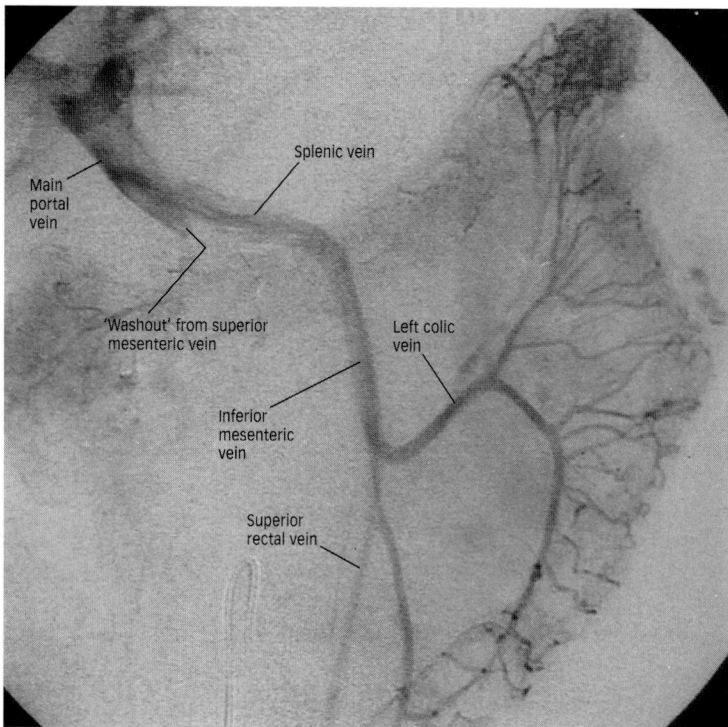

Fig. 19.
Inferior mesenteric venous anatomy.

Fig. 20.
Venous drainage of the stomach after injection of contrast

Gastric veins

The left gastric vein (Fig. 20) parallels the left gastric artery and drains into the splenic vein in approximately 15%, into the confluence of the splenic and superior mesenteric veins in 60% and into the main portal vein in 25%. It drains both the anterior and posterior surfaces of the stomach and the lower oesophagus.

The right gastric vein (Fig. 19) is usually smaller than the left, but may occasionally be larger and provide the major gastric venous drainage. It is rarely seen on angiography except when the left gastric artery is selectively catheterized and even then it is only visible in about a third of patients. It parallels the right gastric artery along the lesser curvature of the stomach and drains into the main or left portal veins or into an intrahepatic portal venous branch, the last of which is likely to be the cause of the 'flow defect', which is relatively frequently seen within the quadrate lobe on computerized tomography during arterial portography.

The short gastric veins drain the gastric fundus and greater curvature into the splenic vein close to the splenic hilum.

The left gastroepiploic vein drains into the splenic vein close to the splenic hilum. It lies along the greater curvature of the stomach and drains both sides of the gastric body and the greater omentum. It is continuous with the right gastroepiploic vein, which drains the inferior portion of the gastric antrum and combines with the middle colic and anterior superior pancreatico-duodenal veins to form the gastrocolic trunk.

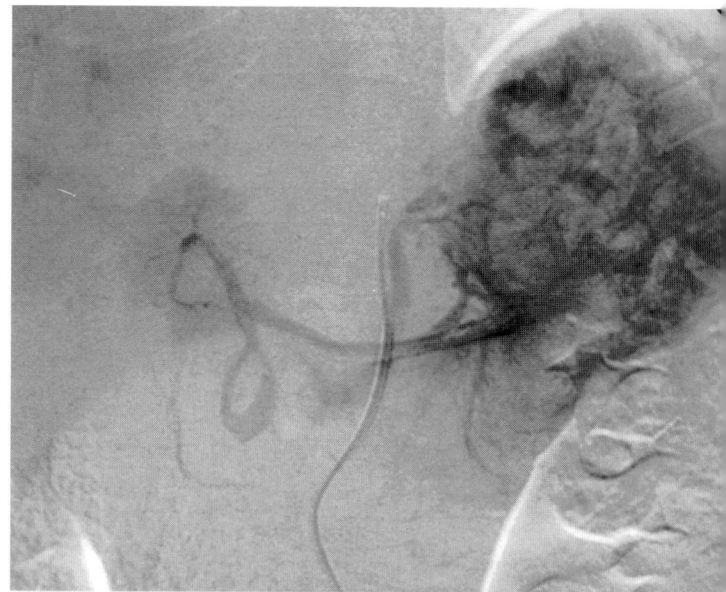

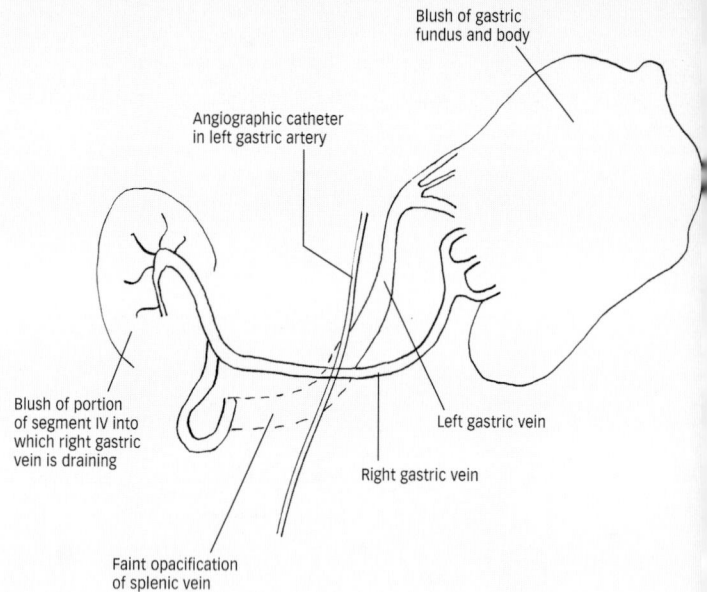

The epiploic veins are tributaries of the gastroepiploic veins and may form a large venous arcade inferiorly in the posterior layers of the greater omentum (venous arcade of Barkow) which assumes importance as a collateral venous return from the spleen when the splenic vein is occluded or stenosed.

Pancreatic veins

Numerous small pancreatic veins drain the body and tail of the pancreas into the splenic vein.

The transverse pancreatic vein courses along the posteroinferior aspect of the pancreatic body and tail and communicates with the dorsal pancreatic vein, which drains into the splenic vein or the confluence of the splenic and superior mesenteric veins. The dorsal pancreatic vein receives tributaries from the pancreatic head, neck and body.

236

The anterior and posterior inferior pancreatico-duodenal veins usually drain into the first jejunal or superior mesenteric veins often as a common trunk. The anatomy of the anterior and posterior superior pancreatico-duodenal veins has been described above.

Cystic vein

A single vein usually drains the anterior portion of the gall bladder, whilst two veins drain its posterior surface. These unite at the gall bladder neck and usually drain into the right branch of the portal vein or the main portal vein.

12

Liver, gall bladder pancreas and spleen

A.W.M. MITCHELL
and R.DICK

Imaging methods

Ultrasound scanning (USS) is the initial investigation of choice for examining the organs of the upper abdomen. A 3.5 MHz probe provides good depth penetration and resolution. However, lower frequency transducers may be necessary in larger patients. A distinct advantage of USS is that tissues can be examined in non-orthogonal planes and, when combined with the modern small transducer heads, organs can be examined through small anatomical windows, e.g. between the ribs. Intraoperative USS, using a 5 MHz probe, is often used for the assessment of surgical resectability of liver masses when the extent of the lesion could not be clearly demonstrated by other imaging methods.

The sonographer should not only examine the liver but use its excellent acoustic properties to obtain optimal views of the retroperitoneal organs, e.g. the pancreas. By changing the position of the probe and altering the position of the liver relative to other organs (e.g. breath holding), an acoustic window to the upper abdomen is created.

Doppler USS is used routinely to examine the blood flow to the organs to the upper abdomen. The coeliac axis, superior mesenteric artery and portal venous system are all amenable to study using pulsed wave real time Doppler scanning. Examination of these vessels demonstrates the velocity and direction of blood flow, as changes in these parameters are of great importance in the assessment of patients with liver disease and portal hypertension.

Computed tomography (CT) and contrast enhanced CT (CECT) demonstrate the organs of the upper abdomen in the axial plane. Helical CT enables the abdomen to be examined rapidly and is often combined with CECT to demonstrate the arterial, venous and mixed phases of hepatic perfusion and enhancement. In order to study selectively the individual vascular supplies of the liver, additional investigations are necessary. Indirect CT portography (computed tomographic arterio-portography, CTAP), is undertaken by catheterizing the superior mesenteric artery prior to CT scanning. During the CT scan a bolus of contrast is injected (at 2 ml/s), into the superior mesenteric artery, which passes into the capiliary bed of the midgut and thence to the portal vein. CT scanning during the phase of portal venous return not only outlines the portal vein but demonstrates the portal venous perfusion and the hepatic veins. Similarly, CT hepatic arteriography is performed by direct catheterization of the hepatic artery and demonstrates the hepatic arterial perfusion. The importance of these methods of investigation is that they distinguish normally perfused tissue from abnormal tissue. Furthermore, many hepatic tumours derive their blood supply from the hepatic artery and will become relatively hyperdense (compared with normal liver parenchyma), with arterial contrast, whereas CTAP produces dense enhancement of normal liver parenchyma and no enhancement of lesions supplied from the hepatic artery, e.g. liver tumours and metastases. Using modern computer software, three-dimensional reconstructions can enable the radiologist and the surgeon to assess the resectability of these lesions.

Magnetic resonance imaging (MRI) provides a useful adjunct to CT, although the extent of its role in imaging the hepato-biliary tree and pancreas is still under evaluation. The inherent tissue contrast and multiplanar image display, combined with the lack of ionizing radiation, suggest that MRI will play a useful role in

(a)

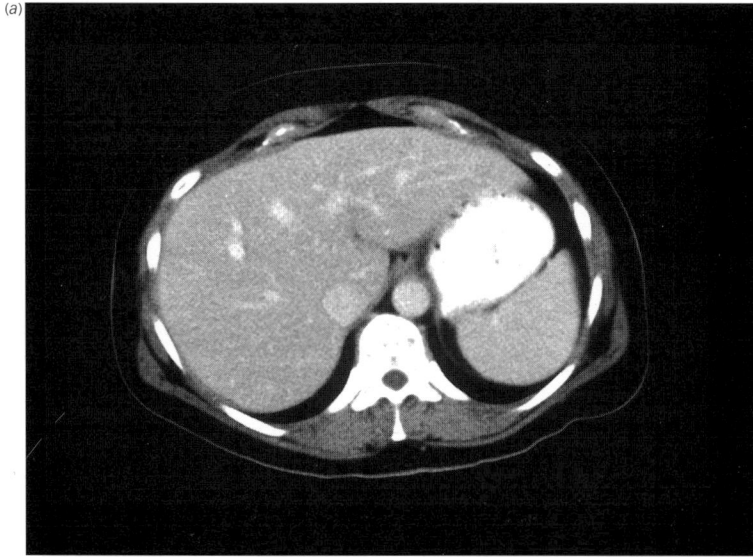

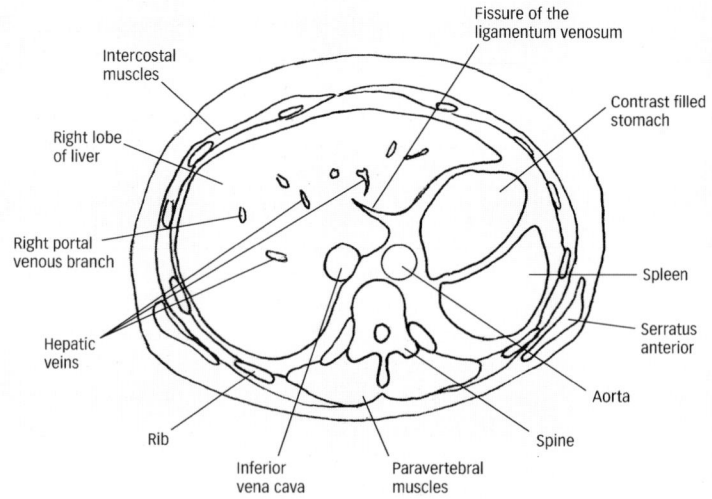

Intercostal muscles

Right lobe of liver

Right portal venous branch

Hepatic veins

Rib

Inferior vena cava

Paravertebral muscles

Fissure of the ligamentum venosum

Contrast filled stomach

Spleen

Serratus anterior

Aorta

Spine

(b)

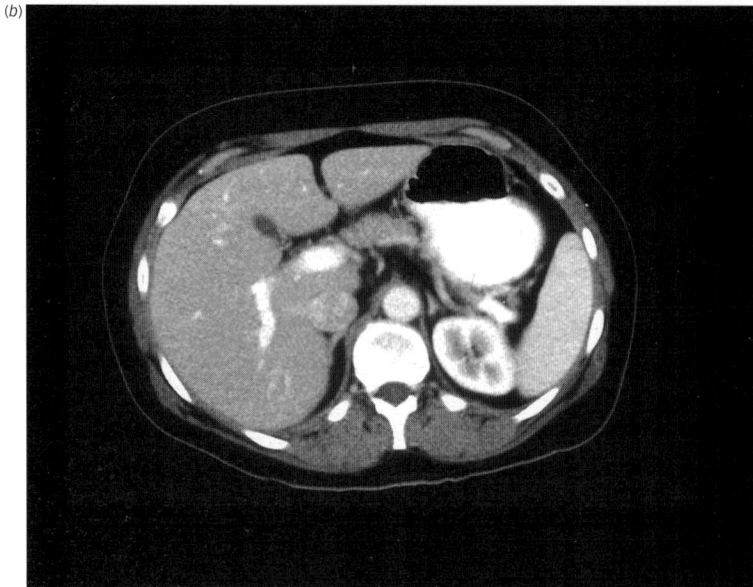

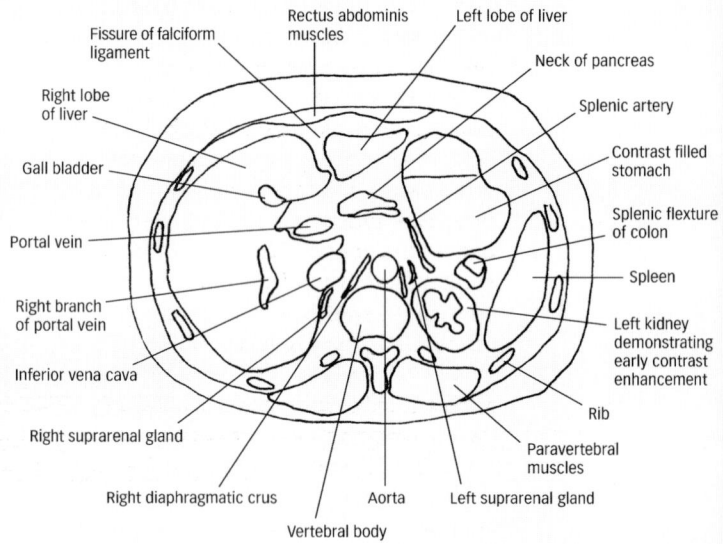

Fissure of falciform ligament

Rectus abdominis muscles

Left lobe of liver

Right lobe of liver

Neck of pancreas

Splenic artery

Gall bladder

Contrast filled stomach

Portal vein

Splenic flexture of colon

Right branch of portal vein

Spleen

Inferior vena cava

Left kidney demonstrating early contrast enhancement

Right suprarenal gland

Rib

Right diaphragmatic crus

Aorta

Left suprarenal gland

Paravertebral muscles

Vertebral body

(c)

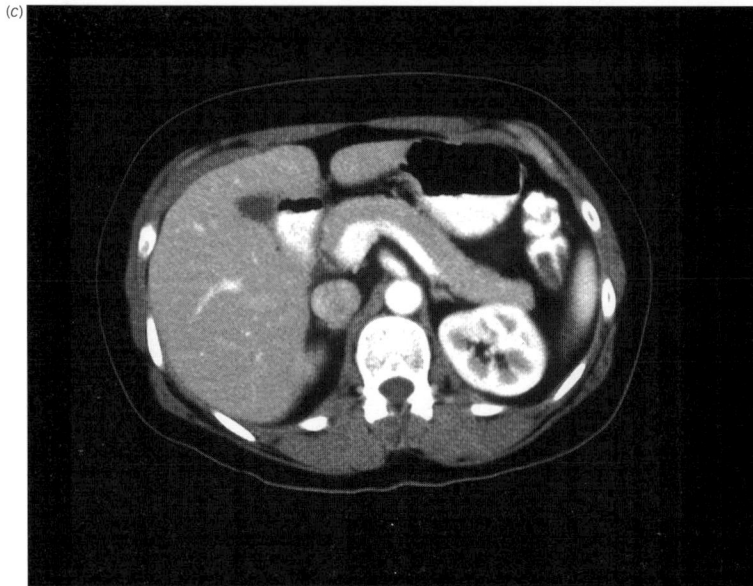

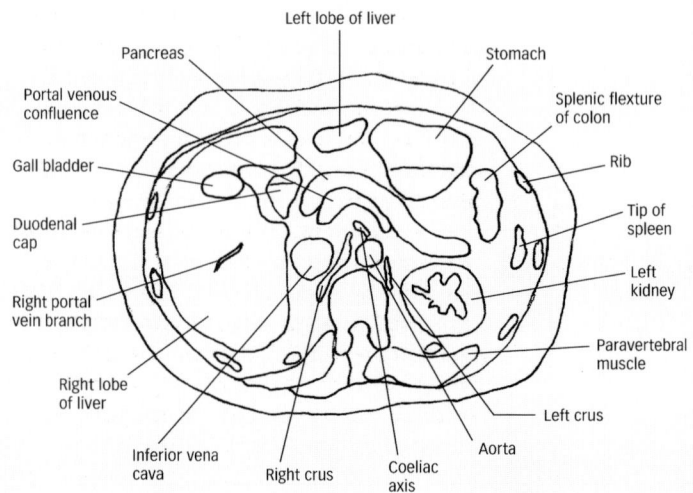

Pancreas

Left lobe of liver

Portal venous confluence

Stomach

Gall bladder

Splenic flexture of colon

Duodenal cap

Rib

Right portal vein branch

Tip of spleen

Right lobe of liver

Left kidney

Inferior vena cava

Paravertebral muscle

Right crus

Left crus

Coeliac axis

Aorta

the future imaging of the liver and upper abdominal organs. Magnetic resonance angiography (MRA) has the potential to supersede conventional angiography; however, its current clinical use is limited. Recently, developed sequences have been described that differentiate the tissue properties of the liver from the bile so as to produce a magnetic resonance cholangiogram.

Nuclear medicine techniques can provide both functional and static information that cannot be obtained by CT or MRI. Often these techniques are very sensitive at the expense of poor spatial resolution. Technetium-labelled *n*-substituted iminodiacetic acid (e.g. Tc99^m HIDA), a compound that is secreted by the hepatocytes, displays the gross anatomy and function of the biliary tree and gall bladder. Technetium 99^m sulphur colloid is taken up by the reticulo-endothelial system, and thus allows assessment of the functional Kupffer cell mass.

The commonest procedures for examining the vasculature of the liver, spleen and pancreas are coeliac and superior mesenteric arteriography. Direct splenoportography is performed by injecting contrast through a fine needle into the splenic pulp, following which the splenic and portal veins are clearly delineated (Fig.12). This test is performed in conjunction with splenic pulp pressure measurements. Transhepatic portography demonstrates the venous return to the liver following the introduction of a fine catheter across the liver substance and into the portal vein. Occasionally, in patients with portal hypertension, it is necessary to catheterize selectively portal venous tributaries so that porto-systemic anastomoses can be demonstrated and treated.

Access to the hepatic veins can be achieved by cannulation of the jugular or femoral veins. The radicles of each of the three major hepatic veins are identified using the balloon occlusion technique. The catheter is designed so that, when the tip is introduced at the origin of the selected hepatic vein, a balloon can be inflated. Contrast is injected into the catheter and fills the hepatic vein without flowing away (Fig.13).

Methods to opacify the biliary tree with contrast medium include oral cholangiography, percutaneous transhepatic cholangiography (PTC), endoscopic retrograde cholecystopancreatography (ERCP), intravenous cholangiography, direct cholangiography performed at laparoscopic or open surgery and T-tube cholangiography. Originally the early techniques, e.g. oral cholangiography were aimed at demonstrating the gall bladder for the detection of gall stones. However, these techniques have been superseded by USS. The current indication for using these methods, which are not without risk, is to assess the biliary and pancreatic ductal systems. Oral and intravenous cholangiography depend upon the hepatocytes taking up the contrast and excreting it into the biliary tree. Poor hepatocyte function, for example, in the jaundiced patient, precludes this method of investigation. The direct studies of PTC and ERCP inject contrast directly into the biliary tree either transhepatically or via the duodenal papilla. In diseased states, where the sphincter of Oddi is lax or where there is an abnormal communication between the biliary tree and the bowel, the biliary tree may be outlined by air.

Anatomy

The liver

The liver is the largest and heaviest organ in the body (1.5 kg) and occupies the upper abdomen and lower thoracic cavity (Fig. 1); the bulk of the liver lies to the right side of the sagittal plane. It has two surfaces; the antero-superior surface, which is convex and smooth and referred to as the diaphragmatic surface, and the visceral surface which is flat and irregular and faces posteroinferiorly.

The liver is divided by the 'principal plane' into two halves of approximately equal size. The principal plane is defined by an imaginary parasagittal line from the gall bladder to the notch posteriorly created by the inferior vena cava. At this point, approximately 4 cm to the right of the midline, the two anatomical halves of the liver are separated. (These are sometimes referred to as the true left and right lobes. To prevent any such confusion, the segments of interest should be described.)

Owing to the convexity and shape of the left lobe of the liver, its visceral relations are posterior. The oesophagus grooves the posterior surface of the liver as it crosses the diaphragm at the level of T10. The stomach is suspended by the lesser omentum which arises from the peritoneal reflections lying in the porta hepatis and the fissure for the ligamentum venosum at the undersurface of the liver. The stomach produces the gastric impression which extends across the inferior surface of the left lobe. Directly posterior to this is the lesser sac, and the body and tail of the pancreas. The visceral relations of the right lobe of the liver are the duodenum, gall bladder, and the hepatic flexure of the colon. On the posterior surface of the liver is a region that is not invested in peritoneum, this region is the *bare area* of the liver. Thus the

Fig. 1. opposite (*a*), (*b*), (*c*). Three CT sections of the upper abdomen.

upper pole of the right kidney, the right suprarenal gland and the distal inferior vena cava are related directly to the liver and have no peritoneal coverings. The importance of this is that free peritoneal fluid cannot be seen anterior to the upper pole of the right kidney and suprarenal gland except in patients that have undergone liver transplants. The diaphragmatic surface of the liver lies on the inferior surface of the diaphragm and can be clearly demonstrated on the frontal chest radiograph.

USS of the liver demonstrates a similar or slightly increased echogenicity when compared to the right kidney (Fig. 2). The portal vein and its branches have echo-reflective (bright) walls which contrast with the walls of the hepatic veins which are poorly seen (Fig. 3(b)). The intrahepatic bile ducts can be demonstrated using higher frequency probes, e.g. 5 MHz, but when they are clearly seen paralleling the portal vein branches (the shotgun sign), and of similar calibre, they should be regarded as abnormal (enlarged).

Most CT operators examine the liver and upper abdomen with standard settings, between a window level of 40–60 HU

(Hounsfield Units) and window width of 350–400 HU using contiguous cuts, e.g. 10 mm cuts at 10 mm intervals. The liver parenchyma (Fig. 1) should appear uniformly grey and of similar density to soft tissue. The relative density is approximately 60 HU and should be at least 10 HU greater than the spleen. The portal vein and vascular structures are not often identified on the unenhanced scans unless they are outlined by low density fat, approximately −70 HU. After the administration of intravenous contrast, various structures within the liver may be identified. Early scan-

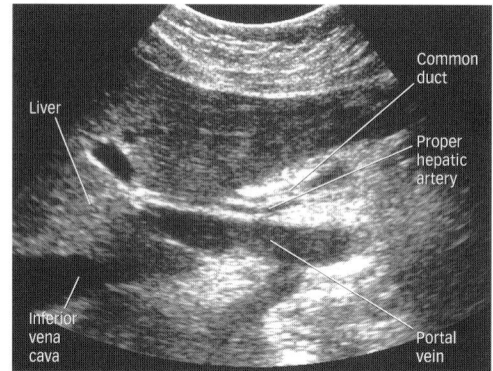

(a)

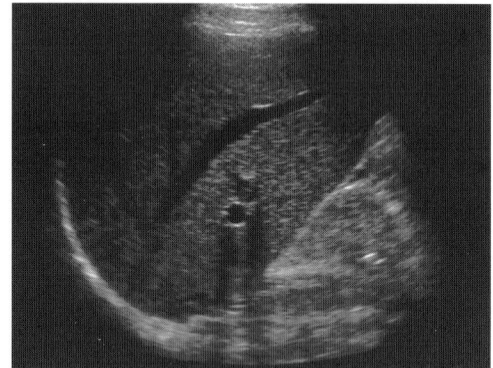

(b) Fig. 3.
(a) USS to demonstrate the portal vein and the relationship to the common duct. Note the hyperecho walls of the portal vein.
(b) USS of the liver to demonstrate the hepatic veins. Compare the echogenicity of the walls with those of the portal vein.

Fig. 2.
Parasagittal USS to demonstrate the relationship of the right kidney to the right lobe of the liver. Note the relative hepatic hyperechogenicity.

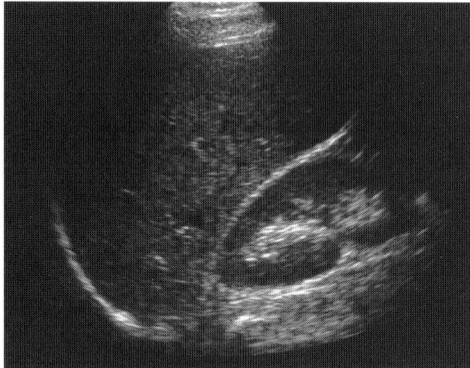

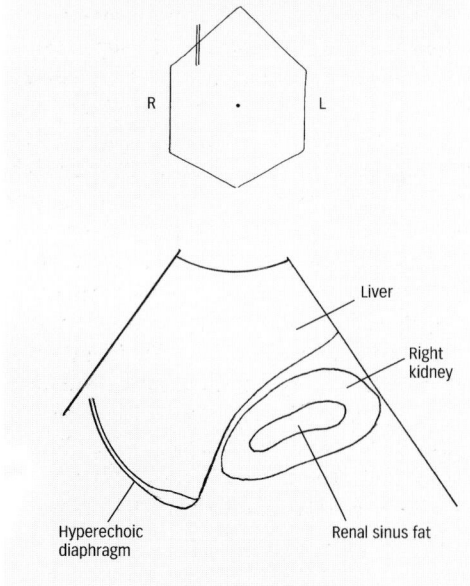

ning, within the first 30 seconds, will demonstrate the arterial perfusion phase. After the first 30 seconds, both the arterial and venous phases of perfusion enhance the liver, which allows the portal vein and hepatic veins to be identified. (A good 'rule of thumb' is to add 10 s to the time it takes the total bolus to be delivered, e.g. 100 ml contrast at 3 ml/s should be imaged at 43 s to demonstrate the portal vein adequately.)

Most primary and secondary hepatic tumours derive their blood supply from the hepatic artery. Certain tumours, for example, primary liver cell carcinoma, preferentially 'take-up' lipiodol (an oil-based contrast agent) when directly injected into the hepatic artery. The importance of this phenomenon is that the size and number of lesions can be clearly demonstrated and monitored. Furthermore, combining cytotoxic agents with lipiodil may enable the radiologist to target cancer chemotherapy.

The segmental anatomy of the liver

The principal plane divides the liver into the true *anatomical* left and right *halves*. The liver is further subdivided into segments (Couinaud, 1957) (Fig. 4). The eight-segment anatomy relates to the hepatic arterial portal and biliary drainage to regions (segments) of the liver. The caudate lobe is defined as segment I, the remaining segments are numbered in a clockwise fashion up to segment VIII (Fig. 4). These features are relatively consistent between individuals. However, in approximately 5–10% of normal females and very rarely in males the right lobe is markedly enlarged and referred to as a Riedel's lobe (Fig. 5). This is not a separate lobe, but is merely an inferior prolongation of the right lobe of the liver. The divisions of the liver can be appreciated on CT and MRI scanning; the caudate lobe (segment I) is situated posterior and to the right of the inferior cava, segments VII, VIII, IV and II run in a clockwise fashion above the portal vein and segments VI, V, IV and III are situated in a similar manner below the portal vein (Fig. 6). Thus, when one visually inspects the liver, the left lobe only comprises segments II and III.

Blood supply

The liver has a dual blood supply, from the hepatic artery and the portal vein. The hepatic artery provides a small volume (15%) of blood at systemic arterial pressure, whereas the portal vein provides the remainder at a lower pressure (<7 mmHg above central venous pressure). Doppler USS of the portal vein, hepatic veins and the hepatic artery demonstrates the direction of flow and provides characteristic waveforms for each of the individual vessels (Fig. 7(a), (b), (c)). The common hepatic artery arises from the coeliac axis at the level of T12/L1 (Fig. 8). The artery passes retroperitoneally and to the right, over the superior border of the head of the pancreas to give off the right gastric artery. Proximal to the opening of the lesser sac, the epiploic foramen (of Winslow), the common hepatic artery divides into the gastroduodenal artery and the hepatic artery. The hepatic artery continues superiorly and lies anterior to the portal vein and to the left of the common bile duct, which is in the free edge of the lesser omentum. At the hilum of the liver, the hepatic artery divides into the left, middle and right main hepatic branches (Fig. 9(a), (b)) which supply the left lobe, the quadrate lobe and the right lobes of the liver, respectively. The caudate lobe (segment I) obtains its blood supply from both left and right branches.

Fig. 4.
The segmental anatomy of the liver. (After Couinaud, 1957.)

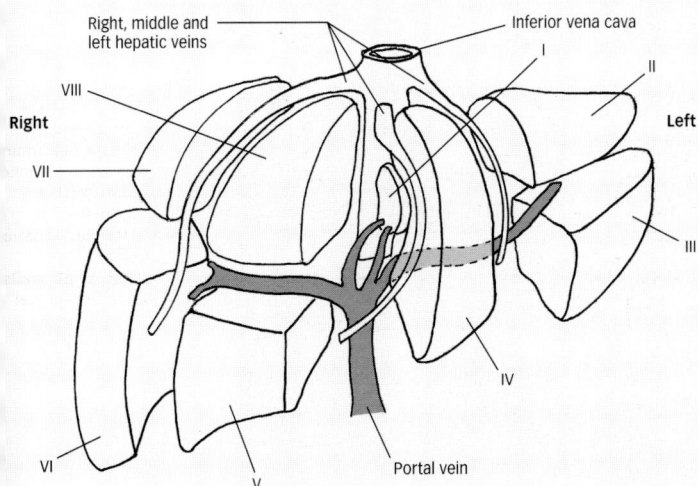

Fig. 5.
An intravenous urogram showing incidentally Riedel's lobe of the liver.

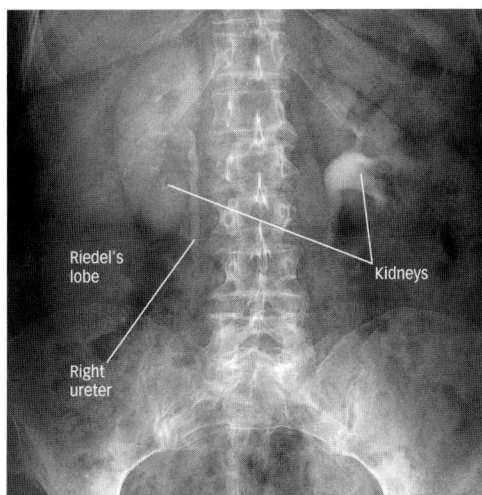

(a)

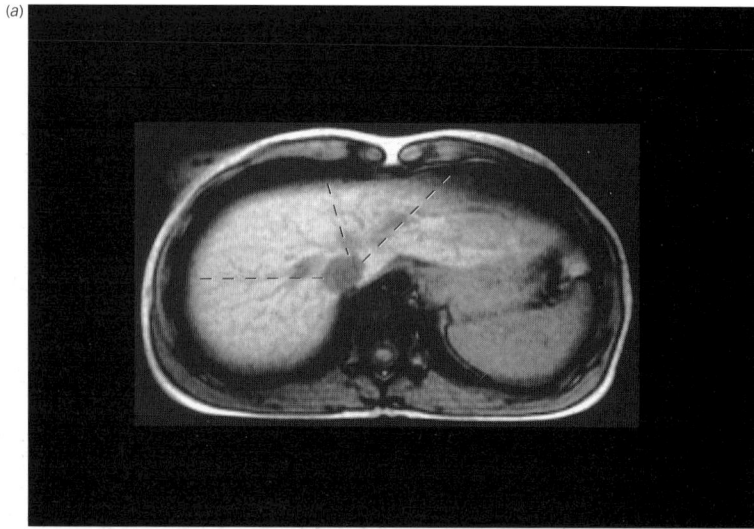

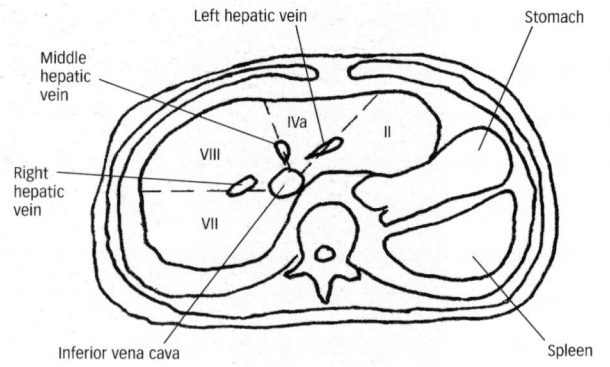

(b)

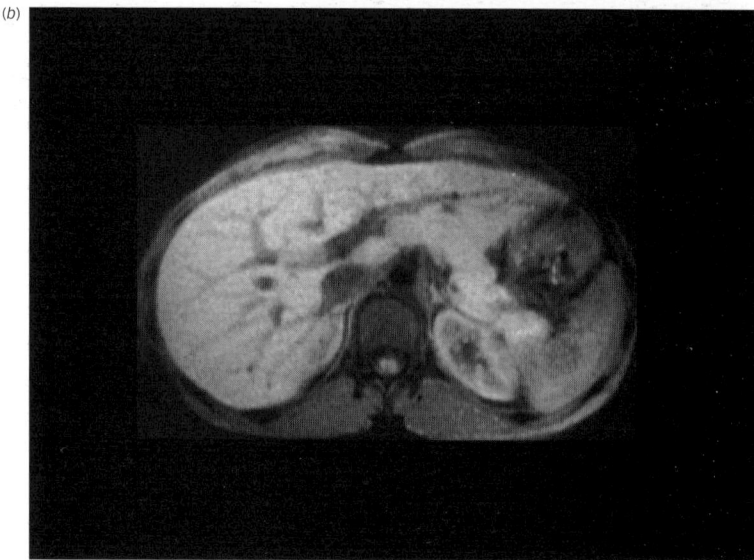

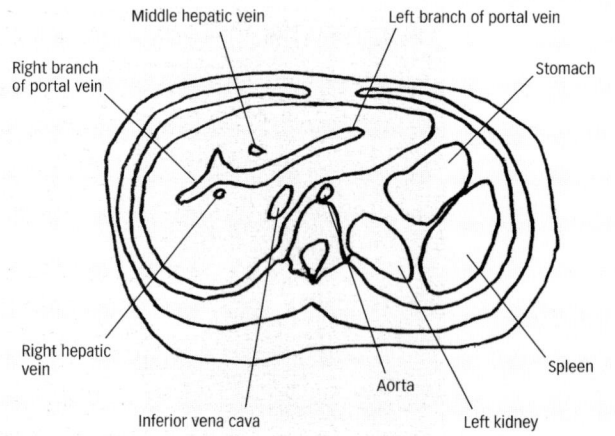

(c)

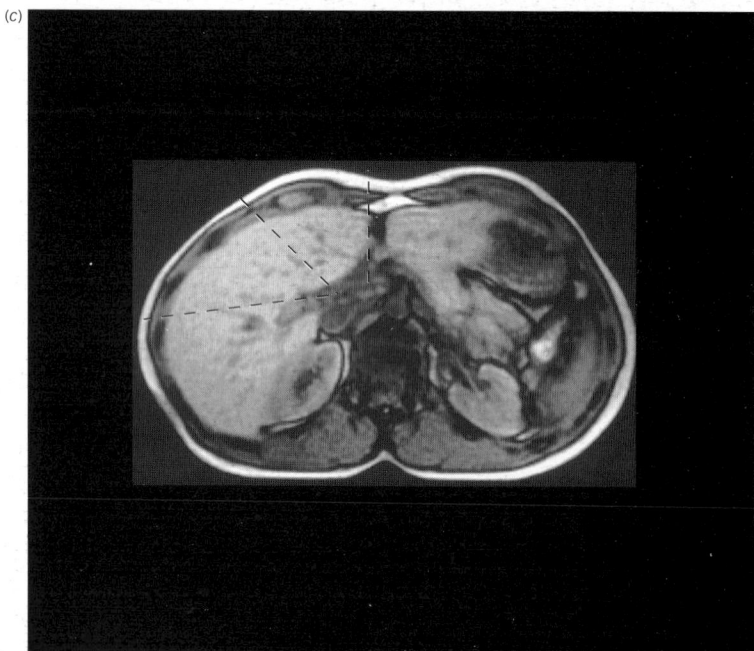

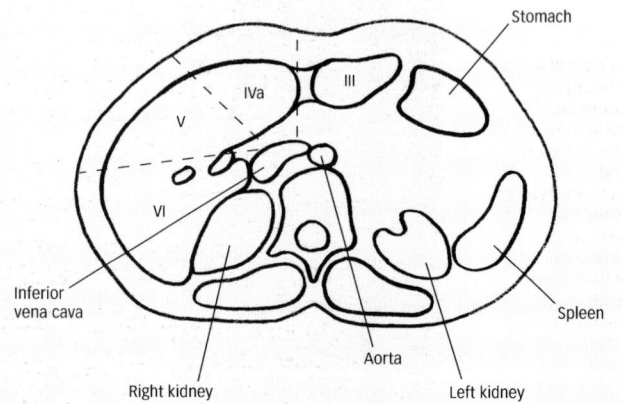

(a)

(b)

(c)

6. opposite

eries of T2W MRI scans
he liver and upper
domen. Note the
ationship of the
gments of the liver to
e portal vein.
A cut above the level of
e portal vein. The
mbers refer to the
gments of the liver above
e level of the hepatic
rtal vein (after Couinard,
57). The hatched lines
present their boundaries.
At the level of the
urcation of the portal
n.
The numbers refer to the
gments of the liver below
e level of the division of
e hepatic portal vein into
right and left branches.

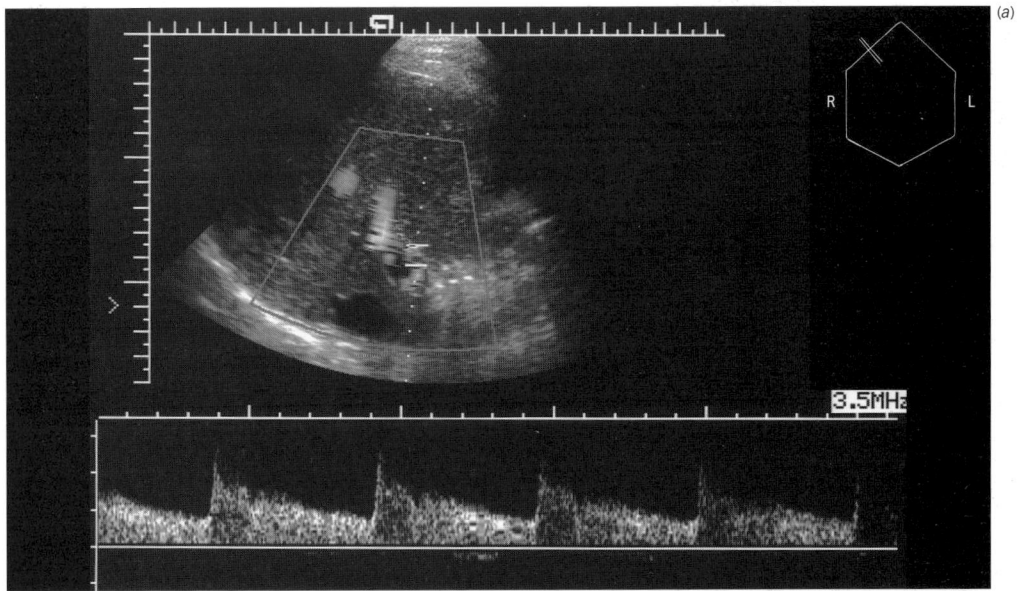

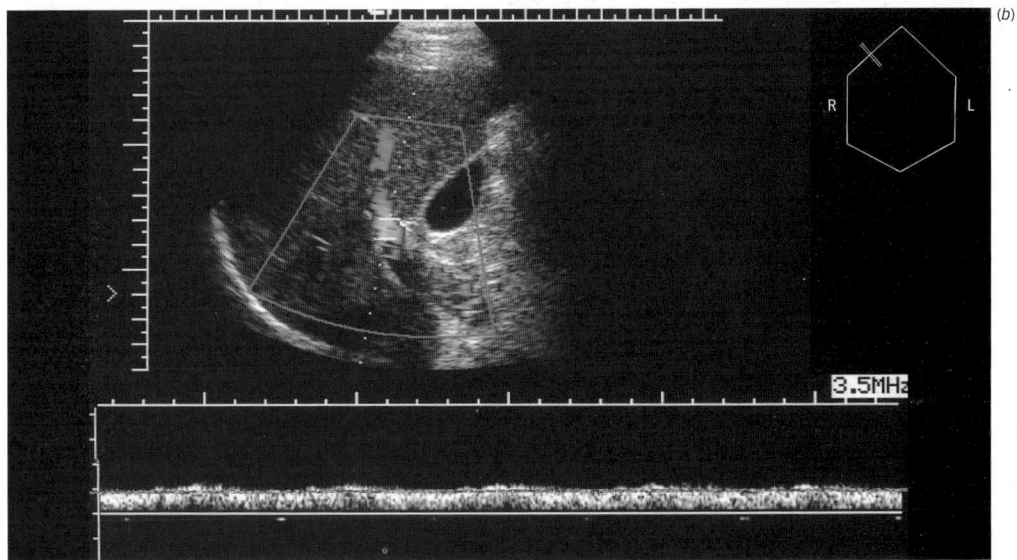

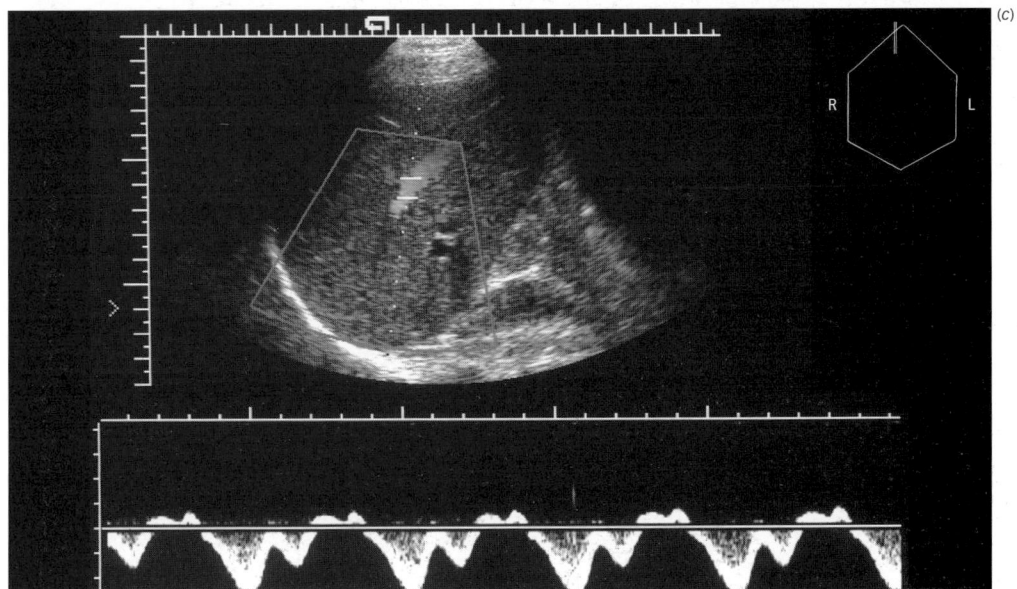

Fig. 7.
(a) Normal hepatic artery
Doppler trace.
(b) Normal portal vein
Doppler trace.
(c) Normal hepatic venous
Doppler trace.

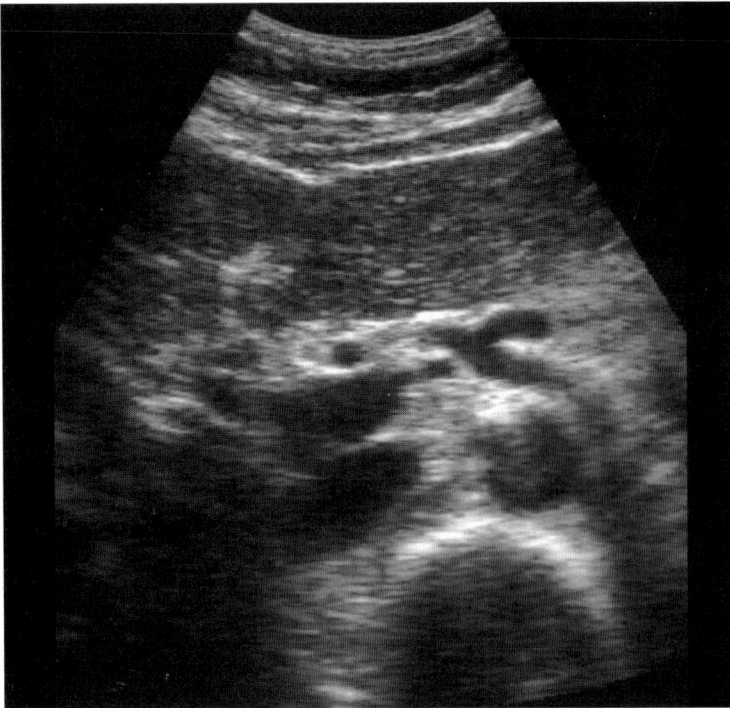

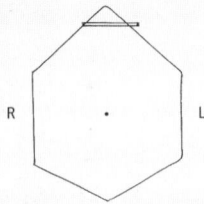

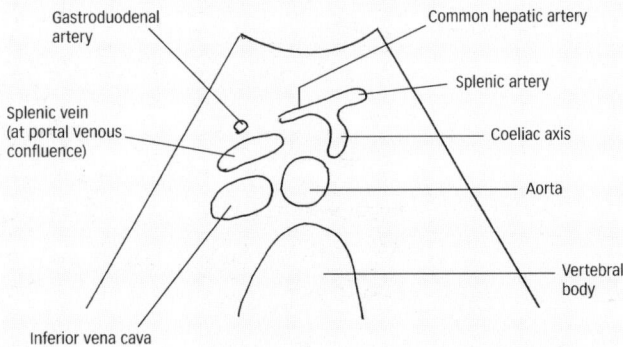

Fig. 8.
Axial USS of the coeliac axis utilizing the liver as an acoustic window.

There are a small number of normal variants which are important to demonstrate angiographically as they may influence surgical and interventional radiological procedures. A vessel which supplies a lobe in addition to its normal vessel is defined as an *accessory artery*. A *replaced* hepatic artery is a vessel that does not originate from an orthodox position and is the sole supply to that lobe. In the majority of individuals the hepatic artery divides into the left and right hepatic arteries. However, in 18.5% of individuals a partially or wholly replaced hepatic trunk emerges from the superior mesenteric artery.

- 10% are replaced right hepatic arteries.
- 6% are accessory right hepatic arteries (Fig. 10).
- 2.5% are replaced common hepatic arteries.

The variants to the left lobe of the liver are demonstrated in 25% of normal individuals and arise from the left gastric artery.

- 13% are accessory left hepatic arteries.
- 12% are replaced hepatic arteries.

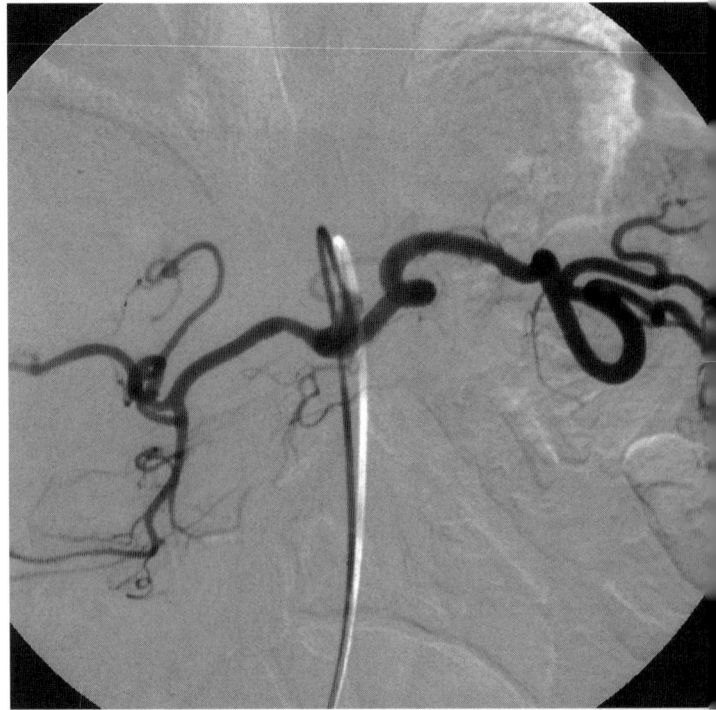

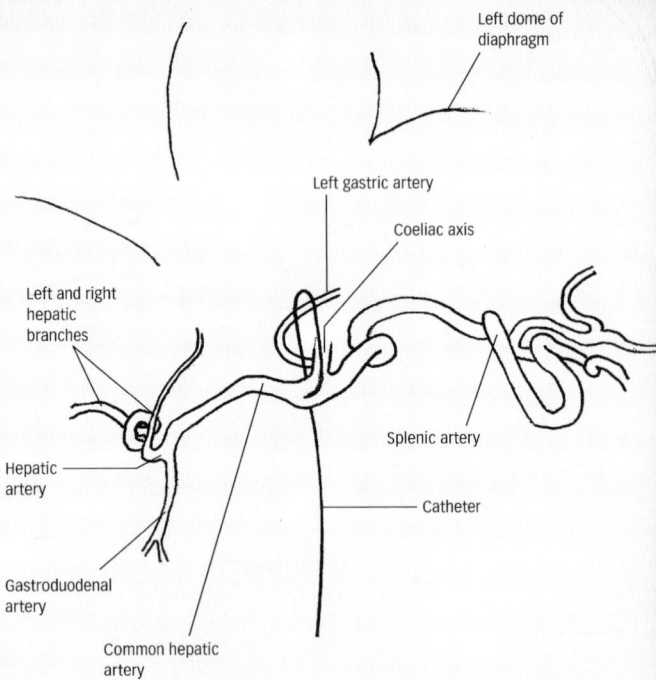

Fig. 9.
(*a*) An angiogram of the coeliac axis demonstrat the three major branche (*b*) A selective hepatic artery angiogram (oppos

246

10

Right rib

Right and left
hepatic branches

Common hepatic
artery

Proper hepatic
artery

Right gastroepiploic
artery

Gastroduodenal
artery

Catheter

Pancreatico-
duodenal
artery

Dome of left
diaphragm

Accessory right
hepatic artery

Superior mesenteric artery

Jejunal branches

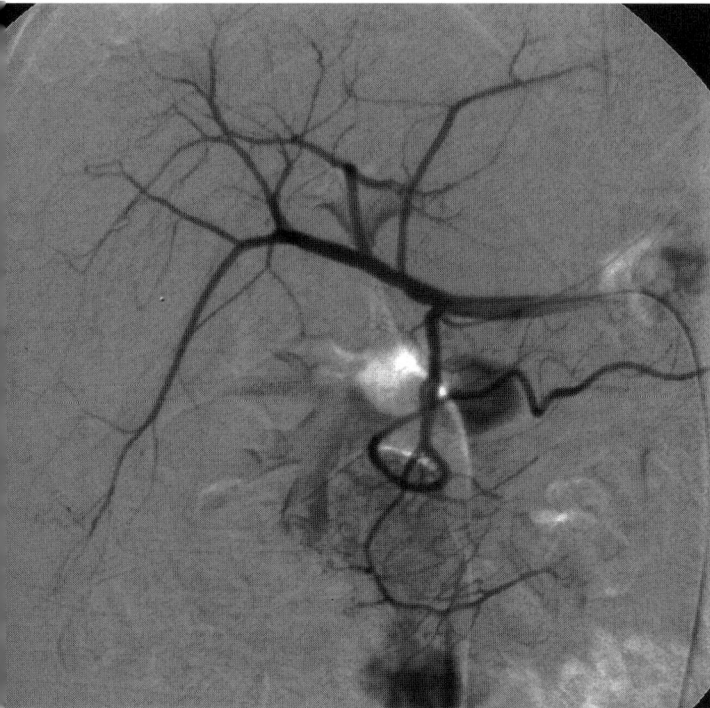

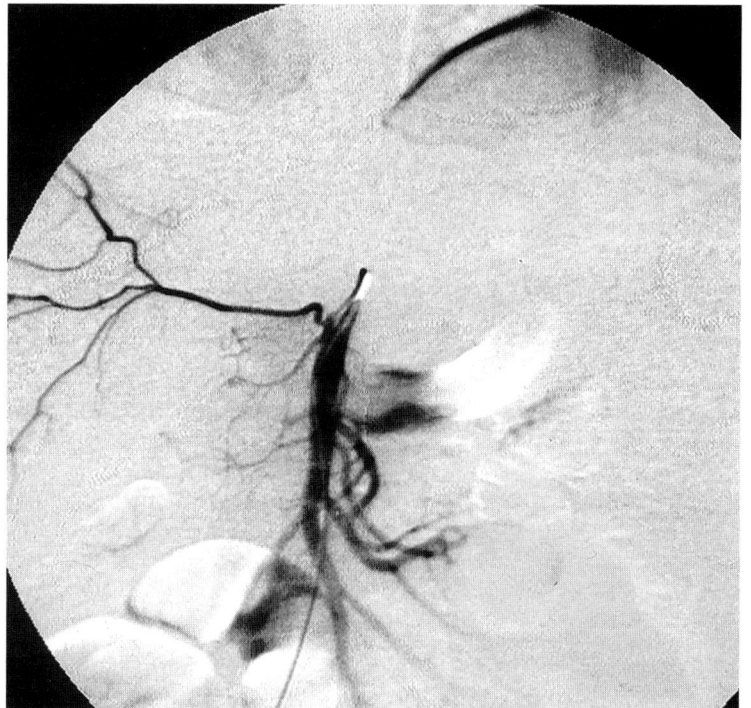

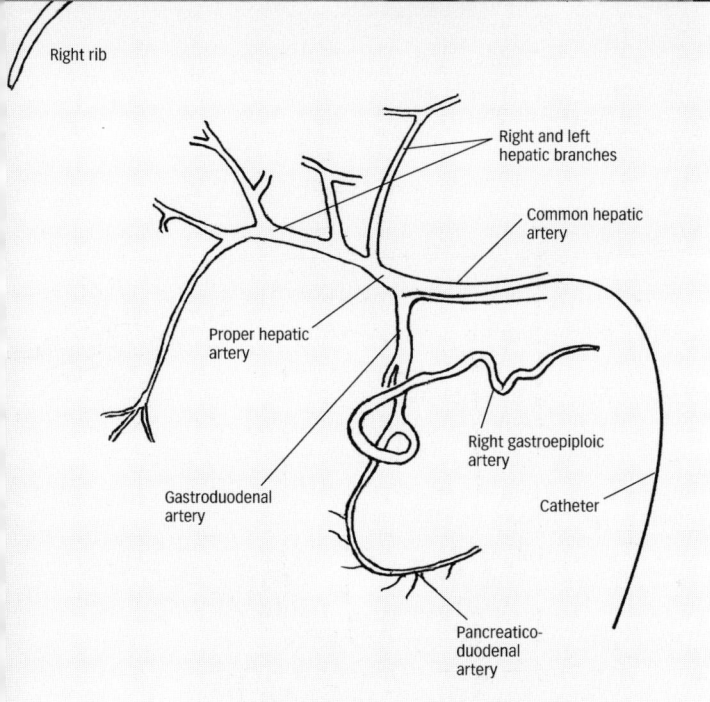

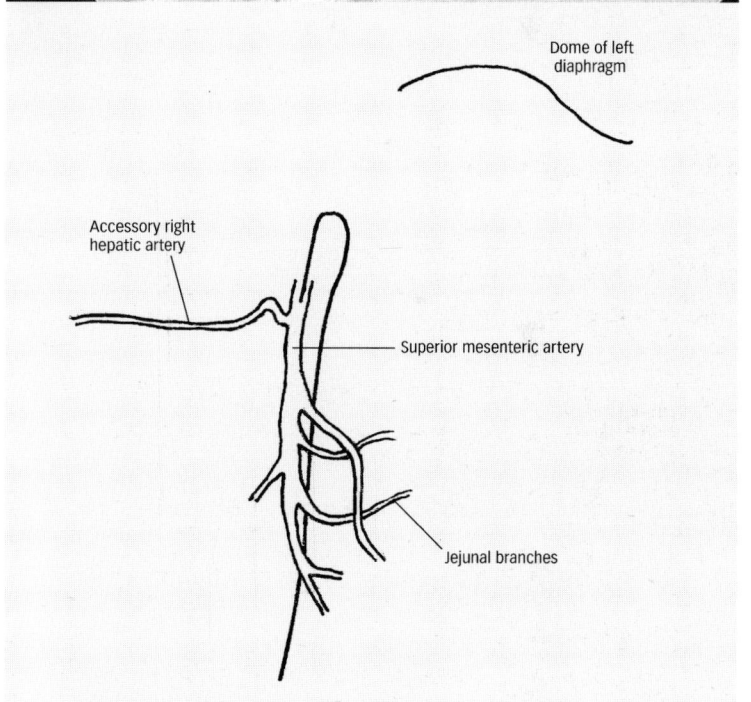

It was believed that hepatic arteries were end arteries; this is not so as tiny anastomoses exist between the vascular territories. It is, however, important to appreciate that accessory hepatic arteries are vital arterial contributors to the hepatic segments they supply.

The venous drainage of the small and large bowel is via the superior and inferior mesenteric veins, which drain their respective arterial territories. The inferior mesenteric vein anastomoses with the splenic vein near to, or at its union with, the superior mesenteric vein. The portal vein is formed by the anastomosis of the superior mesenteric vein and the splenic vein posterior to the neck of the pancreas at the level of the L1/L2 intervertebral disc (Figs. 11 and 12). The portal vein passes superiorly and laterally to the right to run in the posterior aspect of the free edge of the lesser omentum. It is approximately 8 cm long and divides into the main right and left portal venous branches at the porta hepatis. In approximately 10% of normal individuals portal venous perfusion defects can be

Fig. 10.
A selective superior mesenteric angiogram to demonstrate an accessory right hepatic artery.

Fig. 11.
A diagram to demonstrate the normal portal venous system.

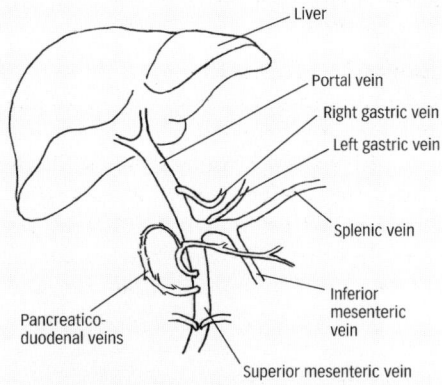

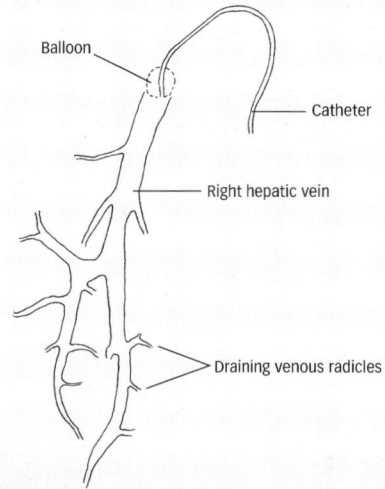

- Liver
- Portal vein
- Right gastric vein
- Left gastric vein
- Splenic vein
- Inferior mesenteric vein
- Pancreatico-duodenal veins
- Superior mesenteric vein

- Balloon
- Catheter
- Right hepatic vein
- Draining venous radicles

Fig. 13.
A wedged hepatic venogram. The catheter balloon is inflated in the origin of the right hepatic vein preventing the escape of contrast.

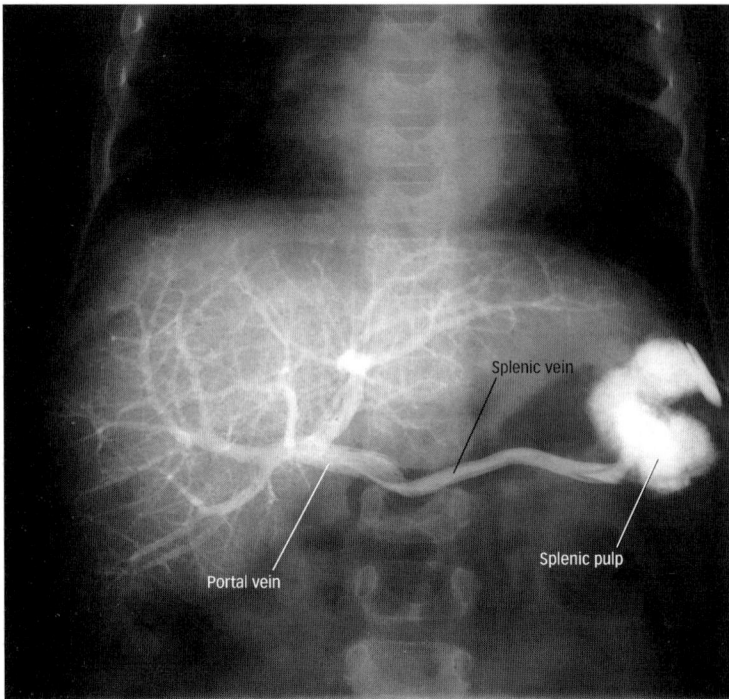

- Splenic vein
- Splenic pulp
- Portal vein

Fig. 12.
A direct splenoportogram.

demonstrated in the caudate and quadrate lobes (segments I and IV) using CTAP. It is important not to misinterpret these defects as metastases. Angiography has demonstrated that these perfusion defects are produced by aberrant venous drainage from the left gastric vein and from the pericardiphrenic vein directly into subsegmental hepatic parenchyma.

The posterior relations of the portal vein are the epiploic foramen and the inferior vena cava. The close relation of the portal vein to the inferior cava is utilized by surgeons when performing porta-caval anastomoses in patients with portal hypertension (Fig. 1).

The venous drainage of the liver is via the right, middle and left hepatic veins. Smaller unnamed accessory veins drain the liver

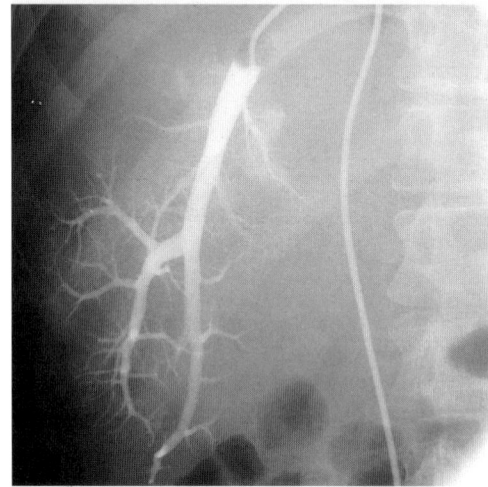

directly into the inferior cava. The intrahepatic course of the right hepatic vein is demonstrated in Fig. 13. The veins unite to join the inferior vena cava at the level of T9, which is in close proximity to the caval diaphragmatic hiatus (Fig. 14(a), (b)). The segmental anatomy is defined by its blood supply from the portal vein and the hepatic artery. However, the hepatic veins drain multiple segments, e.g. the left hepatic vein drains segments II, III and IV.

The caudate lobe of the liver obtains its blood supply from both the right and left hepatic arteries and portal veins and drains directly into the inferior vena cava via small tributaries. This is of clinical significance as in certain pathological states the caudate lobe may preferentially hypertrophy (e.g. Budd–Chiari syndrome).

Lymphatic drainage
The lymphatics of the liver follow the course of the hepatic artery and portal vein towards the hilum of the liver. They continue in the free edge of the lesser omentum where small nodes can normally be demonstrated on

anatomical specimens. Nodes can be demonstrated on CT; however, their transaxial diameter should not exceed 10 mm. The liver drains into pre-aortic nodes via lymphatics along the coelic axis (Fig. 15). Biliary lymphatics are especially important in children with biliary atresia, where they act as the sole route of drainage of bile. The surgery for this condition aims to provide drainage of the lymphatics into a loop of bowel prior to liver transplant (the Kasai procedure).

Nerve supply

The sympathetic nerve supply to the liver is from the coeliac ganglion and the parasympathetic supply is from the left vagal trunk. The nerves travel along the lesser omentum and run with the vessels to the porta hepatis. The capsular supply is via the visceral segmental peritoneal innervation.

Peritoneal attachments

The peritoneal attachments are complex and important as they produce specific compartments within the upper abdomen (see Chapter 10). They limit the direction of flow of peritoneal fluid and may contain fluid collections in pathological states. On the anterior convexity of the liver (Fig. 16(a)) the sickle-shaped falciform ligament passes forwards to the anterior abdominal wall. In its free edge runs the ligamentum teres (see Embryology).

Fig. 14.
(a) USS of the hepatic venous confluence (axial view).
(b) Parasagittal view of the left hepatic vein.

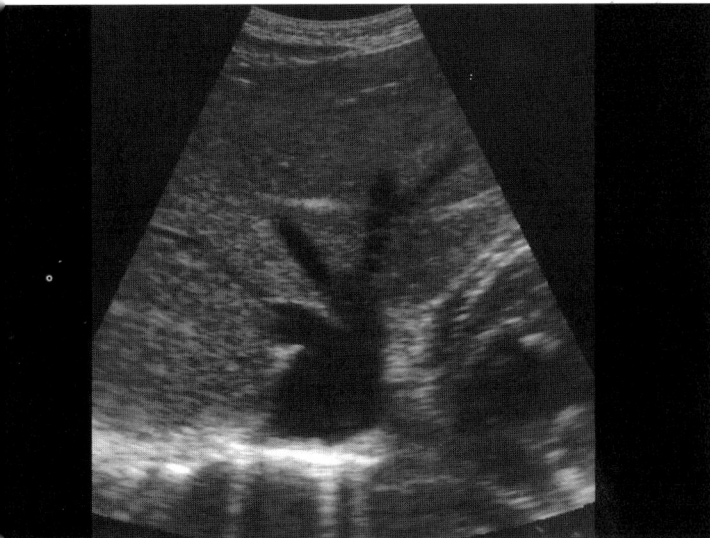

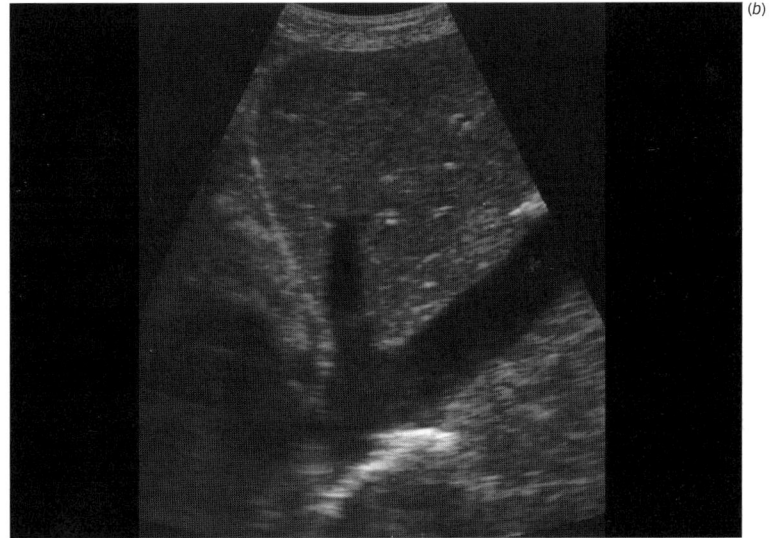

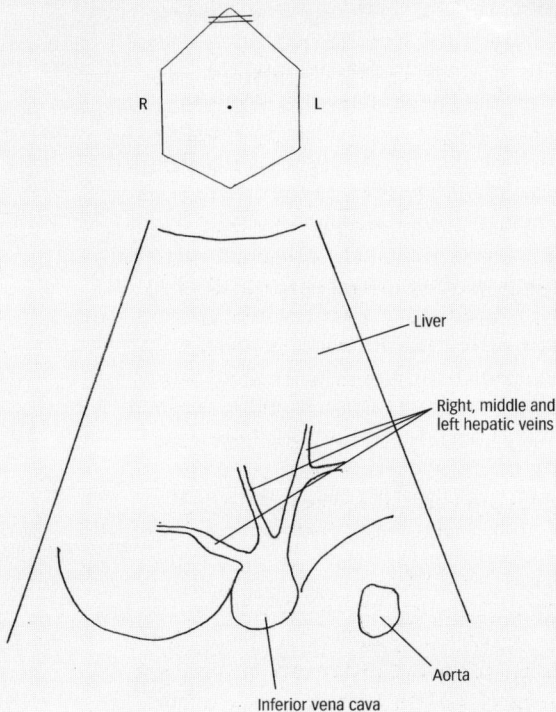

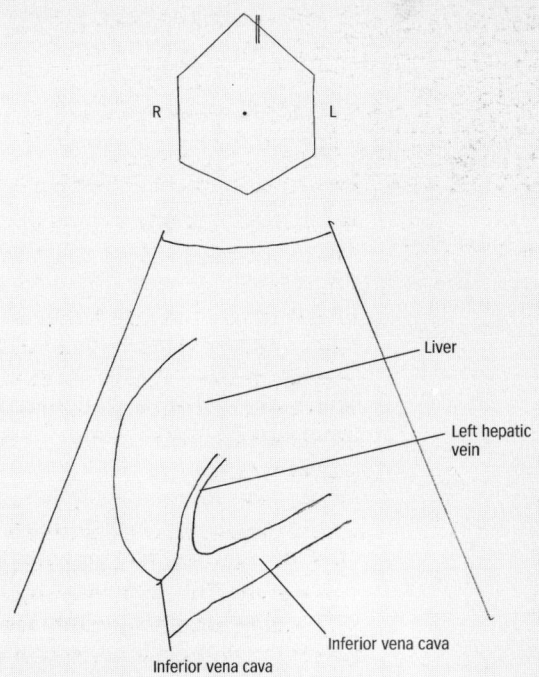

(b)

Liver

Right, middle and left hepatic veins

Aorta

Inferior vena cava

Liver

Left hepatic vein

Inferior vena cava

Inferior vena cava

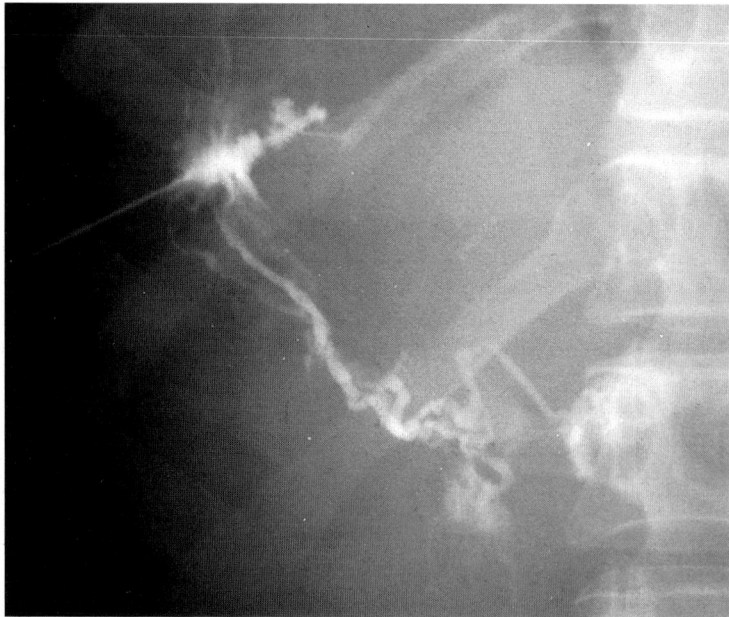

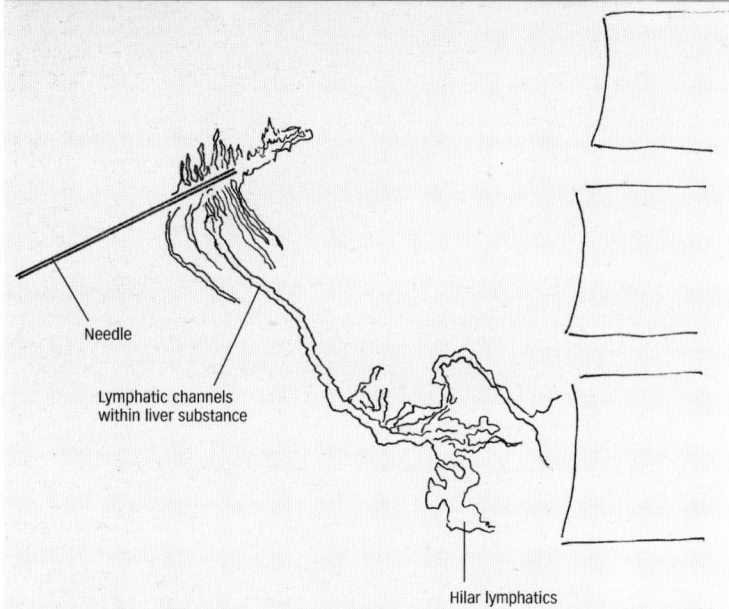

Needle

Lymphatic channels
within liver substance

Hilar lymphatics

Fig. 15.
A transhepatic
lymphangiogram
demonstrating the flow
of lymph towards the
hepatic hilum.

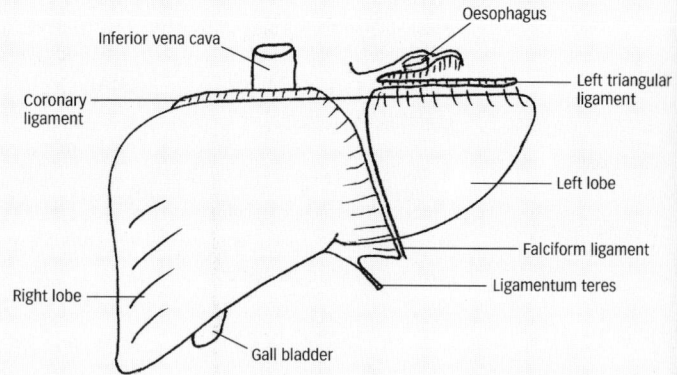

Inferior vena cava

Oesophagus

Coronary
ligament

Left triangular
ligament

Left lobe

Falciform ligament

Ligamentum teres

Right lobe

Gall bladder

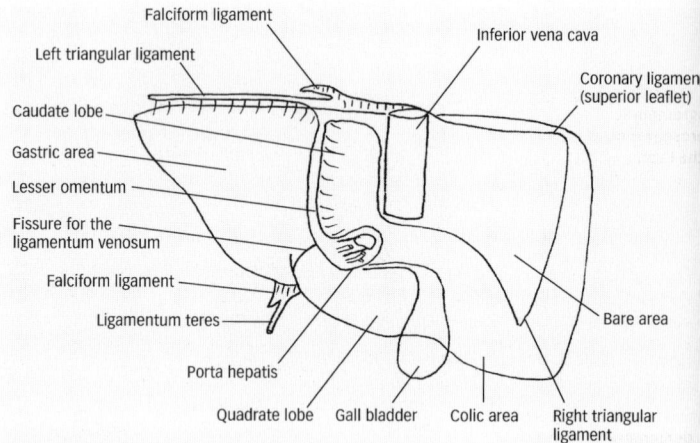

Falciform ligament

Inferior vena cava

Left triangular ligament

Coronary ligamen
(superior leaflet)

Caudate lobe

Gastric area

Lesser omentum

Fissure for the
ligamentum venosum

Falciform ligament

Ligamentum teres

Bare area

Porta hepatis

Quadrate lobe   Gall bladder   Colic area   Right triangular
ligament

Fig. 16.
(a) The diagram
demonstrates the
peritoneal attachments
of the anterior surface
of the liver.
(b) The diagram
demonstrates the
peritoneal attachments
of the posterior surface
of the liver.

Viewing the liver from its posterior aspect (Fig. 16(b)), an area of the right lobe is not covered by peritoneum. This is referred to as the bare area, and is roughly triangular in shape. The base of the triangle is formed by the inferior vena cava, the upper and lower sides by the superior and inferior coronary ligaments and its apex, which lies inferiorly, forms the right triangular ligament. The superior coronary ligament continues medially, crosses the midline along the superior border of the liver and passes to the left of the midline. It unites with the anterior leaflet of the left triangular ligament to form the falciform ligament, which in turn passes anteriorly to the posterior aspect of the anterior abdominal wall. The lesser omentum extends from the lesser curvature of the stomach and is

attached in its superior extent to the hepatic fissure of the ligamentum venosum. The two leaflets of the lesser omentum divide to invest the anterior and posterior gastric surfaces. It can be seen (Fig. 16(b)) that the omental reflections divide the caudate from the quadrate lobe; thus the caudate lobe lies within the lesser sac and the quadrate lobe lies within the greater sac. In order that the liver may maintain its position in the upper abdomen, it is stabilized and suspended by its peritoneal reflections and by the union of the three hepatic veins to the inferior vena cava.

On the visceral surface of the liver, there is a transversely placed central depression through which the portal vein, hepatic artery, common hepatic ducts, autonomic nerves and lymphatics pass. This is the porta hepatis (or hepatic hilum) and is described as the 'the gateway to the liver' (Fig. 17). Anterior to the porta hepatis lies the gall bladder fossa, with the quadrate lobe to the left. Posterior to the porta hepatis the liver is deeply grooved by the inferior vena cava.

It is classically taught that the most posterior structure in the porta hepatis is the portal vein. Anterior to this and to the right lies the common hepatic duct, which is formed by

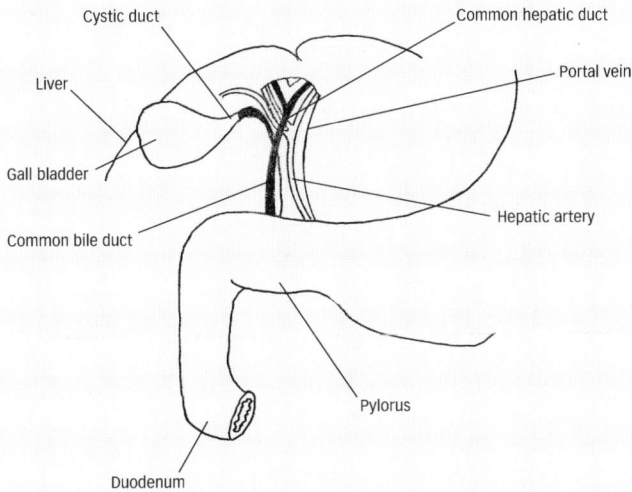

17. above
**grammatic
resentation of the hilum
he liver.**

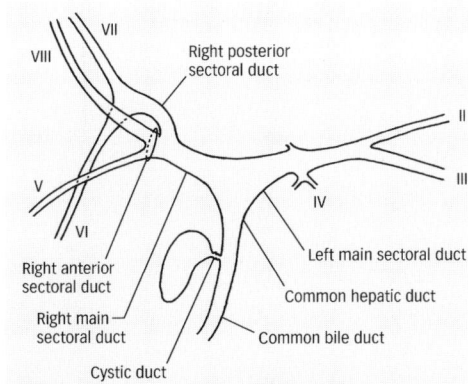

Fig. 18.
**A line diagram to
demonstrate the normal
(57%) segmental biliary
drainage of the liver**

union of the left and right hepatic ducts.
Anteriorly and to the left of the portal vein lies
the hepatic artery, which divides into the left
and right hepatic branches. USS frequently
demonstrates (Fig. 3) the hepatic artery 'sand-
wiched' between the portal vein and common
hepatic duct.

The biliary tree
Bile produced by hepatocytes is collected in
the canaliculi within the hepatic lobules,
which follow a course along the portal canals
to drain into the bile duct tributaries. The
portal vein radicles and the hepatic arterial
branches run with the bile duct tributaries
in the portal triads. Biliary drainage follows
segmental to the anatomy of the liver (Fig. 18).
Access to the biliary tree can be obtained
percutaneously via segment III in the left lobe
of the liver and segment V and VI in the right
lobe of the liver. The segmental ducts unite
to form the major left and right biliary ducts,
which in turn unite at the porta hepatis
forming the common hepatic duct (Fig. 19).
The common hepatic duct lies anterior to the
portal vein in the free edge of the lesser omentum, with the hepatic artery on its left side,

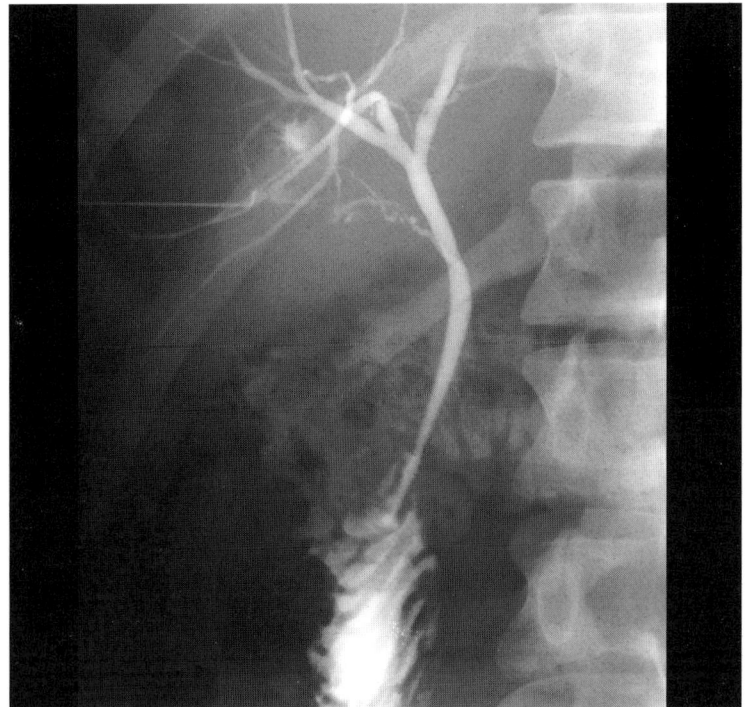

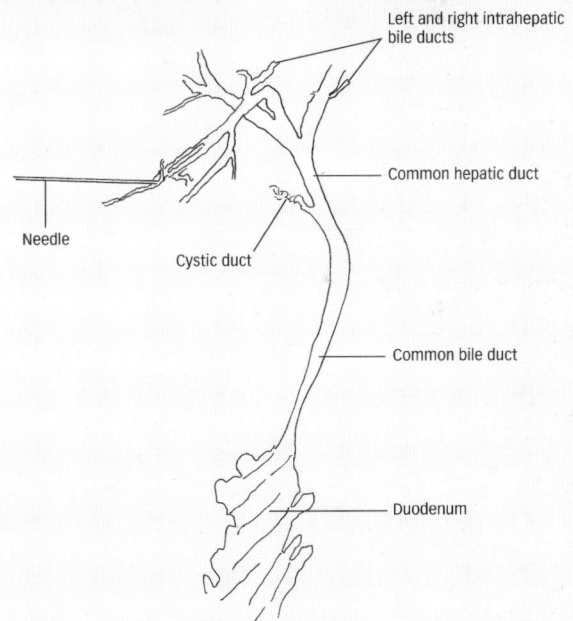

Fig. 19.
**Percutaneous transhepatic
cholangiogram performed
by a right lobe approach.
(The gall bladder has not
filled.)**

and is joined at a variable position by the cystic duct which receives bile from the gall bladder. From this point distally, it is referred to as
the common bile duct. The common bile duct
is divided into three portions.

- *The upper third* is the region from its formation at the hilum of the liver to the first part
of the duodenum.
- *The middle third* passes posterior to the first
part of the duodenum and slopes away to
the right from the portal vein. Its immediate posterior relation is the inferior vena

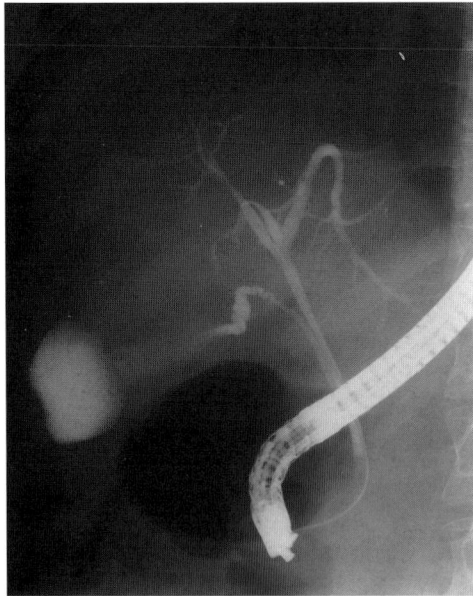

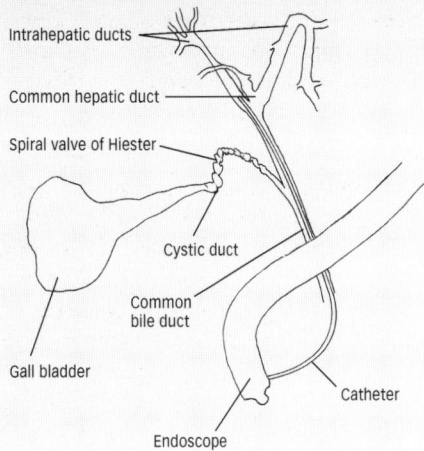

Intrahepatic ducts

Common hepatic duct

Spiral valve of Hiester

Cystic duct

Common
bile duct

Gall bladder

Endoscope

Catheter

also with previous biliary pathology. Thus, in the young an upper limit of 5 mm is normal. However, in the elderly, 10 mm can be normal (a good 'rule of thumb' is 1 mm per decade). Following cholecystectomy, the common bile duct should not enlarge; however, if it was enlarged prior to surgery, its calibre may not decrease post-operatively. At ERCP, an accepted working rule is that the common bile duct and common hepatic duct should be no bigger than the endoscope. This allows for technical considerations and radiographic magnification (Fig. 20).

The gall bladder lies in a depression on the undersurface of the right lobe of the liver, referred to as the gall bladder fossa (Fig. 21). The fundus of the gall bladder has a bulbous blind end which protrudes from the visceral surface of the liver to abut the posterior surface of the anterior abdominal wall at the level of the tip of the 9th costal cartilage in the

Fig. 21.
**USS of the normal
gall bladder**

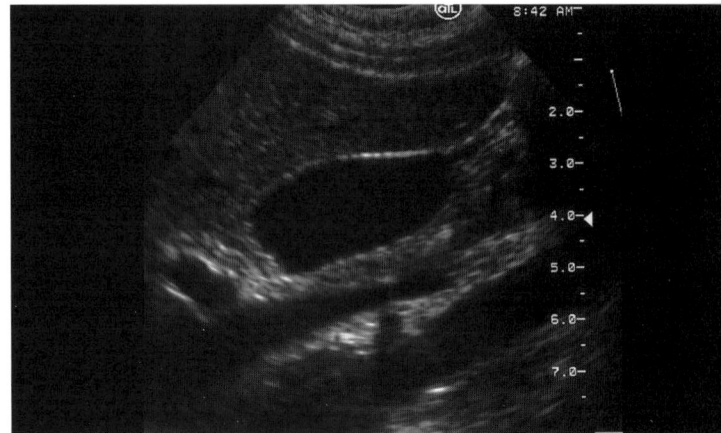

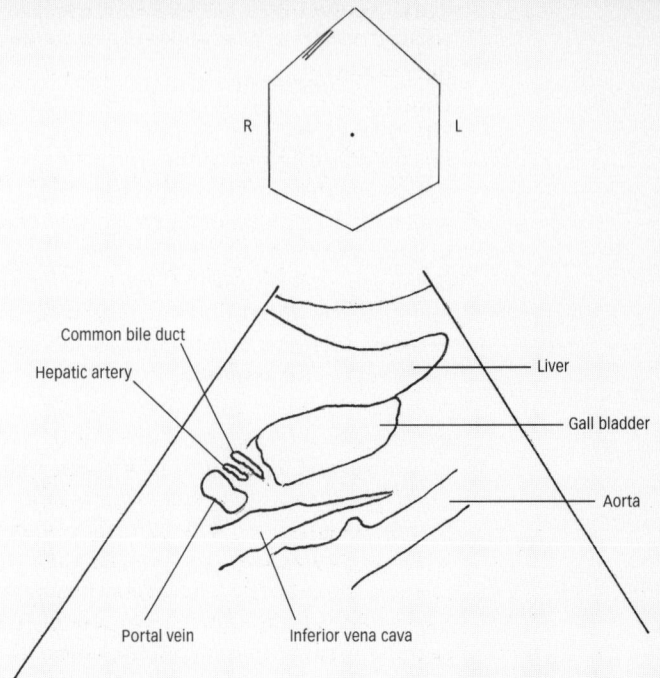

R   L

Common bile duct

Hepatic artery

Liver

Gall bladder

Aorta

Portal vein   Inferior vena cava

cava. Occasionally, on barium studies, the middle third of the common bile duct can be demonstrated to groove the posterior surface of the first part of the duodenum.

- *The lower third* passes inferiorly, and to the right, behind the head of the pancreas. This portion of the common bile duct grooves or tunnels the head of the pancreas passing anterior to the right renal vein. It is joined by the main pancreatic duct to form the ampulla of Vater which opens into the posterio-medial wall of the second part of the duodenum at the duodenal papilla.

The ampulla is surrounded by a circular layer of involuntary muscle which is arranged such that its orifice pouts into the second part of the duodenum. The muscular layer is referred to as the sphincter of Oddi.

The length of the common bile duct is approximately 8 cm, which is, to some extent, dependent upon the level of insertion of the cystic duct. The diameter varies with age and mid axillary line. The body of the gall bladder passes posteriorly and superiorly and can occasionally be demonstrated, during barium studies, to indent the anterior aspect of the first part of the duodenum. The body continues to narrow to form the neck of the gall bladder which is often referred to as Hartmann's pouch (classically Hartmann's pouch only exists in the pathological state when a gall stone is impacted in the neck). The cystic duct arises from the neck of the gall bladder and runs along the visceral surface of the liver to lie against the porta. The duct has a muscular wall which acts so as to regulate the flow of bile (the spiral valve of Hiester). It passes anterior to the right main branch of the hepatic artery and unites with the common hepatic duct to form the cystic duct (Fig. 17). Care should be taken during USS of the neck of the gall bladder, as the highly echogenic wall of the cystic duct may be misdiagnosed as gall stones.

The gall bladder (Figs. 16(*b*), 21) is partially invested in peritoneum in its fossa on the visceral surface of the liver. Occasionally, the gall bladder may hang on its own mesentery, in which case it is susceptible to volvulus. A common variant, encountered in 2–6% of the population, in gall bladder anatomy, is the phyrgian cap. The Phrygian cap is the fundus of the gall bladder that is folded back upon the body of the gall bladder. USS demonstrates this as an apparent septum across an otherwise normal gall bladder. Other anomalies are rare but include agenesis, bilobed gall bladder and gall bladder diverticula.

There are a number of variants of the relations of the cystic duct to the common hepatic duct as demonstrated in 5–10% of operative cholangiograms. These include:

- aberrant intrahepatic duct, which may join the common hepatic duct, the common bile duct, the cystic duct the right hepatic duct or the gall bladder;
- cystic duct entering the right hepatic duct;
- duplication of the cystic duct/common bile duct;
- congenital biliary/respiratory fistula.

Accessory ducts can be demonstrated in approximately 5–10% of the population. Although many of these variants are well known to the surgeons, there has been an increase in iatrogenic damage to the extrahepatic biliary tree associated with laparoscopic cholecystectomy. Demonstration of the extrahepatic biliary tree prior to laparoscopic procedures can be undertaken by three-dimensional CT and cholecystography. Using

tailored MRI sequences, without contrast, three-dimensional images of the biliary tree can be produced.

Blood supply

The cystic artery which supplies the gall bladder commonly arises from the right hepatic artery at the angle between the common hepatic duct and the cystic duct (75%), although in approximately 10% of cases it may arise from the left hepatic artery. Less frequently, the cystic artery may arise from the common hepatic or the superior mesenteric artery. When the hepatic artery arises to the left of the common hepatic duct, it tends to lie anterior to it (Fig. 22). The venous drainage is via cystic veins which pass either directly into the liver or via small tributaries which drain into the portal venous system.

In healthy individuals, ligation of the hepatic artery is of little consequence, whereas in certain disorders of the liver and post-liver transplant, interruption of the hepatic artery can produce necrosis and strictures of the bile ducts.

Lymphatic drainage

The lymphatic drainage is from fundus to neck and follows the same course as the common hepatic and common bile duct. Some of the biliary lymph drains directly into the liver; this is important in malignancy of the gall bladder as it may be necessary to resect local segments of the liver with the gall bladder tumour.

The pancreas

The pancreas is a retroperitoneal structure which measures approximately 15 cm. It is retort shaped and macroscopically is finely lobulated, lying closely applied to the posterior abdominal wall (Fig. 23). The gland is

Fig. 22.
Diagrammatic representation of the cystic artery and its relationships. Note in this diagram the cystic artery arises from the right hepatic artery

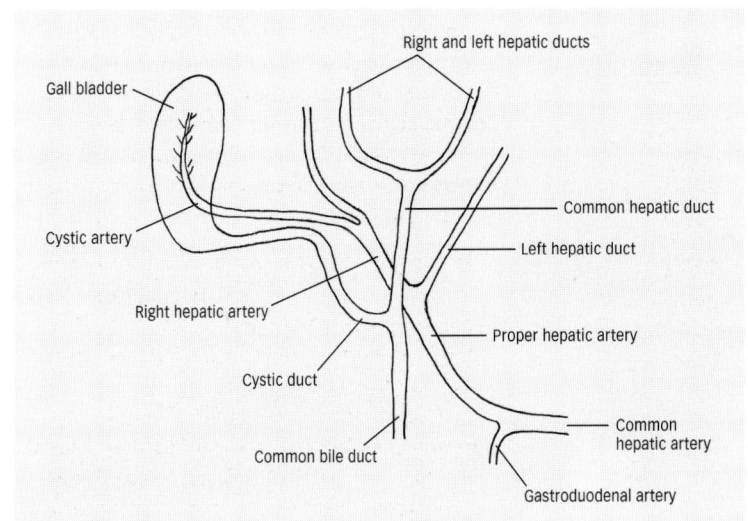

(a)

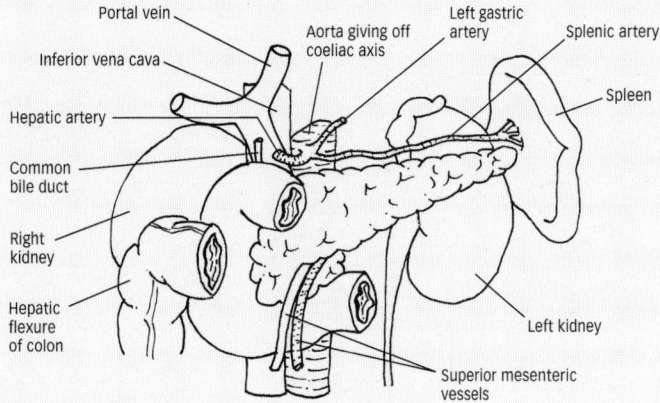

(b)

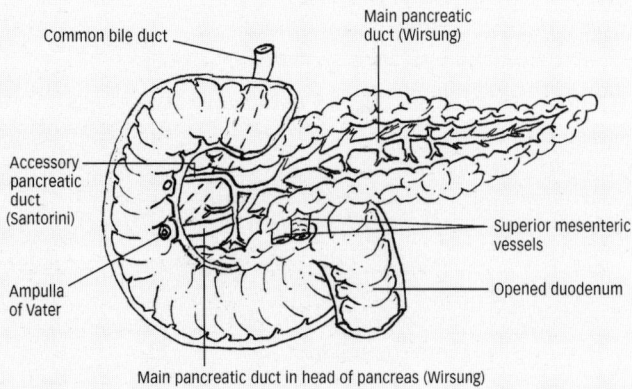

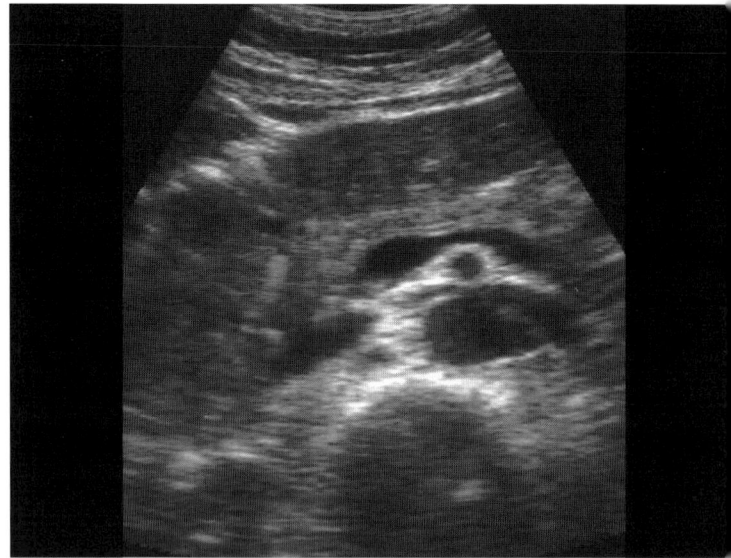

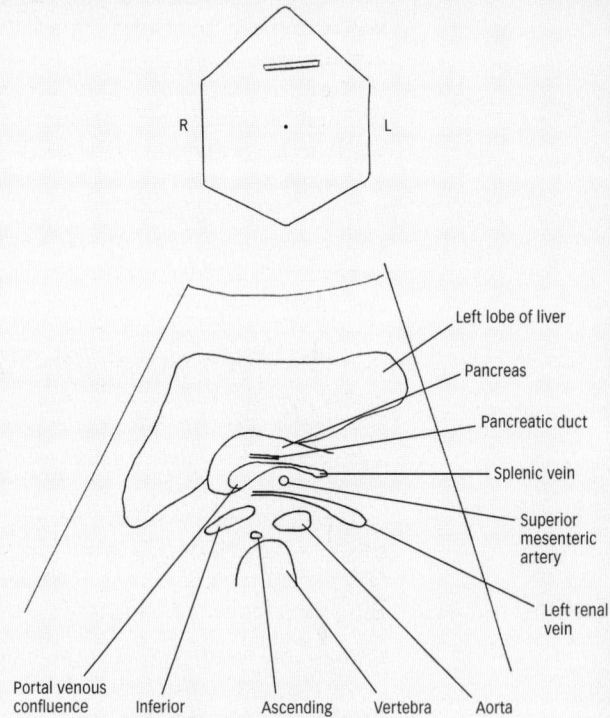

Fig. 23.
**The pancreas:
(a) its relations, and
(b) ductal anatomy**

Fig. 24.
**Transverse USS of the head
and neck of the pancreas.**

angled superiorly from right to left crossing the vertebral bodies at the level of L1 and L2 (Fig. 1). Anteriorly, the transverse mesocolon takes origin from its head, neck and body, and thus most of the gland lies posterior to the lesser sac.

The pancreas consists of four parts, namely, the head, neck, body and tail. The head of the pancreas lies to the right of the midline and has an inferior uncinate (hook-like) process. Anteriorly, it is related to the first part of the duodenum, the lesser sac and transverse colon. Posteriorly, it is related to the common bile duct, inferior vena cava, and right renal vein. The head lies within the C-loop of the duodenum, and thus to its right lies the second part of the duodenum, and inferiorly the third part of the duodenum. The uncinate process arises from the inferior portion of the head and is related anteriorly to the origin of the superior mesenteric artery and the inferior mesenteric vein. Posteriorly, the uncinate process is directly related to the left renal vein.

The head is joined to the neck of the pancreas, which passes anteriorly over the vertebral column. Anterior to the neck lies the gastroduodenal artery, whilst posteriorly the neck is defined by the portal vein as this is formed by the union of the splenic vein and superior mesenteric vein.

The body lies to the left of the midline and is related anteriorly to the lesser sac and to the stomach. Posteriorly lie the splenic vein and the anastomosis of the inferior mesenteric vein to the splenic vein. Behind this lie the aorta, left suprarenal gland and the left kidney.

254

The tail of the pancreas is reflected anteriorly into the lienorenal ligament which passes to the hilum of the spleen (Fig. 1). Using the liver as a US acoustic window, the pancreas can be readily identified in most cases. However, occasionally it may be obscured by bowel gas. The pancreas is hyperechoic compared with liver, although with increasing age the pancreas becomes more echogenic due to progressive accumulation of fat. The size of the pancreas is variable but should not be greater than 30 mm in the transverse axial length in the region of the head. The duct can often be demonstrated in the head, neck and body measuring 3 mm, 2 mm and 1 mm in diameter, respectively (Fig. 24).

On CT scanning, the pancreas is of similar density to the liver, although with increasing age the density is reduced owing to the normal progressive accumulation of fat. After intravenous contrast, the pancreas enhances homogeneously.

The main pancreatic duct unites with the common bile duct to form the ampulla of Vater, which opens into the second part of the duodenum (Fig. 25).

During development, the pancreas is formed from the dorsal and ventral processes (see Embryology). After rotation and fusion of these processes, the ductal systems unite.

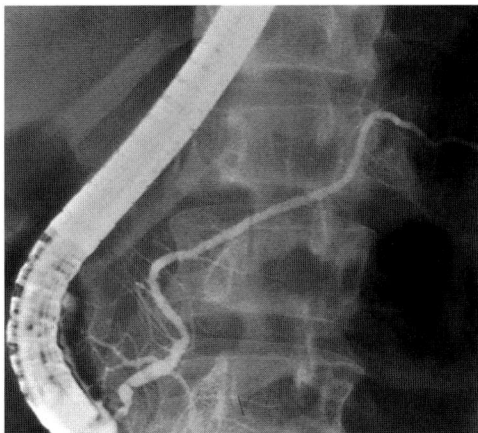

Occasionally the two ductal systems persist to open individually into the second part of the duodenum (Fig. 26). Often there is communication between the two ductal systems. The two systems may be separate in 10% of individuals. In individuals with separation of the ductal systems, the superior and inferior ducts are eponymously named the ducts of Santorini and Wirsung, respectively (Fig. 26). Rarely, there is a failure of complete rotation wherein the second part of the duodenum is gripped by pancreatic tissue and is referred to as the annular pancreas.

Blood supply

The blood supply to the pancreas is mainly from the splenic artery which is a branch of the coeliac axis (Fig. 9(*a*)). The splenic artery is unique in being the only tortuous artery within the trunk. Numerous small branches of the splenic artery run deep into the pancreatic substance as it passes along the superior border of the pancreas. Halfway along the length of the splenic artery, a larger artery, the arteria pancreatica magna, passes deep within the pancreatic substance towards the main pancreatic duct. This anastomoses with the transverse pancreatic artery, which runs beside the duct along the length of the pancreas. The dorsal pancreatic artery arises from the proximal portion of the splenic or coeliac artery to supply the body and neck and anastomoses with the transverse pancreatic artery.

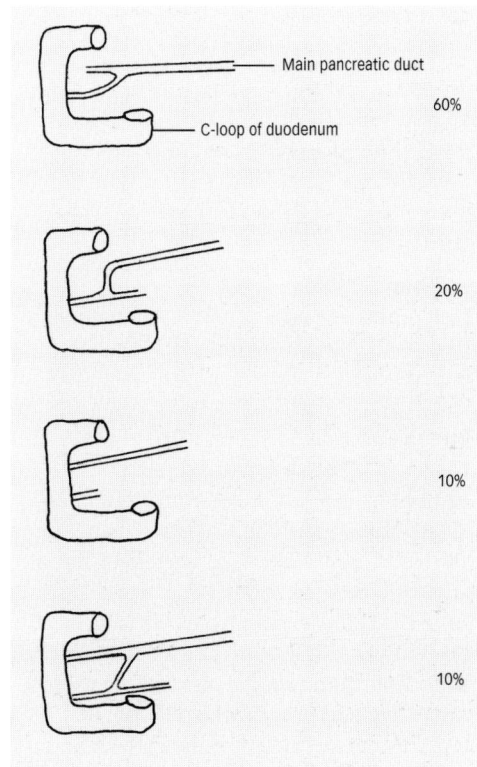

Fig. 25.
The normal pancreatic duct at ERCP.

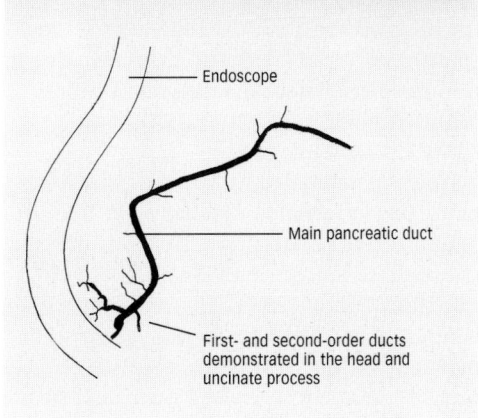

Endoscope

Main pancreatic duct

First- and second-order ducts demonstrated in the head and uncinate process

Main pancreatic duct

60%

C-loop of duodenum

20%

10%

10%

Fig. 26.
The diagram demonstrates the normal variations in pancreatic ductal anatomy

The head of the pancreas has a dual blood supply (Fig. 27(b)). The superior pancreatico-duodenal artery is a branch of the gastroduodenal artery which passes inferiorly to divide into anterior and posterior divisions which encircle the head. The inferior pancreatico-duodenal artery is the first branch of the superior mesenteric artery which, like the superior pancreatico-duodenal artery, divides into anterior and posterior branches which encircle the inferior portion of the head. There are numerous anastomoses between these vessels within the pancreas which allow multidirectional flow.

The venous drainage of the gland is via small vessels which drain directly into the splenic vein, the superior mesenteric vein and, from the head, into the portal vein. Again, flow is multidirectional.

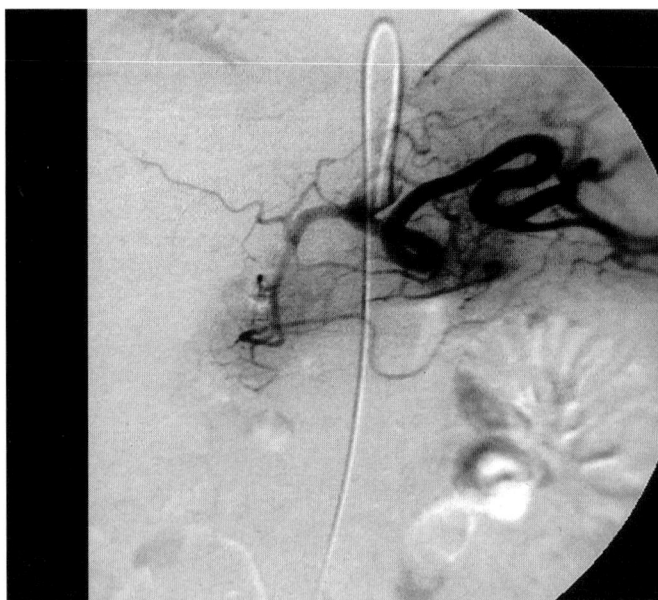

27(b)

27(a)

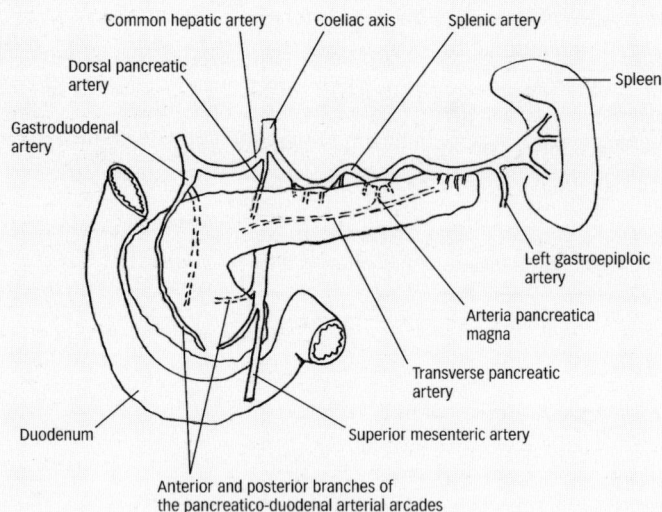

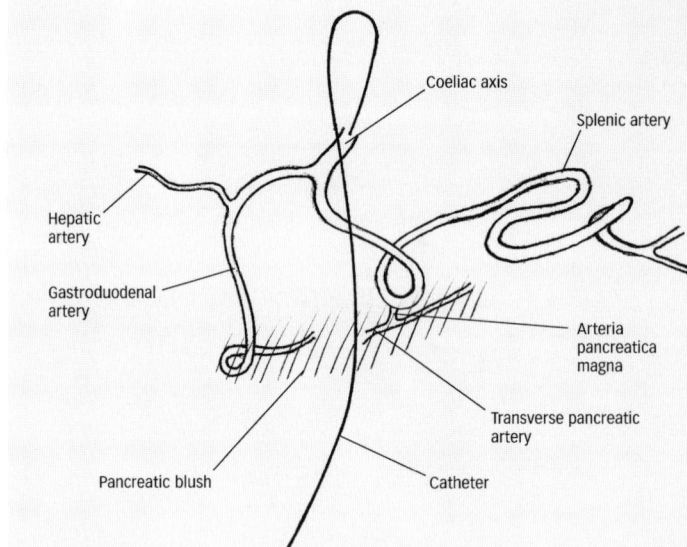

Fig. 27.
(a) A diagram of the normal blood supply to the pancreas.
(b) An angiogram to demonstrate the vasculature of the pancreas.

Lymphatic drainage
The lymphatics of the pancreas drain along its arterial blood supply to pre-aortic coeliac lymph nodes.

The spleen
The spleen is both a lymphoid and a haemopoietic organ. A traditional mnemonic aids retention of anatomical detail using the rule of odd numbers, 1, 3, 5, 7, 9 and 11. Its size is $1 \times 3 \times 5$ inches, it weighs 7 oz, and lies posterior to the axillary line adjacent to the 9th–11th ribs. The spleen is most easily imaged by ultrasound and should measure no more than 14 cm in its longest axis (Fig. 28). Embryologically, it is formed by numerous splenunculi which fuse. Occasionally (10%) unfused and accessory splenunculi are demonstrated by CT and USS, and tend to lie in the region of the hilum or the lienorenal ligament. If the spleen is surgically removed and residual functioning splenic tissue is suspected, a Tc 99^m denatured red blood cell scan will demonstrate any remaining tissue.

The spleen has two surfaces, the diaphragmatic surface which is notched on its inferior border and the hilar surface that lies between the stomach and the left kidney. It is invested by a thin adherent layer of peritoneum, which when split or damaged can produce torrential bleeding, owing to the vascular nature of the organ. Anteriorly, the spleen is attached by the

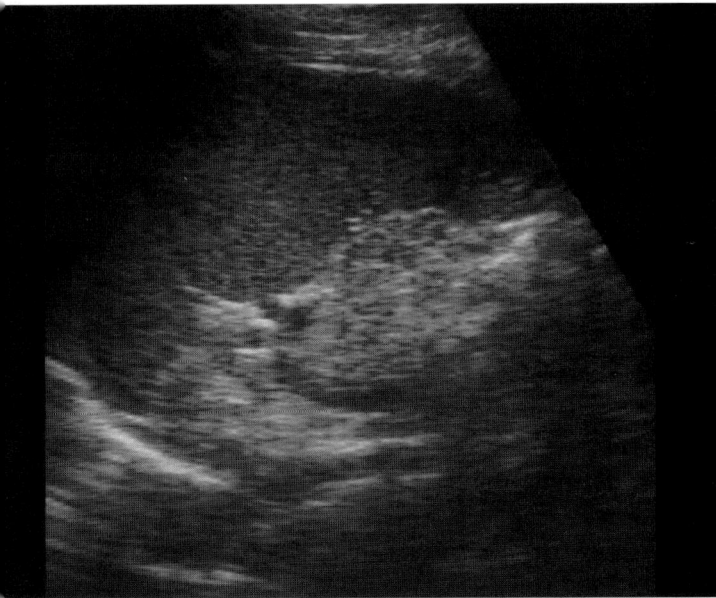

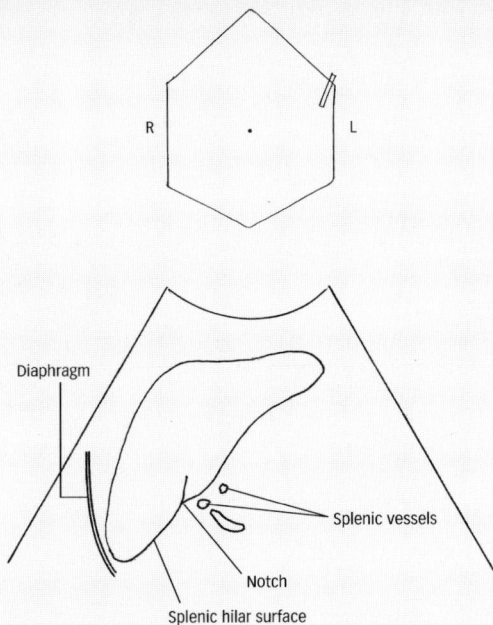

Fig. 28.
USS of the normal spleen.

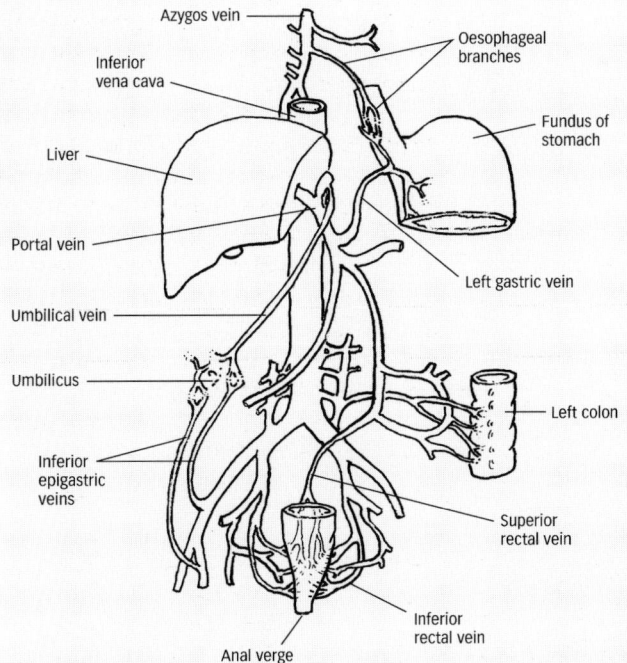

Fig. 29.
The diagram demonstrates the normal portal-systemic anastomoses.

gastrosplenic ligament which is continuous with the greater omentum to the stomach. Posteriorly, the lienorenal ligament attaches the spleen to the kidney and contains the tail of the pancreas and the splenic and short gastric vessels.

The spleen is related medially to the stomach and the tail of the pancreas. Anteriorly, it lies in close proximity to the left colonic flexure (the splenic flexure) and, posteriorly, it is related to the left kidney and a suprarenal gland (Fig. 1).

Blood supply
The blood supply to the spleen is from the splenic artery (Fig. 9(a)). The splenic artery divides near the hilum into four or five main branches that pierce the splenic substance at its hilum. The intrasplenic blood supply is inconsistent. This can be appreciated on CT as inhomogeneous enhancement in the early arterial phase. The venous drainage is into the splenic vein and then to the portal vein (Fig. 12).

Lymphatic drainage
Splenic lymphatics follow the arterial supply to the coeliac axis and pre-aortic nodes.

Portal–systemic anastomoses
In non-pathological states the portal and systemic circulations are separate. When the portal venous pressure is elevated (as in hepatic cirrhosis), tiny collateral vessels open between the two systems. As the disease progresses, they become dilated and varicose possibly leading to rupture and exsanguination, especially in the case of varices at the oesophagogastric junction.

There are four common sites where these anastomoses develop (Fig. 29):

- the lower oesophagus between the left gastric and the azygos veins;
- the inferior and middle rectal veins with the superior rectal veins;
- the paraumbilical (portal) veins and the superficial epigastric veins;
- the colic twigs with the peritoneal veins.

Reference
Couinaud, C. (1957). *Le Foie. Etudes Anatomiques et Chirurgicales.* Vol. 1. Masson, Paris

13

The renal tract and retroperitoneum

J. CROSS

and A.K. DIXON

Development of the urinary tract

(Professor H. Ellis)

The kidney and the ureter develop in the mesoderm on the dorsal wall of the coelomic cavity (Fig. 1). The pronephros, a series of tubules of importance in the lower vertebrates, is transient in man, but the distal part of its duct receives the tubules of the next renal organ to develop, the mesonephros, and is now termed the mesonephric duct. The mesonephros itself then disappears except for some of its ducts, which form the efferent tubules of the testis.

A diverticulum then appears at the lower end of the mesonephric duct, which develops into the metanephric duct (or ureteric bud). On top of the latter, a cap of tissue differentiates to form the metanephros, which will develop into the definitive kidney. The metanephric duct develops into the ureter, pelvis, calyces and collecting tubules. The metanephros develops into the glomeruli and the proximal part of the renal duct system. The mesonephric duct now loses its renal connection, atrophies in the female (remaining only as the epoöphoron), but persists in the

male, to become the epididymis, vas deferens and ejaculatory duct. The seminal vesicle develops as a swelling at the termination of the mesonephric duct.

Initially, the kidney is lobulated and this persists throughout fetal life. Usually, the lobulation disappears during the first year after birth but varying degrees may persist into adult life.

Initially, the metanephric renal rudiment is situated in the pelvis. As the ureteric outgrowth lengthens, it becomes more and more cranially situated to take up its definitive position. During this period of ascent, the kidney receives its blood supply sequentially from adjacent blood vessels, first from the middle sacral and common iliac arteries and then from the aorta. The definitive renal artery develops about the twelfth week of fetal life. It is common for one or more distally placed arteries to persist (aberrant renal arteries) and one may even run to the kidney from the common iliac artery.

Apart from vascular anomalies, other developmental abnormalities are common. Occasionally the kidney will fail to migrate cranially, which will result in a persistent pelvic kidney. The two metanephric masses may fuse in development to form a horseshoe kidney, linked across the midline, with the ureters passing in front of the inter-renal bar. There may be complete failure of development of one kidney (congenital absence), which occurs in about 1 in 2400 births. Congenital polycystic kidneys (autosomal recessive polycystic kidney disease, ARPKD) probably result from cystic dilatations of many of the tubules of the metanephros. The mesonephric duct may give off a double metanephric bud so that two ureters may develop on one or both sides (duplex kidney).

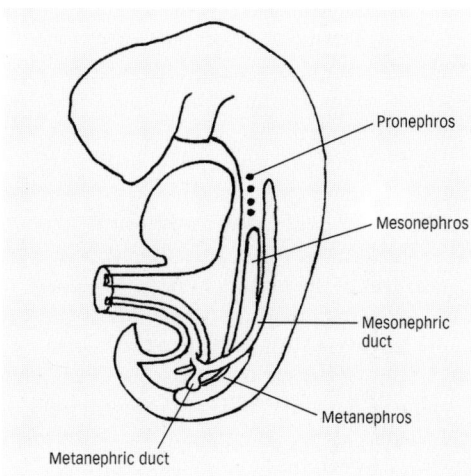

Fig. 1.
Development of the pro-, meso- and metanephric systems.

Pronephros

Mesonephros

Mesonephric duct

Metanephros

Metanephric duct

2(*a*)

Renal cortex
Liver
Renal pyramid
Renal sinus
Psoas

Renal cortex
Portal vein
Renal sinus
Renal vein
Vertebral body
IVC

Liver
Gall bladder containing gall stone
IVC
Right kidney
Superior mesenteric artery
Left renal vein
Aorta

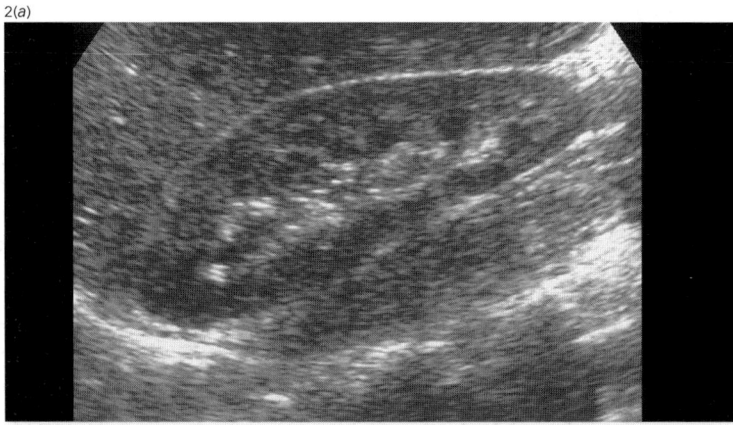

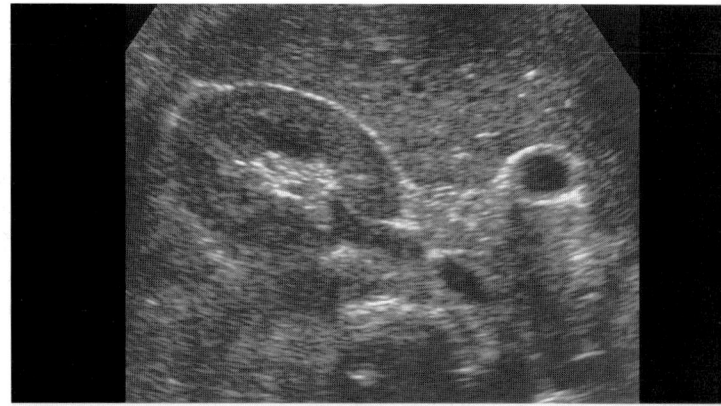

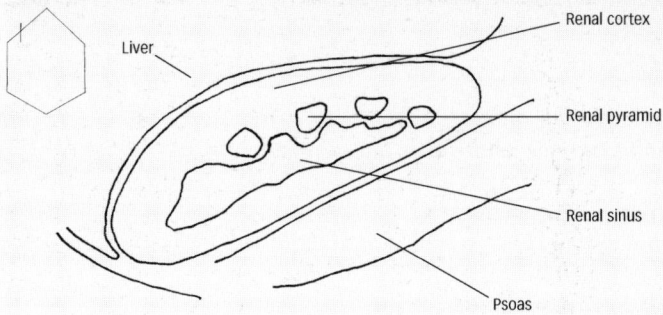

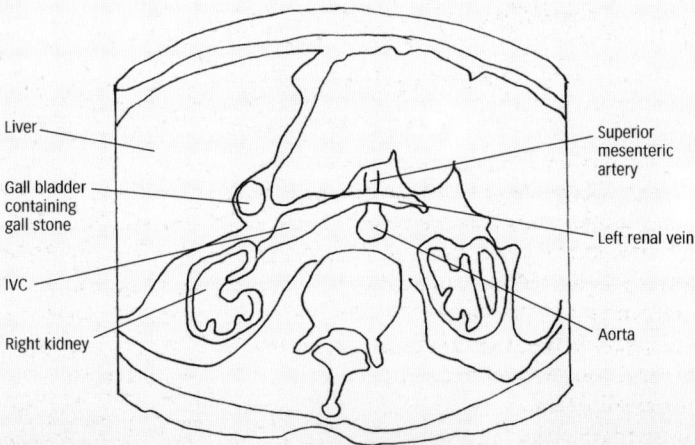

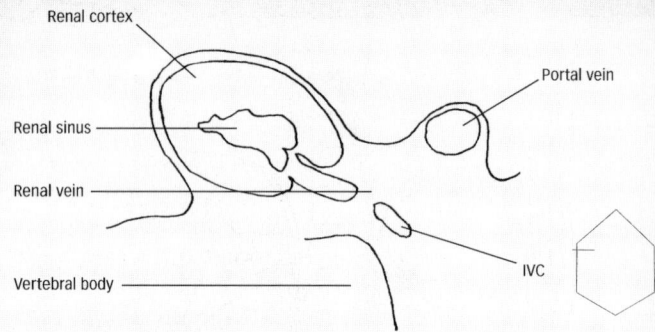

Fig. 2.
Ultrasound images showing the right kidney (*a*) longitudinal and (*b*) axial.

These ureters may fuse into a single duct anywhere along their course or open separately into the bladder (where the upper ureter enters below the lower ureter). Rarely, the extra ureter may open ectopically into the vagina or urethra.

Development of the bladder

The cloaca of the hindgut is divided by the urorectal septum into a posterior compartment, which becomes the rectum, and an anterior primitive urogenital sinus. This continues above with the allantois, a diverticulum of the hindgut, which extends into the umbilicus. Inferiorly the urogenital sinus is bounded by the urogenital membrane. The upper part of the primitive urogenital sinus expands into the bladder, while its lower part develops into the urethra in the male and the urethra and vestibule of the vagina in the female.

The distal portion of the mesonephric ducts, together with their attached ureteric buds, become incorporated into the posterior wall of the bladder between the fourth and sixth weeks of fetal life. This process brings the orifices of the ureters into the bladder wall, while the openings of the mesonephric ducts are carried inferiorly to open, in the male in the prostatic urethra as the ejaculatory ducts. A triangular area of mesonephric duct wall is incorporated on to the posteroinferior wall of the bladder to form the bladder

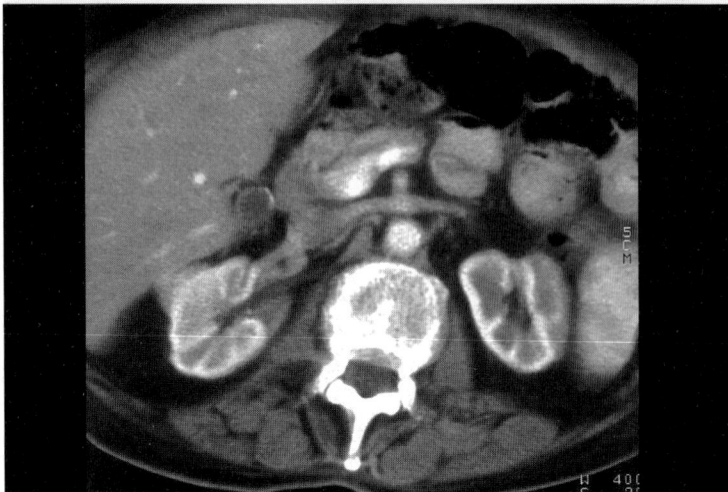

Fig. 3. left
Axial CT image after intravenous contrast medium showing both kidneys.

4(b)

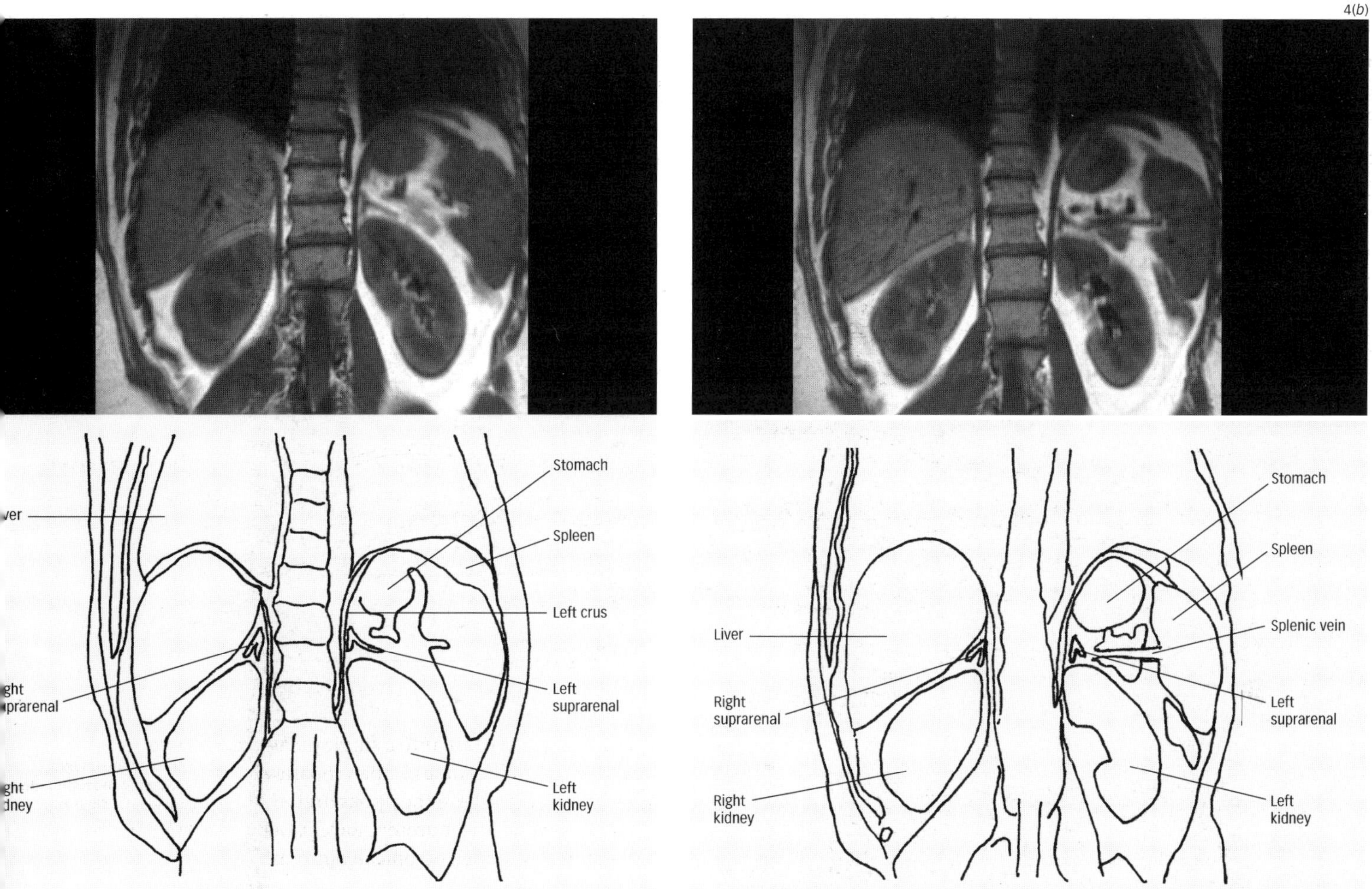
Stomach
Spleen
Left crus
Left suprarenal
Left kidney
Stomach
Spleen
Splenic vein
Liver
Right suprarenal
Left suprarenal
Right kidney
Left kidney

Fig. 4.
Coronal MR images of the retroperitoneum showing: (*a*) suprarenal glands and their relationship to the kidneys and both diaphragmatic crura, (*b*) suprarenal glands, kidneys, spleen and splenic vein, (*c*) hepatic veins draining into the inferior vena cava, (*d*) branches of the abdominal aorta, (*e*) the portal vein.

trigone, a triangular area between the ureteric orifices and the bladder neck. The mesodermal tissue of the trigone is overgrown by epithelium from surrounding bladder, but in the adult the trigone remains visible as a smooth triangle in contrast to the trabeculated remaining bladder mucosa.

Imaging the renal tract

Plain films

A radiograph taken at low kV optimizes the detection of calcification. Movement of the kidney with respiration can be used to demonstrate whether calcification is genuinely renal. Tomograms and oblique projections are also used for this purpose. The renal outline is rendered visible because of the surrounding perirenal fat, although it is frequently obscured by overlying bowel gas (colon, small bowel, stomach on the right, small bowel on the left). The ureters are projected over the tips of the transverse processes of L2 to L5, the sacroiliac joints and within the pelvis over a course which runs laterally to the ischial spines and then medially towards the bladder.

IVU (Intravenous urogram)

This investigation demonstrates the renal outline (nephrogram), the pelvi-calyceal systems, ureters and bladder (urographic phase). In the adult, the kidneys appear approximately three vertebrae in length (11–15 cm) allowing for magnification and diuretic load. The renal outline and calyces may be seen more clearly if tomograms are taken, in which case more posterior cuts are required for the upper poles (and more anterior cuts for the lower poles) because of the orientation of the kidneys with regard to the lumbar lordosis. Because of this obliquity to the coronal plane, the whole length of the kidney can be seen best at slight caudal angulation of the tube, which can be a useful technique in children. Furthermore, a 'lateral' view of the kidney to demonstrate the anterior and posterior surfaces of the kidney is obtained with posterior obliquity (e.g. LPO for left kidney). The ureters may be shown fully or in part of their course; prone views aid mid-ureteric filling.

4(c)

Liver

Liver (left lobe)

Hepatic vein

Aorta

IVC

Small bowel

Liver

Left gastric artery

Coeliac axis

Right renal artery

Inferior mesenteric vein

IVC

Small bowel

Aorta

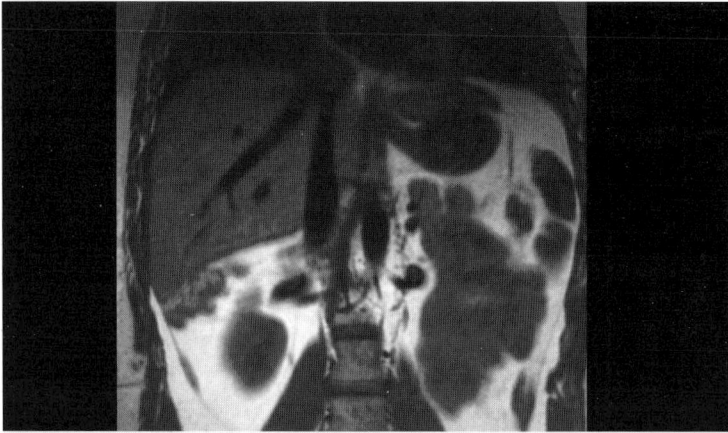

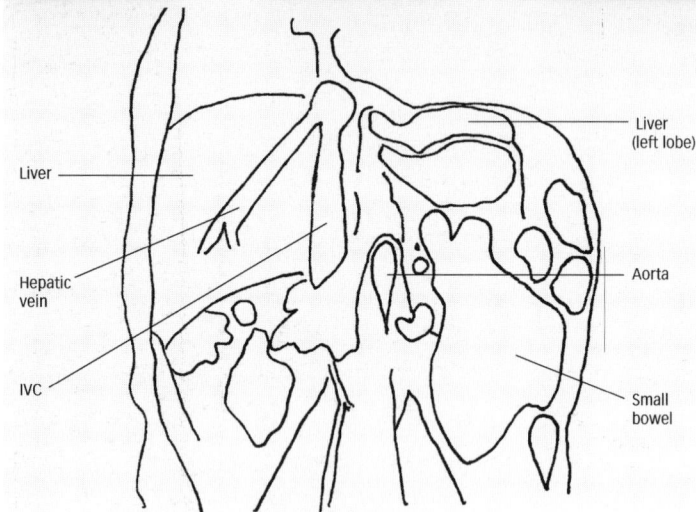

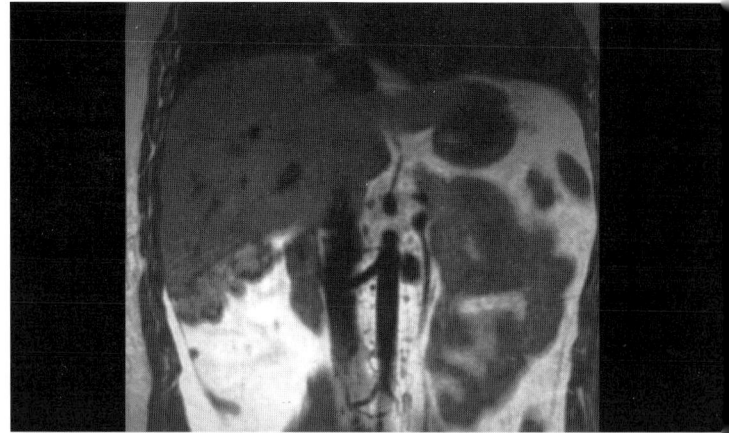

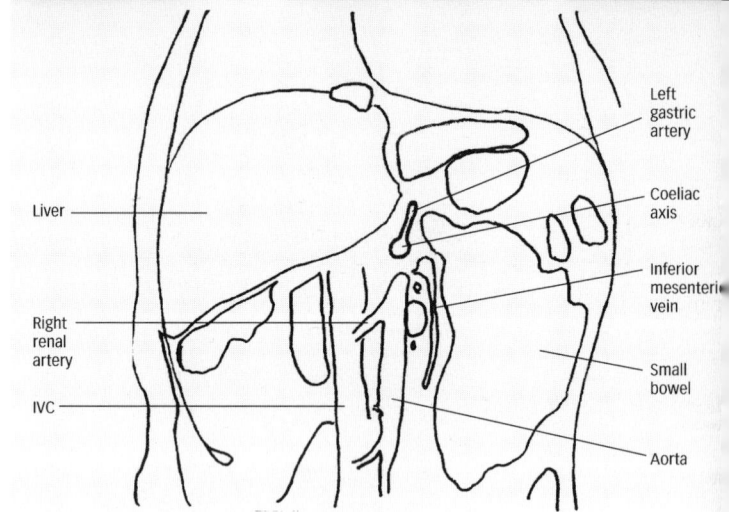

Ultrasound (USS)

This technique is used to assess renal size, cortical scarring, distention of the pelvicalyceal system, calculi and focal renal abnormalities. The right kidney is imaged using the right lobe of the liver as an acoustic window. On the left there is no such acoustic window and bowel loops may obscure the left kidney; thus a posterior approach is used. The cortex is less reflective than the medulla while fat within the renal sinus is highly reflective. The pyramids are less reflective than the medulla (Fig. 2). The proximal and distal ureter may be demonstrated if it is dilated but the rest of the ureter is usually invisible because of overlying bowel gas. Experts can demonstrate flow in renal arteries and veins using Doppler.

CT (Computed tomography)

The kidneys usually lie between T12 and L3 and are well demonstrated along with the perinephric fat. The perinephric fat is most abundant medial to the lower pole of the kidney. Immediately after injection of contrast medium the cortex opacifies and only later do the medulla and pyramids opacify with contrast medium (Fig. 3). At the hilum, the

pyramids are seen from base to tip, but at other levels they are less well defined because of degrees of obliquity. The ureter may be seen and its course is more easily identified when opacified with intravenous contrast medium. Bolus enhanced techniques allow documentation of the patency of renal vessels and when images are acquired in a helical fashion, elegant three-dimensional views of the renal arteries can be obtained.

Magnetic resonance imaging (MRI)

MRI is a non-invasive way of demonstrating the kidneys. The corticomedullary pattern is well seen on T1 weighting without the need for contrast medium (see Fig. 4). Likewise, magnetic resonance angiography (MRA) allows demonstration of renal vessels without contrast medium.

Angiography

This is used to assess the vascularity of tumours and other lesions and to see the renal vein. It is much less frequently used since the advent of CT, US and MRI. Aortography is the definitive test for demonstrating accessory renal arteries and is therefore performed prior

Fig. 6.
MAG3 scintigram.

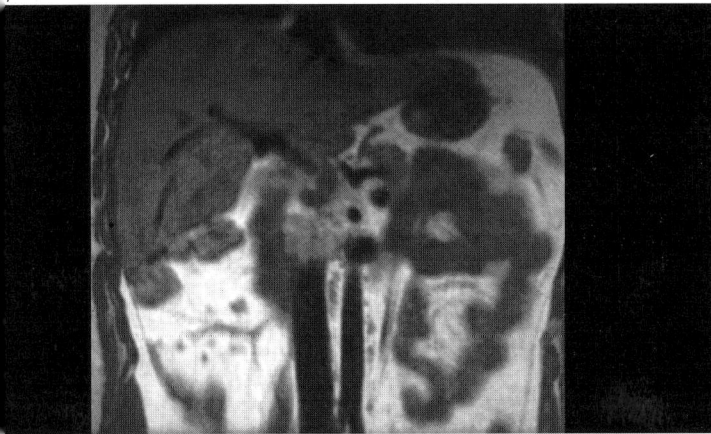

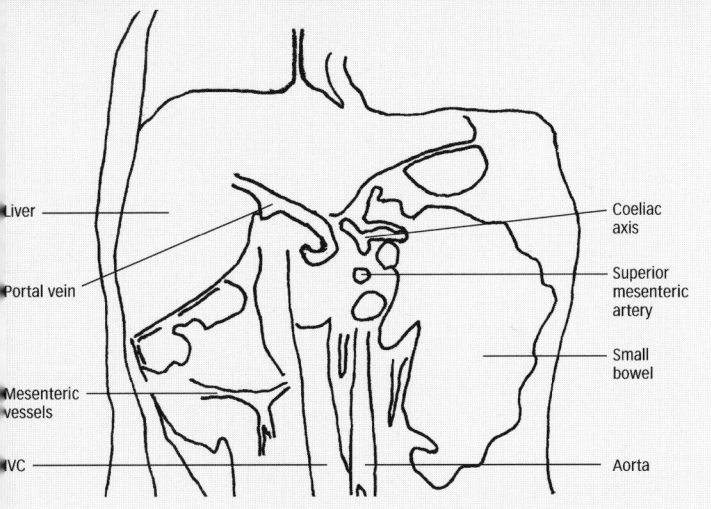

Fig. 5.
DMSA scintigram of both kidneys. This study illustrates the poor anatomical resolution compared to CT or ultrasound. The photopenic area on the oblique images corresponds to the renal sinus. No corticomedullary differentiation is evident.

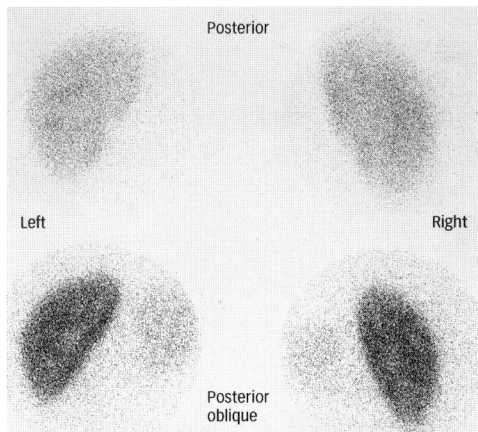

Scintigraphy

This gives information about physiology as well as anatomy. Dimercaptosuccinic acid (DMSA) scintigrams (Fig. 5) provide information about the function of the kidney as well as structure and is used to investigate renal scarring, which areas of the kidney are functioning and percentage function on each side. Diethylene triamine pentaacetic acid (DTPA) or mercaptoacetyltriglycine (MAG3) (Fig. 6) can be used to quantify renal function, but also provides structural information especially reflux of urine from the bladder into the ureter.

The kidneys

The kidneys are retroperitoneal organs lying in the paravertebral gutters of the posterior abdominal wall. Each kidney measures approximately 11 cm in length and weighs 150 gm. The left kidney may be 1.5 cm longer than the right; it is rare for the right kidney to be more than 1 cm longer than the left. The upper poles lie more medially and posteriorly than the lower poles (Fig. 7). The middle third of the medial border contains a hilum, a narrow slit through which travel nerves, fat, the renal vessels, renal pelvis (becoming ureter) and lymphatics.

The kidney is made up of a cortex: the outer one-third and a medulla (the inner two-thirds) surrounded by a fibrous capsule. There are columns of cortical tissue (columns of Bertin) which extend medially within the substance of the kidney, separating the medulla into pyramids (see Fig. 8).

The pyramids consist of a rounded apex, the papilla, a body and a base into which medullary rays radiate from the renal cortex. The papillae project into the calyces, which

to selective studies. The upper pole is supplied by anterior and posterior branches of the renal artery, and the lower pole by an anterior branch.

Venography

This can be performed via the inferior vena cava, but the inferior vena cava and renal veins are nowadays usually very well shown by US, CT and MRI.

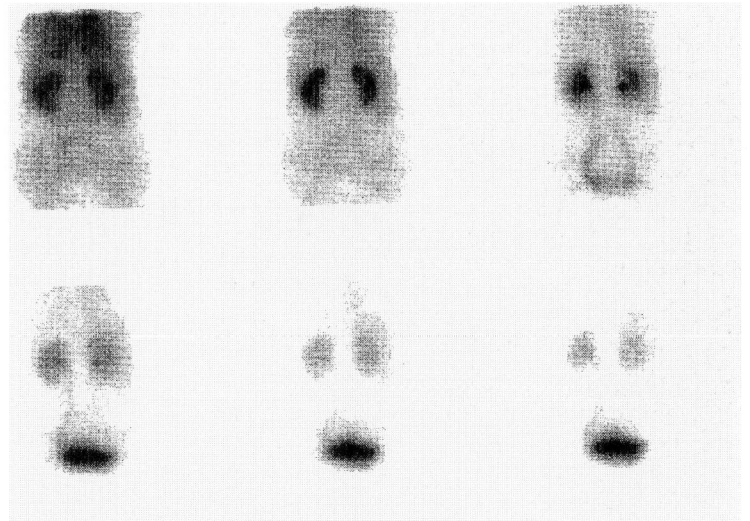

Fig. 7.
**The orientation of the
kidneys in the sagittal,
coronal and transverse
planes.**

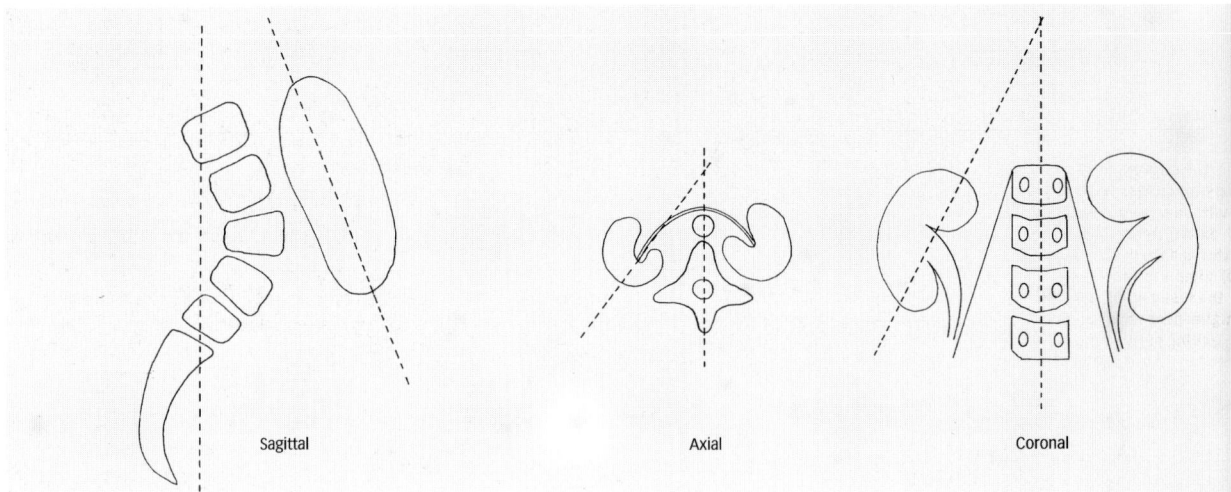

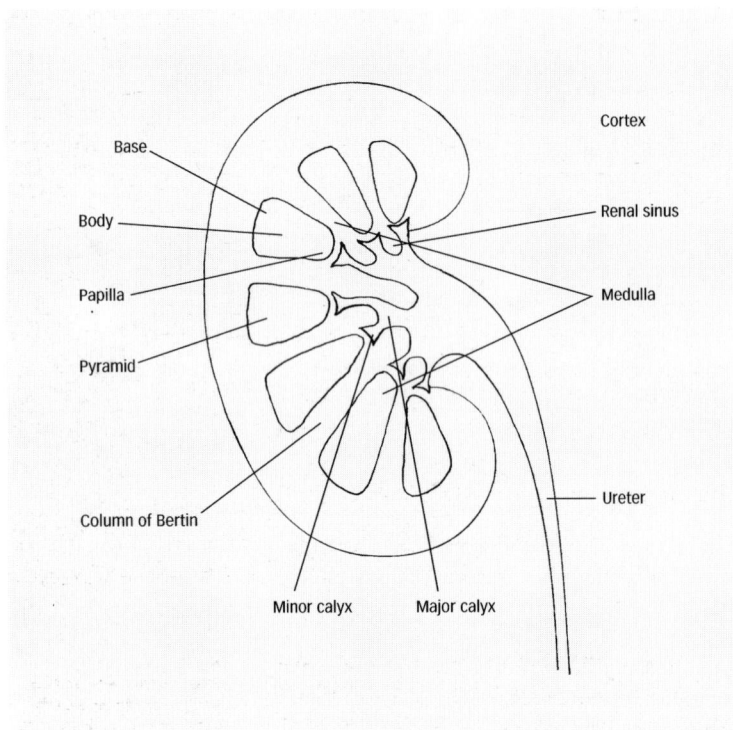

Sagittal

Axial

Coronal

Fig. 8.
The structure of the kidney

9(a)

9(b)

9(c)

9(d)

Fig. 9.
**Anatomical variations of
the kidney and ureters:**
(a) duplex kidney with
partial ureteric duplicati
(b) duplex kidney, ureteri
duplication and ectopic
insertion of ureter
from upper moiety into
proximal ureter.

drain into infundibula. These drain into the
renal pelvis, which lies partly within the renal
sinus, a slit-like space within the kidney, which
also contains a variable amount of fat, vessels
and lymphatic channels. The renal pelvis is
normally formed from the junction of two
infundibula, one from the upper and one from
the lower pole calyces, but there may be a third,
draining calyces in the mid-portion of the kidney. There is considerable variation in the
arrangement of the infundibula and in the extent
to which the pelvis is extrarenal (see Fig. 9).

The calyces of each kidney are arranged
classically in seven pairs (seven ventral and
seven dorsal) although there is wide variation.
These are usually grouped so that three pairs
of calyces drain into the upper pole infundd-

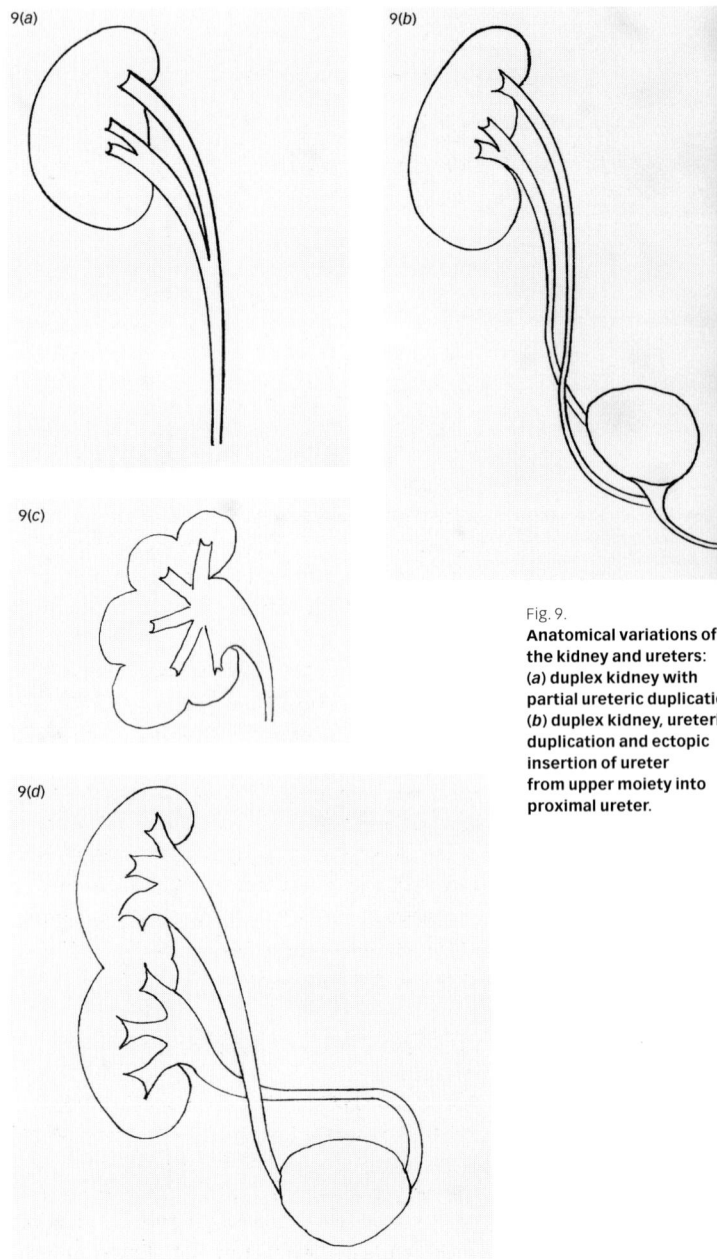

264

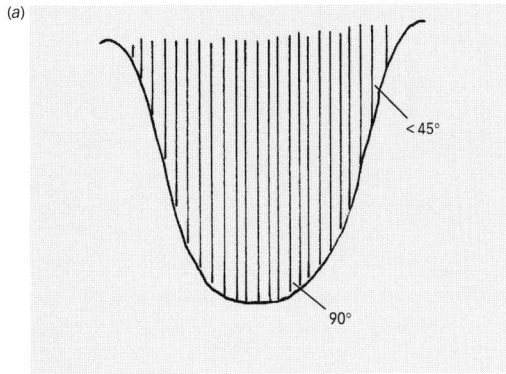

(a)

Fig. 10.
The structure of a renal pyramid: (a) simple calyx with few collecting ducts exiting perpendicular to the surface of the papilla, (b) compound calyx, where the fused papillae have a higher proportion of ducts exiting at right angles to the papilla.

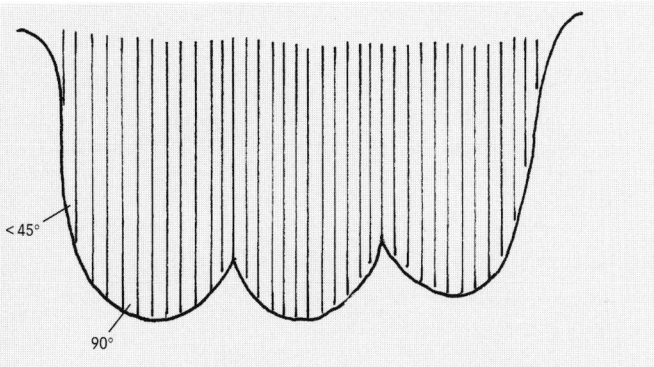

ibulum and four pairs into the lower pole infundibulum. If there is a middle infundibulum, the distribution is normally three pairs at the upper pole, two in the middle and two at the lower pole (Fig. 9).

A simple calyx has just one papilla indenting it, a compound calyx has more than one; compound calyces are less efficient at preventing intrarenal reflux and are thus incriminated in the aetiology of reflux nephropathy (chronic pyelonephritis). The pyramid is designed as a one-way valve to prevent reflux of urine from the renal pelvis into the renal parenchyma (Fig. 10). The collecting ducts open on to the convex surface of the papilla so that, as the pressure within the filling renal pelvis increases, the distal ends of the ducts tend to be squeezed shut. At both poles but especially at the upper pole the papillae are more crowded and compound calyces form in which the valve mechanism is less effective. Intrarenal reflux tends to damage the centre of the papilla because this is where the ducts are most perpendicular to its surface.

Microstructure of the kidney

The kidney is formed of around 1 million nephrons and each nephron is made up of a glomerulus and a uriniferous tubule.

The glomerulus is a loop of capillaries which invaginates the membrane of the blind end of the uriniferous tubule to form a structure resembling a ball in a socket, the renal corpuscle (Malpighian corpuscle). The dilated, blind end of the uriniferous tubule is termed Bowman's capsule. This is connected to the proximal convoluted tubule, the loop of Henle, the distal convoluted tubule and finally the junctional tubule which discharges into the collecting ducts. About 12 collecting ducts open on to the surface of each pyramid.

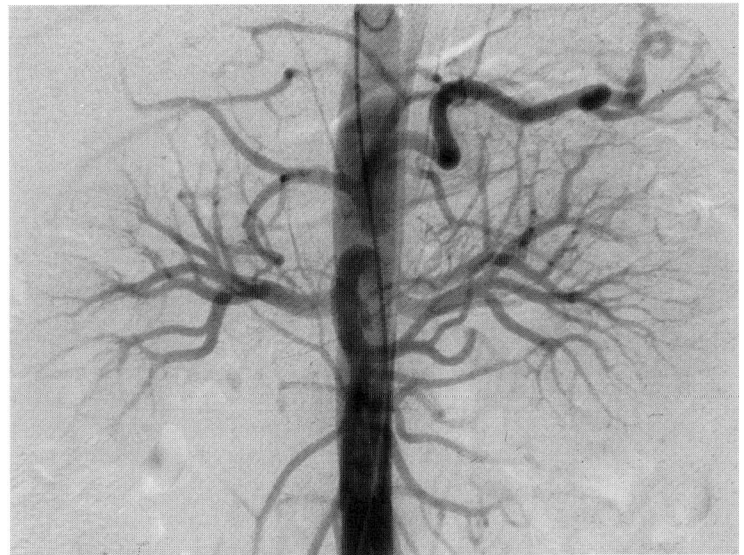

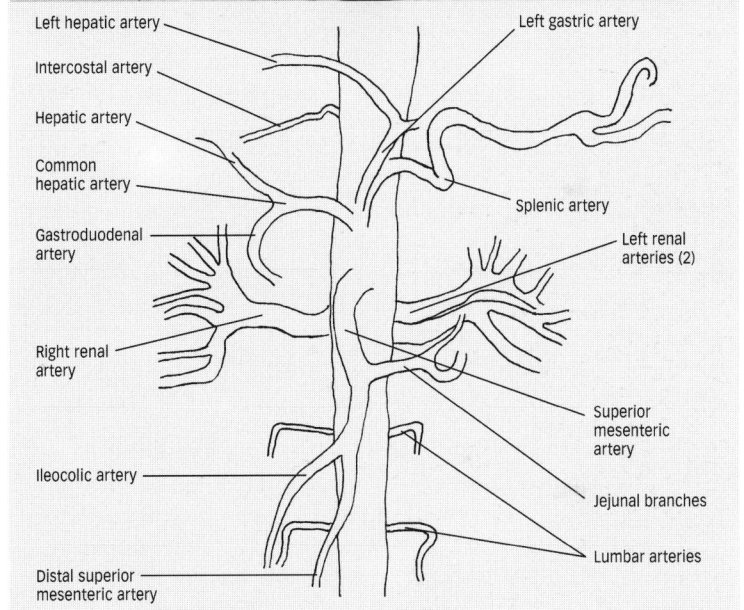

Renal arteries and veins

The renal arteries typically arise from the abdominal aorta at the superior margin of L2, immediately caudal to the origin of the superior mesenteric artery (see Fig. 11). The right renal artery is longer and straighter than the left and courses posterior to the inferior vena cava. Both renal arteries usually have two divisions, which pass anterior and posterior to the

Fig. 11.
Flush aortogram, frontal projection. Note the left hepatic artery arises from the left gastric artery (a variant seen in 25% of normal individuals). This patient has two left renal arteries.

Fig. 12.
**The conventional anatomy
of the intrarenal vessels.**

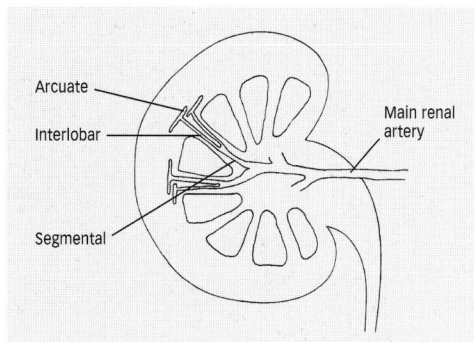

Fig. 12.
The conventional anatomy of the intrarenal vessels.

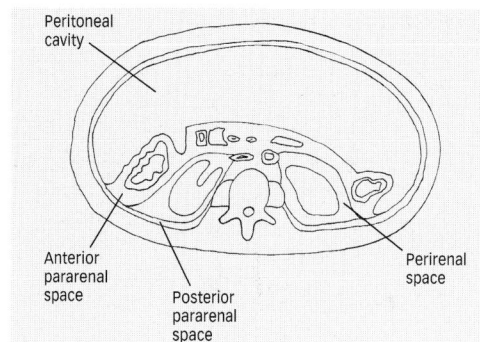

Fig. 13.
The fascial compartments of the retroperitoneum.

renal pelvis. The posterior division supplies the upper and mid-portions of the posterior aspect of the kidney and the anterior division supplies the apex, the anterior aspect of the upper poles and the entire lower pole. Within the renal hilum, the arteries divide inconstantly into five segmental branches which traverse the renal sinus and pierce the medulla between pyramids. These interlobar branches (so-called because they are between pyramids or lobes) pass through the medulla to the cortico-medullary junction where they become arcuate arteries. These arteries form arcs but do not anastomose to form arcades and the arcs run along the bases of the pyramids (see Fig. 12). Their branches, the interlobular arteries, pass to the capsule giving off arteriolar branches (afferent arterioles) to the glomeruli. Distal to the glomeruli are the efferent arterioles, which in turn provide capillaries for the renal cortex and medulla. The capillaries from the efferent arterioles near the capsule supply the convoluted tubules, those from the innermost glomeruli form vasa recta which accompany the loops of Henle and the intermediate capillaries do both.

The earliest tributaries of the renal veins are the stellate venules just deep to the renal capsule. There are extensive anastomoses between the veins inside the kidney. At the hilum there are five or six interlobular veins which join to form the renal vein. This leaves the renal hilum anterior to the renal pelvis. The left renal vein is five times longer than the right and passes anterior to the aorta. Because of the loss of the posterior cardinal vein during fetal development, the left renal vein receives the inferior phrenic vein, the gonadal and the suprarenal vein of that side. There are no extrarenal tributaries to the right renal vein.

The complex embryology of the retroperitoneal venous system leads to numerous normal variants of the left renal vein and inferior vena cava (see above).

The nerve supply of the kidneys

The kidney is supplied by sympathetic nerves, parasympathetic nerves and sensory nerves of root value T12, L1 and L2. The sympathetic pre-ganglionic fibres travel in the thoracic and lumbar splanchnic nerves to the coeliac, renal and superior hypogastric plexuses, and the fibres in the lowest splanchnic nerve travel to the renal plexus. The postganglionic fibres are vasomotor in function and accompany arteries.

Afferent fibres, including those subserving pain, travel with the sympathetic fibres. The fibres pass through the splanchnic nerves to the dorsal roots of T12–L2. Cutting dorsal roots at these levels relieves renal pain but does not interfere with urine production.

There is a parasympathetic supply to the kidneys from the vagus nerve of uncertain function. Indeed, a kidney functions perfectly well with no nerve supply (e.g. after transplantation).

The fascial spaces around the kidneys

Perirenal fat surrounds the capsule of the kidney. This in turn is surrounded by Gerota's fascia (or renal fascia) which has an anterior and a posterior leaf. Thus the retroperitoneum has three compartments: the perirenal space within Gerota's fascia and the anterior and posterior pararenal spaces outside it (see Figs. 13 and 14).

The perirenal space is bounded by the two leaves of Gerota's fascia and contains the kidney, suprarenal gland and perinephric fat. The suprarenals are separated from the kidney by a layer of perirenal fat and there is some debate as to the precise location of the suprarenals to the open superior extent of Gerota's fascia.

The anterior pararenal space lies between the anterior leaf of Gerota's fascia (anterior renal fascia) and the posterior peritoneum. The space extends across the midline to encase the pancreas, duodenum and both the ascending and descending colon.

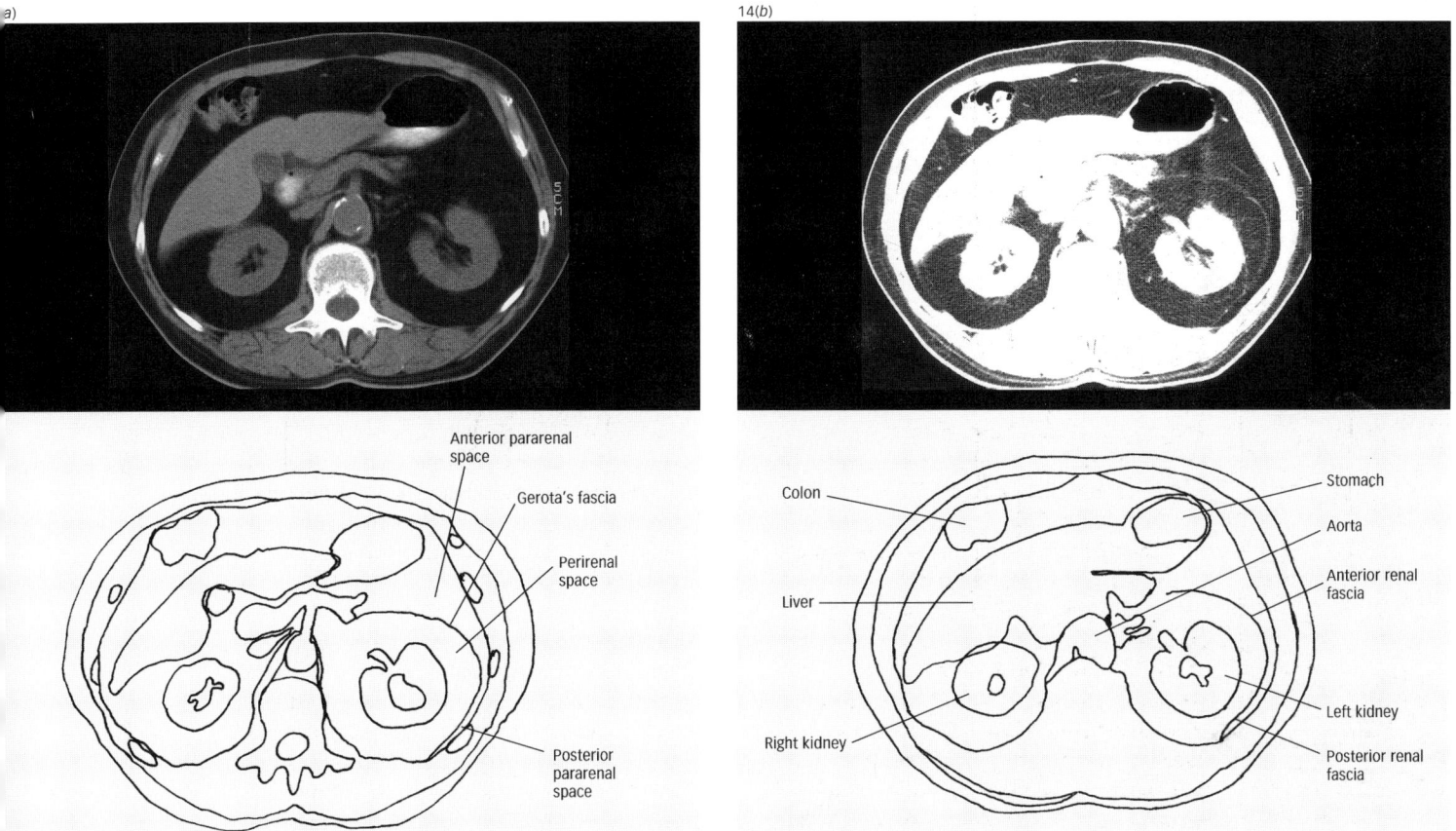

Fig. 14.
Axial CT images:
(a) on soft tissue window
settings to demonstrate
retroperitoneal anatomy
and (b), using narrower
window widths to show
he renal (Gerota's) fascia.

The posterior pararenal space lies between the posterior leaf of Gerota's fascia (posterior renal fascia) and the muscles of the posterior abdominal wall (psoas, quadratus lumborum and transversus abdominis). The space is limited medially by the attachment of the posterior renal fascia to the psoas fascia. Laterally the space is continuous with the extraperitoneal fat deep to transversalis fascia and passes anteriorly towards the umbilicus. Hence a retroperitoneal operation can be performed from an anterior incision.

Lateral to the kidney, the two leaves of Gerota's fascia fuse to form the lateroconal fascia which passes lateral to the colon and medial to the posterior renal space. Superiorly the leaves fade out in the region of the diaphragmatic fascia. Medially they blend with the fascia surrounding the aorta and vena cava which prevents communication between the perirenal spaces across the midline. Inferiorly, the perirenal space remains relatively open, the two layers of fascia approximate to each other so that the perirenal space resembles an inverted cone and blends loosely with the iliac fascia and perirureteric fascia.

The relations of the kidneys

The right kidney is related anteriorly to the liver, the right suprarenal, the second part of the duodenum and the ascending colon. The left kidney is posterior to the stomach, spleen, jejunum, descending colon and pancreas. Posteriorly both kidneys are adjacent to the costodiaphragmatic recess, the twelfth rib, the diaphragm, and the psoas and quadratus lumborum muscles.

The ureter

The ureter is a fibromuscular tube about 25 cm in length which extends from the kidney to the posterolateral angle of the bladder. It may be divided into abdominal, pelvic and intravesical portions. Its narrowest points, and therefore the commonest sites for impaction of a stone, are at the pelviureteric junction, in mid-ureter at the site where it crosses the iliac vessels and the pelvic brim, and at the vesicoureteric junction.

Each ureter passes inferiorly and anteriorly from the renal pelvis within the retroperitoneal areolar tissue to the bifurcation of the common iliac artery. It continues closely related to the internal iliac vessels on the lateral pelvic side walls until it reaches a point anterior to the ischial spines where it turns anteriorly and medially to enter the bladder. During intravenous urography the normal ureter can reach a diameter of 5 mm above the pelvic brim and 7 mm within the pelvis.

The ureters pass anteroinferiorly as they descend the lumbar retroperitoneum as a result of the forward displacement by the psoas muscles, the lumbar lordosis and the

pelvic brim. Having crossed the iliac vessels, the ureters then pass posteriorly to enter the posterior aspect of the bladder.

Because the aorta is left-sided, the left ureter crosses the common iliac artery more obliquely than on the right. The right common iliac artery therefore has a larger extrinsic effect on the ureter. Thus in pregnancy the fetus compresses the right more than the left, which can lead to right-sided hydronephrosis.

Microstructure of the ureter

The ureter is a tube of smooth muscle with an outer adventitial layer and lined internally with mucosa. The smooth muscle fibres are arranged in multiple helices which run in many different directions. The blood supply enters the ureter through the adventitial layer. The mucosa is lined by a transitional epithelium.

The blood supply of the ureter

The upper ureter is supplied by the ureteric branch of the renal artery and the most distal part by branches from the superior and inferior vesical, middle rectal and uterine arteries. The intervening section is supplied by branches from the gonadal artery, often with contributions from the common iliac artery as well.

The nerve supply of the ureter

The ureter receives sympathetic supply from T12–L2 from postganglionic fibres arising in the coeliac and superior hypogastric plexus, although the function of this innervation is unclear since ureteric peristalsis proceeds normally without ureteric innervation.

The lymphatic drainage of the ureter

The abdominal ureter drains to paraaortic nodes and the pelvic ureter to internal iliac nodes on the pelvic side wall. The lymph vessels accompany the relevant arteries.

The relations of the ureter

The ureter lies on the psoas fascia, closely adherent to the posterior parietal peritoneum. Deep to the ureter is the psoas muscle, which separates it from the transverse processes of the lumbar vertebrae. The genitofemoral nerves pass posterior to the ureters on both sides. The ureter usually lies just medial to the tips of the transverse processes. The anterior relations are different on the two sides of the body. On the right the ureter is crossed by the duodenum (2nd part), gonadal, right colic and ileocolic vessels, the root of the mesentery and terminal ileum. On the left the ureter lies deep to gonadal and left colic vessels, loops of

Fig. 15.
The relations of the ureter: (a) in the male and (b), in the female pelvis.

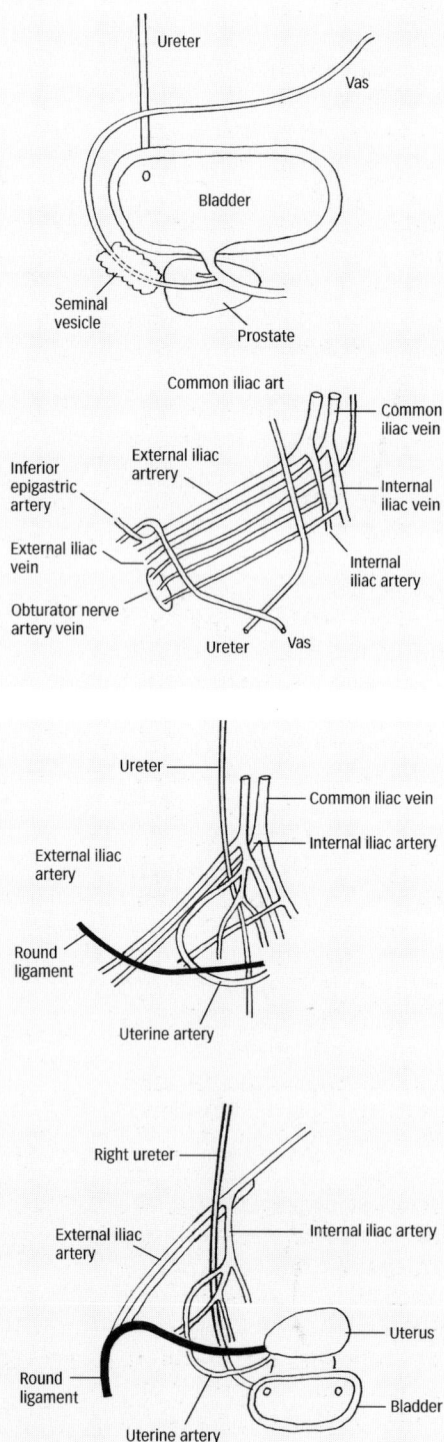

(a)

(b)

268

jejunum and the sigmoid mesocolon. The inferior vena cava is medial to the right ureter while the left ureter lies lateral to the aorta. The inferior mesenteric vein has a long retroperitoneal course lying close to the medial aspect of the left ureter. It crosses the left ureter anteriorly and passes anterior to the left renal vein before joining the splenic vein (see Fig. 4).

Within the pelvis the relations depend on the sex of the individual (Fig. 15). In males the ureter passes anterosuperior to the seminal vesicle and hooks caudal to the vas deferens just before entering the bladder. In the female, the ureter passes close to the lateral fornix of the vagina and is 2.5 cm lateral to the cervix at this point. Before entering the bladder it passes just inferior to the uterine artery in the base of the broad ligament. Here it is in danger during a hysterectomy.

The intravesical part of the ureter, which is about 2 cm in length, passes obliquely through the bladder wall. The bladder wall thus acts as a valve which prevents reflux of urine as the bladder fills.

Normal variants and developmental abnormalities of the renal tract

A duplex ureter and kidney is a common variant of normal anatomy. In the classical duplex kidney the upper pole infundibulum is separated from the middle and lower infundibula. Renal duplication is commoner in females than males and has a prevalence of about 2%. Of subjects with a duplication anomaly, 20% have bilateral abnormalities. Duplication of the ureter is usually incomplete, often with mild constriction where the two ureters unite. Occasionally complete duplication of the ureter may occur, in which case the ureter from the upper moiety may open in an ectopic location (e.g. the floor of the urethra or posterior vagina). Interestingly, the ureter from the lower moiety often runs less obliquely through the bladder wall, thereby predisposing the patient to possible vesicoureteric reflux.

A ureterocele is a dilation of the intramural part of the ureter due to a stenosis of the orifice. This may occur in association with duplication, in which case it affects the ectopic ureter.

Fetal lobulation – The fetal kidney develops from separate lobes which fuse to form the adult kidney: evidence of this normal developmental process may commonly be seen in the adult kidney when it is called persistent fetal lobulation. The appearance can be distinguished from pathological scarring because of the site of the irregularity in the renal surface; in fetal lobulation the divisions lie between calyces whereas in cortical scarring the loss of cortex overlies a calyx. Similarly, because of the lobulation, columns of cortex (named after Bertin) can be infolded within medula causing confusing radiological appearances. Infolded columns of cortex can be elegantly demonstrated in images acquired early during an enhanced CT study.

Abnormalities of migration are the next main group of anomalies. A pelvic kidney occurs in 1 in 1500 deliveries and normally receives its blood supply from the internal iliac artery. Two fused pelvic kidneys are termed a pancake kidney. If there is incomplete fusion of the various components of the diaphragm, the kidney can even ascend into the chest as a thoracic kidney.

There are numerous variations of blood supply with up to four renal arteries possible on each side. These accessory vessels represent persistence of vessels present while the kidney undergoes its embryological ascent.

A horseshoe kidney results if the lower poles of both kidneys fuse and this occurs in 1 in 700 people. The ascent of a horseshoe kidney is usually arrested by the inferior mesenteric artery. Alternatively, the lower pole of a normally situated kidney may fuse with the upper pole of an ectopic contralateral kidney resulting in a condition known as crossed fused ectopia. In cases of abnormal renal migration the suprarenals may have an abnormal discoid shape because of the absence of a normal renal impression during fetal life. However, the suprarenals will nearly always lie in their expected embryological site (right – posterior to the inferior vena cava; left – adjacent to the left crus). Retrocaval ureter is a rare variant in which the right ureter hooks around the inferior vena cava as it runs inferiorly through the abdomen.

Imaging the suprarenal (adrenal) glands

Plain films
The suprarenals are seen if they are calcified, but not otherwise.

CT
Thin (1–2 mm) slices are generally used to produce high spatial resolution images of the suprarenals (see Fig. 18). The thickness of the limbs of the suprarenals can be judged by comparison with the adjacent crus of the diaphragm. There are considerable advantages of spiral techniques which overcome the problems of misregistering small juxtadiaphragmatic lesions.

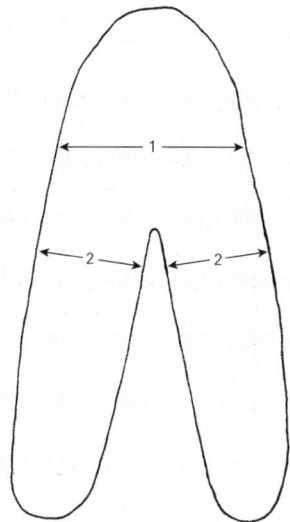

Fig. 16.
The mean dimensions of normal suprarenal glands (cm). (From Vincent *et al.*, 1994.)

	1	2
Right	0.61 (0.2)	0.28 (0.08)
Left	0.79 (0.21)	0.33 (0.10)

USS

The suprarenals are imaged by a posterior approach. The right is situated between the right kidney and liver and the left between left kidney and pancreatic tail. They are particularly well seen in neonates when an anterior approach may be successful (especially on the right).

Venography

This is performed for venous sampling as well as imaging. The right suprarenal vein enters the inferior vena cava 3 cm cranial to the renal vein, near the entry point of the hepatic veins. The left suprarenal vein joins the left renal vein. Care must be taken lest the single suprarenal vein is obstructed, leading to venous infarction.

MRI

This distinguishes suprarenals from neighbouring structures such as vessels and the crura without the need for intravenous contrast medium (Fig. 17). As for CT, the suprarenals are best seen if there is a reasonable quantity of intraabdominal fat.

The suprarenal (adrenal) glands

The suprarenal glands are paired endocrine organs which lie anterior, medial and superior to the superior poles of both kidneys at the level of T12. The right suprarenal is fixed embryologically to the posterior aspect of the inferior vena cava. The left is adherent to the left diaphragmatic crus. Evidence for this comes from studies in patients with horseshoe kidneys; when the kidneys fail to ascend, the suprarenals remain in their correct anatomical position. The suprarenals are separated from the kidneys by the perirenal fat and lie at the superior margin of the perirenal fascia. Both suprarenals can measure up to 50 mm in their crano-caudal dimension and weigh about 5 g. No individual limb should measure much more than 6.5 mm across (usually no more than the width of the adjacent diaphragmatic crus, see Fig. 16). At birth, the suprarenals are about one-third the size of the adjacent kidney, whereas in the adult they are one-thirtieth of the size of the kidney. The mass of the suprarenal is similar in adult life to the mass at birth. The suprarenal atrophies markedly after birth until the end of the second year of life. From this age there is slow growth until puberty when it approaches adult size and little further growth occurs.

The right suprarenal is pyramidal in shape, resembling a cocked hat, and has two well-developed limbs (∧ shaped in cross-section).

The left suprarenal is more of a crescent over the superomedial surface of the upper pole of the left kidney and has three more definite limbs (anterior, posteromedial and posterolateral). Normal suprarenal glands are shown in Figs. 17 and 18.

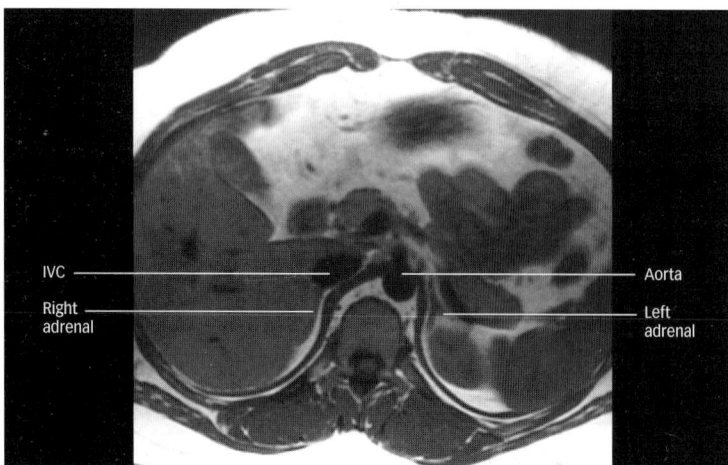

Fig. 17.
Axial T1W MR image showing the suprarenal glands.

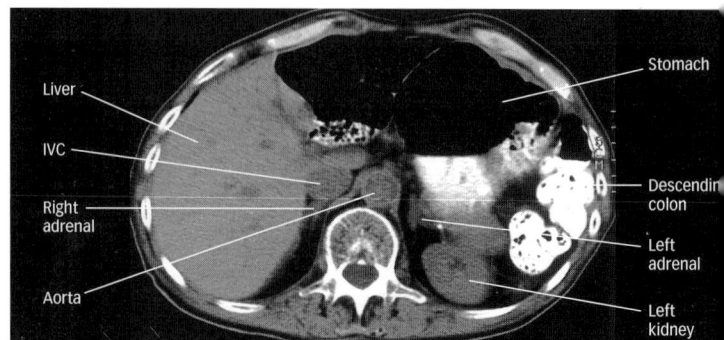

Fig. 18.
Axial CT showing both suprarenal glands

The microstructure of the suprarenals

The suprarenals are composed of an outer cortex (the cells of which are of mesodermal origin) and an inner medulla (derived from neural crest cells). The cortex is rich in lipid and is yellow, while the medulla is darker in colour. The cortex has three layers: the zona glomerulosa is immediately beneath the capsule and contains small rounded groups of cells, the next is the zona fasciculata, the largest of the three containing columns of cells rich in cholesterol and the innermost layer is the zona reticularis which is a network of darkly staining small cells. The medulla contains larger cells with cytoplasmic granules which stain with chromium salts (chromaffin reaction). The medulla is more vascular than the cortex.

The relations of the suprarenal glands

The right suprarenal lies between the crus of the diaphragm (posteromedial aspect), the upper pole of the right kidney (inferiorly, laterally and posteriorly) and the inferior vena cava and right lobe of the liver (anteriorly).

The inferior surface of the right suprarenal is related to the anteromedial surface of the upper pole of kidney and is separated from it by a variable amount of perirenal fat.

The left suprarenal is a crescent between the upper pole of the left kidney and the diaphragm, convex medially and concave laterally. The superior angle is sharp and the inferior rounded. The anterior surface of the left suprarenal has a cranial area covered by the peritoneum of the lesser sac, the cardia of the stomach and the spleen and a more caudal section directly in contact with the splenic vein and pancreas. The posterior surface of the left suprarenal is divided into two by a vertical ridge, the lateral part is related to the left kidney and the medial portion is close to the left crus. The medial surface of the left suprarenal is close to the left coeliac ganglion and the left inferior phrenic and left gastric arteries.

The blood supply of the suprarenal glands

The suprarenals are supplied by numerous branches from three major arteries:

(a) The inferior phrenic artery, a branch of the abdominal aorta, gives rise to the superior suprarenal artery.
(b) The suprarenal artery proper, a branch of the abdominal aorta, gives rise to the middle suprarenal artery.
(c) The renal arteries give rise to the inferior suprarenal arteries.

A large single suprarenal vein leaves the anterior surface of each gland. The right suprarenal vein drains directly into the inferior vena cava and the left into the left renal vein.

The nerve supply of the suprarenal glands

Preganglionic sympathetic fibres in the greater and lesser splanchnic nerves pierce the crura of the diaphragms and synapse in the coeliac ganglion. Postganglionic vasomotor fibres are distributed with the arteries supplying the gland to regulate its blood flow. In addition, preganglionic fibres from the lesser and least splanchnic nerves innervate the cells of the suprarenal medulla, stimulating them to secrete catecholamines.

Normal variants of the suprarenal glands

Cortical bodies (islands of suprarenal cortical tissue) are ectopic crests of chromaffin tissue which may be found in the broad ligament, spermatic cord and epididymis.

Imaging the aorta

Plain films

The aorta is visible on abdominal films if calcified. The amount of calcification increases with age. Calcification is more common in men up to 60; thereafter calcification is often more marked in women.

USS

The aorta can be seen from the point at which it pierces the diaphragm to its bifurcation in most individuals, although the distal aorta may be obscured by bowel gas (Fig. 19). Normally it is 2–3 cm in diameter cranial to the renal arteries and around 60% of this calibre at their origins.

CT

The aorta and its branches can be seen throughout the abdomen. The coeliac trunk and its principal branches, the common hepatic artery, the left gastric artery and the splenic artery are seen cranial to the pancreas. The superior mesenteric artery is normally surrounded by fat which allows it to be easily identified. The inferior mesenteric artery can usually be identified just anterior to the distal aorta close to the bifurcation. The main renal vessels are easily seen and some lumbar arteries may be demonstrated. All these branches are more readily identified following enhancement with intravenous contrast medium. Thin spiral cuts allow three-dimensional reconstructions.

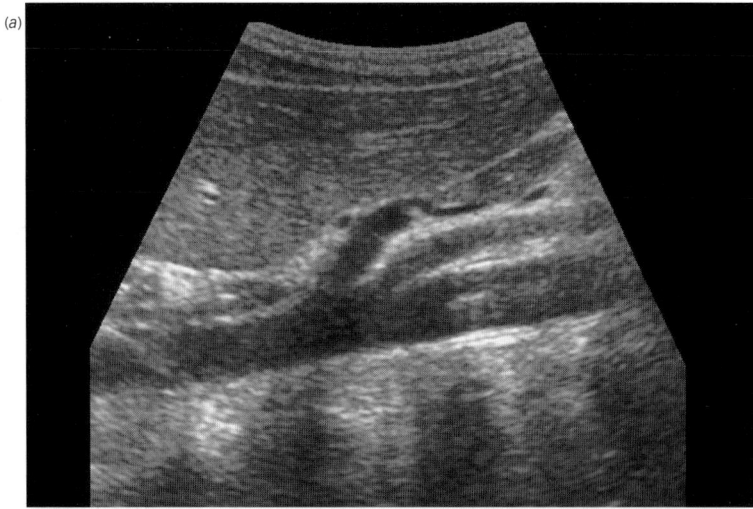

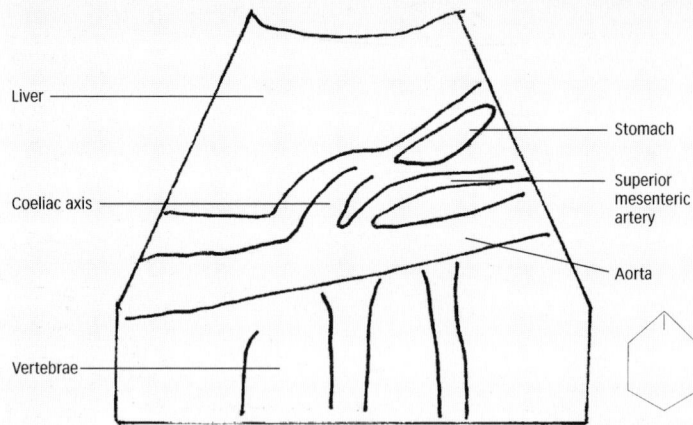

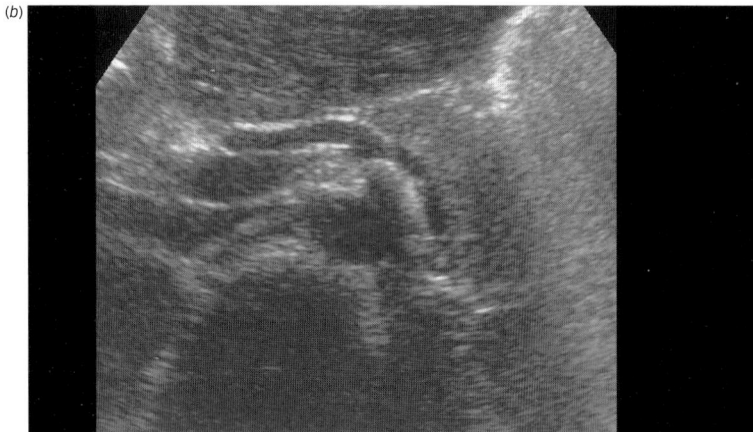

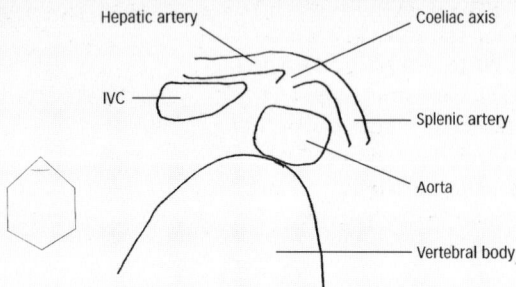

(a)

Liver
Stomach
Coeliac axis
Superior mesenteric artery
Aorta
Vertebrae

(b)

Hepatic artery
Coeliac axis
IVC
Splenic artery
Aorta
Vertebral body

MRI

This technique can produce images of flow in the aorta without intravenous contrast medium and has the advantage over CT of the facility to obtain direct images in any chosen plane (Fig. 4).

Angiography

The aorta is normally demonstrated by a pigtail catheter introduced into the femoral artery, although selective catheterization of specific vessels can be performed.

The abdominal aorta

The aorta traverses the diaphragm deep to the median arcuate ligament of the crura to enter the abdomen at the level of the intervertebral disc between T12 and L1. Having entered the abdomen in the midline, it descends anterior and slightly to the left of the lumbar vertebral bodies, ending at L4 where it bifurcates into the common iliac arteries. Figure 11 shows a normal aortogram.

Branches of the abdominal aorta
Midline, unpaired branches to the GI tract
The usual anatomical sites are:

Coeliac artery	T12/L1
Superior mesenteric artery	L1
Inferior mesenteric artery	L3 (4 cm proximal to the aortic bifurcation and about 2 cm superior to the umbilicus).

Paired branches to kidney, suprarenals and gonads

Superior suprarenal artery	Normally arises from the inferior phrenic artery. May arise directly from the aorta
Middle suprarenal artery	Normally arises from the aorta
Inferior suprarenal artery	Normally arises from the renal artery
Renal arteries	Often multiple
Gonadal arteries	Normally arise from the aorta

All arise close to the level of L1/L2 intervertebral disc

Branches to the diaphragm and abdominal wall

The inferior phrenic artery arises next to the coeliac trunk and passes directly to the diaphragm.

The lumbar arteries (four pairs) pass from the lateral aspect of the aorta to the abdominal wall.

The median sacral artery is a continuation of the aorta, between the two common iliac arteries.

Fig. 19. left
Ultrasound images of the aorta, coeliac axis and superior mesenteric artery (a) longitudinal and (b) axial images.

Imaging the inferior vena cava (IVC)

Ultrasound

The most cranial portion of the inferior vena cava can be seen with ultrasound in the upper abdomen using the liver as an acoustic window (see Fig. 20). More inferiorly in the abdomen, it may be obscured by bowel gas. Patency of the IVC can be confirmed using Doppler. The drainage of the hepatic veins into the inferior vena cava is well seen. The renal veins are less easily seen, but experts are able to demonstrate flow.

CT

The inferior vena cava is seen throughout its length. Contrast medium is used to opacify the cava, but flow artefacts from the renal veins may simulate inferior vena cava thrombosis and a cavagram may be necessary if inferior vena cava obstruction or thrombosis is suspected.

MRI

MRI is used to image the inferior vena cava and is becoming the method of choice to detect flow within the inferior vena cava.

Cavagram

A catheter is introduced into a femoral vein and passed into the inferior vena cava to the level of L1. Contrast medium is injected by a pump and digital subtraction images are obtained.

The course of the inferior vena cava

The inferior vena cava is formed by the confluence of the right and left common iliac veins at the level of L5 posterior to the right common iliac artery. At this level the inferior vena cava lies just posterior to the aortic bifurcation and, having passed cranially anterolateral to the lumbar vertebrae, right crus of diaphragm and right suprarenal gland, it then passes anteriorly to traverse the diaphragm (T12). At this level, the right crus and oesophagus separate the inferior vena cava from the aorta. The inferior vena cava pierces the central tendon of the diaphragm at the level of T8. Anteriorly, from below upwards, it lies behind the right common iliac artery, loops of small intestine and root of mesentery, the horizontal part of the duodenum and head of the pancreas. Above the duodenum, the inferior vena cava is covered by peritoneum in the posterior wall of the epiploic foramen, which separates it from the portal vein, and it then grooves the posterior aspect of the liver before passing through the diaphragm. There is only a very

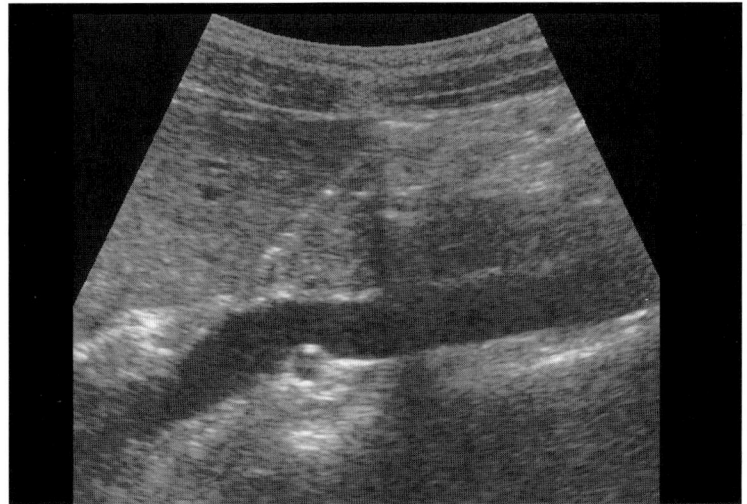

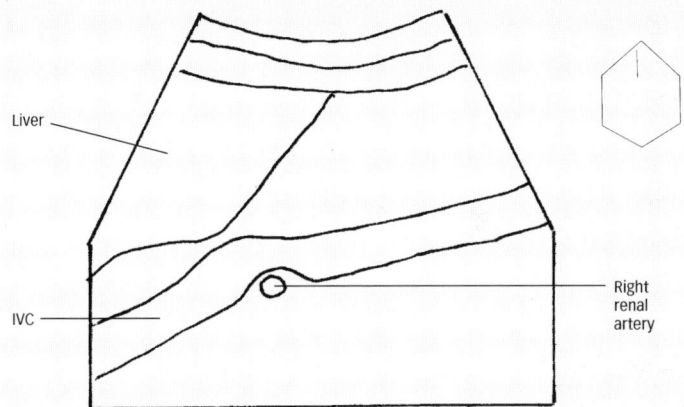

short intrathoracic portion before it enters the right atrium.

Tributaries of the inferior vena cava

(a) Blood from the liver enters the inferior vena cava through three large hepatic veins (see Fig. 4), as well as through a variable number of accessory hepatic veins.

(b) Blood from the three paired glands. On the right the suprarenal vein, the renal and the gonadal vein enter the inferior vena cava separately. On the left, the left renal vein receives the suprarenal and gonadal vein before draining into the inferior vena cava. The entry of the left renal vein into the inferior vena cava is an important anatomical landmark. It demarcates the normal position of the uncinate process of the pancreas.

(c) Blood from the abdominal wall enters the inferior vena cava via the right and left phrenic veins and the third and fourth lumbar veins.

Fig. 20.
Ultrasound image (longitudinal) of the inferior vena cava and right renal artery.

The veins of the posterior abdominal wall

The vertebral venous plexuses drain into the inferior vena cava via segmental lumbar veins. The lumbar veins drain to the inferior vena cava but in addition there is a connection between them – the ascending lumbar veins. These connecting veins extend as far caudally as the lateral sacral veins and iliolumbar veins (which drain into the common iliac veins) and join cranially with the subcostal veins and the azygos/hemiazygos veins. In the event of congenital absence or of acquired inferior vena cava thrombosis, this venous system returns blood from the trunk and lower limbs to the heart via the superior vena cava (SVC). This system also explains the spread of infection or tumours along the vertebral column. Moreover, connections with the pelvic venous plexus probably account for the frequency of metastases from carcinoma of the prostate to the sacrum and lumbar vertebrae.

Imaging of the abdominal lymphatic system

CT

Lymph nodes of 0.5–1 cm (i.e. normal size) can be detected with CT but the internal structure of nodes cannot be seen. Thus abnormal nodes of this size cannot be distinguished from normal ones. Nodes are considered likely to be abnormal on the basis of their size. Nodes of 1 cm in short axis diameter in the retrocrural or left gastric territories are usually abnormal. However, nodes of >1 cm in the external iliac territory are often normal. Intravenous contrast medium can be helpful in distinguishing nodes from normal vessels.

USS

In thin patients the nodal anatomy can be well documented, particularly in the upper abdomen. However, it is often difficult to demonstrate the entire retroperitoneum because of overlying bowel gas.

MRI

Abnormal lymph nodes are again recognized on the basis of size rather than internal structure, although there is some interest in signal intensity and enhancement characteristics. The spatial resolution of MRI is now matching that of CT in the abdomen and better contrast resolution makes it easier to distinguish nodes from the neighbouring normal structures.

Lymphography

Oily contrast medium is injected into a lymphatic vessel in the foot to demonstrate the abdominal lymphatics. Lymph vessels and nodes can be seen and the internal architecture of nodes is shown. This method demonstrates deep inguinal, external iliac, common iliac and paraaortic nodes. However, internal iliac, hepatic, visceral and preaortic nodes are not demonstrated. There are now few indications for this technique with the advent of high-quality CT.

The abdominal lymphatic system

The abdominal lymph nodes are arranged principally around the aorta and are arranged into the following groups:

Preaortic

Coeliac	Gastric
	Hepatic
	Pancreaticosplenic
Sup. and inf. mesenteric	Mesenteric
	Ileocolic
	Colic
	Pararectal

Preaortic nodes

These are arranged around the midline anterior arteries to the gastrointestinal tract and drain lymph from the areas supplied by these arteries, that is the gastrointestinal tract, liver, gall bladder, pancreas and spleen. Before reaching the preaortic nodes, lymph from these organs has already passed through nodes in the intestinal wall, mesentery, porta hepatis and along the course of the arteries supplying them. Lymph from these nodes passes through the intestinal trunks to the cisterna chyli and from there to the thoracic duct.

Preaortic nodes are divisible into coeliac, superior and inferior mesenteric groups, being located at the origins of these arteries.

Coeliac nodes

The coeliac nodes around the origin of the coeliac artery have efferent channels which form the right and left intestinal trunks and receive afferents from three main groups of nodes (which follow the three branches of the coeliac artery): gastric, hepatic and pancreaticosplenic nodes.

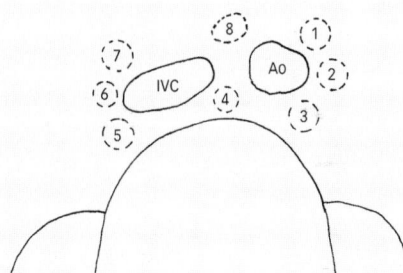

Fig. 21.
The distribution of paraaortic nodes (Dixon *et al.*, 1986).

Gastric group

The gastric nodes accompany the arteries supplying the stomach and are divided into three main groups.

The left gastric group is found on the lesser curvature of the stomach and receives lymph from the stomach and lower oesophagus: superior nodes are near the origin of the left gastric artery, inferior nodes have descending branches along the cardiac aspect of the lesser curve and a paracardial chain surrounds them. Enlarged (>0.8 cm) nodes here often carry grave prognostic significance (e.g. oesophageal neoplasm).

The gastroepiploic group lies near the right gastroepiploic artery on the pyloric part of the greater curve; they drain into pyloric nodes.

A pyloric group of four or five nodes sits in the bifurcation of the gastroduodenal artery which is at the junction between the first and second part of the duodenum. A further node may be found cranial to the duodenum near the right gastric artery. These nodes drain the pylorus and first part of duodenum and receive lymph from the gastroepiploic nodes.

Hepatic group

The hepatic nodes are adjacent to the hepatic arteries and bile ducts in the lesser omentum and are variable in site and number. The most constant are the cystic node (at the junction of the cystic and common hepatic duct) and the node of the anterior border of the epiploic foramen (along the cranial part of the common bile duct). Hepatic nodes drain stomach, duodenum, bile ducts, liver, gall bladder and pancreas.

Pancreaticosplenic group

Pancreaticosplenic nodes follow the course of the splenic artery along the posterosuperior edge of the pancreas and in the gastrosplenic ligament. Stomach, spleen and pancreas supply this group with lymph.

Superior and inferior mesenteric nodes

The superior and inferior mesenteric nodes drain the alimentary tract from the duodeno-jejunal flexure to the upper anal canal. The lymph drains first to mesenteric, ileocolic, colic and pararectal nodes along the mesenteric border of the bowel and then to nodes accompanying the superior and inferior mesenteric arteries.

Mesenteric nodes

There are over 100 nodes in the mesentery, which are said to be in three groups. One follows the upper trunk of the superior mesenteric artery (juxta arterial). Another lies between the loops of the mesenteric arterial arcades (intermediate). A third is near the intestinal wall accompanying the terminal branches of the mesenteric arteries (mural). In practice, when these nodes enlarge they are seen in two main sites, one anterior and one posterior to the plane of the mesenteric vessels (akin to a sandwich).

Ileocolic nodes

A chain of 10–20 nodes accompanies the ileo-colic artery in two main groups, one alongside the artery, near the duodenum and another around the terminal part of the artery at the ileocaecal junction. Dividing with the artery, one group lies along the ileal branch (ileal), another is in the ileocaecal fold (anterior ileo-colic), and the third is in the angle between ileum and ascending colon and partly behind the caecum (posterior ileocolic).

Colic nodes

These are in four groups. The epicolic group are nodules on the colonic wall (sometimes in the appendices epiploicae). The paracolic nodes lie along the mesenteric borders of the transverse and sigmoid and on the medial sides of the ascending and descending colon. Intermediate colic nodes lie along the colic arteries. Preterminal colic nodes are next to the superior and inferior mesenteric arteries.

Perirectal nodes

These are in contact with the muscular wall of the rectum and drain to an intermediate group around the superior rectal artery and from there to the region of the inferior mesenteric artery. Some drain to the common iliac nodes.

Paraaortic nodes

These nodes lie on either side of the aorta (Fig. 21), anterior to the crura, the medial margin of psoas and the lumbar sympathetic trunk. On the right some nodes are lateral and anterior to the inferior vena cava near the termination of the right renal vein. Nodes between the aorta and cava are of particular importance in assessing right testicular lesions.

They receive lymph from the posterior abdominal wall, diaphragm, kidneys, suprarenals and gonads via afferents along the lumbar arteries and outlying nodes near the iliac arteries.

The efferent vessels from the nodes unite to form the right and left lumbar trunks and a few efferents pass to the preaortic and retroaortic nodes.

The lymph from the kidneys, suprarenals, ureter, gonads, Fallopian tubes and upper part of uterus passes directly to the paraaortic nodes, but lymph from the pelvis and posterior abdominal wall passes first to regional nodes around the iliac arteries and their branches. These nodes are in a number of groups including the common, external, internal and circumflex iliac, inferior epigastric and sacral. The paraaortic nodes also drain lymph from both lower limbs since the external iliac nodes receive lymph from the inguinal nodes and the internal iliac nodes from the deep gluteal nodes.

In the upper abdomen the nodes are grouped around the aorta and inferior vena cava as shown in Fig. 21.

Iliac nodes
Common iliac nodes are positioned around the common iliac artery anterior to the L5 vertebra and the sacral promontory. They drain the internal and external iliac nodes and send efferents to the paraaortic nodes. Usually they are grouped into medial, lateral and intermediate chains.

External iliac nodes are in three groups around the artery, medial, lateral and anterior (the anterior is inconstant). The medial nodes collect lymph from the inguinal nodes, the deeper layers of the lower abdominal wall, the adductor compartment of the thigh, the glans penis, the membranous urethra, prostate, upper part of bladder, cervix and upper vagina. Efferents pass to the common iliac nodes. Inferior epigastric and circumflex iliac groups follow their arteries and form part of the external iliac group.

The internal iliac nodes surround the internal iliac artery and serve pelvic viscera as well as draining lymph from the perineum and the gluteal and posterior femoral muscles.

Scaral nodes (along median and lateral sacral vessels) belong to this group. Obturator nodes are best regarded as members of the internal iliac group even though they lie just posterior to the external iliac vessels. On occasions obturator nodes can be difficult to distinguish from ovaries on CT. One distinguishing feature is that there is usually no fat plane between an obturator node and the ilium whereas there is around the ovary.

Cisterna chyli
This thin-walled tube, up to 6 mm wide and 6 cm long lies anterior to the bodies of L1 and L2, posterior to the right crus of the diaphragm and between the right crus and the aorta. After passing through the retrocrural space with the aorta, azygos and hemiazygos veins it becomes the thoracic duct.

Sympathetic trunk

The thoracic sympathetic chain becomes the lumbar sympathetic trunk after passing posterior to the medial arcuate ligament of the diaphragm. The sympathetic trunk continues into the pelvis as the sacral trunk after passing deep to the iliac vessels.

Relations
Both trunks follow the anterior border of the psoas on the vertebral bodies and discs separated from these by the lumbar arteries. The right trunk is overlapped by the inferior vena cava and the left posterolateral to the aorta.

The right trunk is crossed by the right renal artery and the left trunk is crossed by the left renal vessels, left testicular artery and inferior mesenteric vessels.

Distribution
The lumbar trunk normally carries four ganglia but sometimes only three. The chain, along with the splanchnic nerves and the vagus, supplies plexuses around the aorta and its branches, e.g. the coeliac, intermesenteric, hypogastric and renal plexuses. The hypogastric plexus passes anterior to the iliac vessels to supply pelvic viscera via plexuses distributed along branches of the internal iliac artery.

Abdominal sympathetic plexuses

The coeliac plexus consists of two large sympathetic ganglia, one on each side of the roots of the coeliac and the superior mesenteric artery. Although quite large, these ganglia are not well shown because they are essentially of fat attenuation at CT and thus there is little contrast against retroperitoneal fat. Each ganglion receives fibres from the lumbar trunks, the splanchnic, the phrenic and the vagus nerves. From these ganglia, post-ganglionic efferent sympathetic fibres radiate out like the sun's rays (hence solar plexus) to target organs within the abdomen. The ganglia lie on the crura of the diaphragms in the retroperitoneum and hence the right ganglion is related laterally to the right suprarenal and anteriorly to the inferior vena cava while the left ganglion is situated with the left suprarenal laterally and the splenic artery and pancreas anteriorly.

Branches of the coeliac plexus include the phrenic, hepatic, left gastric, splenic, suprarenal, renal, testicular, ovarian, superior mesenteric, intermesenteric and inferior mesenteric plexus.

The superior hypogastric plexus lies in retroperitoneal connective tissue at the bifurcation of the aorta, anterior to the left common iliac vein and L5 vertebra/disc. From this plexus fibres are distributed to pelvic viscera via branches of the internal iliac artery.

The superior hypogastric plexus divides into right and left hypogastric nerves which pass caudally, medial to the internal iliac arteries to form the inferior hypogastric plexus. This is situated lateral to the rectum and the posterior part of the urinary bladder. In males it is related medially to the prostate and seminal vesicles and in females to the vaginal fornix and cervix. The internal iliac vessels, obturator internus, levator ani and coccygeus are lateral to the inferior hypogastric plexus, the sacral and coccygeal plexuses are posterior and the superior vesical and obliterated umbilical artery are superior to it. The inferior hypogastric plexus gives rise to the middle rectal plexus, the vesical and the prostatic plexus as well as the uterine and vaginal nerves.

The posterior abdominal wall

Bones

In the midline are the five lumbar vertebral bodies, intervertebral discs and transverse processes. The 12th rib is the superior margin of the posterior abdominal wall which is divided into a superior and inferior half by the iliac crests. The inferior margin is the pelvic brim.

The vertebral bodies and discs increase in height from L1 to L5. The transverse processes of L1 to L4 extend laterally in the horizontal plane from the upper half of the vertebral bodies, that of L3 projects the furthest. The transverse process of L5 points posterosuperiorly as well as laterally and is conical in shape with a broad base.

The twelfth rib curves downwards and ends in the plane of the second lumbar intervertebral disc. The most cranial part of the iliac crest is at the level of the middle of the body of L4.

Muscles and fascia

The muscles of the posterior abdominal wall are psoas, quadratus lumborum, transversus abdominis, iliacus, intertransversalis and the posterior part of the diaphragm (see Fig. 22).

The psoas major takes its origin from the lateral surface of the bodies and intervertebral discs of all the lumbar vertebrae and T12, immediately posterior to the sympathetic trunk. It contains a readily identifiable central tendon, usually accompanied by a layer of fat. Psoas fascia is part of the fascial sheet that covers the internal layer of abdominal wall musculature. It is thickened superiorly to form the medial arcuate ligament, which forms part of the origin of the diaphragm. Inferiorly, the fascia extends into the thigh, anterior to the psoas and iliacus but deep to the inguinal ligament. The femoral sheath passes deep to the inguinal ligament, and separates the psoas fascia from the ligament, but elsewhere the fascia is adherent to the ligament. The ventral rami of L2–L4 enter the psoas; the lumbar plexus lies within it and the femoral nerve emerges from the lateral border of the psoas, hence the neurological sequelae of a psoas abscess.

Quadratus lumborum attaches to the transverse processes of all the lumbar vertebrae, the twelfth rib, the iliac crest and the iliolumbar ligament. The fascia surrounding quadratus lumborum is thickened superiorly to form the lateral arcuate ligament and inferiorly to form a fibrous band, the iliolumbar ligament (which joins the transverse process of L5 to the iliac crest).

Transversus abdominis is the deepest of the three sheets of muscle which form the bulk of the anterior abdominal wall. Near the lateral border of the quadratus, the muscle becomes aponeurotic and this fibrous sheet splits into two layers which surround the back muscles, the anterior and posterior layers of the thoracolumbar fascia.

Iliacus arises from the iliac fossa and its fibres insert into the anterior and lateral edge

Fig. 22.
The muscles of posterior abdominal wall.

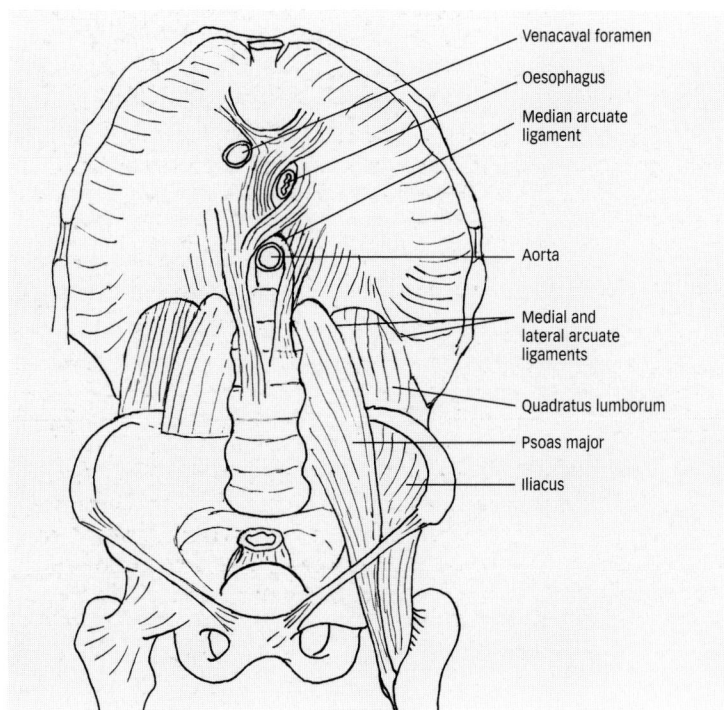

- Venacaval foramen
- Oesophagus
- Median arcuate ligament
- Aorta
- Medial and lateral arcuate ligaments
- Quadratus lumborum
- Psoas major
- Iliacus

of the psoas tendon, the resulting muscle being called the iliopsoas.

The diaphragm is composed of two portions: a peripheral muscular part and a central tendinous area. The muscular part is in three sections: a vertebral component, which includes the crura and medial and lateral arcuate ligaments; a costal section, which attaches to the inferior costal margin; and a sternal part which attaches to the xiphisternum.

The diaphragmatic crura arise from the anterior surfaces of the lumbar vertebrae and intervertebral discs. The right arises from L1–L3 and is slightly longer than the left which attaches to L1–L2 (see Fig. 16). Both crura can be very bulky in muscular individuals. In cross-section they can simulate lymph nodes; they are thicker in inspiration than on expiration. In the midline the crura join to form a tendinous union: the median arcuate ligament.

The medial arcuate ligament is the fascia overlying the psoas muscle which is thickened and gives origin to the diaphragm. The lateral arcuate ligament is fascia overlying the quadratus lumborum.

The central tendinous part of the diaphragm is trefoil in shape and is fused with the pericardium. The inferior vena cava pierces this part of the diaphragm and thus remains patent in all phases of respiration. The aorta passes posterior to the median arcuate ligament in the retrocrural space. The oesophagus passes through a more muscular part of the diaphragm in the region of the right crus.

The retrocrural space is bounded by the vertebral body of T12 posteriorly and is surrounded laterally by the crura and anteriorly by their fused median arcuate ligament. It normally contains aorta, azygos and hemiazygos veins, splanchnic nerves, sympathetic trunk and the thoracic duct. This is a good place to look for abnormal lymph nodes (anything over 8 mm here).

References

Dixon, A.K., Ellis, M. & Sikora, K. (1986). Computed tomography of testicular tumours: distribution of abdominal lymphadenopathy. *Clinical Radiology*, **37**, 519–23.

Lim, J.H., Yoon, Y., Lee, S.W. *et al.* (1988). Superior aspects of the perirenal space: anatomy and pathological correlation. *Clinical Radiology*, **39**, 368–72.

Love, L., Meyers, M.A., Churchill, R.J. *et al.* (1981). Computer tomography of extraperitoneal spaces. *American Journal of Radiology*, **136**, 781–9.

Vincent, J.M., Morrison, I.D., Armstrong, P. & Reznek, R.H. (1994). The size of normal adrenal glands on computed tomography. *Clinical Radiology*, **49**, 453–55.

Vinnicombe, S.J., Norman, A.R., Nicholson, V. & Husband, J.E. (1995). Normal pelvic lymph nodes: evaluation with CT after bipedal lymphangiography. *Radiology*, **194**, 349–55.

14

The pelvis

S. J. VINNICOMBE
and J. E. HUSBAND

Imaging methods

Conventional radiography, ultrasound, computed tomography (CT) and magnetic resonance imaging (MRI) are all capable of providing detailed anatomical information.

The gross bony anatomy of the pelvis, as well as the detailed trabecular pattern of bone, are best demonstrated on conventional radiographs, which have higher spatial resolution than CT or MRI. However, CT with reconstruction of the data using a bone algorithm provides superior information regarding spatial relationships, for example, in the demonstration of bone fragments in pelvic fractures. Although MRI is not capable of demonstrating cortical or trabecular bone, the technique provides unique information regarding bone marrow components such as fat, haemopoietic tissue and bone marrow pathology.

The soft tissues of the pelvis are demonstrated using ultrasound, CT and MRI, which all provide complementary information. Ultrasound and MRI have the advantage of not utilizing ionizing radiation. Transabdominal ultrasound is useful as a basic screen, but requires a full bladder to act as an acoustic window and to displace gas-filled loops of bowel out of the pelvis, whereas endovaginal and transrectal ultrasound, though invasive, can provide exquisite detail of the internal anatomy of the male prostate and seminal vesicles and the female genital tract without the necessity of a full bladder. MRI provides similar detail, either by use of dedicated surface phased array coils or endocavitary coils. However, the hysterosalpingogram (HSG) still has an important role in the evaluation of the uterine cavity and Fallopian tubes.

Although ultrasound (with colour flow and pulsed wave Doppler techniques), MRI and contrast-enhanced CT (particularly helical CT), are able to visualize much of the pelvic vascu-lature, pelvic arteriography remains the gold standard investigation, particularly for delineating the internal iliac arterial tree. The external and common iliac veins can be demonstrated by bilateral lower limb venography, but evaluation of the tributaries of the internal iliac vein may necessitate selective catheterization via the common femoral vein.

The urinary tract is also investigated using contrast studies. These include the intravenous urogram (IVU) and the micturating cystourethrogram (MCUG). The former will normally demonstrate the lower ureters and the full bladder outline; an MCUG demonstrates the entire urethra during micturition, which is particularly important in the investigation of childhood urinary tract disease.

The pelvic floor

CT and MR provide excellent visualization of the muscles of the pelvis and MR is particularly well suited to demonstration of the pelvic floor, with its multiplanar capability. On T1-weighted sequences (T1W) the high signal pelvic fat provides excellent contrast with the low signal pelvic musculature.

The pelvic floor supports the pelvic viscera and is composed of a sling of muscles and fascia pierced by the rectum, the urethra and, in the female, the vagina. The muscle groups are divided into:

(a) the pelvic diaphragm superiorly: levator ani and coccygeus
(b) the superficial muscles of the perineum inferiorly: the urogenital perineum anteriorly and the anal perineum posteriorly.

The levator ani is the most important muscle of the pelvic floor. It arises from the posterior aspect of the pubis, the pelvic fascia over

(a)

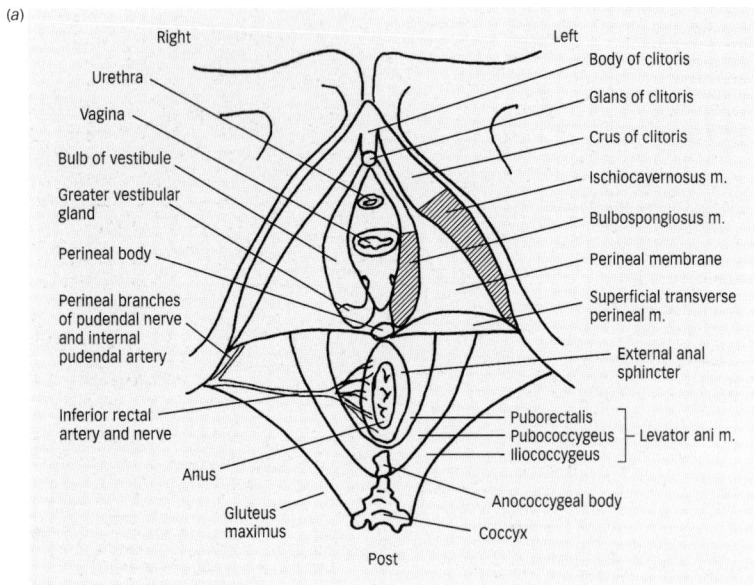

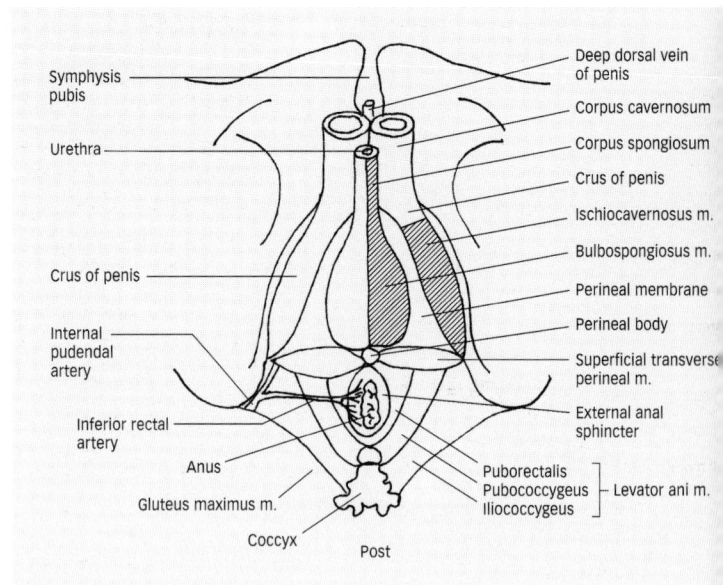

Fig. 1.
Diagrams of (a) the female
and (b) male perineum,
viewed from below. The
cross-hatching indicates
the muscles overlying the
crura and bulb of the clitoris
and vestibule (female) and
the penis (male).

obturator internus and the ischial spine. The fibres sweep downwards and medially to their insertions in three groups:

(a) anterior fibres (levator prostatae or sphincter vaginae) form a sling around the prostate or vagina and insert into the perineal body posterior to the urethra in the male or urethra and vagina in the female;
(b) intermediate fibres (puborectalis) form a sling round the junction of rectum and anal canal and blend with the external anal sphincter;
(c) posterior fibres (pubococcygeus and iliococcygeus) insert into the median anococcygeal body (a fibrous raphe between the anus and coccyx) and the coccyx.

The levatores ani act as a muscular support and have a sphincter action on the anorectal junction and vagina. The deep aspect is related to the pelvic viscera in their extraperitoneal space; the perineal aspect forms the medial wall of the ischiorectal fossa.

The coccygeus muscle is a small muscle which arises from the spine of the ischium as described above. It lies in the same plane as levator ani and aids it in its actions.

The perineum is a diamond-shaped space which lies within the ischiopubic rami and the coccyx. A line drawn between the ischial tuberosities will pass just anterior to the anus, demarcating the urogenital triangle anteriorly and the anal triangle posteriorly (Fig. 1(a), (b)).

The anterior urogenital triangle contains a musculofascial diaphragm, the urogenital diaphragm. The inferior layer of the diaphragm is formed by the tough fascial perineal membrane and is pierced by the urethra in both

sexes and by the vagina in the female. Inferior to the diaphragm is the superficial perineal pouch, in turn enclosed by fatty then membranous (Colles') fascia (Fig. 2). The membranous fascia attaches posteriorly to the posterior border of the urogenital diaphragm and laterally to the public arch. Anteriorly, it is continuous with the fascia of the anterior abdominal wall (Scarpa's fascia) and it is continued over the penis or clitoris and lines the scrotum. The superficial pouch in the male contains: (a) the bulbospongiosus muscle which covers the corpus spongiosum and surrounds the urethra, the whole forming the bulb of the penis; (b) the paired ischiocavernosus muscles which arise from the ischial ramus and cover the corpora cavernosa of the penis; (c) the superficial transverse perineal muscles which run transversely from the perineal body to the ischial rami (Fig. 1(b)).

The same muscles are present in the female although they are less well developed (Fig. 1(a)). In the female, the bulbospongiosus muscles cover the bulb of the vestibule and they are separated in the midline by the vagina and urethra. The pouch also contains the greater vestibular or Bartholin's glands at the posterior limit of each bulb (Fig. 3). The duct of each greater vestibular gland is just under 2 cm in length and opens on each side into the posterior part of the vestibule. In the midline, at the junction of the anterior and posterior perineum, lies the fibromuscular perineal body, to which the anal sphincter, bulbospongiosus, transverse perineal and levator ani muscles are attached.

Deep to the perineal membrane, the deep perineal pouch contains the deep transverse

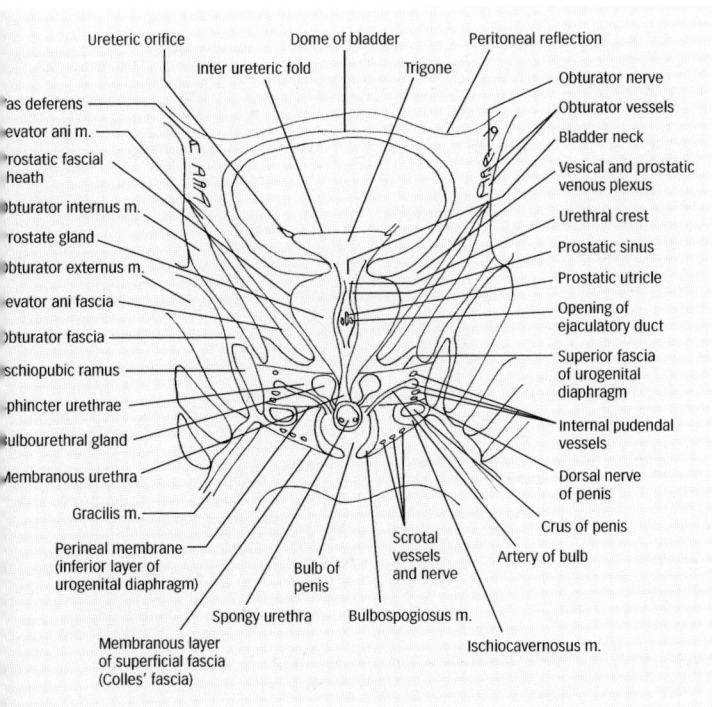

Fig. 2. — Diagram of a coronal section through the male pelvis and perineum.

Labels (Fig. 2): Ureteric orifice · Inter ureteric fold · Dome of bladder · Trigone · Peritoneal reflection · Obturator nerve · Obturator vessels · Bladder neck · Vesical and prostatic venous plexus · Urethral crest · Prostatic sinus · Prostatic utricle · Opening of ejaculatory duct · Superior fascia of urogenital diaphragm · Internal pudendal vessels · Dorsal nerve of penis · Crus of penis · Artery of bulb · Vas deferens · Levator ani m. · Prostatic fascial sheath · Obturator internus m. · Prostate gland · Obturator externus m. · Levator ani fascia · Obturator fascia · Ischiopubic ramus · Sphincter urethrae · Bulbourethral gland · Membranous urethra · Gracilis m. · Perineal membrane (inferior layer of urogenital diaphragm) · Bulb of penis · Scrotal vessels and nerve · Spongy urethra · Bulbospogiosus m. · Membranous layer of superficial fascia (Colles' fascia) · Ischiocavernosus m.

Fig. 3. — Diagram of a coronal section through the female urogenital diaphragm and superficial perineal pouch.

Labels (Fig. 3): Pelvic fascia · Vagina · Levator ani · Obturator internus · Obturator membrane · Sphincter urethrae m. · Dorsal nerve of clitoris · Internal pudendal artery · Artery of bulb · Crus of clitoris · Ischiocavernosus m. · Labial nerves · Bulb of vestibule · Labium majus · Bulbospongiosus m. · Deep fascia of thigh · Labium minus · Greater vestibular gland · Membranous layer of superficial fascia · Artery of crus (deep artery of clitoris) · Perineal membrane (inferior fascial layer of urogenital diaphragm) · Superior fascial layer of urogenital diaphragm

perineal muscles and the sphincter urethrae, formed of voluntary muscle. In the female, this is pierced by the vagina as well as the urethra. In the male, the pouch also contains the paired bulbourethral or Cowper's glands, whose ducts open into the bulbous urethra below the perineal membrane (Figs. 2 and 3).

The whole of the pouch is enclosed superiorly by a second fascial sheath, a condensation of the parietal pelvic fascia. The internal pudendal artery enters the deep perineal pouch on each side and runs anteriorly, giving off the artery to the bulb of the penis or clitoris, the arteries to the crura of the penis or clitoris and, in the male, the dorsal artery of the penis.

The anal triangle, between the ischial tuberosities and coccyx, contains the anus and its sphincters, levator ani and, laterally, the ischiorectal fossae. These lie below and lateral to the posterior fibres of levator ani and are bounded posteriorly by the sacrotuberous ligaments and gluteus maximus. Laterally, they extend to the fascia over obturator internus, in which the internal pudendal vessels and pudendal nerve run, giving off inferior rectal branches. Anteriorly, they are bounded by the urogenital perineum. Their importance lies in their tendency to become infected via the rectum or anal canal, which can result in the development of an ischiorectal abscess.

Behind the anus lies the anococcygeal body, which receives fibres from the anal sphincter and levator ani.

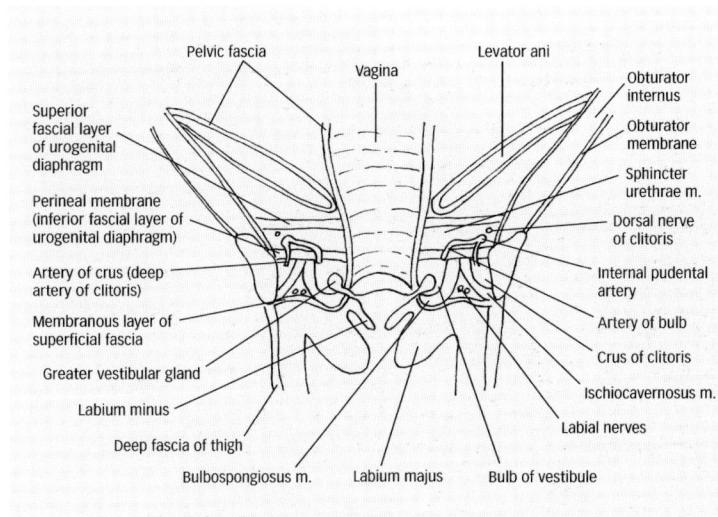

Important nerves of the pelvis

The sacral plexus, formed from the lumbosacral trunk (L4,5) and the ventral rami of the first to fourth sacral nerves, lies on the piriformis muscle, related anteriorly to the parietal pelvic fascia. The largest branch, which is also the largest nerve in the body, is the sciatic nerve, which may be visualized by CT and MR as it passes through the greater sciatic foramen into the gluteal region. The pudendal nerve leaves the pelvis through the greater sciatic foramen to enter the perineum through the lesser sciatic foramen.

The obturator nerve (L2,3,4) runs into the pelvis medial to psoas, then runs along the lateral pelvic wall, where it lies posteromedial to the common iliac vein, to enter the obturator canal.

The femoral nerve (L2,3,4) descends in the groove between psoas and iliacus to pass into the thigh under the inguinal ligament. Both it and the obturator nerve can be identified on MR and occasionally, CT.

The pelvic vasculature

A pelvic arteriogram and venogram are shown in Figs. 4 and 5.

The aorta bifurcates in front of the fourth lumbar vertebral body at the level of the iliac crest into the common iliac arteries, which enter the pelvis on the medial border of the psoas muscles, lying just anterior to the common iliac veins. The common iliac veins are immensely variable in size and the left iliac vein often appears up to twice as large as the right in normal subjects on transaxial sections. This can give a mass-like appearance which should not be confused with lymphadenopathy.

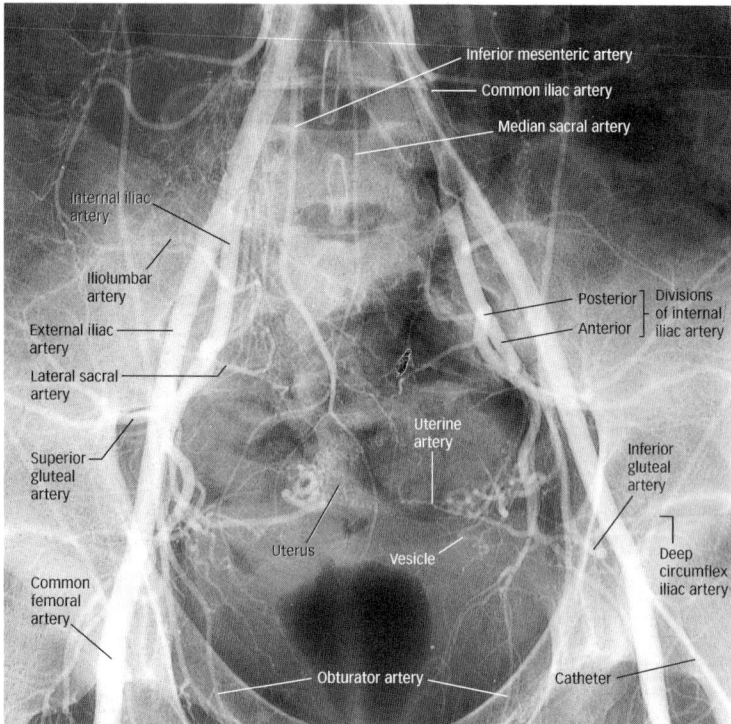

Fig. 4. top left
A normal pelvic arteriogram in a female patient.

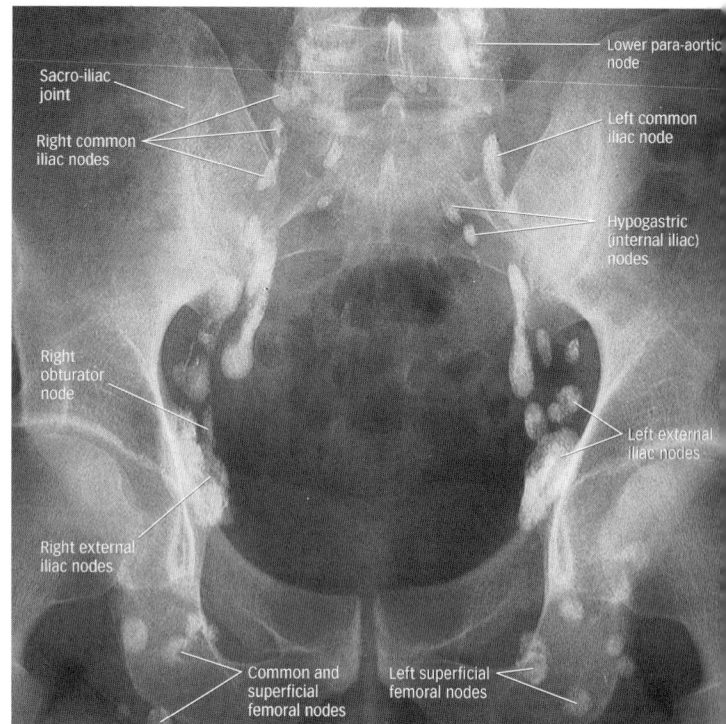

Fig. 6.
Frontal radiograph of the pelvis after bipedal lymphangiography demonstrating the iliac lymph nodes.

The common iliac arteries divide at the pelvic brim anterior to the lower sacroiliac joints into internal and external iliac arteries. On CT, this point is marked by the transition from the convex sacral promontory to the concave sacral cavity.

The external iliac artery runs along the medial border of psoas, passing under the inguinal ligament at a point midway between the anterior superior iliac spine and the pubic symphysis to become the common femoral artery. It is larger than the internal iliac artery except in the fetus, when the internal iliac arteries give rise to the umbilical arteries. Just above the inguinal ligament the external iliac artery gives off:

Fig. 5.
A normal iliac venogram.

(a) the inferior epigastric artery, which runs up on the deep surface of the anterior

abdominal wall to enter the rectus sheath;
(b) the deep circumflex iliac artery, which runs superolaterally to the anterior superior iliac spine under the inguinal ligament to supply the anterior abdominal wall muscles.

The external iliac artery is separated from loops of bowel by the peritoneum. In the male it is crossed by the vas deferens and the testicular vessels; in the female, by the round ligament. The ureter crosses the artery in the region of its origin. The accompanying external iliac vein lies posterior to it superiorly and medial to it near the inguinal ligament.

The internal iliac artery enters the true pelvis anterior to the sacroiliac joint, with the ureter anterior to it. From its origin, it runs inferomedially, anterior to the sacrum, its length varying from 2–5 cm. It has the most variable branching pattern of all the arteries in the body; the commonest pattern is described here. It divides into anterior and posterior divisions at the upper border of the greater sciatic foramen. The anterior division courses down towards the ischial spine and gives off the following branches:

(a) the obturator artery, present as an independent branch in approximately 75% of individuals, passes anteriorly medial to the obturator internus muscle before it exits the pelvis through the obturator canal;
(b) the inferior vesical artery, which supplies the lower bladder, ureter, prostate gland and seminal vesicles;

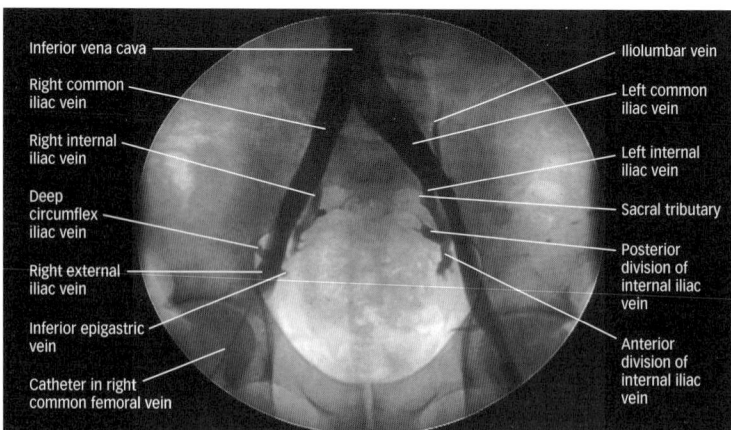

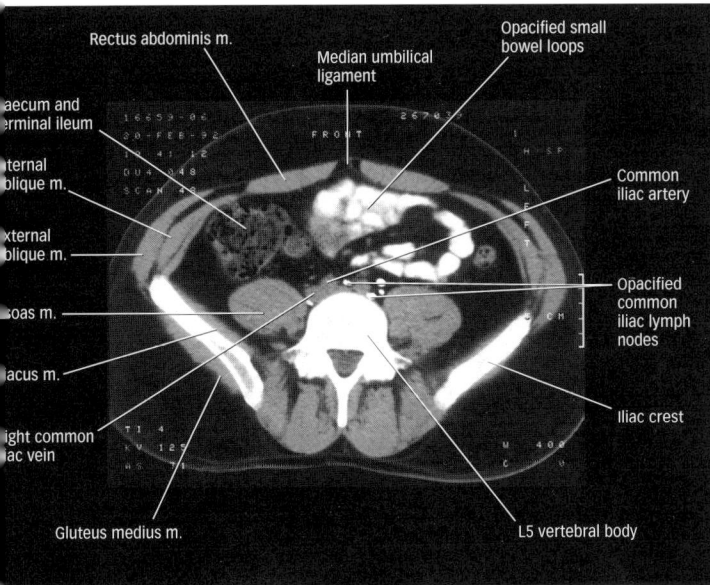

Rectus abdominis m.
Median umbilical ligament
Opacified small bowel loops
aecum and erminal ileum
ternal blique m.
xternal blique m.
soas m.
acus m.
ight common ac vein
Gluteus medius m.
Common iliac artery
Opacified common iliac lymph nodes
Iliac crest
L5 vertebral body

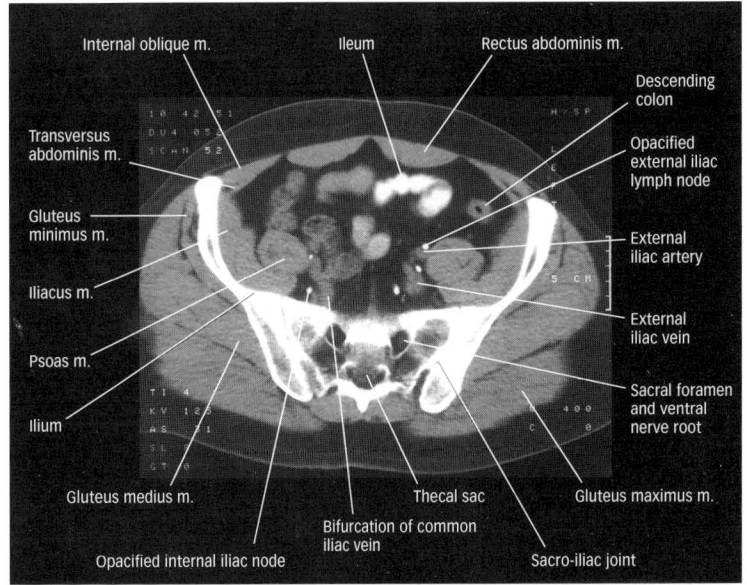

Internal oblique m.
Ileum
Rectus abdominis m.
Descending colon
Transversus abdominis m.
Opacified external iliac lymph node
Gluteus minimus m.
External iliac artery
Iliacus m.
External iliac vein
Psoas m.
Sacral foramen and ventral nerve root
Ilium
Gluteus medius m.
Thecal sac
Gluteus maximus m.
Bifurcation of common iliac vein
Opacified internal iliac node
Sacro-iliac joint

(b)

Fig. 7.
Axial CT of the pelvis following bipedal lymphangiography: (a) at e brim of the false pelvis, (b) 1 cm below the sacral promontory and (c) at the superior acetabulum.

(c) the middle rectal artery, usually arising with the inferior vesical artery, also supplies the prostate gland, seminal vesicles and rectum.

(d) the uterine artery, which pursues a tortuous course in the broad ligament and supplies the uterus, upper vagina, Fallopian tubes and ovary. It is rarely seen on CT images unless it is heavily calcified;

(e) the vaginal artery, equivalent to the inferior vesical artery in the male, supplies the lower vagina;

(f) the internal pudendal artery, which enters the perineum as described above to supply the genitalia. It can be seen coursing along the lateral wall of the ischiorectal fossa, having re-entered the pelvis through the lesser sciatic foramen, particularly in men, in whom it is larger. It gives off the inferior rectal artery;

(g) the superior vesical arteries run medially to supply the upper bladder and are in continuity with the medial umbilical ligaments (see below);

(h) the inferior gluteal artery, which passes through the lower part of the greater sciatic foramen. It is rarely identified at CT or MR unless ectatic, when it may be mistaken for a soft tissue mass. It supplies the sciatic nerve.

The obturator artery arises from the inferior epigastric artery in approximately 25% of individuals and, in a further 5%, there are contributions from both the internal iliac and inferior epigastric arteries.

A further relatively common anatomical variant of radiological importance is the per-

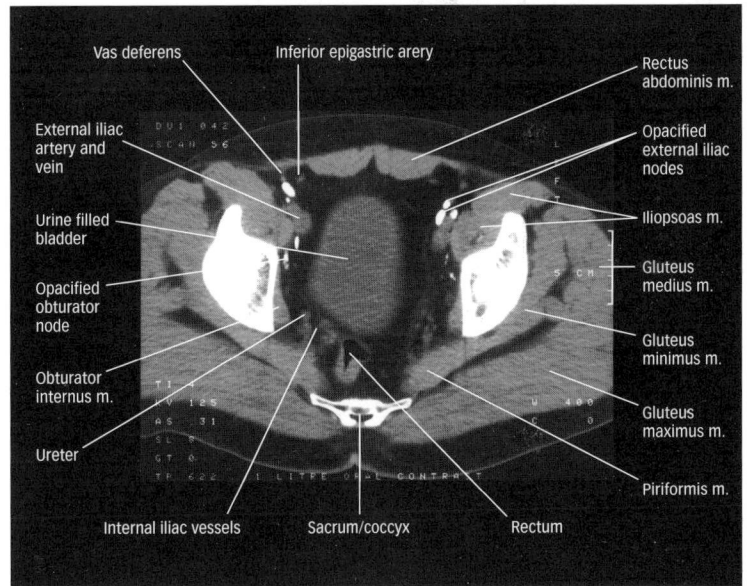

Vas deferens
Inferior epigastric arery
Rectus abdominis m.
External iliac artery and vein
Opacified external iliac nodes
Urine filled bladder
Iliopsoas m.
Opacified obturator node
Gluteus medius m.
Obturator internus m.
Gluteus minimus m.
Ureter
Gluteus maximus m.
Piriformis m.
Internal iliac vessels
Sacrum/coccyx
Rectum

(c)

sistent sciatic artery, present in under 1% of individuals. This is an enlarged inferior gluteal artery that represents a persistence of the fetal vascular supply to the lower limbs. It may be unilateral or bilateral and may be associated with absence of the superficial femoral or profunda arteries. Its posterior location is well demonstrated by a lateral pelvic arteriogram.

The obliterated umbilical artery is the first branch of the internal iliac artery in the fetus. It ascends on the deep surface of the anterior abdominal wall to the umbilicus and after birth, persists as the fibrous medial umbilical ligament, which may be recognized in the presence of a pneumoperitoneum.

Branches of the posterior division of the internal iliac artery are as follows:

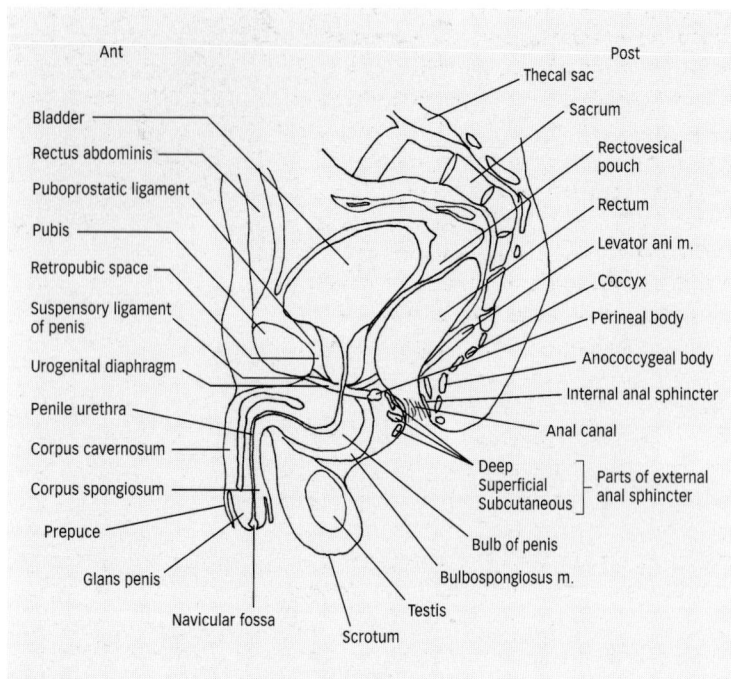

Ant · Post

Bladder
Rectus abdominis
Puboprostatic ligament
Pubis
Retropubic space
Suspensory ligament of penis
Urogenital diaphragm
Penile urethra
Corpus cavernosum
Corpus spongiosum
Prepuce
Glans penis
Navicular fossa
Scrotum
Testis
Bulbospongiosus m.
Bulb of penis
Deep / Superficial / Subcutaneous — Parts of external anal sphincter
Anal canal
Internal anal sphincter
Anococcygeal body
Perineal body
Coccyx
Levator ani m.
Rectum
Rectovesical pouch
Sacrum
Thecal sac

Fig. 8.
Diagram of a mid-sagittal section through the male pelvis.

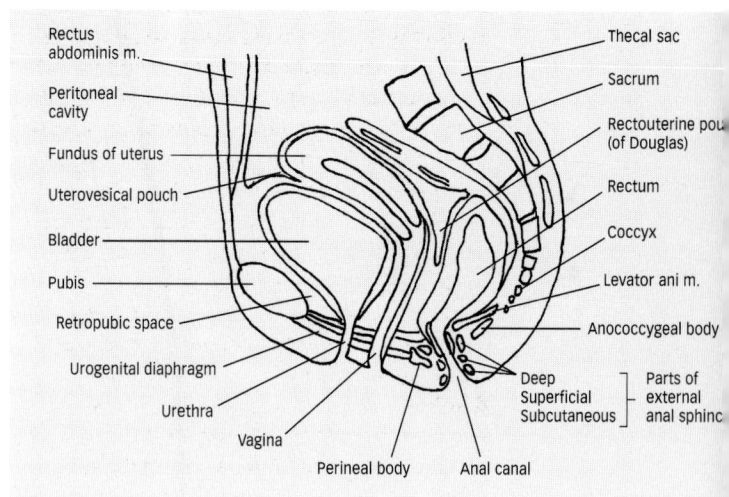

Rectus abdominis m.
Peritoneal cavity
Fundus of uterus
Uterovesical pouch
Bladder
Pubis
Retropubic space
Urogenital diaphragm
Urethra
Vagina
Perineal body
Anal canal
Deep / Superficial / Subcutaneous — Parts of external anal sphincter
Anococcygeal body
Levator ani m.
Coccyx
Rectum
Rectouterine pouch (of Douglas)
Sacrum
Thecal sac

Fig. 9.
Diagram of a mid-sagittal section through the female pelvis.

(a) the iliolumbar artery, which ascends anterior to the sacroiliac joint, dorsal to the external iliac vessels and supplies psoas and iliacus after dividing into iliac and lumbar branches;
(b) the lateral sacral artery, often in superior and inferior pairs, which supplies the sacral canal and the muscles and skin over the back. It anastomoses with the median sacral artery, the last branch of the aorta;
(c) the superior gluteal artery, the largest branch of the internal iliac artery, passing through the greater sciatic foramen above piriformis to the muscles of the pelvic wall and gluteal region. The artery may be recognized at CT, particularly when calcified.

The external and internal iliac veins accompany the arteries. Superiorly, the left common iliac vein passes to the right underneath the left common iliac artery to join the right common iliac vein and form the inferior vena cava, to the right of the aorta. MR, CT and ultrasound can all give information on the pelvic vasculature, though the latter has the disadvantage of being critically dependent on body habitus. However, neither ultrasound nor MR require the administration of intravenous contrast medium.

The lymphatics of the pelvis accompany the vessels and the pelvic lymph nodes are classified accordingly. There are three chains accompanying the external iliac vessels, the most medial of which contains the obturator lymph nodes, related laterally to the obturator internus muscle. These lymph nodes are extremely important in the assessment of the extent of pelvic malignancy. Their short axis diameter rarely exceeds 8 mm. The internal iliac lymph nodes drain to common iliac lymph nodes and thence to para-aortic lymph nodes. Recent research has shown that normal lymph nodes are only very occasionally recognizable at CT unless they have been previously opacified by bipedal lymphangiography, an investigation only rarely performed outside specialist centres. Most external and common iliac lymph nodes have a short axis diameter less than 10 mm. Figures 6 and 7 demonstrate the external and common iliac lymph nodes opacified after bipedal lymphangiography, using conventional radiography and CT, respectively.

The pelvic viscera

The bladder and urethra
The bladder
This is situated behind the pubic bones. In the adult the empty bladder lies entirely within the pelvis. In the child, the empty bladder projects above the pelvic inlet, although it is still extraperitoneal (Figs. 8 and 9).

The empty bladder is pyramidal in shape, with a base, apex, a superior and two inferior surfaces. The apex lies behind the upper border of the symphysis; from here, the urachal remnant passes up to the umbilicus in an extraperitoneal location, forming the median umbilical ligament. The base or posterior surface is triangular and the ureters enter the posterolateral angles. The inferior angle or neck gives rise to the urethra, surrounded by the involuntary internal urethral sphincter. Posteriorly lies the vagina in the female and the vasa deferentia and seminal vesicles in the male. These structures are separated from the rectum by the rectovesical fascia. The superior surface of the bladder is completely covered by peritoneum. In the female, the uterus, also covered by peritoneum, sits on top of the bladder. The two inferolateral surfaces are related anteriorly to the retropubic fat pad with its perivesical venous plexus and further posteriorly, to the obturator internus muscle above and the levator ani below. In the male, the neck of the bladder rests on the prostate gland, whereas in the female it rests directly on the pelvic fascia above the urogenital diaphragm. The bladder thus lies at a lower level within the pelvis in the female. When the bladder fills, it becomes ovoid and the superior surface rises extraperitoneally into the abdomen.

Internally, the bladder wall is trabeculated except at the trigone, the triangular area between the two ureteric orifices superiorly and the urethral orifice inferiorly.

The bladder is anchored inferiorly by condensations of pelvic fascia which attach it to the pubis, lateral pelvic walls and rectum. In the male, the attachment to the prostate renders the bladder more immobile because of the strong puboprostatic ligaments. The peritoneal reflections over the bladder also differ; in the male, the peritoneum over the superior surface of the bladder extends down before passing up over the rectum, forming the rectovesical pouch, the lowest part of the peritoneal cavity. In the female, the peritoneum is reflected up over the anteroinferior surface of the uterus, forming the vesicouterine pouch, before passing off the posterior surface of the uterus and up over the rectum, thus forming the rectouterine pouch of Douglas.

The blood supply to the bladder is from the superior and inferior vesical arteries, described above. The veins of the vesical plexus drain to the internal iliac veins. Lymph drainage is to the internal iliac, thence to the para-aortic lymph nodes.

The distal ureter enters the pelvis anterior to the bifurcation of the common iliac artery. It runs inferoposteriorly anterior to the internal iliac artery and at the level of the ischial spine, turns anteromedially to enter the posterolateral bladder. In the male, the ureters are crossed anteromedially by the vasa deferentia and they lie above the seminal vesicles. In the female, they pass just above the lateral fornices of the vagina, lateral to the cervix and inferior to the uterine vessels within the broad ligament (Fig. 10). In both sexes the intramural ureter courses obliquely through the bladder for approximately 2 cm before entering the bladder cavity.

Imaging On anteroposterior radiographs of the pelvis, the bladder can be seen as a rounded soft tissue mass surrounded by transradiant extraperitoneal fat. Loss of this perivesical fat stripe, particularly unilaterally, is an important sign of pelvic pathology.

The bladder and ureters are opacified after intravenous urography. In women, it is normal to see an impression on the dome of the bladder, often eccentrically placed, produced by the fundus of the uterus. In the male, the prostate gland may protrude up into the bladder base, to produce a 'prostatic impression'. The full bladder outline should be smooth and regular, whereas after micturition, small amounts of contrast medium are seen trapped between the mucosal folds of the empty bladder. The bladder can also be filled with contrast retrogradely, usually as part of a micturating cystourethrogram (MCUG) performed in order to visualize the entire length of the male urethra.

The structure of the bladder wall is best appreciated on ultrasound. When the bladder is full, the thickness of the echogenic wall should not exceed 4 mm. It is also possible to visualize the lower ureters in young children and the use of colour Doppler allows identification of ureteric jets; the contents of the bladder are otherwise transsonic.

On CT, the bladder is best appreciated when filled with urine or contrast. The bladder typically has a rectangular shape and, again, wall thickness should not exceed 4–5 mm. MR is ideal to demonstrate the relationships of the bladder in the coronal and sagittal planes. On T1-weighted (T1W) sequences, the bladder wall and contents are homogeneous, displaying a low signal intensity. On T2 W images, the high signal urine within the bladder contrasts with the low signal bladder wall. Chemical

Fig. 10.
Diagram of the structures of the broad ligament (lateral view). Note the relationship of the ureter to the uterine artery and cervix.

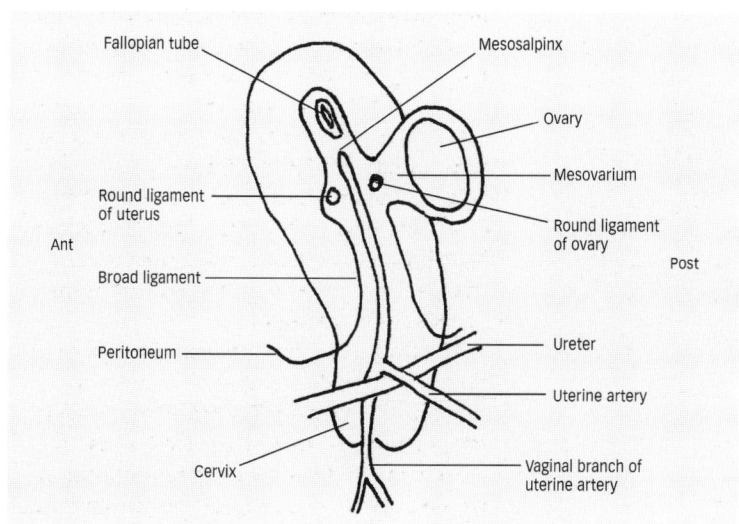

shift artefact in the frequency-encoding direction may produce artefactual high signal within the bladder wall, which should not be misinterpreted as pathology.

The male urethra

The male urethra is approximately 20 cm long and is divided into prostatic, membranous (together making up the posterior urethra) and spongy (anterior) parts. The posterior urethra is 4 cm long and the anterior approximately 16 cm.

The prostatic urethra is 3 cm long. It is the widest part of the urethra. On its posterior wall is a longitudinal ridge, the urethral or prostatic crest (Fig. 2). On each side of this is a shallow groove, the prostatic sinus, into which the prostatic ducts (approximately 15–20 in number) open. In the middle of the crest is a further prominence, the verumontanum, into which the blind-ended prostatic utricle opens. On either side of this, the ejaculatory ducts (the common termination of the seminal vesicles and vasa deferentia) open. The lowermost part of the urethra is fixed by the puboprostatic ligaments and is therefore immobile.

The membranous urethra, 1.5 cm long, runs through the external urethral sphincter within the urogenital diaphragm. This is the narrowest, most fixed and least dilatable part of the urethra. It is therefore most prone to injury, e.g. by pelvic fractures.

The spongy urethra is further subdivided into the bulbous and penile urethra. The bulbous urethra, within the bulb of the penis, has a localized dilatation, the infrabulbar fossa. It is surrounded by the corpus spongiosum. The penile urethra is long and relatively narrow apart from a dilatation within the glans penis, the navicular fossa. The roof of the navicular fossa bears a mucosal fold, the lacuna magna, which must be negotiated during urethral instrumentation. The external urethral orifice is narrow and calculi may lodge at this site.

Imaging The urethra may be outlined with contrast medium retrogradely, with a balloon catheter in the navicular fossa. The anterior urethra is well visualized in this way, but demonstration of the posterior urethra may necessitate catheterization of the bladder followed by micturition. The verumontanum is seen as a filling defect and contrast may occasionally reflux into the utricle and into the ducts of the bulbourethral glands, which open into the membranous urethra. It is also possible to image the anterior urethra with ultrasound, although mucosal detail is poorer (Fig. 11).

The female urethra

This is 3–4 cm in length and extends from the neck of the bladder to the vestibule, where it opens 2.5 cm behind the clitoris. It traverses the urogenital diaphragm (sphincter urethrae) anterior to the vagina. Small paraurethral glands, equivalent to the male prostate, open into the vestibule via small ducts on either side of the urethral orifice. The female urethra may be visualized during MCUG.

The male genital tract
The prostate gland

The prostate gland is a pyramidal fibromuscular gland, 3.5 cm long, which surrounds the prostatic urethra from the bladder base to the urogenital diaphragm (Fig. 2). The base, superiorly, is continuous with the neck of the bladder; the urethra enters it near its anterior border. The anterior wall lies in the arch of the pubis, separated from it by the cave of Retzius (retropubic space). Inferiorly, near the apex, the puboprostatic ligament passes anteriorly to the pubic symphysis. Laterally lie the muscles of the pelvic side wall, the anterior fibres of the levator ani embracing the prostate (levator prostatae).

Posteriorly lie the paired seminal vesicles, in turn separated from the rectum by Denonvillier's fascia, a dense condensation of pelvic fascia. The prostate gland has a thin true capsule, surrounded by a fibrous sheath which is a condensation of the pelvic fascia. Between these two layers lies the periprostatic venous plexus.

The ejaculatory ducts pierce the upper part of the posterior surface of the prostate and open into the prostatic urethra at the lateral margins of the prostatic utricle.

The prostate gland was initially thought to be divided into five anatomical lobes (Lowsley's lobar concept), but it is now recognized that five lobes can only be distinguished in the fetal gland prior to 20 weeks gestation, after which only three lobes are recognizable,

Fig. 11.
Transrectal ultrasound image of the bulb of the penis.

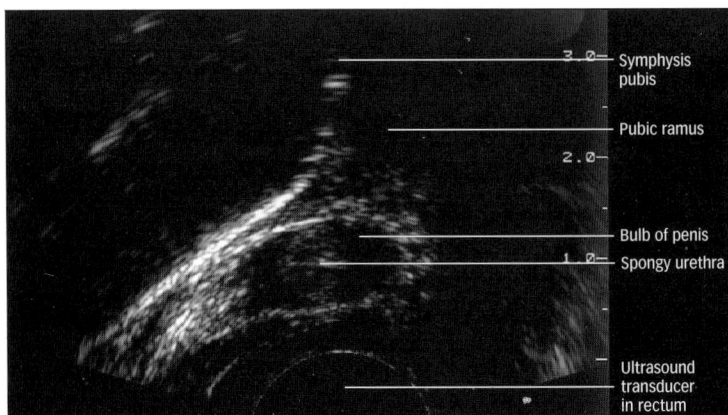

- Symphysis pubis
- Pubic ramus
- Bulb of penis
- Spongy urethra
- Ultrasound transducer in rectum

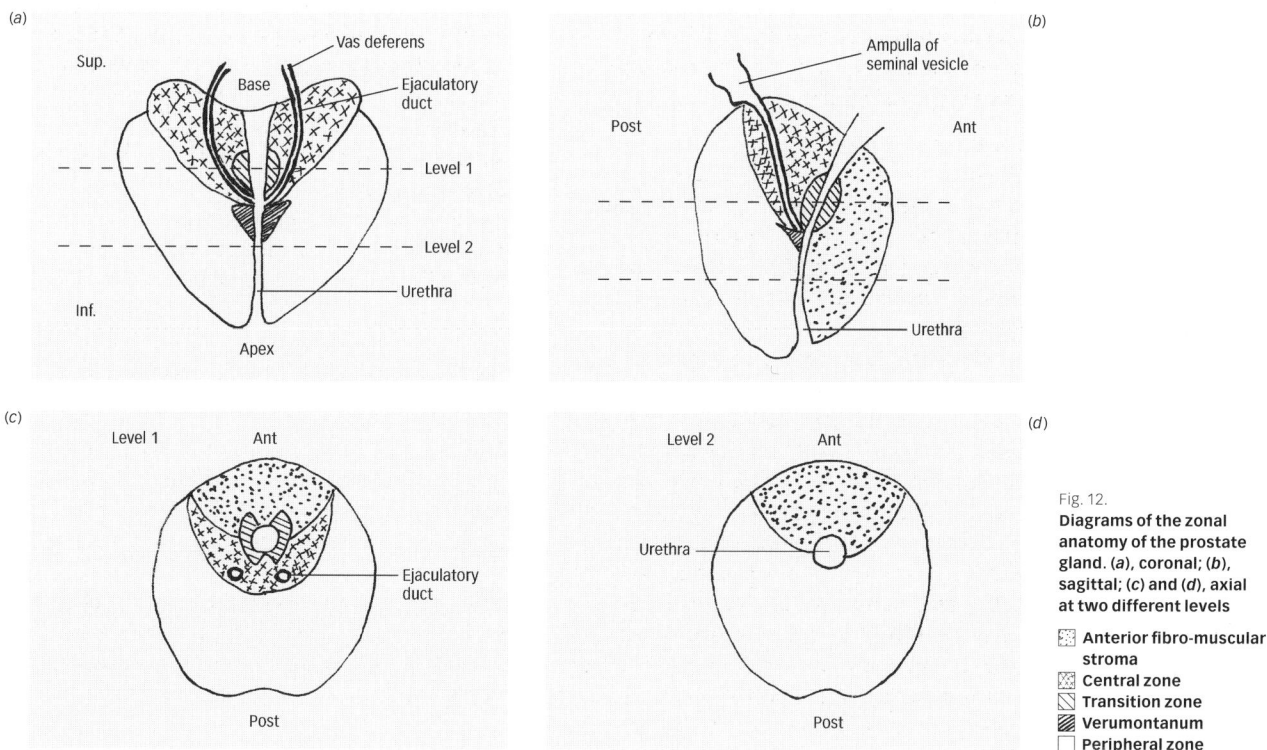

(a) Sup. Base Vas deferens Ejaculatory duct Level 1 Level 2 Urethra Inf. Apex

(b) Ampulla of seminal vesicle Post Ant Urethra

(c) Level 1 Ant Ejaculatory duct Post

(d) Level 2 Ant Urethra Post

Fig. 12.
Diagrams of the zonal anatomy of the prostate gland. (*a*), coronal; (*b*), sagittal; (*c*) and (*d*), axial at two different levels

Anterior fibro-muscular stroma
Central zone
Transition zone
Verumontanum
Peripheral zone

two lateral lobes and a median lobe. In the mature gland, the lobes fuse and the gland is divided into glandular and non-glandular tissue. The glandular tissue is subdivided into three distinct zones: the peripheral zone or PZ (70%), the central zone or CZ (25%) and the transition zone or TZ (5%). The non-glandular tissue comprises the isthmus, which encircles the urethra anteriorly. Figure 12 illustrates the zonal anatomy of the prostate diagrammatically. The CZ surrounds the urethra above the ejaculatory ducts, the narrow TZ lies just inside it, and the PZ makes up the rest of the gland. There is also a small area of glandular tissue composed of periurethral glands. The zonal anatomy is of clinical importance, since most carcinomas arise in the PZ, whereas benign prostatic hypertrophy affects the TZ. The entire inner gland, comprising internal sphincter, periurethral glands and TZ, lies above the verumontanum where the ejaculatory ducts insert. The CZ comprises the base of the prostate and is equivalent to the median lobe of Lowsley but larger, since it surrounds the ejaculatory ducts. The PZ comprises the posterior, inferior and lateral areas of the gland; it and the CZ together form the outer gland.

The arterial supply to the prostate gland is from the inferior vesical and middle rectal arteries. Venous drainage is via the periprostatic plexus to the internal iliac veins and also to the vertebral venous plexus; hence the

propensity of prostatic carcinoma to spread to the vertebrae. Lymphatic drainage is to the internal iliac and obturator lymph nodes.

Imaging The prostate gland can be imaged by transabdominal ultrasound (Fig. 13) but transrectal ultrasound (TRUS) is far superior (Fig. 14). The zonal anatomy may be distinguished to some extent. The central and peripheral zones are generally of uniform low level echogenicity, although slight differences may be appreciated. Surrounding the midline urethra is a less echogenic area that corresponds to the internal sphincter, periurethral glandular tissue and transition zone. The latter enlarges with age and may become the dominant part of the gland. It is often possible to see the ejaculatory ducts coursing to the prostatic urethra on sagittal scans of the gland. The seminal vesicles are seen as hypoechoic sacculated structures superoposterior to the gland.

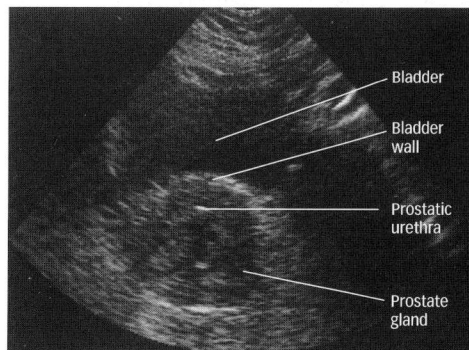

Bladder
Bladder wall
Prostatic urethra
Prostate gland

Fig. 13.
Transabdominal transverse ultrasound of the bladder and prostate gland.

(a)i

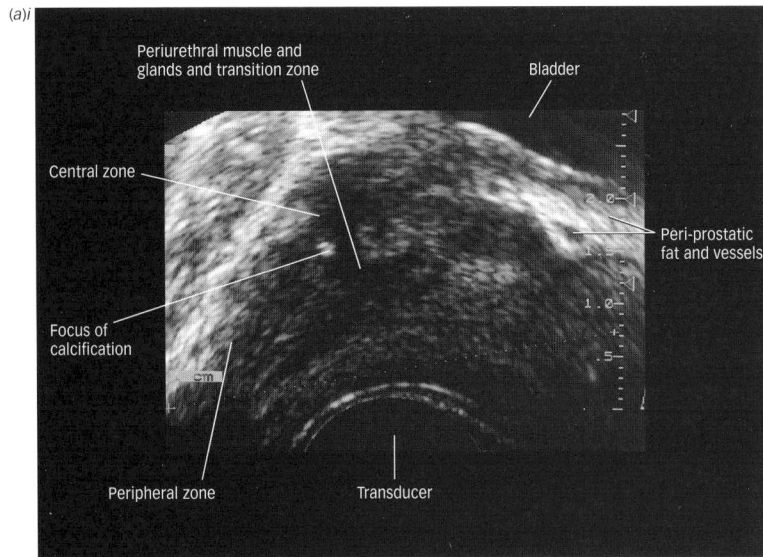

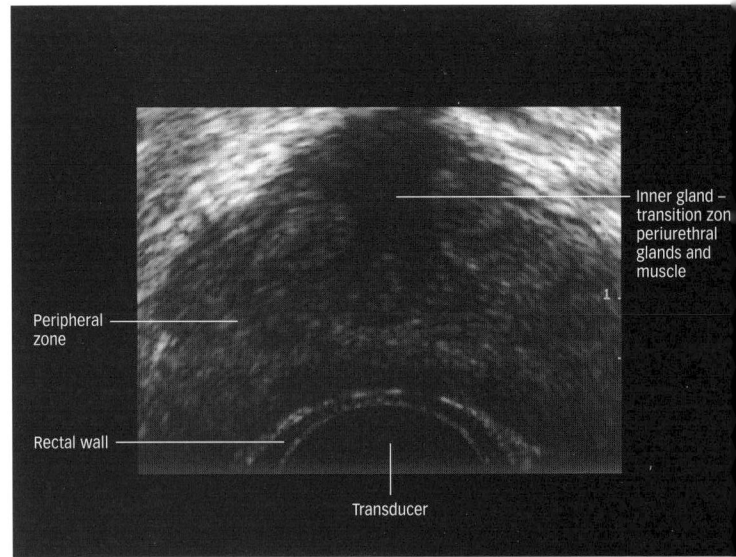

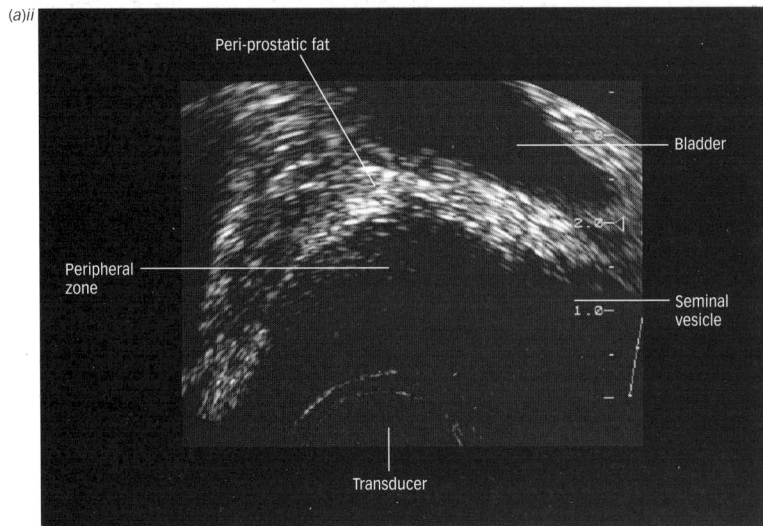

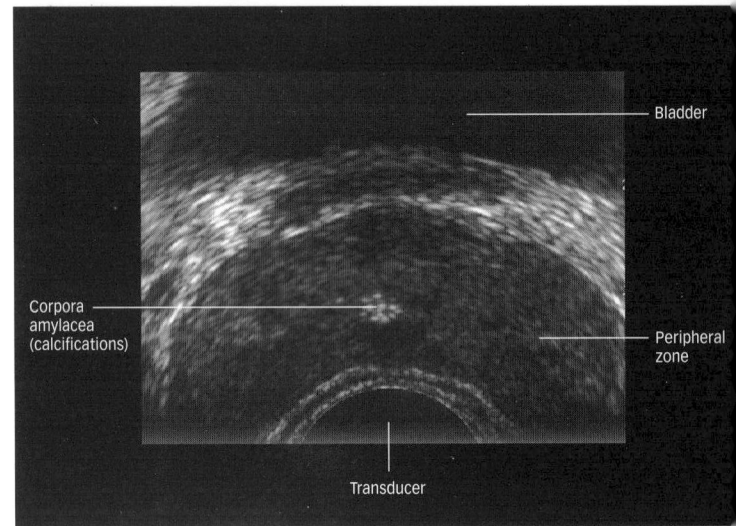

(a) Longitudinal transrectal ultrasound images of the prostate gland: (i) mid-sagittal, (ii), right parasagittal scans.

(a)ii

Fig. 14.

Fig. 14.

(b) Transverse transrectal images of the prostate gland.

There should be a clear tissue plane between the gland and the seminal vesicles.

On CT, the prostate is seen as a rounded soft tissue mass up to 3 cm in diameter, with a well-defined fat plane surrounding it which separates it from the obturator internus muscles (Fig. 15). CT cannot delineate the zonal anatomy of the gland.

On MRI, the appearances vary depending on the type of coil and the sequence used. The gland is of uniformly low signal on T1W sequences, as are the seminal vesicles and periprostatic veins. The neurovascular bundles at 5 and 7 o'clock are seen, outlined by periprostatic fat, as are the pelvic muscles and fascia. On T2W sequences, the zonal anatomy is well demonstrated. The normal PZ has high signal intensity, as does the fluid within the seminal vesicles, whereas the CZ and TZ have relatively low signal. The term 'central gland' is often used to indicate the combined CZ and

TZ, which cannot normally be differentiated other than by knowledge of their respective anatomical locations. The verumontanum may be seen on T2W scans, where it has high signal. The anterior fibromuscular stroma returns low signal on all sequences, in contrast to the anterior periprostatic fascia in the retropubic space. Fat-suppressed T2W sequences give excellent contrast between the high signal peripheral zone and the periprostatic fat. Figures 16, 17 and 18 demonstrate the anatomy of the bladder and male genital tract in the sagittal and coronal planes. Figures 19 and 20 are axial MR images of the male pelvis and the prostate gland, respectively.

The relationship of the zones of the gland normally changes with age. The CZ atrophies, whereas the TZ enlarges secondary to benign prostatic hypertrophy. This often produces a low signal band at the margins between the hypertrophied TZ and the compressed PZ, the

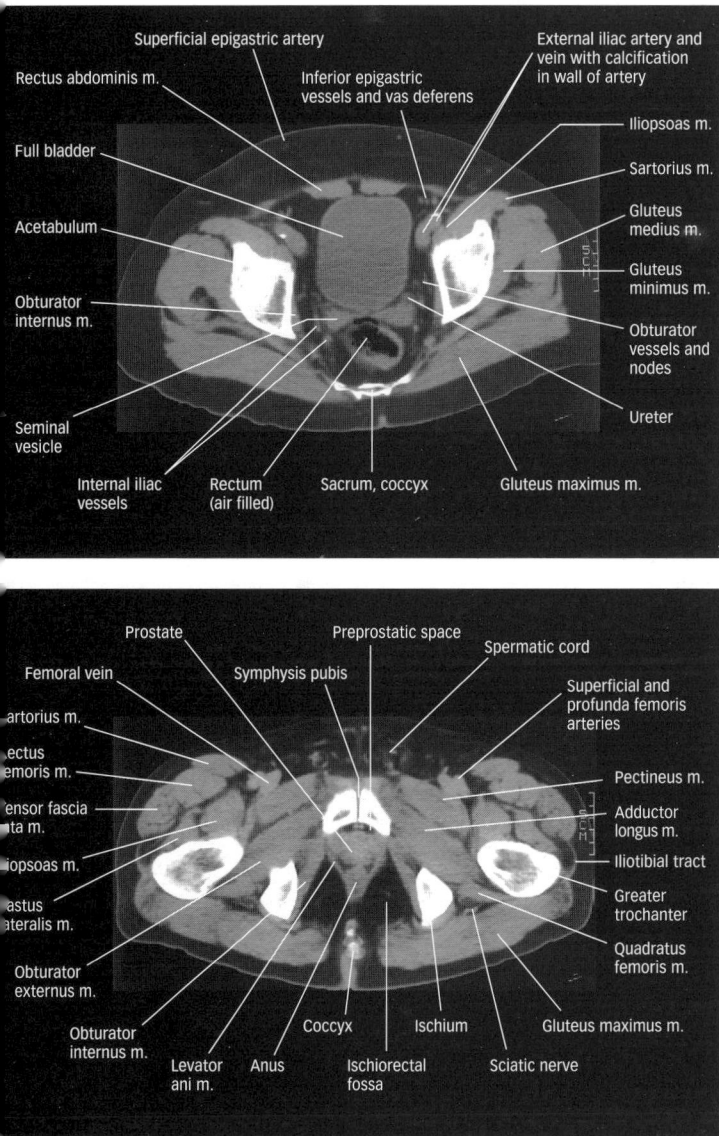

Fig. 15.
Axial CT of the male pelvis: at the levels (a) of the acetabulum and (b) the symphysis pubis.

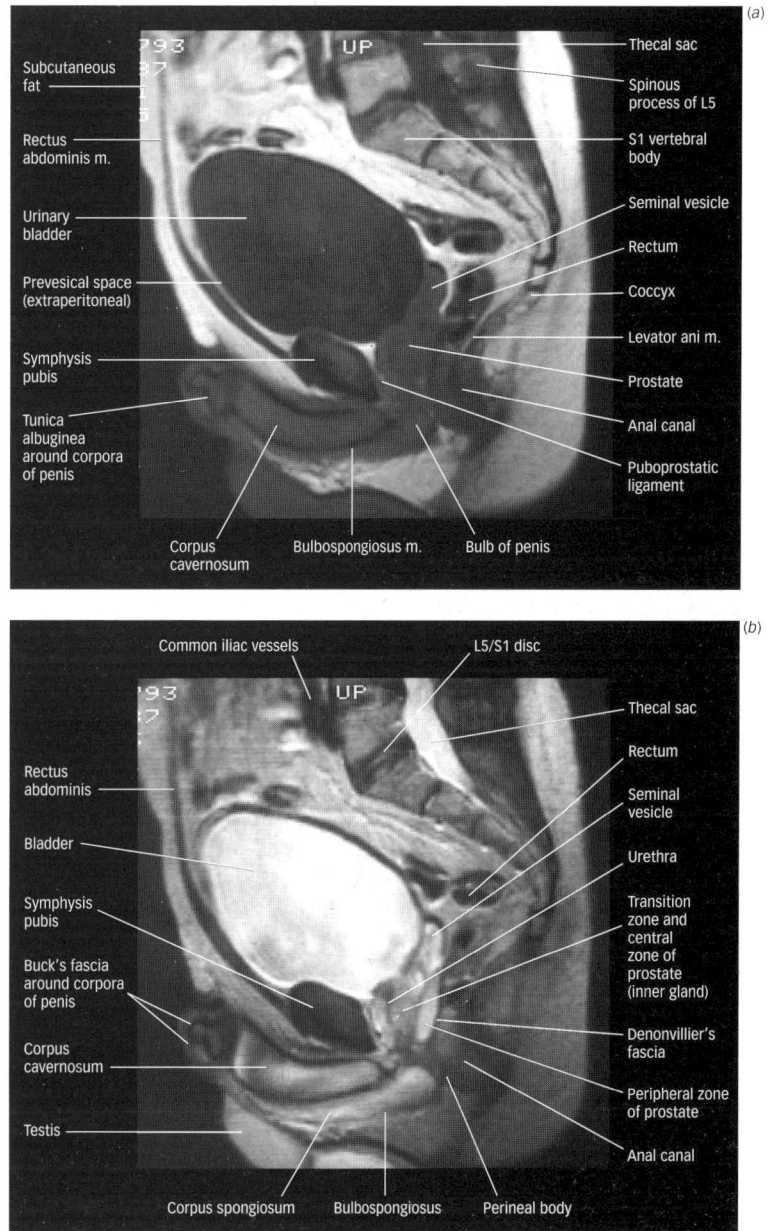

Fig. 16.
Sagittal MR images of the male pelvis, (a) T1 weighted and (b) T2 weighted. (Note chemical shift artefact in superior and inferior bladder walls.)

surgical pseudocapsule. This and the anatomical capsule are well seen on T2W images.

The seminal vesicles and ejaculatory ducts

The seminal vesicles are two lobulated sacs, about 5 cm long, which lie transversely behind the bladder and store semen. Their lower extremities lie close together; medially lie the terminal parts of the vasa deferentia. Posteriorly the seminal vesicles are related to Denonvillier's fascia and the rectum. Inferiorly, each seminal vesicle narrows and fuses with the ampulla of the vas deferens to form the two ejaculatory ducts, each about 2 cm long. These pierce the prostate gland and run obliquely through it to enter the prostatic utricle.

Imaging On TRUS, the seminal vesicles appear as convoluted tubules which contain transsonic fluid (Fig. 21). They are less echogenic than the adjacent prostate. The angle between

the prostate and seminal vesicles is important in the assessment of the spread of prostatic carcinoma, as indicated above.

On CT, the seminal vesicles are of soft tissue attentuation and characteristically form a 'bow tie' appearance in the groove between the bladder base and prostate. There should be a clear fat plane between the bladder base and seminal vesicles (see Fig. 15(i)).However, this is much better appreciated on MR, particularly T1W sagittal sequences where the seminal vesicles return a low signal, in contrast to the surrounding fat. On T2W sequences the fluid – containing seminal vesicles return a high signal and on endorectal high resolution imaging the walls of the vesicles may be seen as low signal intensity structures (Fig. 22).

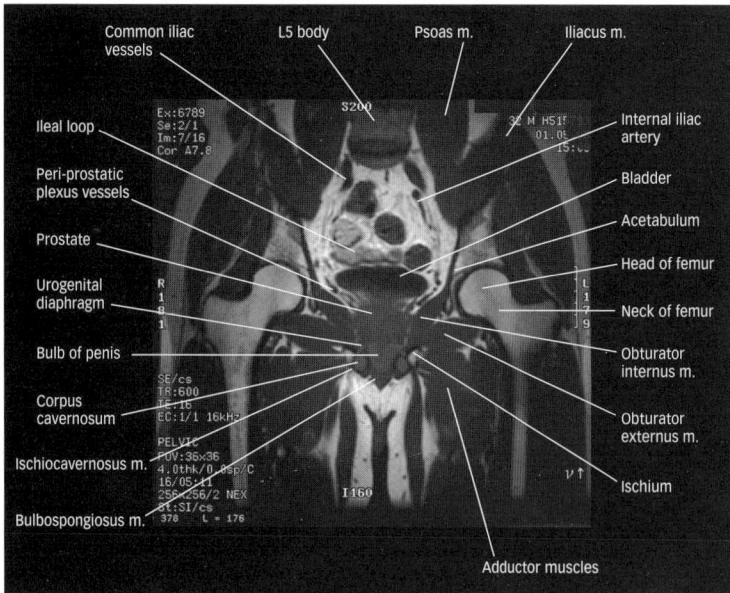

Fig. 17.
Coronal T1 weighted MR image of the male pelvis.

Common iliac vessels — L5 body — Psoas m. — Iliacus m. — Internal iliac artery — Bladder — Acetabulum — Head of femur — Neck of femur — Obturator internus m. — Obturator externus m. — Ischium — Adductor muscles — Ileal loop — Peri-prostatic plexus vessels — Prostate — Urogenital diaphragm — Bulb of penis — Corpus cavernosum — Ischiocavernosus m. — Bulbospongiosus m.

The testis, epididymis, spermatic cord and vas deferens

The testis is an ovoid reproductive and endocrine organ responsible for sperm production (Fig. 23). Each lies within the scrotum, an outpouching of the lower anterior abdominal wall, suspended by the spermatic cord. Each testis has an upper and lower pole and measures 4 cm by 2.5 cm by 3 cm. The left testis lies lower than the right in 85% of subjects. The upper pole of the testis is usually tilted slightly forwards. Each is surrounded by a tough fibrous capsule, the tunica albuginea. This is thickened posteriorly to form an incomplete fibrous septum, the mediastinum of the testis, in which the testicular vessels run. From here, fibrous septa extend into the

gland, dividing it into 200–300 seminiferous lobules, each containing 1–3 seminiferous tubules. The seminiferous tubules drain to the rete testis within the mediastinum, from whence 10–15 efferent ducts pierce the tunica near the upper pole to enter the head of the epididymis. The efferent ducts fuse to form a single convoluted tube which makes up the body and tail of the epididymis.

Each testis is invaginated anteriorly into a double serous covering, the tunica vaginalis. This is continuous with the peritoneum during fetal development via the processus vaginalis, which normally becomes obliterated at birth. It covers the anterior, lateral and medial surfaces of the testis.

The epididymis lies posterior and slightly lateral to the testis, with the vas deferens along its medial side. It has an expanded head

Fig. 18.
Coronal T2 weighted MR images of the male pelvis, (a) to (c), from anterior to posterior. (Note chemical shift artefact from superior and inferior bladder walls, in anterior.)

(a)

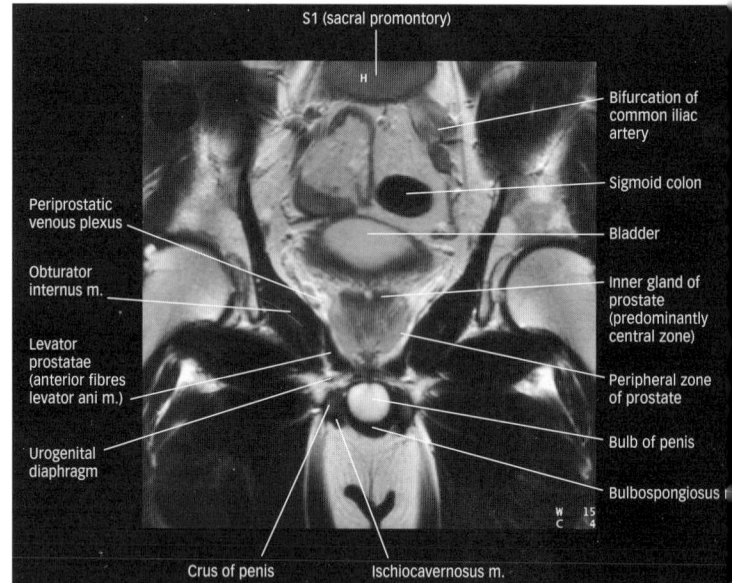

Psoas m. — Iliac arteries — Bowel loops — Urinary bladder — Obturator externus m. — Corpus cavernosum — Ischiocavernosus m. — Bulb of penis — Bulbospongiosus m. — Iliacus m. — Ilium — Acetabulum — Femoral head — Perivesical plexus — Superior pubic ramus — Symphysis pubis — Suspensory ligament of penis — Dorsal vein of penis — Buck's fascia — Penile urethra

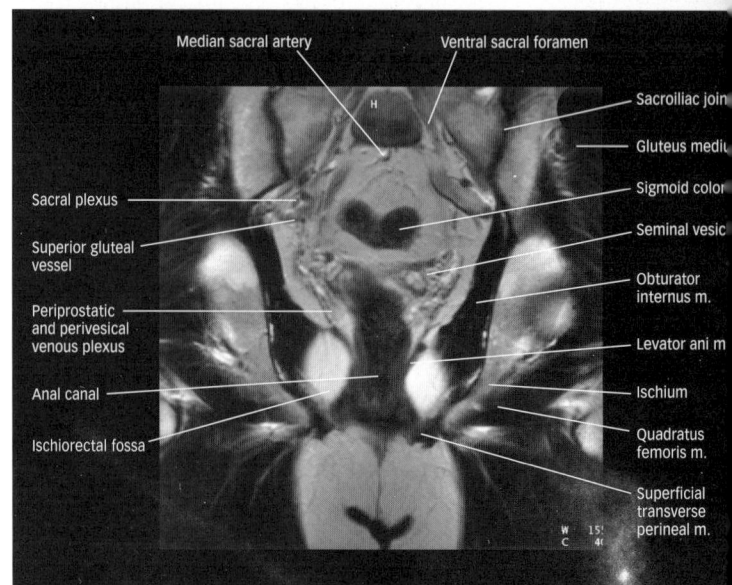

S1 (sacral promontory) — Bifurcation of common iliac artery — Sigmoid colon — Bladder — Inner gland of prostate (predominantly central zone) — Peripheral zone of prostate — Bulb of penis — Bulbospongiosus — Periprostatic venous plexus — Obturator internus m. — Levator prostatae (anterior fibres levator ani m.) — Urogenital diaphragm — Crus of penis — Ischiocavernosus m.

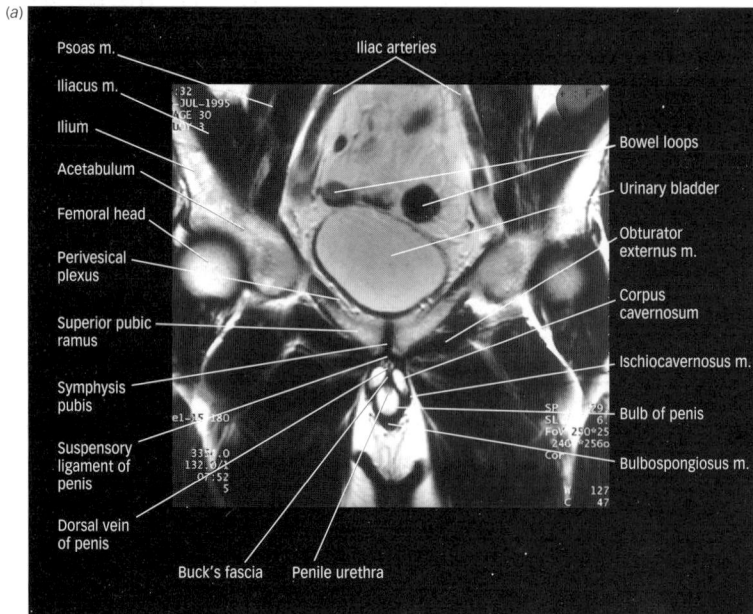

Median sacral artery — Ventral sacral foramen — Sacroiliac join — Gluteus medi — Sigmoid colo — Seminal vesic — Obturator internus m. — Levator ani m — Ischium — Quadratus femoris m. — Superficial transverse perineal m. — Sacral plexus — Superior gluteal vessel — Periprostatic and perivesical venous plexus — Anal canal — Ischiorectal fossa or globus major superiorly, a body (corpus) and tail (caudo or globus minor). Its overall length is 6–7 cm and it consists of the single convoluted ductus epididymis formed by the union of the efferent ducts of the testis. From the tail, the vas deferens ascends medially to the deep inguinal ring, within the spermatic cord. The epididymis is invested by the tunica vaginalis (although the latter is less closely applied than to the testis), except at its posterior margin. Laterally there is a deep groove between the epididymis and the testis, the sinus epididymis. At the upper extremities of the testis and epididymis are two small, stalked bodies, the appendix testis and appendix epididymis. These are developmental remnants of the paramesonephric (Müllerian) duct and the mesonephros, respectively. These are liable to undergo torsion.

Each testis is separated from its fellow by a fibrous median raphe which is deficient superiorly.

The spermatic cord extends from the posterior border of the testis, on its medial side, to the deep inguinal ring. It has three fascial layers, derived from the layers of the anterior abdominal wall; the internal spermatic fascia, the cremasteric fascia and the external spermatic fascia. It contains the vas deferens, the

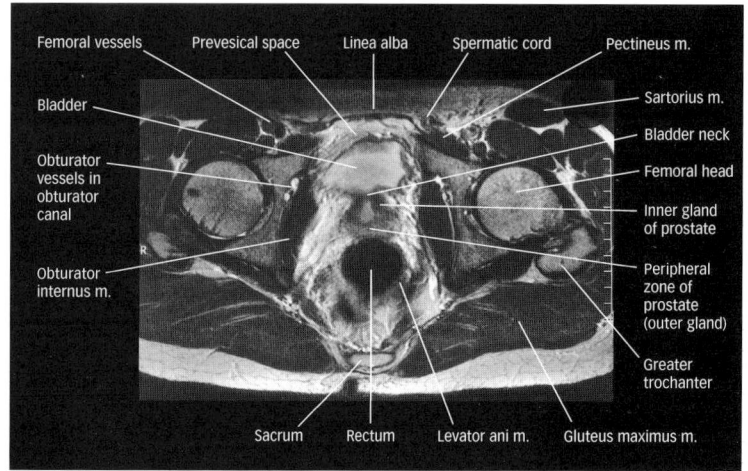

testicular artery and veins in addition to the cremasteric artery (a branch of the inferior epigastric artery), the artery to the vas deferens (from the inferior vesical artery), the genital branch of the genitofemoral nerve and lymph vessels from the testis.

The testicular artery arises from the aorta at the level of the renal vessels. It anastomoses with the artery to the vas (which supplies the vas and the epididymis). The scrotum is supplied by the external pudendal branch of the femoral artery. Venous drainage is via the

Fig. 19.
Axial T2 weighted images of the male pelvis, at the level of the hip joint.

Fig. 20.
High resolution axial T2 weighted MR scans through the prostate gland. Image (*a*), at the verumontanum, is cephalad to image (*b*).

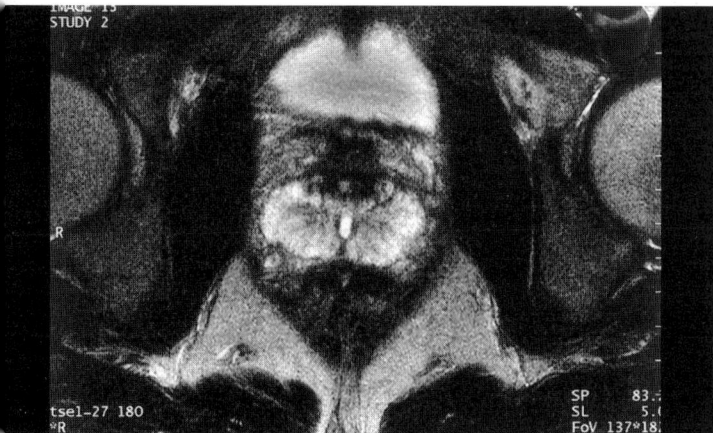

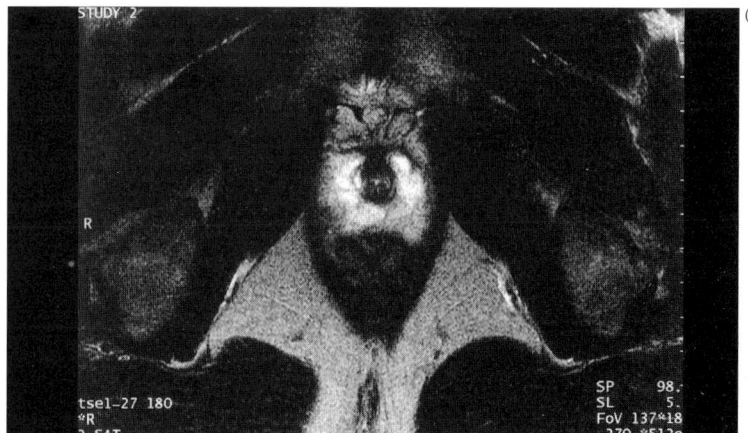

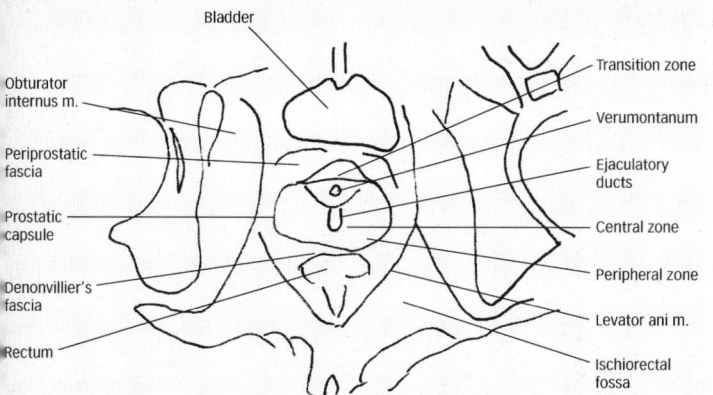

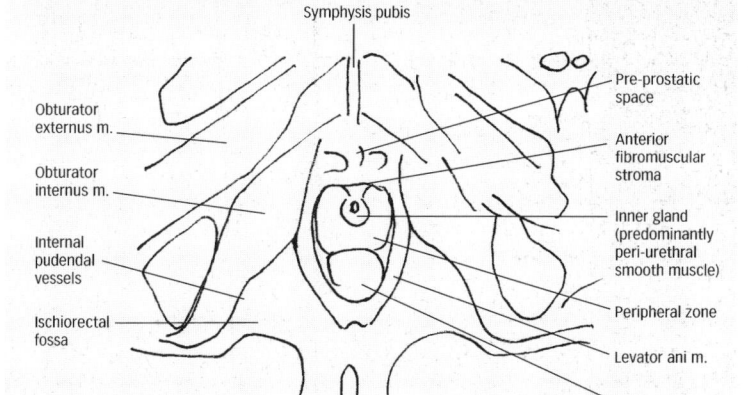

291

Fig. 21.
Transverse transrectal
images of the seminal
vesicles. In a younger
patient, the seminal
vesicles are often larger in
both length and breadth.

(a)

Right
seminal
vesicle

Right
ampulla
of vas

(b)

Left
seminal
vesicle

Left
ampulla
of vas

Rectal
wall

Bladder

Vas deferens

Walls of
seminal
vesicle

Left seminal
vesicle

High signal
from fluid
contents
of seminal
vesicle

Coil in rectum

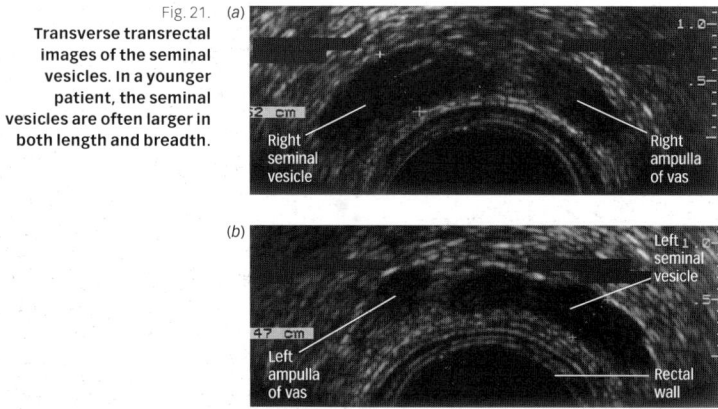

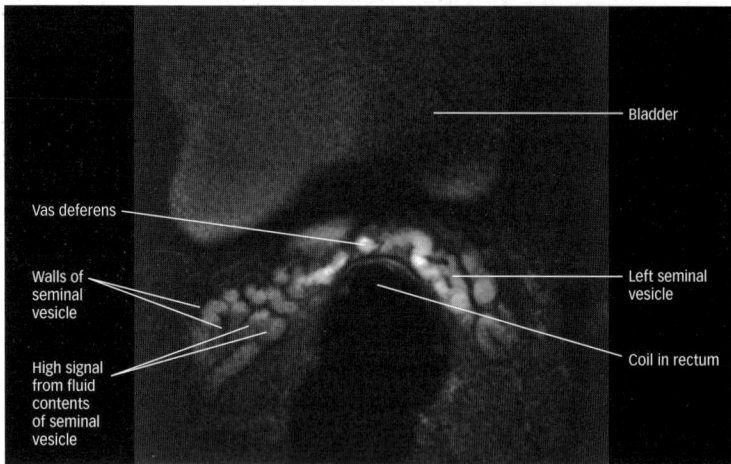

Fig. 22.
Axial T2 weighted MR image
of the seminal vesicles with
an endorectal coil.

(a)

Testicular veins

Testicular artery

Pampiniform plexus

Artery to
vas deferens

Vas deferens

Body of epididymis

Tail of epididymis

Appendix
epididymis

Head of epididymis
(globus major)

Appendix testis

Testis

(b)

Scrotum

Tunica vaginalis

Tunica albuginea

Septulum testis

Lat

Sinus of
epididymis

Epididymis

Mediastinum testis

Testicular artery

Artery to vas

Scrotal septum

Med

Vas deferens

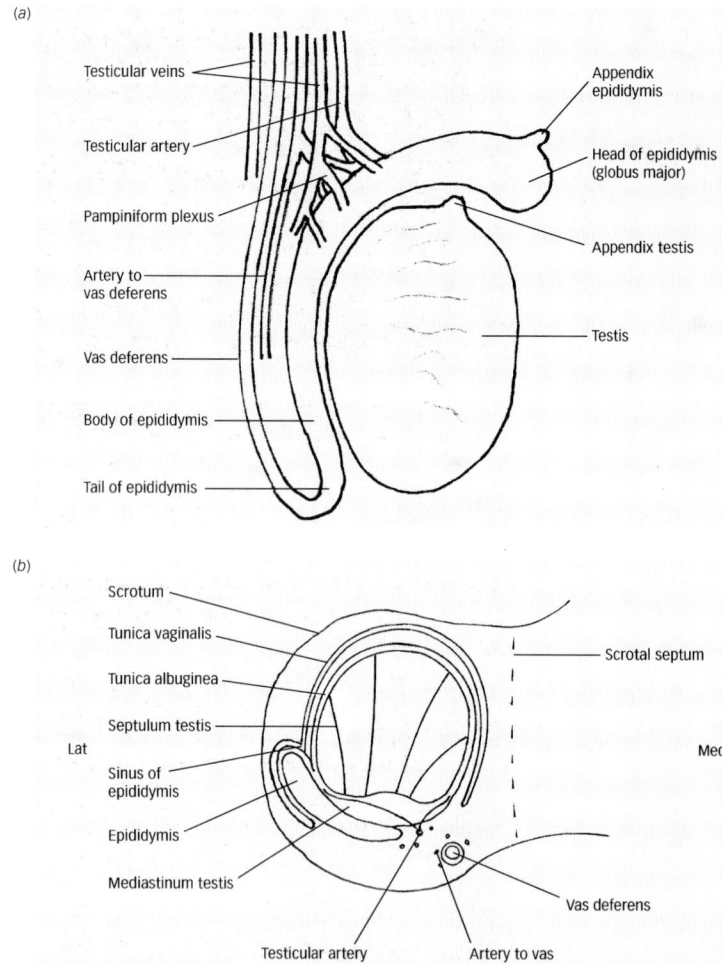

Fig. 23.
Diagrams of (a) sagittal
oblique and (b) transverse
sections through the testis

pampiniform plexus of veins above and behind the testis, which becomes one single vein in the region of the inguinal ring. The testicular vein ascends to the inferior vena cava on the right and the renal vein on the left. Lymphatic drainage accompanies the testicular vessels to paraaortic lymph nodes at the level of L1-2, whereas the scrotum drains to the superficial inguinal lymph nodes.

The vas deferens is a muscular tube, 45 cm long, which conveys sperm to the ejaculatory ducts. The vas traverses the scrotum and spermatic cord to the deep inguinal ring, where it passes round the lateral aspect of the inferior epigastric artery. It then runs back on the lateral pelvic wall to the ischial spine, where it turns medially to the bladder base, looping over the ureter. Its terminal dilatation, the ampulla, joins the seminal vesicle behind the bladder base to form the ejaculatory duct.

Imaging The testis is well suited to examination by ultrasound (Fig. 24). Normal testicular echogenicity is similar to the thyroid with medium level echoes throughout. The tunica albuginea is not routinely seen unless there is an accompanying hydrocele, when it appears highly echoic, but the mediastinum testis can be identified as an echogenic line posteriorly, parallel to the epididymis. Coronal scans show the mediastinum as a line of high echogenicity posteriorly. The septulae testis may be visualized as linear echogenic or hypoechoic bands. Rarely, very small intratesticular tubular structures can be resolved adjacent to the epididymis, representing parts of the rete testis. Small foci of increased echogenicity with or without acoustic shadowing may be seen within the gland, thought to represent spermatic granulomas or phleboliths. The appendix testis may occasionally be seen cephalad to the testis in the presence of a hydrocele (Fig. 24).

The epididymis is of similar, or slightly greater, echogenicity to the testis, although with a coarser echotexture. The globus major, approximately 7–8 mm diameter, rests on the superior pole of the testis and therefore, its identification allows the assessment of the orientation of the testis. It is usual to see a pronounced edge artefact from the inferior margin of the head of the epididymis where it abuts the superior pole of the testis (Fig. 24).

Fig. 24.
Ultrasound images of the
testis. (*a*), longitudinal, (*b*),
transverse and (*c*),
longitudinal scans through
the head of the epididymis
(note typical streak
artefact); (*d*), the appendix
testis in the presence of a
hydrocele.

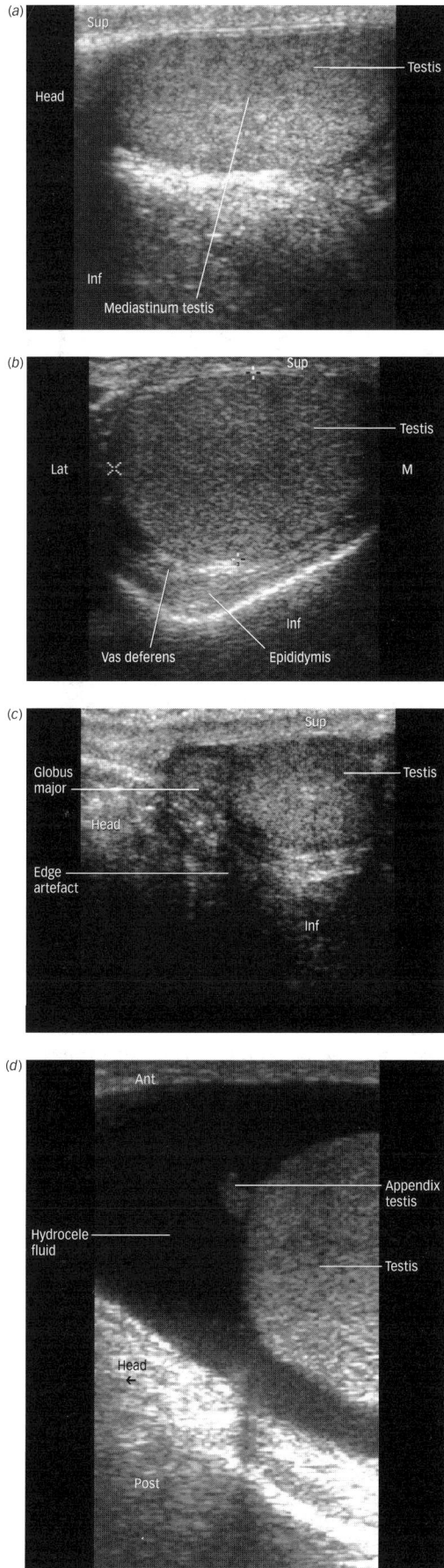

(*a*)

Sup

Head

Testis

Inf

Mediastinum testis

(*b*)

Sup

Lat

Testis

M

Vas deferens

Inf

Epididymis

(*c*)

Sup

Globus
major

Testis

Head

Edge
artefact

Inf

(*d*)

Ant

Hydrocele
fluid

Appendix
testis

Testis

Head

Post

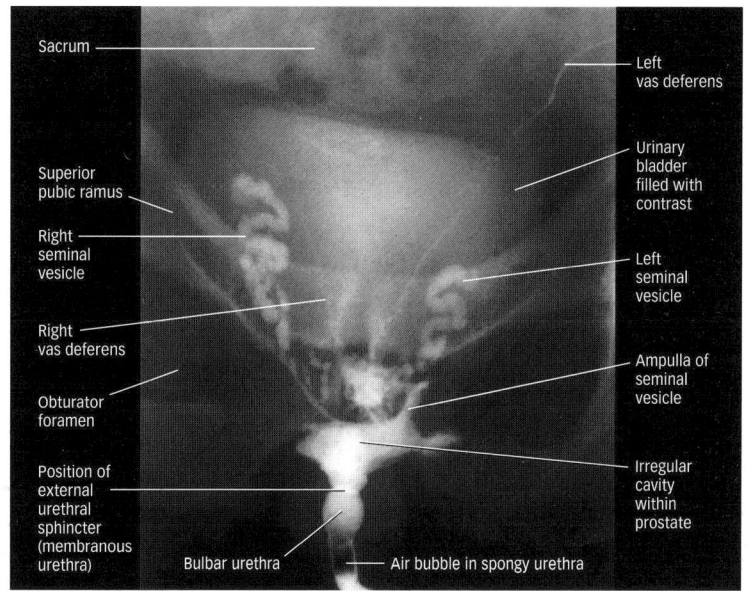

Sacrum

Left
vas deferens

Superior
pubic ramus

Urinary
bladder
filled with
contrast

Right
seminal
vesicle

Left
seminal
vesicle

Right
vas deferens

Ampulla of
seminal
vesicle

Obturator
foramen

Position of
external
urethral
sphincter
(membranous
urethra)

Irregular
cavity
within
prostate

Bulbar urethra

Air bubble in spongy urethra

Fig. 25.
The normal anatomy of the
seminal vesicles and vasa
deferentia (demonstrated
at urethrography after
iatrogenic rupture of the
prostatic urethra). The
normal anatomy of the
prostatic urethra is
totally destroyed.

The body and tail gradually decrease in thickness inferiorly to 1–2 mm and may appear less echogenic than the head of the epididymis. It is not always possible to identify the vas deferens, but it may be visualized as a hypoechoic tubular structure, sometimes with a hyperechoic central stripe, running parallel to the epididymis. Duplex and colour flow Doppler studies can demonstrate flow within the testicular arteries and veins. A small amount of fluid, 1–2 mm thick, within the tunica vaginalis is normal.

At CT, the testes are readily identified as oval structures 3–4 cm in diameter, and the spermatic cord can be seen within the inguinal canal as a thin-walled, oval structure of fat attenuation containing small structures representing the vas and spermatic vessels.

MR with a surface coil also provides excellent detail of the testis. On T1 W images the testis is homogeneous with medium signal intensity, similar to that of the corpora cavernosa and spongiosum and less than that of fat. On T2W images, signal is increased, equal to or greater than that of fat. The fibrous tunica albuginea is of low signal on all sequences. T2W images best depict the lower signal intensity of the mediastinum testis and the septulae testis.

The epididymis has a signal intensity equal to, or slightly lower than, that of the testis on T1W images, not unlike that of fluid, but on T2W images the signal intensity is lower than that of the testis, so that it is readily identifiable. The veins of the pampiniform plexus are seen as signal voids. On T1 W scans the spermatic cord with its fascial coverings is well seen, although it is difficult to identify the structures within the cord. Proximal to the internal inguinal ring, the testicular vessels and vas deferens can be traced with ease.

Vasography involves the injection of contrast medium into the vas deferens, from whence it refluxes into the seminal vesicles via the ejaculatory ducts. It may occasionally be required in the investigation of male infertility, as may testicular venography, in which the testicular vein is selectively catheterized via the femoral vein and inferior vena cava. Figure 25 demonstrates the seminal vesicles and vasa deferentia opacified during a urethrogram after urethral trauma.

The penis

The root of the penis is described in the section on the perineum. The body of the penis comprises three masses of expansile tissue; the two corpora cavernosa dorsally, partially separated by an incomplete fibrous septum, and the ventral corpus spongiosum, which surrounds the urethra. All three corpora are covered by a tough tube of fascia, the tunica albuginea, and Buck's fascia, derived from the deep fascia and the membranous layer of the superficial fascia. Buck's fascia is continuous with the suspensory ligament of the penis, attached to the symphysis pubis. Distally, the corpus spongiosum expands to form the glans penis, which covers the distal corpora cavernosa. The arterial supply to the penis is from the dorsal artery, chiefly supplying the glans, the artery to the bulb and the arteries to the crura, which form the cavernous arteries. Venous drainage is mainly via the cavernous veins; the deep dorsal vein drains the glans. These drain, in turn, to the internal pudendal veins. The superficial dorsal vein drains to the periprostatic venous plexus. Increased arterial flow during sexual excitement compresses the draining veins, resulting in erection. Lymphatic drainage from the body is to the superficial inguinal nodes and the proximal penis also drains to the deep inguinal nodes.

Imaging Ultrasound examination of the penis demonstrates low level echoes within the corpora; the urethra is seen as a circular anechoic structure. Colour flow and pulsed wave Doppler techniques allow visualization of the penile arteries, which is important in the assessment of erectile dysfunction.

Cavernosography involves the injection of contrast medium into the corpora along with agents such as papaverine to induce an erection; this is done in the assessment of erectile dysfunction due to a suspected venous leak.

The MR appearance of the penis is variable, depending on the sequence used and the state of erection (Figs. 16–18). On T1 W sequences the corpora are indistinguishable, returning a signal less than that of fat and higher than that of muscle. The tunica albuginea and Buck's fascia have low signal intensity and can occasionally be distinguished on proton density images. On T2W images, all three corpora have increased signal, in contrast to the tunica albuginea. The corpus spongiosum is of uniform high signal, apart from the low signal intensity urethra, but the corpora cavernosa can return a signal which is very variable and this can be quite heterogeneous, depending on penile blood flow and cavernosal volume. MR can assess the changes in the penis during erection. The corpora increase in size and demonstrate increased signal on T2W images, while the tunica albuginea is thinned. After intravenous gadolinium DTPA, there is an increase in the signal intensity of all three corpora. Since the penis is fully developed at birth, congenital anomalies of the penis are well demonstrated at any age.

The female genital tract
The female perineum, vulva and vagina

The female perineum differs from that of the male in that the urogenital diaphragm is pierced by both the urethra and the vagina (Figs. 1 and 3). The labia majora correspond to the scrotal sac of the male. The vestibular bulbs, the equivalent of the bulb of the penis, lie on either side of the vestibule into which the vagina and urethra open; they have erectile tissue and are covered by the bulbospongiosus muscles, then by the skin of the labia minora.

The vagina is a muscular tube, approximately 8 cm long, which extends up and back from the vulva to surround the cervix of the uterus (Fig. 26). The vagina has anterior and posterior walls, normally in apposition. Superiorly, the cervix divides the vagina into a shallow anterior and deep posterior and lateral fornices.

Fig. 26.
Diagram of a sagittal section through the female pelvis demonstrating the relations of the uterus.

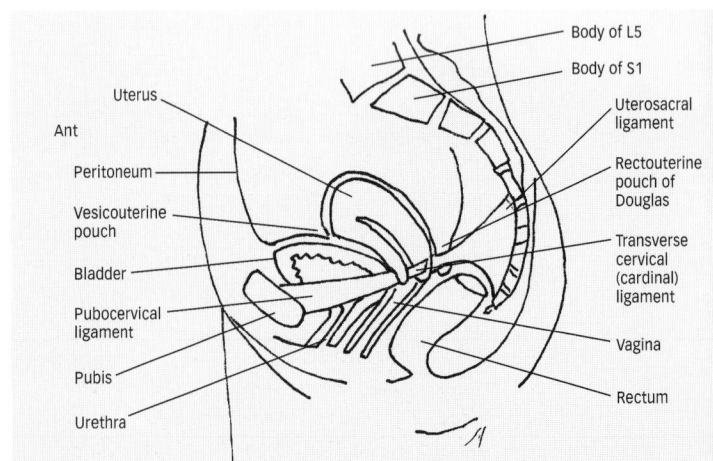

Anterior to the vagina are the bladder base and urethra. Behind the upper third of the vagina is the rectouterine pouch of Douglas, the lowest part of the peritoneal cavity in the erect subject, and behind the middle third the ampulla of the rectum. Behind the lower third is the perineal body. The urethra, vagina and rectum are all parallel to each other and to the pelvic brim.

On either side are the anterior fibres of the levator ani and the pelvic fascia. The ureters pass medially above and lateral to the lateral fornices. Inferiorly the lateral relations are the bulb of the vestibule and the urogenital diaphragm.

Blood supply is via the vaginal artery, a branch of the internal iliac artery, and the vaginal branch of the uterine artery. The vaginal veins form a plexus around the vagina that drains to the internal iliac veins. Lymphatic vessels from the upper third drain to the internal and external iliac nodes; from the middle third to internal iliac nodes and from the lower third to the superficial inguinal nodes.

Following the menopause, the vagina shrinks in length and diameter and the cervix projects into it less so that the fornices virtually disappear.

Superiorly the vagina is supported by the levator ani, the transverse cervical (cardinal), pubocervical and uterosacral ligaments, all attached to the vagina by pelvic fascia (Fig. 26). Inferiorly, support is provided by the urogenital diaphragm and perineal body.

The uterus

The uterus is a pear-shaped muscular organ lying between the rectum and bladder. The non-pregnant uterus is 8 cm long, 5 cm across and 3 cm thick. It has a fundus, body and cervix. The Fallopian tubes enter each superolateral angle (the cornu), above which lies the fundus. The body narrows to a waist, the isthmus, below which lies the cervix, embraced about its middle by the vagina and dividing the cervix into supravaginal and vaginal parts.

The cavity of the uterus is triangular in coronal section, but is a mere cleft in the sagittal plane. The cavity communicates with the cervical canal via the internal os, and the cervical canal opens into the vagina via the external os. This lies approximately in the same horizontal plane as the superior border of the symphysis pubis. The external os is circular in the nulliparous subject but, in parous women, the external os enlarges transversely so that it has anterior and posterior lips, the latter being longer and thinner than the former.

Normally the long axis of the uterus lies horizontally in the sagittal plane, forming an angle of ninety degrees with the vagina. In addition the fundus is flexed anteriorly in relation to the cervix in a position which is referred to as anteverted and anteflexed.

In retroversion, the cervix is directed up and back, though the uterus may still be anteflexed. If retroflexed, the axis of the uterus is directed posteriorly to that of the cervix. These conditions may make visualization of the uterus by ultrasound difficult.

In fetal life, the cervix is much larger than the body of the uterus. In childhood, the cervix remains larger (the infantile uterus), the uterine volume normally being less than 4 ml. By prepuberty, the two are equal in size and postpuberty, the uterus grows disproportionately, so that by adulthood the uterine body is twice the size of the cervix.

Peritoneum covers the entire uterus except below the level of the internal os anteriorly, where it is reflected on to the bladder, and laterally between the layers of the broad ligament. The thick smooth muscle myometrium is related directly to the endometrium with no intervening submucosa. The endometrium is continuous with the mucous membrane of the uterine tubes and the endocervix.

Anteriorly, the uterus is related to the uterovesical pouch and the superior surface of the bladder. Posteriorly it is related to the pouch of Douglas, with coils of ileum and colon within it. Laterally are the broad ligaments and uterine vessels. The supravaginal cervix is closely related to the ureters above the lateral fornices of the vagina.

The main arterial supply of the uterus is the uterine artery, a branch of the internal iliac artery which passes medially to the uterus in the base of the broad ligament, crossing above the ureter and running perpendicular to it to reach the cervix at approximately the level of the internal os. The artery ascends along the uterus within the broad ligament and anastomoses with the ovarian artery. The vein accompanies the artery and drains into the internal iliac vein (Fig. 35). Lymphatic vessels from the fundus accompany the ovarian artery to drain into paraaortic nodes at the level of the first lumbar vertebra. Vessels from the body and cervix drain to internal and external iliac lymph nodes and a few accompany the round ligament of the uterus through the inguinal canal to the superficial inguinal lymph nodes.

Uterine ligaments and supports include: (a) the levator ani muscles; (b) the transverse cervical (cardinal), pubocervical and uterosacral ligaments, all condensations of pelvic fascia; (c) the broad and round ligaments.

The medial edges of the anterior parts of the levator ani are attached to the cervix via the pelvic fascia. The transverse cervical ligaments pass to the cervix and upper vagina from the pelvic side walls. The pubocervical ligaments run from the pubis on either side of the neck of the bladder (pubovesical ligaments) to the cervix and the uterosacral ligaments pass from the cervix and upper vagina to the lower sacrum, forming two ridges on either side of the pouch of Douglas which are covered with peritoneum to form the rectouterine folds.

The broad ligaments are formed by anterior and posterior reflections of peritoneum passing over the Fallopian tubes. They enclose the parametrial connective tissue in addition to the round ligaments, uterine vessels and accompanying lymph channels and ovarian ligaments laterally. The ovary is attached to the posterior layer by the mesovarium. That part of the broad ligament above the mesovarium is known as the mesosalpinx. The round ligament originates at the lateral angle of the uterus and passes through the inguinal canal to the labia majora. It is equivalent to the male gubernaculum testis.

The uterine tubes

Each Fallopian tube is about 10 cm long and lies in the free edge of the broad ligament, extending out from the uterine cornua. They are divided into four parts:

(a) the infundibulum, the funnel-shaped lateral part which extends beyond the broad ligament and overhangs the ovary with its finger-like fimbriae, one of which is attached to the ovary (fimbria ovarica);
(b) the ampulla, a wide, dilated tortuous outer part;
(c) the isthmus, long and narrow, just lateral to the uterus;
(d) the interstitial part, which pierces the uterine wall. All but the latter part are clothed in peritoneum, beneath which are two muscle layers, and the mucosa, which is of columnar ciliated epithelium thrown into numerous folds.

Arterial supply is from the ovarian and uterine arteries and there is corresponding venous drainage. Lymphatic drainage is chiefly to paraaortic lymph nodes.

The ovaries

These paired almond-shaped reproductive and endocrine organs lie in the ovarian fossae, situated in the lateral pelvic sidewalls between the obliterated umbilical artery anteriorly and the internal iliac artery and ureter posteriorly. Each ovary has medial and lateral surfaces, anterior and posterior borders and superior and inferior poles. Their size and appearance varies with age. At birth, the ovaries are relatively large and may contain follicles, under the influence of maternal hormones. In childhood, ovarian volume is less than 1 ml and any follicles are less than 2 mm in diameter (the microcystic ovary). Above the age of 8 years, it is usual to see six or more follicles of greater than 4 mm in diameter (the multicystic or multifollicular ovary). Normal adult dimensions are approximately $3 \times 1.5 \times 2$ cm with a weight of 2–8 g. After the menopause, the ovary atrophies, measuring less than 2 cm in length and weighing only 1–2 g.

Usually the ovary lies with its long axis vertical, but this is dependent on parity and bladder and bowel filling. The ovary is attached to the back of the broad ligament by the mesovarium. It is attached to the infundibulum of the Fallopian tube and its fimbriae by its anterior border. That part of the broad ligament lateral to the mesovarium running to the lateral pelvic wall is known as the suspensory ligament of the ovary (infundibulopelvic ligament) and within it run the ovarian vessels and lymphatics, crossing over the external iliac vessels at the pelvic brim. Further support is provided by the ovarian ligament, a continuation of the round ligament which runs from the medial extremity of the ovary to the side of

Fig. 27.
Longitudinal transabdominal scans of the uterus: (*a*) secretory phase, (*b*) proliferative phase. Note difference in thickness of endometrium

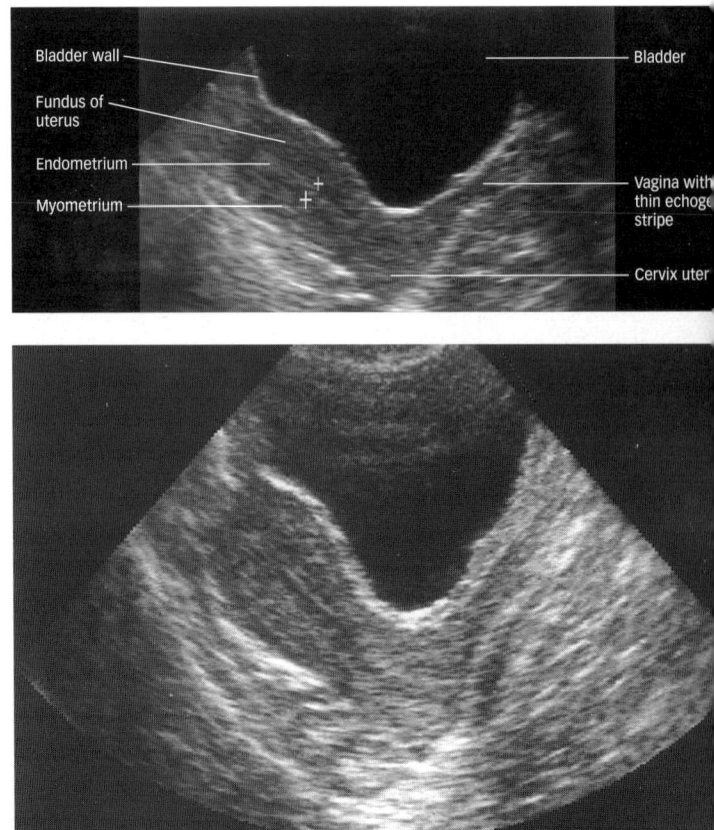

the uterus. The free border of the ovary is directed posteriorly to the ureter and internal iliac vessels. Inferiorly lies the levator ani muscle with its covering of fascia and laterally the parietal peritoneum separates it from the obturator vessels and nerve, crossing the floor of the ovarian fossa.

Arterial supply is by the ovarian artery, which arises from the aorta at L1/2, and enters the ovarian hilum via the mesovarium. Venous drainage is from the pampiniform plexus into the ovarian veins, which drain into the inferior vena cava on the right and the renal vein on the left. Lymph drainage is along the ovarian vessels to preaortic lymph nodes at the level of the first and second lumbar vertebra. The ovary lacks a peritoneal covering. In the adult it consists of a central vascular medulla and an outer cellular cortex, the outer layer of which is condensed to form a fibrous capsule, the tunica albuginea. The neonatal ovary (measuring $1.5 \times 0.5 \times 0.5$ cm) contains up to 750 000 primary ovarian follicles and a surface germinal epithelium. Many of the follicles degenerate from childhood onwards. At puberty, the gland enlarges and then contains follicles, a few of which develop each cycle, 70 000 immature follicles and postovulatory corpora lutea and corpora albicantia (scarred areas marking the site of previously ruptured follicles).

Imaging The commonest method of investigation of the female genital tract is with ultrasound. The full urinary bladder provides an acoustic window through which the uterus, and in 85–90% of patients the ovaries may be visualized. In the adult the myometrium is of uniform low echogenicity and the

endometrium is seen as a highly echogenic stripe on longitudinal images and a central echogenic area on transverse images. The thickness of the central echogenic stripe depends on the phase of the menstrual cycle, being maximal perimenstrually (Fig. 27). In the menstrual and early proliferative phases it measures 2–4 mm, is only mildly hyperechoic and is surrounded by a thin hypoechoic band (representing the inner layer of the myometrium). In the secretory phase it is very echogenic and measures up to 8 mm in thickness. Postmenopausally, the thickness and echogenicity of the endometrium is reduced, unless the patient is on hormone replacement therapy.

The vagina is seen inferiorly on sagittal scans as a highly echogenic stripe making an acute angle with the body of the uterus. The ovaries can usually be identified in the adnexal areas and in the adult it is possible to see up to five or six small transsonic follicles within the low-level echoes of the stroma (Fig. 28). However, if the ovaries lie in the pouch of Douglas, it may not be possible to identify them. It is normal to see a small amount of fluid in the pouch of Douglas towards the end of the menstrual cycle. Endovaginal ultrasound provides much improved resolution with better visualization of the adnexal areas in particular (Fig. 28(*b*)). It is possible to demonstrate the vascular supply of the ovaries, particularly with colour Doppler. The internal structure of the uterus is also better shown with transvaginal ultrasound. Ultrasound is capable of demonstrating most congenital abnormalities of the uterus and recently, ultrasonic contrast agents have been introduced into the uterus *per vaginam* to demonstrate tubal patency.

On CT scans, the uterus is seen as a homogeneous soft tissue mass dorsal to the bladder (Fig. 29). There may be a central area of low attenuation. The pouch of Douglas is readily identified, but it is not usually possible to recognize the ovaries unless they are enlarged or contain cysts. If a vaginal tampon is used, the vagina is seen as a tubular air-filled structure. After intravenous contrast, the adult uterus enhances because of the vascularity of the myomentrium and the ureters can be identified lateral to the cervix. The broad ligament appears as a thin, soft tissue density extending anterolaterally from the uterus to the pelvic sidewalls. It is particularly well seen in the presence of large amounts of pelvic fat or ascitic fluid.

The appearance of the uterus, vagina and ovaries on MR depends on the age and hor-

Fig. 28.
Ultrasound scans of the ovaries: (a) transverse transabdominal, (b) ngitudinal transvaginal. te much greater detail of ovarian structure in the latter.

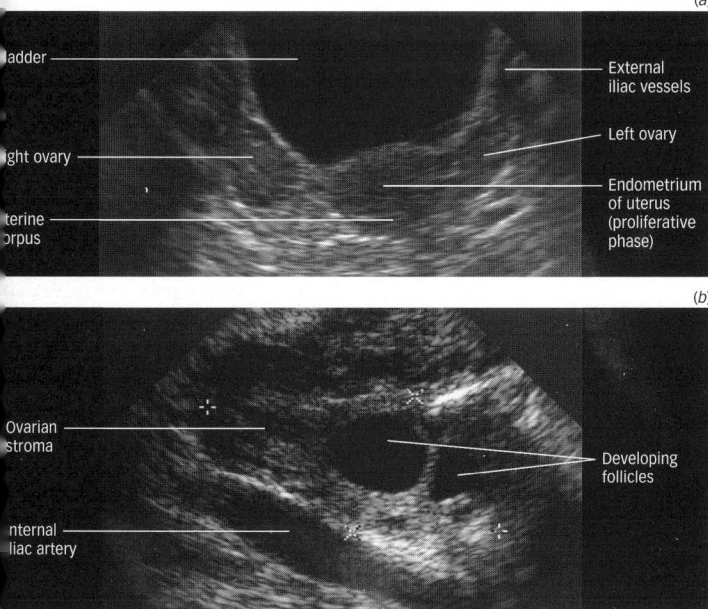

(a)

ladder
External iliac vessels
ight ovary
Left ovary
terine orpus
Endometrium of uterus (proliferative phase)

(b)

Ovarian stroma
Developing follicles
nternal iliac artery

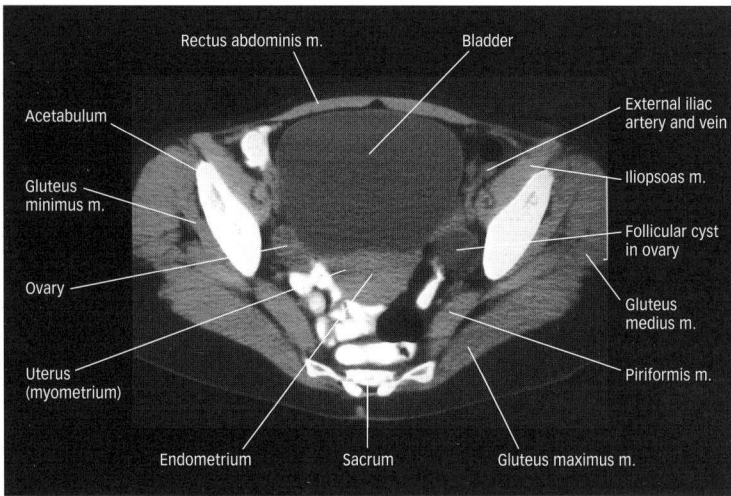

Fig. 29.
Axial CT of the female pelvis at a level above the acetabulum to show the normal uterus and ovaries.

Labels: Rectus abdominis m.; Bladder; Acetabulum; External iliac artery and vein; Gluteus minimus m.; Iliopsoas m.; Ovary; Follicular cyst in ovary; Gluteus medius m.; Uterus (myometrium); Piriformis m.; Endometrium; Sacrum; Gluteus maximus m.

(a)

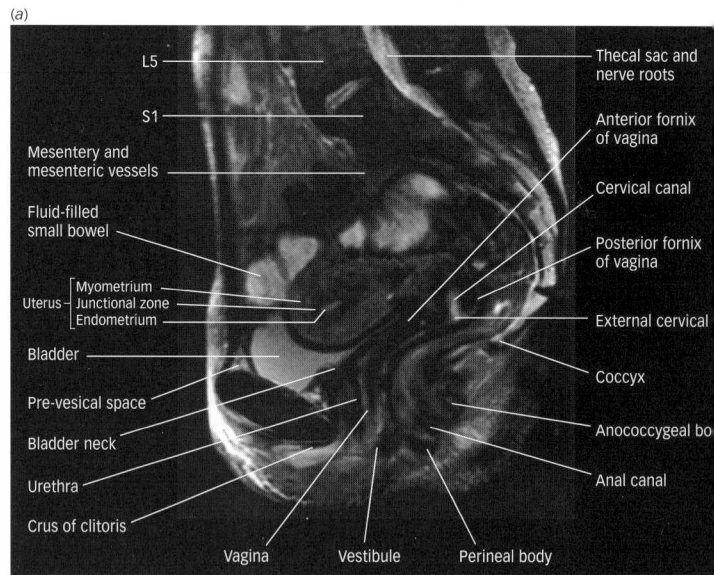

Labels: L5; Thecal sac and nerve roots; S1; Anterior fornix of vagina; Mesentery and mesenteric vessels; Cervical canal; Fluid-filled small bowel; Posterior fornix of vagina; Uterus — Myometrium, Junctional zone, Endometrium; External cervical; Bladder; Coccyx; Pre-vesical space; Anococcygeal bo; Bladder neck; Anal canal; Urethra; Crus of clitoris; Vagina; Vestibule; Perineal body

(b)

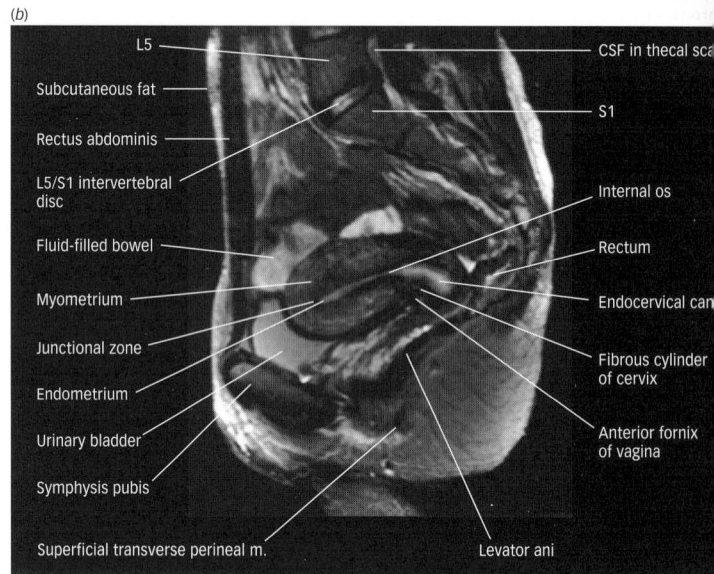

Labels: L5; CSF in thecal sca; Subcutaneous fat; S1; Rectus abdominis; L5/S1 intervertebral disc; Internal os; Fluid-filled bowel; Rectum; Myometrium; Endocervical can; Junctional zone; Fibrous cylinder of cervix; Endometrium; Urinary bladder; Anterior fornix of vagina; Symphysis pubis; Superficial transverse perineal m.; Levator ani

Fig. 31.
Sagittal (*a*) and parasagi (*b*) T2 weighted MR ima of the female pelvis, demonstrating the zona anatomy of the uterus. the chemical shift artef between the superior a inferior bladder wall wi artefactual thinning of inferior wall.

monal status of the patient. The internal anatomy of the vagina can be readily seen, particularly on T2 W axial and sagittal scans. In the early proliferative phase, the vaginal wall returns low signal, whereas the mucosa and mucus is of high signal (Figs. 30 and 31). There is less contrast in the mid-secretory phase, though the vaginal wall and mucus are thickest and have highest signal at this stage. In postmenopausal women, the signal intensity of the mucosa decreases and the central mucus is thinned unless the patient is on hormone replacement therapy. Appearances are similar in prepubertal girls. In pregnancy, especially the third trimester, the vaginal wall, central mucus and surrounding tissues all return medium to high signal on T2W images, so that contrast is lost. The vaginal wall and submucosa enhance after intravenous gadolinium DTPA.

On T1W sequences the uterus has moderate to low signal intensity, but on T2W sequences three distinct zones are seen: the endometrium, junctional zone (JZ) and myometrium. The endometrium and uterine cavity appear as a high signal stripe whose thickness varies with the menstrual cycle, measuring 3 mm in the early proliferative phase and up to 7 mm in

Fig. 30.
Axial T2 weighted MR scans through the female pelvis, above the level of the hip joint.

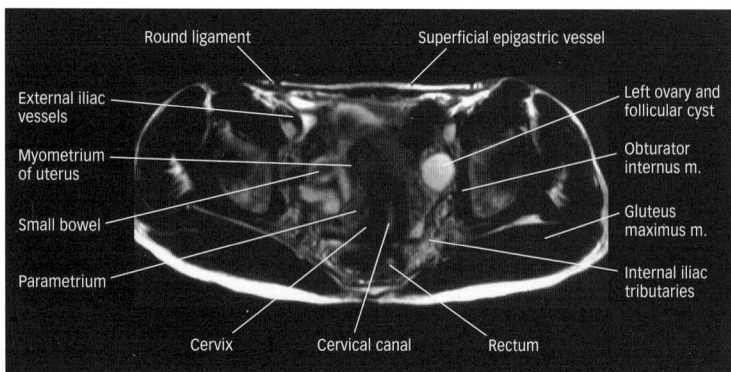

Labels: Round ligament; Superficial epigastric vessel; External iliac vessels; Left ovary and follicular cyst; Myometrium of uterus; Obturator internus m.; Small bowel; Gluteus maximus m.; Parametrium; Internal iliac tributaries; Cervix; Cervical canal; Rectum

the midsecretory phase. The endometrium is bordered by a band of low signal intensity, the JZ. This represents the inner myometrium and, at the level of the internal os, it blends with the low signal band of fibrous cervical stroma. It averages 5 mm in width and is constant in thickness and signal throughout the menstrual cycle. The outer myometrium is of medium signal intensity which increases in the midsecretory phase, when it averages 2.5 cm in width. Figures 32 and 33 are coronal T1- and T2-weighted images, respectively, of the female pelvis.

In prepubertal females, the uterus is smaller (only 4 cm in length) and on T2W images the endometrium is minimal or absent with an indistinct junctional zone. In post-menopausal women, the corpus decreases in size and zonal anatomy is indistinct. The endometrium is 3 mm or less in thickness,

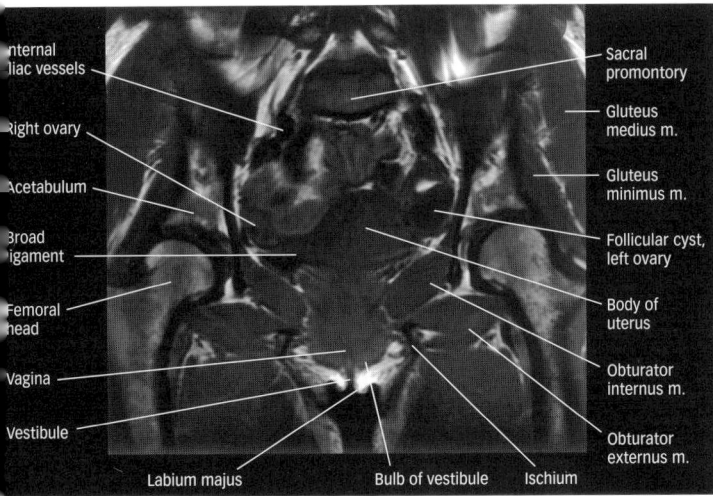

Labels (Fig. 32): Internal iliac vessels, Right ovary, Acetabulum, Broad ligament, Femoral head, Vagina, Vestibule, Labium majus, Bulb of vestibule, Ischium, Sacral promontory, Gluteus medius m., Gluteus minimus m., Follicular cyst, left ovary, Body of uterus, Obturator internus m., Obturator externus m.

Fig. 32.
Coronal T1 weighted image of the female pelvis.

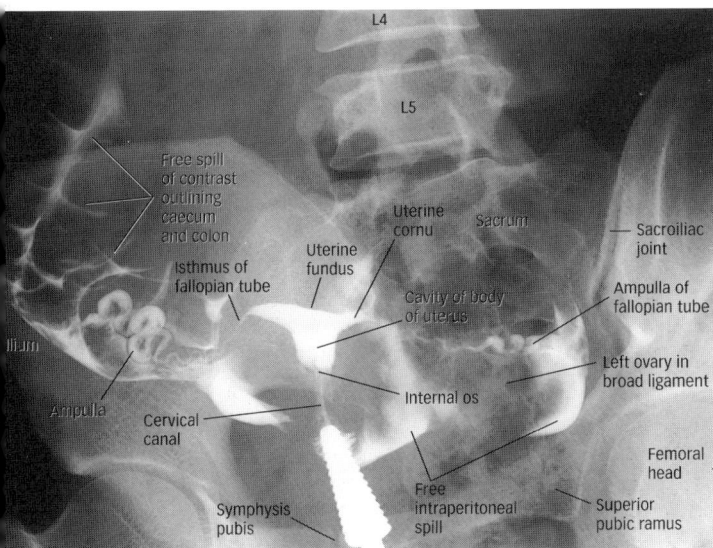

Labels (Fig. 33): Common iliac vessels, Body of L5, L5/S1 intervertebral disc, Uterus (Myometrium, Junctional zone, Endometrium), Bladder, Ischial ramus, Vagina, Vestibule, Urogenital diaphragm, Labia majora, Psoas m., Sacral promontory, Iliacus m., Ilium, Left ovarian follicular cyst, Gluteus medius m., Gluteus minimus m., Acetabulum, Femoral head, Obturator internus m., Obturator externus m.

Fig. 33.
Coronal T2 weighted image of the female pelvis to show the zonal anatomy of the uterus.

the JZ is thinner and indistinct and myometrial signal is decreased so that contrast is diminished.

On T2W images the cervix has an inner cylinder of low signal stroma continuous with the JZ of the uterus. Many patients have an outer zone of intermediate signal continuous with the outer myometrium. The appearances do not change with the menstrual cycle or with oral contraceptives. The central stripe measures 3.8–4.5 mm and the low signal cylinder, 3.8–4.2 mm in width. The external os can be seen protruding into the high signal vaginal canal.

Normal ovaries can be identified in up to 85% of women of reproductive age. They are low to medium signal on T1W images and higher signal on T2W images, where a low signal intensity rim occasionally surrounds them. Follicles stand out as hyperintense foci. After intravenous gadolinium DPTA, when the stroma of the ovary enhances, the low signal follicles are more prominent.

The broad ligament is often identified as a low signal intensity band running laterally, while the round ligament runs anterolaterally to the inguinal canal.

The anatomy of the Fallopian tubes and fine mucosal detail of the uterine cavity are still best demonstrated by hysterosalpingography (HSG) (Fig. 34). The cervical canal is about a third of the length of the uterine long axis. It has longitudinal ridges on the anterior and posterior walls which may have branches running laterally in nulliparae (plicae palmate). Cervical glands can be seen as outpouchings filled with contrast. The isthmus and internal os may occasionally be identified. The uterine cavity is usually triangular and smooth walled, leading to the narrow isthmus of the Fallopian tubes, then the wider, tortuous ampulla. Contrast should spill freely into the peritoneal cavity. Occasionally, the walls of the uterus demonstrate longitudinal folds and if the

Fig. 34.
Normal hysterosalpingogram.

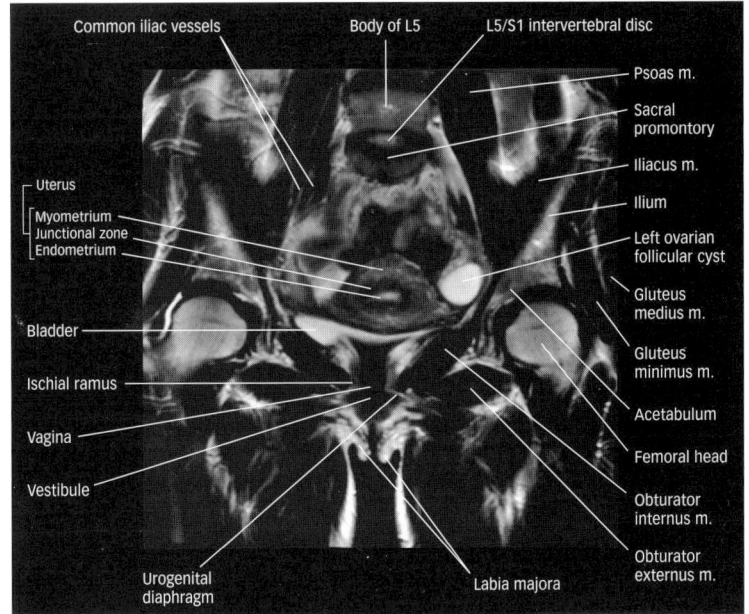

Labels (Fig. 34): L4, L5, Free spill of contrast outlining caecum and colon, Isthmus of fallopian tube, Uterine fundus, Uterine cornu, Sacrum, Cavity of body of uterus, Ilium, Ampulla, Cervical canal, Internal os, Symphysis pubis, Free intraperitoneal spill, Sacroiliac joint, Ampulla of fallopian tube, Left ovary in broad ligament, Femoral head, Superior pubic ramus

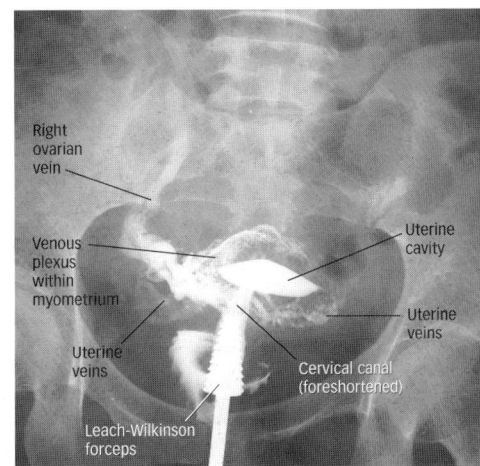

Labels (Fig. 35): Right ovarian vein, Venous plexus within myometrium, Uterine veins, Leach-Wilkinson forceps, Uterine cavity, Uterine veins, Cervical canal (foreshortened)

Fig. 35.
Hysterosalpingography performed on day 9 of the menstrual cycle with venous intravasation. Note the normal venous drainage of the uterus.

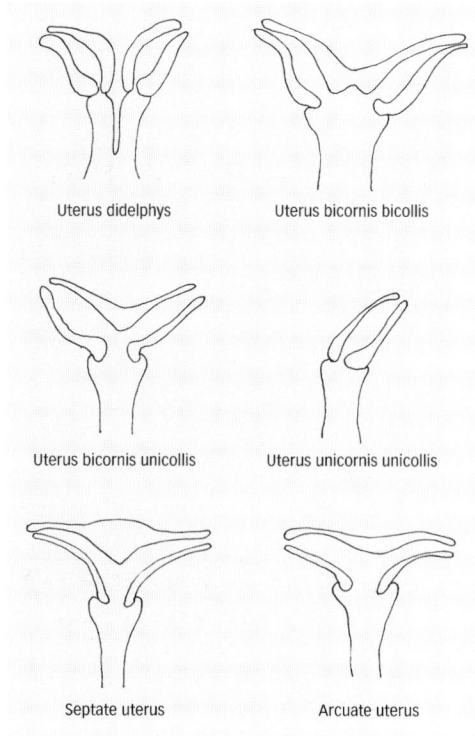

Uterus didelphys

Uterus bicornis bicollis

Uterus bicornis unicollis

Uterus unicornis unicollis

Septate uterus

Arcuate uterus

Fig. 36.
Congenital anomalies of the uterus.

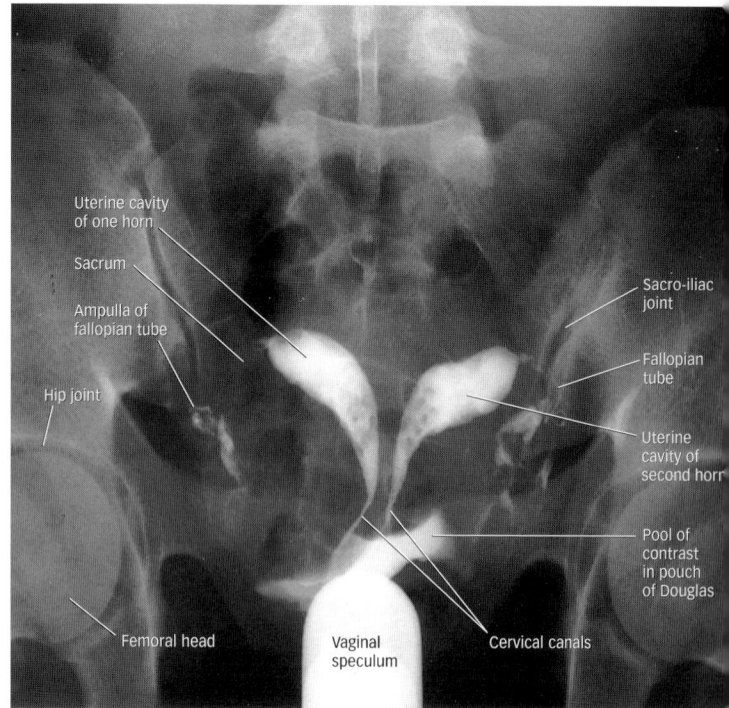

Uterine cavity of one horn

Sacrum

Ampulla of fallopian tube

Hip joint

Femoral head

Vaginal speculum

Cervical canals

Sacro-iliac joint

Fallopian tube

Uterine cavity of second horn

Pool of contrast in pouch of Douglas

Fig. 37.
Hysterosalpingogram in a patient with uterus bicornis bicollis.

study is done in error in the secretory phase, polypoid filling defects and filling of the endometrial glands may be observed. If the study is inadvertently done during menstruation, intravasation of contrast medium may occur (Fig. 35). Figure 36 illustrates the more common congenital anomalies. The HSG appearances of the bicornuate uterus is shown in Fig. 37, but MRI is an excellent non-invasive means of demonstrating congenital anomalies of the uterus and should be the investigation of choice.

Further reading

Hricak, H. & Carrington, B.M. (1991). *MRI of the Pelvis: A Text Atlas*. Koln: Deutscher Arzte-Verlag.

Lowsley O.S. (1912). The development of the prostate gland with reference to the development of other structures at the neck of the urinary bladder. *American Journal of Anatomy*, **13**, 299–349.

McNeal, J.E. (1983). The prostate gland. Morphology and pathobiology. *Monographs in Urology*, **4**(1), 5–13.

Vinnicombe, S.J., Norman, A.R., Nicolson, V. *et al*. (1995). Normal pelvic lymph nodes: evaluation with CT after bipedal lymphangiography. *Radiology*, **194**, 349–56.

15

The vertebral column and spinal cord

S.A.A.SOHAIB
and P. BUTLER

The vertebral column forms the central axis of the skeleton. It is composed of 33 vertebral 'segments', united by cartilaginous discs and ligaments. There are seven cervical, twelve thoracic and five lumbar vertebrae. Caudally, there are five sacral and four coccygeal segments, all of which are fused.

Imaging methods

Plain radiography

Plain radiography is the most commonly performed imaging investigation of the vertebral column, especially following trauma. The spatial resolution of plain radiographs is high and they are simple to acquire. The mineralization of bone and its trabecular pattern are well shown and vertebral alignment is easily assessed. In common with most plain radiographs, soft tissue detail is poor. Conventional tomography has been supplanted largely by computed tomography.

Computed tomography

Computed tomography (CT) provides cross-sectional images of the bony and soft tissue elements of the vertebral column. The attenuation of the X-ray beam passing through tissue is recorded in Hounsfield units (HU). Cerebrospinal fluid and water have an attenuation value of near 0 HU. Fat, which is radiolucent, has lower values of between –60 and –100 HU and therefore appears darker than cerebrospinal fluid. The dural sac has a lower attenuation (5 to 25 HU) than the spinal cord (between 35 and 70 HU). The intervertebral discs and the ligaments have higher attenuation values (between 50 and 100 HU) than the spinal cord (between 35 and 70 HU). The spinal meninges, the dorsal root ganglia and blood vessels enhance following intravenous iodi-

nated contrast medium, whereas the spinal cord, nerve roots and intervertebral discs do not.

All CT images are displayed using a grey scale within a specific range of Hounsfield units. Densities above or below this are displayed as white or black, respectively. Two window settings are used conventionally for spinal imaging (Fig. 1); 'soft tissue' (level 40 HU, width 300 HU) and 'bony' (level 200 HU, width 1500 HU). Dedicated 'bone reconstruction algorithms' maximize the spatial resolution of skeletal structures and so allow the dimensions of the spinal canal to be measured accurately. These are also used to display

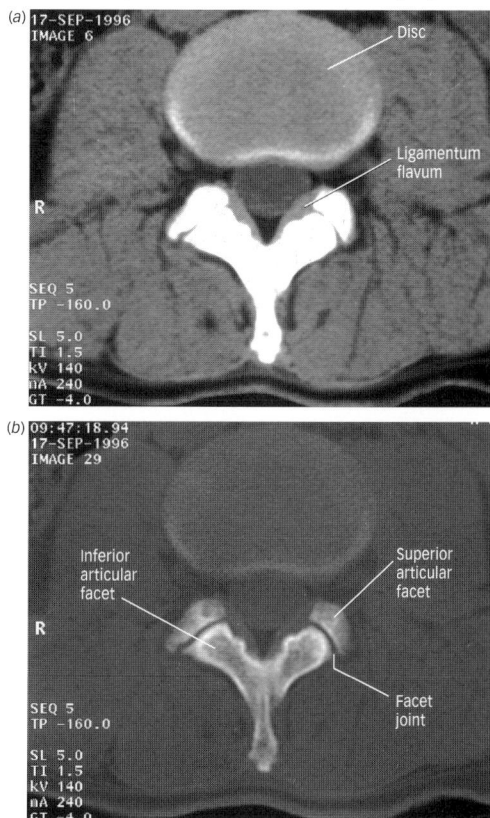

(a) 17-SEP-1996
IMAGE 6
Disc
Ligamentum flavum
R
SEQ 5
TP -160.0
SL 5.0
TI 1.5
kV 140
mA 240
GT -4.0

(b) 09:47:18.94
17-SEP-1996
IMAGE 29
Inferior articular facet
Superior articular facet
R
Facet joint
SEQ 5
TP -160.0
SL 5.0
TI 1.5
kV 140
mA 240
GT -4.0

Fig. 1.
Axial CT L3/4 disc: (*a*) soft tissue, (*b*) bone windows.

images of CT myelography, which is necessary to display intradural structures. Only in the high cervical region, where the subarachnoid space is relatively capacious, can the spinal cord normally be resolved with plain CT.

Magnetic resonance imaging

Magnetic resonance imaging (MRI) is now the primary imaging method for the vertebral column and spinal cord. The advantages of MRI are the multiplanar imaging, superior contrast resolution, and the facility to acquire different images by altering pulse sequences. Unlike plain CT, MRI can demonstrate the entire spinal cord and the nerve roots within the intradural as well as the extradural compartments. MRI will also reveal pathological change in the spinal cord substance, whereas CT myelography only shows any alteration in contour. Grey and white matter within the spinal cord can be distinguished with high-quality axial MRI. On T1W images, the cortical bone of the vertebral bodies appears as an hypointense (dark) rim around the marrow-containing cancellous bone. This hypointensity is shared with the various spinal ligaments and cerebrospinal fluid. The cancellous bone, in the adult, returns a relatively high signal (i.e. appears whiter) because of the high fat content of yellow marrow. The intervertebral discs appear homogeneous and are lighter grey than the vertebral bodies. Fat returns a high signal on T1W images (i.e. appears white) and, in both MRI and CT (where it appears dark owing to its radiolucency), it provides a background against which other structures are more easily visualized.

T2W images have a myelographic effect. Cerebrospinal fluid appears hyperintense (white), whereas the neuraxis and the ligaments are hypointense (dark). The T2W image shows the interface between cerebrospinal fluid and the spinal canal most clearly of all the MRI pulse sequences. The intervertebral discs appear brighter than the vertebral bodies, owing to their water content. T2W images are therefore most sensitive to changes in water content which may, for example, alter in discal degeneration or infection.

Intravenous contrast agents are used more often in MRI than in CT of the vertebral column. The range of structures showing enhancement with MRI is similar to CT (see above), but with some exceptions. For example, although blood vessels may enhance with gadolinium, those in which blood is flowing rapidly will show a signal void. Red marrow within the vertebrae of children, which therefore are relatively hypointense on T1W

images, enhances. Gadolinium-DTPA is used with T1W sequences. It shortens the T1 relaxation time of those structures it causes to enhance, which show a higher signal (i.e. become lighter). This may lead to a loss of contrast with fat and therefore enhancing material can sometimes, paradoxically, be more difficult to appreciate. This can be overcome by using fat-suppression techniques.

Myelography

Myelography is now reserved largely for those cases where non-invasive imaging has proved either inconclusive or is contra-indicated. It is almost always combined with CT. Non-ionic iodinated contrast agent is injected into the subarachnoid space, usually in the lumbar region but occasionally also by high cervical or cisternal puncture.

Before the lumbar puncture, the patient's spine is flexed to maximize the interspinous space. Flexion also causes the lower end of the spinal cord to migrate in a craniad direction by as much as one vertebral segment. The spinal needle is advanced in the midline between the third and fourth lumbar vertebrae until cerebrospinal fluid is obtained. A horizontal line passing through the iliac crests passes through the fourth lumbar vertebra.

A lateral cervical puncture may be performed when lumbar puncture is contraindicated or when an obstruction to the craniad flow of contrast medium is encountered following a lumbar injection. The patient is placed in the prone position with the neck extended. In the upper cervical region the spinal subarachnoid space is capacious. The anteroposterior dimension of the canal at the level of the first and second cervical vertebrae is divided into thirds. Using lateral fluoroscopy, the spinal needle is inserted horizontally into the subarachnoid space at the junction of the middle and posterior thirds, just anterior to the fusion of the laminae (Fig. 2). Lateral puncture can also be accomplished with the patient supine, in which case the needle is directed at a point between the anterior and middle thirds.

Rarely, it may be necessary to inject contrast medium into the cisterna magna. The patient is placed in the lateral decubitus position, with the neck well flexed and supported so that it is parallel to the table top. The needle is introduced in the midline between the external occipital protuberence and the spinous process of the second cervical vertebra and directed towards the glabella. The cisterna magna is usually punctured at a depth of between 5 and 6 cm from the skin surface in the adult.

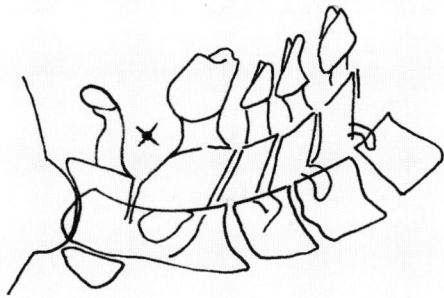

Fig. 2.
Lateral cervical puncture.
X denotes the position of
the spinal needle.

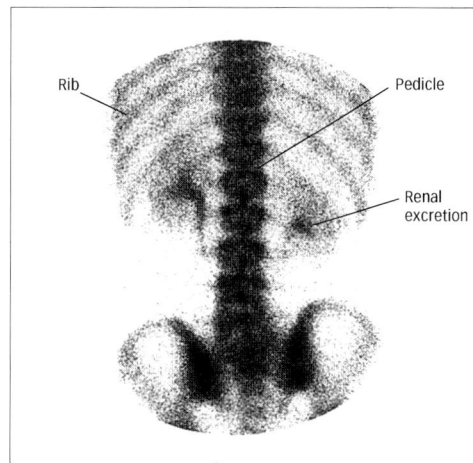

Fig. 3.
Radio-isotope bone scan
of the vertebral column.

Discography

Discography is a somewhat controversial investigation, which involves the injection of a small amount of contrast into the nucleus pulposus of the intervertebral disc. Besides the acquisition of morphological information, discal injections are used for pain provocation in patients with backache, prior to spinal fusion or chemonucleolysis (the enzymatic dissolution of the nucleus pulposus).

Arteriography

Spinal arteriography is now used for vascular malformations and for some tumours where detailed vascular anatomical information is required prior to surgery or embolisation.

Radionuclide bone scanning

Radionuclide studies of the spine are most often performed as part of a whole body scan. They give poor anatomical detail but provide functional information related to local blood flow and the rate of bone turnover in the spine. On bone scans, using ^{99m}Tc methylene diphosphonate, the spine is best seen in the posterior projection with the vertebral bodies, pedicles and spinous processes all visualized (Fig. 3). Spatial resolution can be improved with coned views and with SPECT imaging the vertebral body and neural arch can be discriminated.

Ultrasound

Ultrasound is of limited use in the spinal imaging and is restricted to the evaluation of the fetal spine, infants with posterior spinal defects and intraoperative examination in the adult (see Chapter 20).

The vertebral column

The vertebral column has four curves in the sagittal plane, which increase its strength. The cervical and lumbar curves are convex anteriorly (or lordotic) and the thoracic and sacro-coccygeal (pelvic) are concave anteriorly (or kyphotic). Whereas the thoracic and pelvic kyphoses are primary curves, since they are present in fetal life, the cervical and lumbar lordoses are secondary, or compensatory, curves which develop after birth. The vertebral column also shows a slight lateral curvature most marked in the thoracic region. In most individuals, this is directed towards the right and is referred to as the physiological right lateral scoliosis.

The cervical lordosis extends from the atlas to second thoracic vertebra with its anterior prominence at fourth cervical vertebra. The cervical curve is not fixed and is obliterated in the supine position, with the neck flexed. The thoracic curve begins at the second thoracic vertebra and ends at the twelfth. The most prominent point of this curve dorsally corresponds to the spinous process of the seventh thoracic vertebra. The lumbar lordosis, which extends caudally from the thoracic curve to the lumbosacral angle, is exaggerated in females. The third lumbar vertebra is at its centre. The pelvic curve begins at the lumbosacral junction and ends at the tip of the coccyx.

In the axial plane, the vertebral column can be divided into two compartments, or columns, by the posterior longitudinal ligament. The anterior compartment contains the vertebral bodies, intervertebral discs and the anterior longitudinal ligament. These act as a tension band to limit extension and as a support to prevent excessive flexion. The posterior compartment contains the neural arch and ligamenta flava. These limit flexion and prevent excessive extension, and there is thus a reciprocal response of the two compartments to flexion and extension.

Following injury, complete rupture of the posterior ligament alone is insufficient to cause instability. Disruption of the posterior annulus fibrosus is also necessary. The vertebral column can therefore be considered as a three-column structure (Fig. 4); a middle column being formed by the posterior longitudinal ligament, the posterior annulus fibrosus and the posterior wall of the vertebral body. The posterior column is formed by the neural arch and posterior ligamentous complex. The anterior column is formed by the anterior longitudinal ligament, the anterior annulus fibrosus and the anterior part of the vertebral body (Denis, 1983).

The vertebra

A typical vertebra (Fig. 5) has a body anteriorly and a vertebral (or neural) arch posteriorly, enclosing the spinal canal. The arch consists, on each side, of a pedicle laterally and a lamina posteriorly. The laminae fuse posteriorly to form the spinous process. A transverse process extends laterally on each side at the junction of the pedicle and the lamina.

The pedicles are short processes extending backwards from the posterolateral aspect of the vertebral body. Each is grooved above and below so that adjoining pedicles are separated by an intervertebral (neural) foramen, which transmits the segmental spinal nerves and blood vessels.

The articular processes project superiorly and inferiorly at the junction of the lamina and pedicle. The articular surfaces of the superior facets face posteriorly and those of the inferior facets face anteriorly. The pars interarticularis is that part of the lamina between the superior and inferior articular facets on each side. The vertebral body consists of a mass of cancellous bone surrounded by a cortical rim of compact bone. The cancellous bone is arranged in horizontal and vertebral trabeculae. The vertical, or weight-bearing trabeculae, are between 0.2 and 0.5 mm thick and contribute approximately two-thirds of the mass of cancellous bone. The horizontal, or connecting, trabeculae are somewhat thinner (less than 0.2 mm), and constitute the remaining one-third. The trabecular pattern is well seen on plain radiographs and with CT. Bone marrow contained within cancellous bone is predominantly haemopoietic or 'red' in the young, becoming increasingly fatty ('yellow') with age. The marrow of the young adult contains 30% fat, which increases to 50% after the age of 60 years. The red marrow in children will enhance on T1W MR images, following intravenous gadolinium.

The intervertebral disc

The intervertebral disc forms a secondary cartilaginous joint between adjacent vertebrae. The joint surfaces are lined by hyaline cartilage with an intervening fibrocartilaginous disc and the joint is strengthened by both the anterior and posterior longitudinal ligaments and by fibres arising from the disc. The posterolateral portion of the disc is not reinforced by the posterior longitudinal ligament in the lumbar spine, and it is from this region of the disc that many lumbar discal prolapses arise.

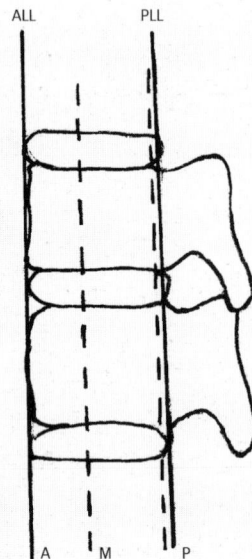

Fig. 4.
The three-column concept of the vertebral column
ALL, anterior longitudinal ligament;
PLL, posterior longitudinal ligament;
A, anterior column;
M, middle column;
P, posterior column.

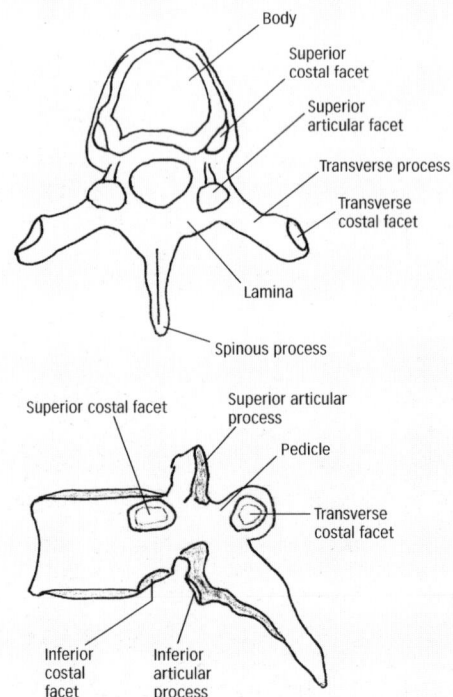

Fig. 5.
A typical vertebra (sixth thoracic).

There are regional differences in the size and shape of the intervertebral discs. In the cervical and lumbar spine the discs are slightly thicker anteriorly and thus contribute to the regional lordosis. The discs are thinnest in the upper thoracic spine and thickest (up to 12 mm) in the lumbar region. The disc accounts for 20% of the height of the vertebral column.

Each intervertebral disc consists of a central nucleus pulposus and a thick margin of fibrous lamellae, the annulus fibrosus. The nucleus pulposus represents the remnant of the notochord. It has a gelatinous structure of proteoglycans, which help retain water, and type II collagen. This collagen is similar to that in hyaline cartilage and hence has ability to resist compressive forces. The nucleus pulposus contains between 85 and 90% water and the annulus comprises 80%. The annulus fibrosus has a fibrillary structure that may be separated into two components known as the internal and external annulus. There are fine fibres in the internal annulus, which insert on the hyaline cartilage of the vertebral end plates. The external annulus has thick (Sharpey's) fibres which insert at the periphery of the end plates around the cartilaginous plate and beyond the vertebral margins. The collagen in the annulus is 'type I', which is similar to the collagen in fibrocartilage.

The intervertebral disc in infants and children has a rich blood supply, which decreases after puberty. By the age of 20 the normal disc is avascular and receives its nutrition by diffusion through the vertebral endplates. In the second and third decade an internuclear cleft develops. This is thought to represent compacted collagenous fibres oriented transversely in the disc, due to invagination of the inner annular lamellae. This internuclear cleft is found in the normal disc, especially in those over 30 years. It may not be present in up to 6% of subjects but, when present, it is seen in all that individual's discs. With increasing age, the disc undergoes progressive dehydration with loss of height. By 80 years of age the nucleus is totally replaced by fibrous tissue. Nerve fibres originating from the vertebral nerves are present in the peripheral 1–2 mm of the disc and the longitudinal ligaments but not within the central zone.

On plain radiographs the disc is represented as the radiolucent space between the vertebrae. CT shows the intervertebral disc as a low attenuation area between the vertebral bodies (Fig. 1). The nucleus pulposus and annulus fibrosus cannot be distinguished. The disc has a slightly greater radiodensity than the thecal sac and, peripherally, each disc is slightly more radiodense than the central portion due to the partial volume averaging and because of Sharpey's fibres. A normal disc does not enhance following intravenous iodinated contrast medium.

MRI demonstrates discal morphology in greater detail. The external annulus is hypointense on T1W or T2W images and can be separated from the composite internal annulus and nucleus pulposus (also known as the central zone or complex). The central zone

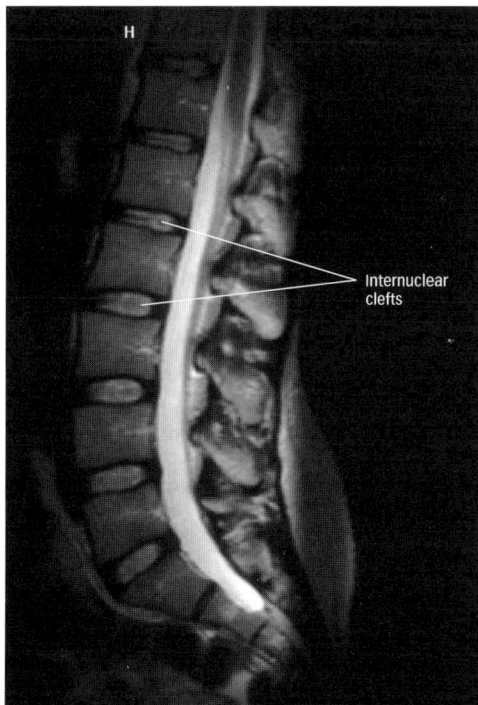

Fig. 6.
T2W MRI, sagittal plane, lumbar internuclear cleft.

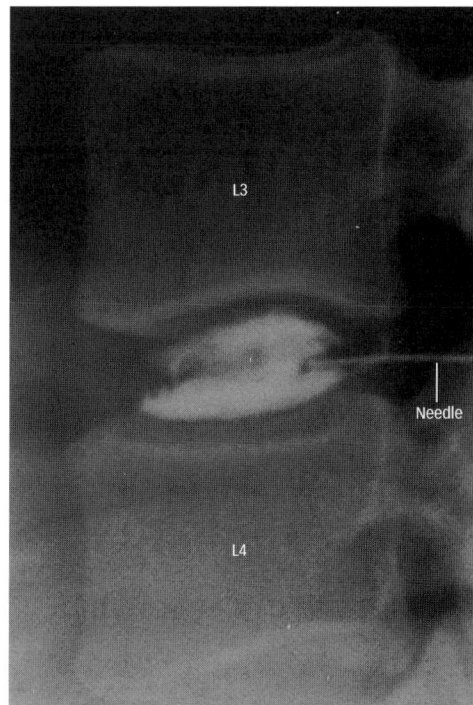

Fig. 7.
Lumbar discogram.

shows a homogenous intermediate signal on T1W and a hyperintense signal on T2W images. The internuclear cleft is seen on T2W sagittal images as a hypointense transverse band across the mid portion of the disc (Fig. 6).

On discography a normal disc has a smooth, central, unilocular or bilocular nucleus and the contrast medium is contained within the annulus. The normal discal nucleus accepts between 1 and 3 ml of contrast medium (Fig. 7).

The ligaments of the vertebral column

The anterior longitudinal ligament extends from the basiocciput to the anterior surface of the upper sacrum. It is firmly attached to the periosteum of the anterior aspect of the vertebral bodies, but less firmly to the discs. It is a flat band which broadens as it passes inferiorly. It is composed of three sets of fibres: the deep layer joins adjacent vertebrae, the intermediate layer is attached to two or three and the superficial layer to four or five contiguous vertebrae (Fig. 8).

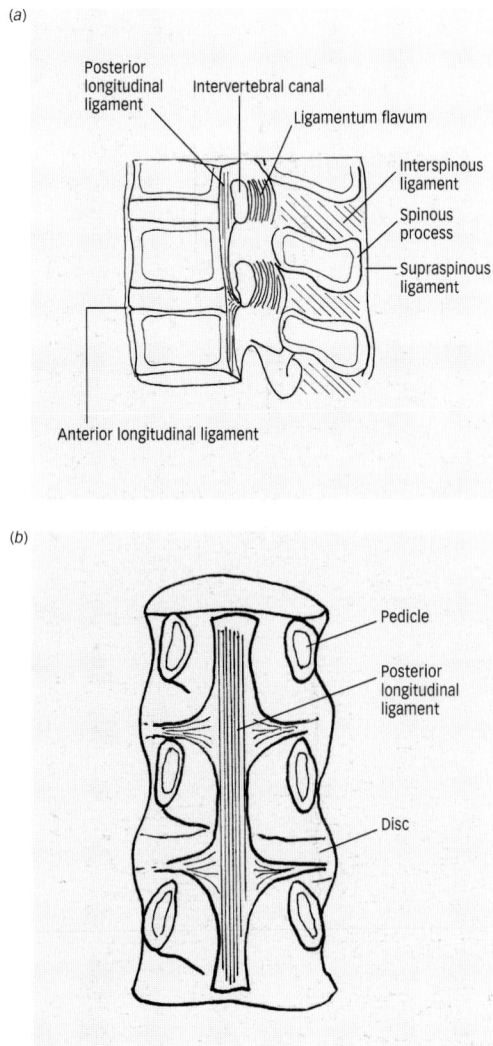

(a)

(b)

Fig. 8.
The ligaments of the
vertebral column, (*a*) lateral
view, (*b*) vertebral bodies
viewed from behind.

The posterior longitudinal ligament extends from the body of the axis to the sacrum. Above the axis it continues as the tectorial membrane. It gradually narrows as it passes downward. It is attached to the intervertebral discs but is separated from each of the vertebral bodies by the emerging basivertebral vein and epidural venous plexus. This ligament is also attached to the dura through an epidural membrane. The posterior longitudinal ligament bulges slightly posteriorly at the level of the intervertebral disc which is evident on myelography particularly of the cervical spine. This bulge is more marked in extension but disappears in flexion.

The supraspinous ligament joins the tips of adjacent spinous processes, from the seventh cervical vertebra to the sacrum. It blends in with adjacent fascia in the back and it is thickest in the lumbar region. Above the seventh cervical vertebra it continues as the ligamentum nuchae which inserts into the external occipital protuberance. The ligamentum nuchae is a bilaminar fibroelastic intermuscular septum.

The ligamentum flavum is made of yellow elastin fibres. It joins the anterior surface of the lamina to the posterior surface of the lamina below. It inserts into the most anterior and lateral aspect of the articular facet hence covering the articulation. On axial section, the ligamentum flavum appears as a V-shaped structure blending with the capsular ligament of the facet joint on each side, and within the limits of the 'V' lies the epidural fat (Fig. 1). This ligament becomes thicker caudally and is best seen in the lumbar region where it is between 3 and 5 mm thick. Unlike the other ligaments, the ligamentum flavum is elastic and extends by up to 35% of its length on flexion. The elasticity of the ligament helps approximate the laminae but with advancing age this elasticity is lost. The ligamentum flavum on T1W MR images has slightly higher signal intensity (i.e. is lighter grey) than the other spinal ligaments and its CT attenuation value is similar to that of muscle.

The interspinous ligaments unite the spinous processes along their adjacent borders. They consist of relatively thin and weak sheets of fibrous tissue that are well developed only in the lumbar region and merge with the supraspinous ligament. The intertransverse ligaments, which join the transverse processes also form a weak, fibrous sheet.

The joints of the vertebral column

These comprise the intervertebral discs (symphyses), the facet joints, which are synovial and fibrous joints (syndesmoses) between the laminae, transverse and spinous processes.

The facet joint

The facet (or apophyseal) joints are small, synovial joints between the articular process on each side of adjacent vertebrae. These joints unite the posterior elements of the vertebral column. The articular process of the vertebra above (its inferior facet) is posterior to that from the vertebra below (its superior facet). The joint surfaces are lined by hyaline cartilage, and a simple capsule is attached beyond the margins of the articular surfaces. The ligamentum flavum and synovial membrane separate the joint from the spinal canal. The facet joint is innervated by the medial division of the posterior primary ramus at the level of the joint and from the level above.

In the cervical spine, the joint is inclined at 45° to the vertical. Menisci are present in the cervical facet joints, which allow more uniform distribution of pressure. The joint capsule is not firmly adherent in this region.

In the thoracic spine, the facet joint is inclined at 60° to the vertical and rotated so that the superior facet faces posteriorly, laterally and superiorly.

In the lumbar spine, the articular facets are curved but near vertical. The lumbar facets lie at 45° to the sagittal plane in the upper lumbar spine but are oriented almost in the coronal plane at the lumbosacral junction. A tough fibrous capsule is present on the posterolateral aspect of the lumbar facet joint but there is no fibrous capsule on the ventral surface. The maximum weight borne by the vertebral column is supported by the lowest two lumbar vertebrae and the facet joints are largest here. The plane of the lumbar facet joints is perpendicular to that of the sacroiliac joint of the same side. The lumbar facet joints are asymmetrical in about 30% of normal individuals.

The intervertebral canal

The intervertebral (or neural) canal (Fig. 9) is situated between adjacent pedicles, which form its upper and lower boundaries. In the thoracic and lumbar regions, each is directed laterally and is limited in front by the lower part of the vertebral body and the intervertebral disc and behind by the facet joint and its capsule. The intervertebral canal is covered on its posterior aspect by the smooth surface of the ligamentum flavum.

The intervertebral canal is widest superiorly, narrowing inferiorly. The superior part is rigid but the inferior part has some mobility and can be distorted slightly. The intervertebral canal narrows with extension as the facets slide over each other, a feature most readily seen in the cervical spine. An inconstant transforaminal ligament is occasionally seen across the lumbar and thoracic intervertebral canal, which may decrease the space for the nerve root. In the thoracic and lumbar regions the neural elements traverse the superior part of the canal. These are supported within the foraminal fat, especially in the lumbar region. The thoracic and lumbar intervertebral canals are directed laterally between transverse processes lying above and below, posteriorly. The upper ten thoracic canals also have the head of the rib articulation as their anteroinferior borders. The intervertebral canal is smaller and more rounded in the thoracic region compared to either the lumbar or cervical regions. The lumbar canals lie between the principal lines of vertebral attachment of the psoas muscle.

The arrangement of the anterior foraminal boundary in the cervical region differs from that of the lumbar and thoracic regions. As the cervical pedicles arise from the vertebral body more inferiorly, a small part of the vertebral body below the disc contributes to the anterior boundary (Fig. 10). The cervical intervertebral canal is orientated anterolaterally at 45° to the sagittal plane and is thus demonstrated using an oblique radiographic projection (Fig. 11).

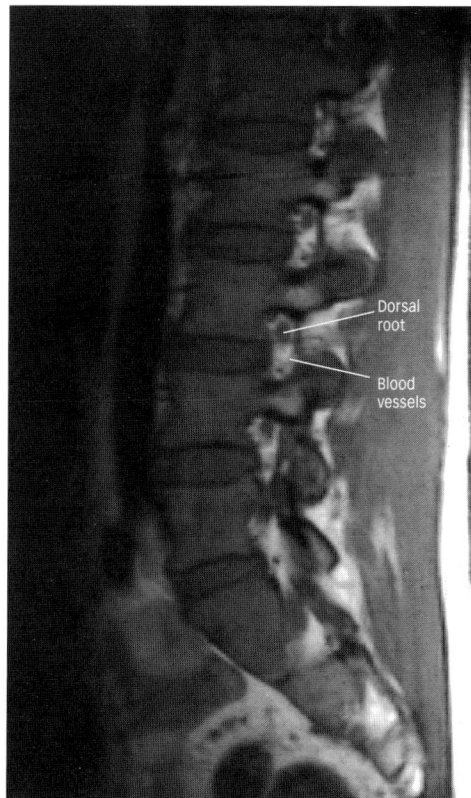

Fig. 9.
T1W MRI, parasagittal plane, the lumbar neural foramina.

Lateral radiographs are appropriate for those of the lumbar and thoracic regions.

The superior part of the cervical canal contains foraminal veins. The nerve root ganglia lie in the inferior part. There is very little epidural fat in the cervical intervertebral canals and it thought that the venous structures play a supporting role for the neural elements in this region.

The dorsal root ganglia, epidural fat, the spinal nerves and blood vessels are found within the intervertebral canal. The ventral root lies anterior and medial to the spinal ganglion in the axial plane and neural elements occupy about 20–25% of the canal.

Fig. 10.
The cervical neural foramen, (*a*) diagram (magnified), and (*b*) T1W parasagittal MRI.

(*a*)

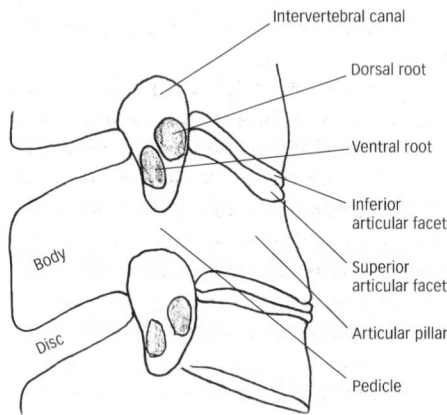

(*b*)

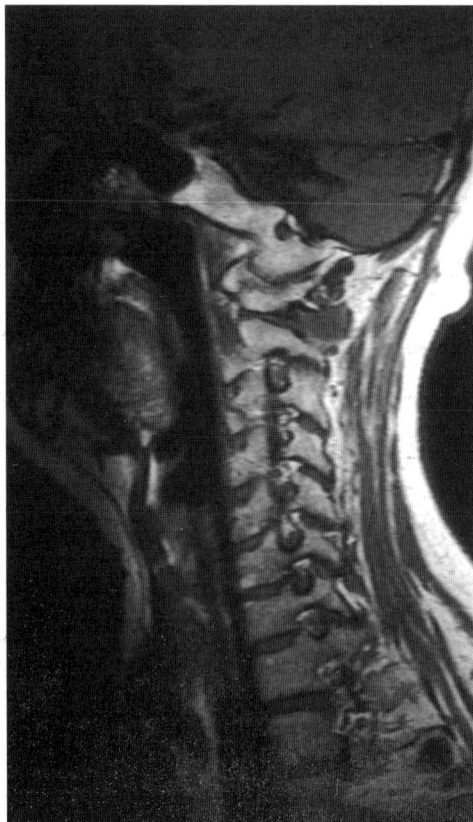

The paraspinous muscles

The paraspinous muscles are well seen on CT and MRI and can be considered as the anterior (or flexor) group and posterior (or extensor) group. The muscles that flex the spine are found in the cervical and lumbar region where there is the greatest mobility. These muscles are supplied by the anterior rami. Muscles constituting this group are the longus capitis, longus colli and rectus capitis in the cervical spine and the psoas muscles in the lumbar region. The psoas muscles also control the degree of lumbar lordosis and contribute to stability of the lumbar spine. The psoas major is attached from the lower border of the bodies of the twelfth thoracic to the fifth lumbar vertebrae and intervening discs to the medial ends of the transverse process of the lumbar vertebrae. Distally, it inserts into the lesser trochanter of the femur. A strong fascia invests the muscle.

The muscles that actually flex the spine are the sternocleidomastoid in the neck and rectus abdominis in the lumbar region. The rectus abdominis acts indirectly by way of the pelvis and thoracic cage. The rotators of the vertebral column are the flank (oblique) muscles, which also act indirectly. The flexor system antagonizes the posterior extensor system to stabilize the spine.

The extensor muscles run the whole length of the vertebral column and are innervated by the posterior rami of the spinal nerves. These muscules lie in the vertebral grooves on each side of the vertebral spines. They are grouped into deep, intermediate and superficial layers. The superficial layer, also known as the erector spinae, is the most powerful group.

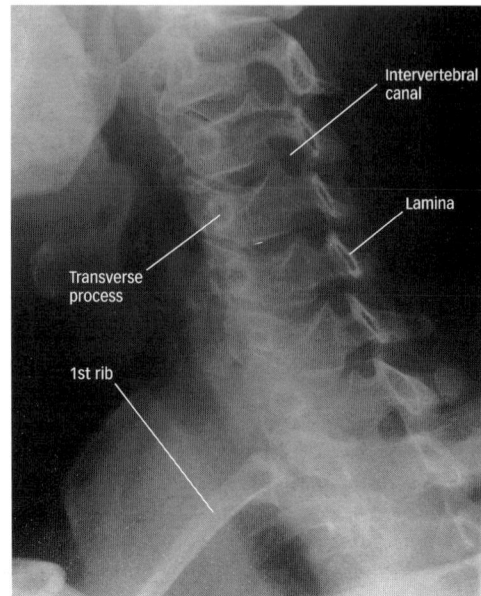

Fig. 11.
Cervical spine radiograph oblique projection.

The extensor muscles are almost all oriented obliquely and thus may act to cause rotation, which is known to accompany idiopathic scoliosis.

The vertebral canal

The transverse diameter of the spinal canal is larger than, or equal to, the sagittal diameter. The distance between the cord and the bony canal (the perimedullary space) varies. Its maximum width, in the cervical region, is about 8 mm and its minimum width, in the thoracic spine, is about 3 mm.

The cervical spinal canal is relatively large and triangular in cross-section except at the level of the atlas vertebra, where it is almost circular. The size of the canal decreases from the first to the third cervical vertebrae, but inferior to this it is relatively constant. In the adult the lower limit of the anteroposterior diameter at the atlas is 16 mm; at the axis, it is 15 mm and in the lower cervical spine it is 12 mm. The upper limit is 27 mm at the atlas and 21 mm in the lower cervical region.

In the thoracic region, the spinal canal is relatively constant in size and round in cross-section. The thoracic dural sac is significantly larger than the cord.

The spinal canal in the superior part of the lumbar spine is round or oval with transverse and anteroposterior diameters approximately equal. The mid and lower lumbar spinal canal is triangular with the base anteriorly. The normal sagittal diameter varies from 15 to 25 mm and is slightly greater caudally. The thecal sac in the lumbar region is close to the vertebral body but occasionally a wide fat-filled space separates the thecal sac at the lumbosacral level. The lateral recess of the spinal canal forms the entrance to the intervertebral foramen. It is the bony groove which gives the spinal canal the characteristic tricorn appearance on axial sections. It is limited anteriorly by the vertebral body, posteriorly by the base of the superior articular facet and laterally by the pedicle (Fig. 12). The lateral recess is larger from above down and is continuous with the neural foramen. Within the recess lies the spinal nerve root, epidural fat and venous plexus.

Movements of the vertebral column

Only limited mobility exists between adjacent vertebrae, owing to restrictions imposed by the facet joints and the limited deformability of the intervertebral discs. However, these small movements augment each other with the result that flexion, extension and abduction (lateral flexion) are possible in the cervical, thoracic and lumbar region. Rotation occurs mainly in the thoracic region. In each region, movement occurs around the nucleus pulposus and the range of movements is determined by the direction of the articular facets on the neural arches.

In flexion, the space between the laminae is increased. The inferior articular process of one vertebra moves superiorly on the superior articular process of the vertebrae below. The anterior longitudinal ligament is lax in flexion, and the anterior portion of the disc is compressed. The posterior part of the disc, and the posterior spinal ligaments, are stretched. Tension of the posterior vertebral muscles limits flexion.

In extension, the vertebrae move back on each other especially in the cervical and lumbar segments. The changes in the ligaments and intervertebral discs are opposite to those in flexion. In lateral flexion, there is compression of the lateral aspect of the disc and rotation causes torsional deformation of the disc.

The type and degree of movements vary in different regions of the spine. In the cervical spine, the inclination of the articular facets allows flexion and extension, aided by the relatively large size of the intervertebral discs. Lateral flexion and rotation occur together in the cervical region.

In the thoracic spine, motion is limited by the adjacent bony structures, the relatively thin discs, and the superior articular facets. However, rotation is possible as the articular facets lie in an arc of circle, the centre of which is near that of the vertebral body. In the lumbar spine, the large intervertebral discs allow considerable flexion and extension but rotation is limited by the articular facets.

Vertebral blood supply

The vertebral column has a segmental blood supply. In the cervical region, segmental branches arise from the vertebral arteries and

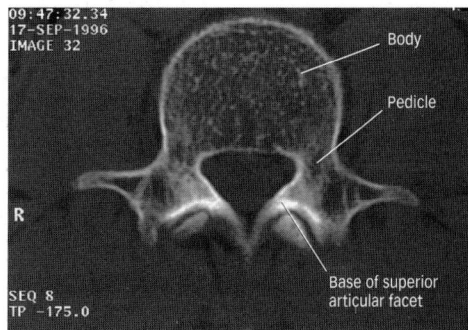

Fig. 12.
Axial CT; the lumbar lateral recess.

Fig. 13.
CT myelogram: (*a*) lumbar;
(*b*) cervical regions to show
the channels for the
basivertebral veins.

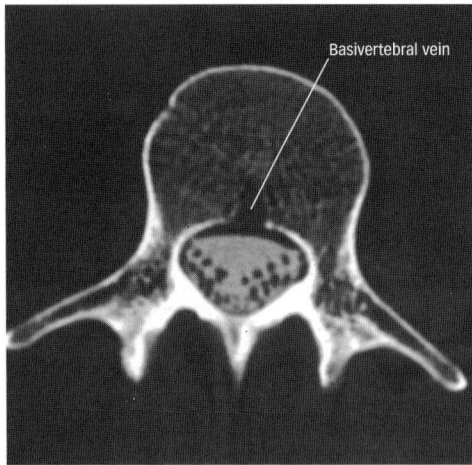

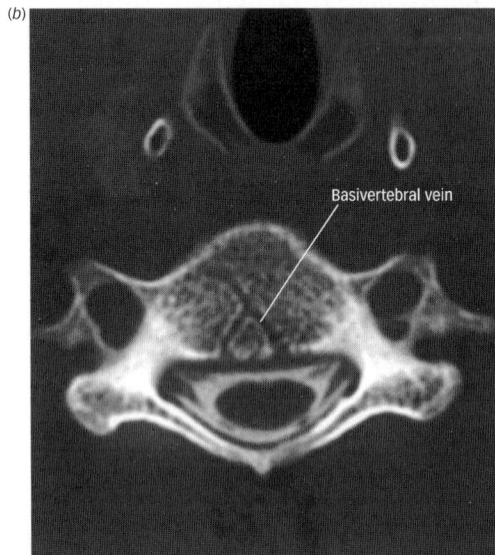

Fig. 13.
CT myelogram: (*a*) lumbar;
(*b*) cervical regions to show
the channels for the
basivertebral veins.

(*a*)

Basivertebral vein

(*b*)

Basivertebral vein

Fig. 14.
T2W MRI, sagittal plane:
the course of the
basivertebral veins.

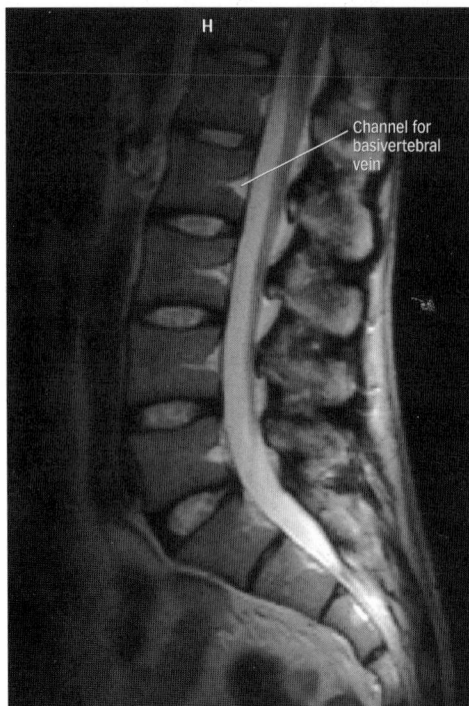

H

Channel for
basivertebral
vein

the costocervical and thyrocervical trunks. The ascending pharyngeal and occipital arteries supply the atlas and axis vertebrae. The thoracic and lumbar parts of the vertebral column are supplied by segmental aortic branches. The lateral sacral artery, which is a branch of the internal iliac artery, supplies the sacrum and sacral nerves. Each segmental artery supplies the corresponding hemivertebra and adjacent musculature. An exception to this arrangement occurs in the upper thoracic vertebrae, where the right intercostal artery also supplies the anterior half of the left side. The left-sided intercostal artery at those levels supplies only the posterior half of the hemivertebra.

The venous drainage of the vertebral body is through a pair of large basivertebral veins into the internal vertebral venous (or epidural) plexus. They penetrate the posterior wall of the vertebral body centrally through a deep notch. The basivertebral vein anastomoses with the anterior epidural vein. The course of the basivertebral vein is seen as a Y-shaped channel within the vertebral body on axial sections (Fig. 13). On MRI, the course of the vein is often shown as high signal due to a combination of slow venous flow and perivenous fat (Fig. 14). Two venous channels are present in the lumbar region, where these veins are best seen, and there may be up to four channels in the thoracic vertebrae. The basivertebral veins are difficult to identify in the cervical region due to their small size and oblique course.

The epidural venous plexuses comprise two, or more, anterior and posterior longitudinal venous channels interconnected at various levels. The anterior veins lie on the posterior surface of the vertebral body and disc. They drain the vertebral bodies. The posterior longitudinal veins lie ventral to the vertebral arch and ligamentum flavum. The vertebral arch and its attached muscles drain into the external vertebral venous plexus. This plexus is intramuscular and almost absent anterior to the vertebral bodies. The internal and external vertebral plexuses drain together into the regional segmental veins. These large, valveless, veins permit reflux of blood draining from the other viscera into the vertebral bodies and are thus a potential route for the haematogenous spread of metastatic neoplasm or infection to the vertebral column.

Within the epidural space, both fat and the venous plexus may appear as high signal on T1W MR scans. The relative amount of epidural fat varies according to the region. Within the cervical spine, for instance, there is very little fat and the epidural venous plexuses are prominent. The latter enhance with intravenous contrast medium on CT and MRI scans.

Ossification of the vertebrae

The vertebral column ossifies in hyaline cartilage. There are three primary ossification centres for a typical vertebra; one in the centrum and one for each half of the neural arch. These appear at 8 weeks gestation. There are two ossification centres in the centrum, which soon fuse. Failure of one-half of this ossification centre to develop results in the formation of a hemivertebra.

The cartilage between the neural arches begins to ossify after birth and ossification is complete by 2 years. The centrum in connected to each half of the neural arch by a synchondrosis or neurocentral joint. The neurocentral joints ossify and fuse by the age of 7 years. The arches unite first in the lumbar region and last in the cervical. Conversely, the centrum unites with the arch in the cervical region first and in the lumbar region last.

The epiphyses for each of the vertebral bodies appear, by puberty, as a bony ring on the upper and lower surface and fuse early in the third decade. Secondary ossification centres also appear at the tips of the spinous processes (two where these are bifid), the tips of the transverse process and mamillary process of the twelfth thoracic vertebra and of the lumbar vertebrae. They also fuse in the early 20s. Failure of fusion of these centres produces accessory ossicles.

Costal elements develop in association with the vertebrae and connect the transverse process with the vertebral body. In the thoracic spine they develop separately to form the ribs. In the cervical and lumbar vertebrae they ossify by direct extension from the neural arch. An occasional centre in the costal elements of the seventh cervical and the first lumbar vertebrae may gives rise to a cervical or a lumbar rib. Weight-bearing costal elements of the sacrum have bony centres which appear at 6 months in utero and fuse with the neural arch at 5 years. They fuse with each other and with the body of the sacrum in the early 20s.

The atlas has three primary ossification centres. The centres for the lateral masses appear at 7 weeks in utero and fuse at 4 years of age. The centre of the anterior arch appears in the first year and fuses at 7 years. Its junction with the lateral mass, on each side, cuts across the anterior part of the upper articular surface and may permanently divide the articular surface.

The axis has two extra centres for the dens (one for each half). These appear at 5 months in utero and fuse 2 months later. The dens unites with the rest of the body at 3 years. Secondary centres for the tip of the dens appear at 3 years and fuse at 12 years. Non-union of the secondary ossification leads to the os odontoideum. An epiphyseal ring appears in the lower part of the body of the axis at puberty and fuses at 25 years. The epiphysis of the dens is V-shaped.

Failure of fusion of the neural arches leads to spina bifida. Defects in the lumbosacral region are very common (in up to 20% of the population) and are almost always less than 4 mm wide. Non-fusion of the posterior arch of the atlas is seen in between 2 and 6% of the population. Occasionally the anterior arch may be unfused in the midline.

Abnormal vertebral segmentation occurs most commonly in the lumbosacral region and usually manifests as a transitional vertebra (see p. 20–21). The absence of segmentation results in the formation of a block vertebra. The block vertebra has biconcave anterior and posterior surfaces and its centre is usually narrow, with a 'waist'. The disc space is usually narrow, but the overall height of the combined vertebral bodies and disc remains close to normal. If the segmentation defect involves the entire articulation, no obvious deformity results.

The craniovertebral junction

The craniovertebral junction is formed between the basiocciput, the atlas and the axis. It held together by strong ligaments and muscles. This region has great mobility. The foramen magnum, within the occipital bone, is oval in shape and, in the normal adult, has a maximum dimension of 37 mm ($\pm$ 6 mm) in the sagittal plane and 30 mm ($\pm$ 4 mm) in the coronal plane. It transmits the neuraxis, the vertebral arteries, the spinal roots of the accessory (XIth) cranial nerve and the spinal arteries and veins, which are all intradural. Meningeal arteries and veins traversing the foramen are extradural in location.

The atlas (the first cervical vertebra)
The atlas (Fig. 15), unlike the other cervical vertebrae, has no vertebral body. It consists, simply, of a ring of bone with two bulky lateral articular masses, united by a short anterior and a longer posterior arch. The superior articular facet is kidney-shaped, which is oriented anteriorly and medially. It is concave superiorly and articulates with the occipital condyle

Fig. 15.
**Atlas (C1) vertebra
(superior view).**

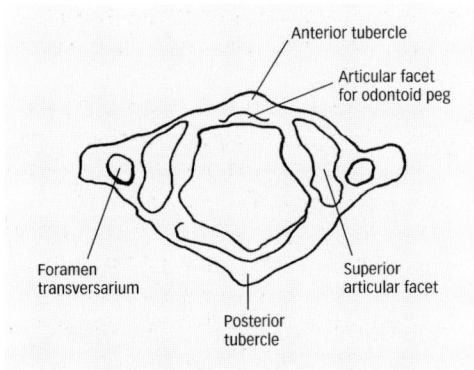

Fig. 15.
**Atlas (C1) vertebra
(superior view).**

Anterior tubercle

Articular facet
for odontoid peg

Foramen
transversarium

Superior
articular facet

Posterior
tubercle

Fig. 16.
**Axis (C2) vertebra (anterior
view).**

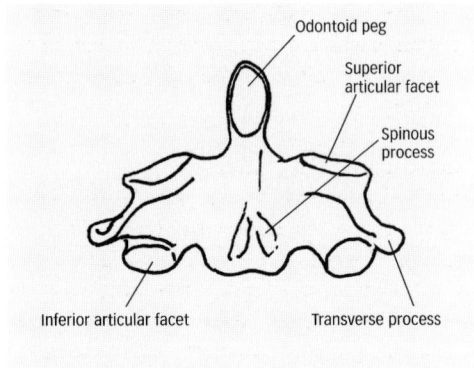

Fig. 16.
**Axis (C2) vertebra (anterior
view).**

Odontoid peg

Superior
articular facet

Spinous
process

Inferior articular facet

Transverse process

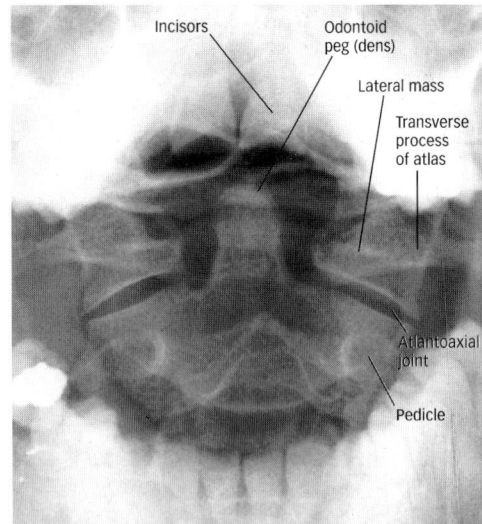

Incisors

Odontoid
peg (dens)

Lateral mass

Transverse
process
of atlas

Atlantoaxial
joint

Pedicle

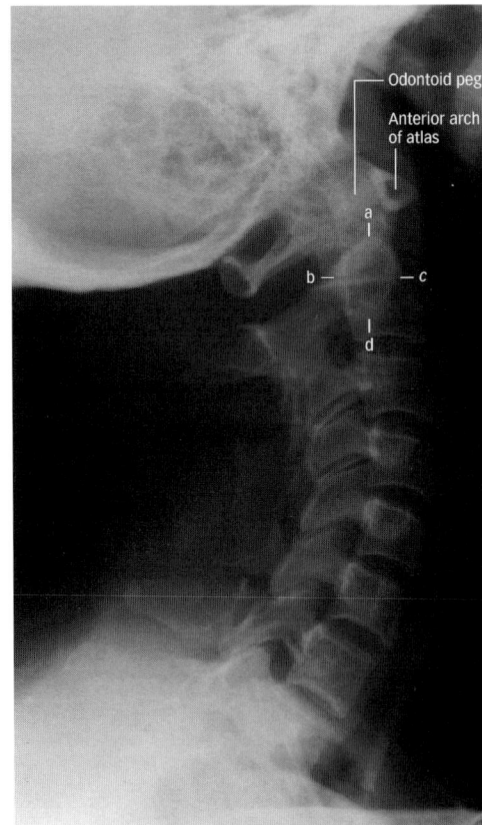

Fig. 18.
**Harris's ring; lateral
radiograph.
a, upper margin of
superior articular facet
b, posterior vertebral bo
c, inferior border of
foramen transversarium
d, pedicle and anterior
body of the axis**

Odontoid peg

Anterior arch
of atlas

a
b — — c
d

on each side. The inferior articular facet is flat
and oriented medially and slightly posteriorly.
It articulates with the axis. The articular facets
are in line with the uncovertebral joints of the
other cervical vertebrae but not with the
neural arches. On the anteromedial aspect of
each lateral mass is a rounded tubercle to
which the transverse ligament of the atlas is
attached.

The anterior arch of the atlas has a tubercle
anteriorly. It has a facet posteriorly for articulation with the dens. The anterior arch is
slightly concave inferiorly.

The posterior arch of the atlas is grooved
superiorly by the vertebral artery behind the
lateral mass. Between the groove and the lateral mass is the attachment for the posterior
atlanto-occipital membrane. Occasionally
there may be calcification of the posterior
atlanto-occipital membrane laterally, which
creates an arcuate foramen, through which
the vertebral artery and the suboccipital nerve
pass. A small midline tubercle is present on
the posterior arch to which the ligamentum
nuchae is attached. A thin posterior arch may
appear discontinuous on axial CT, since it may
fall outside that scan 'slice'. The transverse
processes are long and wide and have no
tubercles. The foramen transversarium,
within each transverse process transmits the
vertebral artery, surrounded by sympathetic
nerve fibres.

The axis (the second cervical vertebra)

The axis (Fig. 16) is the strongest of the cervical
vertebrae. It forms the pivot on which the
atlas and the head turn. The axis has an odontoid process (dens), which represents the body
of the atlas. The dens and the body of the axis
have differing bony architecture. The body of
the axis has a thin cortical layer with well-
developed trabecular bone, similar to the body
of other vertebrae. The dens has relatively
more compact bone than the body of the axis,
although there is individual variation. Due to

its compact bone, the dens shows a lower signal intensity than the body on T1W MR images. The persistent remnant of the subchondral synchondrosis of the dens is seen on T1W images as a dark horizontal band. A variable amount of fat is found between the clivus and the dens.

The superior articular facets of the axis are directed cranially and laterally. They are large, oval and slightly convex in the sagittal plane. The large lateral masses on each side articulate with the atlas and transfer the weight of the skull on to the vertebral column. From the axis, the weight of the skull is transmitted to the vertebral bodies.

On a frontal radiograph, there should be bilateral symmetry of the alignment of the lateral borders of the lateral masses of the atlas and axis vertebrae. In the presence of a con-

genital anomaly of fusion, no more than 2 mm unilateral or bilateral offset are permissible (Daffner, 1996). In children, this offset may be up to 3 mm (Fig. 17).

The anterior surface of the body of the axis is marked by vertical ridges separating two lateral depressions for the insertion of the longus colli muscles. The axis also has a long bifid spinous process. The foramen transversarium of the axis is directed obliquely cranially and laterally and can be seen overlying the anterior aspect of the inferior margin of the body on lateral and oblique radiographs.

On a lateral radiograph, 'Harris's ring' can be identified (Fig. 18) (Harris *et al.*, 1984). The structures which contribute to it are labelled. Disruption of this 'ring' indicates a fracture or fractures.

Craniovertebral ligaments

The skull, atlas and axis are joined by strong ligaments (Fig. 19). The tectorial membrane prolongs the posterior longitudinal ligament up to the anterior margin of the foramen magnum to blend with the dura. Anterior to this is the transverse ligament of the atlas, which passes behind the dens. This ligament is bulky, about 6 mm wide, and divides the atlantal ring. From the midpoint of the transverse ligament, bands pass superiorly to the basiocciput and inferiorly to the body of the axis, forming the cruciform ligament. More anteriorly still, the apical ligament passes from the dens to the anterior midpoint of the foramen magnum. The alar ligaments pass laterally from the dens to the occipital condyles and limit the rotation of the skull on the atlas. The accessory atlantoaxial ligament runs between the atlas and axis. The transverse ligament and both longitudinal ligaments can be seen on MRI.

The craniovertebral joints

The atlanto-occipital joint is a synovial joint between the convex occipital condyle and the concave facet of the lateral mass of the atlas (Fig. 20). Both surfaces are covered with hyaline cartilage and there is a lax, but strong,

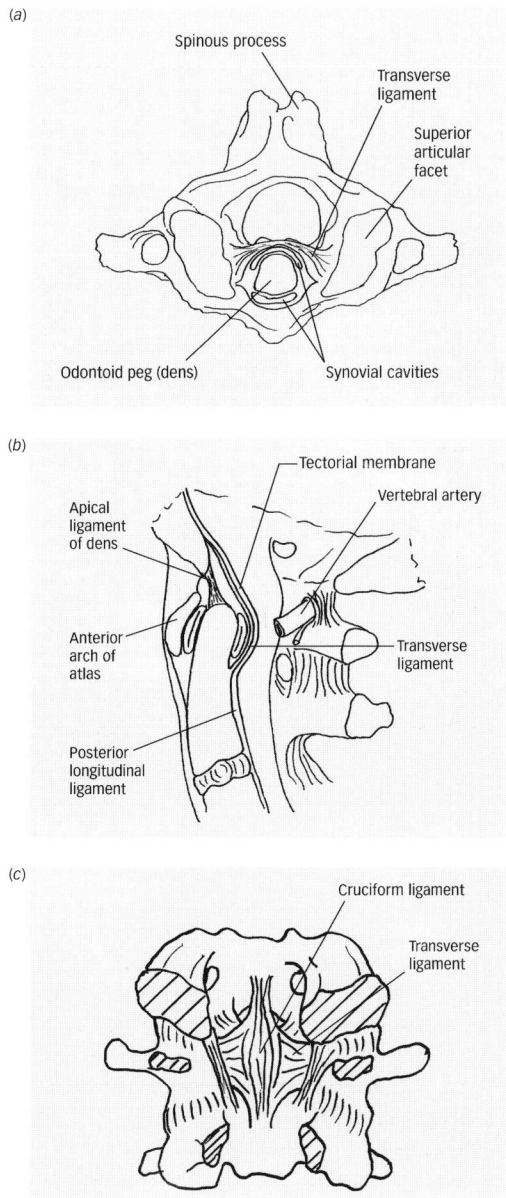

(a)

(b)

(c)

Fig. 19.
The craniovertebral ligaments and atlantoaxial joints viewed (a) from above, (b) in sagittal section and (c) from behind after removal of the posterior arch of C1 and the lamina of C2.

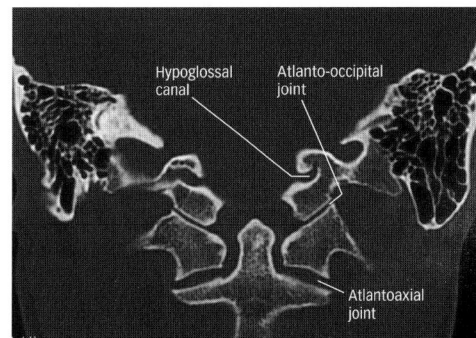

Fig. 20.
The craniovertebral junction: coronal CT reformat.

capsule attached around the articular margins of both bones. The anterior and posterior atlanto-occipital membranes are attached to the upper borders of the respective parts of the arch of the atlas and the outer margin of the foramen magnum. The anterior membrane completely closes the space between the two synovial joints. The posterior membrane is deficient laterally to transmit the vertebral artery and first cervical nerve. The centre of gravity of the skull passes anterior to the joint and the position of the head is maintained by the cervical extensor muscles.

The median atlanto-axial joint is a synovial joint between the anterior arch of the atlas and the dens, held together by the transverse limb of the cruciform ligament. Large synovial bursae are present between the articular surfaces. The lateral atlanto-axial joint is a synovial joint between the respective lateral masses.

The curved surfaces of the atlanto-occipital joint allow the head to flex, extend and undergo lateral flexion, but rotation occurs at the atlanto-axial joint around the vertical axis of the dens. Rotation and lateral flexion produce radiographic changes in the relationship of the axis to the atlas and may alter the distance between the dens and the lateral masses of the atlas on a frontal film. In the early phase of rotation, the axis remains stationary. This rotation is accompanied by a slight vertical descent of the head, due to the oblique character of the articular surfaces. With further rotation, the axis rotates in the same direction. In lateral flexion, the skull and atlas move as a unit and glide from the midline to the side of the tilt. The axis and subjacent vertebrae rotate in the direction of the tilt during lateral flexion. This rotation occurs earlier during lateral flexion than in pure rotation.

The osseous relationship of the spine to the brainstem can be assessed on radiographs (Fig. 21). Chamberlain's line is drawn on the lateral radiograph along the line of the hard palate to the posterior lip of the foramen magnum. Normally, no more than one-third of the total height (or 5 mm) of the dens should be above this line. A modification of this is the McGregor line which uses the inferior surface of the occiput rather than the foramen magnum. In normal individuals, the tip of the dens should be no higher than 7 mm above this line. The bimastoid and digastric lines can be used on the frontal radiograph to assess basilar invagination. The bimastoid line, which joins the tips of the mastoid processes should touch the upper extremity of the dens. The digastric line joining the digastric notches of the skull is normally 1 cm above the atlanto-occipital joints. On the lateral film a line bisecting the long axis of the clivus should normally pass through the tip of the dens.

The gap between the anterior surface of the dens and the posterior aspect of the anterior arch of the atlas (the anterior atlanto-dental interval or 'AADI') is maintained by the transverse atlantal ligament. It is less than 3 mm in adults and less than 5 mm in children on a lateral film with a target – film distance of 180 cm, in any lateral view whether in flexion, extension or in a neutral position.

On midline sagittal MRI scans, the anterior lip of the foramen magnum is taken as the signal void due to the cortical bone at the posteroinferior lip of the clivus (basion). The posterior margin is taken as the anterior limit of the occipital squame (the opisthion), although the interface between the signal void of the compact bone and hypointense cerebrospinal fluid on T1W images may not be easy to identify. It is clear that minor degrees of tonsillar

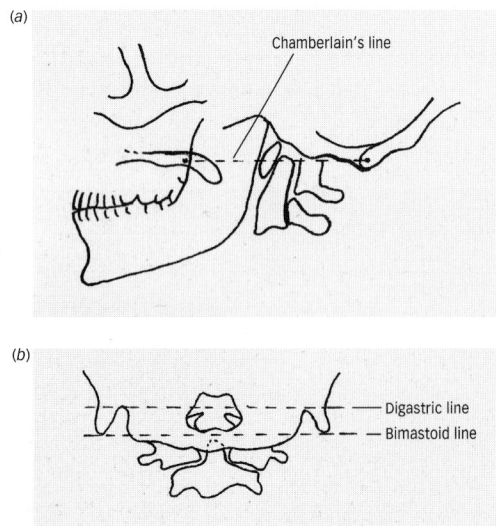

Fig. 21.
The craniovertebral junction: Chamberlain's line, the bimastoid and digastric lines.

(a)

Chamberlain's line

(b)

Digastric line
Bimastoid line

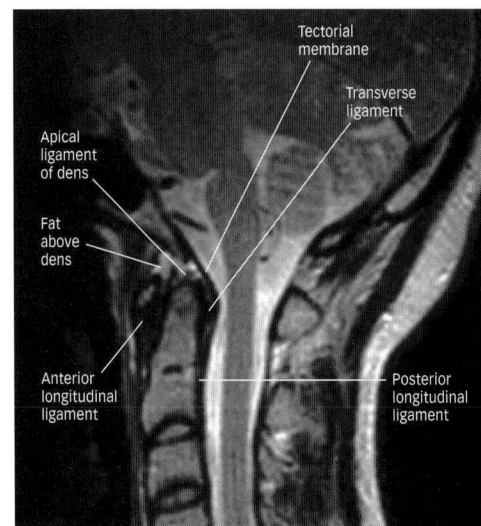

Fig. 22.
T2W MRI, midline sagittal plane, the craniovertebral junction.

Tectorial membrane

Transverse ligament

Apical ligament of dens

Fat above dens

Anterior longitudinal ligament

Posterior longitudinal ligament

descent (of up to 3–5 mm) into the spinal canal is seen without evidence of brainstem compression (Fig. 22).

Cervical spine

The third to seventh cervical vertebrae are broadly similar in configuration (Fig. 23). The small, oval vertebral bodies progressively increase in size from above down. On each side of the superior aspect of the cervical vertebral bodies is the uncinate process, which is a bony ridge projecting superiorly from the lateral margin. These ridges articulate with a bevelled notch on the posterolateral surface of the vertebra above to form the uncovertebral, or neurocentral joints of Luschka (Figs. 24, 25(*a*)). Whether or not these are true synovial joints is a matter of academic controversy. The uncinate process, which is not present at birth, lies in the same axial plane as the intervertebral disc and behind the uncinate process lies the nerve root.

The transverse processes are short and wide and end laterally with an anterior and a posterior tubercle. These tubercles are connected by the intertubercular lamella. The sixth cervical vertebra has the largest anterior tubercle, whereas it is virtually absent in the seventh. This facilitates their identification on axial CT sections. The transverse process encloses the foramen transversarium, which is round or oval in shape, slightly larger on the left side and occasionally double. It transmits the vertebral artery and its accompanying veins and sympathetic nerves. The foramen trans-

versarium of the seventh cervical vertebra is small or absent and usually transmits only the vertebral veins.

The articular masses (or 'pillars') are dense, heavy, rhomboid-shaped structures, bounded by the superior and inferior articular facets. The articular facets are large, rounded and relatively flat. The superior articular facet faces anterosuperiorly and the inferior process posteroinferiorly. On a lateral radiograph a line can be drawn connecting the posterior margins of the superior and inferior articular facets (Fig. 25(*b*)). This slightly convex line is formed by the posterolateral cortex of the articular mass. Due to superimposition, the lateral cortical margins of the articular masses appear, on the frontal radiograph, as a continuous, smoothly undulating, sharply defined lateral margin of the spine. This gives the appearance of a solid column of bone, the so-called 'lateral column'. Distortion of this implies changes in the vertebral arch.

Fig. 25.
Cervical spine radiographs:
(*a*) anteroposterior,
(*b*) lateral projections.

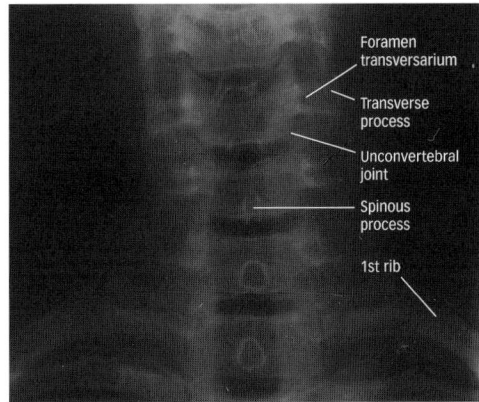

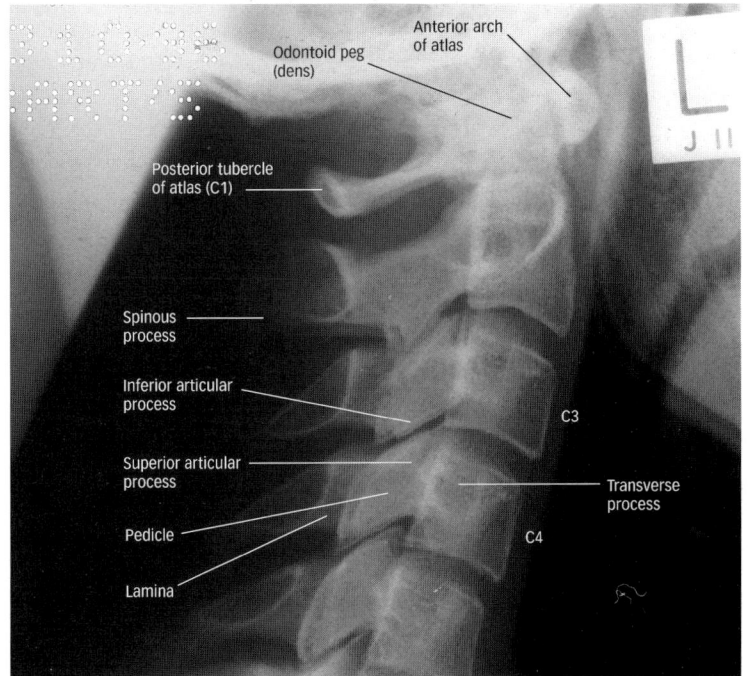

Fig. 23.
A cervical vertebra.

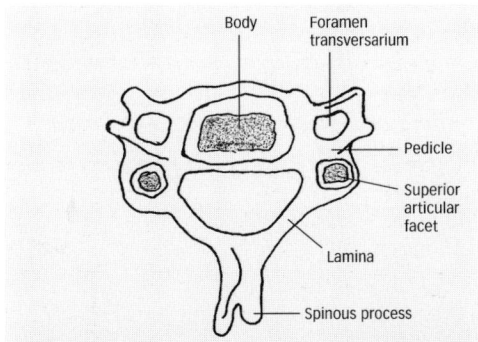

Fig. 24.
Cervical CT myelogram demonstrating the uncinate processes and the neurocentral joints of Luschka.

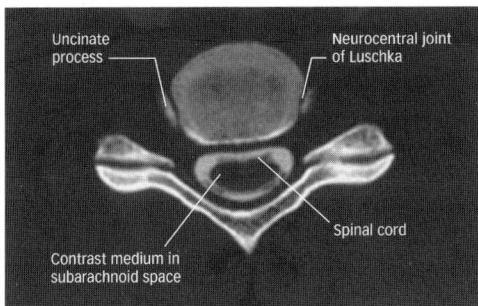

315

Fig. 26.
Lateral cervical spine
radiograph with the neck
in flexion showing the
'stepped' pattern (see text).

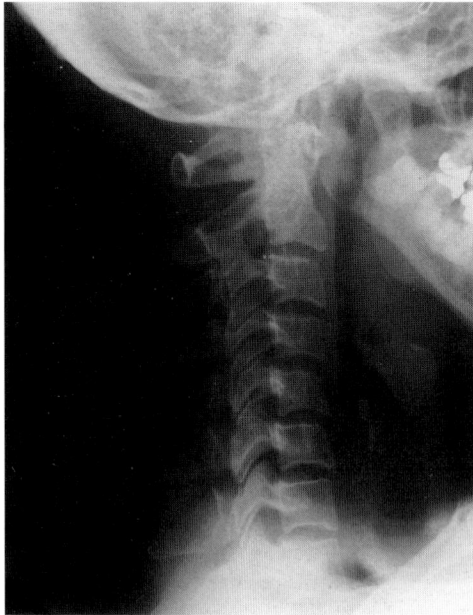

Fig. 26.
Lateral cervical spine radiograph with the neck in flexion showing the 'stepped' pattern (see text).

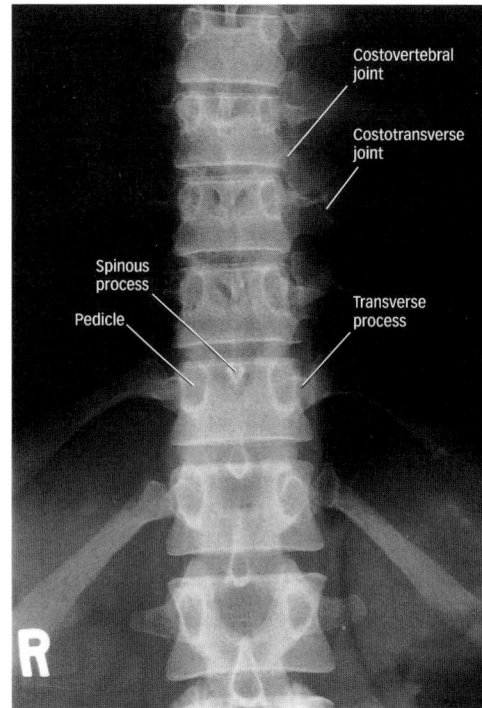

(a) Fig. 27.
Thoracic spine radiograph (a) anteroposterior, (b) lateral projections

Costovertebral joint

Costotransverse joint

Spinous process

Pedicle

Transverse process

R

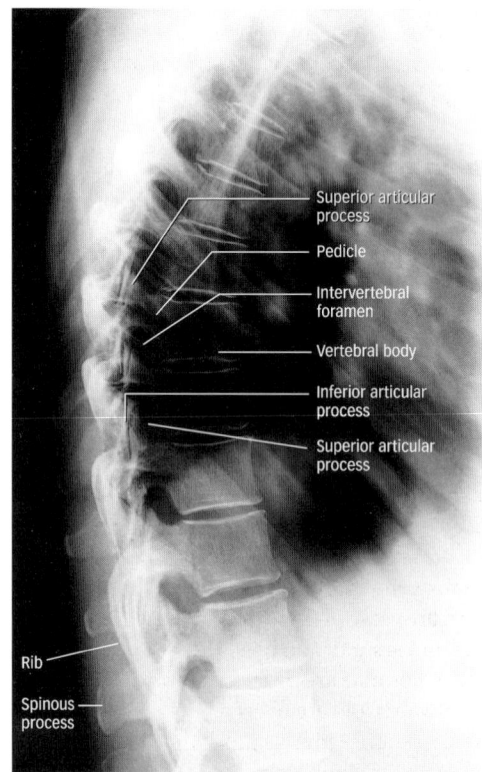

(b)

Superior articular process

Pedicle

Intervertebral foramen

Vertebral body

Inferior articular process

Superior articular process

Rib

Spinous process

The paired laminae are posteromedial extensions of the articular masses and form the posteromedial aspect of the spinal canal. The thin vertical strip of internal cortex at the base of the spinuous process forms the posterior laminal line visible on lateral radiographs. This represents the posterior boundary of the spinal canal. In the oblique projection the laminae are seen 'end-on' with the lamina of the vertebra above covering the lamina of that below (Fig. 11).

The spinous processes are small and bifid except for the seventh cervical vertebra (the 'vertebra prominens'), which has a long, non-bifid spinous process to which is attached the lower extremity of the ligamentum nuchae.

A cervical rib results from the prolongation of the costal elements of the seventh cervical vertebra and may be present in up to 6% of the normal population. It may be truly rib-like or be represented by a fibrous band passing to the first rib, in which case the anterior tubercle of the transverse process, at that level, is enlarged. The subclavian artery and the first thoracic nerve root may be compressed from below by the cervical rib.

The alignment of the cervical spine can be assessed on the lateral radiograph. The anterior and posterior longitudinal lines form parallel smooth lordotic curves from the base of the skull to the first thoracic vertebra. The spinolaminar (posterior laminal) line follows the same curve except at the level of the second cervical vertebra, where a posterior displacement of up to 2 mm is normal due to the long spinous process. The sagittal dimension of the spinal canal, measured between the pos-

terior longitudinal and the spinolaminar lines, should be greater than 13 mm.

The prevertebral soft tissue has a sharp anterior margin, formed by the posterior wall of the pharynx. In the upper cervical spine of the adult (from the atlas to the interspace between the fourth and fifth cervical vertebrae), its maximum sagittal dimension is

3 mm, with a film-target distance of 180 cm. In children, this retropharyngeal soft tissue may be up to 7 mm. Below the fourth cervical vertebra, the oesophagus contributes to the soft tissue shadow, which may be up to 22 mm wide in adults. In children, it should be no more than 14 mm. In the lower cervical spine, the sagittal dimension of the prevertebral soft tissue should not exceed that of the adjacent vertebral body.

Flexion and extension views of the cervical spine show the change in relationship of adjacent vertebrae may occur in one of two ways (Fig. 26). The forward translation of each vertebra may be continuous so that a line connecting the posterior cortical margins of the vertebral body on the lateral radiograph is smoothly concave anteriorly. Alternatively, flexion may occur as each successively higher segment translates anteriorly a short distance through a series of anterior increments. On the lateral radiograph the vertebral bodies will have a stepped pattern. The posterior cortical margin of each cervical vertebra is offset from the adjacent segment by a distance that is normally less than 3 mm. In extension, the movements are reversed, but again the offset should not exceed 3 mm.

Thoracic spine

The thoracic vertebrae (Fig. 27) have wedge-shaped bodies, which contribute to the thoracic kyphosis. The thoracic vertebral bodies become progressively larger caudally, although the width decreases from the first to the third thoracic vertebrae before increasing again. The lateral margins of the vertebral bodies are slightly concave.

The pedicles arise from the upper half of each vertebra. The transverse processes are directed laterally, posteriorly and slope downwards. They decrease in size progressively towards the thoracolumbar junction and the transverse process of the twelfth thoracic vertebra is small and irregular.

The laminae are broad. They slope downwards and are overlapped in a similar manner to the spinous processes. The spinous processes are longer and more slender than in cervical or lumbar region. Those in the lower thoracic vertebrae are orientated near horizontally.

The superior articular facets face posteriorly and laterally, although those in the upper thoracic spine face superiorly also. The articular facets of the first to the tenth thoracic vertebrae lie in coronal plane and therefore resist anterior translation (Fig. 28). Those of the

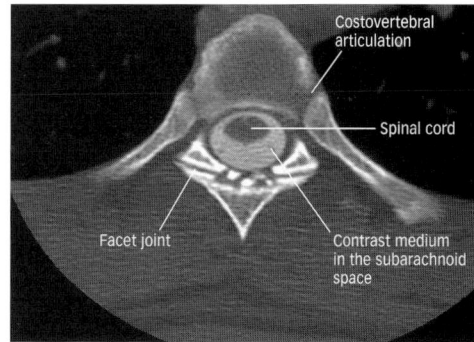

Fig. 28.
Thoracic CT myelogram showing the facet joints.

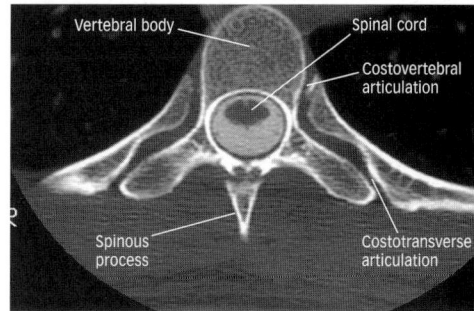

Fig. 29.
Thoracic CT myelogram showing the rib articulations.

eleventh and twelfth resemble the orientation of the lumbar vertebral facet joints.

The thoracic spine bears the ribs and their articulations (Fig. 29). The second to the tenth thoracic vertebrae have superior and inferior demifacets for the ribs on each side. The first thoracic vertebra has a complete facet superiorly and a demifacet inferiorly. A single complete facet is present on each side of the eleventh and twelfth thoracic vertebrae. These facets articulate with the heads of the ribs and form synovial costovertebral joints. The crest of the head of the rib is joined at the intervertebral disc by an intra-articular ligament, which lies parallel to the plane of the intervertebral disc and divides the joint into two compartments. The rib articulation identifies the plane of the intervertebral disc on axial CT scans.

The tubercles of the ribs articulate with articular facets on the anterior surface of the ends of the transverse processes, except at the eleventh and twelfth thoracic vertebrae. They form synovial costotransverse articulations, and the capsule of these joints is strengthened by the accessory costotransverse ligament.

The lateral border of the paravertebral soft tissue is covered with pleura and forms the paraspinal line on a frontal radiograph. The paraspinal space contains lymph nodes, intercostal vessels, sympathetic nerves and fat (see Chapter 6 'Chest').

Lumbar spine

The lumbar vertebral bodies are kidney-shaped in axial section, and the transverse dimension of each exceeds its anteroposterior dimension (Fig. 30). Each vertebral body has convex anterior and lateral margins. The posterior, superior and inferior margins are flat or slightly concave. The third lumbar vertebra is the largest and has the longest transverse processes (Fig. 31).

The articular facets face each other in the sagittal plane (Fig. 32). The posterior surface of each superior articular facet has a rounded mamillary process. The laminae are short and, unlike the thoracic vertebrae, do not overlap. The region of the lamina between the articular facets is the pars interarticularis. This is represented as the 'collar of the Scotty dog', seen on the oblique radiograph (Fig. 33). On axial section the pars interarticularis lies at the vertebral body level, while the facet joint lies in the same axial plane as the intervertebral disc.

The pedicles are directed backwards from the upper part of the vertebral body and each has a deep notch on its inferior surface. Both pedicles and spinous processes consist mainly of dense cortical bone. The interpedicular distance increases progressively caudally. Pedicle 'thinning' with a slight increase in the interpedicular distance at that level is normal at the thoracolumbar junction in about 7% of the population. The 'thinned pedicles' may have a concave medial border.

The fifth lumbar vertebra is atypical. Its body is wedged-shaped and taller anteriorly. Its transverse process is shorter than those of the other lumbar vertebrae and pyramidal in shape. It arises from the lateral aspect of the pedicle and vertebral body and may articulate with the adjacent sacrum and iliac bone. The inferior articular facet of the fifth lumbar vertebra faces forwards, which prevents forward translation on the sloping surface of the sacrum.

(a) Fig. 31.
Lumbar spine radiographs
(a) anteroposterior,
(b) lateral projections

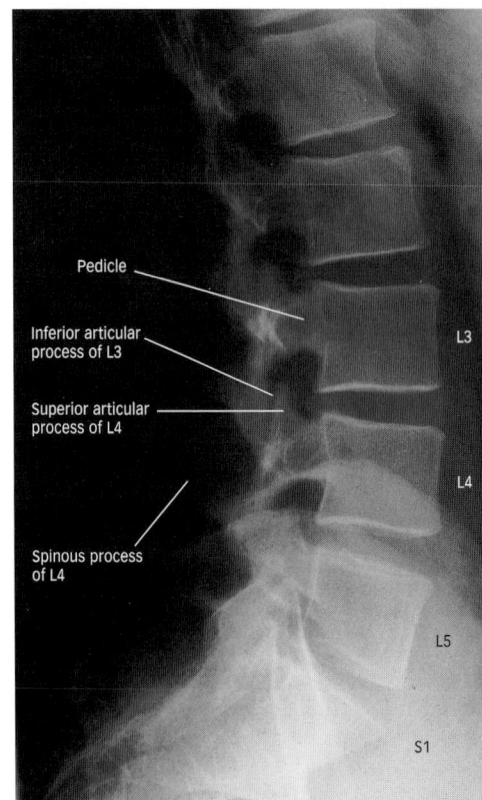

Fig. 30.
A typical lumbar vertebra.

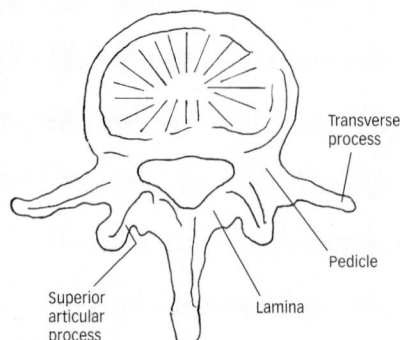

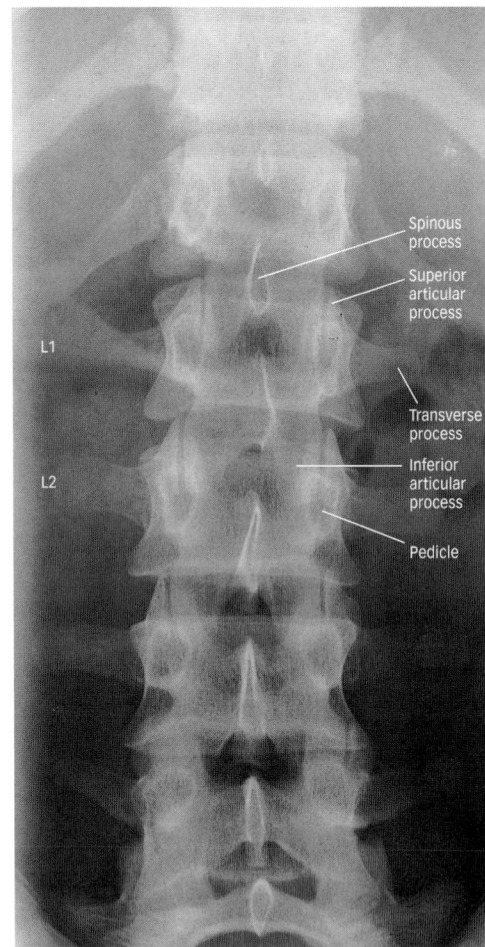

Fig. 32.
Lumbar spine: (*a*) axial CT,
(*b*) T1W axial MRI to show
the facet joints.

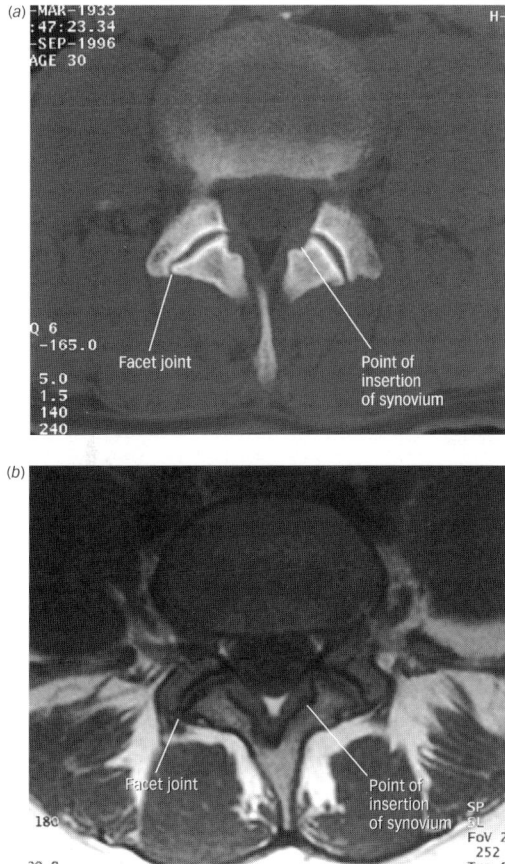

Facet joint

Point of insertion of synovium

(*b*)

Facet joint

Point of insertion of synovium

Fig. 33.
Lumbar spine radiograph, oblique projection.

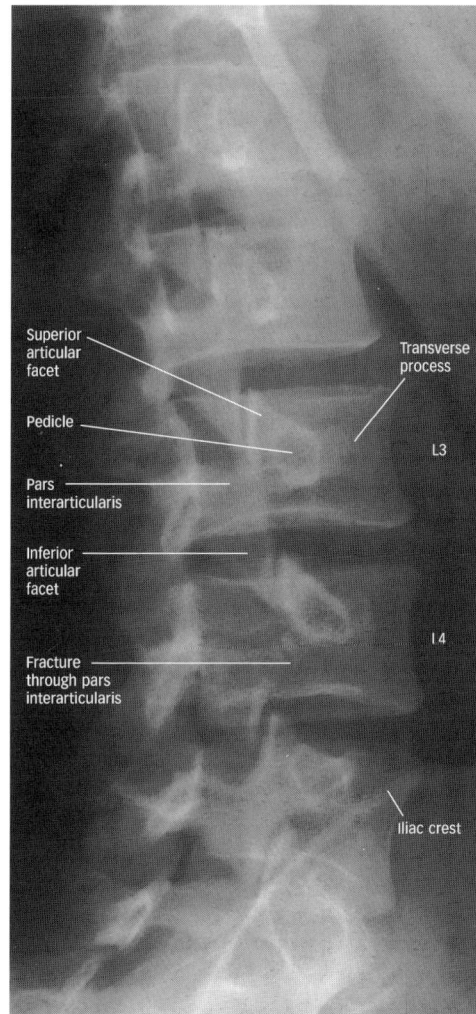

Superior articular facet

Pedicle

Pars interarticularis

Inferior articular facet

Fracture through pars interarticularis

Transverse process

L3

L4

Iliac crest

Fig. 34. below
Lateral radiograph of the lumbosacral junction.

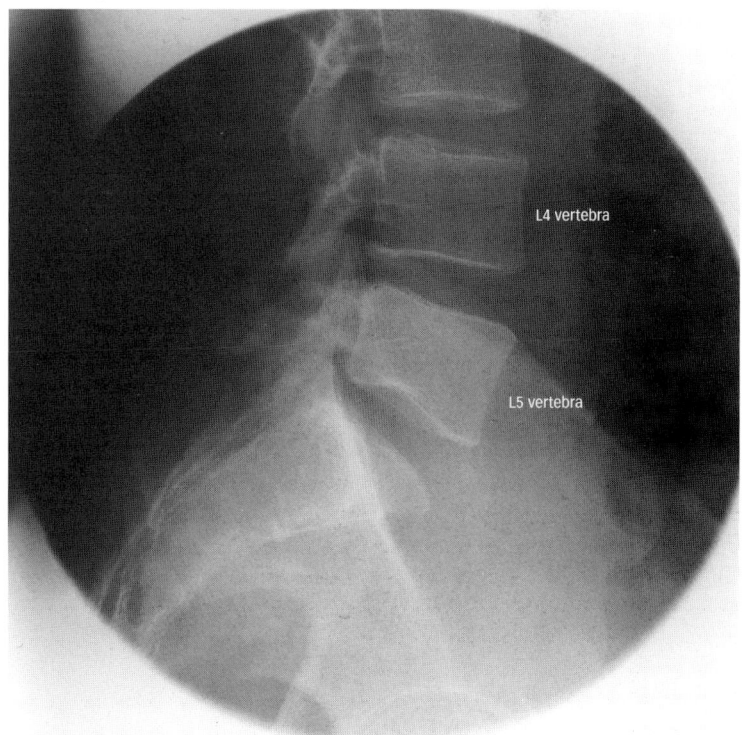

L4 vertebra

L5 vertebra

The lumbosacral junction

The junction between the fifth lumbar vertebra and the sacrum is inclined to the horizontal at an angle of between 25° to 55° in the supine position (Fig. 34). It increases by between 8° and 12° in the erect position. The articulations between the fifth lumbar vertebra and the sacrum resemble those elsewhere in the vertebral column but an additional ligament, the iliolumbar ligament, extends from the anterior inferior part of the fifth lumbar vertebral transverse process and passes laterally to the pelvis. The lower band of the iliolumbar ligament (the lumbosacral ligament) inserts on to the rough surface of the lateral part of the first sacral segment and blends with the ventral sacroiliac ligament. The upper band passes to the iliac crest. The iliolumbar ligament may occasionally calcify.

The heights of the intervertebral discs increase progressively from above down, but the lumbosacral disc is smaller than the other lumbar discs. It is usually less than 10 mm and often less than 5 mm in height. The shape of the disc in the axial plane is also different in that it has a straight or convex posterior margin, whereas the other lumbar discs are concave posteriorly. There may be a substantial amount of anterior epidural fat at the lumbosacral junction in some normal individuals (Fig. 35). This is readily identified by MRI but the appearance may resemble that of a prolapsed disc at myelography. At this level the thecal sac may have a straight rather than convex anterior border in the axial plane, as the paired first sacral nerve roots appear from the thecal sac. An anterior indentation of the sac at the lumbosacral discal level is abnormal. Prominent epidural veins may appear as 'soft tissue' on MRI or CT especially at the level of the fourth and fifth lumbar vertebrae and should not be mistaken for extruded disc. The veins will enhance after intravenous contrast medium.

Failure of segmentation at the lumbosacral region is seen in up to 6% of normal individuals. This usually manifests as a transitional vertebra. Absence of segmentation may be complete or a pseudoarthrosis may form between one or both transverse processes and the sacral ala. A transitional fifth lumbar vertebra, in which one or both transverse processes, as well as the inferior aspect of the body, is partly fused with the sacrum, is regarded as 'sacralized'. With incomplete sacralization, there is narrowing of the lumbosacral space, and hemisacralization of the fifth lumbar vertebra may mimic a bony exostosis on axial sections. When the first sacral segment is significantly separated from the remainder of the sacrum, it is referred to as 'lumbarized'. Lumbarization of the first sacral segment is less common than sacralization of the fifth lumbar vertebra. It is

Fig. 35.
Lumbar spine, T1W sagittal MRI showing prominent caudal epidural fat.

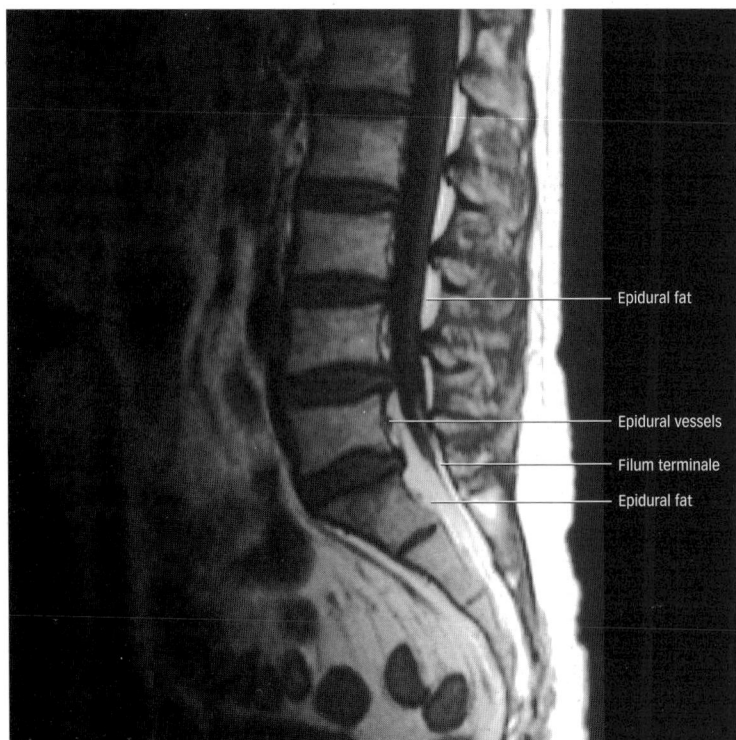

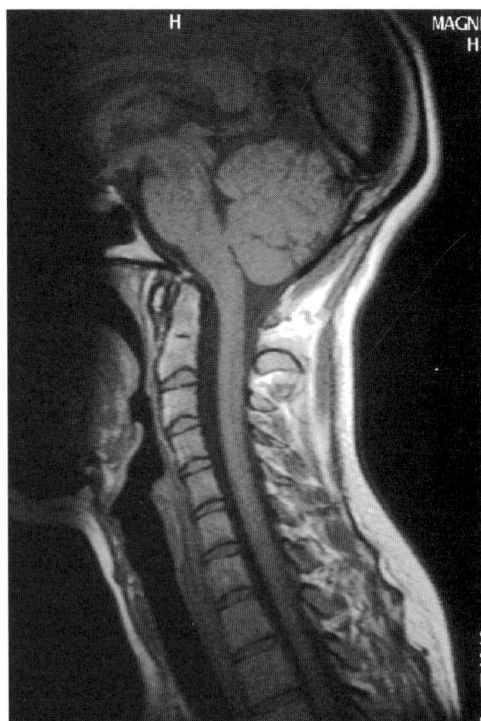

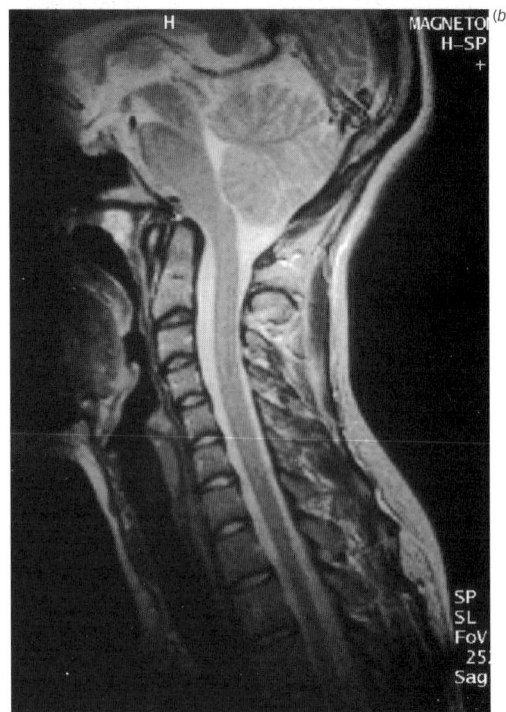

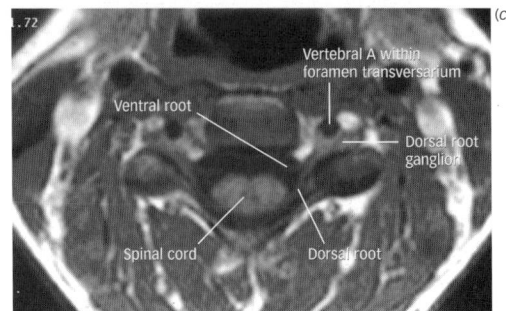

Epidural fat

Epidural vessels

Filum terminale

Epidural fat

Fig. 36.
Cervical spine: (*a*) T1W, (*b*) T2W sagittal MRI, (*c*) T1W, (*d*) T2W axial MRI, (*e*) myelogram, lateral projection. Thoracic spine (*f*) T1W, (*g*) T2W sagittal MRI, (*h*) T1W, (*i*) T2W axial MRI, (*j*) myelogram, frontal projection, and (*k*) lateral projection to show the conus medullaris.

Vertebral A within foramen transversarium

Ventral root

Dorsal root ganglion

Spinal cord

Dorsal root

not infrequent to see six lumbar vertebrae and, in such cases, the distal lumbar segment is referred to as the first presacral vertebra. To identify precisely the nature of any segmentation defect, the entire vertebral colum should be examined radiographically. In practice, however, this is rarely necessary.

The sacrum and sacroiliac joint are described in Chapter 17.

The spinal cord

The spinal cord extends from the foramen magnum to the level of the first or second lumbar vertebrae (Fig. 36). In flexion, its lower end may ascend by as much as one vertebral segment. Because of their different respective lengths, the segments of the spinal cord do not correspond to those of the vertebral column. There is a difference of one segment in the lower cervical spine, two segments at the upper thoracic and three in the lower thoracic regions.

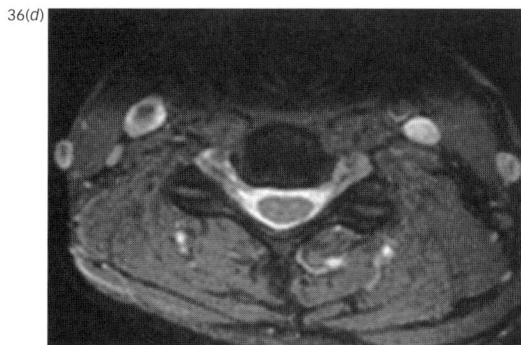

36(d)

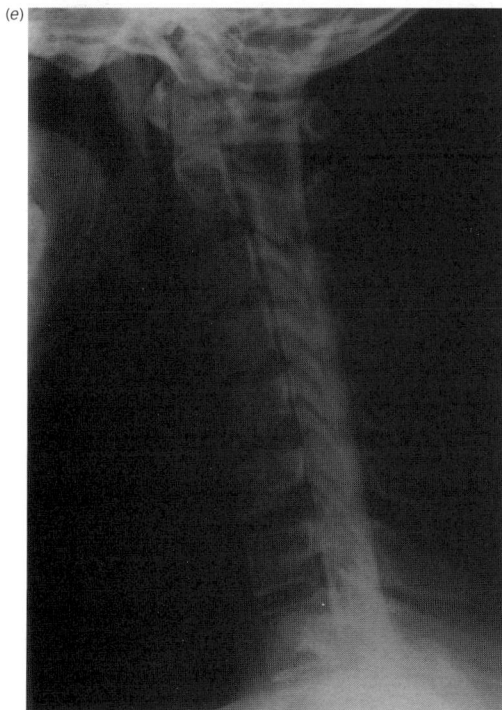

(e)

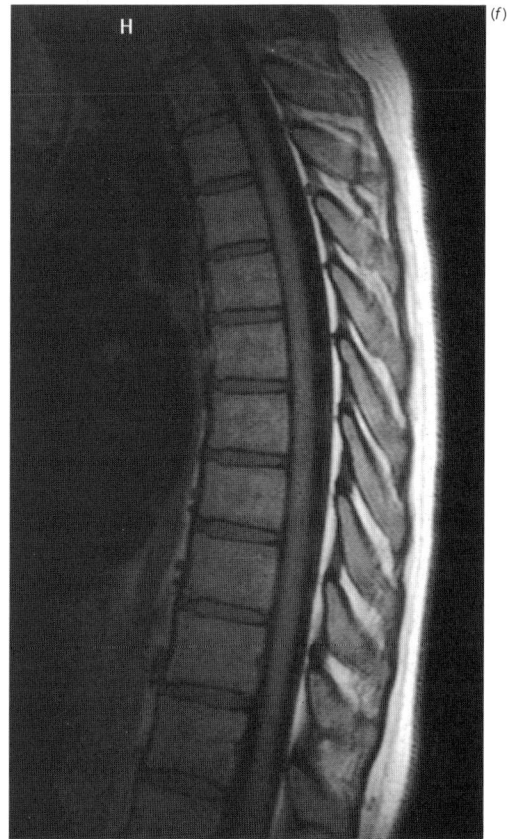

(f)

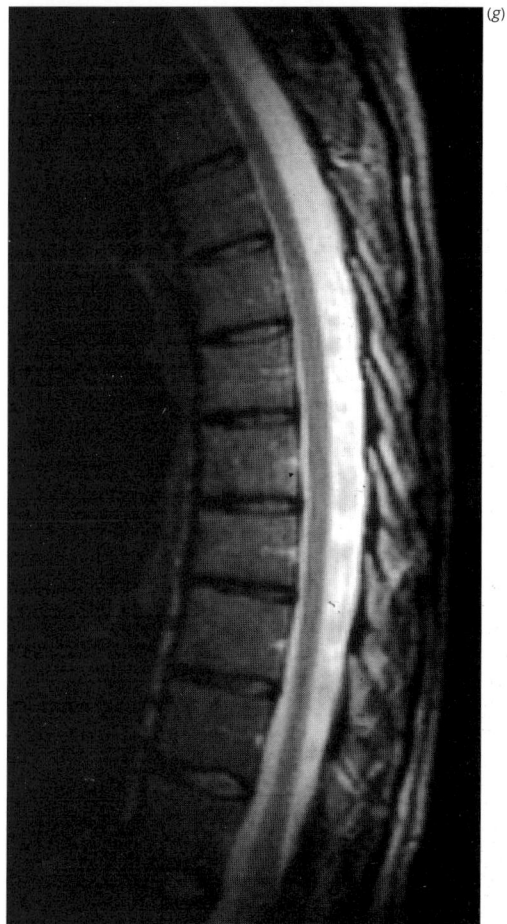

(g)

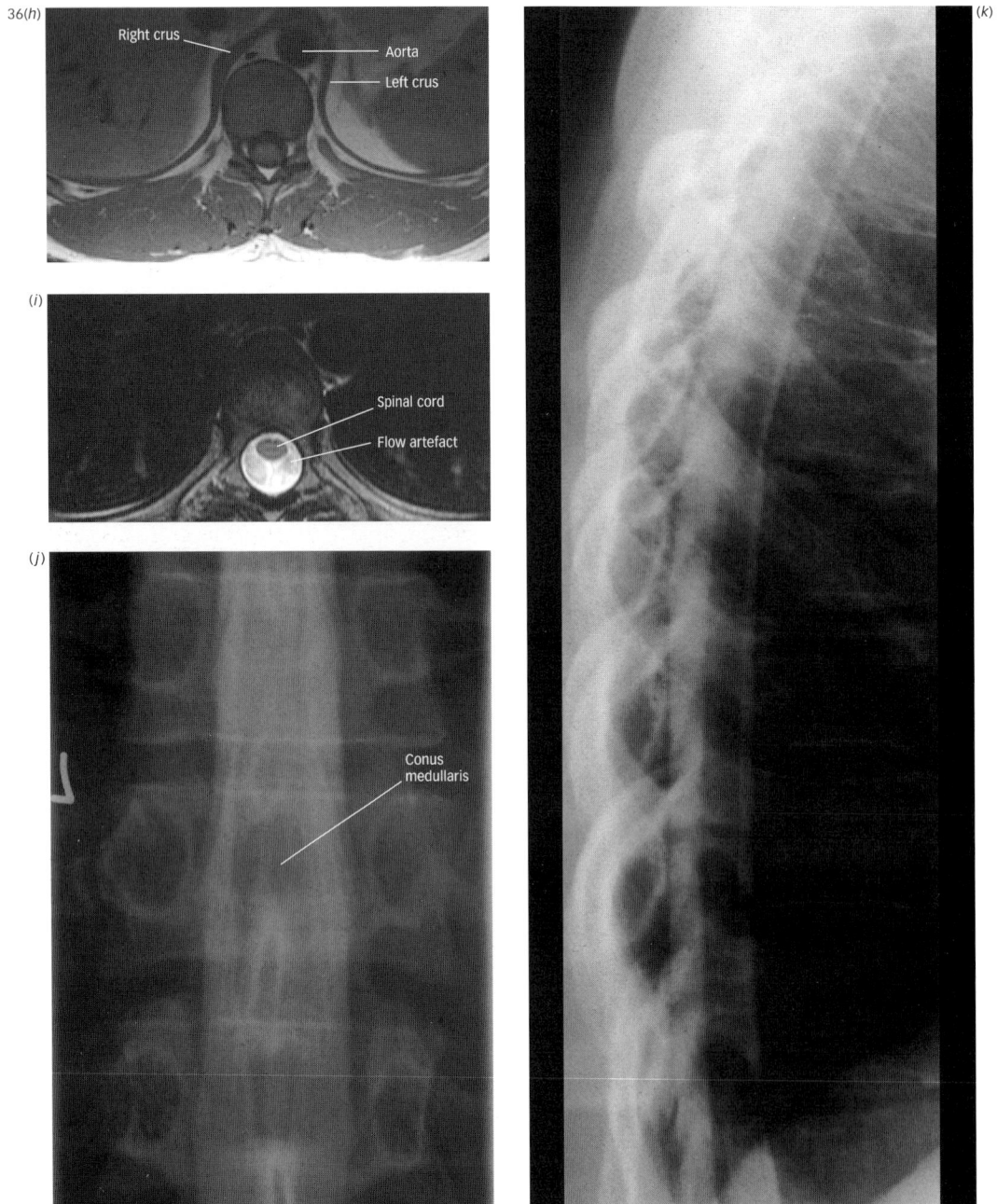

36(h)

Right crus
Aorta
Left crus

(i)

Spinal cord
Flow artefact

(j)

Conus medullaris

(k)

The spinal cord is flattened in axial section, the transverse dimension exceeding the anteroposterior. Its lower end tapers to form the conus medullaris (Figs. 14, 36). There is a deep, anterior midline groove known as the anterior median fissure, and a shallow posterior median sulcus from which the posterior median septum extends into the cord. Spinal nerve rootlets emerge from anterolateral and posterolateral sulci on each side. The calibre of the spinal cord increases in two regions, known as the cervical and lumbar expansions. The cervical expansion includes that region between the fifth cervical and first thoracic cord segments, where the roots forming the brachial plexus emerge. The cervical expansion is found within the spinal canal from the third to the seventh cervical vertebrae.

The nerve roots which form the lumbosacral plexus emerge from the lumbar expansion between the second lumbar and the third sacral spinal cord segments inclusive. These are situated within the spinal canal from the tenth thoracic to the first lumbar vertebrae. These enlargements result from the increase in mass of motor neurones in the anterior horns of the grey matter.

The central canal of the cord is lined by ependyma. It is continuous with the fourth ventricle above and extends 5–6 mm into the

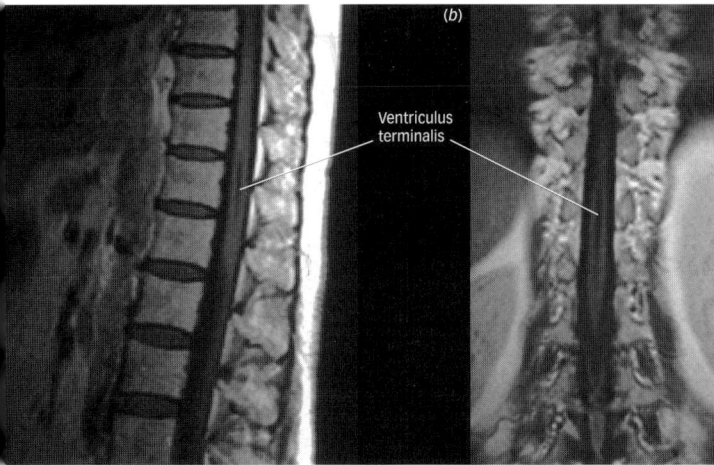

Fig. 37.
Terminal ventricle: T1W MRI, (*a*) sagittal, (*b*) coronal scans

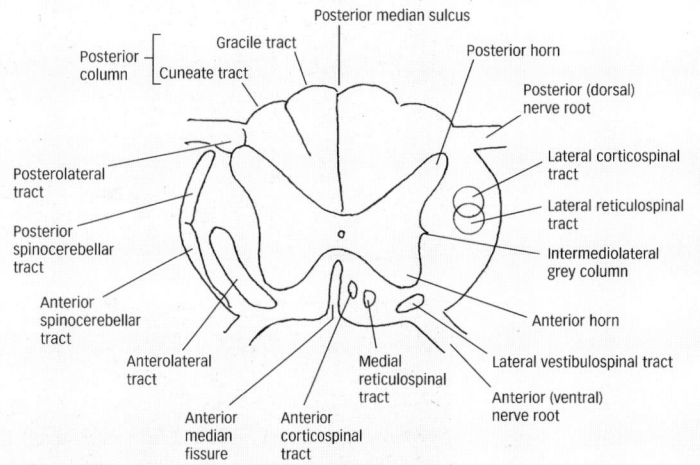

Fig. 38.
The internal structure of the spinal cord.

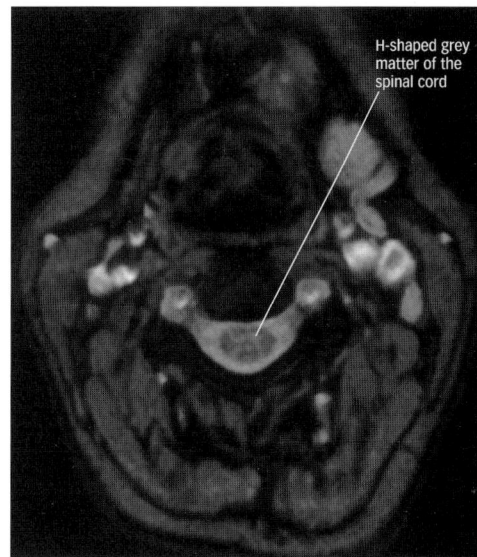

Fig. 39.
Gradient echo T2W axial MRI of the cervical spinal cord to show discrimination of grey and white matter.

filum terminale inferiorly. It is anterior to the midline in the cervical and thoracic cord, central in the upper lumbar cord and posterior to the midline in the conus. The terminal ventricle, also known as the 'fifth ventricle', is a fusiform dilatation of the central canal in the conus (Fig. 37). On MRI it is seen in 2.6% of children less than 5 years of age and measures about 22 mm × 4 mm × 4 mm (Coleman, Zimmerman & Rorke, 1995). It is encountered rarely in adults.

Internal structure

The spinal cord consists of a central mass of grey matter, containing the cell bodies, surrounded by white matter, which consists of myelinated nerve fibres (Figs. 38 and 39). It is incompletely divided, in the sagittal plane, into two halves by the anterior median fissure and the posterior median septum. There are both grey and more anterior, white commissures connecting the grey and white matter across the midline.

The grey matter of the spinal cord surrounds the central canal and is H-shaped in cross-section. The anterior horns contain the cell bodies of the motor neurones. The posterior horns contain the cells of the sensory pathways. The thoracic and upper lumbar sections of the spinal cord also contain a lateral horn, containing the cell bodies of the sympathetic neurones.

The white matter is divided into three columns by the anterior and posterior horns and their emerging nerve rootlets. The anterior white column lies between the anterior horn and the anterior median fissure. The posterior column lies between the posterior median septum and the posterior horns of the grey matter. The lateral column is between the anterior and posterior horns. The fibres within

the white matter are grouped into ascending, descending and intersegmental tracts. The following is a brief description of some of the important pathways.

Ascending tracts

The afferent (sensory) pathways convey impulses from the periphery to the cerebral cortex. The main ascending tracts are the posterior (dorsal) columns and anterolateral tracts. The posterior column tracts are associated with the sensation of light touch, vibration and proprioception. Their fibres are large and myelinated, and the cell bodies lie in the dorsal root ganglia. The posterior column is laminated so that fibres from the lowest part of the body lie nearest to the midline and the incoming fibres are added progressively laterally. These terminate in the lower medulla at the gracile and cuneate nuclei. The axons then decussate to form the medial leminscus which ascends through the brainstem to reach the

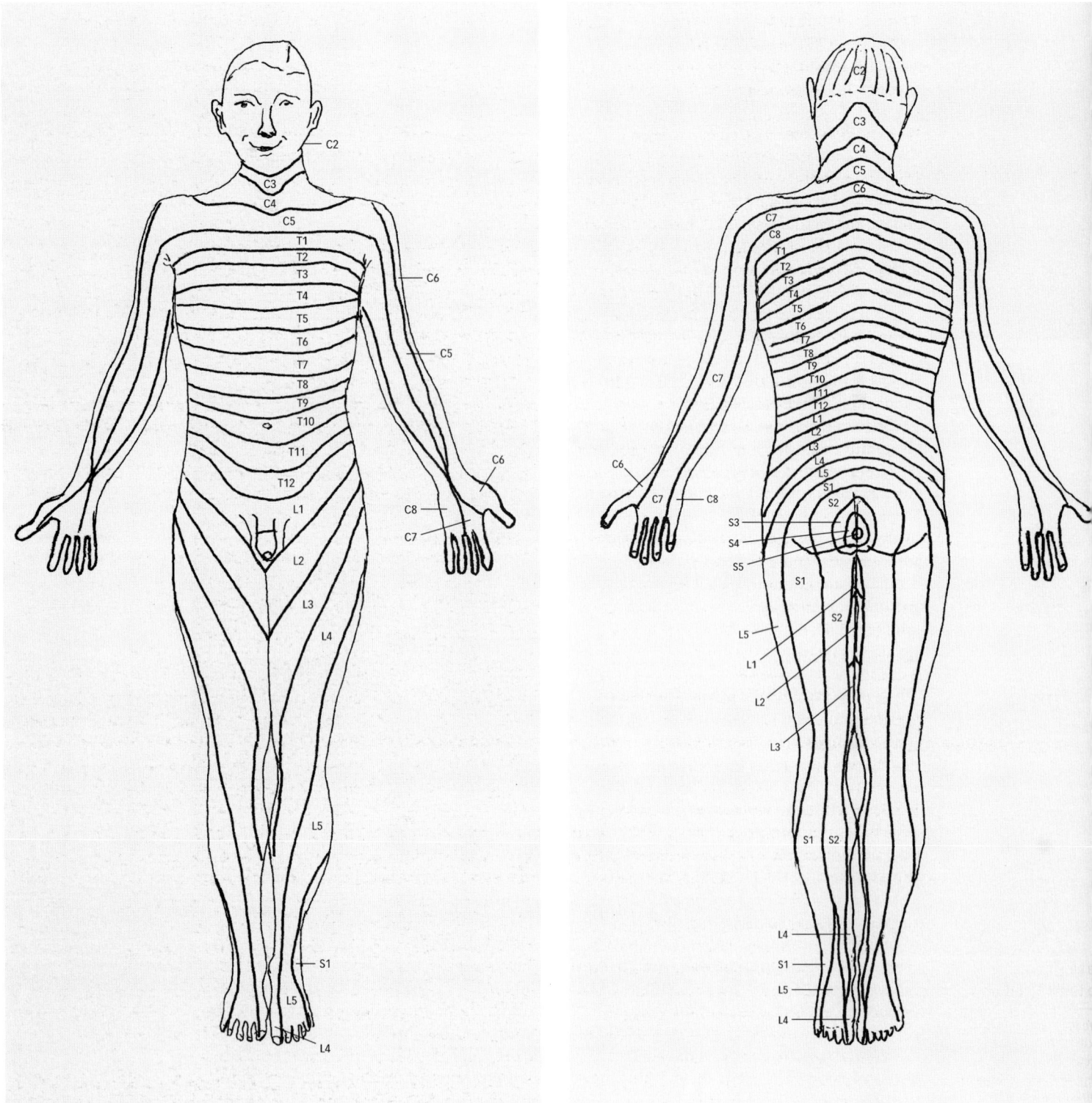

Fig. 40.
The principal dermatomes.

thalamus. From there, the fibres project on to the cerebral cortex via the internal capsule.

The anterolateral tract conveys sensations of pain, temperature and crude touch. It is a combination of the anterior and lateral spinothalamic tracts. This tract is also laminated, with those fibres from the sacral regions lying laterally and those from the cer-

vical lying medially. Nerve fibres conveying painful stimuli from the peripheral nerves enter the spinal cord via the posterior nerve roots. They traverse the posterolateral tract and synapse with the cell bodies of the substantia gelatinosa. These nerves then pass over to the opposite side, crossing in front of the central canal, to the anterolateral tract. The anterolateral tract fibres then pass to the thalamus via the spinal lemniscus in the brainstem.

The fibres of the spinocerebellar tract ascend in the lateral column, and are concerned with proprioception.

Descending tracts

The efferent (motor) pathways convey stimuli from the cerebral cortex to the peripheral nervous system. They comprise the pyramidal and extrapyramidal systems. The pyramidal, or direct corticospinal, pathway consists of upper and lower motor neurones. The cell bodies of the upper motor neurones lie in the cerebral cortex and the fibres pass via the pyramids in the medulla to the anterior horn cells of the spinal cord. The lower motor neurones are the anterior horn cells and their axons extend to the motor end plates.

The lateral corticospinal tract is the most important of the descending tracts and lies in the lateral column, posterior to the attachment of the denticulate ligament. The tract becomes smaller distally as fibres progressively leave to synapse with cell bodies in the anterior horn. The anterior corticospinal tract is adjacent to the anterior median fissure and terminates in the upper thoracic region of the spinal cord. These nerve fibres leave the tract and decussate near the segmental level, which they innervate.

The extrapyramidal system or 'indirect corticospinal tract' is the name given to the groups of fibres from the motor cortex which pass via the subcortical nuclei to the anterior horn cells. As their name implies, these fibres do not pass through the pyramid of the medulla. The main extrapyramidal pathways are the rubroreticulospinal and vestibulospinal tracts.

Spinal nerve roots

There are 31 segmental nerves (eight cervical, twelve thoracic, five lumbar, five sacral and one coccygeal). The cutaneous distribution of the nerve roots is shown in Fig. 40. The root values of the tendon reflexes are shown in Table 1.

The first to the seventh cervical spinal nerves exit above the pedicle of the corresponding vertebrae, whereas all the other roots exit below the pedicles (Fig. 41). As examples, a posterolateral prolapse of the intervertebral disc between the fourth and fifth lumbar vertebrae would be expected to compress the fifth lumbar root. A posterolateral prolapse of the disc between the fourth and fifth cervical vertebrae may compress the fifth cervical root, and so on. It should be remembered that the eighth cervical root exits between the seventh cervical and first thoracic vertebrae.

The ventral spinal roots carry somatic motor fibres, along with sympathetic fibres within the first thoracic to the second lumbar roots and parasympathetic fibres within the

TABLE 1

tendon reflexes

e jerk	L2,3,4
le jerk	S1,2
eps jerk	C6,7
eps jerk	C5,6
inator jerk	C5,6

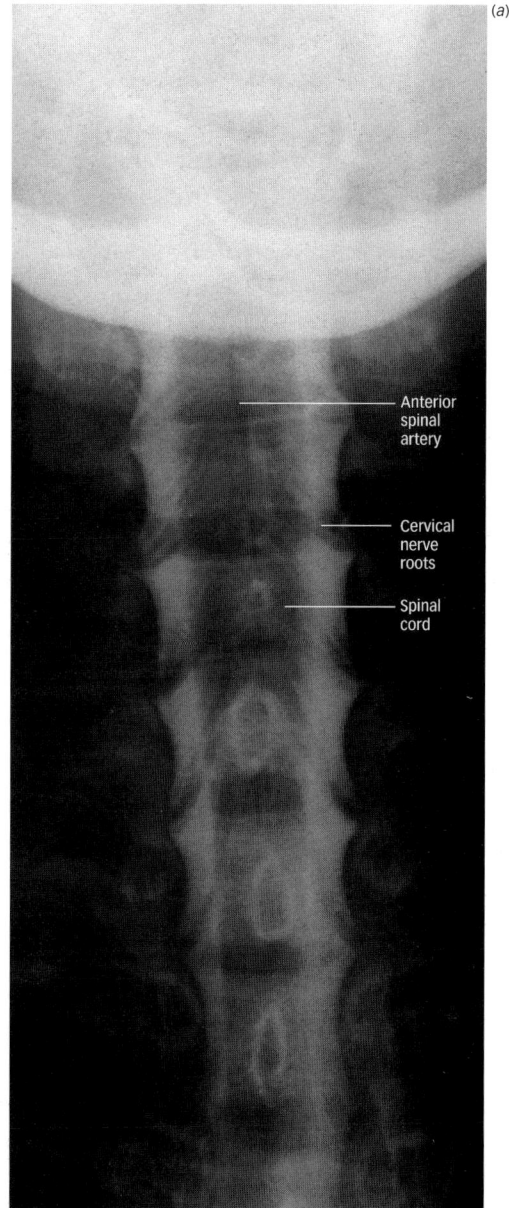

(a)

- Anterior spinal artery
- Cervical nerve roots
- Spinal cord

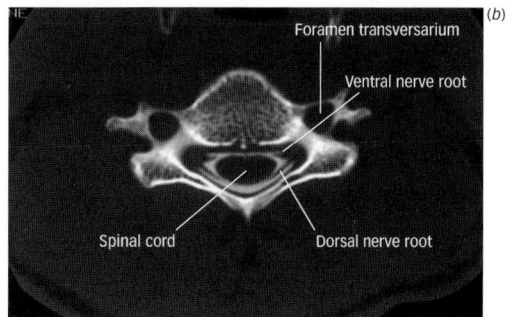

(b)

- Foramen transversarium
- Ventral nerve root
- Spinal cord
- Dorsal nerve root

Fig. 41.
Cervical myelogram: (a) AP projection, (b) postmyelogram CT.

second to the fourth sacral roots. The dorsal nerve roots carry both somatic and visceral afferent sensory fibres.

Each ventral nerve root is formed from three or four rootlets, which arise from the anterolateral sulcus of the cord. Each dorsal root is formed from several rootlets arising from the posterolateral sulcus of the cord. The dorsal and ventral roots at each level pass to the intervertebral canal (Fig. 41(*b*)), where each emerges from the dura separately before uniting to form the mixed spinal nerve in the canal. From the first cervical to the first lumbar segments, the ventral and dorsal nerve roots pass in front of and behind the denticulate ligament, respectively.

The dorsal nerve root ganglion is situated in the intervertebral foramen within the tubular evagination of the dura and arachnoid, immediately before the point of union of the ventral and dorsal nerve roots. The cervical dorsal root ganglia are just lateral to the neural foramen, lying between the vertebral artery anteriorly and the superior articular facet posteriorly. The cervical dorsal root ganglia are not easily identified, unlike those in the lumbar region (Fig. 42).

Because the spinal cord is shorter than the vertebral column, the nerve roots take a progressively more oblique course caudally. The upper cervical roots are horizontal. The upper thoracic roots first slope down to the point where they emerge from the meninges. They then incline upward to reach the foramen. Below the first lumbar vertebra, the nerve roots pass almost vertically downwards

through the subarachnoid space to form the cauda equina (Fig. 43). The lumbar spinal nerve roots normally separate from the theca just below the intervertebral disc, except for the first sacral root, which usually separates above the lumbrosacral disc. The first sacral

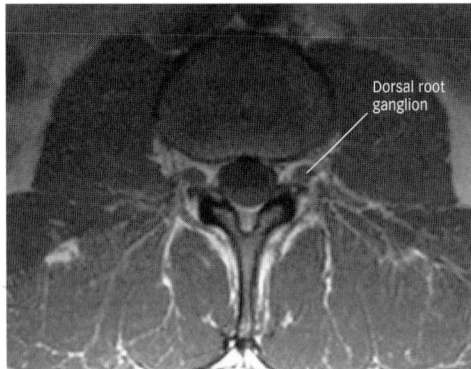

(*a*) Fig. 43.
The cauda equina: (*a*) T2W sagittal MRI, (*b*) lumbar myelogram, oblique projection.

Fig. 42. (*a*)
The lumbar dorsal root ganglion; axial MRI, (*a*) T1W, (*b*) T2W.

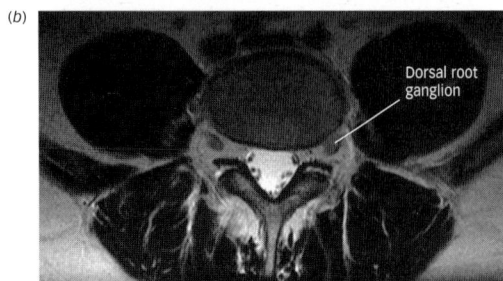

Dorsal root ganglion

(*b*)

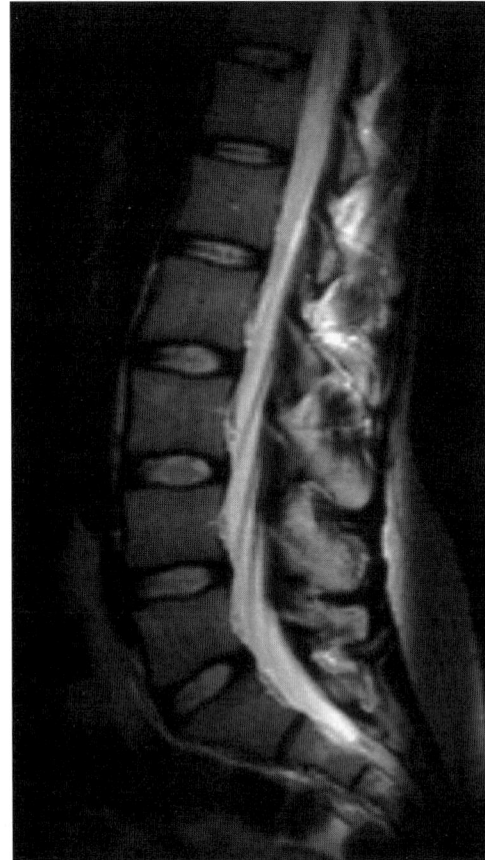

Dorsal root ganglion

(*b*)

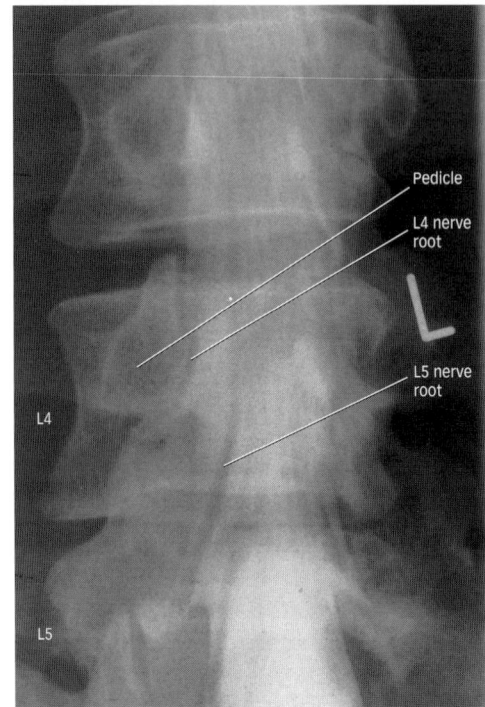

Pedicle

L4 nerve root

L5 nerve root

L4

L5

Fig. 44.
1W coronal MRI to show
ve roots exiting beneath
the pedicles.

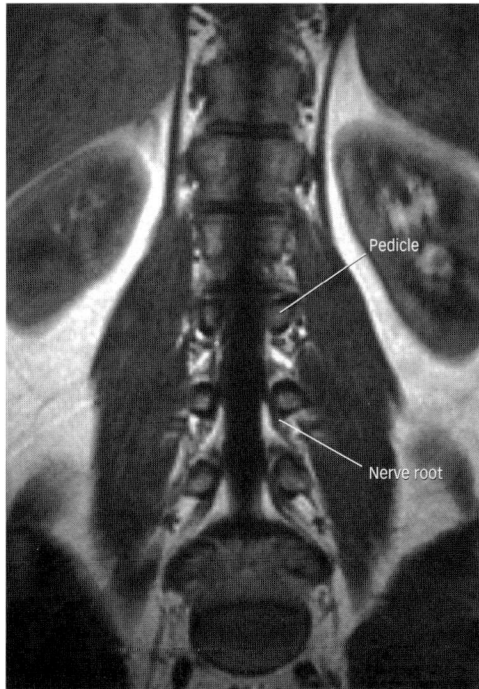

Fig. 45.
Lumbar myelogram to
show a conjoined root.

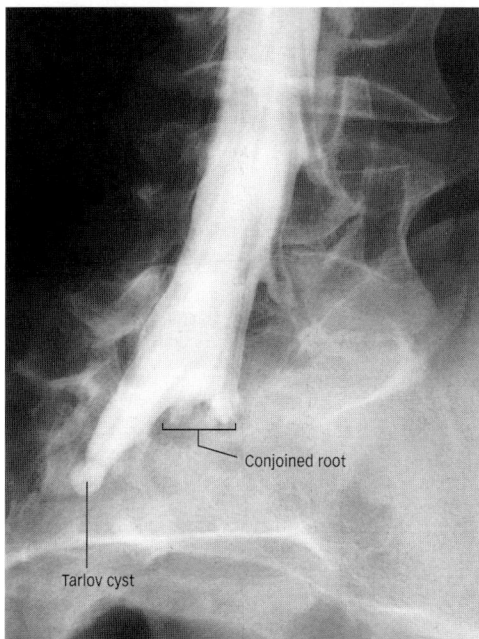

Fig. 46.
Perineural (Tarlov) cysts.
Lumbar myelogram.

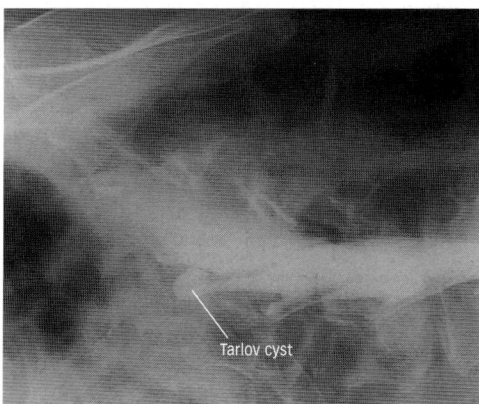

root, in particular, may not separate from the thecal sac at the same level on each side. Each nerve root therefore, lies initially above the neural foramen through which it exits (Fig. 44).

Two adjacent spinal roots may penetrate the dura at a single intervertebral level, forming a conjoined nerve root. The root sheath above is then absent. The conjoined root sleeve is large and composite, and is usually clearly seen at myelography (Fig. 45). The conjoined nerve root separates into single roots distal to the neural foramen. Occasionally, the conjoined root accompanies the nerve root below through its intervertebral canal. Conjoined nerve roots occur in about 1% of the population. They are usually unilateral and may occur at multiple levels. They usually occur at the lumbosacral level but may, less commonly, involve the first and second sacral roots.

Perineural cysts (of Tarlov) develop at the junction of the dorsal nerve root with the ganglion (Figs. 45, 46), between the perineurium (from the arachnoid) and the endoneurium (from the pia). They occur secondarily to enlargement of the arachnoid along the dorsal nerve roots. The walls of the cyst contain nerve fibres. They may be isolated or multiple and occur most commonly, but not exclusively, in the sacral region.

The spinal meninges

The spinal meningeal sheath encloses the spinal cord and accompanies the nerve roots into the intervertebral foramina. It forms a single covering for the neuraxis in continuity with the cerebral meninges, the spinal dura mater (or 'theca') being a continuation of the inner layer of the cerebral dura.

The spinal dural 'sac' extends from the posterior cranial fossa to the second segment of the sacrum. It is attached firmly to the tectorial membrane and posterior longitudinal ligament of the body of the axis but is free of bony or ligamentous attachments elsewhere. The outer periosteal layer of the dura is represented by the periosteum of the vertebrae and between these two dural layers is the extradural (or epidural) space. The spinal meninges extend laterally along the spinal nerve for a short distance beyond the intervertebral foramina and merge with the epineurium of the peripheral nerve. The extradural space contains a venous plexus and fat, the latter extending into the intervertebral foramina accompanying the nerve root within its dural sheath. The extradural space is capacious posteriorly in the cervical and thoracic spine, but only a potential space exits anteriorly. In the lower lumbar and sacrum regions, the extradural space may occupy more than half the cross-sectional area of the spinal canal.

The avascular arachnoid mater, within the dura, is connected to the pia mater by numerous fine, filamentous processes. The arachnoid is particularly well developed in the posterior midline, where it forms an incomplete posterior median septum, the cribriform septum. This septum is most prominent in the thoracic region. The spinal subarachnoid space, between the arachnoid and pia mater, contains approximately half of the total volume of cerebrospinal fluid (75 ml of the total 150 ml). It surrounds the nerve roots for a short distance into the intervertebral foramina. The spinal subdural space, as well as its intracranial equivalent, is a potential space between the arachnoid and dura.

The pia mater is a vascular membrane, applied to the surface of the spinal cord. It is prolonged over the spinal nerve roots and blends with their epineurium. At the distal end of the dural sheath or 'sleeve', surrounding each of the nerve roots, the three meningeal layers fuse. Inferiorly the pia is thickened with glial tissue to form the filum terminale. In some normal individuals, this may contain fat (Fig. 47). The filum terminale perforates the theca at the second sacral segmental level to descend to the coccyx, where it fuses with the periosteum of the first coccygeal segment.

The denticulate ligament partially divides the spinal subarachnoid space into an anterior and a posterior compartment from the foramen magnum to the conus medullaris. It is continuous with the pia medially and dura laterally (between the exiting nerves). The first lumbar nerve root lies at the lowest denticulation. The denticulate ligament, filum terminale and the attachment of the nerve roots together serve to stabilize the spinal cord within the dura.

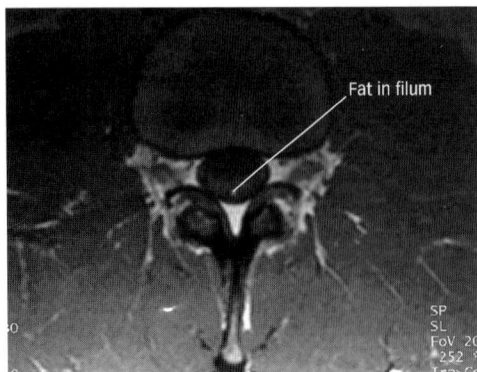

Fat in filum

Fig. 47.
T1W axial MRI showing fat in the filum terminale.

The dura and arachnoid mater are usually obscured by the bright signal from cerebrospinal fluid on T2W and from fat on T1W conventional MRI. However, the dura can be seen on T2*, (T2 'star'), gradient echo image. Rarely, the denticulate ligament and vessels are seen in the subarachnoid space.

The blood supply to the spinal cord

Arterial supply

The spinal cord is supplied by one anterior and two posterolateral spinal arteries, with important contributions from the segmental radicular arteries. The anterior spinal artery runs in the midline, in the anterior median fissure, and is formed at the level of the foramen magnum by the union of the anterior spinal branch of each vertebral artery. It usually arises from the intracranial segment of the vertebral artery on each side, but occasionally both arise from one vertebral artery or one may arise from an anastomotic channel joining the vertebral arteries. These branches unite with the upper end of the anterior spinal artery high in the cervical region. Embryologically, the anterior spinal artery commences as a paired structure which undergoes fusion during development, sometimes leaving persisting paired segments and sometimes becoming very attenuated or discontinuous, particularly in the thoracic region. Its calibre, in the cervical cord, may also vary. Caudally, the anterior spinal artery divides and anastomoses with the posterolateral arteries to form an anastomotic loop around the conus medullaris. Arteries ascending from the filum terminale and cauda equina also join this anastomosis. These ascending arteries arise from the lumbar arteries and/or the internal iliac arteries via their lateral sacral branches and from the medial sacral artery. The anterior spinal artery supplies the whole of the spinal cord with the exception of the posterior horns of grey matter and the dorsal columns (which approximates to two-thirds of its cross-sectional area).

The radicular arteries enter the spinal canal through the intervertebral foramina and penetrate the meninges to run alongside the nerve root (Fig. 48). In the cervical region, radicular arteries usually arise from branches of the vertebral or deep cervical arteries. Occasionally, they may arise from the costocervical trunk and, rarely, one may originate from the thyrocervical branch of the subclavian artery. These vessels may therefore be filled with contrast medium during thyroid or parathyroid angiography, with the potential risk of spinal cord damage. In the thoracic region the two supreme intercostal branches of the subclavian artery and the aortic intercostal arteries give rise to the radicular branches. Radicular branches to the lumbosacral region are supplied by the lumbar and the medial and lateral sacral arteries. The radiculomedullary arteries are radicular arteries, which contribute to the anterior spinal artery. The anterior spinal artery is, in effect, a composite of anastomosing ascending and descending branches of a limited number of anterior radiculomedullary arteries. The origin and number of radiculomedullary arteries are very variable but there are usually between six and ten. These ascend before hooking over to enter the anterior median sulcus at an increasingly steep angle for branches arising at lower at lower aortic levels. The anastomosing vessels vary considerably in calibre and some of them may be so narrow as to be virtually non-functioning. Flow throughout the entire length of the anterior spinal artery may not be maintained if one of the radiculomedullary arteries is occluded.

The posterior aspect of the spinal cord is surrounded by a network of arteries, forming a plexus in which two posterolateral spinal arteries can be identified. The posterolateral spinal arteries arise from one or two branches on each side, which may arise, in turn, from the posterior inferior cerebellar arteries. Each posterolateral spinal artery forms a long trunk that runs behind the posterior nerve rootlets along the length of the cord. They gain numerous arterial inputs from the posterior radiculomedullary arteries. The two posterior arteries supply the posterior white matter columns and the dorsal horns of the spinal cord. The posterolateral circulation is well developed in the cervical and lumbar region and some, often poorly developed, anastomoses exist between the three main spinal arteries.

Three major vascular territories of the spinal cord can be identified. The superior territory includes the cervical cord and the upper two thoracic segments. Three radiculomedullary arteries usually supply this region, accompanying the third, sixth and eighth cervical nerve roots. The sixth cervical radiculomedullary artery is called the artery of the cervical enlargement and is the largest of the three.

The intermediate territory corresponds to the third to the eighth thoracic cord segments. This region is rather poorly vascularized but is supplied from one of the upper intercostal arteries.

The inferior territory of the spinal cord extends from the eighth thoracic segment to the filum terminale. The main arterial supply to this region is provided by the artery of the lumbar enlargement, the arteria radicularis magna (of Adamkiewicz). It usually arises between the ninth thoracic and first lumbar segments, most commonly from the tenth or eleventh thoracic radicular arteries. It arises from the left side in 80% of cases. When it originates below the second lumbar, or above the eighth thoracic radicular arteries, a second major arterial contribution to the anterior spinal artery complex will be found. The morphology of the radiculomedullary junction with the anterior spinal artery varies with the spinal cord segment. The classic hairpin bend is seen at the thoracolumbar level (Fig. 49), but a Y-shaped junction is seen in the cervical segments.

The inconstancy of the origin of the artery of Adamkiewicz is a relevant factor when paraplegia occurs as a complication of aortography. The lumbar arteries extend posterolaterally from the aorta and varying amounts of hyperosmolar contrast medium

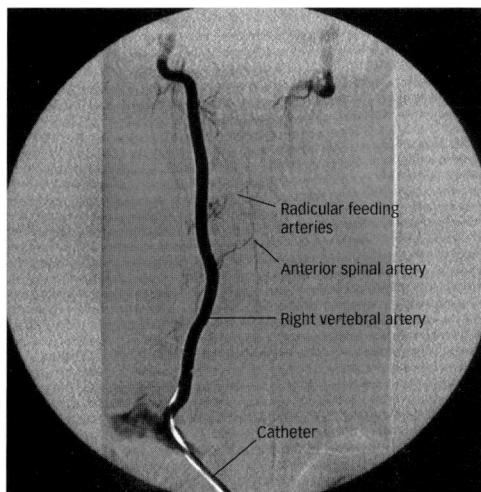

Fig. 48.
Vertebral angiogram showing the anterior spinal artery and radicular arteries.

Radicular feeding arteries

Anterior spinal artery

Right vertebral artery

Catheter

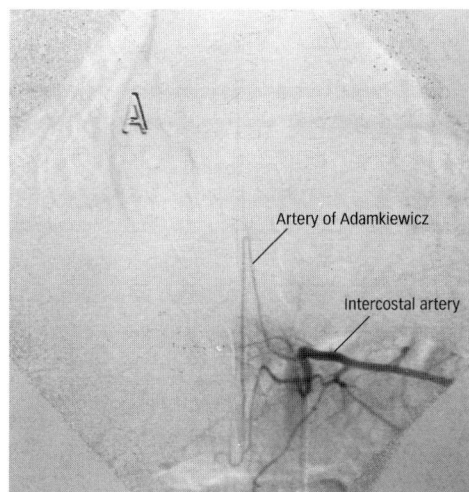

Artery of Adamkiewicz

Intercostal artery

Fig. 49.
The artery of Adamkiewicz arising from the intercostal artery on the left at the level of the ninth thoracic vertebra.

will be directed towards these arteries and hence the spinal arteries. This is especially likely in cases of aortic stenosis, and spinal cord dysfunction may result.

An anterior radiculomedullary artery may arise from a conjoined trunk together with one of the bronchial arteries, and this variant should be specifically sought before therapeutic embolization of a bronchial artery is performed.

The anterior spinal artery provides several sulcocommissural vessels to each spinal segment. These each provide multiple perforating arteries to each side of the spinal cord in an alternating fashion. The circulation from the arteries on each side of the spinal cord splay in the longitudinal axis of the cord with significant overlap, so that occlusion of a single vessel may not produce ischaemia. The intramedullary circulation arises from the anterior spinal artery centrally and from the posterolateral arteries peripherally, with the pial network of vessels around the cord. The anterior spinal artery has sulcal branches at each segmental level of the cord. These sulcal arteries supply the anterior portion of the cord. The arterial vasa corona (lateral pial network) is a plexus of smaller arteries within the pia, which connects the posterolateral and the anterior spinal arteries. A posterior pial network lies in the midline and supplies the posterior spinal cord bilaterally. Radial perforating arteries, originating from the pial network, penetrate the white matter and supply the periphery of the spinal cord.

Small glomus-like structures of uncertain function are present where the dorsal nerve roots penetrate the dura mater. They are supplied by the posterior radicular and radiculomedullary arteries. They are important because shunting of blood through them into the perimedullary venous plexus may be an important factor in the causation of dural arteriovenous fistulae.

Venous drainage

The veins of the spinal cord substance drain radially to the cord surface, where they form the perimedullary or coronal venous plexus. This pial network collects into longitudinal venous channels. The posterior spinal vein is the largest of these and receives all the venous blood from the lateral surface. The anterior spinal vein runs parallel to the anterior spinal artery. It is usually a single vein in the lumbar region, but there are two in the cervical and thoracic regions.

The intrinsic venous system within the cord consists of a capillary network anastomosing in the axial plane and following the grey and white matter tracts vertically. The perimedullary venous plexus is valveless and drains into the epidural plexus which, in turn, drains into the paraspinal veins through the intervertebral foramina. The basivertebral veins also drain into the epidural plexus.

An arteriovenous fistula entering any of the communicating veins around the spinal cord may increase pressure and flow throughout the perimedullary venous plexus and induce spinal cord dysfunction.

References

Coleman, L.T., Zimmerman, R.A. & Rorke, L.B. (1995). Ventriculus terminalis of the conus medullaris: MR findings in children. *American Journal of Neuroradiology*, **16**, 1421–6.

Daffner, R.H. (1996). *Imaging of Vertebral Trauma*. 2nd edn. Philadelphia: Lippincott Raven.

Denis, F. (1983). The three column spine and its significance in the classification of acute thoracolumbar spinal fractures. *Spine*, **8**, 817–31.

Harris, J.H., Burke, J.T., Ray, R.D. *et al.* (1984). Low (type III) odontoid fracture: a new radiographic sign. *Radiology*, **153**, 353–6.

Further reading

Epstein, B.S. (1976). *The Spine*. 4th edn. Philadelphia: Lea & Febiger.

Manelfe, C. (ed.) (1992). *Imaging of the Spine and Spinal Cord*. New York: Raven.

16

The musculoskeletal system 1: the upper limb

A.W. M. MITCHELL
and C. W. HERON

Roentgen produced the first radiological image on November 8th 1895, which was of his wife's hand. Since those early days, radiographic imaging techniques have been developed and refined but the mainstay of skeletal imaging is still the plain radiograph.

Classical plain film radiography gives information about the bones, joints and to a lesser extent the soft tissues. Satisfactory demonstration of these structures requires appropriate radiographic technique, precise positioning and correct choice of views. Appreciation of the normal changes with age and common variants is also needed for accurate interpretation.

Newer sophisticated imaging methods can provide complementary anatomical information that could previously only be obtained by direct inspection.

Anatomy

Anatomical descriptions of the upper limb structures are based on the 'standard anatomical position'. Radiographs are not obtained in this manner, but aim to demonstrate the region in question so that the components are opti-

mally visualized. The three-dimensional perspective of bone and soft tissue is lost on the two-dimensional radiograph; therefore, structures may be superimposed or not appreciated. Standard radiological practice is to obtain two views, usually at 90 degrees to each other; occasionally supplementary views may be required, e.g. of the scaphoid bone.

The growth and development of all bones are determined by genetic and mechanical factors. In both axial and longitudinal planes, growth is asymmetrical. It is important to

(b)

Fig. 1.
The scapula. The diagram demonstrates the three views of the scapula: (*a*) anterior, (*b*) posterior, (*c*) lateral.

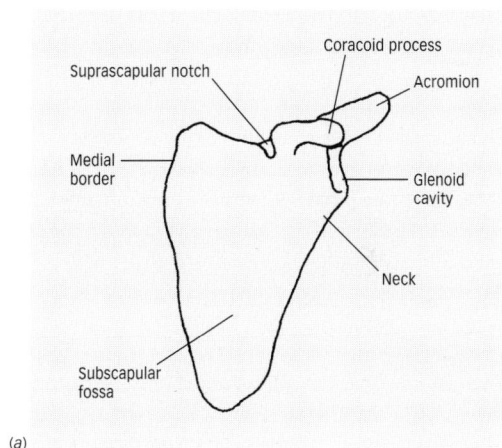

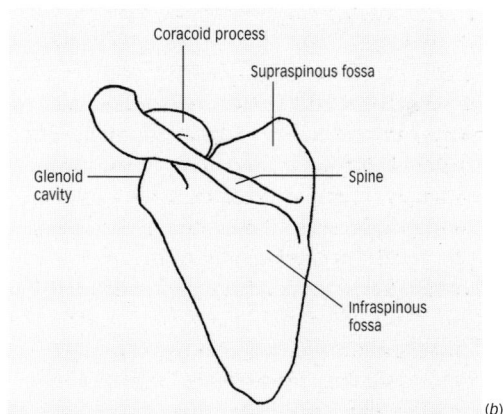

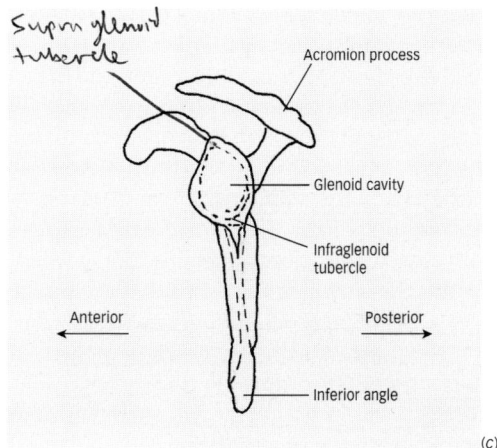

(a)

(c)

(a)

Anterior

Labels (anterior diagram):
- Coracobrachialis and short head of biceps
- Pectoralis minor
- Coracoid process
- Supraspinatus (lesser tubercle) [handwritten: greater]
- Subscapularis (greater tubercle) [handwritten: lesser]
- Latissimus dorsi
- Pectoralis major
- Teres major
- Deltoid
- Subscapularis
- Serratus anterior
- Triceps long head
- Coracobrachialis
- Brachialis
- Brachioradialis
- Pronator teres
- Extensor carpi radialis longus
- Common extensor origin
- Common flexor origin
- Flexor digitorum superficialis
- Brachialis
- Biceps (bicipital tuberosity)
- Pronator teres

Posterior

Labels (posterior diagram):
- Levator scapulae
- Supraspinatus
- Trapezius
- Deltoid
- Infraspinatus ⎫ Greater tubercle
- Teres minor ⎭
- Rhomboid minor
- Long head triceps
- Infraspinatus
- Teres major
- Rhomboid major
- Lateral head triceps
- Deltoid
- Latissmus dorsi
- Teres minor
- Triceps medial-head
- Medial supracondylar ridge
- Lateral epicondyle
- Medial epicondyle
- Anconeus
- Triceps insertion
- Olecranon
- Radial head

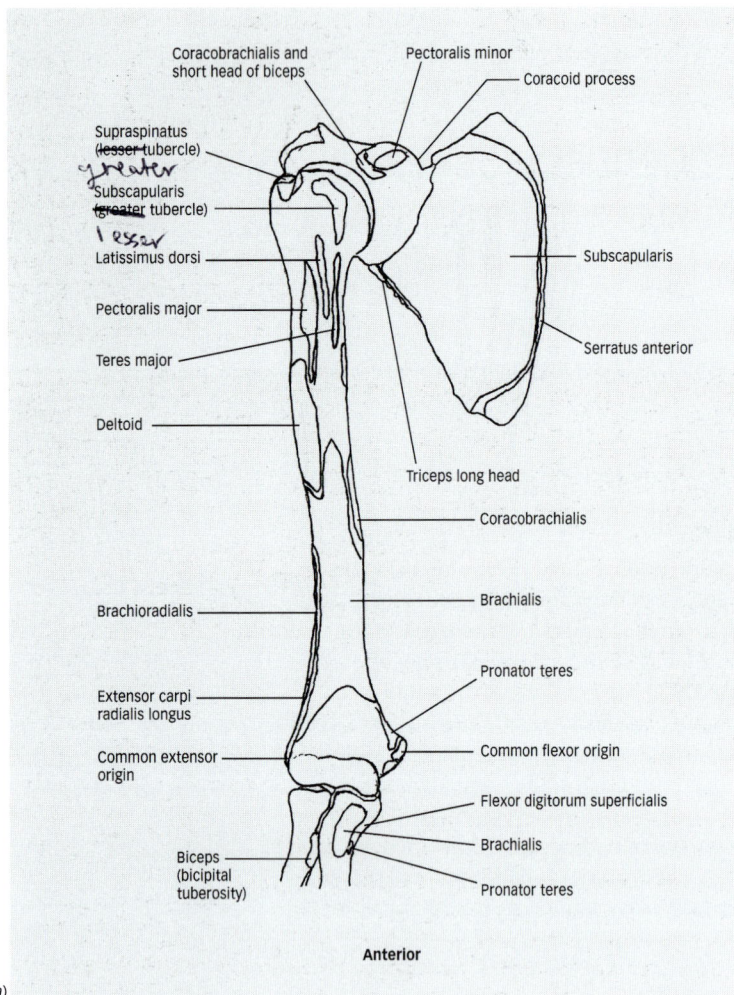

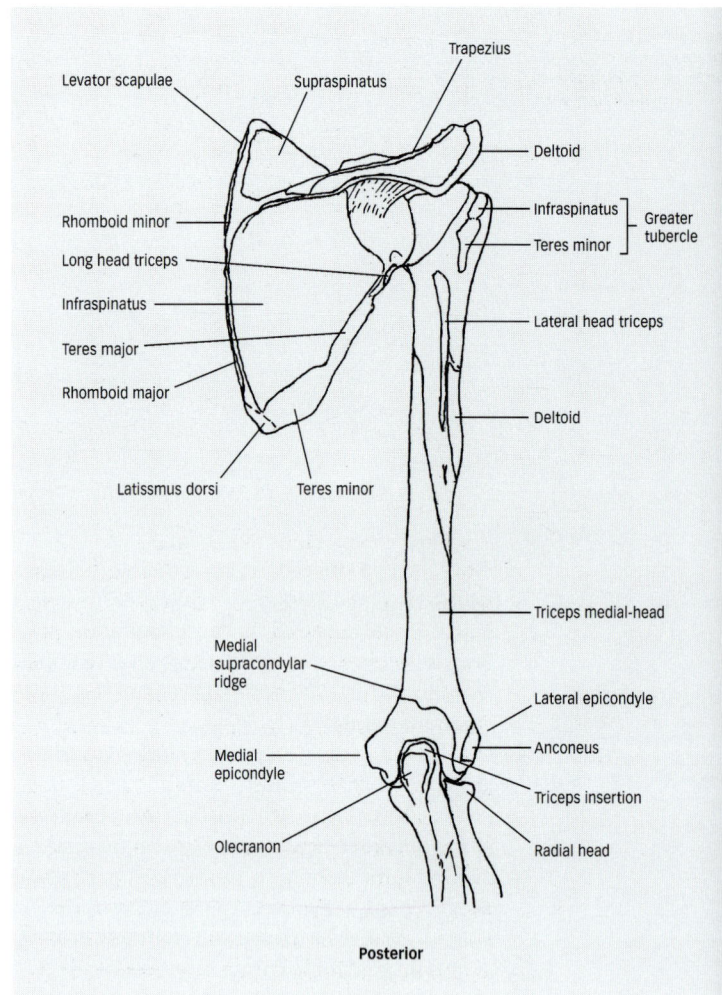

Fig. 2.
Muscular attachments of the shoulder girdle. The anterior (*a*) and posterior (*b*) diagrams demonstrate the origins and insertions of the muscles that provide movement and stability about the shoulder joint.

appreciate the effect of this differential growth as the nutrient arteries, which originally enter the mid-shaft of the bone in the fetus, run obliquely through the cortex in the adult and can be mistaken for fractures (a useful *aide-mémoire* for the direction of the nutrient artery is 'to the elbow they go: from the knee they flee').

The scapula

The scapula (Fig. 1) is a triangular bone whose apex lies inferiorly. It has two surfaces, a costal and a dorsal surface, which are curved to fit the contour of the posterior thoracic wall. The body (or blade) of the scapula is thin and flat from which the glenoid cavity and the coracoid process project laterally. At right angles to the body of the scapula, the spine projects posteriorly, separating the suprascapular from the infrascapular fossa. The spine continues laterally to form the acromion process, under which passes the tendon of the supraspinatus muscle. In the anatomical position, the inferior angle of the scapula lies approximately over the lower border of the seventh rib posteriorly, which is a useful guideline for centring when obtaining the chest radiograph.

Ossification

Ossification of the scapula is first demonstrated in the eighth week of fetal life. The ossification centre of the coracoid process is seen in the first year and fuses with the scapula at 14 years. Further secondary ossification centres are seen around the time of puberty in the acromion, two within the glenoid fossa and a further two centres on the medial border and inferior pole of the scapula fusing at approximately 25 years. An os acromiale may be demonstrated in the axial view and is present in 10% of the normal population.

Scapulothoracic joint

The scapula is able to undertake a complex series of movements against the thoracic wall. Attached to its borders are a series of muscles which suspend and anchor the scapula to the axial and appendicular skeleton whilst permitting freedom of movement (Fig. 2(*a*), (*b*)).

The Clavicle

The clavicle (Fig. 3) is an S-shaped bone between the scapula and the manubrium. It contains no medullary cavity because of its mesenchymal

Fig. 3.
he clavicle. The diagrams
present two views of the
vicle: (a) superior aspect,
(b) inferior aspect.

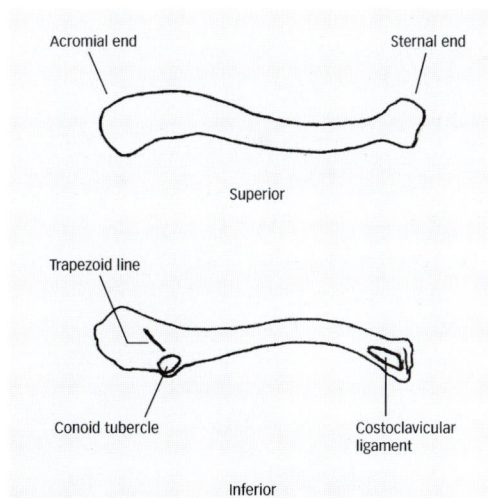

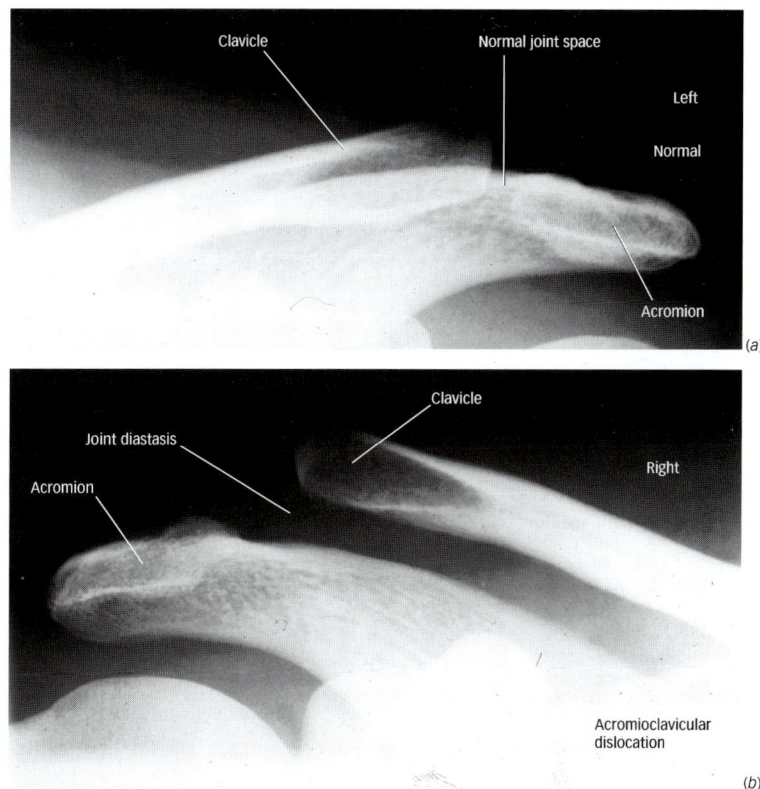

Fig. 4.
Radiograph of the acromioclavicular joint. (a) Normal left acromioclavicular joint. In the normal subect, the acromioclavicular relationship is maintained. (b) Right acromioclavicular joint dislocation. Note the discontinuity of the acromioclavicular line implying disruption of the weak acromioclavicular and coracoacromial ligaments.

developmental origin. Occasionally, it may appear fenestrated in the mid-portion where the supraclavicular nerves from the cervical plexus traverse the diaphysis. The medial end of the bone is enlarged to allow a wide range of movement at the manubriosternal joint about the rhomboid ligament which acts as a fulcrum. The rhomboid ligament (costoclavicular ligament) is attached to the inferomedial aspect of the clavicle and inserts on to the first costal cartilage. In approximately 5% of individuals, an irregular groove in the clavicle, termed the rhomboid fossa, is present at the site of origin of the rhomboid ligament and should not be mistaken for a pathological entity. The lateral aspect of the clavicle is flattened and slightly tapered to provide a surface to articulate with the acromion process at the acromioclavicular joint. Two further ligaments, the conoid (medially) and the trapezoid (laterally), take origin from the inferolateral surface of the clavicle, providing a second fulcrum of movement about their point of insertion at the base of the coracoid process, to make up the coracoclavicular ligament.

Radiographically, the clavicles are always demonstrated on the frontal chest radiograph; their medial ends are projected over the posterior aspects of the fourth ribs.

Ossification
This is the first bone to ossify and is formed in membrane, appearing after the first fetal month. Secondary centres appear at approximately 16 years at the medial end and fuse at 25 years. Occasionally, small pits may be demonstrated within the diaphysis of the clavicle and are related to the passage of the supraclavicular nerves through the bone rather than anterior to it.

The acromioclavicular joint
The acromioclavicular joint (Fig. 4(a)) is a complex synovial joint between the lateral end of

the clavicle and the medial border of the acromion. An incomplete fibrocartilaginous disc is often present; it crosses the joint cavity which is surrounded by a poorly formed sleeve or capsule known as the acromioclavicular ligament. The conoid and trapezoid ligaments provide the principal stability of the joint. Together they constitute the coracoclavicular ligament. In order to assess the integrity of the joint and the ligaments, plain radiographs of the joints (i.e. left and right) should be obtained in the erect position with weight-bearing and non-weight-bearing views as disruption of the acromioclavicular ligament will result in widening of the joint space when stressed (Fig. 4(b)). Injuries resulting in disruption of the conoid and trapezoid ligaments will produce superior subluxation of the lateral end of the clavicle and further joint space widening.

Radiologically the acromioclavicular joint is important because it has a close superior relationship to the supraspinatus muscle and tendon (Fig. 5). Arthropathic conditions, e.g. osteoarthritis, affecting the inferior aspect of the joint may cause impingement on the tendon and damage to it. Imaging plays a crucial role in the diagnosis and the management of the tendinous lesions. Specific views of the joint examine the inferior aspect *en face* (30 degrees tube-angled cephalad (Fig. 6)) and tangentially (30 degrees angled caudally), centred about the joint, provide valuable information about the bony contours and tendon calcification.

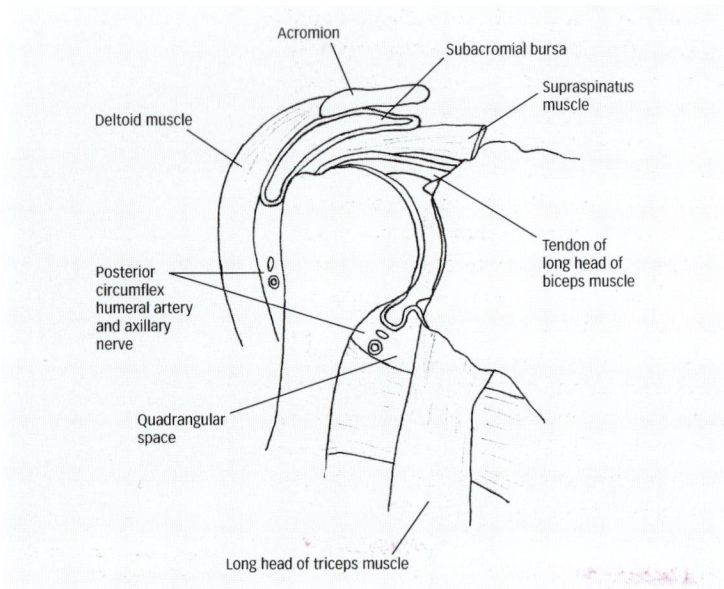

Fig. 5.
Coronal section of the subacromial region and the shoulder joint. The section demonstrates the relationship of the subacromial–subdeltoid bursa to the supraspinatus tendon. The subacromiosubdeltoid bursa does not communicate with the glenohumeral joint unless the supraspinatus tendon is ruptured.

There is some variability in the normal distance between the superior aspect of the humerus and the inferior margin of the acromion. However, a distance of less than 5 mm is indicative of a tear in the supraspinatus tendon.

The axilla

The axilla is the anatomical region between the lateral aspect of the chest wall and the upper limb. It takes the shape of a truncated pyramid and thus has six sides.

Apex

The apex forms the junction between the posterior triangle of the neck and the arm. It is bounded by the scapula, the middle third of the clavicle and the outer border of the first rib.

Anterior wall

This is formed by the pectoralis major, pectoralis minor, subclavius and the clavipectoral fascia.

Fig. 6.
Radiograph of the acromioclavicular joint. (Radiograph: 30 degree cephalad beam.) The angulation demonstrates the joint en face.

Posterior wall

The posterior wall is formed by the subscapularis, latissimus dorsi, and teres major.

Medial wall

The medial wall is bounded by the serratus anterior and intercostal muscles.

Lateral wall

This is much narrower than the other sides of the axilla. It is formed by the intertubercular (bicipital) groove of the humerus. In the floor of the intertubercular groove runs the tendon of the long head of biceps and about its borders are the pectoralis major, latissimus dorsi and pectoralis minor, which insert on to the lateral lip of the groove, the floor and the medial lip, respectively.

Base

The base is formed by the axillary fascia, the subcutaneous tissues and skin.

The contents of the axilla are the axillary artery and vein, the cords and terminal branches of the brachial plexus, the coracobrachialis and biceps muscles, the axillary lymph nodes, lymphatics and fat.

The axillary artery, as it passes through the axilla, is surrounded by the cords and branches of the brachial plexus (see below). The axillary vein lies medial to this neurovascular bundle, all of which are enclosed within the axillary sheath. The axillary sheath is a continuation of the prevertebral fascia and forms an important compartment. The axillary artery is occasionally used to obtain vascular access; any extravization of blood into this space can compress the cords of the brachial plexus and produce a neuropraxia.

The axilla contains numerous lymph nodes that receive lymph from the upper limb, the

Fig. 7.
The shoulder joint.

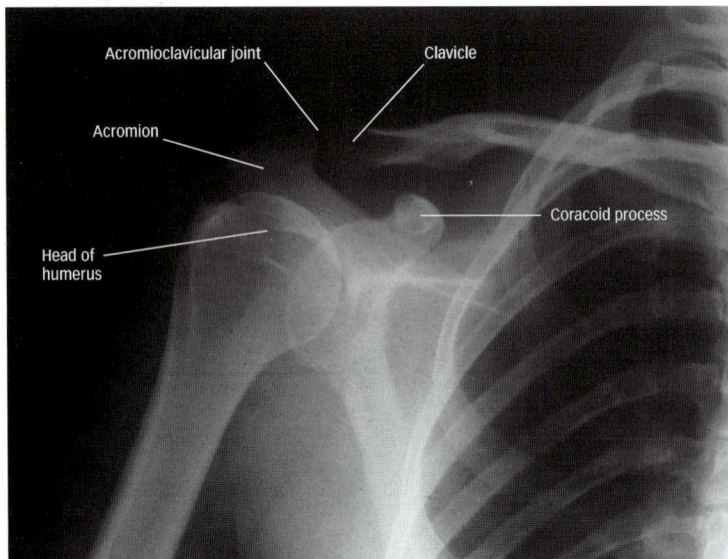

Acromioclavicular joint · Clavicle · Acromion · Coracoid process · Head of humerus

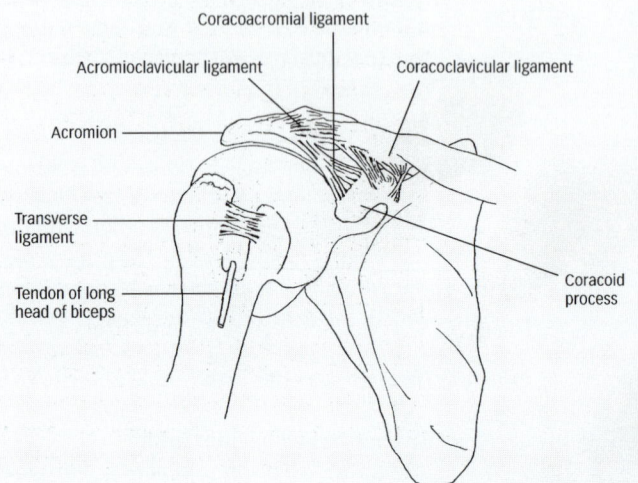

Coracoacromial ligament · Acromioclavicular ligament · Coracoclavicular ligament · Acromion · Transverse ligament · Tendon of long head of biceps · Coracoid process

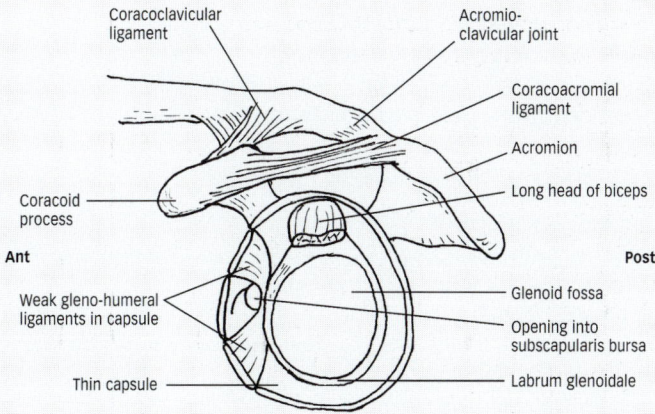

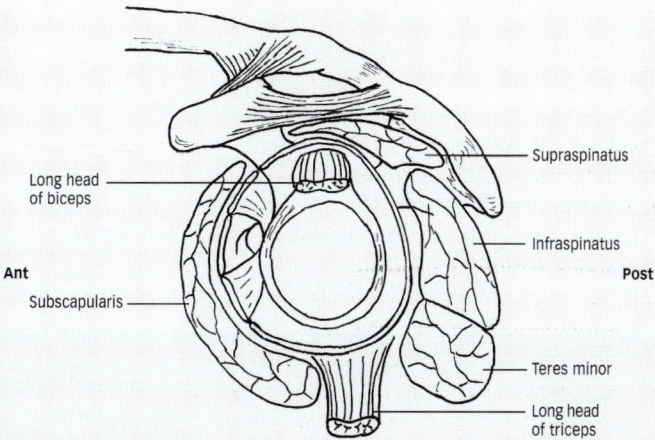

Coracoclavicular ligament
Acromio-clavicular joint
Coracoacromial ligament
Acromion
Long head of biceps
Coracoid process
Glenoid fossa
Opening into subscapularis bursa
Ant
Post
Weak gleno-humeral ligaments in capsule
Labrum glenoidale
Thin capsule

Long head of biceps
Supraspinatus
Infraspinatus
Ant
Post
Subscapularis
Teres minor
Long head of triceps

Fig. 8.
The shoulder joint: oblique parasagittal view. The diagrams show the close relationship of the muscles of the rotator cuff to the shoulder joint. (a) Left shoulder joint: its ligaments are shown after removal of the humerus (b) As (a) but with the addition of the surrounding muscles.

orly by the three glenohumeral ligaments (Fig. 8). The coracohumeral ligament also passes between the under surface of the coracoid process to the lesser tubercle and continues to form the intertubercular or transverse ligament under which runs the long head of the tendon of biceps. The synovial membrane is attached around the glenoid labrum and to the anatomical neck of the humerus. The tendon of the long head of biceps is enclosed within the synovium and passes through the joint and beneath the intertubercular ligament. The subscapular bursa lies deep to the subscapularis muscle, separating it from the neck of the scapula and the shoulder joint, and is formed by a herniation of the shoulder joint synovial membrane through a defect in the glenohumeral ligament. A subacromial–subdeltoid bursa is situated superior to the

breast and the chest wall. The superficial lymphatics of the upper limb tend to accompany the veins, whereas the deep lymphatics accompany the arteries. The nodes are arranged into five groups, namely, the pectoral, the lateral, the subscapular, the central and the apical groups. The apical nodal group receives lymph from all the groups. Most of the lymph from the upper limb is to the lateral group of axillary nodes with the exception of the first web space and thumb, which drain to the infraclavicular nodal group. MRI and CT may detect enlarged nodes and are therefore of value in the assessment of certain disease processes.

The shoulder joint

The shoulder joint is a ball and socket synovial joint (Fig. 7). The capsule of the shoulder joint is strong but is lax inferiorly. It is attached proximally to the glenoid labrum, which is a fibrocartilaginous ring that deepens the glenoid fossa, and distally to the anatomical neck of the humerus, encroaching inferiorly on the neck of the bone. The effect of the fibrocartilaginous ring is to enlarge the articular surface by two thirds. The capsule is thickened anteri-

Fig. 9.
MRI oblique parasagittal view. T1 weighted image.

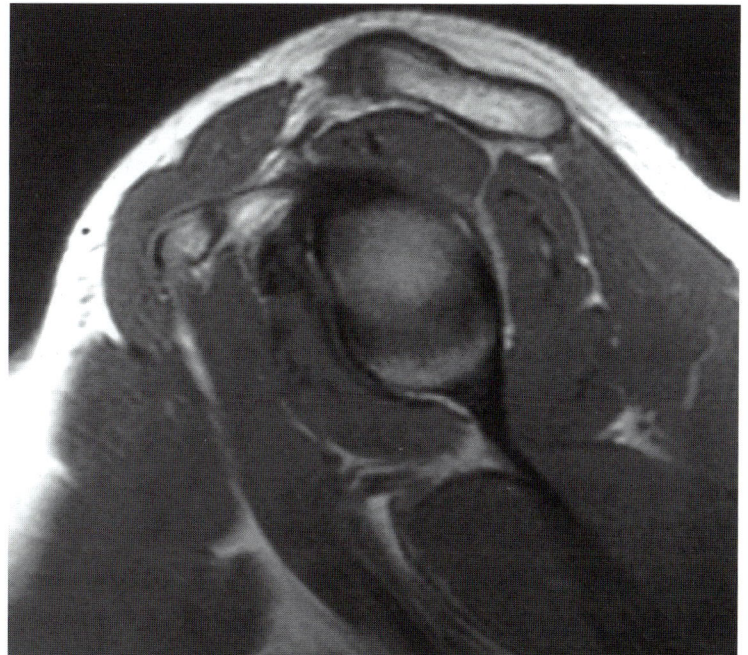

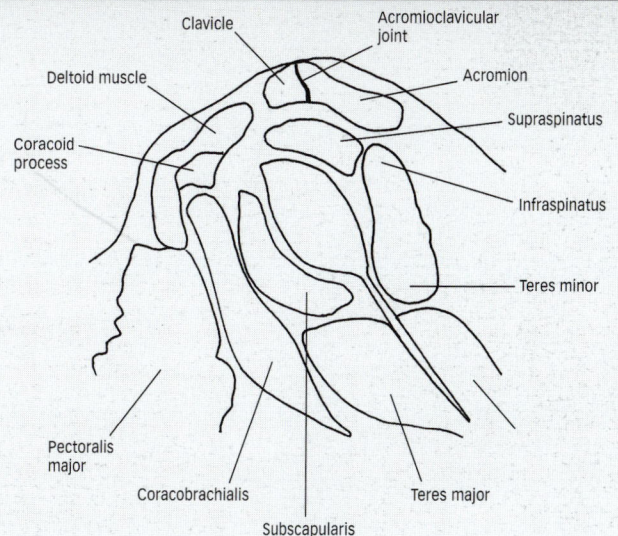

Clavicle
Acromioclavicular joint
Deltoid muscle
Acromion
Coracoid process
Supraspinatus
Infraspinatus
Teres minor
Pectoralis major
Coracobrachialis
Teres major
Subscapularis

supraspinatus muscle and tendon and inferior to the coracoacromial arch and the deep surface of the deltoid muscle (Fig. 7). There is no communication with the shoulder joint unless the supraspinatus tendon is ruptured.

The principal muscles involved in the stability and movement of the shoulder are referred to as the rotator cuff muscles. The four muscles which form the rotator cuff are (Fig. 9):

- The **subscapularis** which is attached to the costal surface of the scapula and the lesser tubercle of the humerus.
- The **supraspinatus** which is attached to the supraspinous fossa of the scapula and the superior facet of the greater tubercle of the humerus.

- The **infraspinatus** which is attached to the infraspinatus fossa of the scapula and the middle facet of the greater tubercle of the humerus.
- The **teres minor** which is attached to the lateral border of the scapula and the inferior facet of the greater tubercle of the humerus.

Further movement, power and stability are provided by the biceps muscle, latissimus dorsi, teres major, deltoid and the pectoralis major muscles (Fig. 2(a), (b)).

The standard plain radiographic views are the anteroposterior and the axial projections (Fig. 10(a), (b)). If, following trauma, shoulder abduction is limited and the axial view cannot be obtained, further views should be performed by alternative means. The Strip view provides a 'pseudo' (or near) axial view and is obtained in the seated position. The patient holds the film above the shoulder and leans backwards by 15 degrees. The tube is positioned on the ground and directed cephalad. The trans-scapular projection (Fig. 10(c)) centres the X-ray beam through the head of the humerus and the long axis of the scapula. Thus three congruous semicircles can be

Fig. 10.
Standard radiographic projections of the shoulder (a) Anteroposterior view. (b) Axial view. (c) Transscapular view. The three curved lines of congruence the superior aspect of the glenoid fossa, the head of the humerus and the inferior borders of acromion process and clavicle.

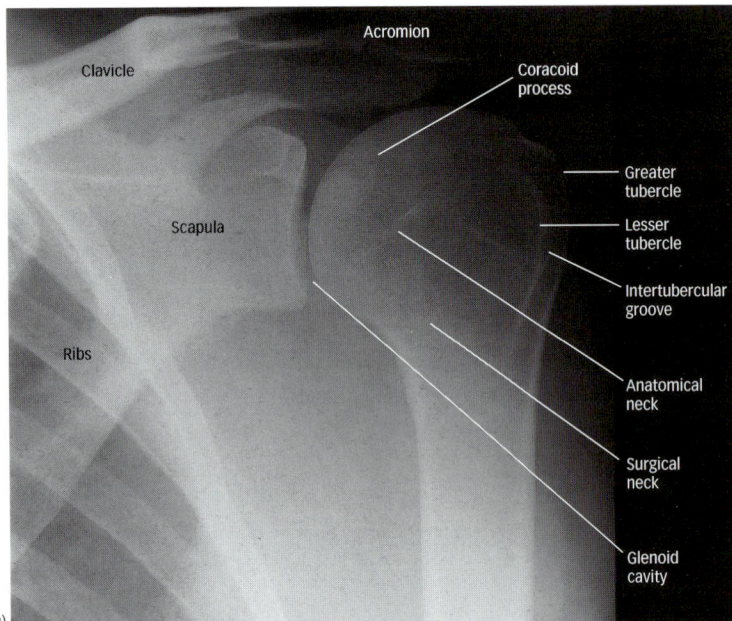

(a)

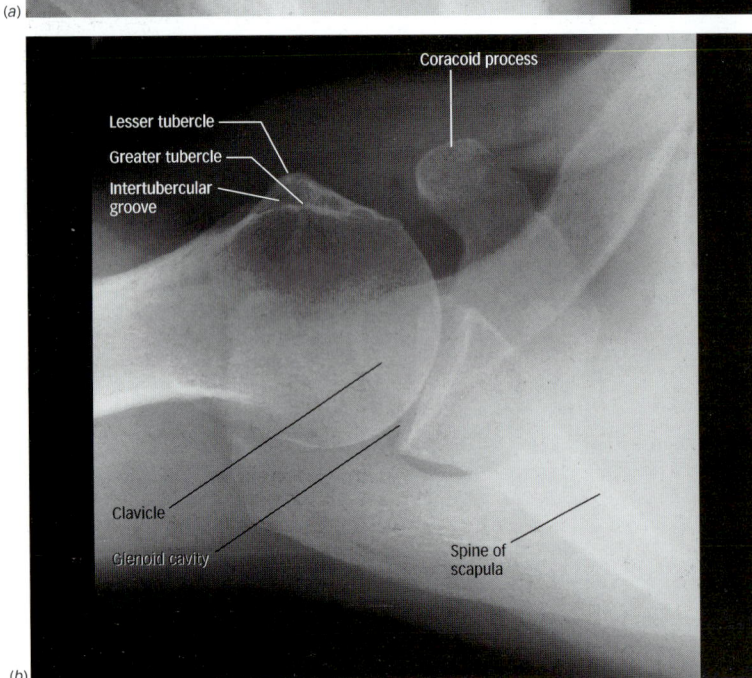

(b)

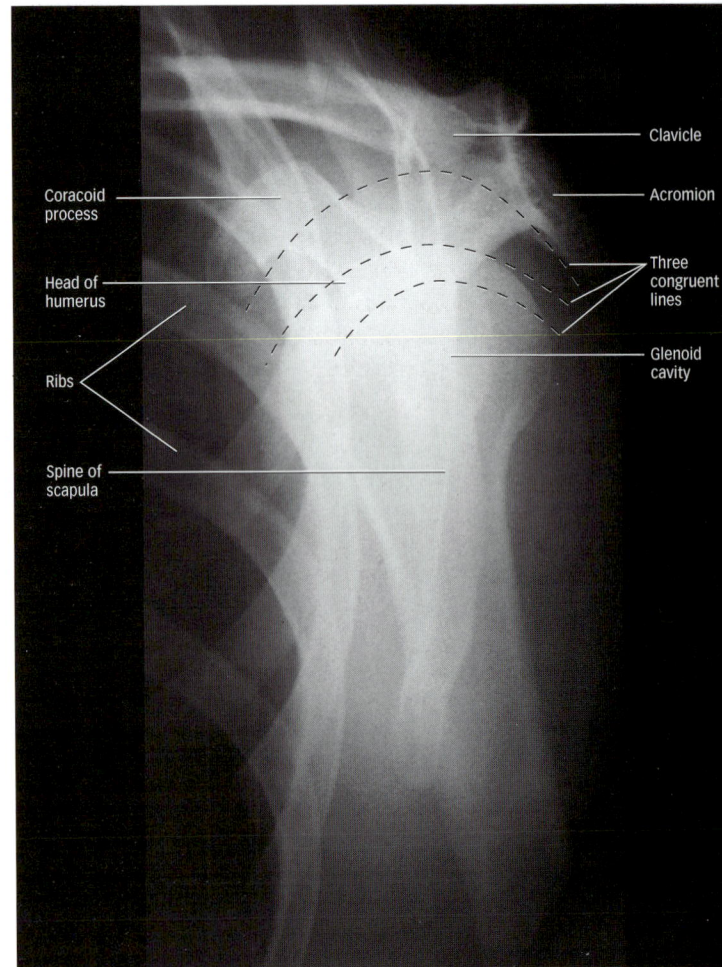

Coracoid process

Humeral head

Acromion

Glenoid cavity

Acromio-clavicular joint

Clavicle

Rib

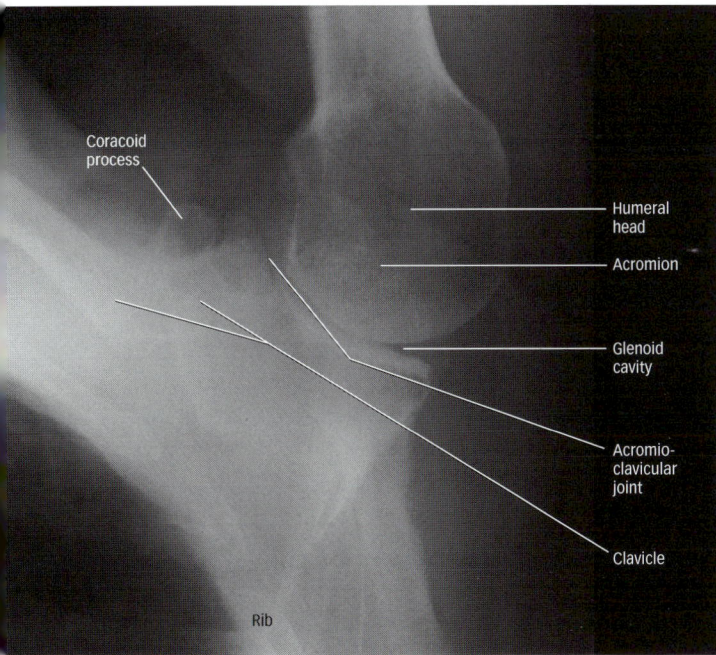

Fig. 11.
Striker's view of the shoulder. This view demonstrates the posterior aspect of the humeral head. The view is obtained by a 25 degrees cephalad beam with the patient supine and the humerus at 90 degrees to the table.

(a)

Internal rotation

Subscapularis bursa

Tendon of long head of biceps

Fig. 12.
Shoulder arthrograms. Contrast and air are introduced into the shoulder joint. The films demonstrate the axillary fold, the tendon of the long head of biceps and the inferior margin of the supraspinatus. (a) Internal rotation. (b) External rotation.

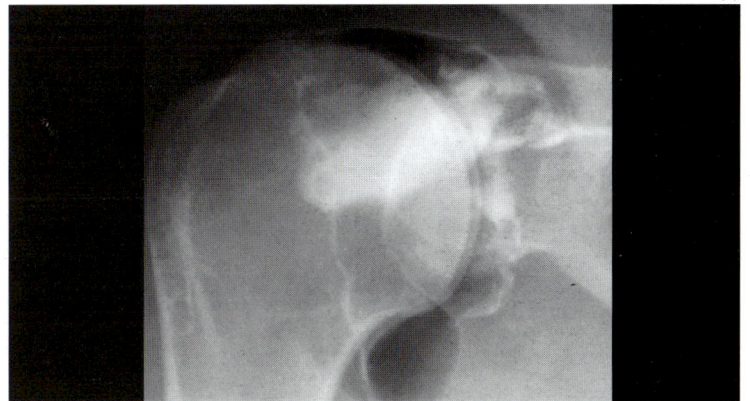

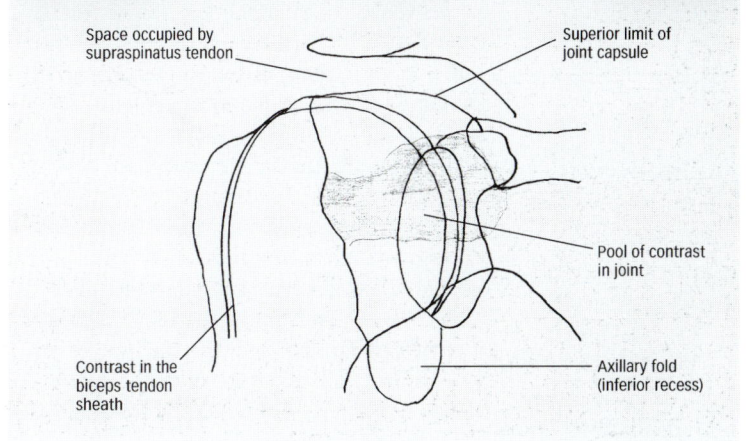

(b)

Space occupied by supraspinatus tendon

Superior limit of joint capsule

Pool of contrast in joint

Contrast in the biceps tendon sheath

Axillary fold (inferior recess)

demonstrated namely, the glenoid, the head of the humerus and the arc formed by the acromion process and the acromioclavicular joint. To demonstrate the posterior aspect of the head, and visualize cortical defects that may occur with anterior shoulder dislocation (i.e. the Hill–Sachs lesion), a Strikers' view is performed. The patient is supine with the humerus 90 degrees to the table, the tube is centred on the humeral head and angled 25 degrees cephalad (Fig. 11).

Double contrast arthrography (air and water-soluble contrast medium), was principally employed to demonstrate the integrity of the rotator cuff. In this role, it has largely been superseded by MRI. CT arthrography is of value in the assessment of the integrity of the glenoid labrum. Fine sections (2 mm) are obtained in the axial projection through the joint. Traditionally, the patient has been positioned in the supine position, but the prone oblique projection has been shown to provide further information about the posterior aspects of the glenoid labrum and the capsular attachments, which are important structures in the assessment of patients with previous posterior dislocations of the shoulder joint.

Arthrography, in combination with CT or MRI may be used to assess the following structures (Figs. 12 and 13):

- the bony configuration of the humeral head and glenoid;
- supraspinatus tendon: if contrast passes from the shoulder joint into the subacromial–subdeltiod bursa disruption of the tendon/muscle is implied (Fig. 7);

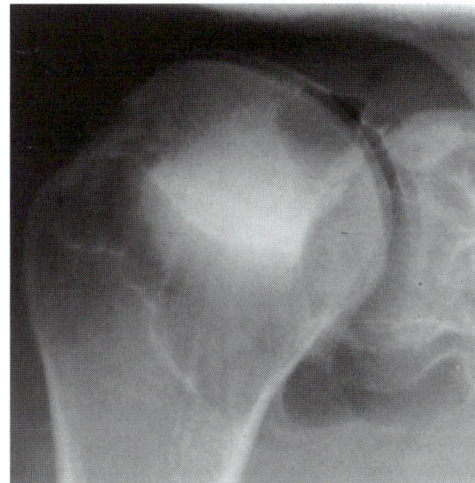

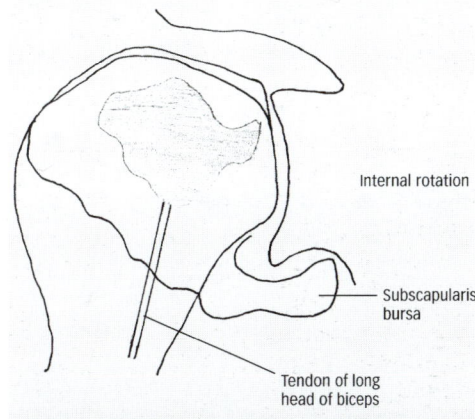

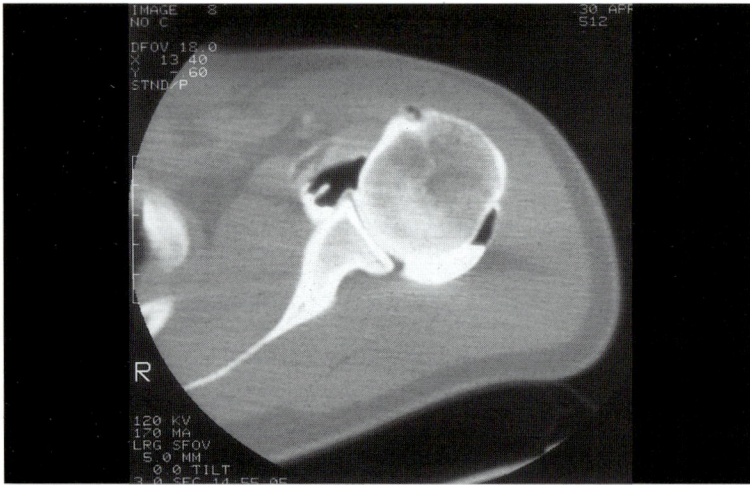

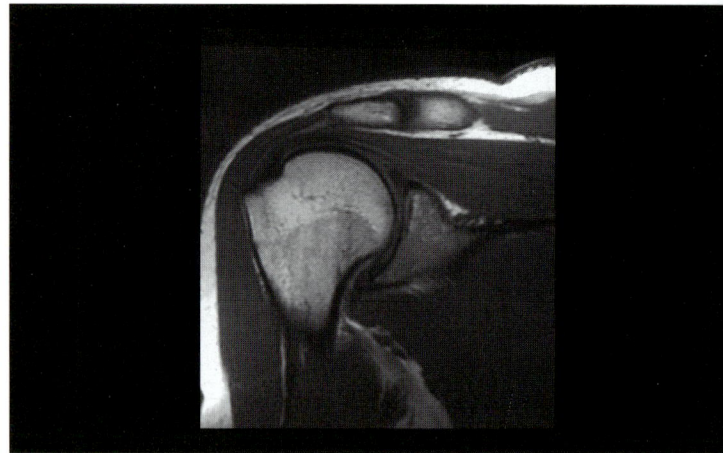

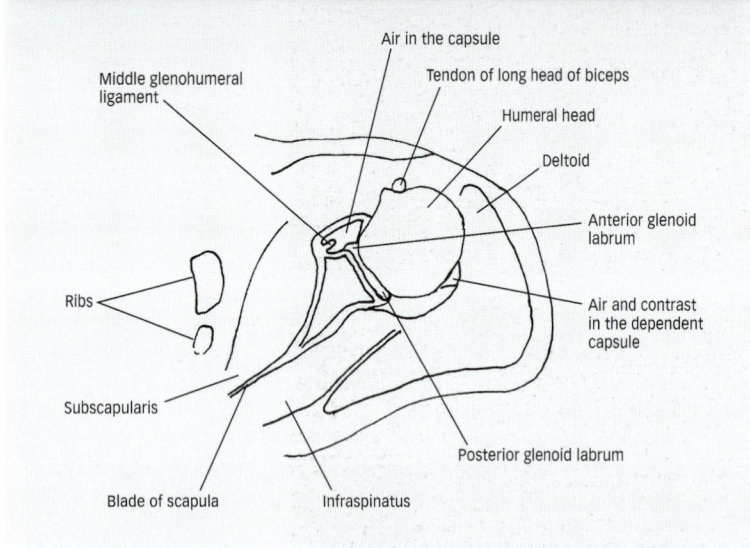

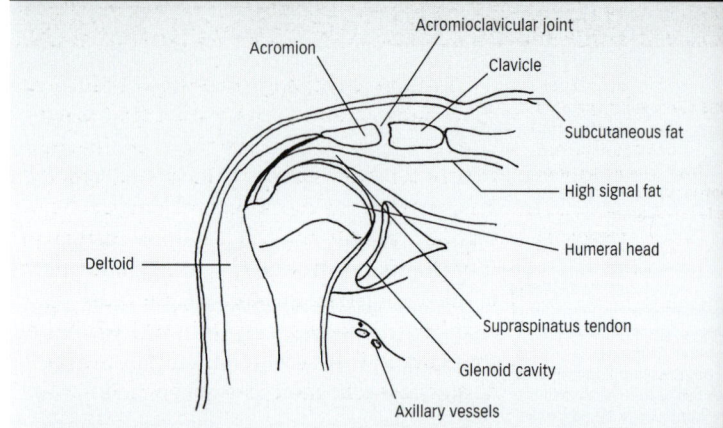

Fig. 13.
CT arthrogram. In the supine position, the contrast collects in the posterior aspect of the joint and outlines the margins of the glenoid fossa and labrum.

- the tendon of the long head of biceps, which passes through the joint and continues in the bicipital groove;
- the subscapularis tendon;
- the axillary recess, which represents a loose fold of synovium inferiorly;
- the subscapularis bursa (which is present in 70–80% of the normal population);
- the volume of the joint space.

Direct visualization of the soft tissues and bony detail, described above, is possible using MRI (Fig. 14). The supraspinatus tendon is best evaluated in the oblique coronal plane, whereas the glenoid labrum, glenohumeral ligaments and capsular structures are best appreciated in the axial plane. The T1W (T1-weighted) images generally provide anatomical information, whereas the T2W (T2-weighted) images and STIR (short tau inversion recovery) fat suppression sequences can identify tears in the tendon. Axial images provide information about the glenoid labrum, the glenohumeral ligaments and the osteochondral articular surfaces.

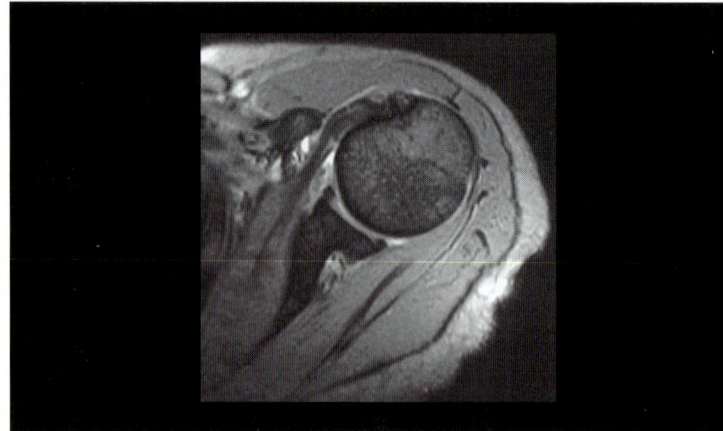

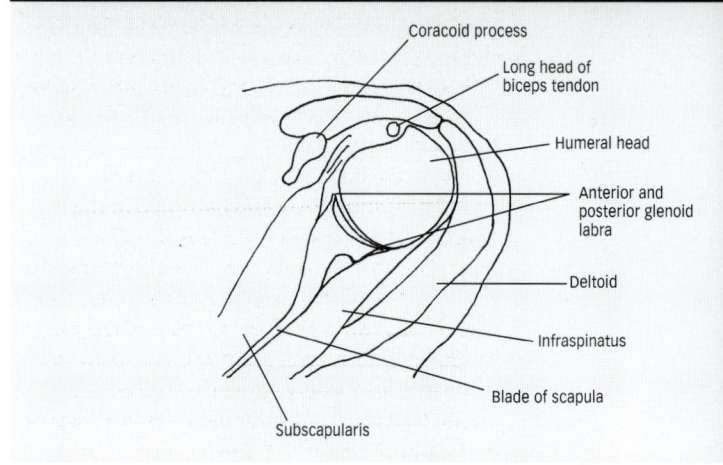

Fig. 14. (right)
MRI of the shoulder. (*a*) Oblique coronal view. T1 weighted image. (*b*) Axial view. Gradient echo sequence.

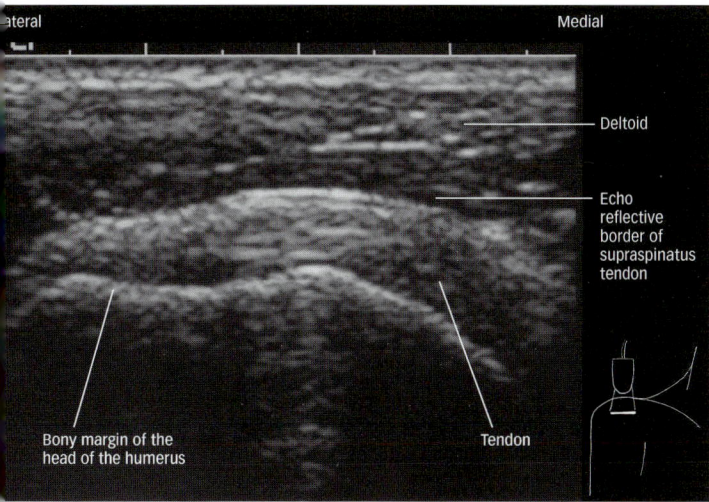

Fig. 15.
USS of the supraspinatus tendon. The scan demonstrates the hyperechoic superior border of the tendon and the less echogenic body of the tendon.

Ultrasound scanning can provide useful 'real time' information about the muscles and tendons of the rotator cuff and their relationship to the coracohumeral arch during movement. The length of the supraspinatus muscle and tendon may be easily visualized and changes in the reflectivity can be used to assess the integrity of the tendon (Fig. 15). Rotating the arm enables the operator to examine the whole of the echoreflective tendinous margin and the darker, less echogenic, central portion.

Humerus

The proximal aspect of the humerus includes the head and the greater and lesser tubercles. The head is smooth and hemispherical and bounded by the anatomical neck of the bone, which is to be distinguished from the surgical neck which lies inferiorly and is at right angles to the cortical margins. A greater and a lesser tubercle are situated on the anterolateral aspect of the head. The greater tubercle lies laterally and slightly posterior to the lesser tubercle and both are separated by the intertubercular groove. There are three facets on the greater tubercle, into which the supraspinatus tendon is attached superiorly, the infraspinatus on the middle facet and the teres minor on the inferior facet. The subscapularis is attached to the lesser tubercle, and the tendon of the long head of biceps passes through the intertubercular groove.

The body (Fig. 16(a), (b)) of the humerus is cylindrical superiorly and flattened in the anteroposterior aspect towards the elbow joint. The radial groove runs inferiorly and laterally on the posterior aspect of the bone and within this runs the radial nerve and the profunda brachialis artery (Fig. 17). The nerve and the artery are closely applied to the bone and bound by a fibrous attachment. Thus fractures in the midshaft of the humerus stretch and

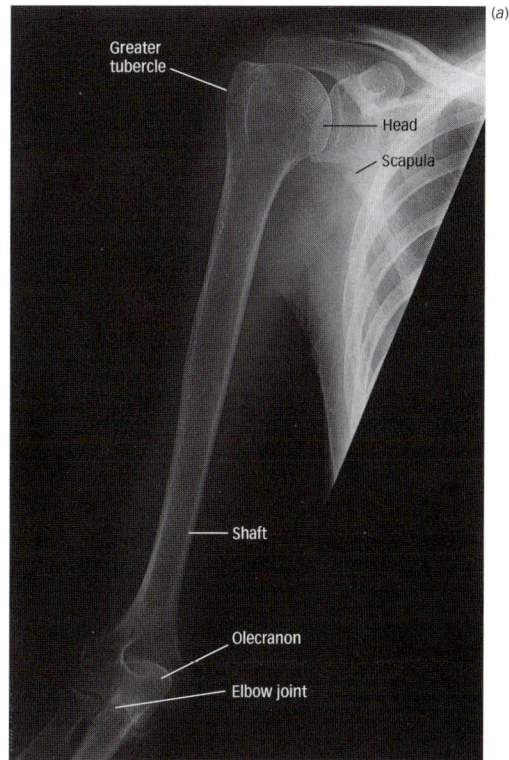

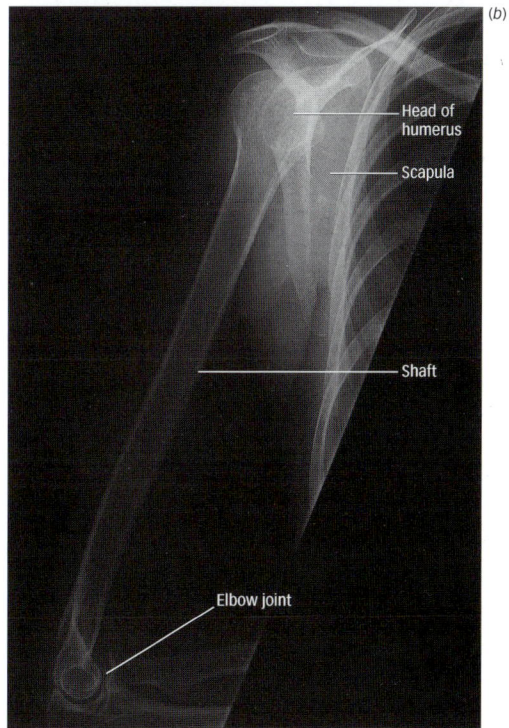

Fig. 16.
The humerus.
(*a*) Anteroposterior view.
(*b*) lateral view.

distort the nerve with the potential to cause neuropraxia. At the lower end of the shaft, the medial and lateral supracondylar ridges extend to the epicondyles. Below lie the articular surfaces of the elbow joint, the capitulum laterally and the trochlea medially. Superior to the trochlea, the bone is excavated posteriorly to form the olecranon fossa. In 5% of Caucasians (double in Afro-Caribbeans) the olecranon

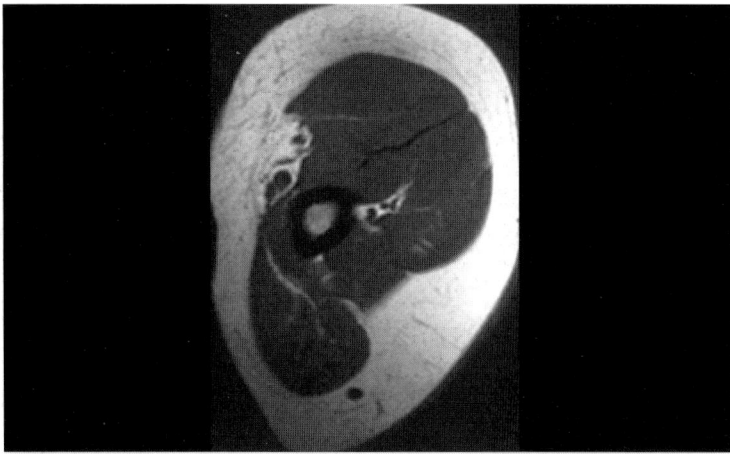

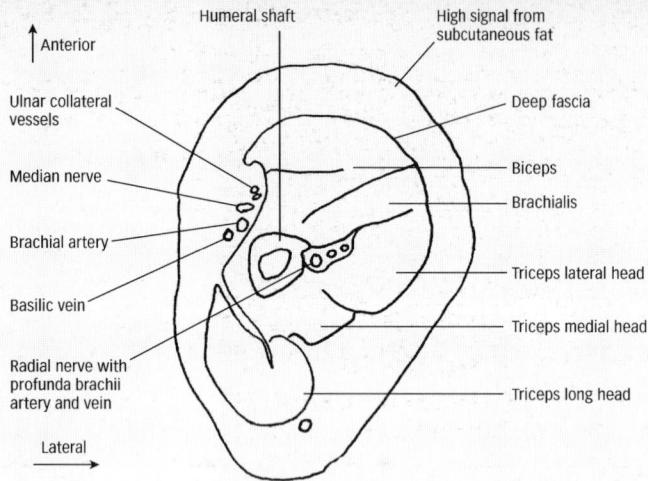

Fig. 17.
MRI Cross-section of the arm. T1 weighted image.

Oblique view *(a)i*

Lateral view *(a)ii*

Anteroposterior view *(b)i*

Lateral view *(b)ii*

Fig. 18.
Radiographs of the secondary ossification centres of the elbow.
(*a*) 2 years, (*b*) 5 years,
(*c*) 5 years, (*d*) 10–11 years
(*e*) 12 years.

fossa is fenestrated and is termed the olecranon or supratrochlear foramen. Anteriorly, the distal humerus has two further depressions, the radial fossa laterally and the coranoid fossa medially which deepen the potential articular surfaces in flexion.

In less than 1% of individuals, a supracondylar spur can be demonstrated anteromedially about 5 cm proximal to the medial epicondyle. Morphologically, this is formed from the inferior portion of the coracobrachialis muscle. From this spur, a ligament (the ligament of Struthers) may pass to the medial epicondyle, beneath which the median nerve and brachial artery may run and be compressed, producing a median nerve palsy.

The upper arm is divided into two compartments by the medial and lateral intermuscular septa which extends to the investing layer of deep fascia (Fig. 17). The anterior compartment contains the flexor muscles, namely the biceps, coracobrachialis and brachialis. The posterior compartment contains the extensors, which are essentially the medial and lateral heads of the triceps and the long head, which originates from the inferior aspect of the glenoid fossa.

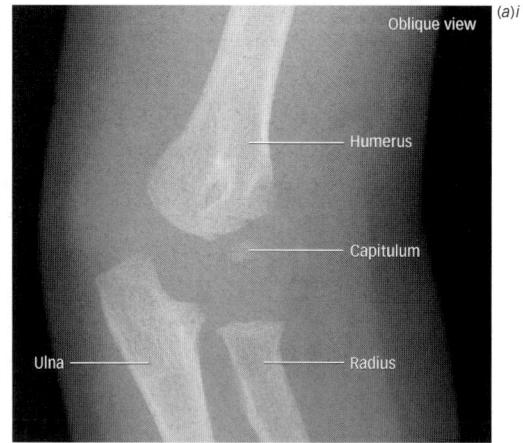

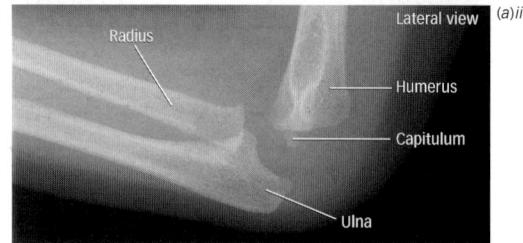

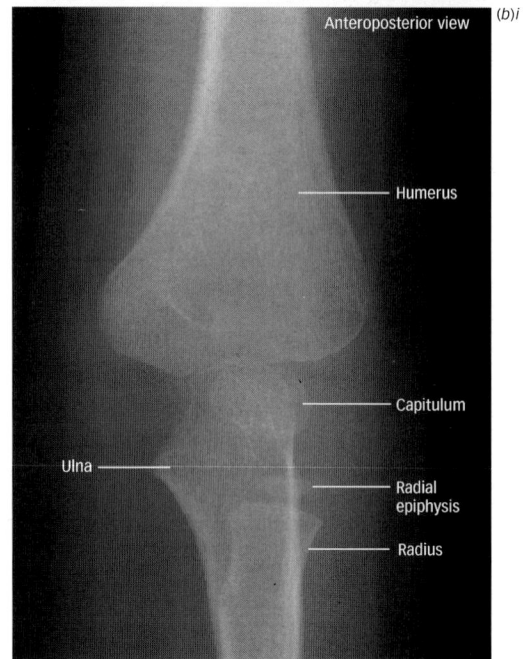

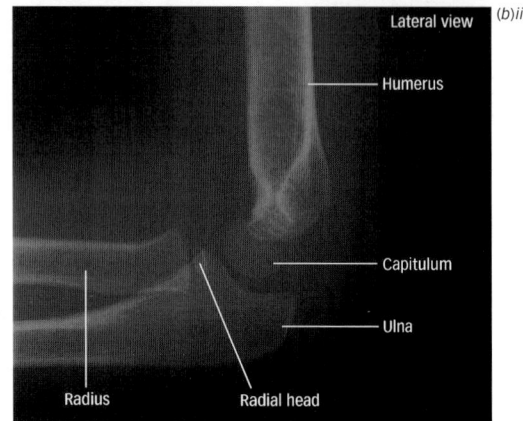

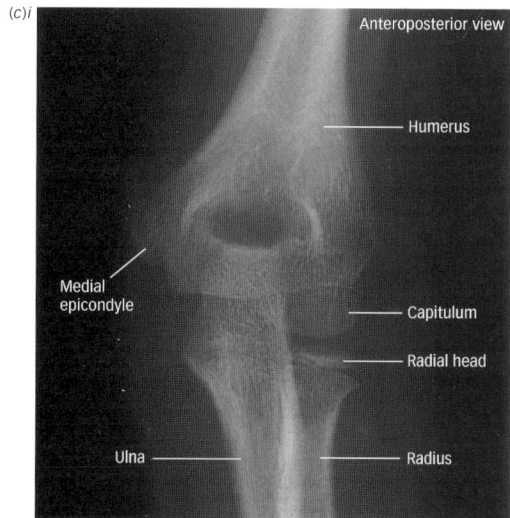

(c)i
Anteroposterior view
Humerus
Medial epicondyle
Capitulum
Radial head
Ulna
Radius

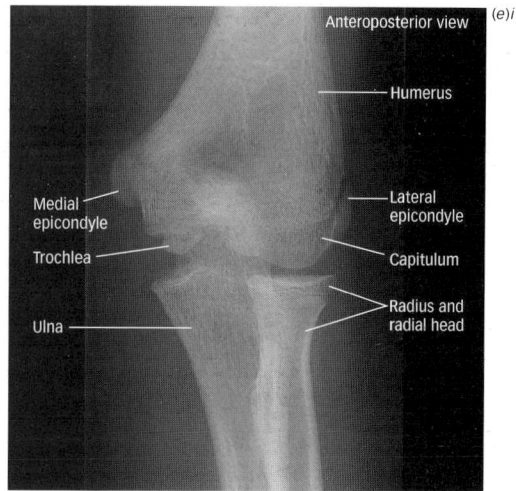

(c)ii
Lateral view
Humerus
Medial epicondyle
Capitulum
Ulna
Radius
Radial head

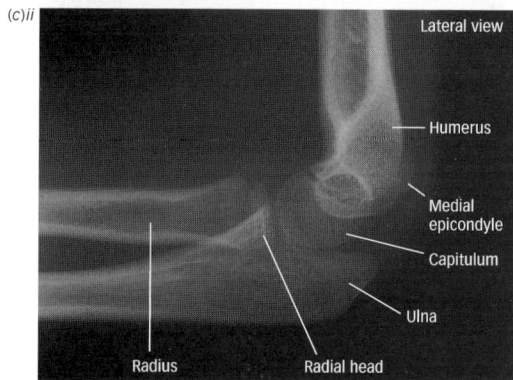

(d)i
Anteroposterior view
Humerus
Capitulum
Trochlea
Radial head
Ulna
Radius

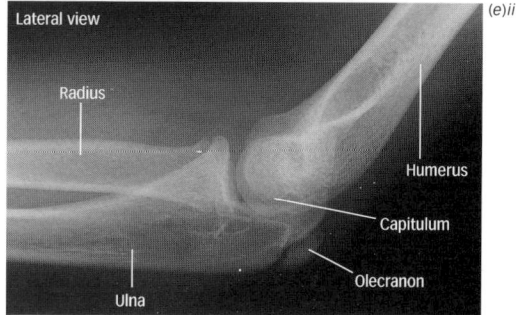

(d)ii
Lateral view
Humerus
Radius and head
Capitulum
Olecranon

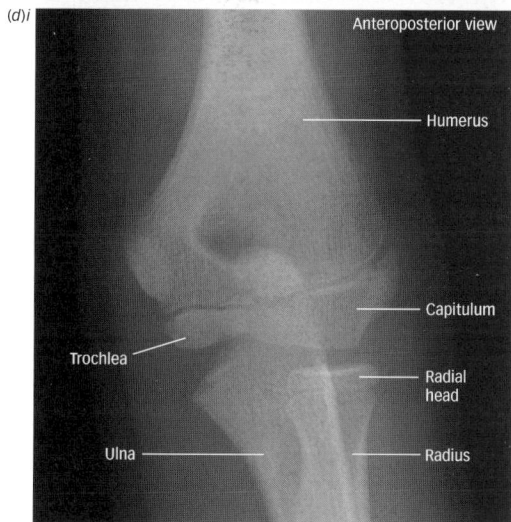

(e)i
Anteroposterior view
Humerus
Medial epicondyle
Lateral epicondyle
Trochlea
Capitulum
Ulna
Radius and radial head

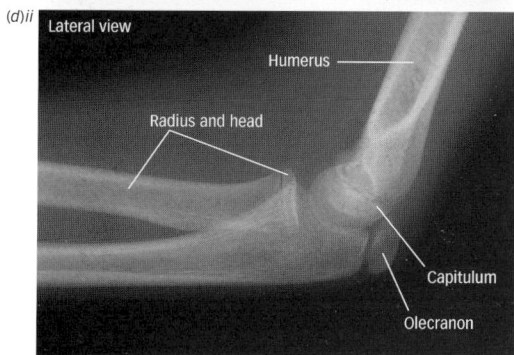

(e)ii
Lateral view
Radius
Humerus
Capitulum
Olecranon
Ulna

Sectional imaging is able to define the muscles and muscular compartments. Providing there are good fat planes, the neurovascular bundles and lymph nodes are seen. The superior soft tissue contrast and lack of ionizing radiation mean that MRI is now the technique of choice in the assessment of soft tissue abnormalities of the muscle groups (Fig. 17).

Ossification

The primary ossification centre forms in the mid-shaft of the humerus in the second month of fetal life. Secondary centres appear in the head, greater tubercle and lesser tubercle at 1, 3 and 5 years of life, all fusing together at 6 years and with the shaft at 20 years.

Distally, the situation is more complex and may lead to confusion in the unfused skeleton. It is best to consider the ossification around the elbow joint as a single unit, which can be remembered by the mnemonic CRITOL (Fig. 18). Thus, the secondary centre for the Capitulum appears at 1 year, the Radial head and Internal (medial) epicondyle at 5 years, the Trochlea at 11 years, the Olecranon at 12 and the Lateral epicondyle at 13 years. These bones fuse with each other and the humerus between 15 to 17 years. Furthermore, notches may be seen between 10 and 15 years on the medial aspects of the proximal and distal humerus and the distal radius. These notches are normal variants and represent irregular metaphyseal growth.

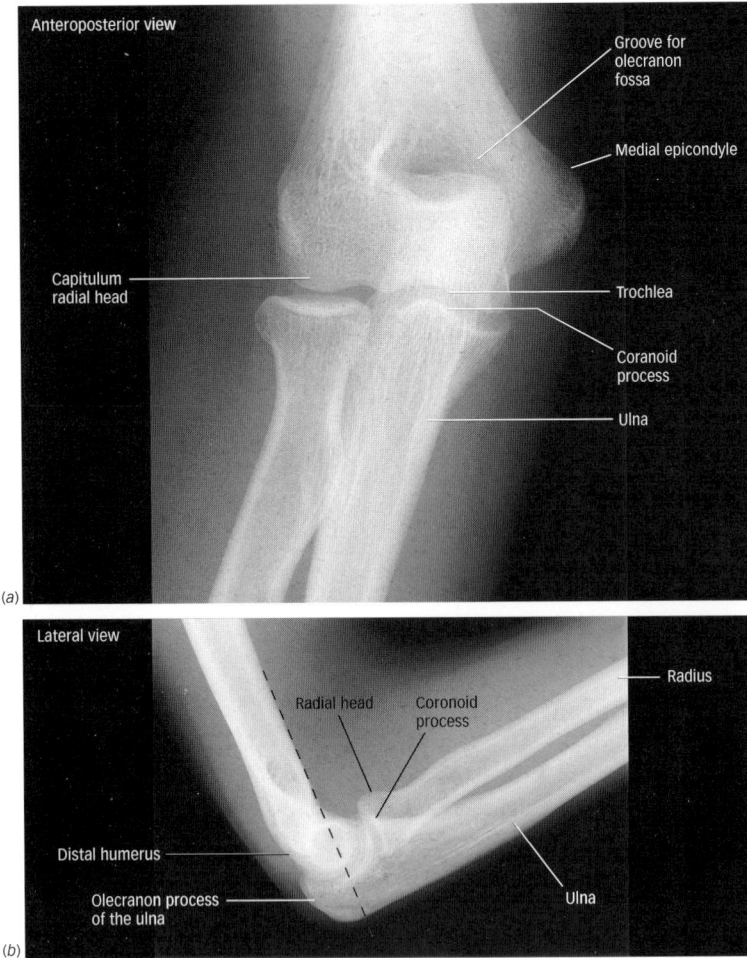

Anteroposterior view

Groove for olecranon fossa

Medial epicondyle

Capitulum radial head

Trochlea

Coranoid process

Ulna

(a)

Lateral view

Radius

Radial head

Coronoid process

Distal humerus

Olecranon process of the ulna

Ulna

(b)

Fig. 19.
Radiographs of the elbow.
(a) Anteroposterior view,
(b) lateral view

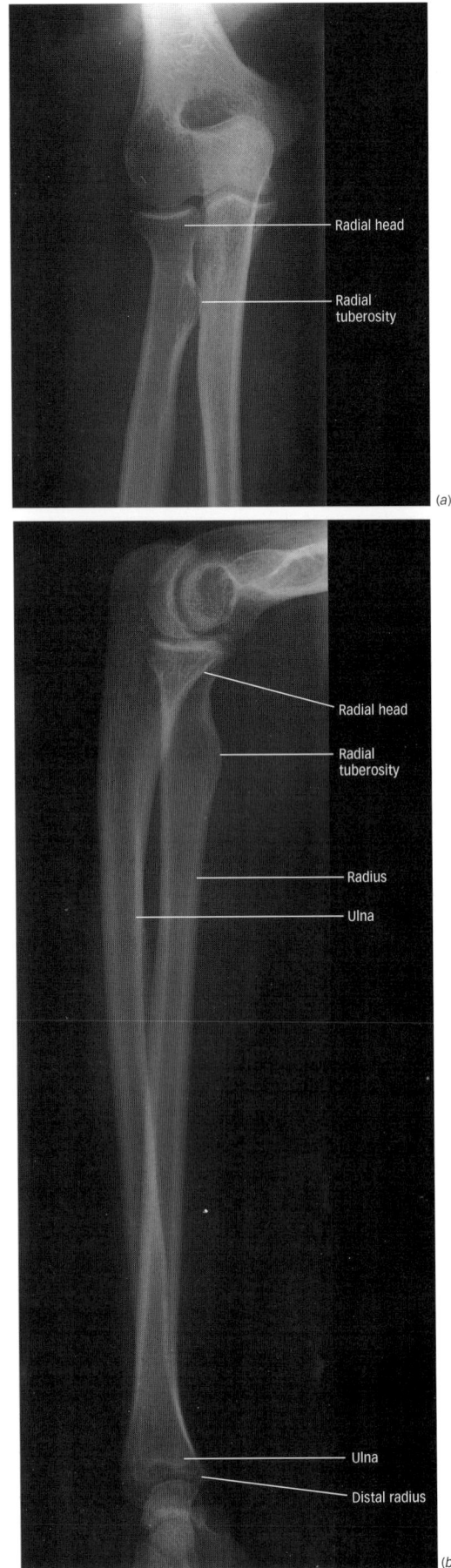

Fig. 20.
Radiographs of the radius and ulna.
(a) Anteroposterior view,
(b) lateral view.

Radial head

Radial tuberosity

(a)

Radial head

Radial tuberosity

Radius

Ulna

Ulna

Distal radius

(b)

The elbow joint

The distal aspect of the humerus expands laterally and medially to form the medial and lateral epicondyles. Inferiorly, the round capitulum and the trochlea articulate with the head of the radius and the trochlear notch of the ulna, respectively (Fig. 19(*a*), (*b*)). The joint capsule is attached along the superior borders of the olecranon, the coronoid and radial fossae of the humerus. Inferiorly, it is attached to the olecranon and coronoid process blending with the superior portion of the annular ligament of the proximal radioulnar joint.

Within the capsule, fat pads are interposed between the synovial membrane and the capsular ligament in the olecranon and coronoid fossae. In the presence of a joint effusion the fat pads are displaced anteriorly and posteriorly, respectively. The effusions become visible as triangular lucency on the lateral radiography. A prominent anterior fat pad may be seen as a normal variant in up to 15% of individuals. The posterior fat pad is only identifiable in cases of joint effusion.

Posteriorly, the tendon of the triceps muscle inserts on to the superior aspect of the olecranon and provides a powerful elbow extensor.

Anteriorly, the brachialis muscle arises from the anterior aspect of the humerus and inserts onto the coronoid process. The biceps muscle crosses the elbow joint and divides into two tendons, which insert into the bicipital tuberosity of the radius and the deep fascia of the forearm. The latter forms the bicipital aponeurosis. The bicipital aponeurosis separates the more superficial median cubital vein from the deeper brachial artery and was referred to by the physician 'blood letters' as the *grâce à dieu* for obvious reasons.

The ligaments of the elbow are the radial and ulnar collateral ligaments and the annular ligament. The radial collateral ligament is a thickening of the capsule which blends with the annular ligament, whereas the ulnar collateral ligament is more anatomically complex, although it is only identified as a single structure on MRI. The annular ligament surrounds the head of the radius in a horseshoe manner and is attached medially to the ulna and laterally to the fibres of the radial collateral ligament.

Plain radiographs consist of anteroposterior and lateral views (Fig. 19(a), (b)). On the lateral view, a line may be drawn that passes inferiorly from the anterior cortical line of the humerus to divide the capitulum. If more than one-third of the thickness of the capitulum lies anterior to this line, a fracture of the epiphysis or a supracondylar fracture should be suspected. Supplementary views may be obtained with the forearm pronated and supinated. The radial head may also be demonstrated using the oblique projection. The arm is rotated laterally or the beam angled in order to project the radial head clearly away from the ulna.

Radius and ulna

The radius carries the hand and is stabilized against the ulna for pronation and supination and against the humerus for flexion and extension (Fig. 20(a), (b)). Superiorly, the bone has a cylindrical head, which tapers into a narrow neck. Distally, the shaft thickens as it curves towards its larger lower extremity, which bears a prominent larger styloid process on its lateral distal aspect. In the region of the radial neck there is an oval prominence, the bicipital tuberosity, which projects towards the ulna. This prominence provides attachment for the biceps tendon. Continuing distally, there is a fine medial ridge which provides attachment for the interosseous membrane. The lower extremity expands to form the articular surface, which articulates with the wrist joint and the ulna.

The ulna stabilizes the forearm and allows the radius to rotate about its axis. The superior aspect has a saddle-shaped articular surface, the trochlear notch, which provides articulation with the trochlea. From the anterior portion of this (saddle-shaped) articular surface projects the coronoid process, which is notched laterally to articulate with the head of the radius. The shaft is angled laterally resulting in a carrying angle, which is measured in full extension and supination. The normal angle is 168 degrees in males and two degrees greater in females. The lateral border of the ulna forms a prominent ridge, which provides the attachment for the interosseous membrane. The distal end of the bone expands into a small, rounded prominence referred to as the head of the ulna. The ulnar styloid process projects distally from the posteromedial side of the head.

The forearm is divided into an anterior and posterior compartment by the interosseous membrane, which may be visualized by CT and MRI (Fig. 21). Anteriorly, there are three

Fig. 21.
MRI Cross-section of the mid forearm. T1 weighted image.

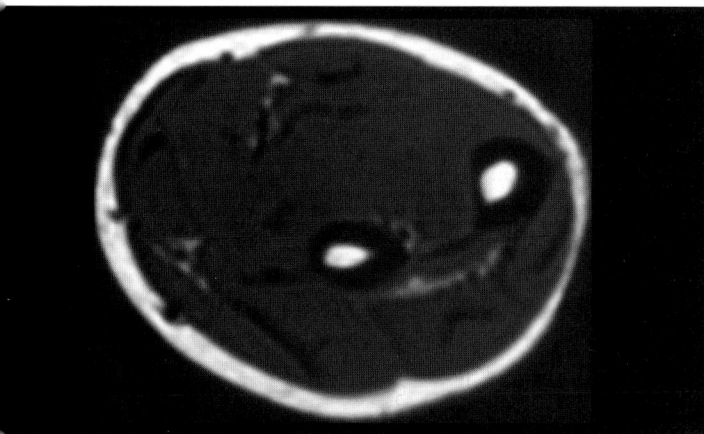

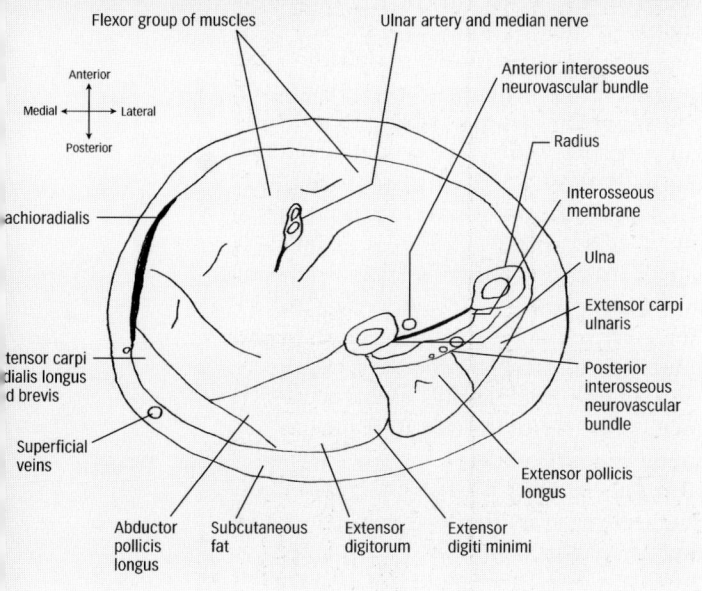

Flexor group of muscles — Ulnar artery and median nerve — Anterior — Medial ← → Lateral — Posterior — Anterior interosseous neurovascular bundle — Radius — Interosseous membrane — Ulna — achioradialis — Extensor carpi ulnaris — Posterior interosseous neurovascular bundle — tensor carpi dialis longus d brevis — Extensor pollicis longus — Superficial veins — Abductor pollicis longus — Subcutaneous fat — Extensor digitorum — Extensor digiti minimi

(a)

Trapezium

Trapezoid

Capitate

Scaphoid

Radius

Metacarpals

Hook of hamate

Hamate

Lines of congruence

Triquetral

Pisiform

Lunate

Ulna

Fig. 22.
Radiographs of the wrist.
(a) Anteroposterior view.
The congruent lines drawn
are formed by the proximal
and distal margins of the
radiocarpal joint and the
midcarpal joint.
(b) The lines represent the
relationship of the radius to
the lunate and the lunate to
the capitate.

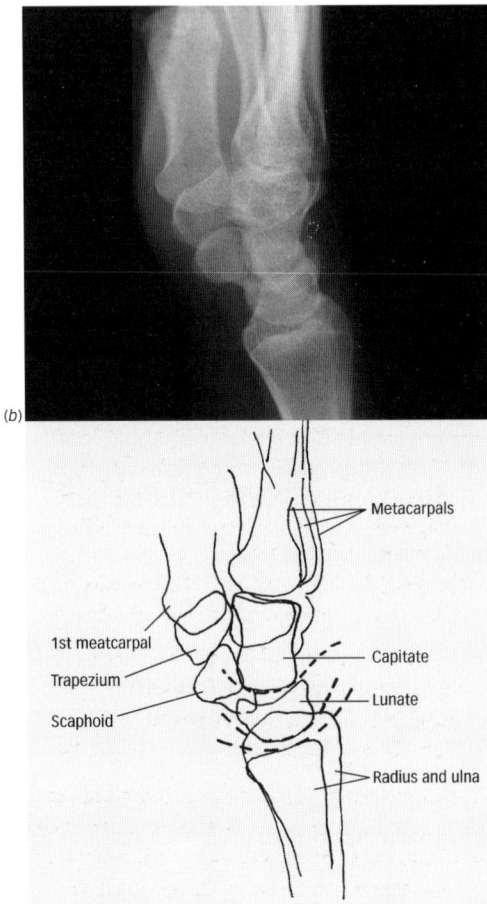

(b)

1st meatcarpal

Trapezium

Scaphoid

Metacarpals

Capitate

Lunate

Radius and ulna

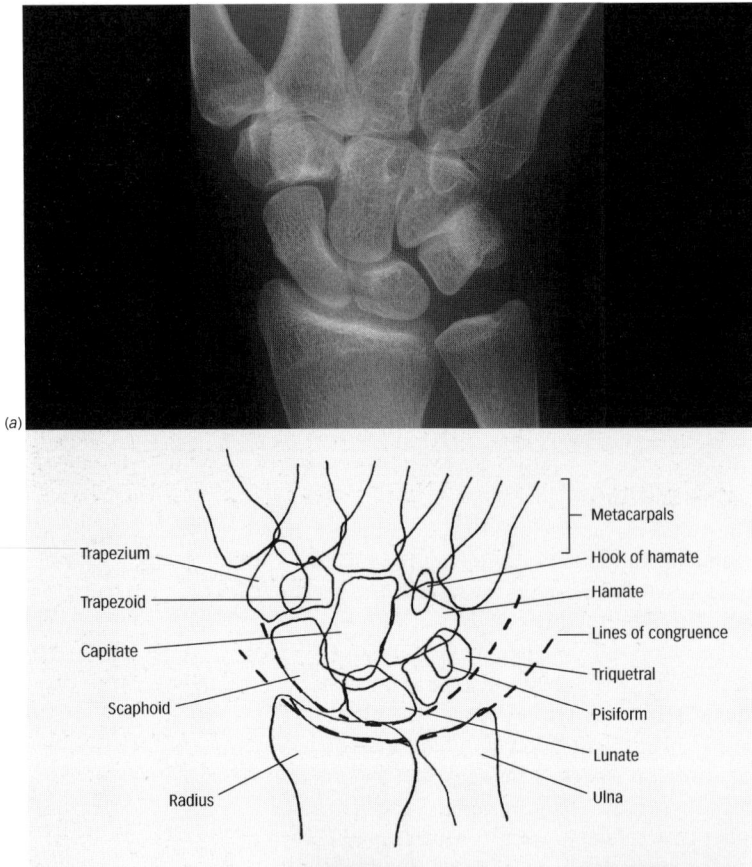

groups of muscles, namely those which produce movement of the radius and ulna, e.g. pronator teres and pronator quadratus, those which produce movement at the carpus, e.g. flexor carpi ulnaris, flexor carpi radialis and including the long flexors, and those which provide movement of the fingers and thumb, e.g. flexor digitorum superficialis, flexor digitorum profundus and flexor pollicis longus. Posteriorly, there are 12 muscles that occupy the extensor compartment. These muscles have an antagonistic action with the flexor muscles. The muscles that can be visualized in the mid-forearm are the extensor pollicis longus, extensor carpi ulnaris, extensor digiti mimini, extensor digitorum, abductor pollicis longus, the extensor carpi radialis group and brachioradialis.

Ossification

The primary ossification centre of the radius appears in the eighth week of fetal life. The distal secondary centre appears in the first year and fuses at approximately 20 years.

The primary centre of the ulna, like the radius, appears in the eighth week of fetal life. The secondary centre appears in the distal ulna at 5 years and fuses at 17 years.

The inferior radioulnar joint

The inferior radioulnar joint is a pivot synovial joint. It has no communication with the carpal joints and thus, if communication is demonstrated by arthrography, its triangular fibrocartilaginous ligament must be disrupted. The capsule of this joint extends superiorly between the radius and ulna to form the recessus sacciformis.

The wrist and carpus

The radius enlarges distally and laterally to form the articular surface with the carpus. On its distal surface there are facets for the lunate and scaphoid bones. The radius only articulates with the triquetral bone in ulnar deviation of the wrist. The distal ulna appears shorter than the distal radius on the plain radiograph of the wrist (Fig. 22(a), (b)). An imaginary line drawn between the styloids subtends an angle of 7–10 degrees from the axis of the line of carpal flexion. Joint congruity is maintained by a fibrocartilaginous disc, which projects laterally from the ulna styloid to the medial aspect of the distal radius, thus no carpal bone articulates with the head of the ulna. The radiocarpal (wrist) joint is an ellipsoid synovial joint. The distal end of the radius and the triangular fibrocartilaginous disc articulate with the scaphoid, lunate and tri-

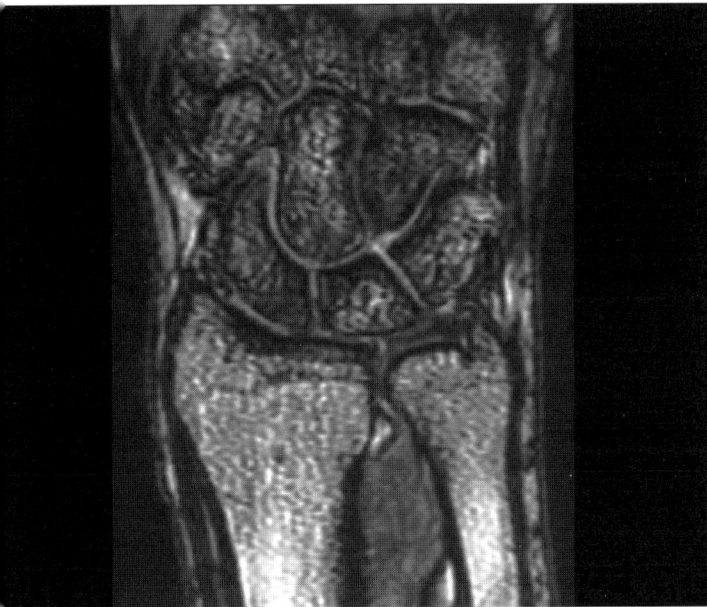

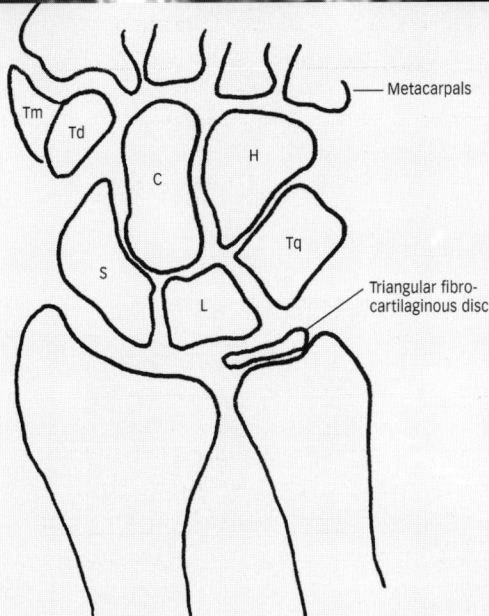

Fig. 23.
Coronal MRI of the wrist.
Gradient echo sequence.
Tm, trapezium, Td,
trapezoid, H, hamate, C,
capitate, L. lunate, Tq,
triquetral, S, scaphoid.

Fig. 24.
Arthrograms of the wrist.
R, radius, U, ulna. TFCD,
triangular fibro-
cartilaginous disc

quetral bones. The capsule is attached to the articular margins of the joint, and the synovial membrane lines the non-articular surfaces.

The carpal bones are arranged in two rows of four bones. The proximal row, from lateral to medial, are the scaphoid, lunate and triquetral bones, with the pisiform articulating on the anterior aspect of the triquetral bone. The distal row is formed by the trapezium, trapezoid, capitate and hamate bones. The intercarpal joints are all synovial joints and the joint between the proximal and distal rows of the carpal bones is called the midcarpal joint (Fig. 23). The midcarpal joint is separated from the radiocarpal joint by a series of interosseous ligaments across which there is no communication. A series of complex palmar and dorsal ligaments provide support. Single contrast arthrography (Fig. 24) is ideally conducted in three stages so

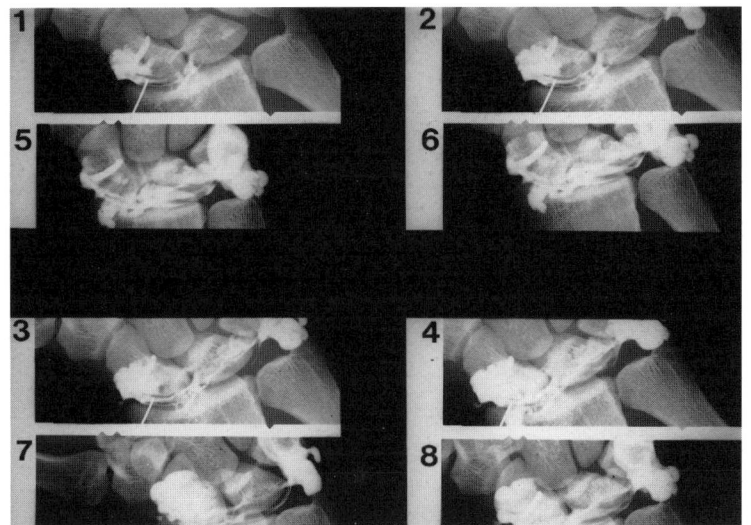

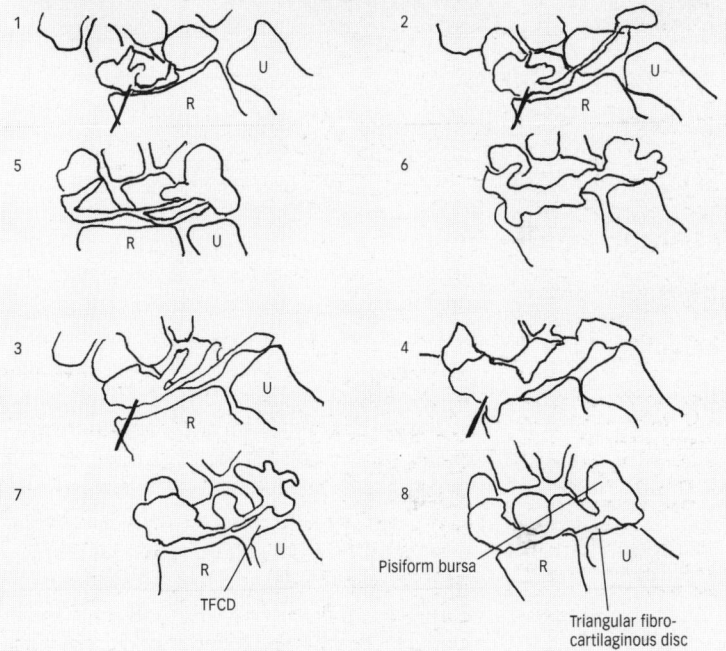

as to demonstrate the three compartments. Current research has demonstrated that communication between the compartments of the carpal bones, in normal individuals, occurs most commonly at the radioulnar and radiocarpal joints (30%), the radiocarpal and midcarpal joint (50%) and from the radioulnar joint to the pisiform bursa (50%).

On the AP radiograph of the wrist three congruous curves are formed by (Fig. 22(a)):

- the distal radius and ulna;
- the proximal cortical margins of the scaphoid, lunate and triquetral;
- the midcarpal joint.

The lunate bone is the key to understanding the lateral radiograph of the wrist. The proximal, convex, surface articulates with the distal surface of the radius, whereas the capitate

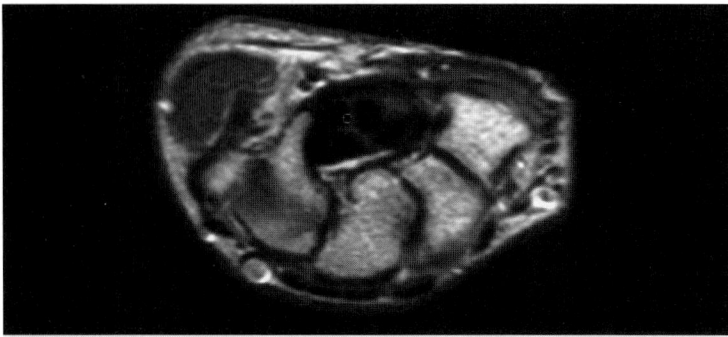

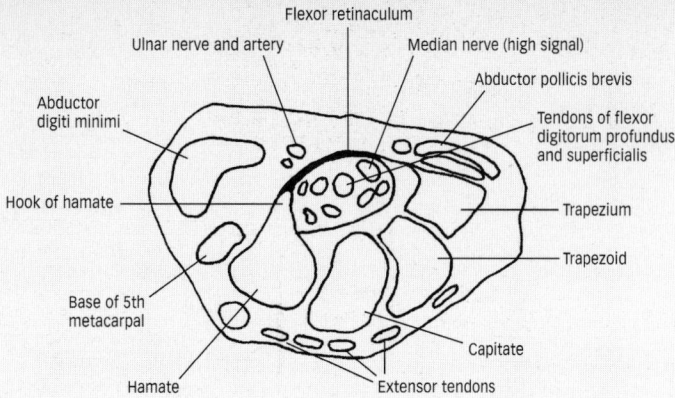

Fig. 25.
**MRI of the carpal tunnel.
T1 weighted image.**

Fig. 26.
The flexor retinaculum.

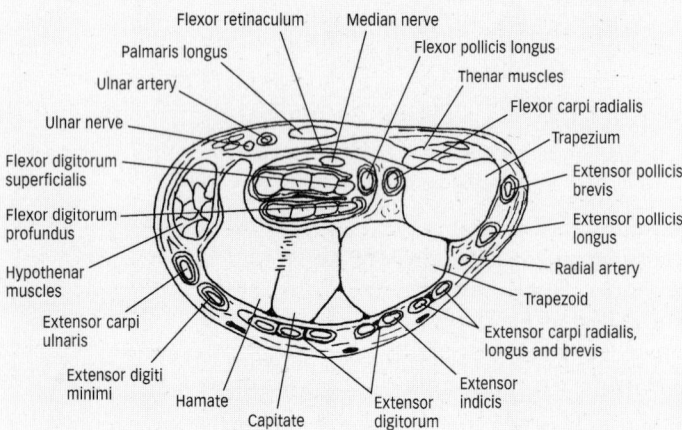

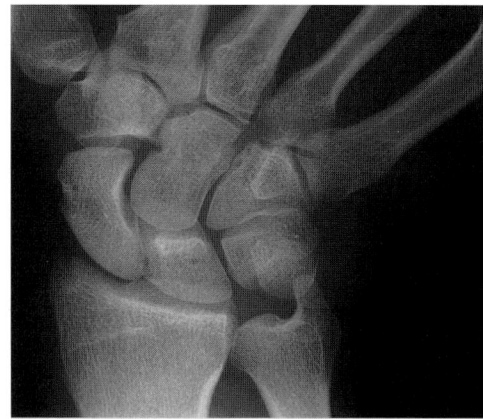

(a)

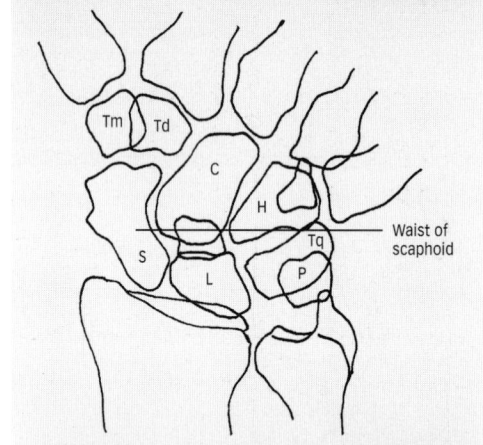

(b)

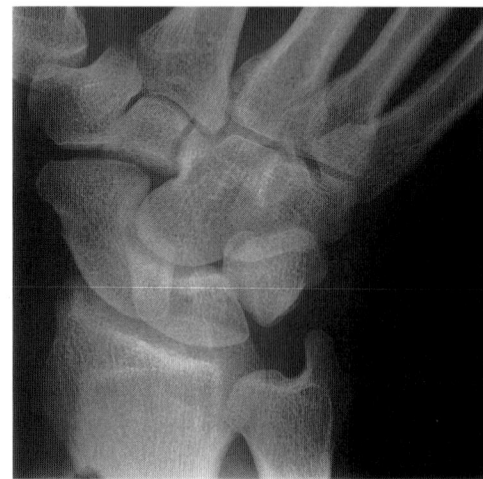

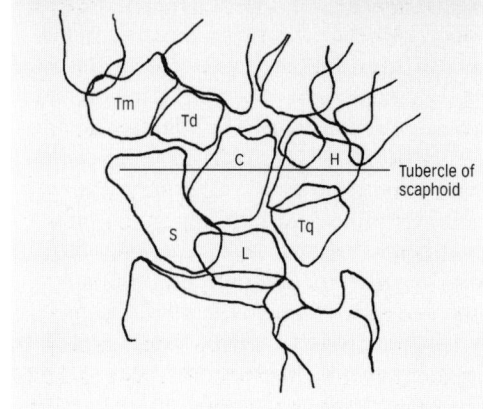

Fig. 27.
Radiographs of the scaphoid.
(a) Anteroposterior view
(b) 30 degree anteroposterior view. Tm, trapezium, Td, trapezoid, C, capitate, H, hamate, L, lunate, P, pisiform, Tq, triquetral, TS, scaphoid.
(c) Lateral view.
(d) scaphoid centred view

articulates with the concave distal surface of the lunate (Fig. 22(*b*)). Close inspection of the lateral radiograph reveals an anterior tilt, of approximately 86 degrees, of the distal radius. It is important to the stability of the joint that this angle is maintained. If this angle is lost, a distal radial fracture should be suspected.

The sides of the carpal bones are angled so as to produce an anterior concavity. The hollow formed by these bones (Fig. 25) is bounded anteriorly by the flexor retinaculum, which is attached to the pisiform bone, hook of hamate, the scaphoid tubercle and the ridge of the trapezium. It is approximately the size of a postage stamp. Within this 'D'-shaped cavity (Fig. 26) lies the carpal tunnel containing the

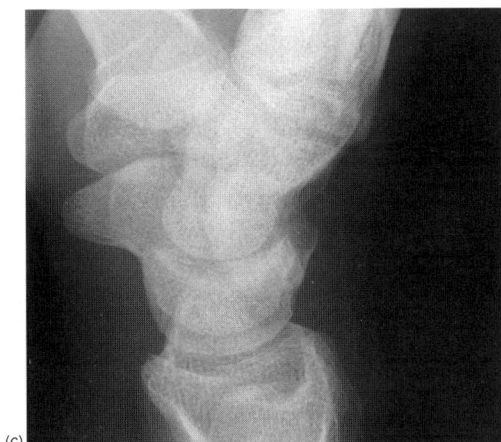

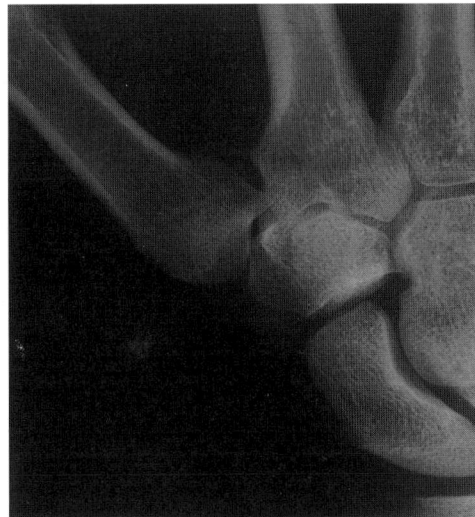

(c)

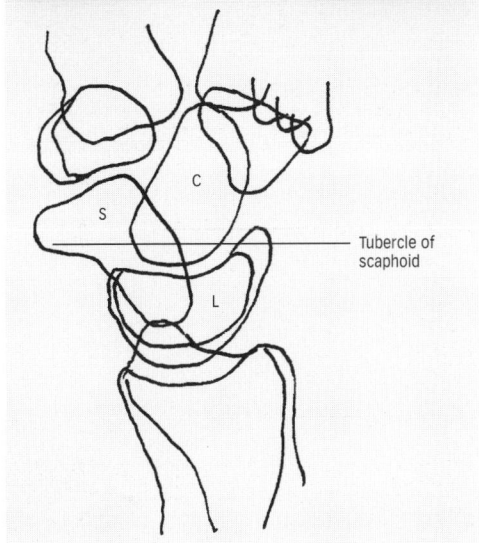

(d)

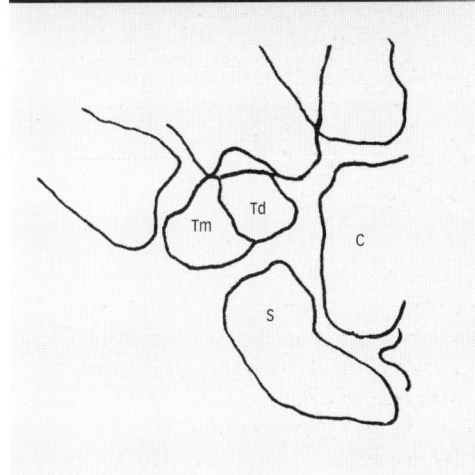

tendons of flexor pollicis longus, the four long tendons of flexor digitorum superficialis and flexor digitorum profundus. The median nerve passes immediately deep to the flexor retinaculum. The tendon of flexor carpi radialis grooves the trapezium and lies in a separate compartment of the carpal tunnel. The ulnar artery is situated superficial to the flexor retinaculum and lateral to the ulnar nerve.

The muscles and tendons of the forearm cross the carpal bones to provide long and short finger extensors and flexors. The exception is flexor carpi ulnaris, which attaches to the pisiform.

On the posterior aspect of the wrist joint lie the extensor tendons in six fibro-osseous tunnels bound by the extensor retinaculum. The small muscles of the hand, including the thenar and hypothenar eminences take their origins from the carpal bones and the flexor retinaculum and insert into the metacarpal bones and phalanges of the thumb and little fingers, respectively.

The most important bone both clinically and radiologically is the scaphoid. Four standard views are necessary in most cases as fractures

are easily missed (Fig. 27). In approximately 15% of individuals, the blood supply to the scaphoid bone is solely supplied from nutrient arteries which pass from distal to proximal. Thus, fractures across the waist of the scaphoid can produce ischaemic necrosis of the proximal portion. Increased uptake on MDP Tc99^m bone scanning may indicate bone damage when the pain radiograph is equivocal.

Ossification

The capitate and hamate ossify in the first year, the triquetral in the second year, the lunate in the third year, the scaphoid, trapezium and trapezoid in the sixth year and the pisiform at the twelfth year (Fig. 28).

The metacarpals and phalanges

Traditionally, these bones have been numbered from lateral to medially (Fig. 29). However, this system is a potential cause of confusion. Therefore, each ray should be named, e.g. thumb, index finger, middle finger, ring finger and little finger, so as to avoid this complication. The metacarpals apart from the first, which articulates solely with the trapezium,

Fig. 28.
Radiographs of carpal ossification. The films demonstrate the changes from the first year of life to the age of 12 years. It should be appreciated that the bones do not always ossify in order and that there is considerable variation as shown. (*a*) 1 year, (*b*) 3 years, (*c*) 5 years, (*d*) 7 years, (*e*) 12 years. Tm, trapezium, Td, trapezoid, S, scaphoid, H, hamate, C, capitate, Tq, triquetral, P, pisiform, L, lunate.

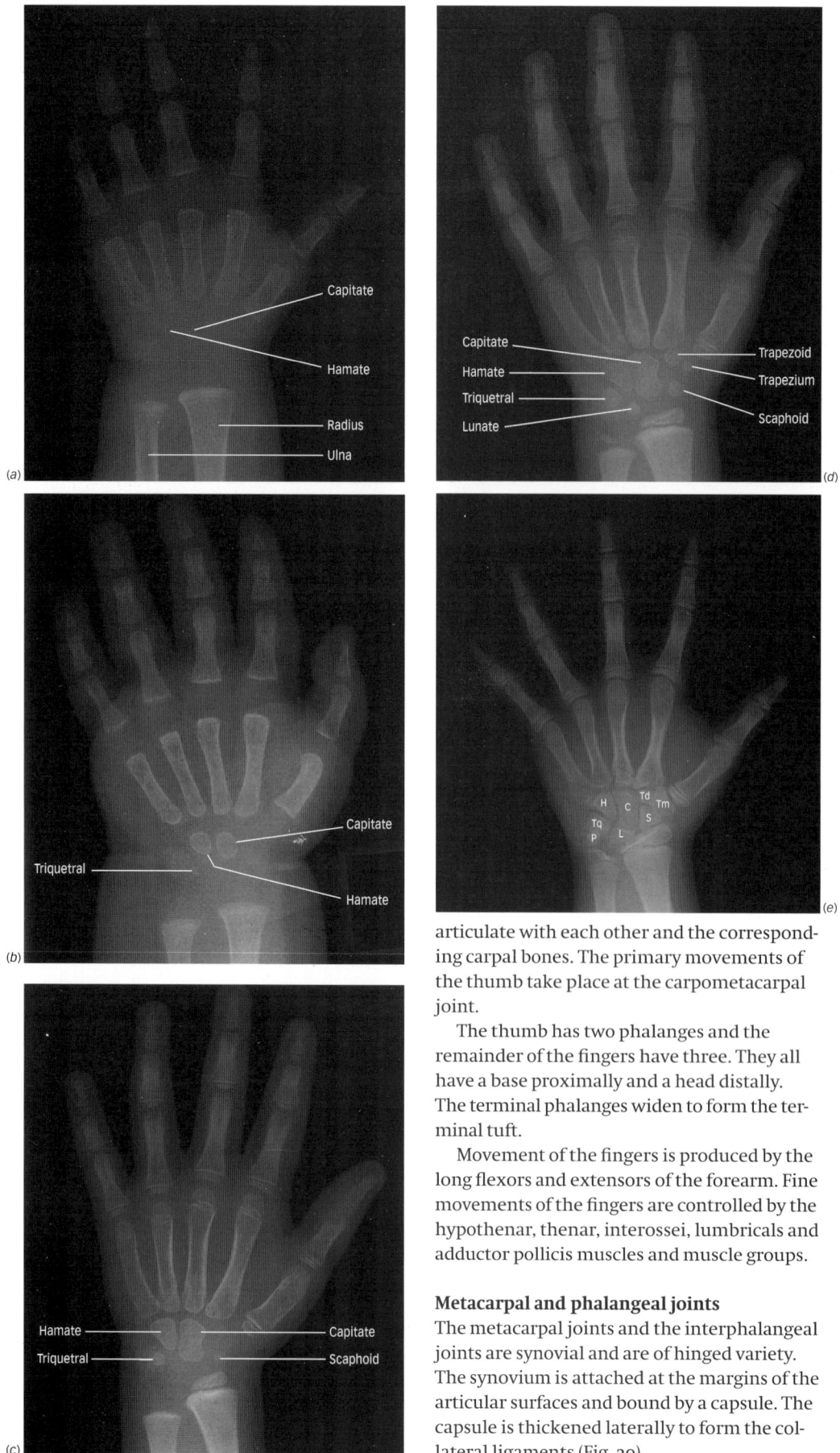

(*a*)

(*d*)

(*b*)

(*e*)

(*c*)

articulate with each other and the corresponding carpal bones. The primary movements of the thumb take place at the carpometacarpal joint.

The thumb has two phalanges and the remainder of the fingers have three. They all have a base proximally and a head distally. The terminal phalanges widen to form the terminal tuft.

Movement of the fingers is produced by the long flexors and extensors of the forearm. Fine movements of the fingers are controlled by the hypothenar, thenar, interossei, lumbricals and adductor pollicis muscles and muscle groups.

Metacarpal and phalangeal joints

The metacarpal joints and the interphalangeal joints are synovial and are of hinged variety. The synovium is attached at the margins of the articular surfaces and bound by a capsule. The capsule is thickened laterally to form the collateral ligaments (Fig. 29).

Reference
Greulich, W. W. & Pyle, S.I. (1976). *Radiographic Atlas of Skeletal Development of the Hand and Wrist*. Stanford, CA: Stanford University Press.

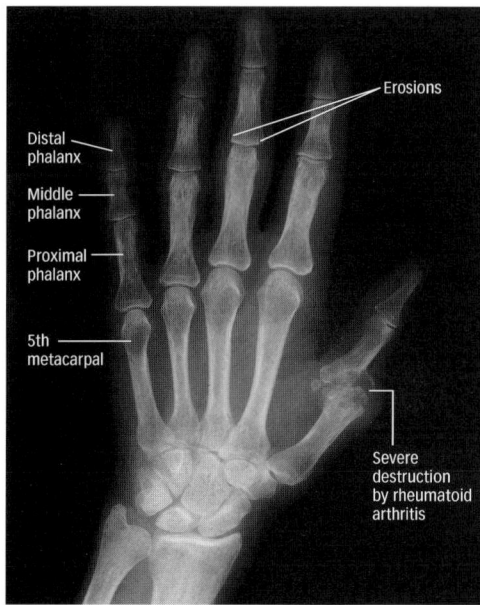

29.
...iograph of the hand. The ...iograph demonstrates ...ere rheumatoid arthritis ...st marked in the thumb. ...umatoid arthritis ...ses synovial ...liferation and erodes the ...rgins of the bone at the ...es of synovial ...achment.

Erosions

Distal phalanx

Middle phalanx

Proximal phalanx

5th metacarpal

Severe destruction by rheumatoid arthritis

Supernumerary bones

Most of the supernumeraries in the hands are sesamoid bones. The commonest is the sesamoid in the tendon of flexor pollicis brevis, which is demonstrated close to the carpometacarpal joint of the thumb. Further supernumerary bones may be found around the wrist joint. The commonest supernumerary bone, in the region of the wrist joint, is the os radiale externum, which lies immediately distal to the radial styloid.

Bone age

Estimation of bone age is of great importance as it can be used to assess the development and maturity of the growing skeleton in relation to the chronological age of the child. Radiographs of the left hand are obtained for bone age assessment by comparing certain features such as epiphyseal development and growth of the hand with standards, e.g. Greulich and Pyle.

The nerve supply to the upper limb

The brachial plexus is described in Chapter 5.

The axillary nerve

This is a branch of the posterior cord of the brachial plexus which supplies the deltoid muscle and the skin in the mid-lateral region of the arm. The nerve passes posteriorly around the surgical neck of the humerus in the muscular quadrilateral space. Thus, an inferior dislocation of the humerus may produce paresis in the deltoid muscle by damaging the nerve.

The radial nerve

The radial nerve is a branch of the posterior cord, which passes obliquely posteriorly to the humerus to run in the spiral groove. It lies between the medial and lateral heads of the triceps and is bound to the bone by tight fascia. The nerve pierces the lateral intermuscular septum, leaving the posterior compartment to enter the anterior compartment.

At the elbow the nerve branches to form the posterior interosseous nerve, which supplies the muscles of the posterior compartment of the forearm. The radial nerve continues in the forearm deep to brachioradialis muscle to supply the skin over the dorsum of the hand.

The median nerve

The median nerve is formed from the medial and lateral cords of the brachial plexus. Superiorly in the arm it lies lateral to the brachial artery; however, at the level of the mid-humerus it crosses the artery anteriorly to lie medial to it. At the elbow it crosses the cubital fossa and runs deep to the flexor digitorum superficialis and at the wrist passes beneath the flexor retinaculum. The anterior interosseous nerve is a branch of the median nerve originating in the cubital fossa. The median nerve supplies most of the muscles of the flexor compartment of the forearm and some of the small muscles of the hand, i.e. those of the thenar eminence and the two radial lumbricals.

The ulnar nerve

The ulnar nerve is derived from the medial cord of the brachial plexus. It descends in the anterior compartment of the arm and pierces the medial intermuscular septum to enter the posterior compartment. The nerve passes behind the medial epicondyle and between the heads of the flexor carpi ulnaris to continue deep to this muscle in the forearm. The ulnar nerve supplies flexor carpi ulnaris and the ulnar half of flexor digitorum profundus in the forearm and mainly innervates the small muscles of the hand, with the exception of those supplied by the median nerve.

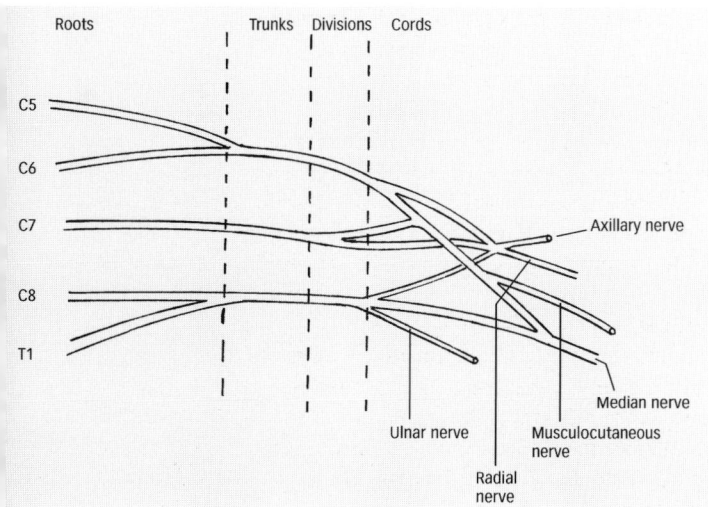

30.
...ematic diagram of the ...chial plexus.

Roots   Trunks Divisions Cords

C5

C6

C7

C8

T1

Axillary nerve

Median nerve

Ulnar nerve

Musculocutaneous nerve

Radial nerve

17

The musculoskeletal system 2: the lower limb

A. NEWMAN-SANDERS
and A. L. HINE

Imaging methods

The bony pelvis and lower limb are increasingly examined using the full armoury of imaging modalities as these become more widely available. Plain radiography remains as important as ever, and its more detailed applications will be discussed further in the relevant anatomical subsections.

Computed tomography (CT)

Scanning is now available in the majority of hospitals, finding particular favour in the further examination of complex skeletal trauma, where it is often capable of contributing valuable additional information.

Magnetic resonance imaging (MRI)

This is revolutionizing the investigation of bone, joint and soft tissue abnormalities. Multiplanar imaging capability and high contrast resolution mean that the presence and extent of pathology can be defined far more accurately. This capacity is enhanced with the use of phased array surface detection coils, which greatly improve the signal-to-noise ratio (SNR).

The exact choice of sequences and imaging planes varies greatly, depending on the clinical problem, the anatomical location and individual radiological preference. In bony structures, the relatively high signal of bone marrow fat may mask pathology on T2-weighted images, so the use of techniques for abolishing the signal from fat is a valuable adjunct. Increasingly, chemical fat saturation techniques are available in conjunction with T2-weighted imaging. Alternatively, STIR (short tau inversion recovery) sequences may also be used. The principal limitation of MRI is that cortical bone and calcification have no signal at all, which can make abnormalities difficult to interpret. More specific applications of MRI will be dealt with in the appropriate sections.

Ultrasound

Ultrasound is commonly used to investigate the musculoskeletal system. High frequency (7.5–10 mHz) probes can obtain excellent resolution of the internal architecture of tendons and muscles. Other applications include the detection of fluid collections around joints and the initial assessment of soft tissue masses and cysts.

Nuclear medicine

[99m] Technetium methylene diphosphonate is the commonest isotope in routine use and is administered intravenously. A three-phase study is composed of immediate vascular phase images (0–3 minutes), a blood pool phase (3–5 minutes) and the delayed static (4 hours) images. The patient is encouraged to remain well hydrated and to empty the bladder frequently during this time. Detailed images of the localized areas can be achieved using pinhole collimation. The bone scan is very sensitive to the presence of any pathology but is relatively non-specific. Areas of increased uptake ('hot spots') are due to both increased blood supply and increased osteoblast activity and may be seen in fractures, malignancy, soft tissue and bony infection, and joint disease.

The bony pelvis and pelvic walls
(with Dr S. J. Vinnicombe)

The bony pelvis consists of a ring formed by the paired innominate bones, the sacrum and the coccyx (Fig. 1). The ring is completed by the paired sacroiliac joints posteriorly and the pubic symphysis anteriorly. The symphysis pubis is a secondary cartilaginous joint. Each articular surface is covered with a layer of hyaline cartilage enclosing a fibrocartilaginous

Fig. 1.
Frontal radiograph of an adult female pelvis.

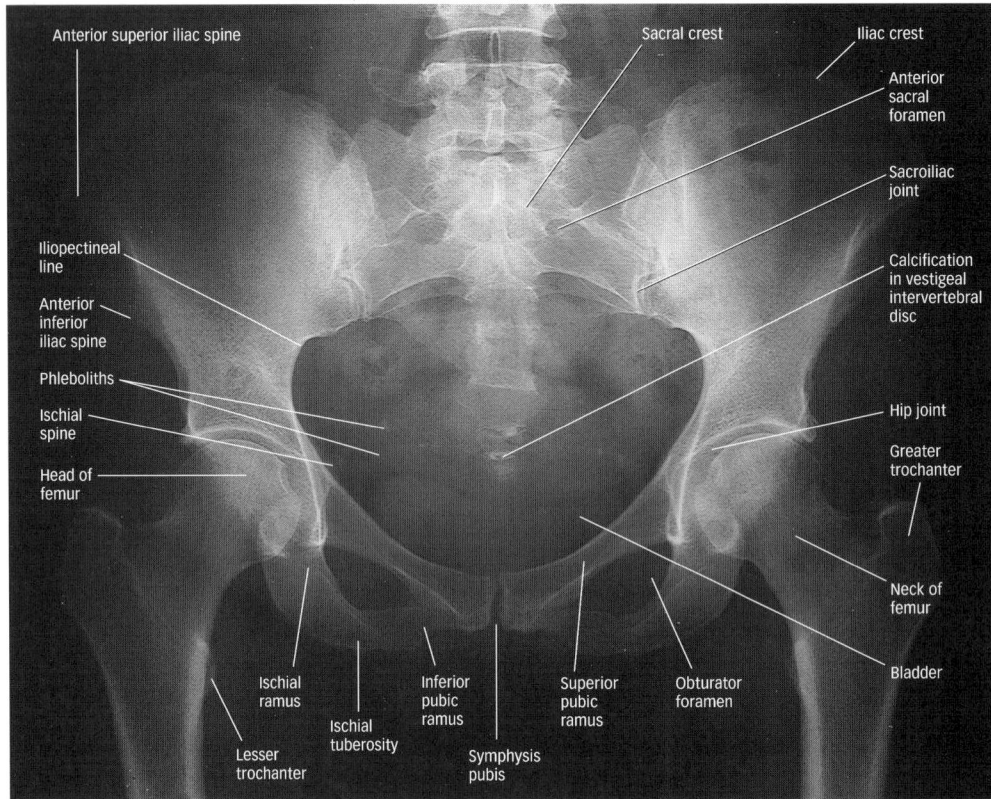

Anterior superior iliac spine
Sacral crest
Iliac crest
Anterior sacral foramen
Sacroiliac joint
Iliopectineal line
Anterior inferior iliac spine
Calcification in vestigeal intervertebral disc
Phleboliths
Ischial spine
Hip joint
Head of femur
Greater trochanter
Neck of femur
Ischial ramus
Inferior pubic ramus
Superior pubic ramus
Obturator foramen
Bladder
Ischial tuberosity
Lesser trochanter
Symphysis pubis

Fig. 2. below
Frontal radiographs of a juvenile pelvis demonstrating the appearances of the ischiopubic synchondrosis (a) before and (b) during fusion.

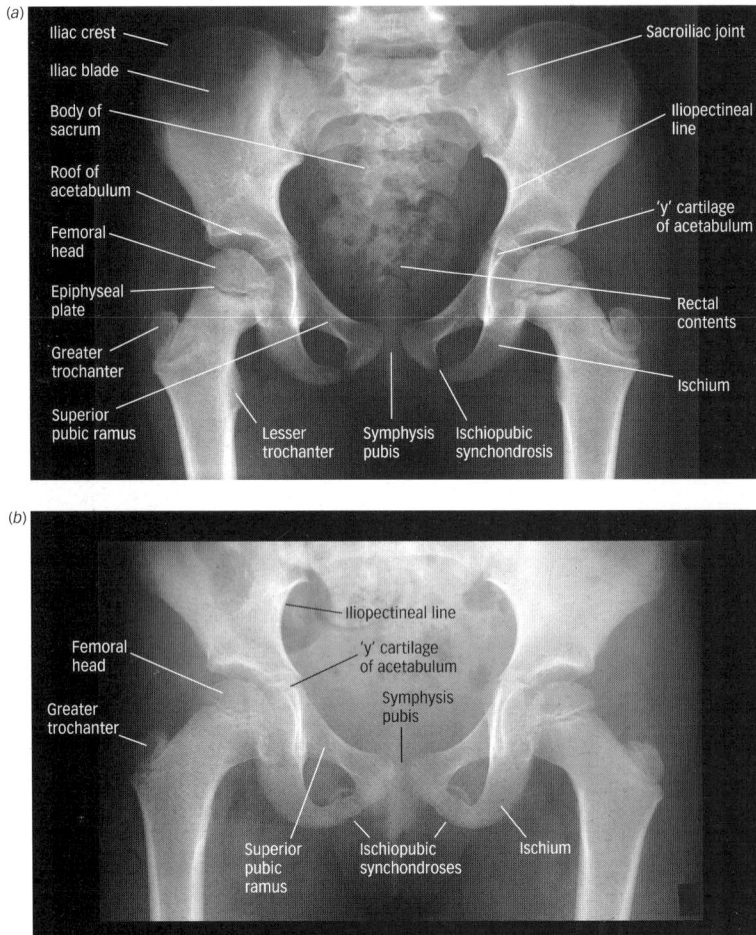

(a)
Iliac crest
Iliac blade
Body of sacrum
Roof of acetabulum
Femoral head
Epiphyseal plate
Greater trochanter
Superior pubic ramus
Sacroiliac joint
Iliopectineal line
'y' cartilage of acetabulum
Rectal contents
Ischium
Lesser trochanter
Symphysis pubis
Ischiopubic synchondrosis

(b)
Femoral head
Greater trochanter
Iliopectineal line
'y' cartilage of acetabulum
Symphysis pubis
Superior pubic ramus
Ischiopubic synchondroses
Ischium

disc. The whole joint is covered by dense ligaments, which are particularly strong superiorly and inferiorly. Virtually no movement is possible at the joint and, in the adult, the width of the joint should not exceed 7 mm on AP radiographs of the pelvis.

The innominate bones are composed of three parts: the ilium, ischium and pubis. These meet at the triradiate cartilage, visible in the immature skeleton as a Y-shaped irregular lucency at the acetabulum. Two or more centres of ossification appear in this cartilage at puberty and fuse at the age of 20 years.

The ilium is a curved, flat bone with the iliac crest superiorly. At either end of the crest are the anterior and posterior superior iliac spines, below which lie the anterior and posterior inferior iliac spines. The iliac crest has a separate secondary ossification centre, which appears at the age of puberty and fuses from 20 years onwards. This should not be mistaken for a fracture. There is also a separate ossification centre for the anterior inferior iliac spine, which appears at a similar age. This is the origin of the straight head of the rectus femoris muscle, and it is common for 'tug' lesions to develop at this site, causing an irregular appearance. The inner surface of the ilium is smooth and bears a prominence, the iliopectineal line. This, together with the sacral promontory posteriorly and the pubic symphysis anteriorly, forms the pelvic brim which separates the false or greater pelvis from the true or lesser pelvis inferiorly. In the erect posture, the pelvic inlet forms an angle of 50–60° and the outlet approximately 15° to the horizontal plane (Fig. 9).

The ischium has a vertically orientated body with a tuberosity inferiorly. From this, the ischial ramus runs anteriorly to join the inferior pubic ramus at a synchondrosis, which fuses at the age of 7 years (Fig. 2). The synchondrosis may have a bizarre appearance at the time of fusion, which may simulate a healing fracture. The ischial tuberosity has a separate secondary ossification centre, which appears at puberty and fuses at around 20 years. Posteriorly, the ischial spine demarcates the greater and lesser sciatic notches superiorly and inferiorly, respectively.

The pubis consists of a body and superior and inferior pubic rami. The obturator foramen is bounded by the bodies and rami of the pubis and ischium.

The false pelvis has little clinical or radiological significance and should be regarded as part of the abdominal cavity. It contains loops of small bowel and the ascending, descending and sigmoid colon. The true pelvis, bounded above by the pelvic brim or inlet and below by the pelvic outlet, contains the genital tracts and the lower parts of the intestinal and urinary tracts. The outlet is bounded by the coccyx posteriorly, the ischial tuberosities laterally and the pubic arch anteriorly. The pelvic cavity so enclosed is short and curved, with a shallow anterior wall and a deep posterior wall.

There are some gender differences in the appearance of the pelvis visible on plain radiographs. The male pelvic inlet is narrower with more prominent ischial spines and the angle of the pubic arch is smaller. The alae of the sacrum are relatively narrow in comparison to the body of the sacrum, when compared with the female, and the sacral promontory is more prominent. The sacrum is longer and the true pelvic cavity is deeper than in the female. Muscle attachments are generally more pronounced than in the female (Fig. 3).

Important ligaments extend from the various bony landmarks of the pelvis and define the pelvic cavity. These include: the sacrotuberous ligaments, running from the ischial tuberosity to the side of the sacrum and coccyx and to the posterior inferior iliac spine (which defines the posterior limit of the lesser sciatic foramen) and the triangular sacrospinous ligament, with its apex at the ischial spine and its base at the sides of the sacrum and coccyx. This is covered by the coccygeus muscle and

separates the greater and lesser sciatic foramina. It defines the inferior limit of the greater sciatic foramen. A further ligament, the iliolumbar ligament, extends from the transverse process of the fifth lumbar vertebra to the iliac crest. All these ligaments may calcify in the normal ageing population.

The paired psoas muscles run into the pelvis on either side of the vertebral column. As they descend, they run alongside the anteromedial aspect of the iliacus muscles arising from the inner ilium. The combined iliopsoas muscles then run anterolaterally to the lesser trochanter of the femur, passing under the inguinal ligament.

Within the true pelvis, the piriformis muscles arise from the anterior sacrum and pass laterally through the greater sciatic foramen, inserting on to the greater trochanter of the femur, so forming part of the posterior wall of the pelvis, along with their parietal fascial covering.

Laterally, the tough obturator membrane almost completely fills the obturator foramen. A small deficiency anteriorly forms the obturator canal, through which the obturator vessels and nerve pass to enter the thigh. The obturator internus muscle arises from the pelvic surface of the obturator membrane and the adjacent ischium and pubis. The fibres converge on a tendon, which runs through the lesser sciatic foramen to insert on the greater trochanter of the femur.

The aponeurosis of the external oblique muscle of the anterior abdominal wall inserts on to the pubic crest on the superior surface of the superior pubic ramus. A thickening of the aponeurosis forms the inguinal ligament, running from the pubic tubercle to the anterior superior iliac spine.

Fig. 3.
Frontal radiograph of an adult male pelvis. Note the differences between this radiograph and that of the female pelvis illustrated in Fig 1.

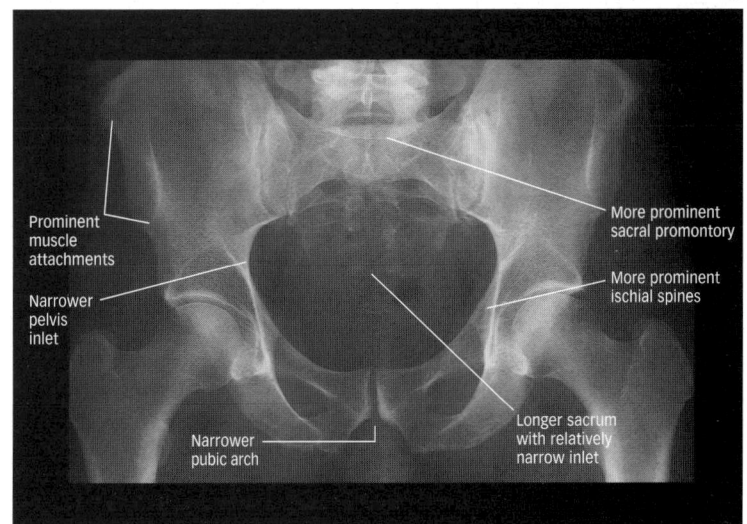

Prominent muscle attachments

Narrower pelvis inlet

Narrower pubic arch

More prominent sacral promontory

More prominent ischial spines

Longer sacrum with relatively narrow inlet

The sacrum

This triangular bone is formed by the fusion of the five sacral vertebrae (Fig. 4). Its broad base lies superiorly and forms a cartilaginous joint with the inferior surface of the body of the fifth lumbar vertebra. Its concave anterior surface forms a hollowed posterior wall to the true pelvis. Four pairs of anterior sacral foramina communicate with the sacral canal and transmit the ventral rami of the first four sacral nerves. The dorsal surface bears a median sacral crest from which arise four sacral tubercles. Lateral to these are the four pairs of dorsal sacral foramina through which pass the dorsal rami of the first four pairs of sacral nerves. The superior articular processes of the first sacral vertebra protrude above the superior foramina, their articular surfaces facing backwards to articulate with the inferior articular surfaces of the fifth lumbar vertebra. The articular surfaces of the remaining sacral segments are visible only as small tubercles just medial to the sacral foramina, which collectively are called the intermediate sacral crest. The lateral sacral crests lie lateral to the foramina, sometimes bearing transverse tubercles which are the vestigial transverse processes. The sacral hiatus is a horseshoe-shaped deficiency in the lower end of the posterior wall of the sacral canal.

The lateral surface of the sacrum is occupied superiorly by the auricular ('ear-shaped') surface for articulation with the ilium. Below this, the lateral surface narrows and curves medially tapering towards the inferior surface, which articulates with the coccyx, a triangular bone formed from the fusion of the four coccygeal vertebrae (occasionally three or five).

The sacroiliac joint

This is a synovial joint between the auricular surfaces of the sacrum and ilium. The irregularities in both joint surfaces, which are reciprocal, add to the strength of the joint. The iliac surface is covered with hyaline cartilage, the sacral surface by fibrocartilage. In later life, adhesions and synostosis may occur. The joint is strengthened by the ventral and dorsal sacroiliac ligaments and by the interosseous sacroiliac ligament which occupies the area immediately above and behind the joint beneath the dorsal sacroiliac ligament. It is the strongest ligament in the body and provides the main strength of the joint. A small amount of rotatory movement occurs at the joint, which is increased in pregnancy and child-bearing.

Ossification

The centre for the ilium appears at 8 weeks of fetal life and those for the ischium and pubis at 18–22 weeks. At birth, the iliac crests, acetabular floor and the inferior surface of the innominate bone are unossified. The pubis and ischium fuse at 7–8 years. The triradiate cartilage of the acetabular floor ossifies from two centres which appear at puberty and fuse

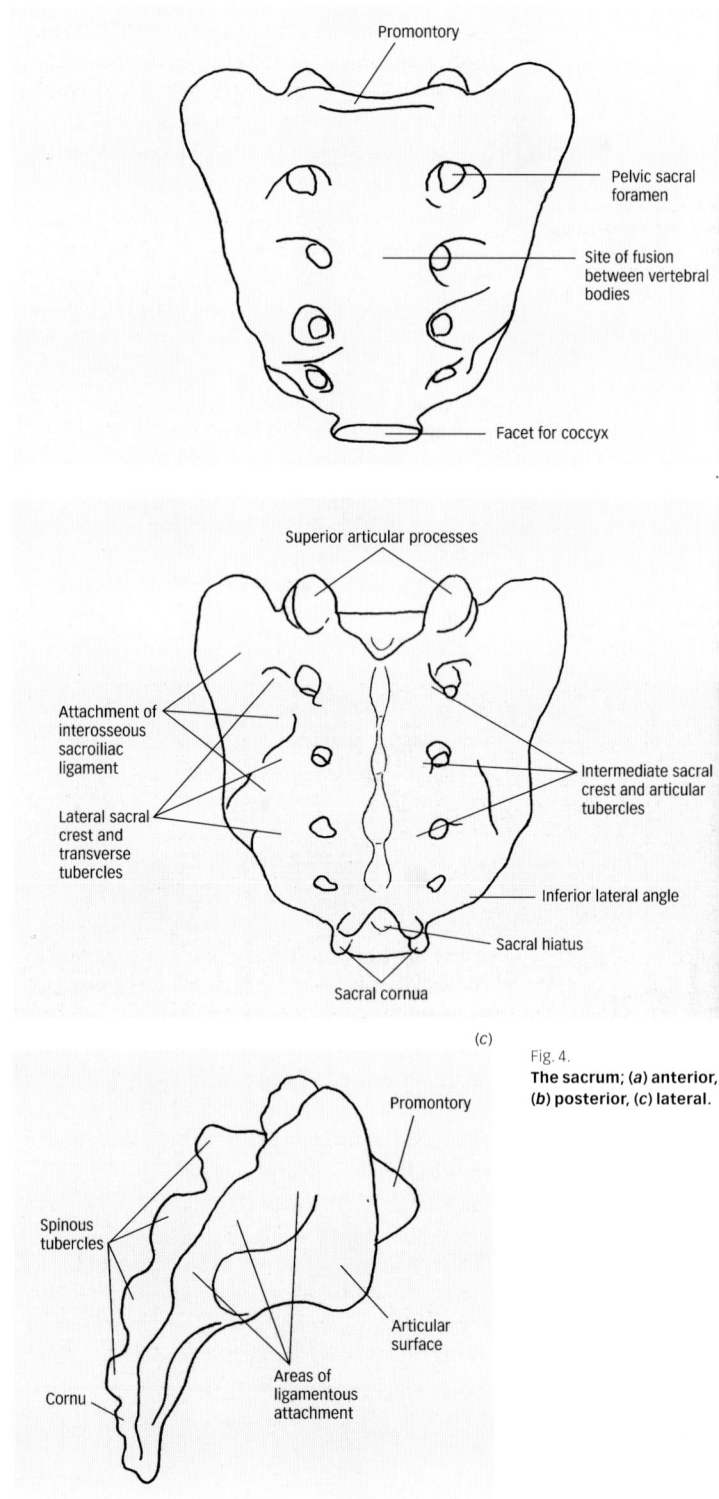

Fig. 4.
The sacrum; (*a*) anterior, (*b*) posterior, (*c*) lateral.

at 20–25 years. The centres for the iliac crest and for the inferior surface of the innominate bone likewise appear at around puberty and fuse with the remainder of the bony pelvis at 20–25 years (Fig. 5). The sacrum ossifies in an analogous manner to the remainder of the spine, centres for the vertebral body and each half of the vertebral arch appearing at 10–20 weeks of fetal life. The vestigial costal elements (above and lateral to the sacral foramina) appear at 6 to 8 months of fetal life. After birth, the costal and vertebral elements unite at about 5 years and fusion with the vertebral body and with the vertebral arch of the other side occurs at 8 years. From puberty onwards,

Fig. 5.
Ossification of the bones of the pelvis. The secondary centres (hatched) start to ossify at puberty and fuse at 20–25 years.

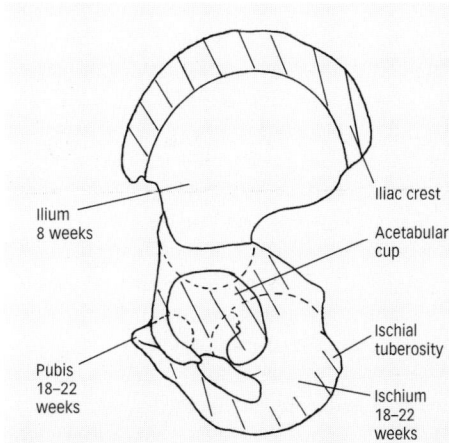

6.
Axial MRI of the pelvis demonstrate the muscles around the hip joint.

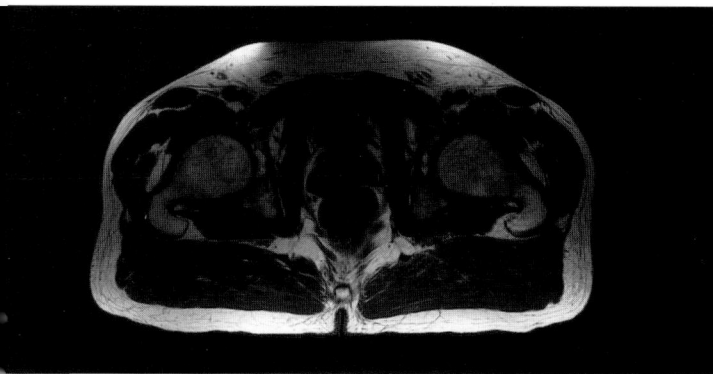

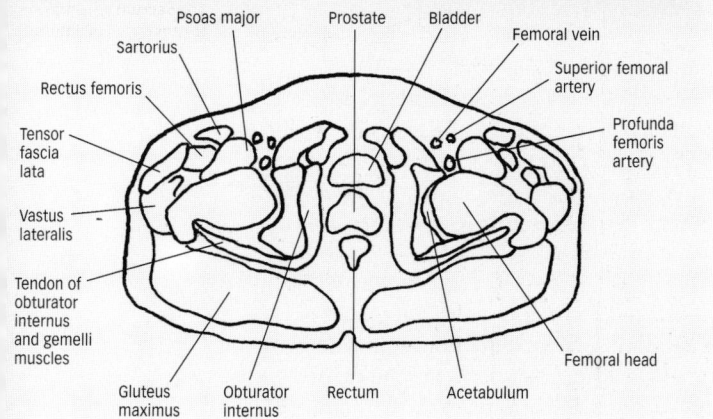

the lateral costovertebral elements of the sacral segments fuse from below upwards and the end plate epiphyses of the bodies begin to ossify. These also fuse from the twentieth year onwards.

The muscles of the pelvic girdle

A brief outline of the attachment of the most important muscles of the lower limb is given below to supplement the images and diagrams of the cross-sectional anatomy (Fig. 6). Relevant details of the actions of the muscles are given in the section on the corresponding joint. *Gluteus maximus* arises from the superior part of the posterior surface of the ilium including the crest, the side of the sacrum, coccyx and sacrotuberous ligament. The majority of the muscle converges as a tendinous sheet to merge with the iliotibial tract. The deeper fibres attach to the gluteal tuberosity of the femur. *Gluteus medius* arises deep to, and below, gluteus maximus and attaches to the lateral aspect of the greater trochanter. *Gluteus minimus* arises below, and deep to, gluteus medius and is completely covered by it. It is attached to the anterior surface of the greater trochanter.

Piriformis arises from the front of the sacrum and from the gluteal surface of the ilium. It passes out of the pelvis through the greater sciatic foramen and inserts on the upper border of the greater trochanter.

Obturator internus arises from the pelvic surface of the medial part of the obturator membrane and the surrounding bone and passes though the lesser sciatic foramen. Its tendon receives the fibres of the *gemelli muscles* (gemellus superior arises from the ischial spine, gemellus inferior from the ischial tuberosity), and inserts at the medial surface of the greater trochanter.

Obturator externus takes its origin from the outer surface of the obturator membrane and the surrounding bone and passes below the hip joint to insert into the trochanteric fossa at the base of the medial surface of the greater trochanter.

Quadratus femoris lies between gemellus inferior and adductor magnus, passing from the ischial tuberosity to the trochanteric crest, at the quadrate tubercle.

Imaging modalities
Plain radiography relies mainly on the anteroposterior (AP) view (Figs. 1, 3). This is taken with the legs rotated internally 10–15° to compensate for the anteversion of the femoral neck. Figure 7 shows the auricular or paragle-

Fig. 7.
AP radiograph of the pelvis to show the paraglenoid sulcus.

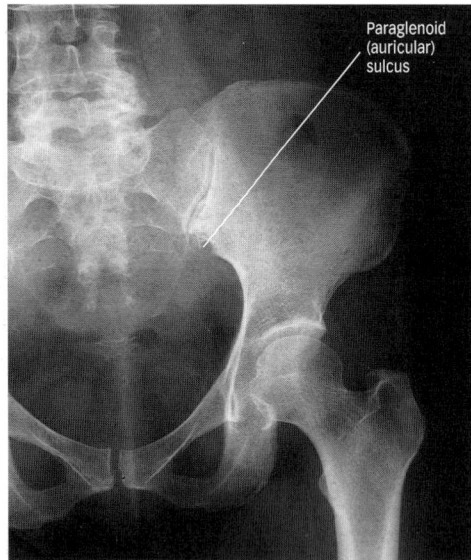

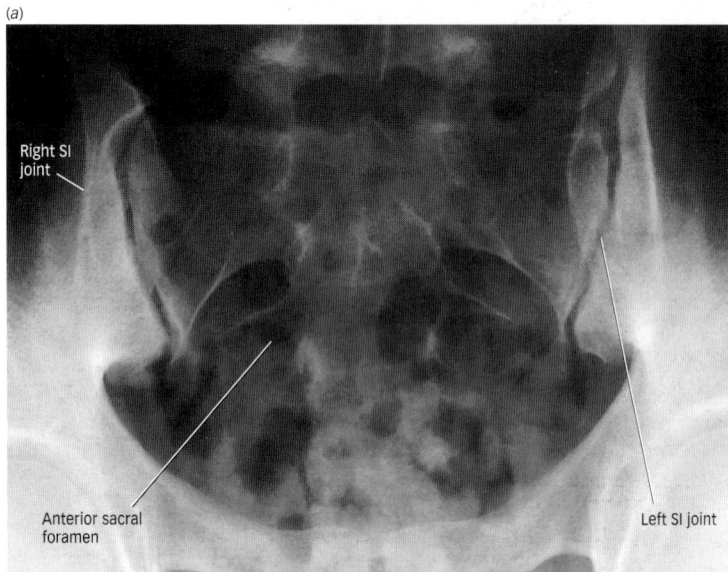

Fig. 8.
(a) PA radiograph of both sacroiliac joints, (b) oblique AP radiograph of the left sacroiliac joint.

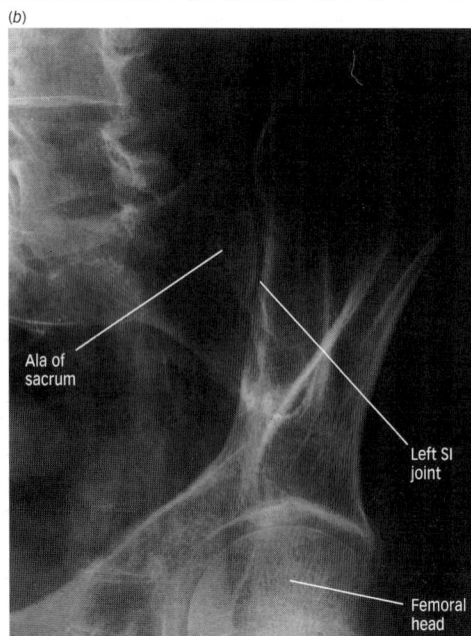

noid sulcus which transmits the superior branch of the gluteal artery and is a feature of the female pelvis. Shenton's line (Fig. 13(a)) is visible on the anteroposterior radiograph of the pelvis as an arc running from the medial aspect of the femoral neck to the superior border of the obturator foramen. It should be a smooth curve. The iliopectineal line is a smooth, curved line sweeping anteriorly from the medial border of the ilium marking the junction of ilium and pubis.

The posterior and anterior rims may be identified. The acetabular 'teardrop' has its borders formed by the quadrilateral plate of the iliac bone medially, the inferior part of the acetabular fossa inferiorly and the anterior part of the acetabular fossa laterally. Kohler's 'teardrop distance' (Fig. 13(a)) should be less than 11 mm, and there should not be a difference of more than 2 mm between the two sides. The sacrum may be better seen on an anteroposterior projection with 35° of cephalad angulation (Ferguson's view). Oblique views (Judet's views) of the acetabulum and femoral heads will often give additional information about the anterior (iliopubic) and posterior (ilioischial) columns of the acetabulum if a fracture is suspected. The 'stork' view, to assess pubic symphysis instability, is taken standing alternately on each leg. A change in the alignment of the superior surface of the pubic rami of more than 3 mm is abnormal.

Because the sacroiliac joint planes diverge in the posteroanterior direction, the joints are often better profiled with a posteroanterior radiograph because the diverging beam is more nearly parallel to the joint surfaces. Oblique anterioposterior views of each sacroiliac joint may be required to see them optimally (Fig. 8).

CT is particularly useful for assessing complex fractures, the sacroiliac joints and intra-articular fragments. MRI has superseded it in the assessment of soft tissue injuries and medullary bone abnormalities.

Pelvimetry
It is occasionally necessary to assess the female pelvis radiologically to assess the likelihood of difficulties in labour. The commonest indications during pregnancy are a persistent breech delivery confirmed by ultrasound at 36 or more weeks gestation in a previously untried pelvis where a vaginal delivery is envisaged. Following a difficult labour or Caesarian section, if further vaginal deliveries are envisaged, pelvimetry may be carried out before a subsequent pregnancy. CT and MRI are now widely used for pelvimetry.

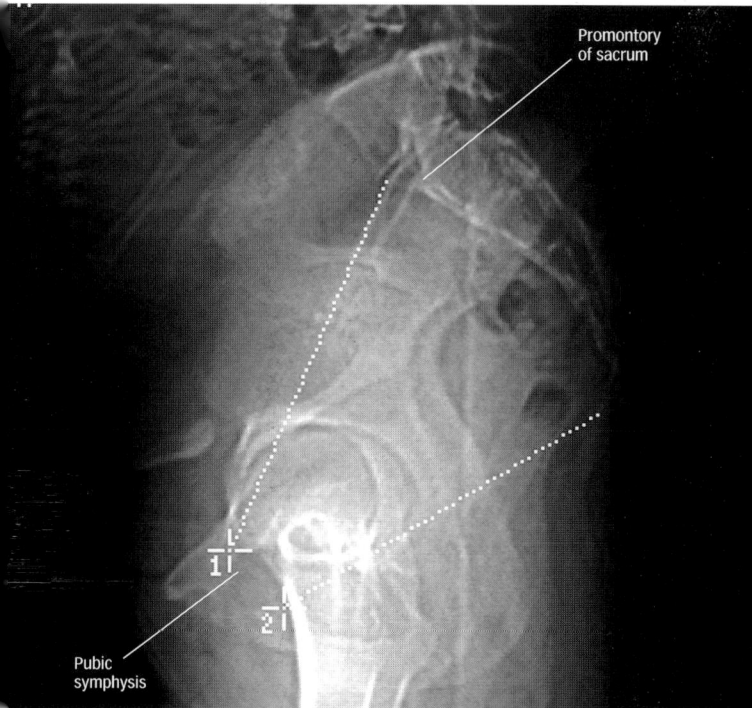

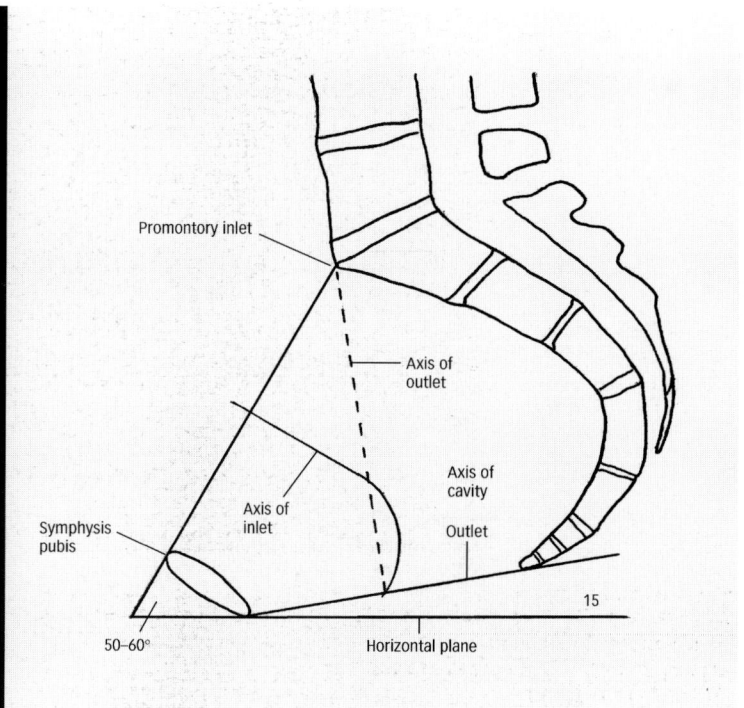

Fig. 9. above
 pelvimetry showing the
AP inlet (conjugate) and
outlet.

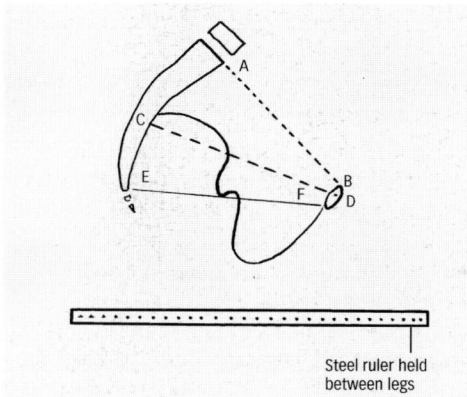

Fig. 10.
The technique of lateral pelvimetry.

MRI should be used if available as it imparts no radiation dose. MR pelvimetry in pregnancy is performed using a lateral scout view and measuring the inlet and outlet diameters in the sagittal plane. In the non-pregnant woman this may be supplemented by an AP scout view. Alternatively, two sections may be obtained, one at the pelvic inlet and one at the outlet, or even a single section at the level of the femoral heads (Fig. 9).

If MR or CT are not available, conventional pelvimetry in pregnancy is carried out by taking a true lateral radiograph of the pelvis while the patient holds a metal ruler between her legs (Fig. 10). A higher kV (90–95 kV) is used as this reduces the absorbed dose. If an anteroposterior view is required, a correction is needed to allow for magnification.

The most important measurement is the AP inlet or conjugate diameter, which is the smallest AP diameter between the posterior margin of the symphisis pubis and the anterior aspect of the sacrum. The normal value varies between 11.0 and 12.5 cm. Values of less than 10.5 cm indicate increasing likelihood of cephalopelvic disproportion.

If there is a breech presentation, values in the upper half of the range are needed to predict safe vaginal delivery at term.

On the anteroposterior view, both the transverse diameter of the inlet (average value = 13.0 cm) and the interspinous distance (between the ischial spines; average value = 11.0 cm) can be measured. It is generally accepted that the minimum values for safe vaginal delivery are a transverse inlet diameter of 11.0 cm and a bispinous diameter of 10.0 cm. The pelvic outlet dimensions are probably less important because of the considerable increase in the outlet diameter of up to 4 cm that may occur during delivery due to relaxation of the symphysis and rotation of the sacroiliac joints. The average value for the transverse outlet diameter (between the ischial tuberosities) is 10.5 cm.

The hip joint

This is a synovial articulation of the 'ball and socket' type between the head of the femur and the acetabulum. The articular surface of the femoral head is thickest at the centre of the head. The fovea capitis, where the ligament of the head (ligamentum teres) is

Fig. 11. (a)
The ligaments of the right hip joint, (a) anterior, (b) posterior.

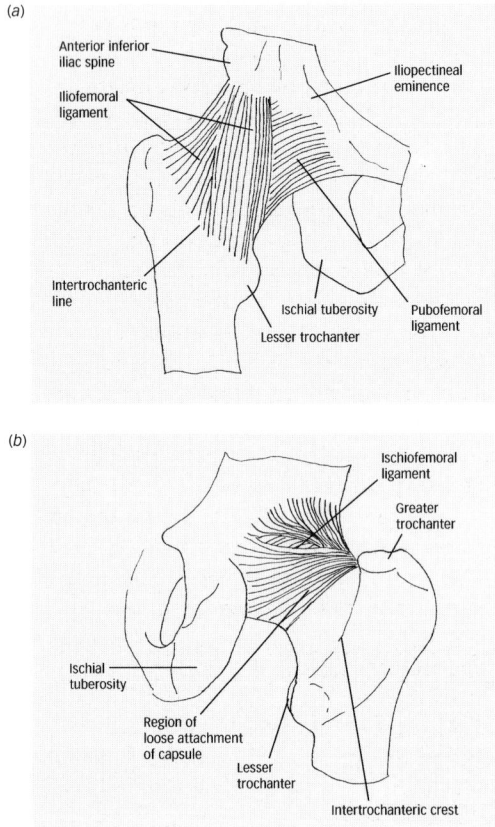

Fig. 11. (a)
The ligaments of the right hip joint, (a) anterior, (b) posterior.

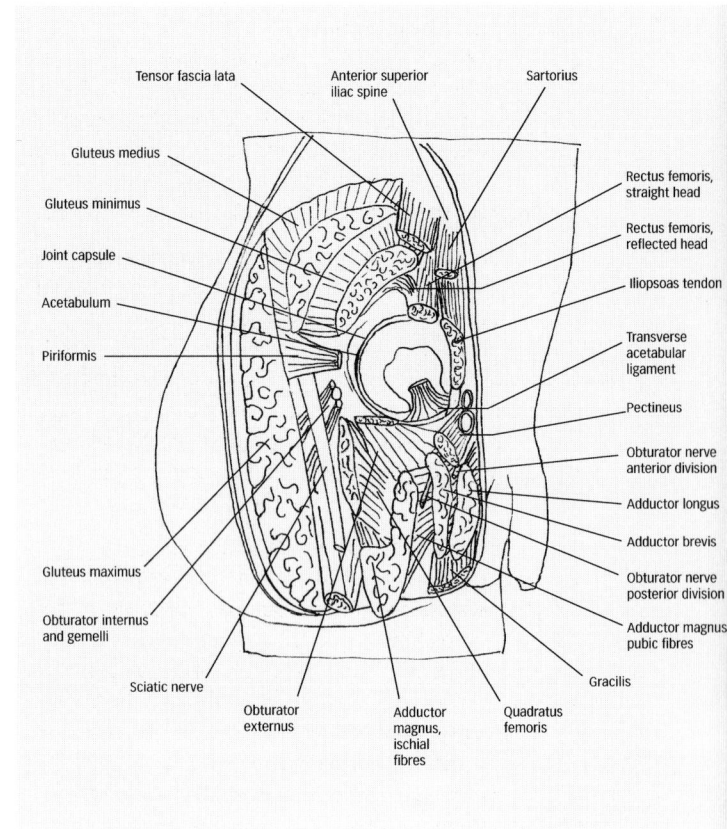

Fig. 12.
The relations of the right hip joint (the femur has been removed).

attached, is not covered in cartilage. The articular (lunate) surface of the acetabulum is deficient inferiorly over the acetabular notch and centrally where the floor of the acetabulum is filled with a fibrofatty pad. The articular cartilage is thickest and broadest superiorly where the weight is borne. The fibrocartilaginous acetabular labrum serves to deepen the articular cup formed by the lunate surface. It bridges the acetabular notch as the transverse acetabular ligament.

The fibrous capsule is attached around the rim of the acetabulum and inferiorly to the transverse acetabular ligament. Its femoral attachments are to the base of the neck; anteriorly to the inter-trochanteric line and posteriorly 10 mm above the trochanteric crest. The capsular retinaculum is made up of fibres that are reflected proximally along the neck carrying part of the blood supply to the head and neck.

The fibrous capsule is thickest and strongest anteriorly and superiorly. The synovium arises from the margins of the articular cartilage of the femoral neck and covers the intracapsular femoral neck, the inner surface of the capsule, the acetabular labrum, the fibrofatty pad filling in the floor of the acetabulum and is reflected as a tube sheathing the ligamentum teres. It may communicate with a bursa beneath the tendon of psoas major through a deficiency in the fibrous capsule and iliofemoral ligament.

The fibrous capsule is reinforced by three ligaments (Fig. 11).

The *iliofemoral ligament* (of Bigelow) is an inverted, V-shaped band, which is attached superiorly to the anterior inferior iliac spine and inferiorly to the lower and upper ends of the intertrochanteric line. It is very strong and intimately blended with the fibrous capsule.

The *pubofemoral ligament* is a triangular band reinforcing the inferior capsule with its base attached to the iliopectineal line, superior pubic ramus and obturator membrane and its apex to the base of the femoral neck. The *ischiofemoral ligament* is a thickening of the posterior capsule by fibres spiralling from the ischium upwards and forwards over the back of the femoral neck to be inserted into the greater trochanter. The transverse acetabular ligament and the ligament of the femoral head have been mentioned above.

The relations of the hip joint (Fig. 12), are:

• Anteriorly from medial to lateral: pectineus with the femoral vein overlying it, iliopsoas tendon with the iliacus bursa deep to, and the femoral artery and nerve superficial to it, rectus femoris with the iliotibial tract lying deep to it;

- Superiorly: reflected head of rectus femoris, gluteus minimus;
- Posteriorly, from above down: piriformis, obturator internus and gemelli tendons separating the joint from the sciatic nerve, the tendon of obturator externus with quadratus femoris overlying.
- Inferiorly: pectineus and obturator externus.

The blood supply is derived from branches of the obturator, medial circumflex femoral and superior and inferior gluteal arteries. The nerve supply is from branches of the femoral, obturator, superior gluteal and inferior gluteal nerves and the nerve to quadratus femoris. For a more detailed description of the blood supply to the femoral head, see 'The Femur'.

The movements of the joint are:

- flexion: iliacus, psoas (principally), pectineus, rectus femoris and sartorius;
- extension: gluteus maximus and the hamstrings;
- abduction: gluteus medius and minimus, tensor fascia lata and sartorius;
- adduction: adductor longus, brevis and magnus, pectineus and gracilis;
- medial rotation: anterior fibres of gluteus medius and minimus, tensor fasciae latae;
- lateral rotation: obturator muscles, gemelli, quadratus femoris, piriformis, gluteus maximus and sartorius.

Imaging modalities

On an anteroposterior radiograph (Fig. 13), the foreshortening of the femoral neck is minimized by internally rotating the leg 10–15°. The medial border of the neck should form a smooth curve (Shenton's line) continuous with the inferior border of the superior pubic ramus (superior boundary of the obturator foramen), and a line drawn along the lateral border of the neck should transect the lateral part of the femoral head. A lateral film is often required, usually a groin lateral using a horizontal beam. A 'frog' lateral is sometimes obtained using an AP radiograph with the hip abducted and externally rotated so that the knee is lying nearly on the table top.

The frog lateral is particularly useful in assessing the femoral capital epiphyses in children and comparing one side with the other. Von Rosen's view is obtained with the hips abducted to about 45° and internally rotated. In the normal hip, the lines of the femoral shafts bisect the acetabulum and intersect with each other in the midline at the level of the lumbosacral junction. This view is useful in the assessment of congenital dislocation of the hip in infants and small children if ultra-

sound scanning is not possible. (The radiological features of the immature hip are dealt with in the chapter 'Paediatrics'.)

Normal appearances that may simulate pathology include a large fovea capitis, superimposition of the acetabulum on the femoral head, especially the lucent interval between anterior and posterior rims and the os acetabuli, an accessory ossicle at the upper outer lip of the acetabulum. Although often visible, the fat planes around the joint are not a reliable indicator of a joint effusion if displaced.

Ultrasound is often able to detect small amounts of fluid within the joint; the anterior surface of the femoral neck within the joint capsule is accessible to high resolution scanning. CT is particularly useful in the evaluation of complex bony injuries. MRI is increasingly being used to make the early diagnosis of avascular necrosis, a condition for which MR has a high sensitivity and specificity. It is also

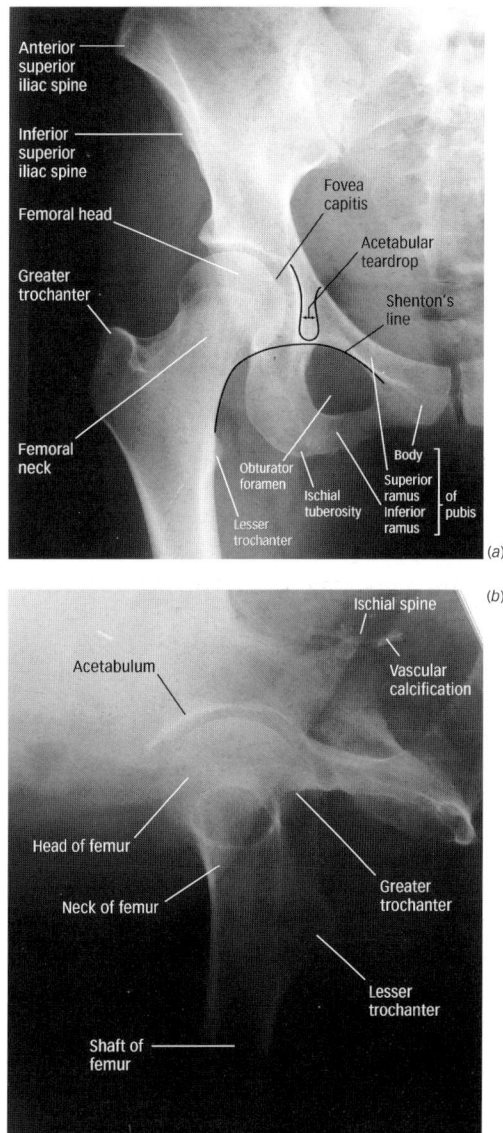

Fig. 13.
AP and lateral Radiographs of the right hip, (a) anteroposterior, (b) lateral.

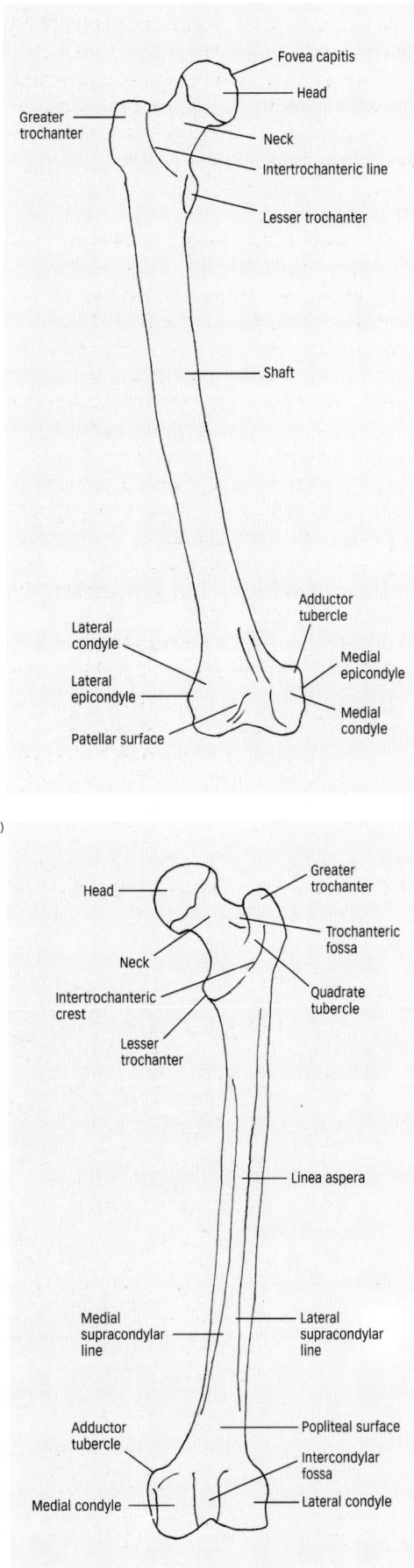

Fig. 14. (a)
**The right femur,
(a) anterior, (b) posterior.**

The thigh

The femur

The femur (Fig. 14) consists of a shaft, whose superior portion is angled medially to form the neck, and a head which articulates with the acetabulum. The greater and lesser trochanters lie at the junction of shaft and neck. The lower end of the shaft is expanded to form two condyles for articulation with the tibia.

The head is a little more than half a sphere and is directed upwards, medially and slightly forwards to articulate with the articular surface of the acetabulum. It has a central pit or fovea where the ligamentum teres is attached. The neck is about 5 cm long and makes an angle of 125–135° with the shaft and is also anteverted by about 8°. In children, the degree of anteversion is much greater; up to 50° in the first year, up to 30° at 2 years, 25° at 3–5 years, 20° at 6–12 years, 17° at 13–15 years and 11° up to 20 years of age.

The junction of the neck with the shaft is marked anteriorly by a prominent roughened intertrochanteric line and posteriorly by a more rounded intertrochanteric crest. The greater trochanter is a large projection at the upper end of the intertrochanteric line, which projects upwards and slightly medially, so that its medial surface, the trochanteric fossa, is concave. It gives attachment to most of the muscles of the gluteal region. The lesser trochanter projects posteromedially from the lower end of the junction of shaft and neck. Iliopsoas tendon inserts into it.

The blood supply of the femoral head merits description because of its importance in relation to fractures of the femoral neck, their sequelae and the implications for clinical management. A small supply to the central part of the head is provided from the artery of the ligamentum teres, which in turn is derived from the obturator and medial circumflex femoral arteries. The terminal medullary branches of the shaft of the femur also contribute. The principal supply, however, is from a vascular ring around the femoral neck at the level of attachment of the fibrous capsule lying largely within the cap-

able to characterize the soft tissues, ligaments and acetabular labrum. Arthrography is rarely necessary, although it is often helpful if combined with manual or digital subtraction techniques in the assessment of hip prostheses, especially in the context of possible loosening. MR or CT arthrography may be useful in the assessment of acetabular labral tears.

sule anteriorly and outside it posteriorly. The trochanteric anastomosis lies in the trochanteric fossa and provides most of the supply to the vascular ring. It is formed from ascending branches of the lateral and medial circumflex femoral arteries, a descending branch of the superior gluteal artery and frequently a branch of the inferior gluteal artery. The cruciate anastomosis lies at the level of the middle of the lesser trochanter and is formed from transverse branches of the medial and lateral circumflex femoral arteries, an ascending branch of the first perforating branch of the profunda femoris, and a descending branch of the inferior gluteal artery. From the vascular ring, retinacular arteries pierce the capsule and run beneath the reflected synovial membrane to supply the head. Two-thirds of the supply to the femoral head is from lateral epiphysial branches which run along the posterior superior surface of the neck. The practical consequence of this arrangement is that intracapsular fractures of the femoral neck compromise the blood supply of the femoral head with a high incidence of avascular necrosis of the femoral head or non-union.

The shaft of the femur is angled medially forming an angle of about 10° with the vertical axis of the tibia in men. This degree of normal valgus is slightly more pronounced (about 14°) in women. The lower part of the shaft is angled backwards by about 17° on the upper part. The linea aspera is a roughened ridge on the posterior aspect of the shaft, to which are attached the adductor muscles and the short head of biceps femoris. The nutrient artery, usually single but may be double, enters the bone on the linea aspera in a proximal direction ('flee from the knee') and may be mistaken for a fracture on the lateral view. Below the linea aspera the posterior part of the shaft forms a flattened triangular popliteal surface.

The lower end of the shaft is expanded into medial and lateral condyles, which are continuous with each other anteriorly but separated by the intercondylar fossa posteriorly. The medial condyle is larger and projects more posteriorly and inferiorly, so that the inferior surface of the femur is nearly horizontal despite the obliquity of the shaft. Its most medial projection is the palpable medial epicondyle. The lateral condyle bears the majority of the patellar articulation. It is grooved posterolaterally by the tendon of popliteus.

The patella is a flattened sesamoid bone within the quadriceps tendon. It is roughly triangular with its apex pointing inferiorly and a rounded base superiorly. The apex normally lies 1 cm above the knee joint in the erect position. Its posterior articular surface is divided by a smoothly rounded ridge into a large lateral facet and a smaller medial facet for articulation with the corresponding femoral condyles.

A fabella is frequently found in the lateral head of gastrocnemius.

Ossification

The shaft of the femur starts to ossify at the seventh week of fetal life (Fig. 15). The distal femoral epiphysis starts to ossify at 9 months of fetal life and forms the medial and lateral condyles. The femoral head is cartilaginous at birth and starts to ossify in the first 6 months. The centre for the greater trochanter begins to ossify in the fourth year and that for the lesser trochanter at puberty. These centres fuse with the shaft at 18–20 years. The patella ossifies from several centres which appear at 3–6 years and merge. This may give rise to a very irregular appearance of the normal unfused patella. A bipartite patella is a normal variant in which the superolateral part of the patella fails to unite with the rest (Fig. 16). It appears as a well-defined lucent line running obliquely across the upper outer corner of the patella, which may be difficult to differentiate from a fracture. The separated upper outer part may consist of two or more fragments, in which case it is called a tripartite or multipartite patella. If present, these normal variants are usually bilateral, but may rarely be unilateral. Very rarely, a bipartite patella may appear as a horizontal cleft.

Fig. 15. top
Ossification of femur. The secondary centres fuse with the shaft at 18–20 years.

Fig. 16. below
Bipartite and multipartite patellae.

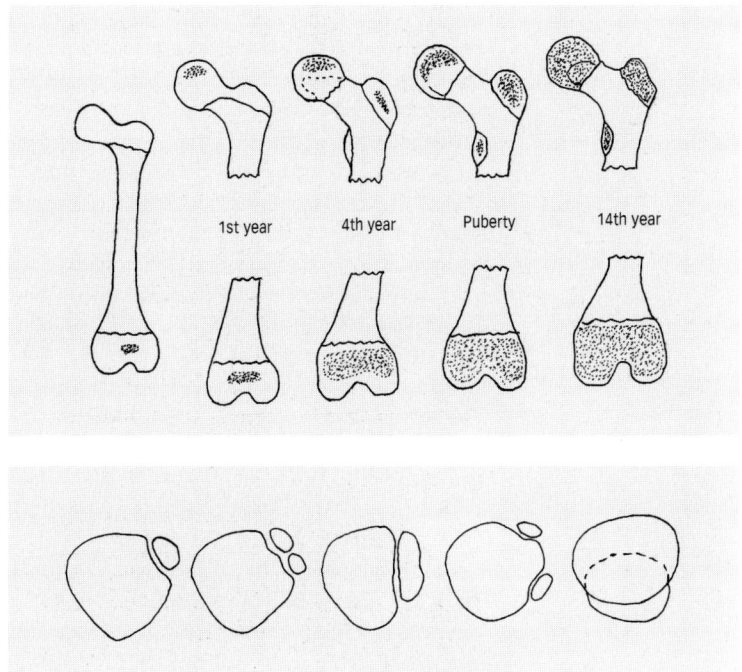

1st year   4th year   Puberty   14th year

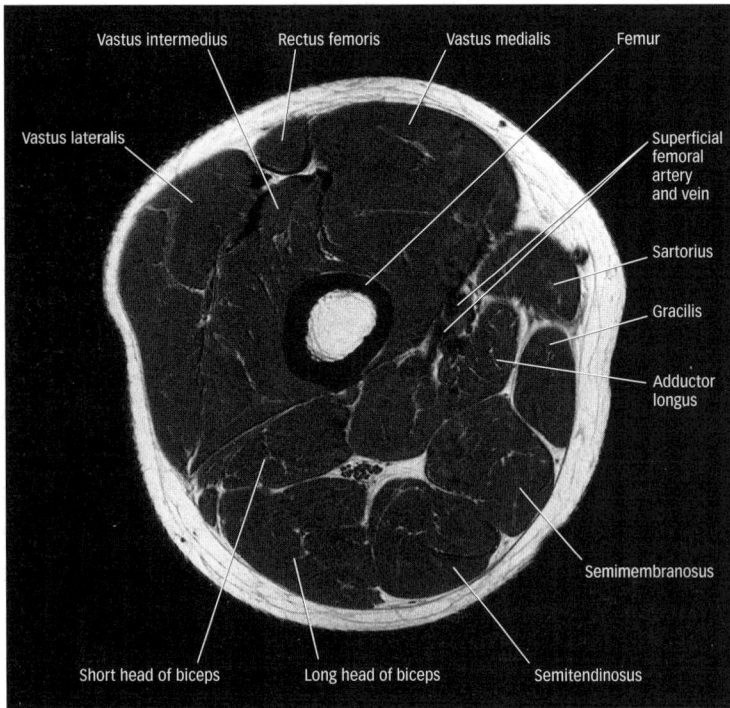

(a)

Vastus intermedius | Rectus femoris | Vastus medialis | Femur

Vastus lateralis

Superficial femoral artery and vein

Sartorius

Gracilis

Adductor longus

Semimembranosus

Short head of biceps | Long head of biceps | Semitendinosus

Vastus medialis

Vastus lateralis

Shaft of femur

Adductor magnus

Gracilis

Sartorius

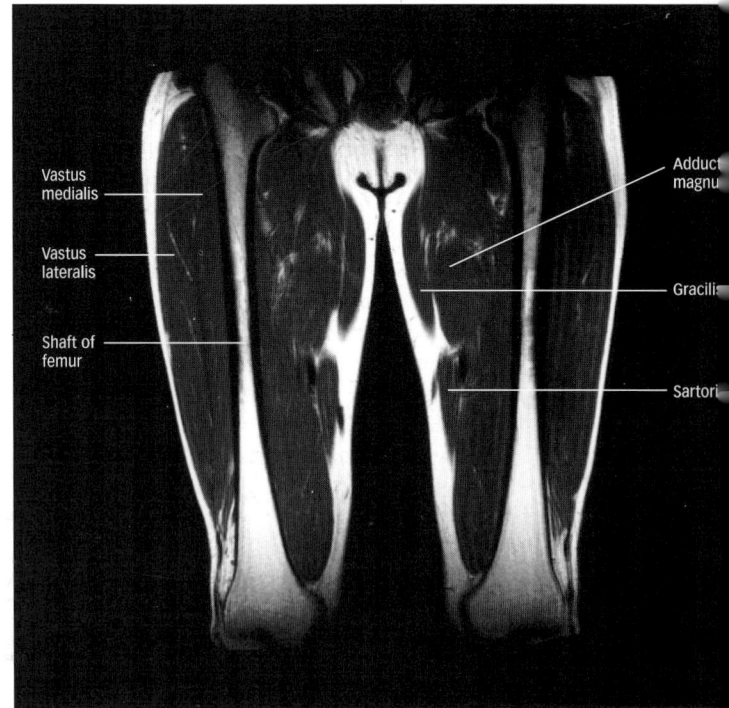

Fig. 17.
T1W MRI of the right thigh: (a) axial scan through mid-thigh and (b) coronal image.

The muscles of the thigh

Anterior femoral muscles

Psoas major arises from the lower body of the twelfth thoracic vertebrae and the bodies, transverse processes and intervertebral discs of all the lumbar vertebrae. It descends along the pelvic brim, under the inguinal ligament to form a tendon that passes anterior to the hip joint receiving the majority of the fibres from iliacus to insert into the lesser trochanter.

Tensor fascia lata arises from the anterior superior iliac spine (ASIS) and is inserted into the iliotibial tract, a strong thickened band of the deep fascia of the lateral aspect of the thigh (fascia lata), which is attached distally to the lateral condyle of the tibia. *Sartorius*, a narrow strap muscle arising from the ASIS descends diagonally across the front of the thigh to the medial aspect of the knee where it inserts via an aponeurosis to the medial tibial condyle.

Quadriceps femoris is made up of four components. *Rectus femoris* arises by a straight head from the anterior inferior iliac spine (AIIS) and a reflected head from the superior margin of the acetabulum and the capsule of the hip joint. Irregularity of the bone at the site of origin of the reflected head may mimic an osteosarcoma. Its tendon inserts into the superior border of the patella. *Vastus intermedius* arises from the anterior surface of the femoral shaft and inserts into the base of the patella deep to the tendon of rectus femoris *Vastus lateralis* arises from the greater trochanter and

the upper part of the linea aspera. A broad aponeurosis becomes a flattened tendon inserting into the outer border of the patella and blends with the iliotibial tract. *Vastus medialis* arises from the lower part of the greater trochanter, the spiral line, the linea aspera and the medial supracondylar line. Its tendon inserts into the medial side of the patella.

The adductor muscles

Gracilis arises from the body and inferior ramus of the pubis and passes down the medial aspect of the thigh over the medial femoral condyle to insert into the medial surface of the tibia below the condyle. *Pectineus* is a flat, quadrilateral muscle arising from the pecten pubis; it passes posterolaterally to insert between the lesser trochanter and the linea aspera. *Adductor longus* arises from the front of the body of the pubis and is inserted by a broad aponeurosis on to the linea aspera. *Adductor brevis* takes origin from the inferior ramus and body of the pubis behind pectineus and is attached between the lesser trochanter and the linea aspera. *Adductor magnus* arises from the inferior ramus of the pubis and the ramus of the ischium and is attached along the linea aspera, the medial supracondylar line and by a strong tendon to the adductor tubercle of the medial femoral condyle. Its distal attachment is interrupted by the adductor hiatus through which the femoral vessels pass to reach the popliteal fossa, as the popliteal artery and vein.

362

The hamstrings

Semimembranosus arises by a flattened 'membranous' tendon from the ischial tuberosity. It has a complex distal attachment to the medial tibial condyle and the medial surface of the tibia with tendinous expansions over the popliteus muscle to the lateral femoral condyle (the oblique popliteal ligament).

Semitendinosus takes origin from the ischial tuberosity. Inferiorly, its extremely long tendon passes round the medial tibial condyle and over the medial collateral ligament to attach to the medial surface of the tibia posterior to the insertions of gracilis and sartorius.

Biceps femoris arises by a long head from the ischial tuberosity and a short head from the linea aspera and forms a single tendon which inserts on to the head of the fibula.

The knee joint

The knee is a synovial modified hinge joint and is the largest joint in the body. Although contained within a single joint cavity, the knee effectively comprises two condylar joints betwee the femoral and corresponding tibial condyles and a saddle joint between the patella and the femur. The tibiofemoral articulations are each divided by a fibrocartilaginous meniscus. The tibial articular surfaces are both slightly concave; the lateral is smaller and more rounded, the medial larger and ovoid. The three components of the femoral articular surface are continuous. The condylar surfaces, when viewed from below, correspond roughly in shape to the corresponding tibial surface, although they are not congruent. The normal tibiofemoral joint space on a plain radiograph is 3–8 mm. The patellar surface, which covers the anterior surface of the condyles, is divided into a larger lateral and a smaller medial facet. The articular surface of the patella corresponds to the femoral surface with a larger lateral and a smaller medial facet. The normal patello-femoral joint space is 3 mm. In the erect person, the lower limit of the patella lies approximately 1 cm above the line of the knee joint. The patellar tendon is the continuation of the quadriceps tendon joining the apex of the patella to the tibial tuberosity. It is normally equal in length to the maximum longitudinal diameter of the patella itself.

The fibrous capsule is attached around the margins of the articular surfaces. Posteriorly, it is attached above the intercondylar fossa and around the margins of the condyles, to the lateral borders of the patella and around the tibial condyles and head of the fibula. Anteriorly, it extends downwards to include the tib-ial tuberosity. Posteriorly, the capsule is strengthened by the two heads of gastrocnemius and by the oblique popliteal ligament. Medially, the capsule blends with the medial collateral ligament and with the outer edge of the medial meniscus. The component of the capsule which helps to tether the meniscus to the tibial condyle is known as the coronary ligament. Anteriorly, the capsule is reinforced by expansions of the tendons of vastus medialis and lateralis and by the iliotibial tract on the lateral side. These expansions are the patellar retinaculae. Laterally, the capsule blends with the lateral margin of the lateral meniscus but the lateral (fibular) collateral ligament is separate from it. Posterolaterally, the capsule is pierced by the tendon of popliteus (Fig. 18).

Fig. 18.
The capsule and ligaments of the knee joint:
(*a*) antero-medial, (*b*) posterior.

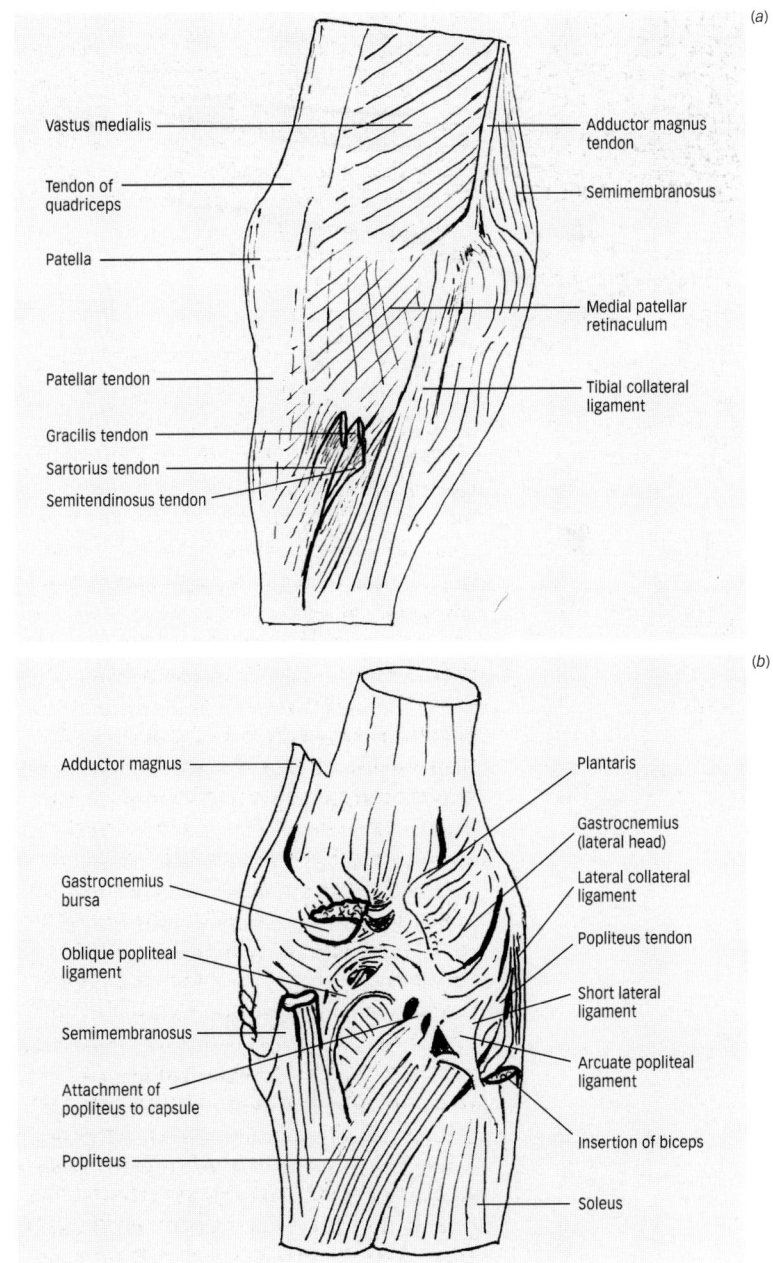

(*a*)

Vastus medialis — Adductor magnus tendon
Tendon of quadriceps — Semimembranosus
Patella
Medial patellar retinaculum
Patellar tendon
Gracilis tendon — Tibial collateral ligament
Sartorius tendon
Semitendinosus tendon

(*b*)

Adductor magnus — Plantaris
Gastrocnemius (lateral head)
Lateral collateral ligament
Gastrocnemius bursa — Popliteus tendon
Oblique popliteal ligament — Short lateral ligament
Semimembranosus — Arcuate popliteal ligament
Attachment of popliteus to capsule — Insertion of biceps
Popliteus — Soleus

The synovial membrane is complex (Fig. 19). It lines the fibrous capsule, but does not cover the surfaces of the menisci. It lines the suprapatellar bursa, which may be regarded as part of the knee joint and lies beneath quadriceps femoris, extending to a hand's breadth above the upper border of the patella. Below the patella, the synovium is separated from the patellar tendon by the infrapatellar fat pad. At this point, two infoldings of synovium, the alar folds, unite as a central infrapatellar fold and pass to the front of the intercondylar fossa. The synovium also forms a subpopliteal recess beneath the tendon of popliteus. Posteriorly, the synovium is reflected anteriorly from the fibrous capsule to cover both cruciate ligaments on their anterior and lateral aspects.

Several bursae surround the knee (Fig. 20):

- Anteriorly: the suprapatellar bursa, the subcutaneous prepatellar bursa, the deep infrapatellar bursa and the subcutaneous infrapatellar bursa;
- Posterolaterally: lateral gastrocnemius, biceps femoris (between the muscle tendon and the fibular collateral ligament) and the popliteus bursa (bursa of the popliteus tendon) between the muscle tendon and the lateral femoral condyle);
- Posteromedially: medial gastrocnemius–semimembranosus bursa between the medial head of gastrocnemius and the tendon of semimembranosus. Further variable bursae may be found deep to the medial collateral ligament and between the tendons of semimembranosus and semitendinosus.

Of the above, the knee joint only communicates with four bursae. The suprapatellar bursa, although a separate bursa in the fetus, almost invariably communicates with the joint in later life and is better regarded as an extension of the joint cavity. It may possess an oblique septum. The popliteus bursa (bursa of the popliteus tendon) usually communicates with the joint. The medial gastrocnemius–semimembranous bursa is said to communicate with the knee joint in 50% in surgical studies. The rate of communication quoted in arthrographic studies is higher but still variable. The lateral gastrocnemius bursa occasionally communicates with the joint.

If the medial gastrocnemius–semimembranosus bursa becomes swollen or inflamed, it is known as a popliteal or Baker's cyst. It is easily seen on ultrasound scanning as an anechoic rounded area that may be seen to connect with the knee joint.

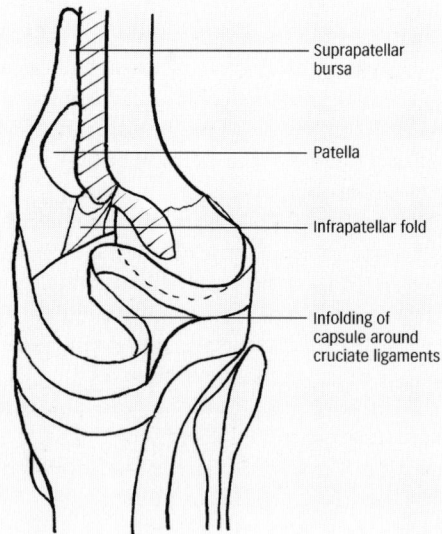

Fig. 19. left
The synovium of knee joint.

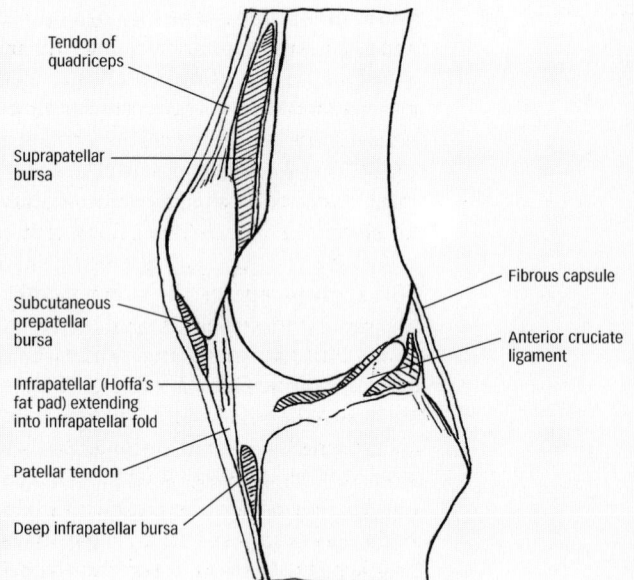

Fig. 20.
Bursae of the knee joint (sagittal section).

Ligaments

In addition to the capsule and its various thickenings, the knee joint is strengthened by five main ligaments (Figs. 18 and 21). The medial (tibial) collateral ligament is attached to the medial epicondyle of the femur and to the medial tibial condyle. It is a flattened band which blends posteriorly with the fibrous capsule but anteriorly may be separated from it by a bursa. The lateral (fibular) collateral ligament is a cord-like structure between the lateral epicondyle of the femur and the head of the fibula. It is separated from the capsule by the popliteus tendon. The oblique popliteal ligament is an expansion of the tendon of semimembranosus and forms part of the floor of the popliteal fossa.

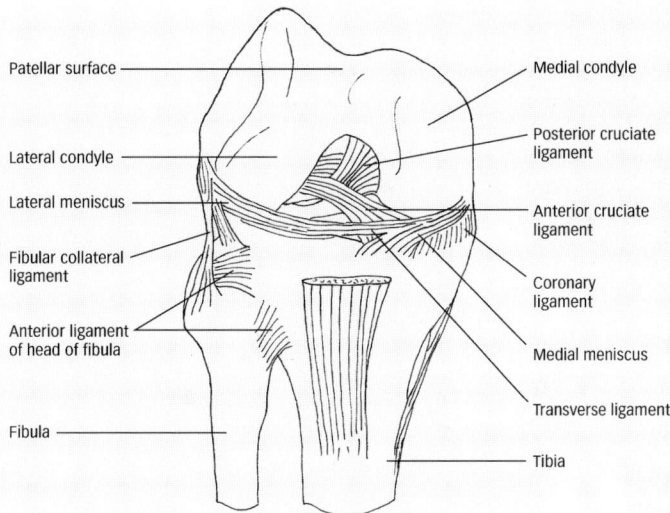

Fig. 21.
Ligaments of the knee joints.

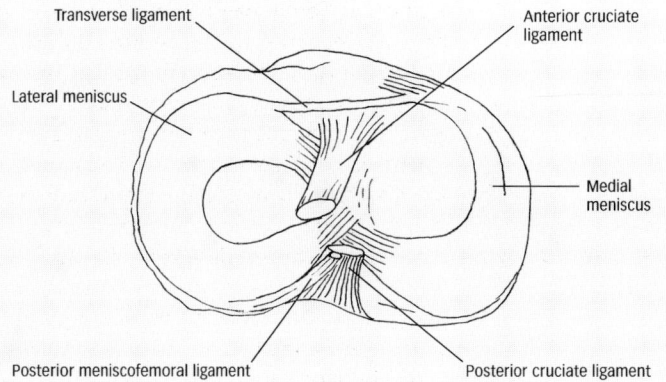

Fig. 22.
The menisci and ligaments of the knee and their attachments.

The anterior cruciate ligament (ACL) is found within the capsule. It passes from the medial part of the anterior intercondylar area of the tibia upwards, backwards and laterally to insert into the posterior part of the medial surface of the lateral femoral condyle. It prevents the femur moving backwards on the tibia. It is easily visible on sagittal MRI as a broad straight band of low signal intensity on T_1- and T_2- weighted images.

The posterior cruciate ligament (PCL) is attached to the posterior intercondylar area of the tibia and passes forwards, upwards and medially to insert into the anterior part of the lateral surface of the medial femoral condyle. It is stronger and shorter than the ACL and is also easily visible on sagittal MRI. It limits posterior sliding of the tibia on the femur. Both cruciate ligaments are taut in all positions of the joint. They are both covered by synovium on their anterior and lateral surfaces by an infolding of synovium from the posterior joint capsule. There may be a synovial bursa interposed between them from the lateral side.

The menisci
These are two semilunar fibrocartilages which deepen the concavity of the tibial articular surfaces and cover approximately two-thirds of the corresponding articular surface (Fig. 22). The medial meniscus is larger and more semicircular. It is broader and thicker posteriorly. The lateral is smaller, thicker and forms a nearly complete ring. Either meniscus may occasionally be discoid, with the thickened periphery extending into the normally thinning centre.

The anterior and posterior horns of the menisci are attached to the corresponding intercondylar areas (see the description of the tibia). The posterior horn of the lateral meniscus is commonly attached to the medial condyle of the femur by the meniscofemoral ligament. This commonly divides to pass either side of the posterior cruciate ligament. If the dominant part is anterior it is known as the anterior meniscofemoral ligament of Humphrey; if posterior to the posterior cruciate ligament, it is known as the posterior meniscofemoral ligament of Wrisberg.

The outer margin of the medial meniscus is blended with the fibrous capsule and the deep surface of the medial collateral ligament. The lateral surface of the lateral meniscus is grooved by, and blends with, the tendon of popliteus, which separates it from the fibular collateral ligament. The transverse ligament joins the anterior ends of the menisci.

The relations of the knee joint are (Fig. 23):

- Anterior: quadriceps femoris, patellar retinacula and suprapatellar bursa;
- Posteromedial: sartorius and gracilis tendons;
- Posterolateral: biceps femoris with the common peroneal nerve on its medial side;

Fig. 23.
The relations of the knee joint.

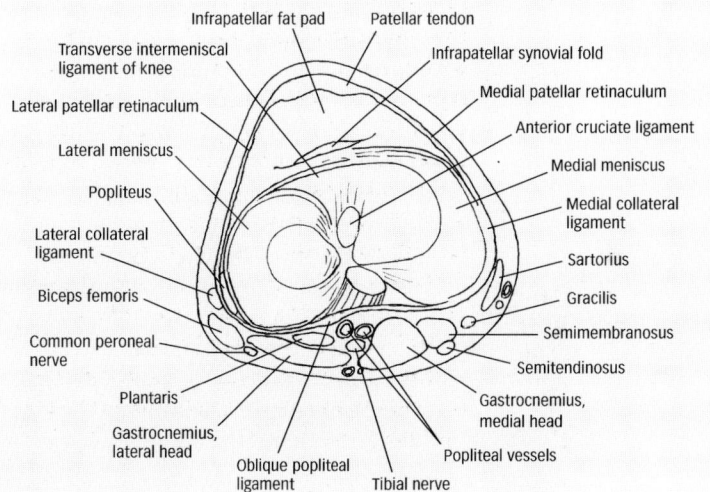

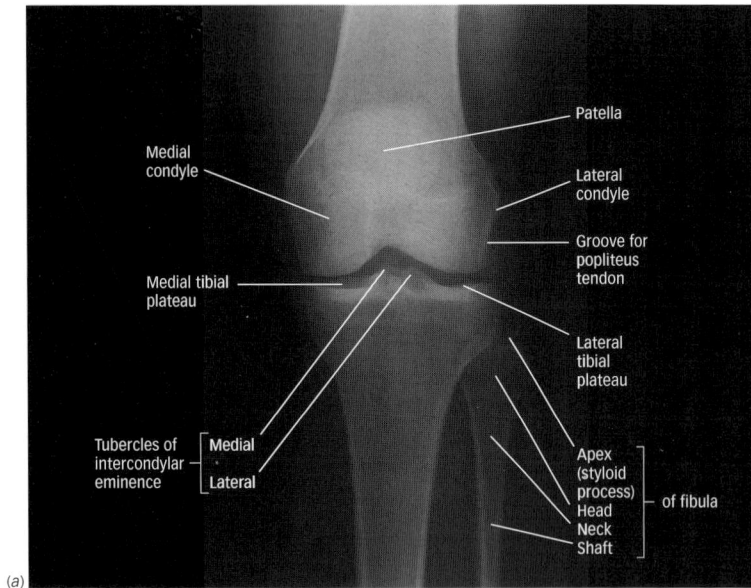

Fig. 24.
(a) AP, and (b) lateral radiographs of the knee.

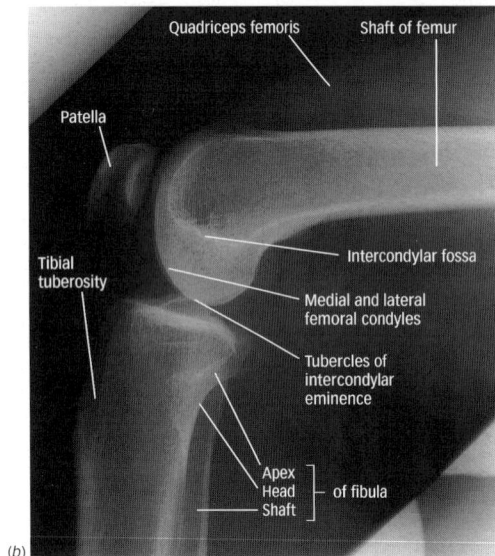

- Posterior: oblique popliteal ligament, popliteus, popliteal artery with vein posterior (superficial) and the tibial nerve posterior to both; lymph nodes; heads of gastrocnemius, lower ends of semimembranosus and semitendinosus.

Movements
- Flexion: biceps, semitendinosus, semimembranosus. The extended knee is unlocked prior to flexion by popliteus, whose action is to rotate the femur laterally on the fixed tibia;
- Extension: quadriceps femoris;
- Medial rotation of the flexed leg: popliteus, semimembranosus and semitendinosus;
- Lateral rotation of the flexed leg: biceps femoris.

Imaging modalities
Plain radiography (Fig. 24) is able to demonstrate the bony contours of the joint space. The fat around the joint enables visualization of the ligamentum patellae, and allows an assessment of the presence or absence of a joint effusion. If a horizontal beam lateral radiograph is taken, a fat-fluid level (lipo-haemarthrosis) in the suprapatellar bursa indicates a fracture within the joint. Occult fractures are usually of the tibial plateau. These may be demonstrated by coronal tomography or by thin slice axial CT with coronal reformatting.

If an abnormality of the patella is suspected, it should be imaged by the 'skyline' view, a tangential view taken with the knee flexed (Fig. 25).

The intercondylar fossa of the lower femur may be imaged by the 'tunnel' view (Fig. 26), which is used to detect clinically suspected intra-articular loose bodies.

Arthrography of the knee (Fig. 27) is much less commonly used but may still be useful in detecting loose bodies within the joint.

MRI is much the most useful imaging technique. It demonstrates the joint cavity, menisci, ligaments and articular cartilage very well. Sagittal images are most useful for the menisci and cruciate ligaments. The meniscofemoral ligaments may often be seen (Fig. 28). Coronal images demonstrate the collateral ligaments and also give useful supplementary information about the menisci (Fig. 29). Spin echo (SE) and gradient echo (GE) sequences are employed. Meniscal abnormalities are best demonstrated on T1-weighted, proton density or gradient echo scans. By obtaining a volume acquisition with GE sequences, it is possible to obtain very thin slices of 1–2 mm. GE sequences, especially with fat suppression, are also useful for hyaline cartilage evaluation.

A discoid meniscus is a congenital anomaly found usually in the lateral meniscus but very rarely in the medial meniscus. The incidence is approximately 0.8%. A meniscus is said to be discoid if there is continuity between anterior and posterior thirds ('bow tie' appearance) on five or more contiguous 3 mm sagittal MRI slices (Fig. 30). Discoid menisci are often symptomatic and are more prone to tear.

Dynamic scanning of the knee is also possible with modern scanners allowing assessment of patellar tracking. Axial images are particularly helpful for assessment of the patellofemoral joint and soft tissue abnormalities around the knee (Fig. 31).

Ultrasound scanning may be used to assess the patellar tendon, the collateral ligaments and meniscal and popliteal cysts.

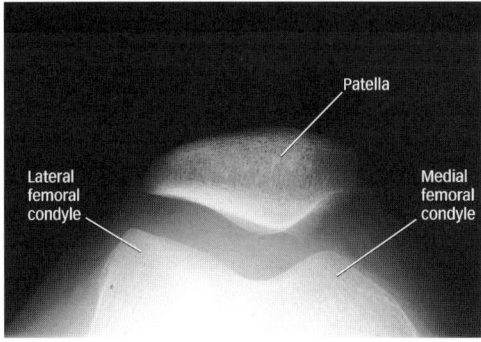

Fig. 25.
A Skyline view of the patella. Note how the lateral femoral condyle projects more anteriorly, tending to prevent lateral patellar dislocation.

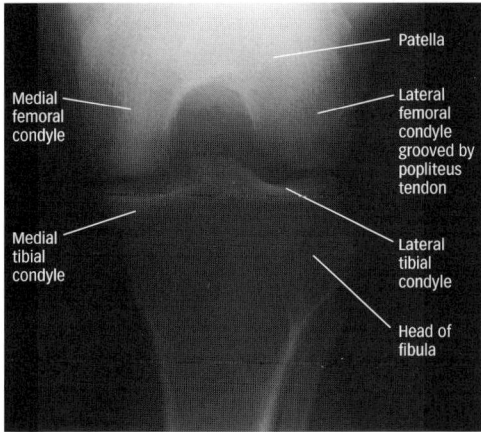

Fig. 26.
Intercondylar view of the knee.

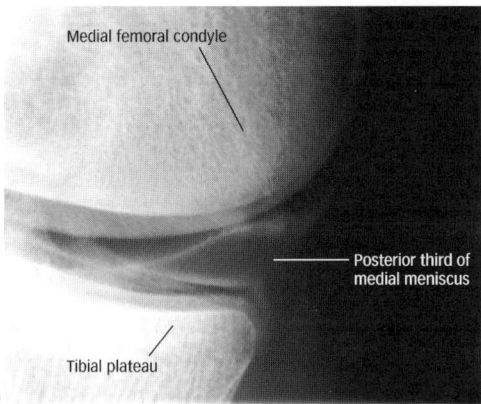

Fig. 27.
Arthrogram of the knee: (a) lateral view demonstrating posterior third of meniscus, (b) AP view demonstrating medial meniscus.

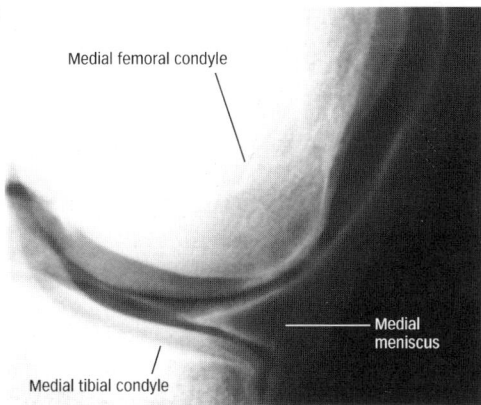

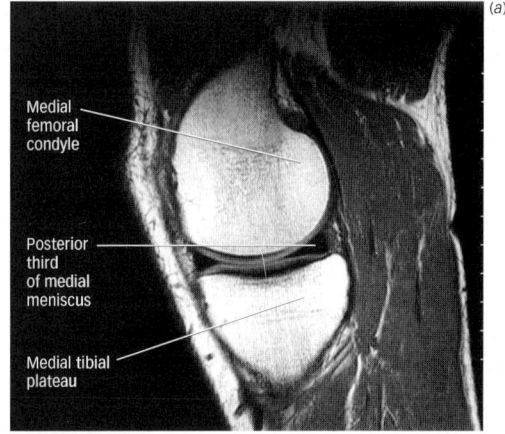

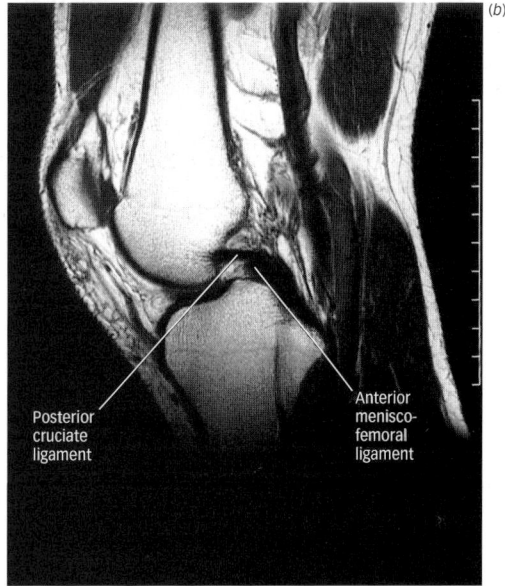

Fig. 28.
T1W sagittal MRI of the knee demonstrating (a) the normal medial meniscus, (b) the posterior cruciate ligament and anterior meniscofemoral ligament, and (c) the anterior cruciate ligament.

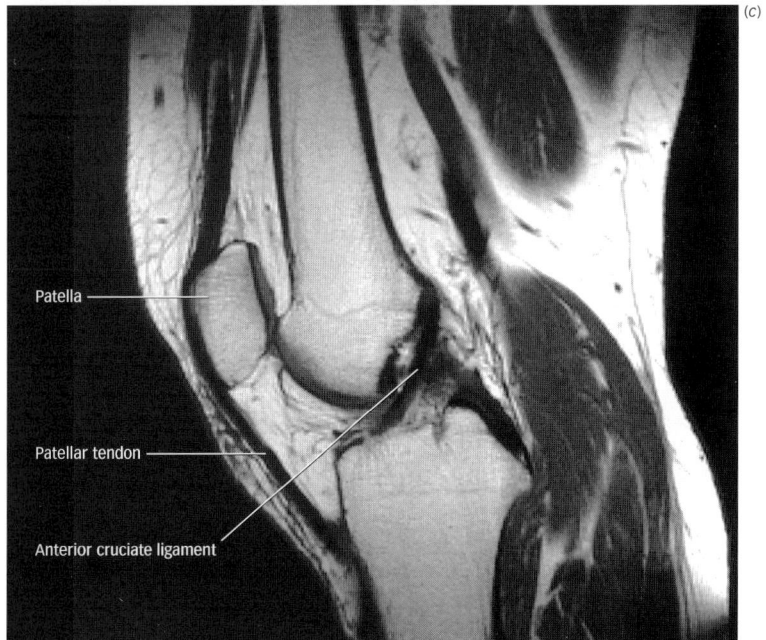

(a)

Medial collateral ligament

Lateral — Meniscus
Medial —

(b)

Medial — Femoral condyle
Lateral —

Lateral meniscus

Lateral collateral ligament

Head of fibula

Lateral — Tibial condyle
Medial —

Lateral femoral condyle

Lateral (discoid) meniscus

Lateral tibial condyle

Lateral head o gastrocnemiu

Patella

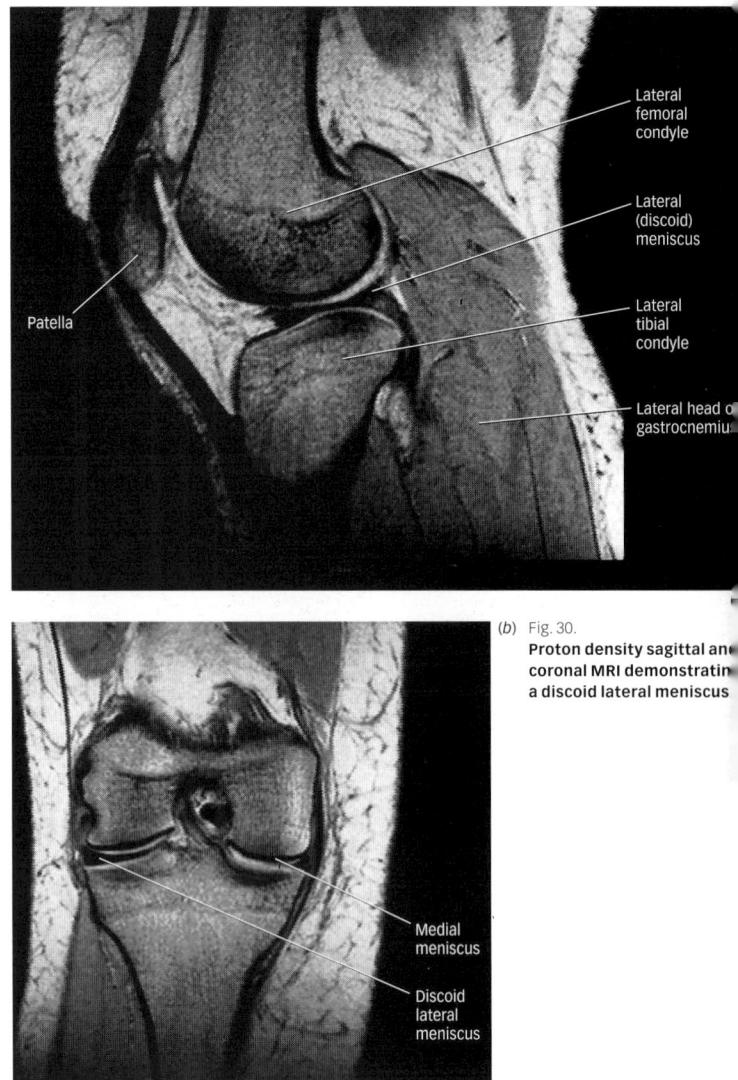

(b) Fig. 30.
Proton density sagittal an coronal MRI demonstratin a discoid lateral meniscus

Medial meniscus

Discoid lateral meniscus

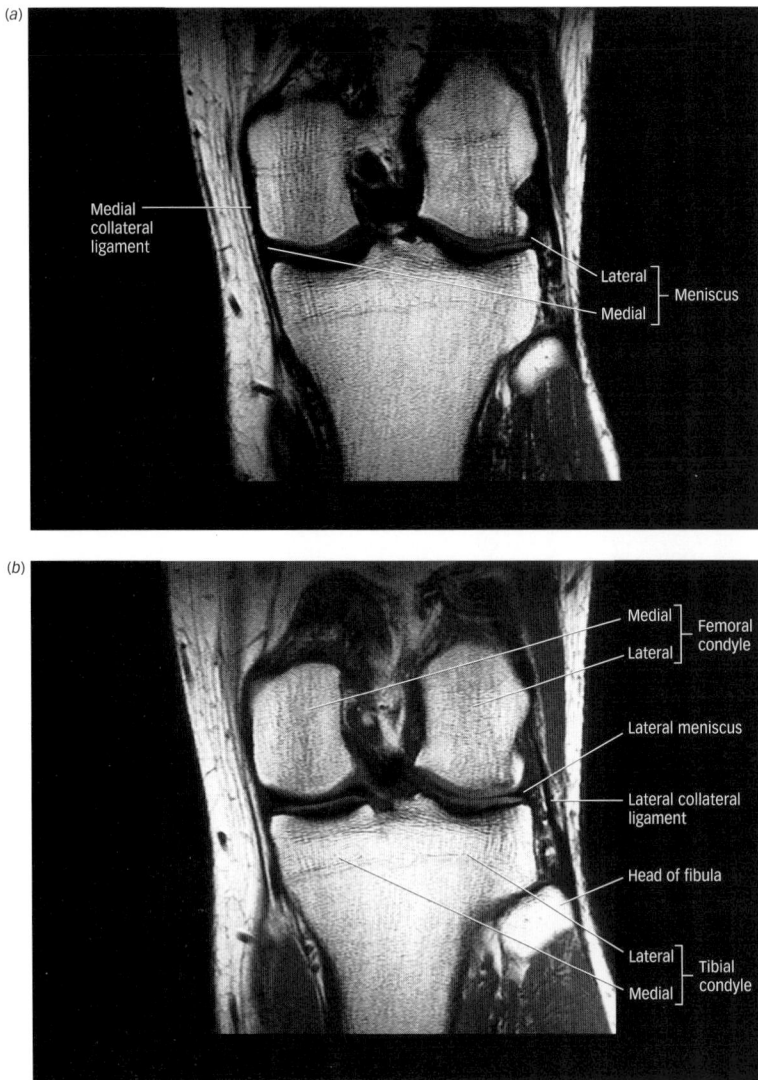

Fig. 29.
T1W coronal MRI of the knee showing the collateral ligaments and menisci.

The leg

The tibia

The tibia is made up of a stout shaft which is expanded superiorly into medial and lateral condyles (Fig. 32). The medial condyle is the larger, but does not project posteriorly as much as the lateral condyle. Its articular surface is oval and concave and its lateral rim covers the medial intercondylar tubercle. The lateral condyle has a smaller almost circular, superior articular surface whose medial rim covers the lateral intercondylar tubercle. Beneath the posterior overhang of the lateral condyle is a facet directed downwards and a little posterolaterally for articulation with the fibula.

The articular surfaces of the condyles are separated by a roughened intercondylar area, which, in its narrow middle part, is raised to form the intercondylar eminence with its medial and lateral tubercles. The anterior intercondylar area gives attachment to the anterior horn of the medial meniscus with the lower end of the anterior cruciate ligament gaining attachment just behind it. The anterior and posterior horns of the lateral meniscus are attached, respectively, anterior and posterior to the intercondylar eminence. The posterior horn of the medial meniscus attaches just behind the medial intercondylar tubercle and the posterior intercondylar area gives rise to the lower end of the posterior cruciate ligament.

The tibial tuberosity is a prominent roughened area which receives the insertion of the patellar tendon. It lies anteriorly at the upper end of the anterior surface of the shaft.

The shaft is triangular in cross-section and has medial, lateral and posterior surfaces. The sharp anterior border and medial surface are subcutaneous. The lateral or interosseous surface gives rise to the interosseous membrane. The posterior surface is crossed in its superior

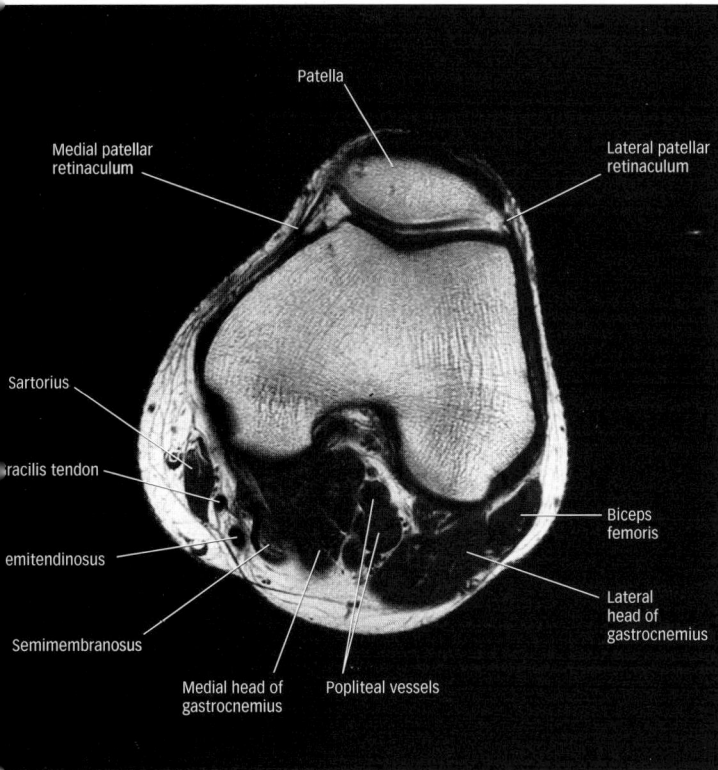

Fig. 31.
**T1W axial MRI of
patellofemoral joint**.

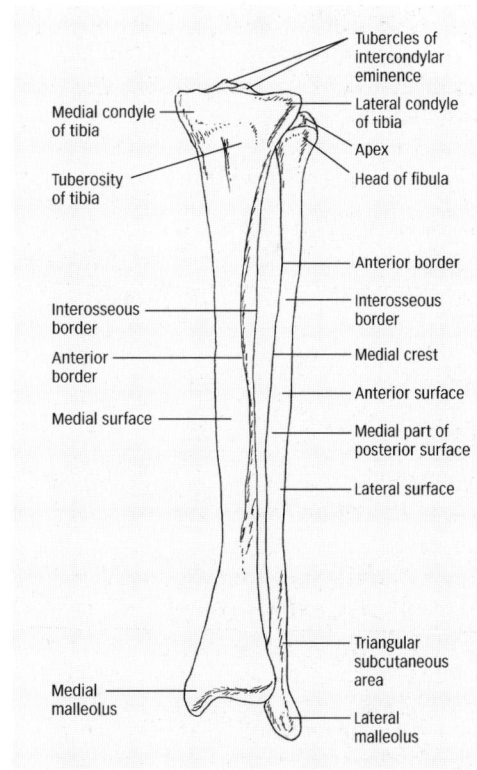

(a) Fig. 32.
**The tibia and fibula;
(a) anterior, (b) posterior.**

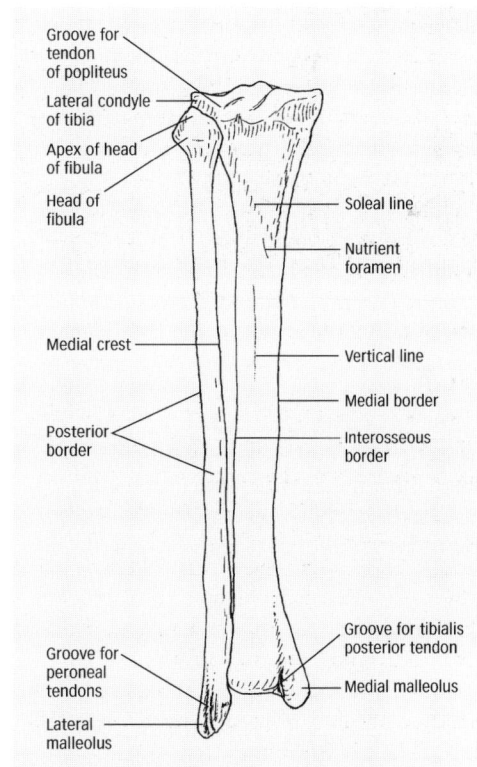

(b)

part by a diagonal ridge, the soleal line, which descends in a medial direction and gives rise to the soleus muscle. Below the soleal line arise the bellies of flexor digitorum longus medially and tibialis posterior laterally. The lower end of the tibia is expanded to form a broad inferior surface, wider anteriorly, with a short medial and inferior projection, the medial malleolus, which, together with the inferior tibial surface, articulates with the talus.

The fibula

The lateral bone of the lower leg is slender. The shaft is slightly expanded superiorly to form the head. This bears a circular facet for articulation with the inferior surface of the lateral tibial condyle. The common peroneal nerve winds round the neck of the fibula posterolaterally. The lower end of the shaft is expanded to form the lateral malleolus. This projects more inferiorly and lies more posteriorly than the medial malleolus. Its inner (medial) surface articulates with the lateral surface of the talus. Just above this, the surface of the bone is slightly roughened by the attachment of the interosseous ligament of the inferior tibiofibular joint.

Ossification

The centres for the shafts of both bones appear at 7–8 weeks of fetal life (Fig. 33). The epiphysis for the upper end of the tibia is usually present at birth. The centres for the lower ends of both bones appear in the first year and that for the upper end of the fibula at 3–4 years. At 7 years the medial malleolus arises as a downward extension of the lower epiphysis, although it may arise as a separate centre. At 10 years the epiphysis of the upper end begins to extend downwards over the anterior surface of the shaft to form the tibial tuberosity. Occasionally, this also arises as a separate centre fusing with the upper epiphysis at 12 years. The lower ends of both bones unite with the shafts at 15–17 years and the upper ends fuse at 16–18 years.

The tibiofibular joints

The superior tibiofibular joint is a plane synovial joint between the head of the fibula and the articular surface under the lateral tibial condyle. It is strengthened by a fibrous capsule and anterior and posterior ligaments. The inferior tibiofibular joint is a fibrous joint (syndesmosis) between the lower end of the fibula and the fibular notch of the tibia. It is reinforced by the interosseous ligament of the joint and the anterior and posterior inferior tibiofibular ligaments. Movements at both joints are extremely limited.

The muscles of the lower leg
Anterior compartment

Tibialis anterior takes origin from the upper part of the anterior surface of the tibia and adjacent interosseous membrane and forms a tendon which descends anterior to the ankle joint, with the anterior tibial vessels and nerve laterally, deep to the extensor retinaculum to attach to the medial cuneiform and the base of the first metatarsal (Fig. 34).

Extensor hallucis longus (EHL) arises from the anterior surface of the fibula lateral and deep to tibialis anterior, initially lateral to the neurovascular bundle. Its tendon crosses to the medial side of the vessels under the extensor retinaculum and inserts on to the dorsum of the base of the distal phalanx of the hallux.

Extensor digitorum longus arises above and lateral to EHL from the anterior surface of the fibula. Distally, it divides into four tendons which pass under the extensor retinaculum and insert via a dorsal expansion onto the dor-

sum of the middle and distal phalanges of the lateral four toes. *Peroneus tertius* arises from the anterior surface of the fibula and inserts into the shaft of the fifth metatarsal.

The lateral (peroneal) compartment

Peroneus longus is the more superficial of the two muscles in this compartment and arises from the upper lateral surface of the fibula. The common peroneal nerve passes through a hiatus in its attachment as it winds round the neck of the fibula. Distally, its tendon passes behind and grooves the lateral malleolus beneath the peroneal retinaculum, passes forwards lateral to the calcaneus, swings under the tarsus and grooves the cuboid before inserting on the base of the first metatarsal and the adjacent medial cuneiform.

Peroneus brevis arises from the lower part of the lateral fibula and its tendon descends anteriorly to that of peroneus longus under the lateral malleolus but then passes superior to the peroneal tubercle to insert on the tuberosity on the base of the fifth metatarsal. Both peroneal muscles share a common synovial sheath beneath the peroneal retinaculum but as they pass forward on the lateral surface of the calcaneum they are invested with separate forward prolongations. A second synovial sheath invests the tendon of peroneus longus as it crosses beneath the cuboid.

The posterior compartment

Gastrocnemius, the most superficial of the muscles of the calf, arises by two heads from the posterior surfaces of the medial and lateral femoral condyles. Inferiorly, its tendon unites with that of soleus to form the Achilles' tendon (tendo calcaneus), the thickest and strongest tendon in the body.

Fig. 33.
Ossification of the tibia and fibula. The distal and proximal epiphyses fuse with the shaft at 16–18 years.

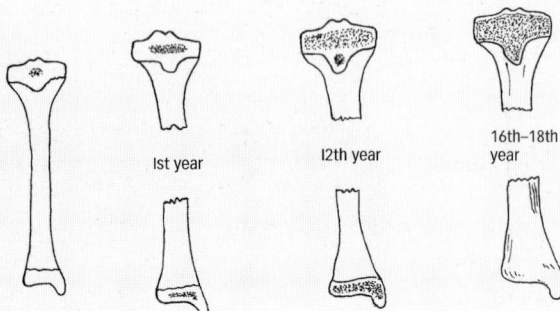

Ist year | 12th year | 16th–18th year

Fig. 34.
T1W axial MRI of the mid-calf.

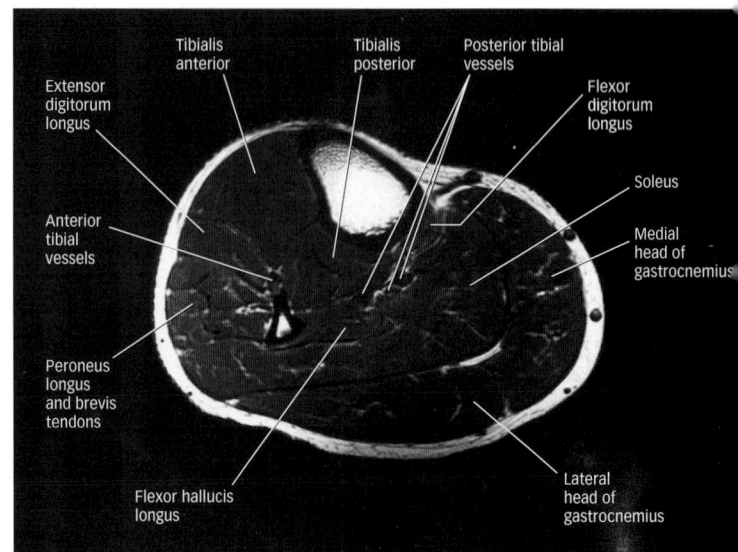

370

Soleus arises from the head and upper posterior surface of the fibula, from the soleal line and from the middle third of the medial border of the tibia.

Plantaris is a slender muscle arising from the lateral supracondylar line and oblique popliteal ligament. It inserts into the dorsal aspect of the calcaneus. It is a vestigial muscle and may be absent.

Popliteus is the triangular muscle that forms the floor of the lower part of the popliteal fossa. It arises from the posterior surface of the tibia above the soleal line and sweeps superolaterally behind the knee joint, where its fibres blend with the capsule to insert by a rounded tendon at the anterior end of the groove on the lateral femoral condyle, having pierced the capsule of the joint. Some of its fibres blend with the edge of the lateral meniscus.

Flexor hallucis longus (FHL) takes origin from the lower two-thirds of the posterior surface of the fibula. Its tendon grooves the back of both the tibia and the talus lateral to flexor digitorum longus and tibialis posterior. Having passed under and grooved the sustentaculum tali, it passes forward into the fibrous sheath of the hallux and attaches to the base of its distal phalanx.

Flexor digitorum longus (FDL) arises from the medial side of the posterior aspect of the tibia below the soleal line medial to FHL. Its tendon descends behind the medial malleolus and then passes under the sustentaculum tali into the foot, crossing the tendon of FHL and giving four slips to the distal phalanges of the lateral four toes.

Tibialis posterior arises from the interosseous membrane and the adjacent posterior aspects of the tibia and fibula. Its tendon shares a groove under the medial malleolus with that of FDL and attaches to the tuberosity of the navicular, giving a variable number of slips to the other tarsal bodies (except the talus) and the bases of the second, third and fourth metatarsals.

The ankle joint

The ankle joint (Fig. 35) is a synovial hinge joint between the trochlear surface of the talus and the concavity formed by the medial and lateral malleoli, the inferior articular surface of the tibia and the inferior transverse tibiofibular ligament, an accessory ligament of the joint.

The articular surfaces are described in the description of the talus, tibia and fibula.

The fibrous capsule is attached around the articular margins except anteriorly, where its

attachment extends down the anterior surface of the neck of the talus. The synovial membrane lines the fibrous capsule.

The deltoid or medial collateral ligament is attached above to the medial malleolus and below to the tuberosity of the navicular (tibionavicular), the sustentaculum tali of the calcaneum (tibiocalcaneal) and the medial side of the talus and its medial tubercle (posterior tibiotalar). The anterior component of the ligament also blends with the plantar calcaneonavicular (spring) ligament. The ligaments on the lateral side of the joint are three: the anterior talofibular ligament, joining the lateral malleolus to the neck of the talus, the calcaneofibular ligament, joining the lateral malleolus to the tubercle on the lateral side of the calcaneum (which is crossed by the tendons of peroneus longis and brevis), and the posterior talofibular ligament, which passes backwards from the lateral malleolus to the lateral tubercle of the posterior process of the talus.

Relations
- Anterior, from medial to lateral (Fig. 36): great saphenous vein, the tendons of tibialis anterior and flexor hallucis longus, anterior tibial vessels and deep peroneal nerve, the tendon of extensor digitorum longus, peroneus tertius;

Fig. 35. top pair
The ankle joint showing the ligaments: (*a*) medial, (*b*) posterior.

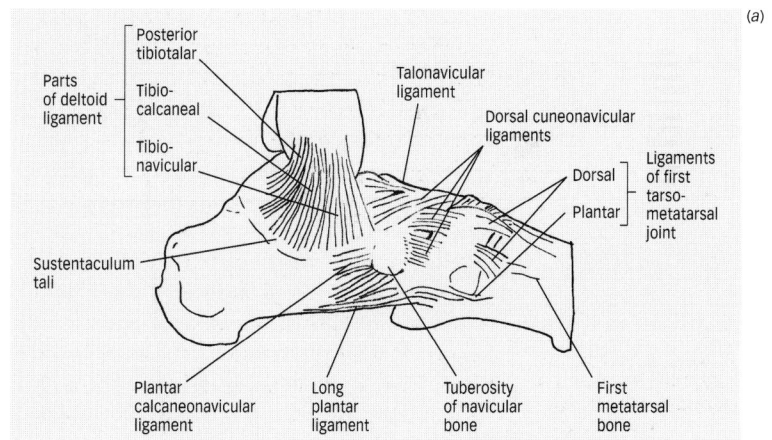

(*a*)

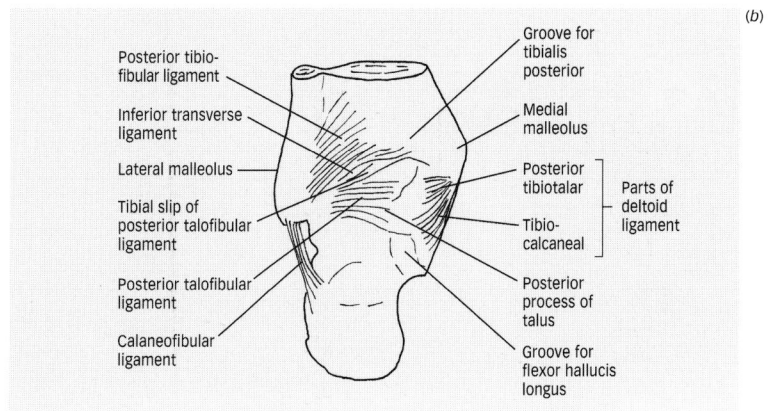

(*b*)

- Posterior, from medial to lateral: tendons of tibialis posterior and flexor digitorum longus, posterior tibial vessels and tibial nerve (deep to the vessels), and tendon of flexor hallucis longus;
- Laterally, behind the fibular malleolus: tendons of peroneus longus and brevis with the short saphenous vein behind.

The movements of the joint are dorsiflexion, produced by tibialis anterior, extensor digitorum longus, extensor hallucis longus and peroneus tertius, and plantarflexion produced in the main by gastrocnemius and soleus but assisted by the three other muscles of the posterior compartment of the leg.

The foot

The tarsus

The tarsus consists of seven bones arranged in three rows: proximally the talus and calcaneus and distally the medial, intermediate and lateral cuneiform bones medially and the cuboid laterally. Between these two rows on the medial side of the foot, the navicular is interposed between the talus and the cuneiforms. Laterally, the calcaneus articulates directly with the cuboid.

The talus

This bone, which bears no muscle attachments, is made up of a head, neck and body (Fig. 37).

The head is directed medially and inferiorly and its distal surface is smoothly convex for articulation with the navicular. Its inferior (plantar) surface has three facets, the anterior and middle calcaneal articular surfaces and, medial to these, a facet for the plantar calcaneonavicular (spring) ligament. The anterior of the calcaneal articular surfaces is continuous with the navicular surface anteriorly and with the middle calcaneal surface posteriorly.

The neck is the slightly narrowed part of the bone joining the head to the body. It is directed inferiorly and medially, making an angle of 150° with the body. The long axis of the talus in the adult and child older than 5 years points along the first metatarsal. In the

Fig. 36.
T1W axial MRI: (a) throug[h] the ankle joint, and (b) ju[st] above the ankle joint.

(a)

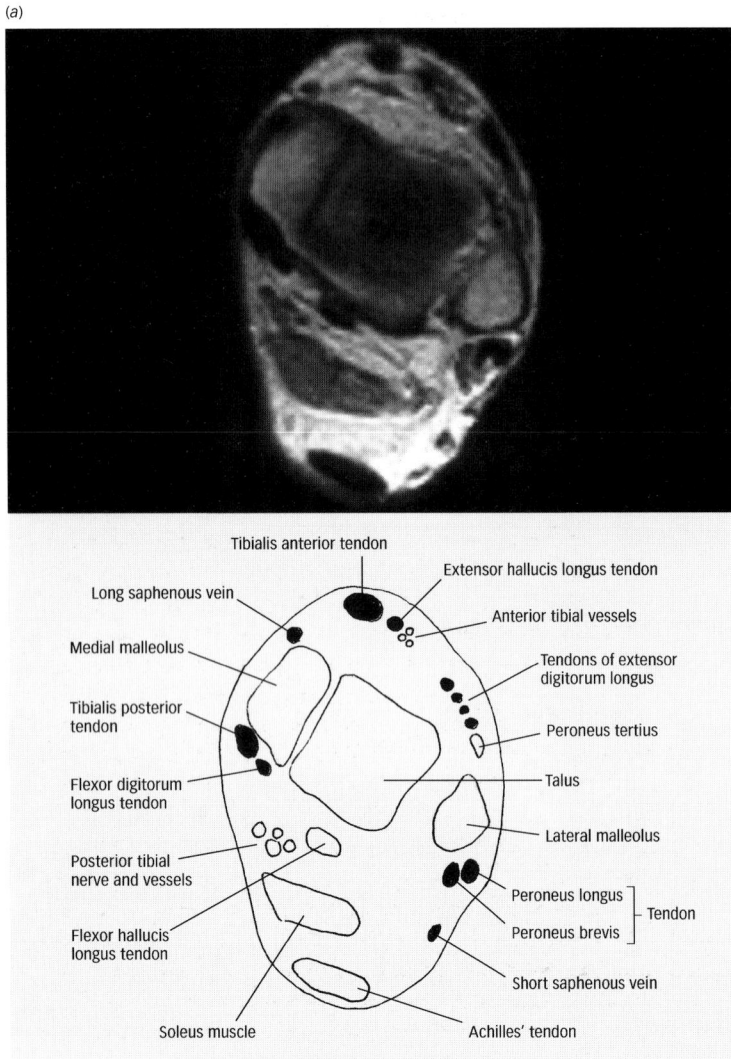

(b)

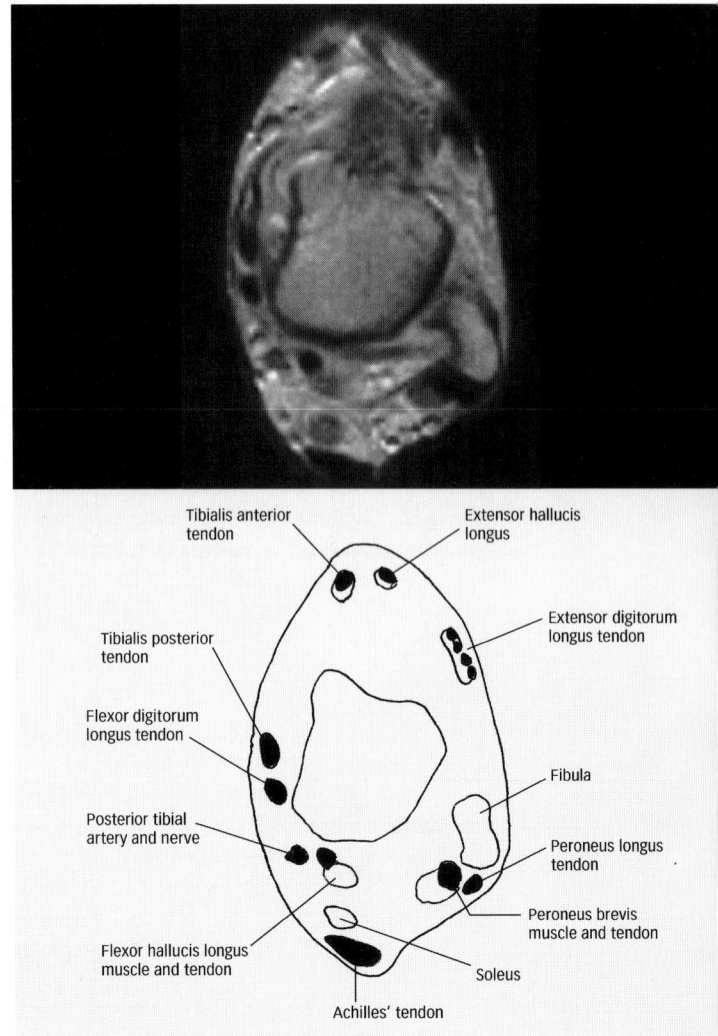

372

infant the neck makes a smaller angle (130–140°) with the body so that the long axis of the talus points below the first metatarsal. Its plantar surface bears a deep groove, the sulcus tali, which separates the middle talocalcaneal articular surface of the head from the large oval posterior talocalcaneal articular facet which lies on the plantar surface of the body.

The body lies between the malleoli and has a superior trochlear surface, which articulates with the inferior surface of the lower end of the tibia and is continuous medially and laterally with the surfaces that articulate with the respective malleoli. Posteriorly, the posterior process is grooved between lateral and medial tubercles. Inferiorly, the plantar surface bears the posterior of the three talocalcaneal articular surfaces.

The calcaneum

The largest of the tarsal bones is irregularly cuboidal in shape with its long axis directed forwards upwards and slightly laterally (Fig. 38).

The dorsal (superior) surface is made up of a roughened posterior third, a middle third bearing the posterior surface for articulation with the plantar aspect of the body of the talus and an anterior third, which has a medial

shelf-like projection, the sustentaculum tali, which bears the middle articular surface for the talus. Anterior and lateral to this on the body of the bone is the anterior surface for articulation with the talus. As with the corresponding surfaces on the talus, the anterior and middle surfaces may be continuous. However, the middle and posterior surfaces are separated by a groove, the sulcus calcanei, which, together with its fellow, the sulcus tali, forms the sinus tarsi (see subtalar joint).

The anterior surface is covered by the articular surface for the cuboid.

The posterior surface gives attachment to the Achilles' tendon. Above this attachment a bursa and fat lie between tendon and bone. Below this attachment the posterior surface is continuous with the calcaneal tuberosity which lies at the posterior end of the inferior surface and is divided into lateral and medial processes. The inferior surface bears an anterior tubercle behind the navicular articulation, which gives rise to the long plantar ligament.

The medial surface has the sustentaculum tali projecting from the anterior part of its superior border. Superiorly, this bears the middle surface for articulation with the talus. The lateral surface bears a peroneal tubercle.

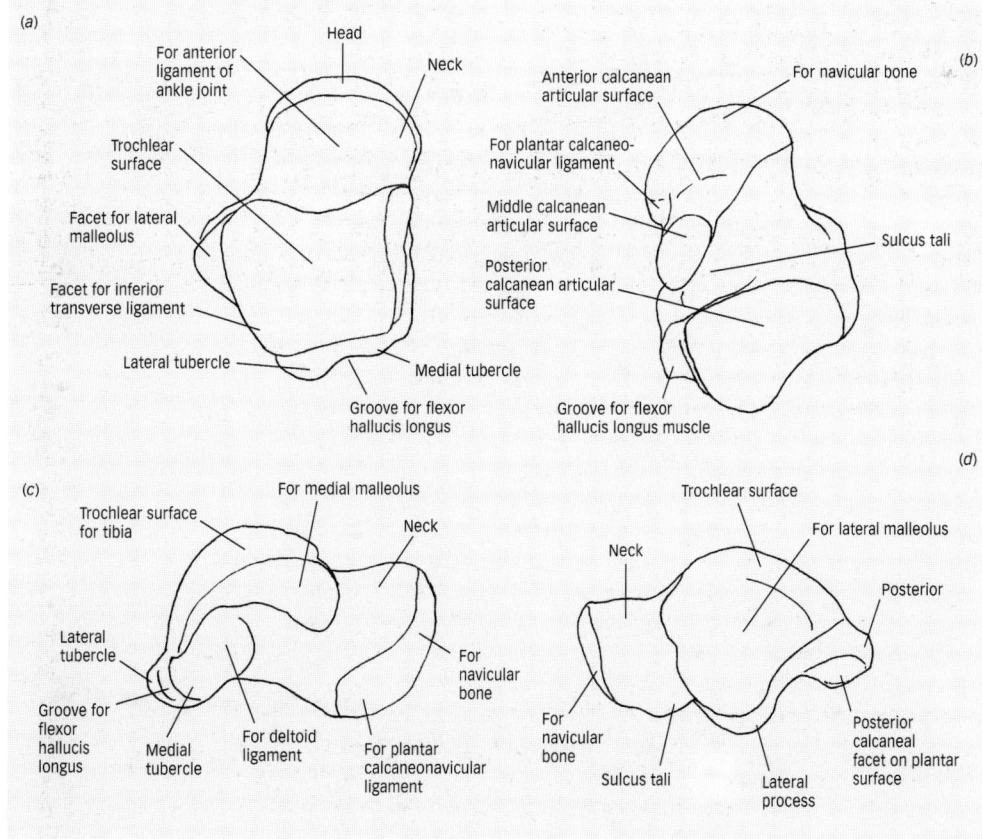

(a)
Head
Neck
For anterior ligament of ankle joint
Trochlear surface
Facet for lateral malleolus
Facet for inferior transverse ligament
Lateral tubercle
Medial tubercle
Groove for flexor hallucis longus

(b)
Anterior calcanean articular surface
For navicular bone
For plantar calcaneo-navicular ligament
Middle calcanean articular surface
Sulcus tali
Posterior calcanean articular surface
Groove for flexor hallucis longus muscle

(c)
For medial malleolus
Trochlear surface for tibia
Neck
Lateral tubercle
For navicular bone
Groove for flexor hallucis longus
Medial tubercle
For deltoid ligament
For plantar calcaneonavicular ligament

(d)
Trochlear surface
For lateral malleolus
Neck
Posterior
For navicular bone
Sulcus tali
Lateral process
Posterior calcaneal facet on plantar surface

The navicular
The proximal surface articulates with the talus. The distal surface is divided into three facets for articulation with the three cuneiform bones. The lateral surface may have an articular surface for the cuboid. The medial surface bears a tuberosity, which is the principal insertion of tibialis posterior.

The cuneiform bones
These are three wedge-shaped bones lying between the navicular and the bases of the first three metatarsals. The medial cuneiform is the largest of the three and articulates with the base of the first metatarsal. It is wedge-shaped, its plantar surface being broader, whereas the other cuneiforms are broader dorsally, which help to maintain the transverse arch of the foot. The intermediate cuneiform is the smallest of the three and articulates distally with the base of the second metatarsal.

The lateral cuneiform articulates distally with the third metatarsal bone and also with the medial part of the base of the fourth metatarsal. The proximal part of its lateral surface articulates with the cuboid.

The cuboid
The most lateral of the distal row of the tarsus articulates proximally with the distal calcaneum and distally with the bases of the fourth and fifth metatarsals. The medial surface articulates with the lateral cuneiform and sometimes with the lateral surface of the navicular. The lateral and plantar surfaces are grooved by the tendon of peroneus longus.

The metatarsal bones
The five metatarsal bones each possess a proximal base, a shaft or body and a distal head. The bases articulate with the distal row of the tarsus and with each other. The heads articulate with the proximal phalanx of the corresponding digit. The first metatarsal is the shortest and thickest. Its head bears two articular facets on its plantar surface for articulation with the two sesamoid bones, which are always found in the tendon of flexor hallucis

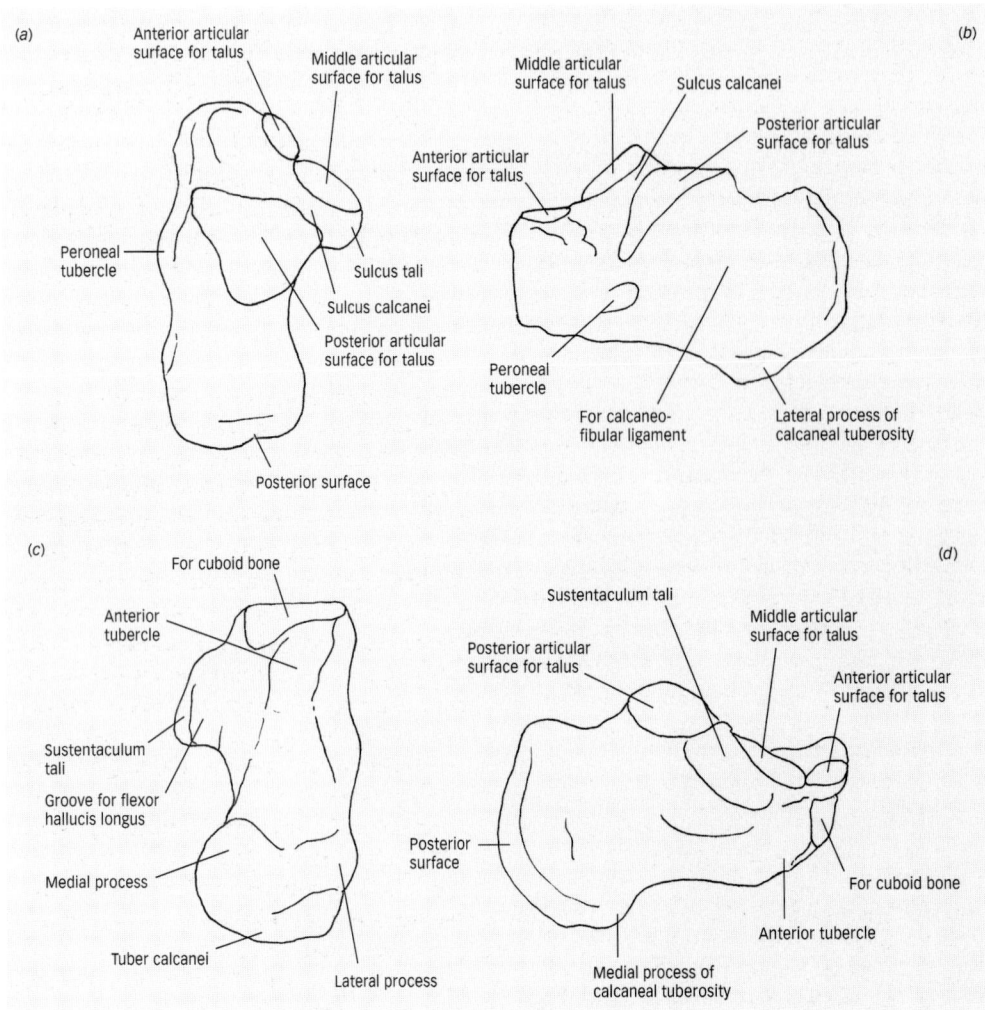

Fig. 38. The calcaneum: (*a*) dorsal, (*b*) lateral, (*c*) plantar, (*d*) medial.

brevis. Both may be duplicated, mimicking fracture. The second metatarsal is the longest.

The base of the fifth metatarsal bears a styloid process on its lateral aspect to which is attached the tendon of peroneus brevis and part of the plantar aponeurosis. It may form from a secondary ossification centre, in which case the epiphyseal line runs parallel to the lateral border of the foot. If it is fractured, which is not uncommon in acute inversion injuries, the fracture line tends to be more perpendicular to the lateral border of the foot.

The phalanges

As in the hand, there are two phalanges in the first digit (hallux) and three in the others. A minor degree of valgus in the great toe is often seen. In infants, the hallux is often adducted (metatarsus adductus) but this is physiological and usually corrects with weight bearing.

Ossification

The centre for the calcaneum appears at 5 months of fetal life with a separate crescentric centre for its posterior surface appearing at 6–8 years, uniting at 14–16 years. The talus begins to ossify next at 6 months of fetal life with the centre for the cuboid appearing just before birth in the ninth month of fetal life. The lateral cuneiform appears at 1 year, the intermediate at 2 years and the medial at 3 years. The navicular also begins to ossify in the third year of life and may ossify from several centres. The centres for the shafts of the metatarsals appear at 9–10 weeks of fetal life, for the distal phalanges at 9–12 weeks of fetal life, for the proximal phalanges at 11–15 weeks of fetal life and the intermediate phalanges after 15 weeks of fetal life. The epiphyses of the heads of the second to fifth metatarsals and the base of the first metatarsal appear at 3–4 years. The first metatarsal may also have a separate epiphysis for its head. The epiphyses for the bases of the proximal phalanges ossify between the second and eighth year; of the intermediate phalanges between the third and sixth years and of the distal phalanges in the sixth year. The epiphyses of all the metatarsals and phalanges unite by the eighteenth year.

Sesamoid and accessory ossicles

The almost constant sesamoid bones in the tendon of flexor hallucis brevis have already been mentioned. Sesamoid bones are also found less frequently over the other metatarsophalangeal joints (Fig. 39). The os peroneum (Fig. 40(*a*)) is seen in 20% of people in the tendon of peroneus longus as it grooves the inferior surface of the tubercle of the cuboid. The

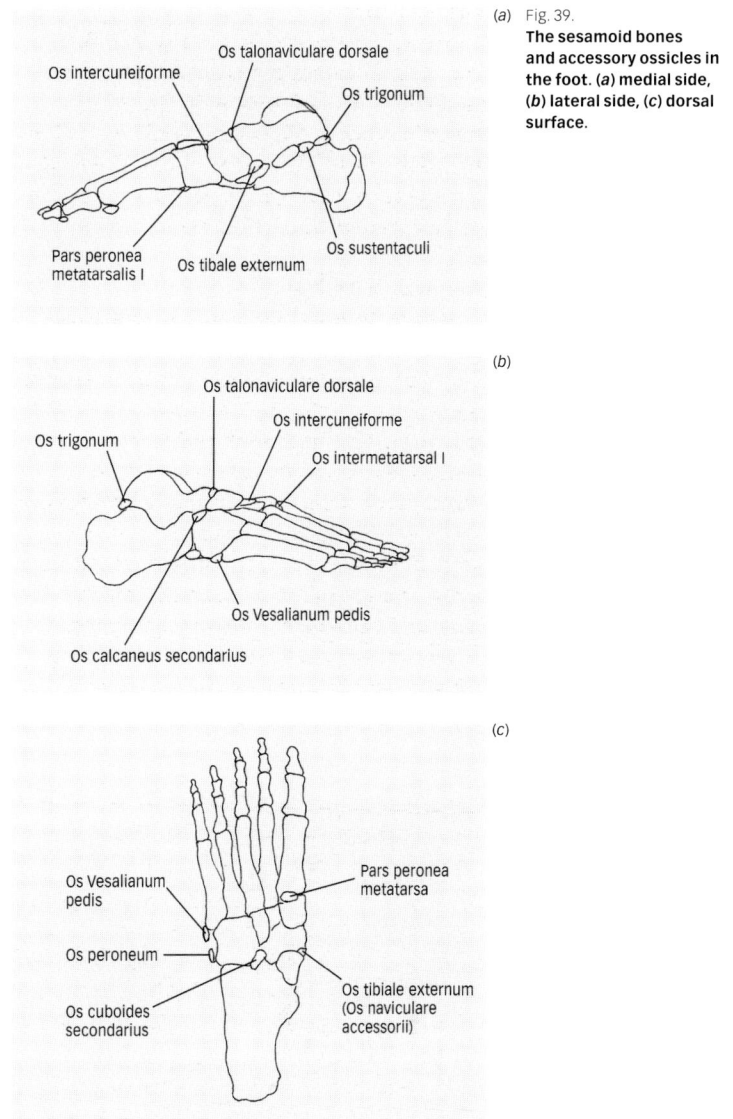

(a) Fig. 39.
The sesamoid bones and accessory ossicles in the foot. (*a*) medial side, (*b*) lateral side, (*c*) dorsal surface.

os Vesalianum pedis is found in the tendon of peroneus brevis proximal to the base of the fifth metatarsal. Sesamoid bones may also be found in the tendon of tibialis anterior, where it slides over the medial surface of the medial cuneiform, and in the tendon of tibialis posterior where it is in contact with the medial surface of the talus. They may also be found in the tendons of psoas major, gluteus maximus and, as has already been mentioned, in the lateral head of gastrocnemius (the fabella). As with sesamoid bones anywhere, they frequently bear articular cartilage and may be associated with a bursa.

Additionally, a number of accessory ossicles are found in the foot. The os tibiale externum (Fig. 40(*b*)) is a separate ossification centre for the tuberosity of the navicular and is seen in 5% of cases. It may be confused with a sesamoid bone in the tibialis posterior tendon, which is seen in 25% of cases. The os trigonum

Fig. 40.
Radiographs of accessory
ossicles: (*a*) Os peroneum,
(*b*) Os tibiale externum,
(*c*) Os trigonum.

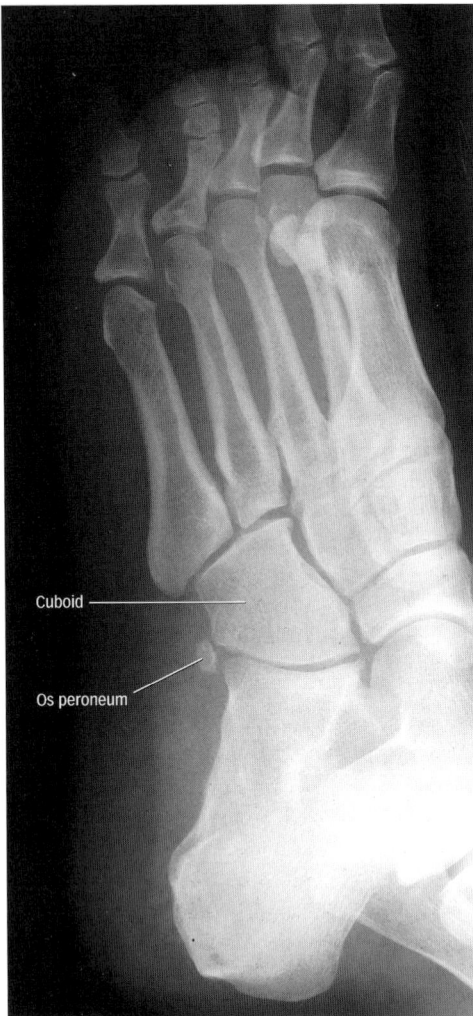

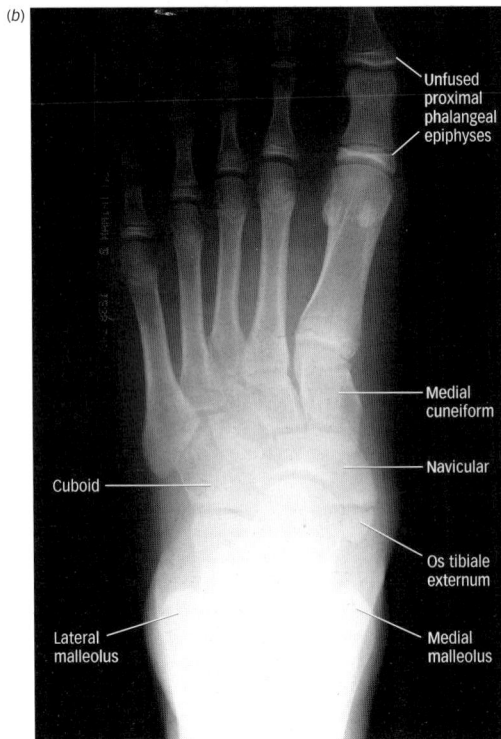

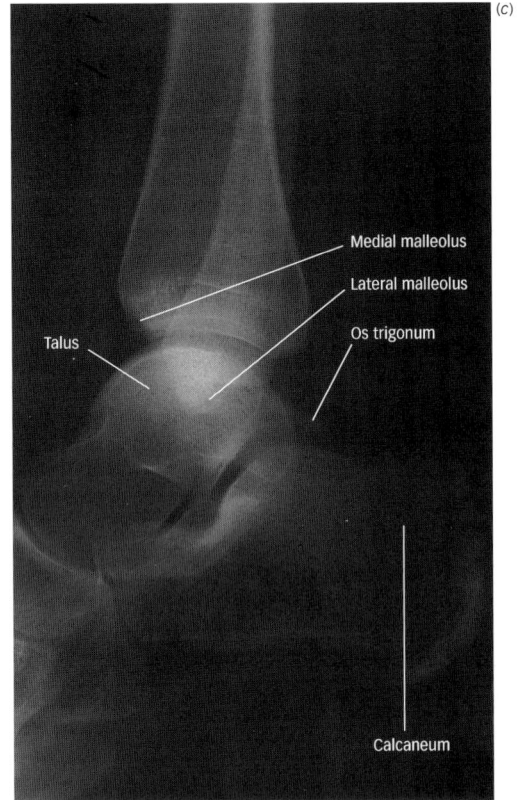

Fig. 40.
Radiographs of accessory
ossicles: (*a*) Os peroneum,
(*b*) Os tibiale externum,
(*c*) Os trigonum.

(Fig. 40(*c*)) is a separate ossification centre for the posterior process of the talus which does not unite. It is present in 8% of people and it is bilateral in two-thirds of these. The os subtibiale is an uncommon accessory bone just below the medial malleolus. The importance of these bones is that they may be mistaken for fractures.

The subtalar joint

This is functionally a single unit composed of two articulations between the talus and the calcaneum, although it is often taken to refer only to the posterior of these components (Fig. 41). The posterior talocalcaneal joint is the articulation between the posterior of the three facets on the inferior surface of the talus and the corresponding surface on the upper surface of the calcaneum posterior to the sinus tarsi (see the descriptions of the respective bones). It is reinforced by medial and lateral talocalcaneal ligaments and by the interosseous talocalcaneal ligament, which joins the sulcus tali to the sulcus calcanei filling in the sinus tarsi. The talocalcaneonavicular joint is the articulation between the head of the talus and the concave posterior surface of the navicular anteriorly and the anterior two facets on the upper surface of the calcaneum together with the plantar calca-

376

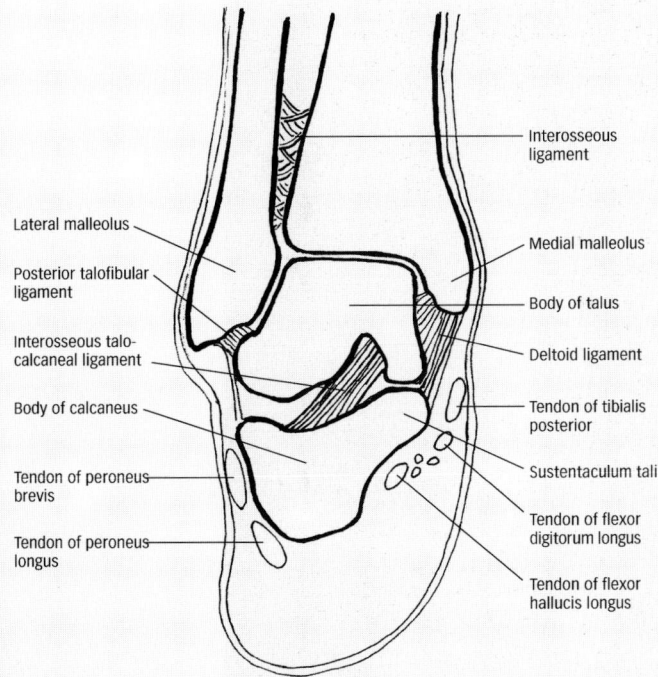

Fig. 41.
Coronal section of ankle
and subtalar joint.

neonaviular (spring) ligament. This ligament connects the anterior margin of the sustentaculum tali with the plantar suface of the navicular bone. In addition to the fibrous capsule and spring ligaments, the joint is strengthened by the talonavicular ligament connecting the neck of the talus to the dorsum of the navicular and by the calcaneonavicular component of the bifurcated ligament.

Inversion of the forefoot, which is also associated with plantar flexion is produced by tibialis anterior and posterior and is limited by tension in the peronei and the lateral components of the interosseous talocalcanean ligament. Eversion which is associated with dorsiflexion is produced by peroneus longus and brevis and limited by tibialis anterior and posterior and by the medial collateral (deltoid) ligament.

The calcaneocuboid joint

This is a saddle-shaped articulation between the anterior surface of the calcaneum and the posterior surface of the cuboid. It permits limited gliding movement in association with the other joints of the foot and ankle. The fibrous capsule is strengthened by the calcaneocuboid component of the bifurcated ligament (see above), by the long plantar ligament, which joins the plantar surface of the calcaneum to

the tuberosity on the plantar surface of the cuboid and by the short plantar ligament, which joins the anterior tubercle of the calcaneum to the adjacent plantar surface of the cuboid.

The remainder of the joints of the foot are of less clinical interest and will not be described.

Imaging modalities

Plain radiography permits assessments of the bony structures and may detect soft tissue swelling. If stress views are used, it can give indirect information about ligamentous disruption. The ankle joint is routinely imaged using anteroposterior and lateral radiographs (Fig. 42). The normal joint space is 3 mm. The foot is normally radiographed in dorsiplantar and oblique projections (Fig. 43). On the dorsiplantar view, the midline of the foot, which passes through the centre of the calcaneum and the head of the third metatarsal, should make an angle of 15° with the axis of the talus, which passes through the head of the first metatarsal. On a lateral view, the lines of the talonavicular joint and that between the navicular and first cuneiform should be parallel and perpendicular to the line of the dorsal surface of the three bones.

Bohler's angle may be measured on a lateral radiograph (Fig. 44(a)). It is the angle subtended by two lines, one joining the posterior lip of the posterior articular surface for the talus with the anterior lip of the anterior surface, the other joining the posterosuperior extremity of the bone with the posterior articular surface of the talus. It normally measures 28–40° and is characteristically reduced in crush fractures of the calcaneum. An erect weight-bearing lateral view may be used to assess the plantar arch. The calcaneal pitch should not be greater than 30° (Fig. 44(b)).

It is also possible to measure the thickness of the heel pad on a non-weight-bearing lateral radiograph, measured from the posteroinferior tip of the calcaneum to the skin surface along a line perpendicular to a line drawn between the anterior and posterior extremities of the superior surface of the calcaneum. The upper limit of normal is 21.5 mm in females and 23 mm in males and is increased in acromegaly, obesity, myxoedema and following injury and infection (Fig. 44(c)).

Common normal variations include a bipartite navicular bone and a bipartite medial cuneiform. A bony bridge may exist between calcaneum and cuboid, and there may be congenital fusion of the cuboid and the lateral cuneiform.

Fig. 42.
(*a*) Anteroposterior (AP)
and (*b*) lateral radiographs
of the ankle.

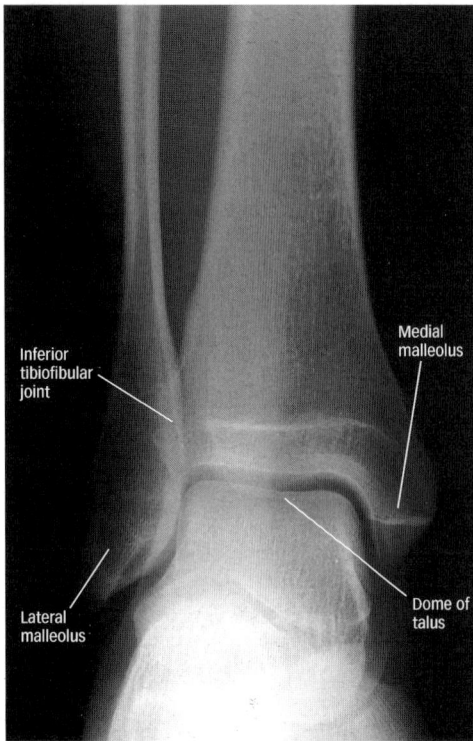

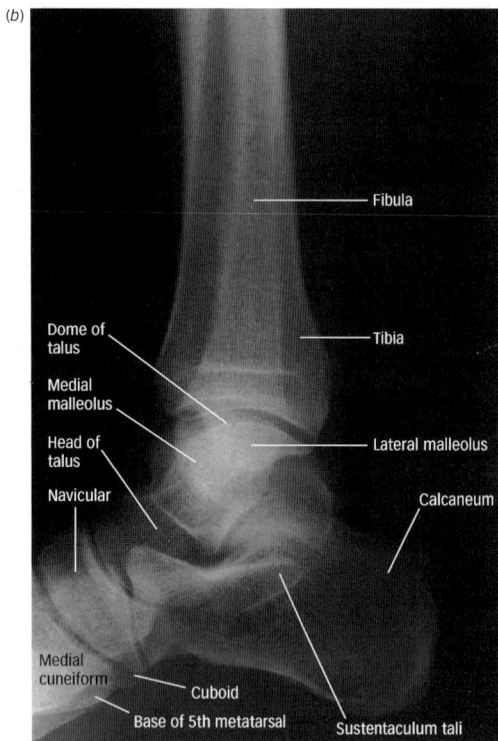

(*a*) Fig. 43.
(*a*) Oblique, and (*b*)
dorsiplantar radiographs
of the foot

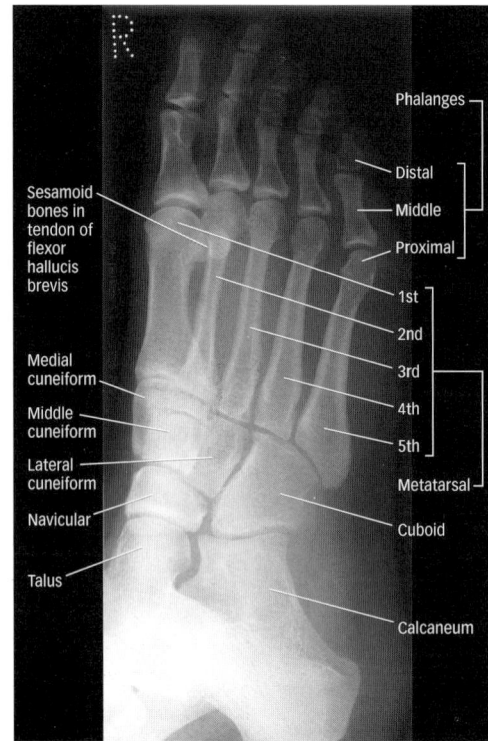

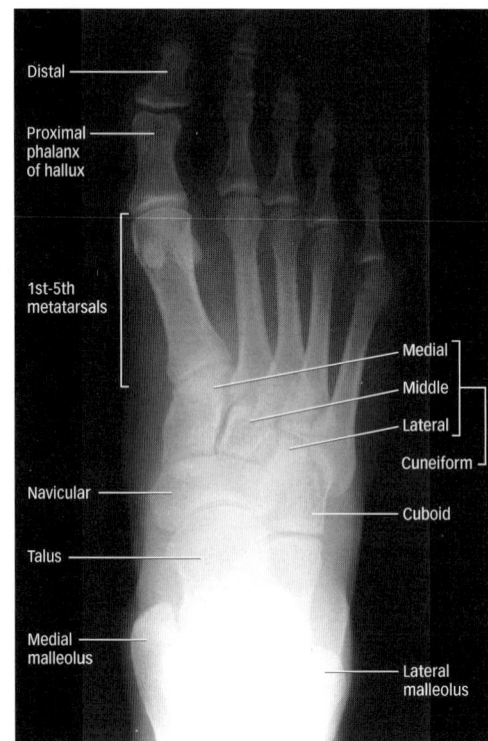

The subtalar joint is imaged optimally with a series of oblique radiographs with the foot internally rotated. These projections are also useful for demonstrating the congenital tarsal coalitions, particularly fusion of the calcaneum with the navicular (calcaneonavicular coalition). Fusion of the talus with the calcaneum (talocalcaneal coalition) is demonstrated with a medial oblique as well as a lateral projection and posterior tangential view of the calcaneum. Tarsal coalitions may be fibrous, cartilaginous or osseous. CT is often required to evaluate these abnormalities and coronal scanning is particularly useful in demonstrating the subtalar joint (Fig. 45). CT may also give valuable additional information

Fig. 44.
Lateral diagrams of the ankle demonstrating: (*a*) Bohler's angle, (*b*) calcaneal pitch and (*c*) heel pad thickness.

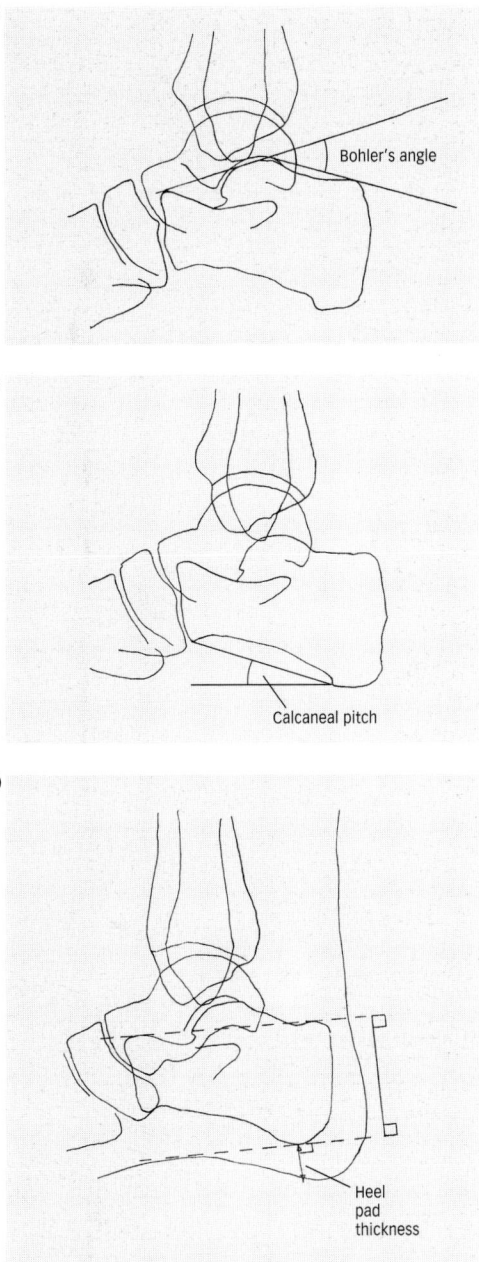

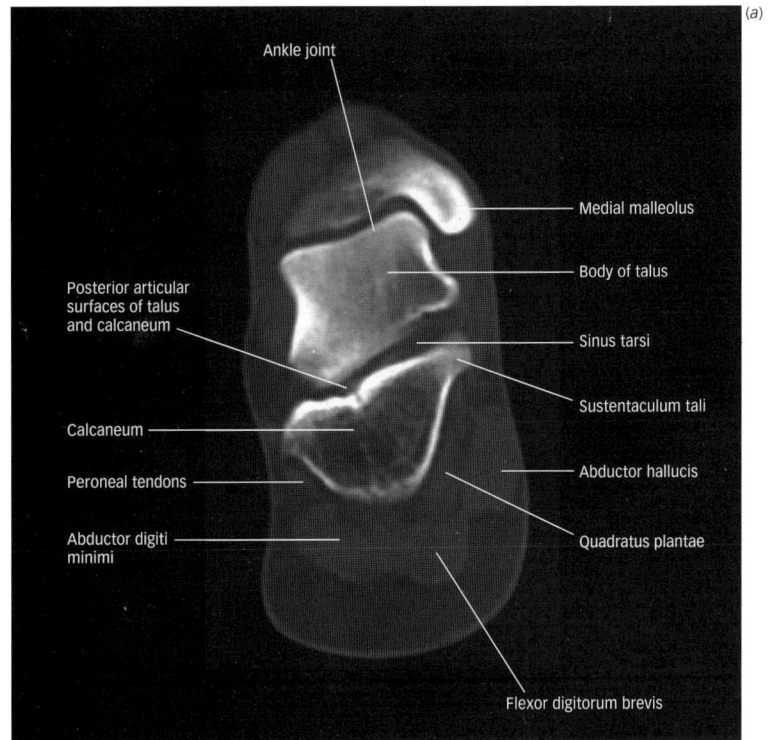

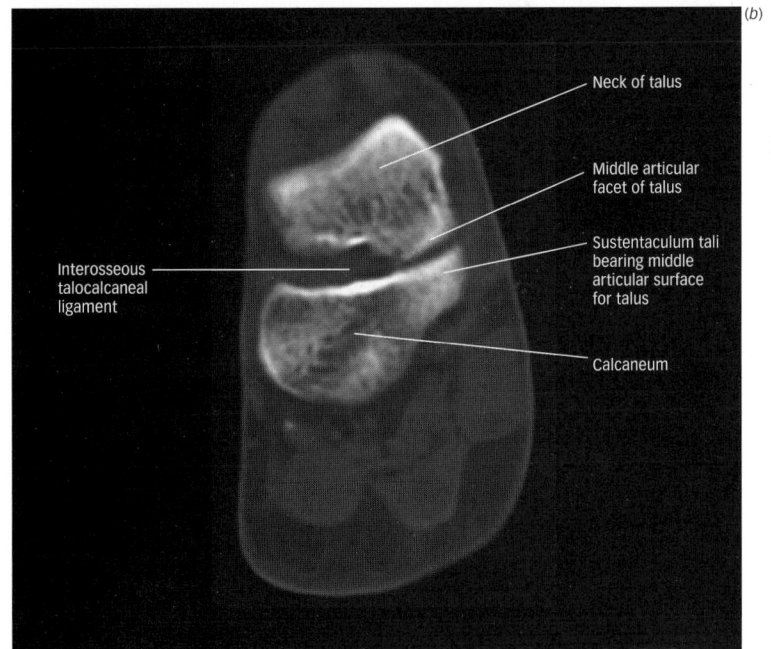

(*a*) Bohler's angle

(*b*) Calcaneal pitch

(*c*) Heel pad thickness

(*a*) Ankle joint; Medial malleolus; Body of talus; Sinus tarsi; Sustentaculum tali; Abductor hallucis; Quadratus plantae; Flexor digitorum brevis; Posterior articular surfaces of talus and calcaneum; Calcaneum; Peroneal tendons; Abductor digiti minimi

(*b*) Neck of talus; Middle articular facet of talus; Sustentaculum tali bearing middle articular surface for talus; Calcaneum; Interosseous talocalcaneal ligament

with subtle plain film abnormalities, for example, in osteoid osteoma.

US scanning may be used to assess the Achilles' tendon and other tendons of the foot and ankle. US is also employed in the evaluation of the plantar fascia and soft tissue masses in the foot.

MRI in various planes, depending on the precise part of the ankle or foot, can be performed to demonstrate all the tendons and most of the ligaments as well as cartilage and medullary bone (Fig. 46). In general, the tendons are most reliably imaged in cross-section, so the imaging of flexor hallucis longus requires axial scans in the lower leg and coronal scans in the foot.

Tenography, injecting contrast into the synovial sheaths, particularly of the peroneal tendon sheaths, is occasionally performed to assess the integrity of the tendons.

Fig. 45.
Coronal CT of the subtalar joint: (*a*) posterior and (*b*) middle of the joint.

(a)

Medial malleolus

Tibialis posterior tendon

Flexor hallucis longus tendon

Head of first metatarsal

Abductor hallucis

(b)

Tibialis anterior tendon

Extensor hallucis longus tendon

Talonavicular joint

Lateral cuneiform

Tibia

Soleus

Long flexor muscles of foot

Posterior talocalcaneal joint

Achilles' tendon

Sinus tarsi

Anterior talocalcaneal joint

Calcaneum

Abductor digiti minimi

Flexor digiti minimi

Peroneus longus tendon

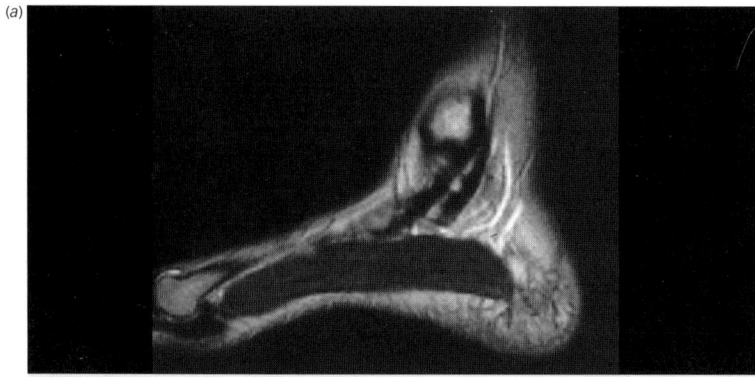

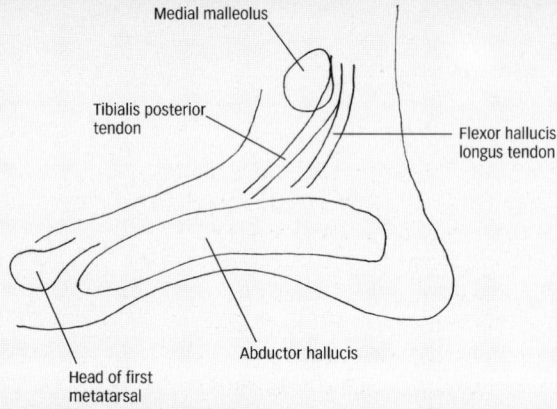

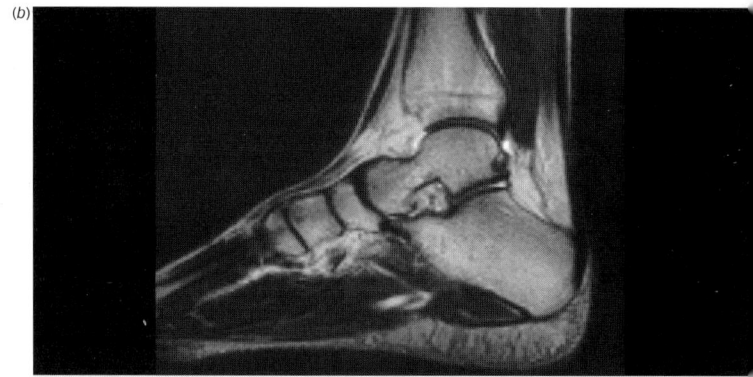

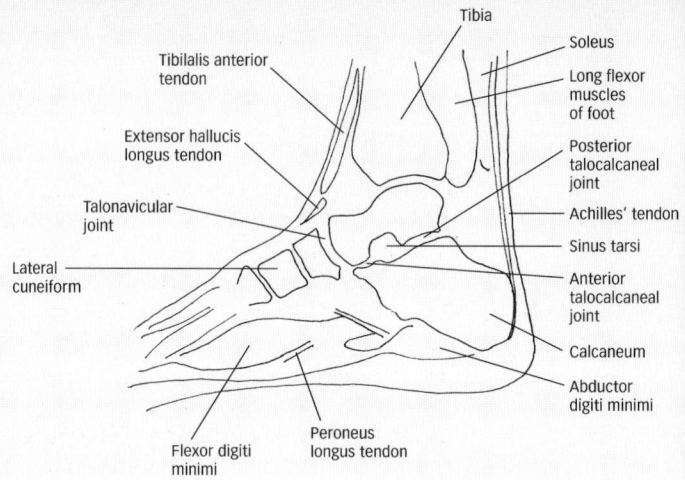

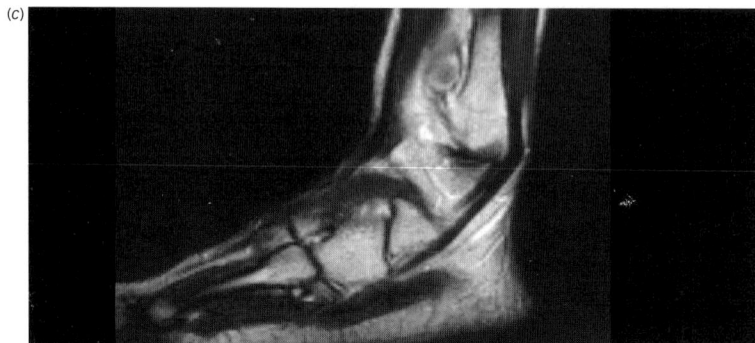

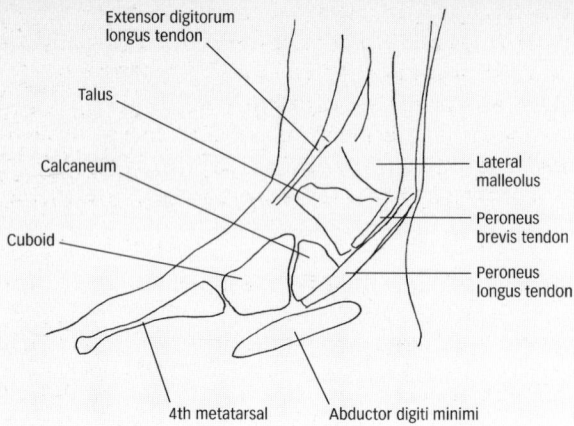

Fig. 46.
T1W sagittal MRI of the ankle joint: (*a*) through the medial malleolus, (*b*) through the mid-ankle, and (*c*) through the lateral malleolus.

(c)

Extensor digitorum longus tendon

Talus

Calcaneum

Cuboid

Lateral malleolus

Peroneus brevis tendon

Peroneus longus tendon

4th metatarsal

Abductor digiti minimi

380

18

Limb vasculature and the lymphatic system

M. EASTY
and O. CHAN

Arterial imaging

Although a variety of newer methods are available, including ultrasound, CT and MRI, catheter angiography remains the gold standard for demonstration of arterial anatomy. Conventional film/screen, digital or digital subtraction methods may be employed. Using digital subtraction angiography (DSA), images of the arteries may be obtained directly by intra-arterial injection of iodinated contrast medium (IA DSA), or indirectly following intravenous injection of larger volumes of contrast agent (IV DSA).

Access to the arterial system is usually obtained by needle puncture of the common femoral artery using the Seldinger technique (Fig. 1). It is therefore important for the angiographer to understand the anatomy of the inguinal region (Fig. 2).

The inguinal ligament extends from the anterior–superior iliac spine to the pubic tubercle. The upper parts of the common femoral artery and vein lie in a vascular com-

partment behind the inguinal ligament and between the iliopsoas and pectineus muscles.

The iliopsoas and femoral nerve lie laterally; the femoral artery lies lateral to the femoral vein, and medial to this lies the femoral canal. The vessels are enclosed in the femoral sheath, formed anteriorly by the transversalis fascia and posteriorly by the fascia iliacus. The sheath tapers and fuses with the vessel walls after approximately 2 cm. The femoral canal is situated anterior to the pectineus muscle and contains fat and lymphatics.

The femoral artery is punctured at its point of maximum pulsation, usually as it passes over the medial third of the femoral head at the mid-inguinal point (halfway between the anterior superior iliac spine and the pubic tubercle). This point often corresponds to the inguinal crease, except in obese patients where the crease may have descended. X-ray screening of the groin to enable the common femoral artery to be entered as it passes over the femoral head may be useful in order to avoid 'high' or 'low' punctures. High punctures, above the inguinal ligament, may result in a retroperitoneal haematoma, as the artery is difficult to compress without the support of

1 high puncture
2 Ideal puncture
3 Low puncture

The artery is punctured at the site of maximal pulsation. A soft-tip guide wire is passed through the needle.

The needle is withdrawn over the guide wire and a catheter advanced over the wire into the artery.

The guide wire is withdrawn.

Fig. 1.
The Seldinger technique. (*a*) 1 high puncture, 2 ideal puncture, 3 low puncture. (*b*) The artery is punctured at the site of maximal pulsation. A soft-tip guide wire is passed through the needle. (*c*) The needle is withdrawn over the guide wire and a catheter is advanced over the wire into the artery. (*d*) The guide wire is withdrawn.

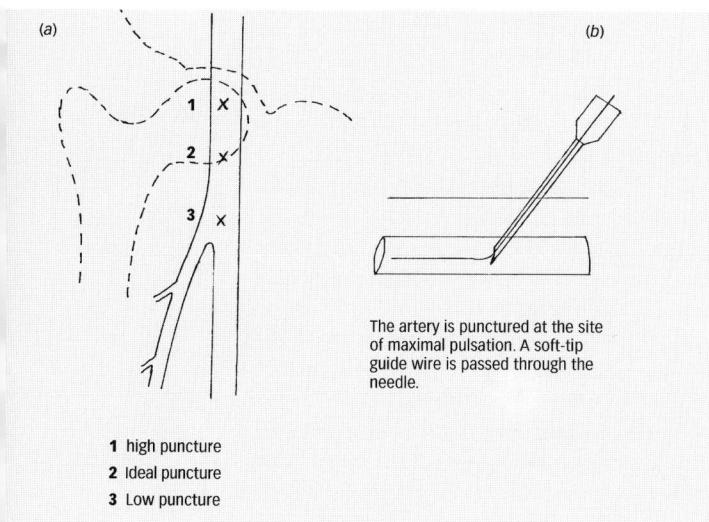

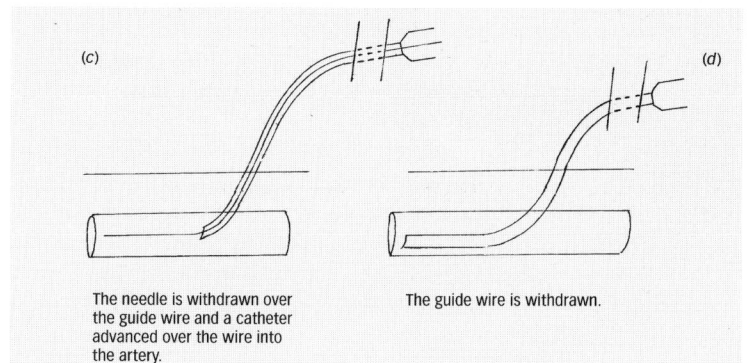

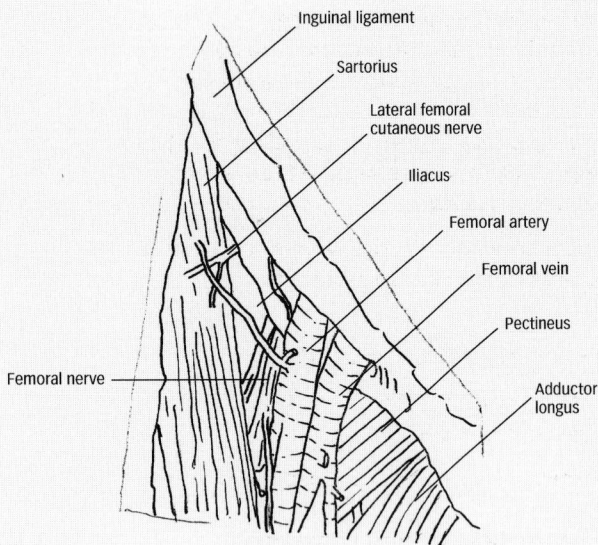

Fig. 2.
The inguinal region.

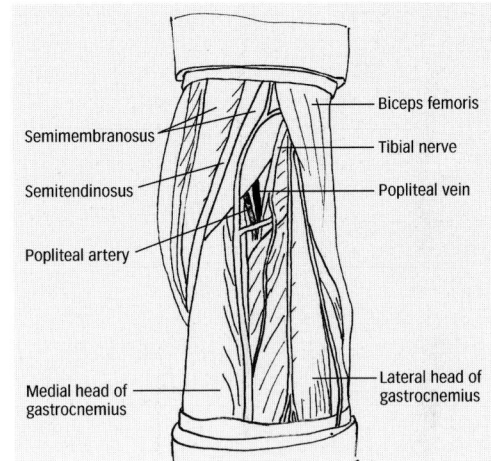

Fig. 3.
The relations of the popliteal artery. The popliteal artery lies deep to the popliteal vein, thus popliteal arterial puncture may lead to an arteriovenous fistula.

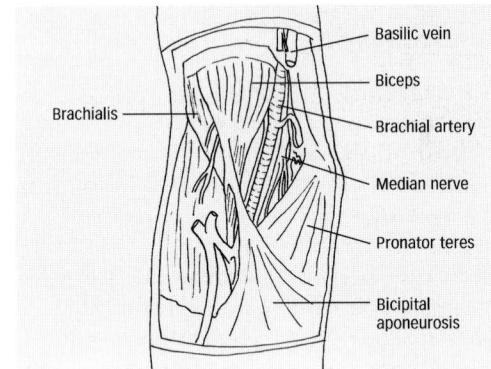

Fig. 4.
The antecubital fossa.

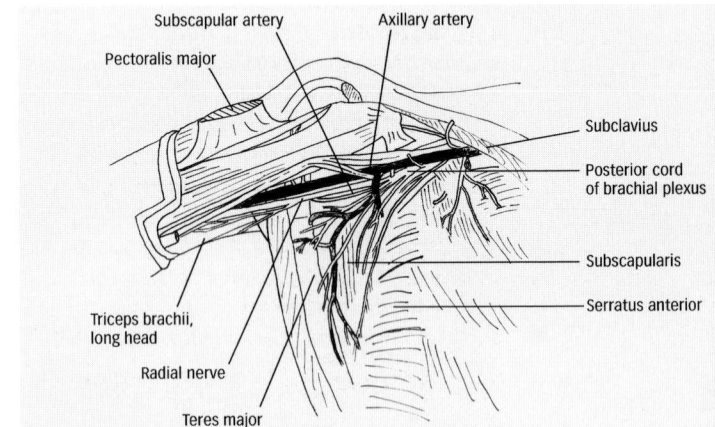

Fig. 5.
The axillary artery.

the femoral head. Low punctures may result in pseudo-aneurysm formation, or inadvertent puncture of the profunda femoris artery with an increased risk of arteriovenous fistula formation. This occurs as the artery and vein are both punctured.

Very rarely, femoral artery punctures result in femoral nerve damage or neural compression by a large haematoma. It is important to bear in mind the proximity of the femoral nerve, which lies just lateral to the artery.

For diagnostic studies of the lower limb, a retrograde puncture of the femoral artery is used, so that the iliac and femoral arteries of both limbs may be examined. An antegrade puncture allows catheters to be directed distally for interventional procedures. Alternatively, retrograde puncture with manipulation of the catheter over the aortic bifurcation into the contralateral femoral artery can be used.

Retrograde popliteal artery puncture may prove valuable for percutaneous transluminal angioplasty of the superficial femoral artery. The relations of the popliteal artery are shown in Fig. 3.

For diagnostic angiography of the upper limbs, the catheter is manipulated from the femoral artery into either the aortic arch or selectively into the subclavian arteries.

Alternative approaches for angiography include puncture of the radial, brachial or axillary arteries.

Punctures of the brachial or axillary arteries are undertaken if the femoral arteries are occluded. If possible, the distal axillary artery or proximal brachial artery should be punctured and the left arm is preferred. This approach avoids manipulation across the origins of the great vessels. Because axillary and brachial artery catheterization can be associated with damage to the nerves of the upper limb, careful single wall punctures and small catheters are used (Figs. 4 and 5).

Radial artery catheterization is increasingly employed, and small catheters (three French gauge) are used. There is a risk of radial nerve damage, and spasm of the artery may jeopardize circulation in the hand unless a good collateral ulnar artery circulation is present. This is assessed by Allen's test, where ulnar arterial pulsation should be palpable when the radial pulse is obliterated by manual compression.

The translumbar approach to the aorta has largely been abandoned in favour of the other routes for arterial access, which permit

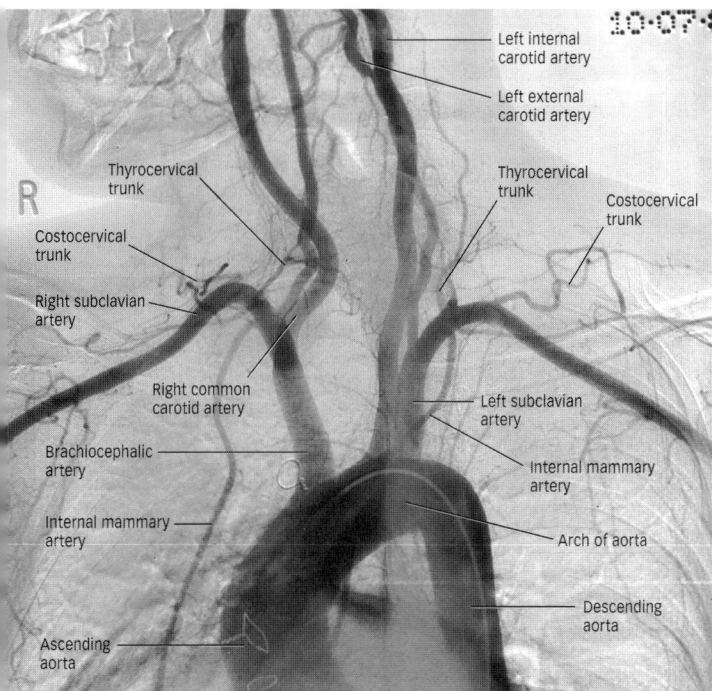

Fig. 6.
An arch aortogram.

greater flexibility for catheterization and percutaneous therapy.

IV DSA studies are performed using a Seldinger technique via an antecubital vein (preferably the basilic vein), or via the common femoral vein. The cephalic vein should be avoided if possible, because the angle at which the vein pierces the clavipectoral fascia may make manipulation of the catheter tip into the superior vena cava difficult. The catheter tip is positioned either in the superior vena cava or the right atrium. The procedure requires larger amounts of contrast medium than IA DSA. The quality of the resultant images of the arterial system are influenced by the patient's cardiac output and by his ability to remain still during image acquisition.

The arterial supply to the upper limb

The subclavian artery
The right subclavian artery arises from the brachiocephalic trunk where it divides behind the sternoclavicular joint to form the right common carotid and subclavian arteries (Fig. 6). On the left, the subclavian artery arises directly from the arch of the aorta, passing upwards behind the left sternoclavicular joint. The subclavian artery grooves the superior surface of the first rib posterior to the subclavian vein and the scalenus anterior muscle and ends at its lateral border where it continues as the axillary artery and enters the arm (Fig. 5).

The subclavian arteries are conventionally divided into three parts by the scalenus anterior muscle.

- The first part is medial to scalenus anterior and arches over the apex of the lung.
- The second part passes behind the scalenus anterior muscle separating it from the subclavian vein.
- The third part passes from the lateral aspect of the scalenus anterior muscle to the outer border of the first rib.

Cervical ribs or fibrous bands may compress the subclavian artery causing claudication in the arm.

Branches of the subclavian artery

First part The branches of the first part of the subclavian artery are:

- The vertebral artery (as discussed in Chapter 5).
- The internal thoracic (the internal mammary) artery arises from the inferior aspect of the subclavian artery and descends just lateral to the sternal border, ending in the sixth intercostal space by dividing into the superior epigastric and musculophrenic arteries. It lies between the costal cartilage and the intercostal muscles and pleura and supplies the chest wall, sternum, anterior pericardium, anterior mediastinum and diaphragm via anterior intercostal arteries and perforating cutaneous branches. It is used in coronary artery bypass grafting. The superior epigastric artery enters the rectus sheath and anastomoses with the inferior epigastric artery from the external iliac artery.
- The thyrocervical trunk is a short vessel which divides into the inferior thyroid, superficial cervical and suprascapular arteries. The inferior thyroid artery passes superiorly towards the inferior pole of the thyroid gland. It lies behind the common carotid artery and sympathetic chain and anterior to the vertebral artery and prevertebral fascia. It supplies the pharynx, larynx, oesophagus, trachea and thyroid gland.

A small branch of the ascending cervical artery and a small branch of the inferior thyroid artery enter the vertebral canal through the intervertebral foramina to contribute to the supply of the spinal cord, membranes and vertebral bodies. The ascending cervical artery anastomoses with the vertebral, ascending pharyngeal, occipital and deep cervical arteries.

The transverse cervical and suprascapular arteries pass laterally over the scalenus muscles and phrenic nerve and supply the muscles of the shoulder girdle, forming an anastomosis around the scapula.

- The left costocervical artery arises from the first part of the subclavian artery. It passes posteriorly over the dome of the pleura, reaching the neck of the first rib where it divides into the deep cervical and superior intercostal branches. The deep cervical branch passes above the neck of the first rib and supplies the posterior vertebral muscles before ascending towards the occiput. A spinal branch enters the vertebral canal between the seventh cervical and first thoracic vertebra.

The superior intercostal branch passes behind the pleura, downwards in front of the neck of the first and second ribs. It gives rise to the first and second intercostal arteries.

Second part The branch of the second part of the subclavian artery is:

- The dorsal scapular artery which arises lateral to the scalenus anterior muscle. It passes laterally and posteriorly over the brachial plexus, deep to the levator scapulae muscle. It supplies the muscles attached

to the medial border of the scapula and takes part in the scapular anastomosis.

The subclavian artery is subject to a number of variations in its course and origin. The right subclavian artery may arise above or below the sternoclavicular level. It may arise separately from the aortic arch and may be either the first or last branch from the arch (aberrant right subclavian artery).

The left subclavian artery is occasionally combined at its origin with the left common carotid artery.

The dorsal scapular artery may arise from the transverse cervical artery and suprascapular arteries may arise from the thyrocervical trunk or separately from the subclavian arteries.

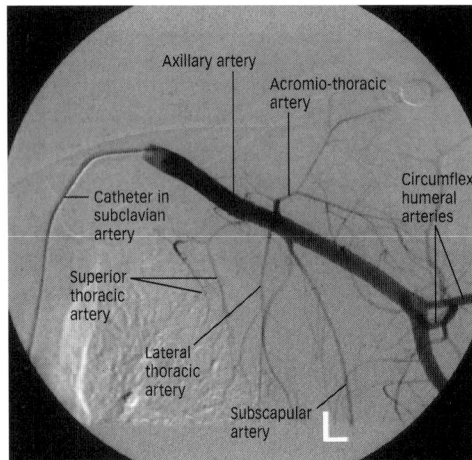

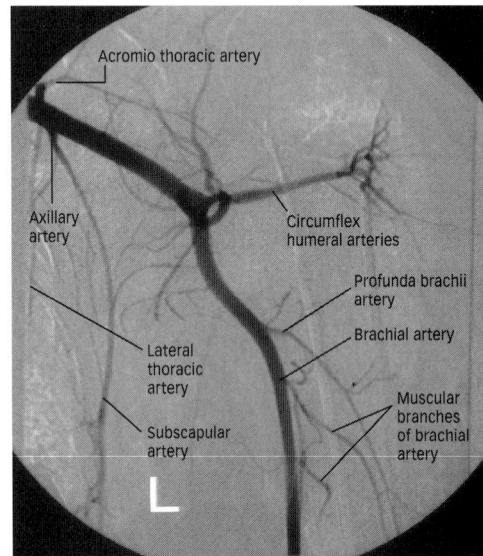

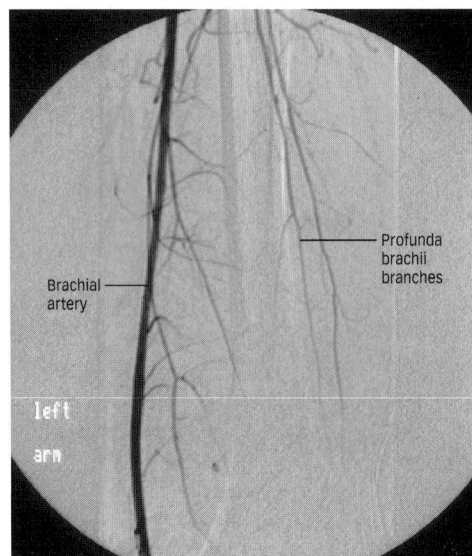

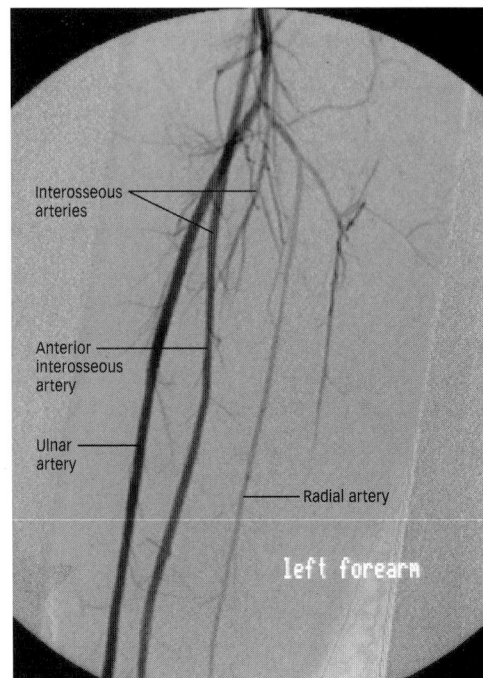

Fig. 7.
The upper limb arteries and arteriography.

The axillary artery

The subclavian artery continues as the axillary artery at the lateral border of the first rib, which, in turn, extends to the lower border of teres major, where it becomes the brachial artery (Fig. 7).

The axillary artery lies lateral to the vein and both are crossed anteriorly by the pectoralis minor muscle which traditionally divides the axillary artery into three parts (Fig. 5).

Relations

The axillary vein lies medially and slightly anteriorly along its whole length. The artery crosses from the medial to the lateral wall of the axilla and therefore, the first intercostal space, the serratus anterior muscle and the long thoracic nerve of Bell are posterior to the first part of the axillary artery.

The cords of the brachial plexus surround the second part of the axillary artery on three sides and separate it from the axillary vein and the adjacent muscles.

The cords of the brachial plexus are named by their relation to the axillary artery: lateral, posterior and medial.

The last or third part of the axillary artery is covered only by skin and fascia and is therefore palpable and may be used for arterial puncture.

Branches of the axillary artery

Six main branches of the axillary artery supply the wall of the axilla.

- The subscapular artery runs downwards on the posterior axillary wall to reach the inferior angle of the scapula and takes part in the scapular anastomosis.
- The circumflex scapular artery: a large branch of the subscapular artery passes through the triangular space, adjacent to the lateral border of the scapula. This space is formed by the subscapularis muscle superiorly, the triceps brachii laterally and the teres major inferiorly.
- The superior thoracic artery supplies the chest wall.
- The lateral thoracic artery aids in the supply of the chest wall.
- The acromiothoracic artery passes over the pectoralis minor to reach the anterior chest wall and gives branches to the deltoid muscle, pectoralis muscles and the acromioclavicular joint.
- The anterior and posterior circumflex humeral arteries encircle the surgical neck of the humerus and supply the shoulder joint. They anastomose with each other and with branches from the suprascapular and

acromiothoracic arteries. The subclavian artery is linked to the third part of the axillary artery via arteries forming the scapular anastomosis, namely the suprascapular and transverse cervical branches of the subclavian artery and the circumflex scapular from the axillary artery.

The brachial artery

The brachial artery extends from the lower border of the teres major to the level of the neck of the radius where it divides into the radial and ulnar arteries (Fig. 7).

The main branch of the brachial artery is the profunda brachii which arises just distal to the teres major and accompanies the brachial nerve as it passes backwards in the radial groove on the posterior surface of the humerus. The profunda brachii gives off a further branch, which passes upwards and anastomoses with the arteries surrounding the shoulder joint. It gives off two lower medial branches, which descend towards the elbow joint on its medial side and take part in the anterior and posterior anastomosis around the elbow.

The brachial artery is superficial along its whole course until overlapped by the bicipital aponeurosis at the elbow and can be compressed against the medial surface of the humerus. It may be used for access in angiography, either by a high brachial approach or in the antecubital fossa where it lies medial to the biceps tendon and lateral to the median nerve.

The brachial artery divides at the neck of the radius into the radial artery, which passes inferiorly and laterally, lying on the tendon of the biceps brachii. High take-off of the radial artery from the brachial artery is a common anatomical variant. The ulnar artery passes down and medially, deep to pronator teres. Within the antecubital fossa, the ulnar and radial arteries give off recurrent branches to the elbow joint. The ulnar artery gives off the common interosseous artery 2 cm below its origin, which further divides into the anterior and posterior interosseous arteries.

The anterior interosseous artery runs downwards on the anterior surface of the interosseous membrane. It supplies the deep muscles of the forearm, reaching the posterior compartment by means of perforating branches. Above pronator quadratus, the anterior interosseous artery gives off an anterior carpal branch and then pierces the interosseous membrane to terminate on the dorsum of the wrist.

The posterior interosseous artery anastomoses with the anterior interosseous artery and branches of the radial and ulnar arteries in the wrist.

The ulnar artery gives off muscular branches as it runs down the forearm and at the wrist it gives off palmar and dorsal carpal branches. The deep branch of the ulnar artery anastomoses with the radial artery in the hand. The superficial palmar arch arises from the ulnar artery.

The radial artery passes down the forearm deep to brachioradialis and is then subcutaneous over the distal radius. It then passes through the anatomical snuffbox and between the first and second metacarpals into the palm.

The radial artery gives off a recurrent branch at the elbow, muscular branches in the forearm and a superficial palmar branch which enters the palm superficial to the flexor retinaculum. It gives off palmar and dorsal carpal branches. The deep palmar arch is a continuation of the radial artery.

Arteries of the lower limb

The aorta trifurcates anterior and to the left of the body of the fourth lumbar vertebra into the common iliac arteries and the median sacral artery. The common iliac arteries divide at the sacroiliac joints into the internal and external iliac arteries (Fig. 8).

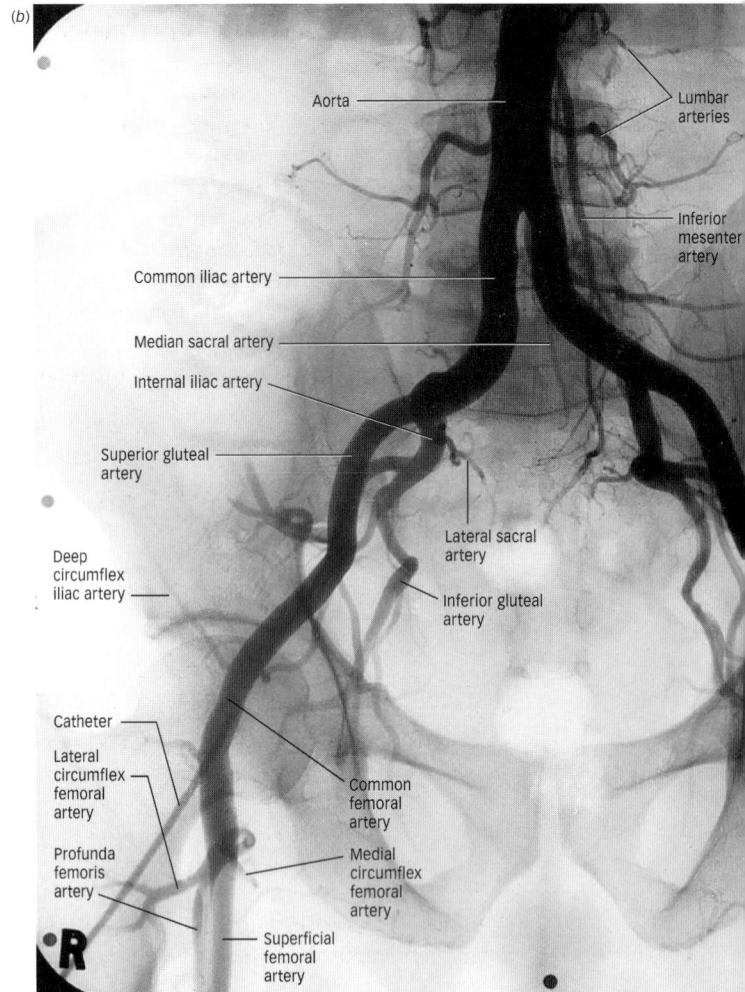

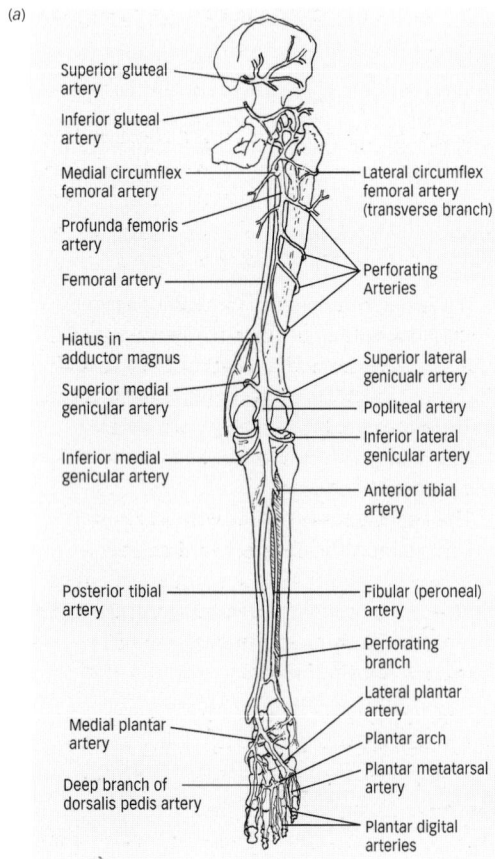

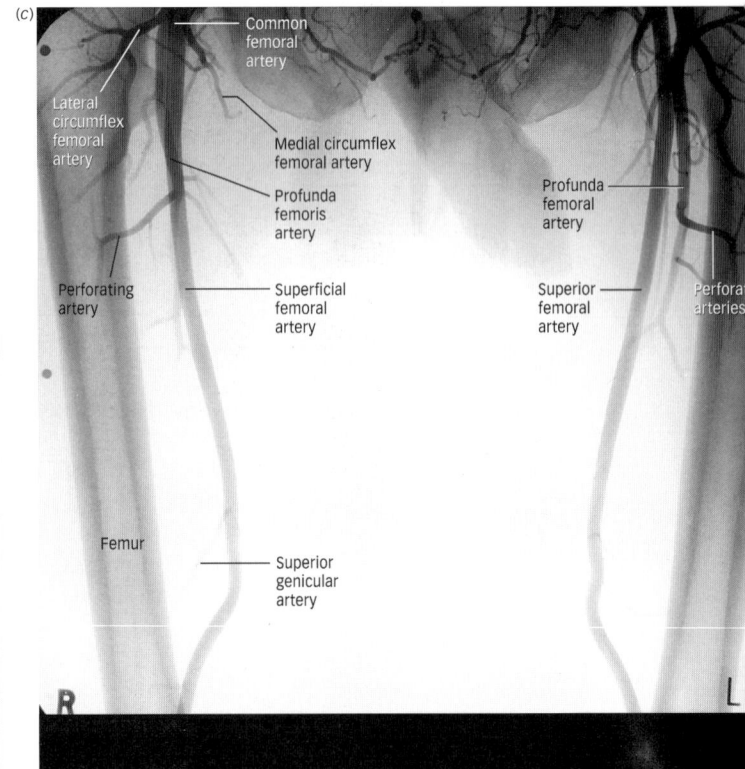

Fig. 8.
The lower limb arteries and arteriography

The right common iliac artery is 5 cm long and lies in front of the fourth and fifth lumbar vertebrae. The ureter lies anteriorly; the common iliac veins, the lumbosacral trunk, the obturator nerve, the iliolumbar artery and the sympathetic trunk lie posterior to the artery. The left common iliac artery is 4 cm in length and lies anterolateral to the left common iliac vein. Its relations are similar to those of the right common iliac artery, and in addition, the superior rectal artery and the preaortic autonomic plexus pass anteriorly.

The common iliac veins lie slightly medially and posterior to the arteries.

The common iliac arteries descend and divide at the level of the lumbosacral intervertebral disc to form the external and internal iliac arteries.

The internal iliac artery (see also Chapter 14 'The Pelvis')

This artery arises in front of the sacroiliac joint at the level of the lumbosacral disc. It descends to the sciatic foramen where it divides into an anterior trunk and a posterior trunk. Anterior to the internal iliac artery are the distal ureters, and, in the female, the ovary and fallopian tube. The internal iliac vein lies posterior to the artery and the external iliac artery and psoas muscle lie laterally. The branches of the anterior and posterior trunks of the internal iliac artery are discussed in Chapter 14.

8(d)

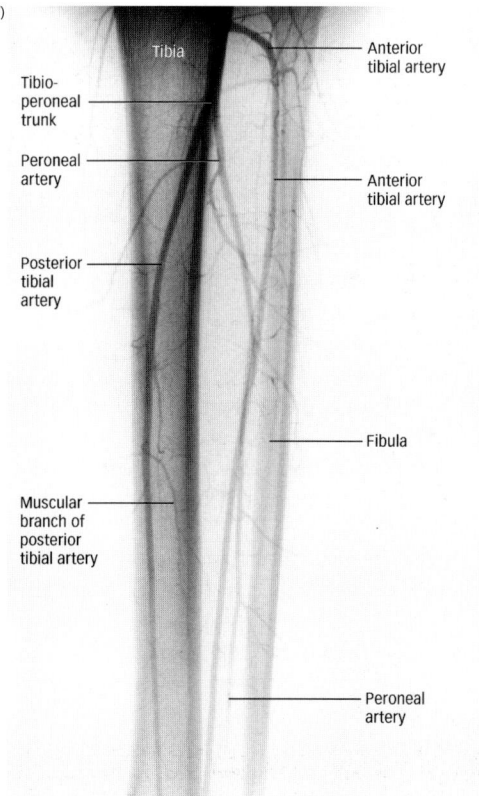

Tibia

Tibio-peroneal trunk

Peroneal artery

Posterior tibial artery

Muscular branch of posterior tibial artery

Anterior tibial artery

Anterior tibial artery

Fibula

Peroneal artery

The external iliac artery

This runs caudally from the pelvic brim on the medial border of the psoas muscle to a point midway between the anterior superior iliac spine and the pubic symphysis; the midinguinal point, where it becomes the femoral artery. The external iliac artery is crossed anteriorly by the ureter, the vas deferens and the testicular vessels in the male, and the ureter, ovarian vessels and round ligament in the female.

Branches of the external iliac artery

There are two branches which arise just above the inguinal ligament.

- The inferior epigastric artery; this ascends medial to the deep inguinal ring, running on the posterior surface of the anterior abdominal wall. It enters the rectus sheath, supplies the rectus abdominis muscles and anastomoses with the superior epigastric artery (branch of the internal thoracic artery). The inferior epigastric artery also gives off a pubic branch to the periosteum of the superior pubic ramus. This anastomoses with the pubic branch of the obturator artery. When the obturator artery is absent (in 30% of cases), this anastomosis is opened up to form an artery known as the abnormal obturator artery.
- The deep circumflex iliac artery; this passes laterally towards the iliac crest and supplies the muscles in this region.

The femoral artery

The common femoral artery is a continuation of the external iliac artery and can be felt pulsating at the mid-inguinal point. It enters the thigh below the inguinal ligament and gives off four superficial branches at this point.

- The superficial epigastric artery runs superomedially to enter the rectus sheath in the anterior abdominal wall. It anastomoses with the superior epigastric artery.
- The superficial circumflex iliac artery passes laterally towards the anterior superior iliac spine.
- The superficial external pudendal artery runs medially to supply the skin and superficial tissues of the external genitalia.
- The deep external pudendal artery emerges more medially to supply the skin of the external genitalia.

The common femoral artery passes inferiorly and slightly posteriorly through the femoral triangle, deep to the sartorius muscle and enters the adductor canal (the subsartorial canal or Hunter's canal). Its main branch, the profunda femoris artery arises 5 cm distal to the inguinal ligament. It passes backwards and downwards and lies posterior to the femoral artery.

The profunda femoris has six branches:

- The medial femoral circumflex artery passes posteriorly between the psoas and pectineus muscles and through successive layers of muscles to the back of the thigh, where it divides into transverse and ascending branches which anastomose with the gluteal arteries to supply the hip joint.

The trochanteric anastomosis provides the main blood supply to the femoral head. It is formed by the anastomosis of the descending branch of the superior gluteal artery with the ascending branches of both the lateral and medial femoral circumflex arteries. The inferior gluteal artery commonly joins the anastomosis. The medial femoral circumflex artery also takes part in the cruciate anastomosis at the level of the lesser trochanter (joined by the transverse branch of the lateral femoral circumflex artery, and ascending branch of the first perforating artery and a descending branch of the inferior gluteal artery).

- The lateral femoral circumflex artery passes laterally, deep to the sartorius and rectus femoris muscles where it divides into ascending and transverse branches which take part in the anastomosis in the glutei and back of the thigh. It also has a descending branch which takes part in supplying the knee.
- Four perforating arteries supply the muscles of the thigh and anastomose with the circumflex arteries in the back of the thigh. The lowest perforating artery anastomoses with branches of the popliteal artery.

The common femoral artery continues as the superficial femoral artery after giving off the profunda femoris artery and has no major branches in the thigh. It passes between vastus medialis, the adductor muscles and sartorius in the adductor canal. In the lower third of the thigh, it passes posterior and medial to the shaft of the femur through the adductor hiatus and becomes the popliteal artery. Prior to entering the adductor hiatus, it gives off a descending genicular branch to supply the knee.

The popliteal artery
The popliteal artery lies deep to the popliteal vein on the fat covering the lower surface of the femur and on the popliteus muscle. At the lower border of the popliteus muscle, it divides into two terminal branches.

Within the popliteal fossa, the popliteal artery gives off seven branches:

- superior and inferior muscular branches.
- medial superior and inferior genicular branches.
- lateral superior and inferior genicular branches.
- middle genicular branch.

These branches supply the adjacent muscles and take part in the anastomosis around the knee joint.

The terminal branches are the anterior and posterior tibial arteries.

- The anterior tibial artery begins posteriorly at the lower border of the popliteus, passes forwards through an opening in the interosseous membrane and runs downwards on the membrane between tibialis anterior medially and extensor hallucis longus laterally. In the lower leg, the artery lies anterior to the tibia and ankle joint, passes deep to the extensor retinaculum and is crossed by the tendon of the extensor hallucis longus. The artery lies midway between the malleoli where it can be palpated lateral to the tendon of the extensor hallucis longus muscle. It continues as the dorsalis pedis, passing to the first intermetatarsal space and then into the sole of the foot. The dorsalis pedis artery gives off branches to the medial and lateral sides of the foot, and before passing to the plantar aspect, gives off the cruciate artery, which passes to the lateral border of the foot. Metatarsal arteries from the cruciate artery supply the toes and communicate with branches on the sole of the foot.
- The posterior tibial artery runs down the leg, deep to the soleus muscle and lies on the tibialis posterior muscle. Lower down, the artery is superficial and lies medial to the Achilles tendon. It passes deep to the flexor retinaculum and abductor hallucis, where it divides into its terminal branches, the lateral and medial plantar arteries. The artery can be palpated posterior to the medial malleolus. High take-off of the posterior tibial artery is a common anatomical variant.

  The posterior tibial artery gives off a branch which winds around the fibula to join in the genicular anastomosis and several muscular branches. It also supplies the nutrient artery to the tibia and takes part in the ankle anastomosis. Its largest branch is the peroneal artery which arises at the upper end of the fibula and passes down, close to the fibula towards the lateral aspect of the ankle where it anastomoses with the vessels supplying the ankle. The peroneal artery gives off the nutrient artery to the fibula and supplies the muscles on the lateral and posterior side of the leg.

Venous imaging

Lower limb venography is most commonly undertaken using a conventional film/screen technique, although digital or digital subtraction imaging may be used.

A tourniquet is applied to the ankle and a 'butterfly' needle is inserted into a vein in the dorsum of the foot, the needle being directed towards the toes to prevent filling of superficial veins. The patient is positioned in a semi-erect position on a tilting table to aid deep vein filling, and standard views of the deep venous system in the calf, thigh and pelvis are obtained. The paired posterior tibial veins are normally the first to fill, followed by the peroneal and anterior tibial veins. The muscular venous arcades draining the soleus muscle and gastrocnemius muscle often fill later.

Films are taken in the posteroanterior and lateral positions to include the veins from the ankle to the knee. A further lateral view of the popliteal vein is then obtained followed by posteroanterior views of the superficial femoral vein, common femoral vein, iliac veins and inferior vena cava. The Valsalva manoeuvre is employed to enhance filling of the iliac vessels and lower inferior vena cava.

Some segments of the venous system in the lower limbs are difficult to demonstrate fully.

(a) The anterior tibial vein is occasionally occluded by the ankle tourniquet. Releasing the pressure enhances filling.
(b) The deep femoral vein or profunda femoris vein fills in only 50% of patients, either as a result of a loop connection with the superficial femoral vein or by retrograde filling during the Valsalva manoeuvre.
(c) The Valsalva manoeuvre is used to fill the internal iliac veins.
(d) If the pelvic veins or lower inferior vena cava are not adequately demonstrated, bilateral pedal injections of contrast may be used.

Upper limb venography is undertaken in a similar manner, via an injection into a vein in the dorsum of the hand. IV DSA is used to image rapid flow in dialysis fistulae in the arm.

Contrast is injected into a vein in the hand, and both the venous and arterial limbs of the shunt may be assessed if a tourniquet is applied to the upper arm and inflated above systolic blood pressure.

Ultrasound may be used to visualize and confirm the patency of relatively short segments of arteries or veins in the limb (Fig. 9). Ultrasound may also be employed to assist in localization of veins prior to placement of central venous catheters.

Magnetic resonance angiography currently has limited applications in imaging the arterial or venous systems in the limbs. Its role is likely to expand once technical difficulties are resolved.

Normal venous architecture

Like arteries, veins have three-layered walls: an endothelium-lined tunica intima, a muscular tunica media and an external tunica adventitia, which is mainly connective tissue. A major difference lies in the comparative weakness of the venous tunica media, which has a lesser amount of muscle and elastic fibres due to lower venous pressure.

Most veins have valves to prevent reflux of blood composed of an inward projection of the intima strengthened by elastic fibres and collagen. The valves are semilunar cusps. Their concave margins are directed with the current but, when blood flow reverses, the valve closes. In the legs, where venous return is against gravity, valves are important in venous flow. Valves are absent in very small and in very large veins.

Arteries and veins usually accompany each other in fascial planes. This proximity probably aids venous return. Paired veins usually

Fig. 9.
Ultrasound scans of the (a) femoral artery, B mode ultrasound and Doppler, (b) femoral vein, B mode ultrasound and Doppler study.

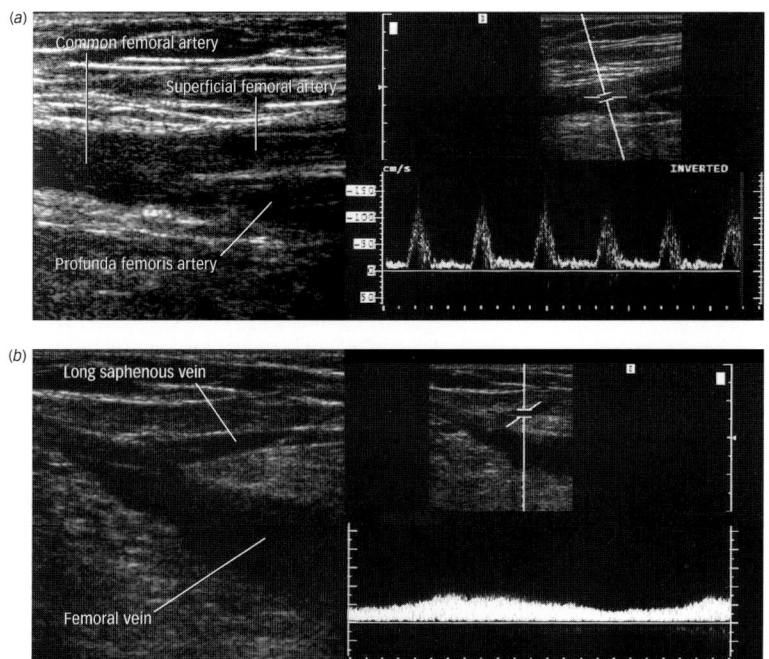

(a) Common femoral artery; Superficial femoral artery; Profunda femoris artery; INVERTED

(b) Long saphenous vein; Femoral vein

accompany a single artery as venae comitantes, although veins such as the cephalic vein or long saphenous vein are unaccompanied by arteries.

Veins of the upper limb

The veins of the upper limb are variable in number and position. In the hand are two sets of veins: deep and superficial (Fig. 10). The deep set follows the arteries, travelling as paired venae comitantes (paired veins following their homonymous arteries). The superfi-

cial veins of the hand and forearm are drained by the cephalic and basilic veins.

Haemodialysis arteriovenous fistulae are generally constructed by joining the cephalic veins to the radial artery at the wrist.

The cephalic vein begins on the lateral aspect of the wrist by draining blood from the venous plexus on the dorsum of the hand. It runs along the lateral side of the forearm and upper arm in the superficial fascia. As the vein drains cranially, it receives tributaries from the anterior and posterior aspects of the forearm. At the elbow, in the cubital fossa, the cephalic vein lies anterolaterally in the superficial fascia and gives off the median cubital vein which joins with the basilic vein. The median vein of the forearm ends in the medial cubital vein. The medial cutaneous nerve of the forearm, usually already branched, is both deep and superficial to the basilic vein. Deep to the deep fascia of the cubital fossa, the three main structures from lateral to medial are the tendon of the biceps

Fig. 10.
The upper limb veins, diagram and venography.

(a)

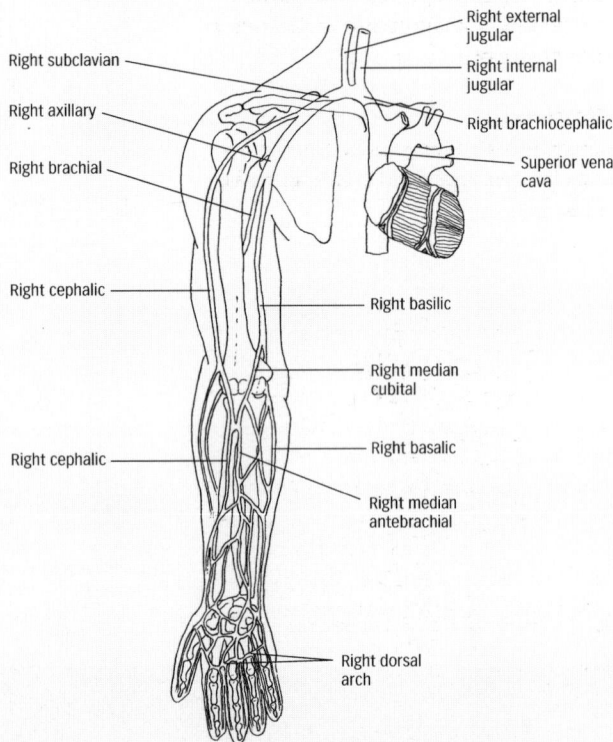

(b)

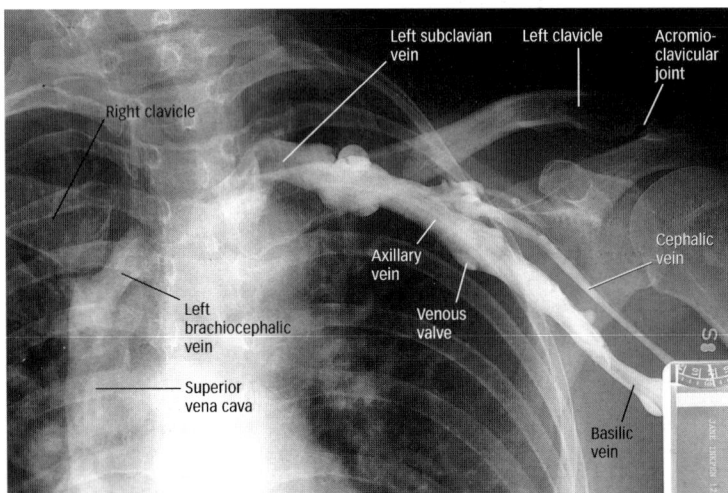

(c)

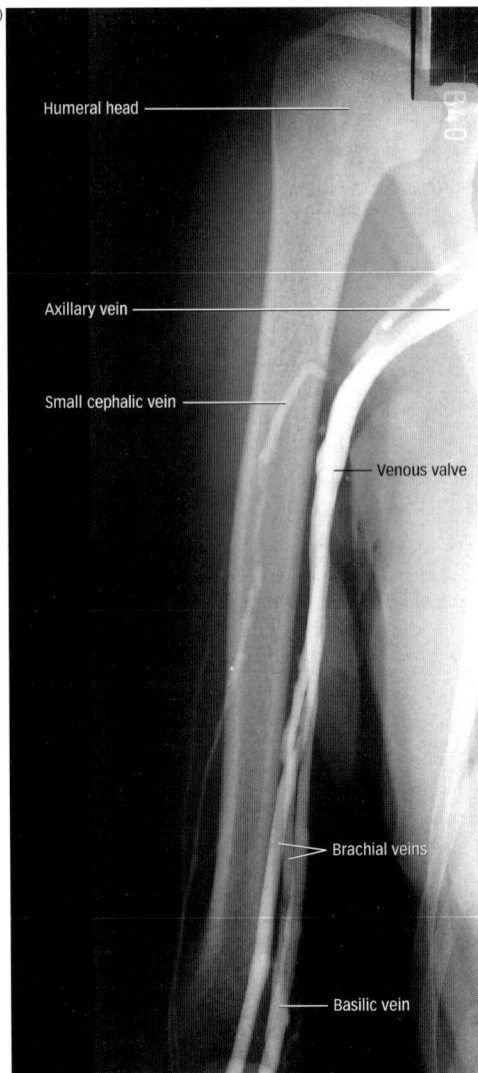

brachii, the brachial artery and the median nerve. The cephalic vein continues superficially in the upper arm, on the lateral side of the biceps muscle. It passes into the deltopectoral groove and then pierces the clavipectoral fascia to drain into the axillary vein.

The basilic vein begins on the medial side of the wrist and drains the medial part of the venous plexus on the dorsum of the hand. The vein passes upwards on the medial side of the fore-arm receiving anterior and posterior tributaries and passes to the anteromedial aspect of the elbow where it receives the median cubital vein.

The basilic vein continues on the medial aspect of the biceps brachii until it pierces the deep fascia to run cranially, medial to the brachial artery. It joins the brachial vein and becomes the axillary vein at the lower border of teres major. Spontaneous thrombosis of the axillary vein occasionally occurs following excessive and unaccustomed movements of the arm at the shoulder joint. The axillary vein lies medial to the axillary artery and becomes the subclavian vein at the outer border of the first rib. The subclavian vein lies anterior and inferior to the subclavian artery and is sepa-rated from it by the scalenus anterior muscle. The clavicle lies anterior to the vein.

On the right side, the phrenic nerve lies between subclavian vein and scalenus ante-rior. On the left, the nerve is more medial and lies between the vein and artery.

The main tributary of the subclavian vein is the external jugular vein which drains superficial veins of the head and neck. The subclavian vein ends by joining the internal jugular vein to form the brachiocephalic vein. These, in turn, drain into the superior vena cava.

Veins of the lower limb

The veins may be divided into superficial and deep with intercommunicating or perforating veins (Fig. 11). Valves are found in the larger veins and in the communicating veins, the valves being arranged so that blood passes from superficial to deep. The valves and the soleal pump help to propel blood to the heart. There are no valves in the common iliac veins or inferior vena cava.

Superficial veins

These drain the subcutaneous tissues through two main channels; the short and long saphe-nous veins.

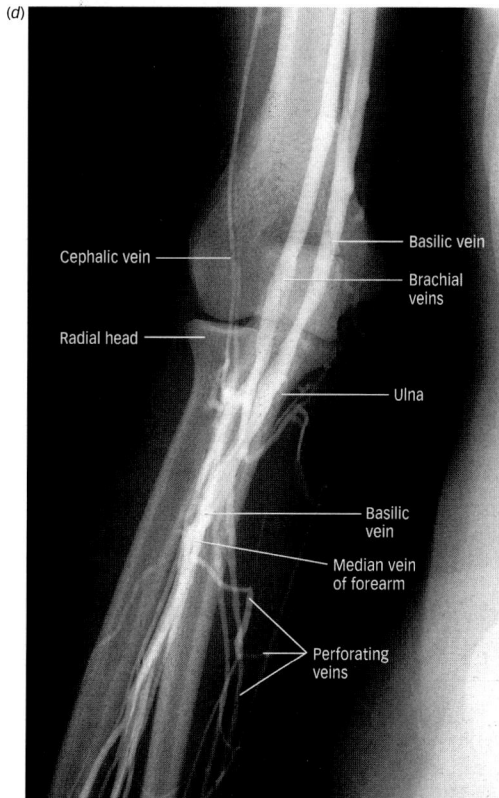

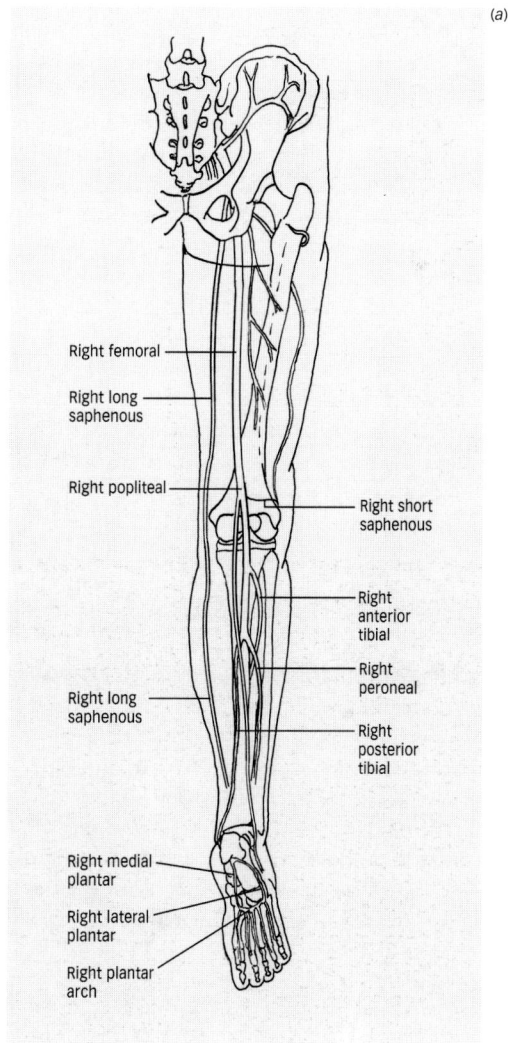

(d)

Cephalic vein — Basilic vein

— Brachial veins

Radial head —

— Ulna

— Basilic vein

— Median vein of forearm

Perforating veins

(a)

Right femoral —

Right long saphenous —

Right popliteal —

— Right short saphenous

— Right anterior tibial

— Right peroneal

Right long saphenous —

— Right posterior tibial

Right medial plantar —

Right lateral plantar —

Right plantar arch —

Fig. 11(a).
The lower limb veins, diagram and venography.

11(b)

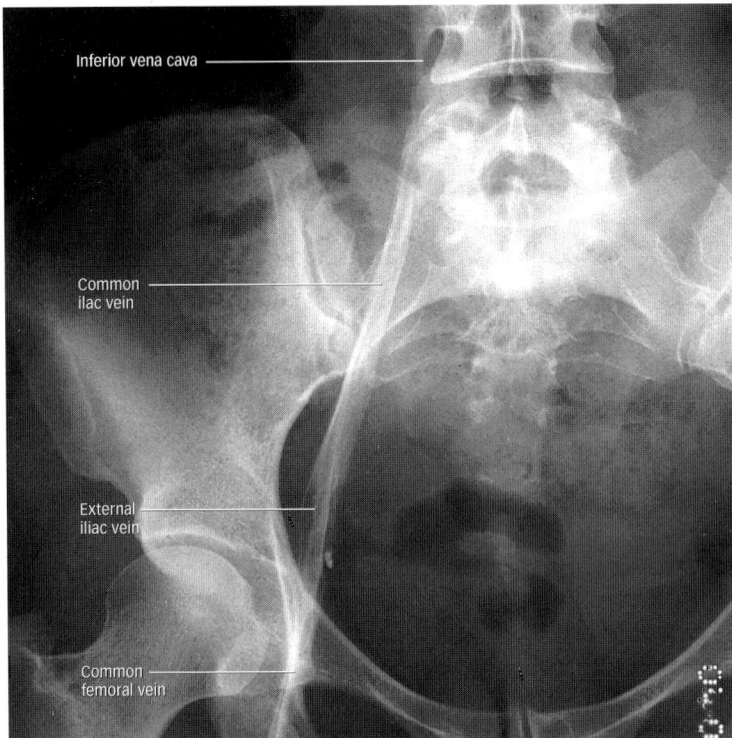

11(c)

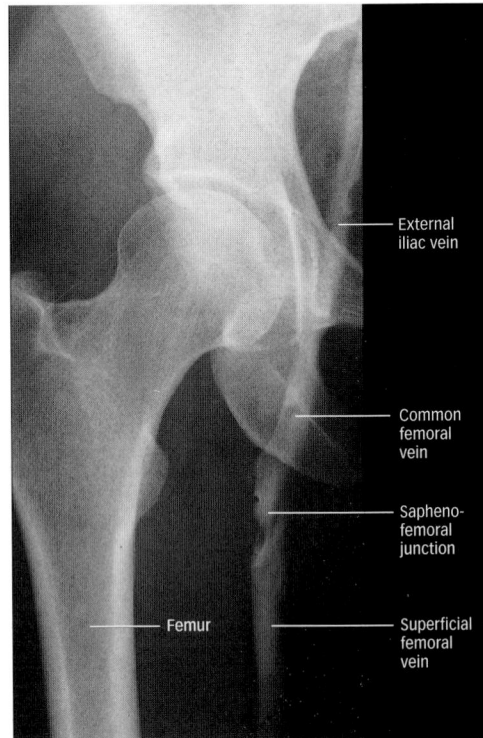

- The short saphenous vein originates from the lateral side of the dorsal venous arch of the foot. It passes behind the lateral malleolus, travels up the back of the calf and pierces the fascia of the popliteal fossa to drain into the popliteal vein at the saphenopopliteal junction. Communicating veins from the short saphenous may continue proximally to drain into the anteromedial and posterolateral veins of the thigh; the long saphenous and profunda femoris veins.

- The long saphenous vein arises from the medial side of the dorsal venous arch. It passes anterior to the medial malleolus, ascends on the medial aspect of the leg and drains into the femoral vein, passing through the saphenous opening in the lower part of the inguinal triangle.

    The long saphenous vein receives a number of tributaries in the leg and thigh but the perforating veins communicating with the deep veins are the most important. The communicating veins are variable in number and position, but constants are found above the medial aspect of the ankle and above the knee in the medial aspect of the thigh.

    The long saphenous vein is commonly used in cardiac surgery as a vascular autograft.

Deep veins

The deep veins of the leg generally follow the arteries as paired venae comitantes. They begin as digital and metatarsal veins in the sole of the foot and form medial and lateral plantar veins. These form the posterior tibial veins. The anterior tibial veins begin as continuations of veins running with the dorsalis pedis artery. They pass backwards through the upper interosseous membrane and join the posterior tibial veins to form the popliteal vein.

The popliteal vein passes through the adductor hiatus, forming the superficial femoral vein which becomes the external iliac vein above the inguinal ligament. The deep femoral or profunda femoris veins drain the back of the thigh and drain into the common femoral vein.

There may be large communications between the profunda femoris and superficial femoral veins.

Iliac veins

The internal and external iliac veins accompany the arteries. They lie posteromedial to the arteries and have similar relations.

The common iliac vein forms anterior to the sacroiliac joint by the union of the internal and external iliac veins. It ascends obliquely and unites with its opposite on the right side of the fifth lumbar vertebra to form the inferior vena cava. It lies posterior and to the right of the common iliac artery. The left vein is

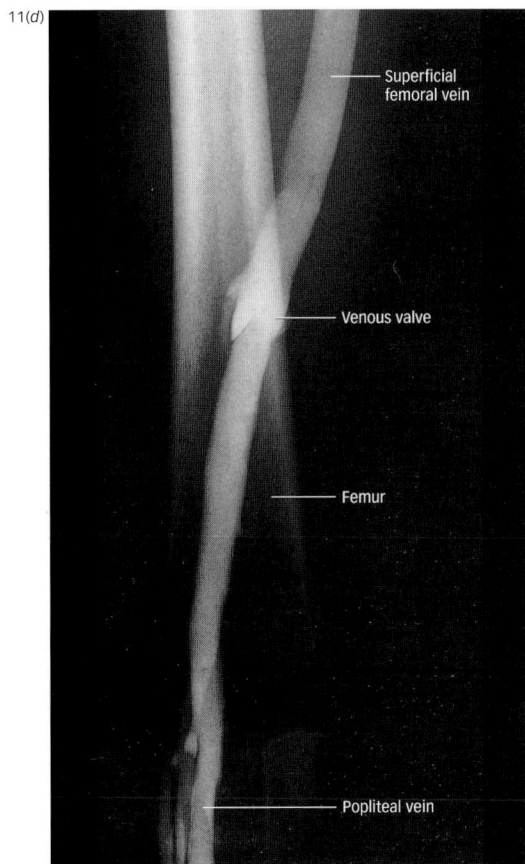

11(d)

- Superficial femoral vein
- Venous valve
- Femur
- Popliteal vein

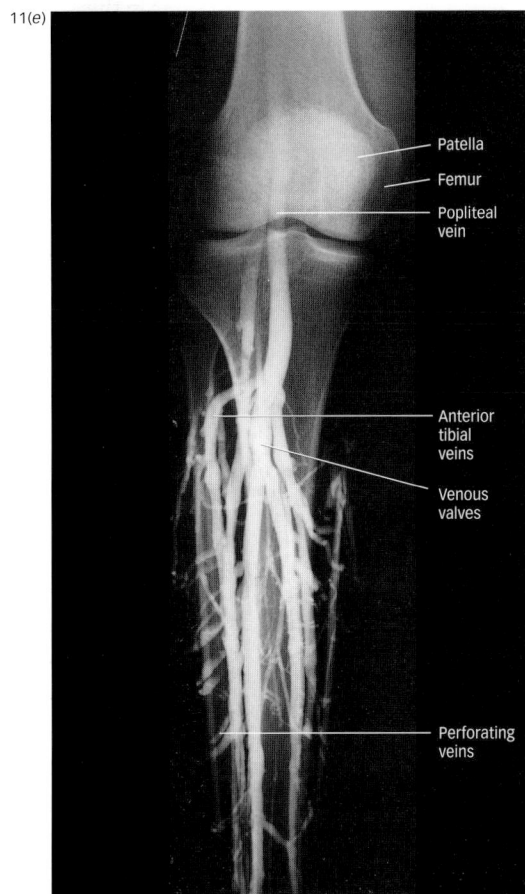

11(e)

- Patella
- Femur
- Popliteal vein
- Anterior tibial veins
- Venous valves
- Perforating veins

longer than the right and is crossed by the right common iliac artery. During venography, flow phenomena may occur in the left common iliac vein by compression from the right common iliac artery causing apparent filling defects. These appearances are a normal variant and the site is known as Cockett's point. The tributaries of the iliac veins match those of the arteries.

The embryology of the major veins and congenital anomalies

Initially, the cardinal veins form the main venous drainage system in the embryo (Fig. 12). They consist of the anterior cardinal veins, which drain the cephalic part of the body and the posterior cardinal veins which drain the remainder. The anterior and posterior cardinal veins join before entering the sinus horn to form the short, common cardinal veins. During the fourth week, the cardinal veins form a bilaterally symmetrical system.

During the fifth to the seventh week of embryological life, additional veins are formed: the subcardinal veins, which drain mainly the kidneys; the sacrocardinal veins which drain the lower extremities and the supracardinal veins which take over the function of the posterior cardinal veins to drain the body wall.

During formation of the vena caval system, anastomoses between the left and right sides form, so that blood from the left is channelled to the right side.

The anastomosis between the anterior cardinal veins develops into the left brachiocephalic vein. The superior vena cava is formed by the right common cardinal vein and the proximal right anterior cardinal vein.

The anastomosis between the subcardinal veins is formed by the left renal vein. The left subcardinal vein disappears with only its distal portion remaining as the left gonadal vein. The right subcardinal vein therefore develops into the renal segment of the inferior vena cava.

The anastomosis between the sacrocardinal veins is formed by the left common iliac vein. The right sacrocardinal vein finally becomes the sacrocardinal segment of the inferior vena cava. When the renal segment of the inferior vena cava connects with the hepatic segment (derived from the right vitelline vein), the inferior vena cava is complete. It consists of a hepatic segment, a renal segment and a sacrocardinal segment.

The obliteration of the posterior cardinal veins causes the supracardinal veins to become more important. The fourth to eleventh right intercostal veins empty into the right subcardinal vein, which, together with a portion of the posterior cardinal vein, form the azygos vein. The left fourth to seventh intercostal veins enter the left supracardinal vein. A connecting vessel develops between the two supracardinal veins; the left supracardinal vein enters the azygos vein and is then named the hemiazygos vein.

This complex development of the venae cavae accounts for the relatively frequent devi-ations from the normal pattern. It has been estimated that approximately 1% of normal subjects have anomalies of the inferior vena cava or its tributaries.

A double inferior vena cava may occur at the lumbar level when the left sacrocardinal vein fails to lose its connection with the left subcardinal vein. This anomaly occurs between 0.2 and 3%. The right cava is usually larger. The left cava rejoins the right cava via the left renal vein (Fig. 13).

Failure of the right subcardinal vein to make its connection in the liver leads to absence of the inferior vena cava. The lower body drains via the azygos system and superior vena cava to the heart. The hepatic vein drains directly to the heart. An absent inferior vena cava is commonly associated with cardiac abnormalities.

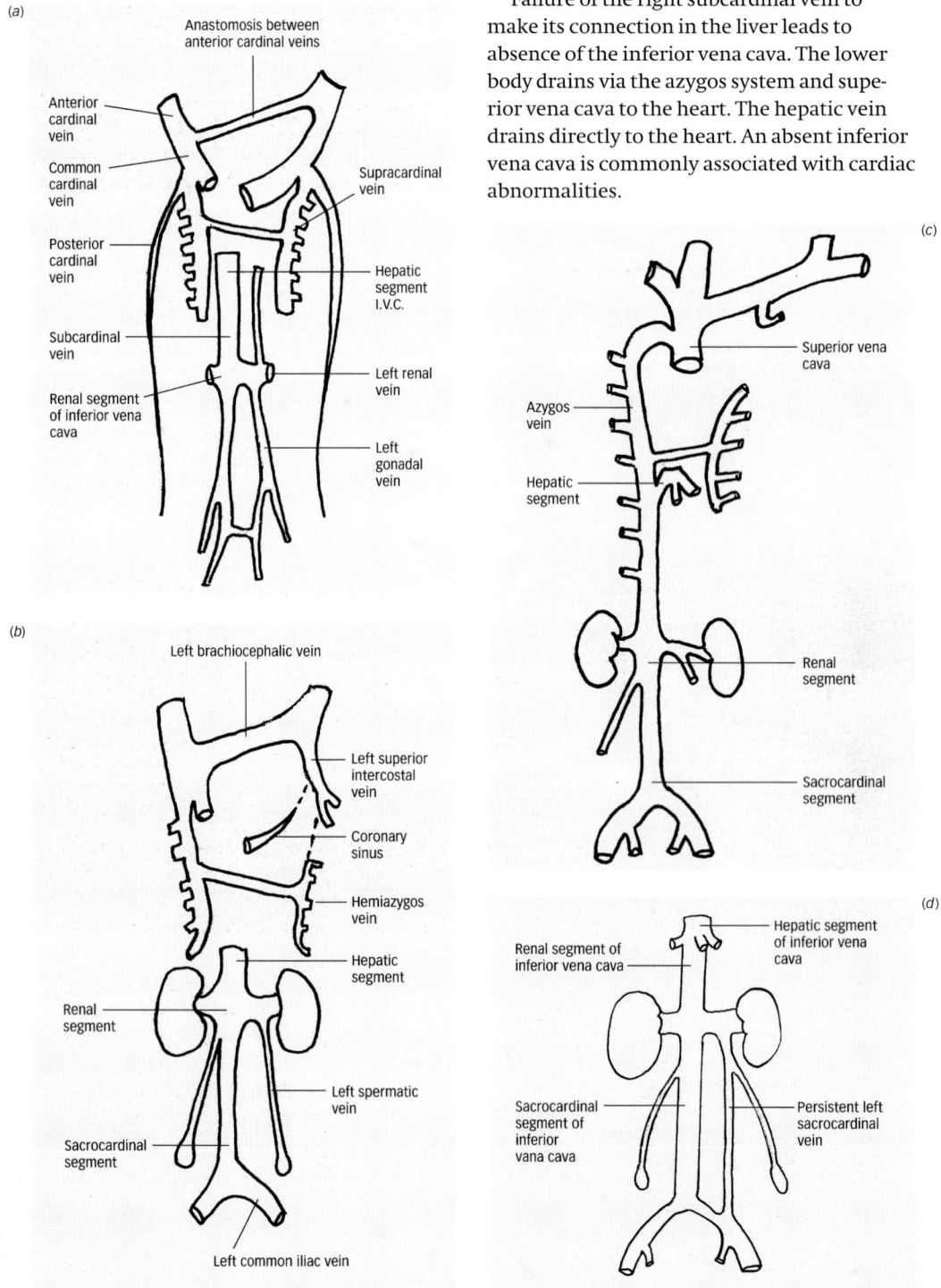

Fig. 12.
The embryology of the venous system and congenital anomalies of the inferior vena cava: (*a*) and (*b*), normal development, (*c*) absence of the inferior vena cava, (*d*) double inferior vena cava.

A persistent left-sided vena cava results from a persistent left sacrocardinal vein and has an incidence of between 0.2 and 0.5%. Cross-over to the right inferior vena cava occurs at the level of the left renal vein.

Imaging of the lymph nodes and lymphatics

The lymphatic system may be imaged using ultrasound, CT, MRI, lymphography and lymphoscintigraphy. Ultrasound is a useful

Fig. 13.
Axial CT (*a*)–(*d*), inferior to superior, double inferior vena cava. (Courtesy of Dr J. Cross and Professor A.K. Dixon.)

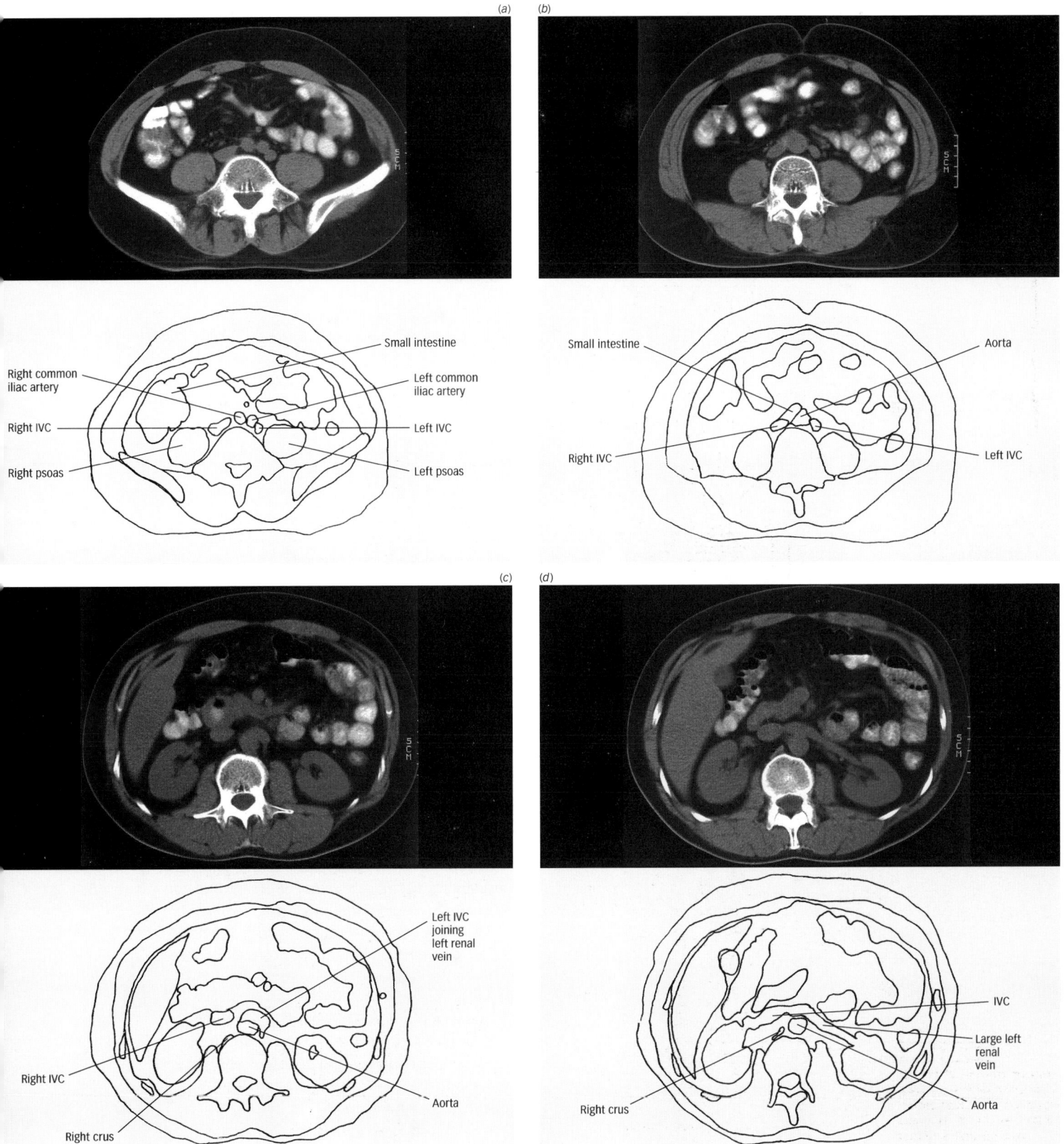

(a)

(b)

Labels for (a): Small intestine; Right common iliac artery; Left common iliac artery; Right IVC; Left IVC; Right psoas; Left psoas

Labels for (b): Small intestine; Aorta; Right IVC; Left IVC

(c)

(d)

Labels for (c): Left IVC joining left renal vein; Right IVC; Aorta; Right crus

Labels for (d): IVC; Large left renal vein; Right crus; Aorta method to detect large superficial nodes but may not always visualize normal-sized nodes.

The lymphatic system may be imaged directly using contrast lymphography.

With aseptic technique, local anaesthetic is infiltrated into the web space between the first and second toes. Patent blue dye is then injected subcutaneously. Oily contrast medium (lipiodol) is injected into the chosen lymphatic, rendered visible by the prior injection of patent blue dye. Images of the lymphatics are taken while injecting contrast. If contrast is inadvertently injected into a vein, globules of contrast are seen (the caviar sign of Kinmouth, Fig. 14). Twenty-four hours following the lymphangiogram phase, the lymphadenogram phase is used to image the lymph nodes. Oily lipiodol is retained within lymph nodes for approximately 12 months and thus contrast lymphography is still used in specialized oncology units to monitor nodal

size following therapy. It is still the only means of imaging the internal architecture of lymph nodes, although new MRI contrast media are being developed which may render contrast lymphadenography obsolete.

Lymphoscintigraphy using ^{99m}Tc-nanocolloidal albumin is a useful method for assessing the lymphatic system if high resolution anatomical detail is not required, for example, in the initial assessment of lymphodoema. Dynamic scanning delineates the lymphatic vessels, and delayed images may be used to assess the nodes (Fig. 15).

Lymphatic drainage of the upper limb

There are superficial and deep lymphatic vessels.

The superficial vessels follow the large superficial veins, the cephalic and basilic. The lymphatic vessels from the hand and forearm pass dorsally and then pass anteriorly to join the vessels on the front of the arm. The superficial lymphatics drain into the lateral nodes of the axilla along the axillary vein, although some from the medial aspect of the hand go to the supratrochlear nodes and some run with the cephalic vein to drain into the infra clavicular nodes (between deltoid and pectoralis major).

The deep lymphatics follow the main blood vessels and go to the lateral axillary nodes; those from the scapula travel to the posterior axillary nodes.

The axillary nodes converge to the apical group and from there into the right lymphatic duct and the thoracic duct. Both ducts drain into the subclavian veins at the jugulosubclavian junctions (see Chapter 16 'Upper Limb').

The lymphatic drainage of the lower limb

CT and MRI have almost completely superseded lymphography in the assessment of lymph node enlargement. The majority of lymph nodes assessed by CT should measure less than 10 mm. The short axis of retrocrural nodes should measure no more than 6 mm, but paraaortic and subcarinal nodes may be up to 12 mm in the normal individual.

The tissues of the lower limb are drained by either superficial subcutaneous lymphatic vessels or deep vessels related to the main blood vessels.

The superficial vessels either accompany the long saphenous vein and drain into the superficial inguinal lymph nodes or follow the short saphenous vein and drain into the popliteal lymph nodes. At lymphography, between 5 and 15 lymphatics can be seen to radiate into the deep inguinal nodes. A num-

Fig. 14.
Lower limb lymphangiogram, demonstrating the 'caviar' sign of Kinmouth (arrow).

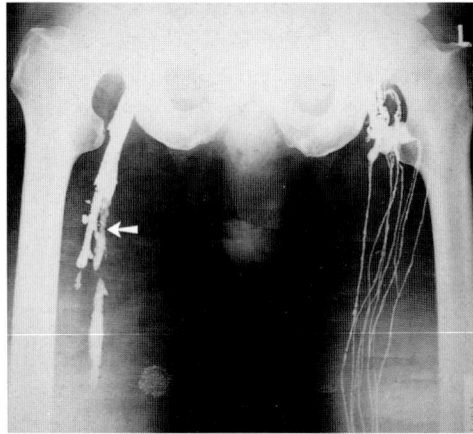

Fig. 15.
Lymphoscintigram

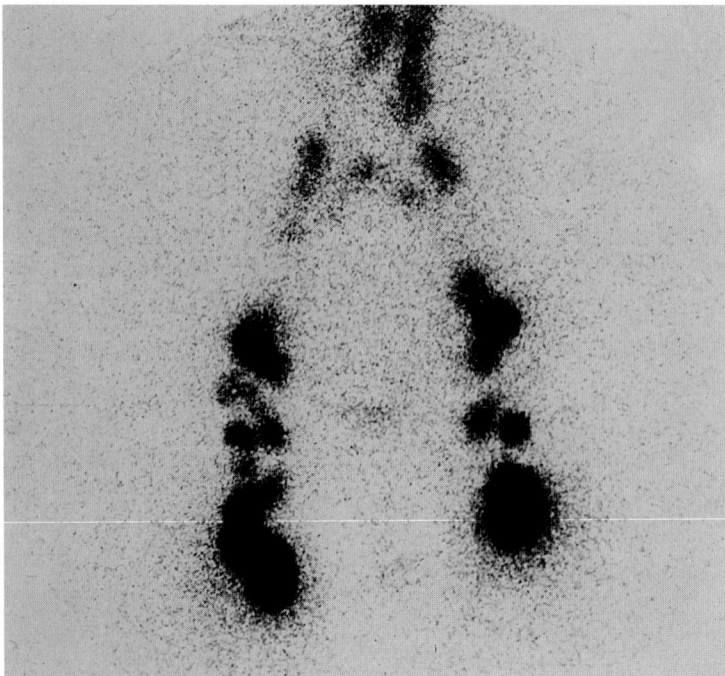

ber less than 5 is suggestive of lymphatic hypoplasia. Fibrofatty filling defects may be seen in the superficial inguinal nodes at lymphadenography due to repeated trauma to the feet and are not considered abnormal. The upper superficial inguinal lymph nodes drain lymph from the lower abdominal wall below the umbilicus, the gluteal region, the anal canal, external genitalia and perineum. They pass into the lower superficial inguinal group and both efferents pass to the deep inguinal group through the saphenous opening. The deep inguinal group comprises between one and three nodes and the efferent vessels pass to the external iliac nodes.

The vessels from the deep tissues of the lower limb end near the femoral vein in the deep inguinal nodes. The vessels from the deep tissues of the buttock drain into the internal iliac nodes in the pelvis. At the level of L3/4, non-opacification of nodes is commonly seen at lymphography (the lumbar gap). Of patients, 50% demonstrate cross drainage at this level, the lymphatics crossing from right to left.

Both internal and external iliac nodes drain into the common iliac nodes and then into the paraaortic nodes (Fig. 16). Efferent vessels from these nodes unite to form the right and left lumbar trunks which drain into the cisterna chyli.

Lymph vessels in the abdomen travel with the arteries and drain into four groups of nodes surrounding the abdominal aorta.

- Preaortic nodes are arranged around the coeliac, superior mesenteric and inferior mesenteric arteries. They drain the areas supplied by the vessels.

- Right and left paraaortic nodes which lie just anterior to the lateral aspect of the psoas. They drain lymph from the organs supplied by the paired branches of the aorta including the diaphragms and posterior abdominal wall. These nodes unite to form the right and left lumbar lymphatics.
- The retroaortic nodes lie behind the aorta and aid in drainage from the paraaortic nodes.

The cisterna chyli is a thin-walled sac, 0.5 cm wide and between 4 and 6 cm in length. It lies on the right crus of the diaphragm to the right of the aorta, in front of the first and second lumbar vertebral bodies. The cisterna chyli receives the right and left lumbar trunks, the intestinal trunk and the descending intercostal trunks.

The upward continuation of the cisterna chyli is the thoracic duct, which enters the thorax through the aortic opening in the diaphragm. It ascends in front of the vertebral column, posterior to the oesophagus and to the left of the azygos vein. At the level of the fifth thoracic vertebra, it passes to the left, posterior to the oesophagus and continues upwards to the seventh cervical vertebra where it arches laterally behind the carotid sheath and then forwards over the subclavian artery to drain into the left subclavian vein at the jugulosubclavian junction. The thoracic duct drains all the body below the diaphragm, the posterior part of the right chest wall and the left of the body above the diaphragm. The right lymph duct drains the remainder (see Chapter 6 'Chest').

Fig. 16.
Lymphangiogram, nodal phase.

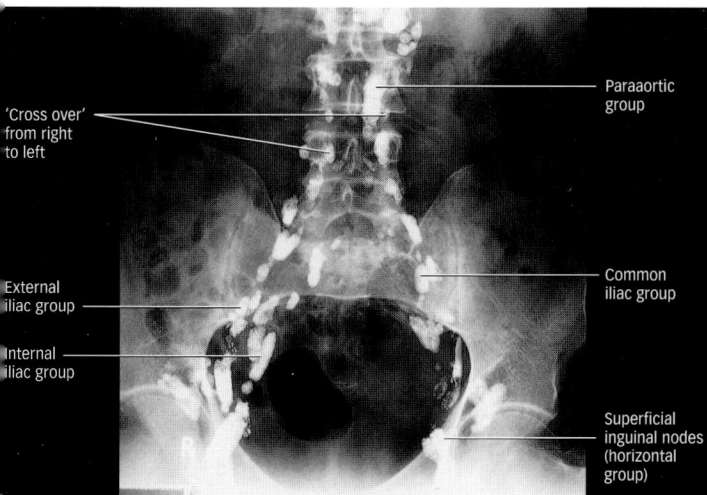

'Cross over' from right to left

External iliac group

Internal iliac group

Paraaortic group

Common iliac group

Superficial inguinal nodes (horizontal group)

19

Obstetric anatomy

A. D. G. WOOD
and K. C. DEWBURY

Imaging methods

Ultrasound provides virtually all the imaging of the fetus and the pregnant uterus. This modality is uniquely suited to the challenge presented by a baby moving in a random fashion, producing high resolution images in any plane. Routine ultrasound is regarded as completely safe for the developing fetus throughout pregnancy from the point of the first missed period. Energy is, however, imparted by the ultrasound beam and this is greater with Doppler examinations and so, as a general principle, it is important that examinations are clinically indicated and that examination time is optimal (Table 1).

Ultrasound is used in the first trimester to establish that the pregnancy is intrauterine and viable, to show the fetal number and to estimate gestational age. In the second and third trimesters, ultrasound is again used to estimate gestational age, and to detect structural fetal anomalies. Fetal lie (the relationship of the long axis of the fetus to the long axis of the uterus), and presentation (the presenting fetal part closest to the cervix), are also determined, and the position of the placenta recorded. The examination is also used to estimate fetal weight and amniotic volume. In the third trimester high risk pregnancies can be monitored serially to assess growth and well-being by use of the biophysical profile which assesses amniotic volume and monitors fetal movement and reactivity. Doppler waveforms in the umbilical artery may also be added to this assessment to help determine the optimum time for delivery.

Magnetic resonance imaging currently has a limited role in evaluation of the placenta and maternal pelvis. Real-time MR examination of the fetus will be possible in the future for selected cases, although the greater avail-

TABLE 1
Developmental timetable

Gestational age	Features visible
4 weeks	Gestational sac first visible by transvaginal (TV) scanning.
5 weeks	Yolk sac visible by TV scanning, gestational sac visible by transabdominal (TA) scanning.
5–6 weeks	Embryo discernible and cardiac activity visible on TV scan.
7 weeks	Embryo discernible and cardiac activity visible on TA scan.
6.5–10 weeks	(Subsequent scanning is by transabdominal route) Crown–rump length is useful measurement of gestational age.
8 weeks	Head, body and limb buds visualized.
12 weeks	Prominent lateral ventricles clearly visible. BPD becomes valid measurement of gestational age (to 24 weeks). Ossification of femur progressing.
14 weeks	Closure of 'physiological umbilical hernia'. Bladder and stomach visible.
18–20 weeks	Routine time for assessment. *CNS.* Cerebral cortex and structure of lateral ventricles visible. Structure and shape of cerebellum visible. Spine assessed. *Trunk.* Four-chamber view of heart and connection of major vessels. Stomach, kidneys, suprarenals, bladder, liver, gall bladder and portal venous connections routinely visible. Abdominal circumference, diaphragm, gender assessed. *Limbs.* Femur length as measurement of gestational age. Relationships of forearm, leg, hand and foot bones.
Third trimester	Assessment of placental position. Biophysical profile (amniotic volume, fetal breathing, fetal body movement, fetal tone, umbilical artery Doppler).

ability and improving resolution of ultrasound will ensure that this remains the main investigation.

First trimester appearances

The oöcyte is fertilized by sperm in the Fallopian tube to produce a zygote. Cleavage proceeds so that a morula (a ball of about 16 cells), is produced, before the conceptus reaches the uterine cavity.

Fluid passes into the morula from the endometrial cavity, separating the embryonic cells into an outer layer (trophoblast), which eventually forms the chorionic membrane and fetal part of the placenta, while the inner cell mass later forms the embryo, amnion, cord and secondary yolk sac.

This cystic structure, the blastocyst, then invades the endometrial wall. Implantation is completed by the end of the first week of development, 3 weeks after the onset of the last normal menstrual period (LNMP). Chorionic villi develop; human chorionic gonadotrophin (HCG) is produced and the pregnancy test becomes positive. The primary yolk sac and amniotic cavity develop. The primary yolk sac involutes as the secondary yolk sac develops. The embryonic disc now lies between the amniotic cavity and the secondary yolk sac. During the third week of development (5 LNMP weeks), the chorionic cavity develops and contains most of the fluid which can be recognized ultrasonographically and is known as the 'gestational sac'. The mean sac diameter (MSD) of the gestational sac is calculated by measuring the length, width and height of the sac and dividing by three.

The gestational sac can be detected by transvaginal scanning at about 2–3 mm MSD (approximately 4 weeks, 3 days post-LNMP) (Fig. 1). A sac with MSD of 5 mm (35 days; 5 menstrual weeks), can be detected transabdominally. When the gestational sac reaches an MSD of 15 mm (40–45 days post-LNMP) a 'double bubble' appearance of the yolk sac and amniotic sac is seen, with a line of echoes in between representing the embryo. By the time the embryo reaches a crown–rump length of 5 mm (approximately 6.5 weeks post-LNMP, gestation sac 15–18 mm) the cardiac pulsation within the embryo can be seen consistently. The cardiac pulsation is therefore visible before any more detailed morphology of the embryo can be seen.

Fig. 1.
Tiny gestational sac demonstrated at the fundus of the uterus by transvaginal ultrasound. Sac diameter (4 mm) corresponds to gestational age of approximately 4 weeks (second week of development). No features are discernible within the sac at this stage.

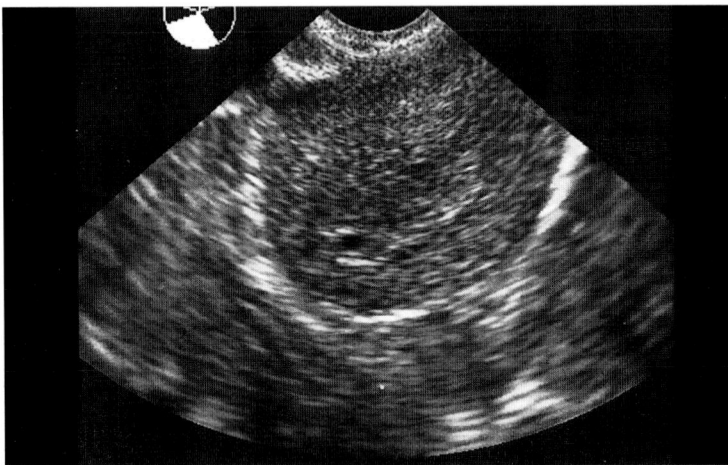

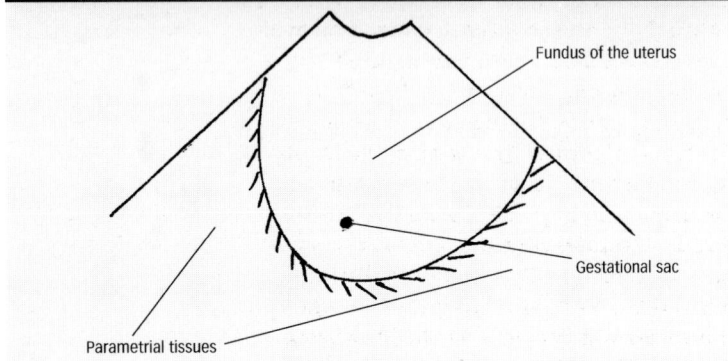

Fig. 2. top
Amniotic and chorionic cavities (approximately 8 weeks).

Fig. 3. below
Amniotic cavity and placenta (approximately 12 weeks).

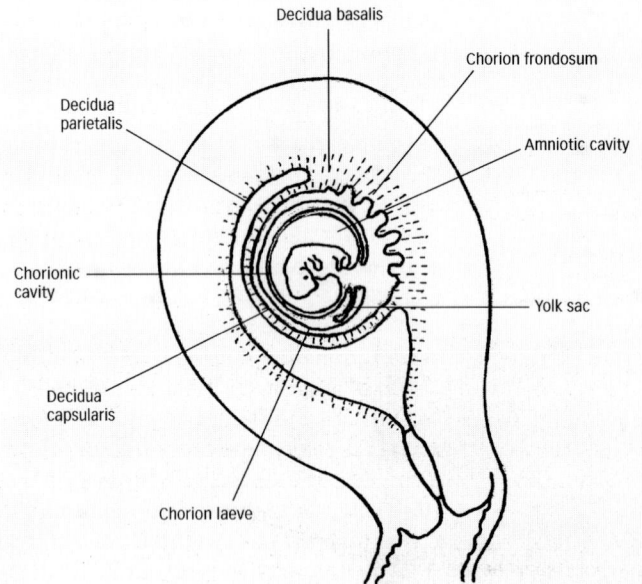

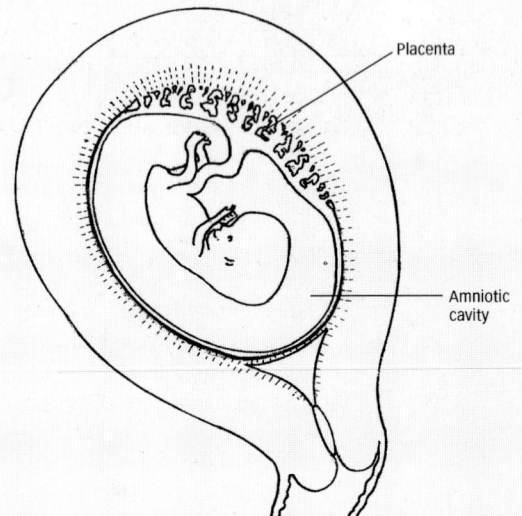

The decidua which healed over the top of the implanting blastocyst is known as the decidua capsularis (Fig. 2). As the blastocyst grows an area of chorion devoid of villi, the chorion laeve, becomes the chorionic membrane. The gestational sac enlarges and the decidua capsularis comes into contact with decidua lining the uterine cavity (decidua parietalis). These layers fuse and the endometrial cavity is obliterated. The decidua capsularis degenerates and the chorion fuses with the decidua parietalis in turn. Meanwhile, the chorion frondosum forms progressively larger villi and eventually forms the early placenta (Fig. 3).

The chorion and placenta therefore have identical origins and are inseparably linked. The edge of the placenta can be found by following the chorion. The amnion surrounds the fetus and is continuous with the umbilical cord where it joins the placenta.

Crown–rump length (CRL) is an accurate determinate of gestational age between 6.5 and 10 menstrual weeks, although sources of inaccuracy exist, particularly since no anatomical marker exists for the crown or rump, and the longest measurement is therefore taken as the most valid. When the CRL is 10 mm, the head can be discriminated from the torso. Following this, limb buds, umbilical cord, primary ossification centres for maxilla mandible and clavicle can be seen (Fig. 4). At

the beginning of the second trimester, biological variation in CRL becomes more marked and it becomes a less accurate determinant of gestational age. From 19 weeks of development (eleventh menstrual week) the terminology fetus rather than embryo is used (Fig. 5).

Second trimester appearances

Skull

The skull vault is composed of the frontal, parietal, temporal, sphenoid wing and supra-orbital bones. The principal sutures can be named from their adjacent bones (frontoparietal, parietooccipital and parietotemporal), although the nomenclature coronal, lambdoid and squamosal is more commonly used. The parietal bones are separated by the sagittal suture. Anteriorly, the metopic suture lies in the midline between the two components of the frontal bone. The small mendosal suture lies in the occipital bone. The metopic and mendosal sutures are normally closed at birth, but may persist, being demonstrated as normal variants on skull radiogrpahy. The other sutures are widely open at birth, 3 mm being the upper limit of normal. The anterior

Fig. 5.
Longitudinal view of the fetus at 12 weeks gestation, clearly showing the head and the structure of the brain within it.

Fig. 4.
Transabdominal ultrasound. The crown–rump length measures 15 mm equivalent to eight weeks gestation. The head can be distinguished from the body and tiny limb buds are beginning to be visualised.

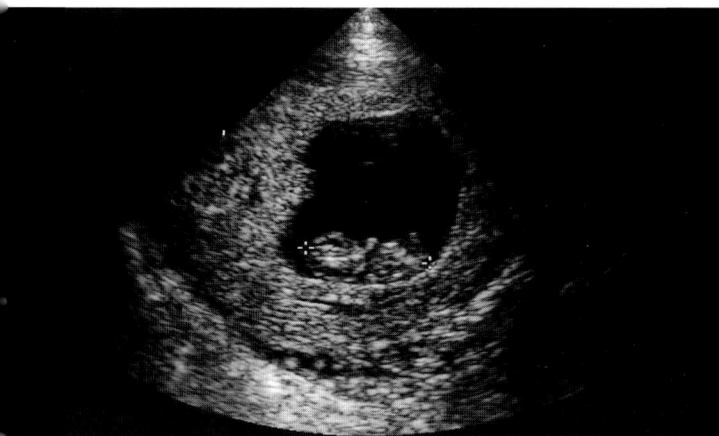

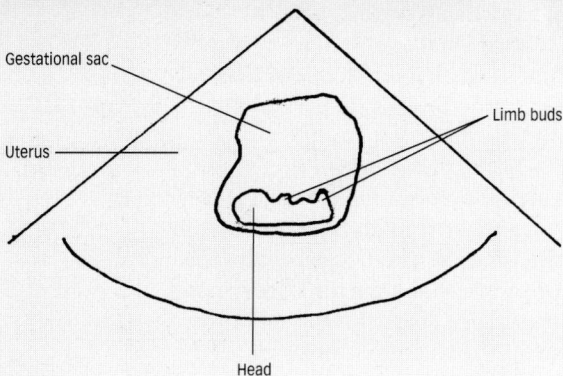

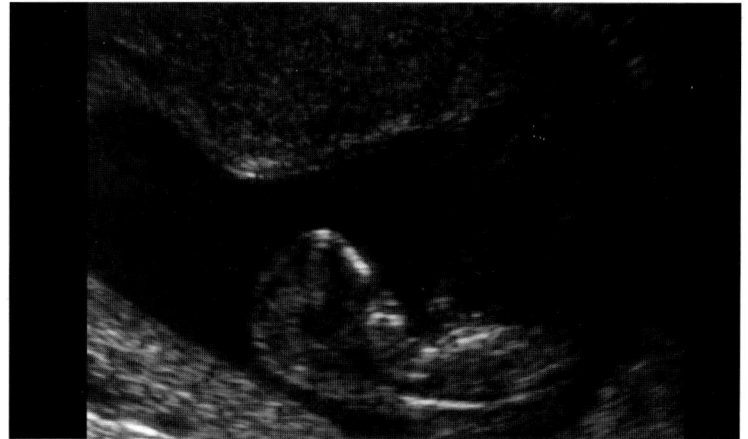

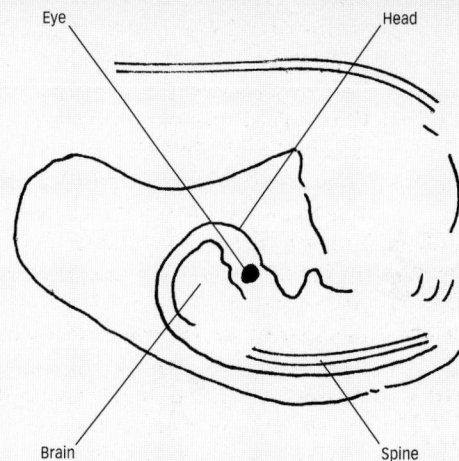

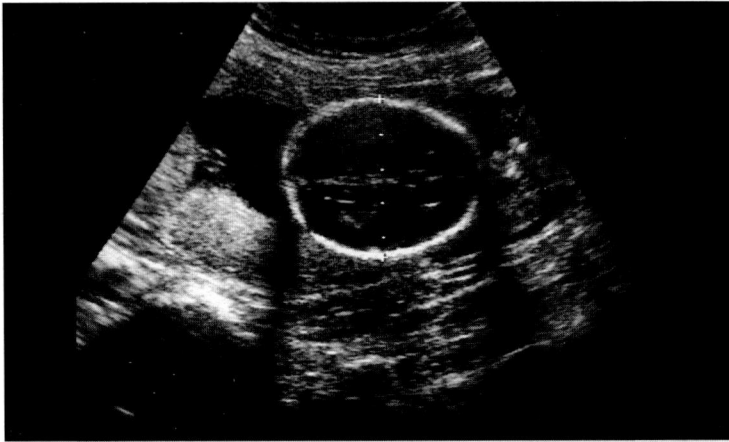

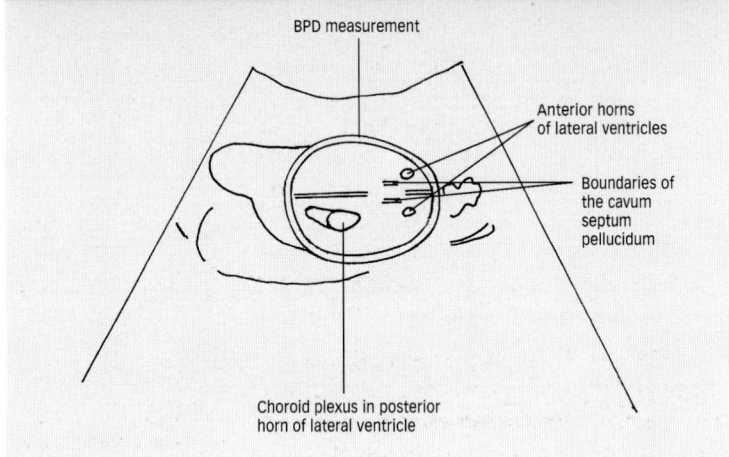

Fig. 6.
Axial section of the brain at 19 weeks gestation, demonstrating the cavum septum pellucidum. The lateral ventricles are seen. This section is the ideal one for measurement of the biparietal diameter.

Central nervous system

The neural plate, a thickened area of embryonic ectoderm, develops approximately 18 to 20 days post-conception. The neural tube forms from the neural plate (motor cells), and neural crest (sensory and autonomic cells), by a process of invagination. Fusion occurs at the seven somite stage (somites are paired cubes of mesoderm), opposite the fourth to sixth somites. The brain forms cranial to this point of fusion and the spinal cord caudally. Fusion then extends in both directions, the anterior neuropore closing before the posterior neuropore.

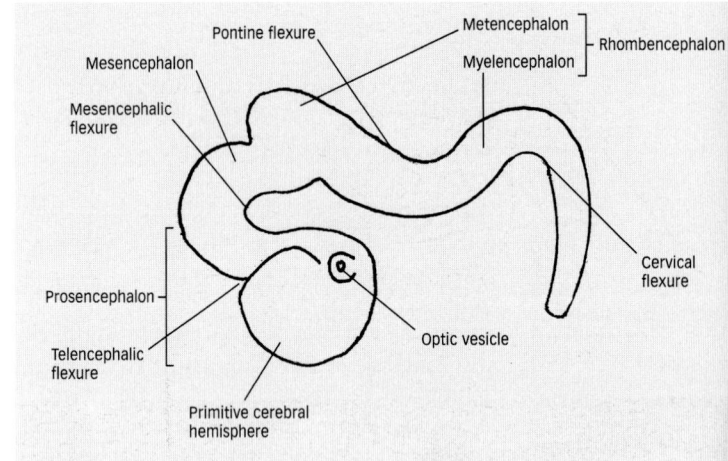

Fig. 7.
Diagram of the developing brain (approximately 6 weeks).

fontanelle is situated at the junction of the sagittal and coronal sutures, and closes at between 18 and 24 months of age. The posterior fontanelle lies at the junction of the sagittal and lambdoid sutures and closes by 3 months of age. The anterolateral fontanelle lies at the junction of the coronal, squamosal and frontosphenoidal sutures and also closes by 3 months of age.

Much of the sphenoid bone is preformed in cartilage, but the other bones of the skull are formed in membrane from multiple ossification centres. Measurements of the biparietal diameter (BPD) as an assessment of fetal age can be made before ossification has reached the top of the head. BPD estimation is made in the axial plane at the widest portion of the skull, with the thalamus positioned in the midline. The distance from the outer edge of the part of the skull nearer to the transducer to the inner edge of the vault further from the probe is measured (Fig. 6). The skull should have an ovoid shape, the BPD being 80–90% of the occipitofrontal diameter (OFD) and narrower in the frontal than in the occipital region. The BPD/OFD ratio may be lower in a breech presentation.

The cranial end of the neural tube differentiates into three primary brain vesicles, the prosencephalon (forebrain) mesencephalon (midbrain) and rhombencephalon. The forebrain buds laterally to each side to form the lateral ventricles and overlying cerebral hemispheres, while the original cavity forms the third ventricle and the diencephalon (thalamus). The hind brain thickens in its upper part to give rise to the pons and cerebellum, while the lower part forms the medulla oblongata.

The familiar brain shape is a result of these dilatations and also the ventral (cervical and mesencephalic) flexures and dorsal (pontine and telencephalic) flexures. The telencephalic flexure in particular is important for its role in throwing the cerebral hemispheres over the diencephalon, which is buried as the cerebral hemispheres grow to meet the cerebellum posteriorly (Fig. 7).

The fetal head can be distinguished when the fetus attains a crown–rump length of about 10 mm. In the second trimester, substantial changes take place in the telencephalon, although from this point the rest of the brain shows little change in appearance apart from enlargement. The lateral ventricles are a prominent feature in the early second

Choroid plexus

Lateral ventricle   Skull vault   Amniotic cavity

Vermis of
cerebellum

Cisterna
magna

Cerebellar hemispheres

Cerebral cortex   Choroid plexus   Lateral ventricle

thickened. The distance from the midline to the lateral wall of the anterior horn is usually under 9 mm in a second trimester brain. Measurements are made from the midline, since the medial wall of the lateral ventricle is difficult to see, and are made using the hemisphere furthest from the probe since the near hemisphere tends to be obscured by reverberation artefact.

The surface of the brain is smooth until about 20 weeks, with few sulci or gyri (Fig. 9). Gyri and sulci extend over the brain surface as the brain grows and are fully developed at term. The lateral sulcus (Sylvian fissure) develops between the insula medially and the temporal operculum. The temporal operculum may be seen as a highly reflective line on scanning, and should not be confused with the lateral wall of the ventricle.

The medial walls of the lateral ventricles are formed by the septum pellucidum. This double membrane contains a cavity (cavum septum pellucidum), which is visible ultrasonographically throughout gestation and remains visible on neuroimaging in a small proportion of adults. The septum pellucidum is seen as two highly reflective lines close to the midline, just posterior to the echoes from the lateral walls of the anterior horns, about one-third of the distance from frontal to occipital calvarium. The third ventricle lies posteroinferiorly between the thalami and is rarely seen in the normal fetus.

Fig. 8. top left
Axial view of the fetal head at 17–18 weeks of gestation. Choroid plexus, which is easily discerned because of its high reflectivity, is almost filling the lateral ventricles.

Fig. 9. below left
Axial section of brain at 19 weeks gestation. Detail of the brain surface distant from the transducer is clearly shown: the surface of the brain is smooth with no visible sulci or gyri at this stage.

Fig. 10. top right
Posteriorly angled section of the brain at 28 weeks gestation to show the cerebellum and cisterna magna. The cerebellum has a slightly greater reflectivity than the cerebral cortex.

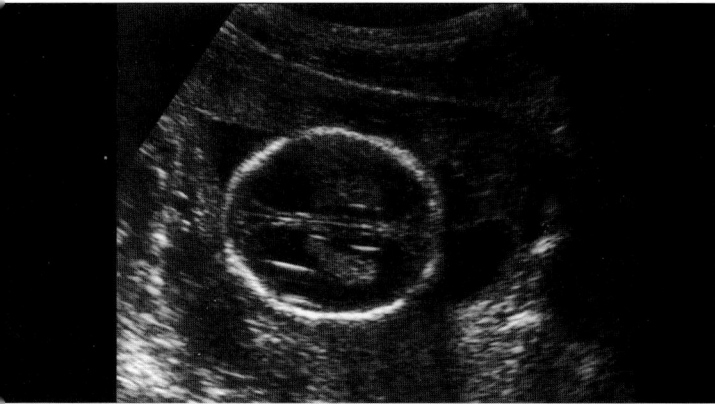

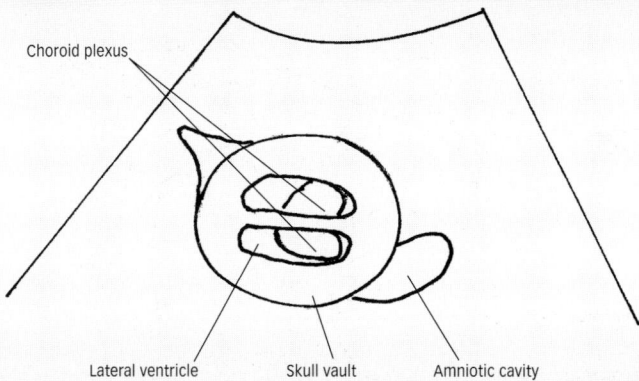

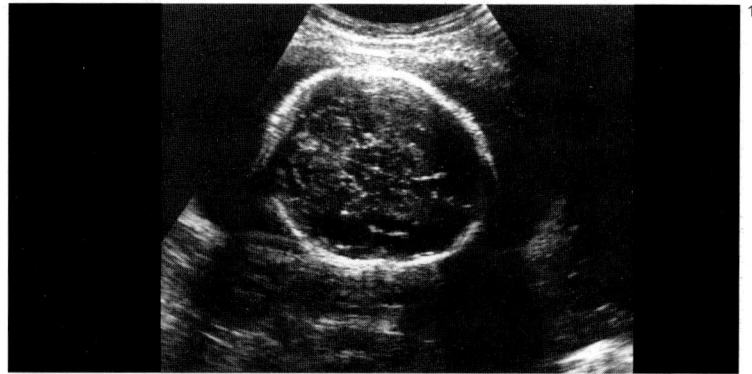

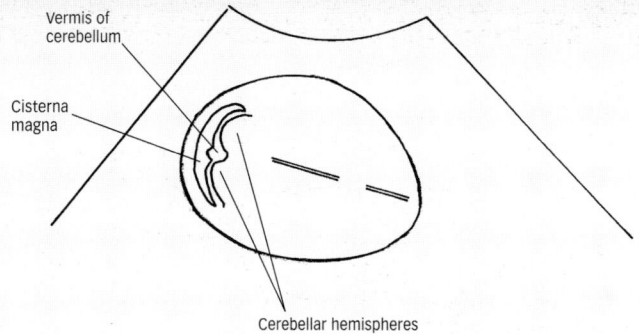

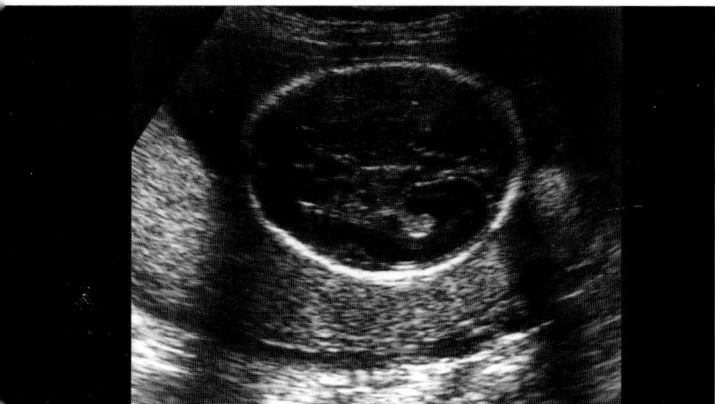

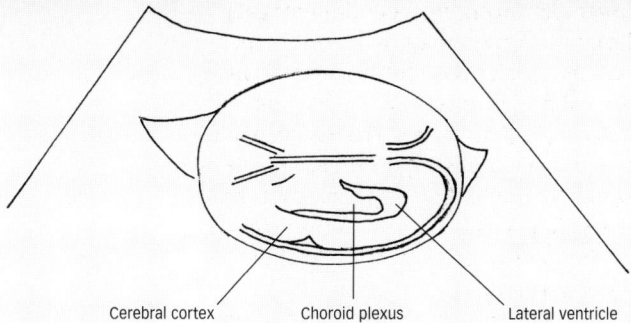

trimester, and these are filled by choroid plexus, apart from their anterior horns (Fig. 8). At 16 weeks the lateral ventricles consist of an anterior horn, body and small inferior horn. By 18 weeks, the mantle of cortical tissue has

Liver
Ossification centres for laminae
Stomach
Rib
Ossification centre for vertebral body

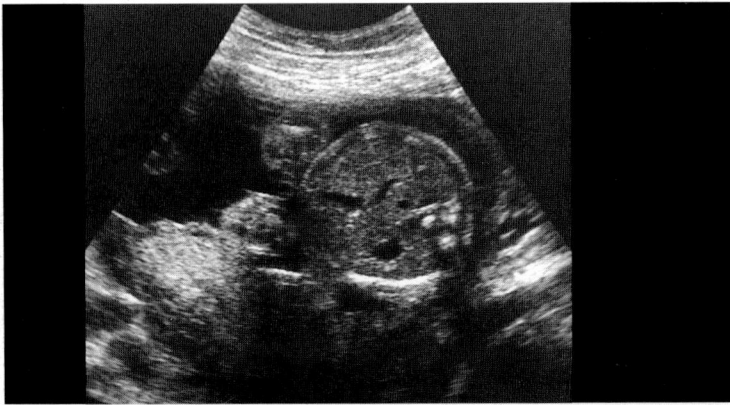

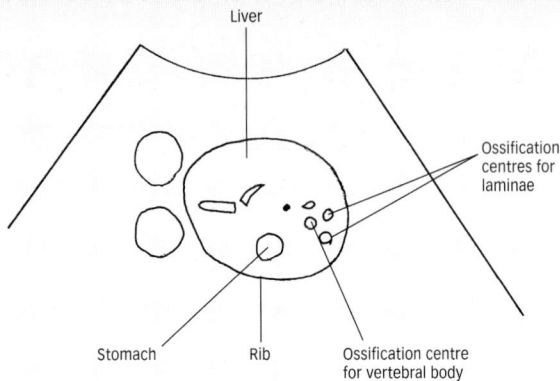

Fig. 11.
Transverse section through the upper abdomen at 19 weeks gestation. The three ossification centres of the upper lumbar vertebrae are identified with the base of the triangle lying posteriorly.

Ossification centres for laminae
Vertebral body ossification centres

Iliac wings
Ribs
Ossification centres for laminae
Vertebral body ossification centres

At 18 weeks, the cerebellar hemispheres are seen as round structures of low reflectivity with a highly reflective ring around them, separated by the highly reflective vermis. The cerebellar hemispheres become more triangular in cross-section as pregnancy progresses. The normal cisterna magna is seen as an anechoic space between the cerebellum and the occipital bone (Fig. 10).

Spine

The spinal cord is formed as a result of growth of the caudal part of the neural plate. By 3 months the bone and cartilage of the vertebral column is growing faster than the cord, so that at birth the cord is opposite L3.

The vertebrae are formed from three ossification centres, one in the vertebral body and one in each lamina (Fig. 11). The spinous process ossifies after birth. In the cervical, thoracic and upper lumbar spine the three centres are orientated as a triangle with its base posterior. In the lower lumbar spine the laminar echoes are more widely spaced, a V-shape is normal, but divergence of the laminar echoes is abnormal. The spinal neural tissue is generally of low reflectivity, but occasionally echoes may be seen from the conus medullaris, the craniocervical junction, the leptomeninges and even the central canal (Figs. 12 and 13).

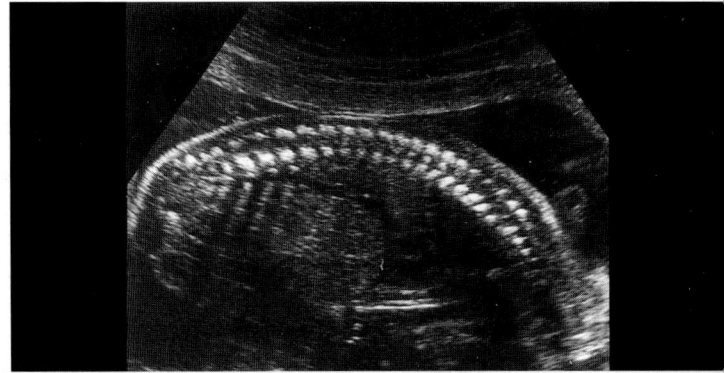

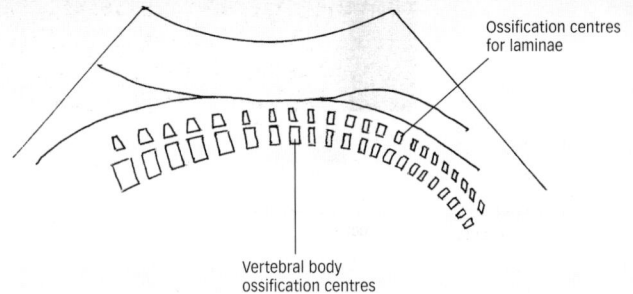

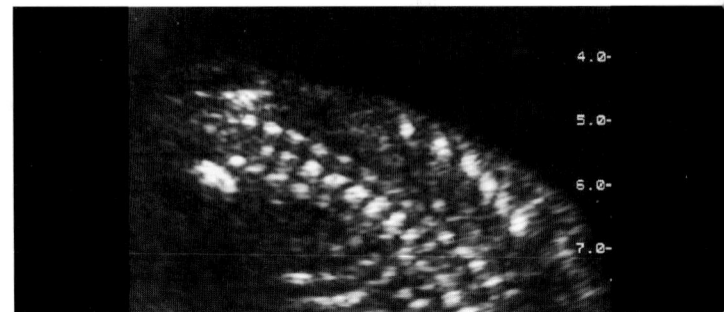

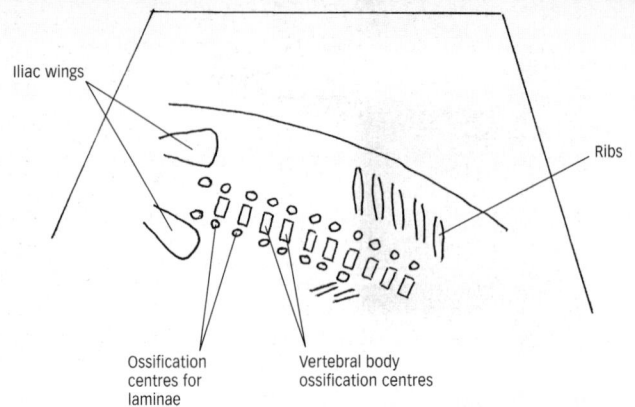

Face

The face is formed as a result of fusion of the frontonasal prominence, which forms the forehead, dorsum and apex of nose and the most medial part of the upper lip, the maxillary prominences, which form the cheeks, and the mandibular prominence forming the mandible. Failure of fusion between the premaxillary part of the frontonasal prominence

Fig. 12. top
Sagittal section of the fetal spine at 19 weeks gestation.

Fig. 13. below
Coronal view of the fetal spine at 19 weeks gestation.

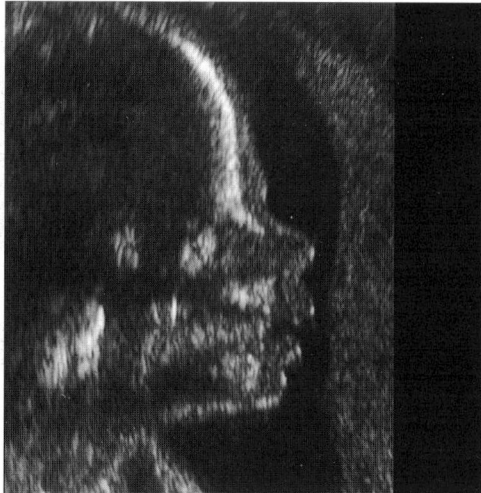

Fig. 14.
Sagittal view showing the profile of the fetal face at 32 weeks gestation. The forehead, nose, lips and chin can all be identified, the hard palate is also seen.

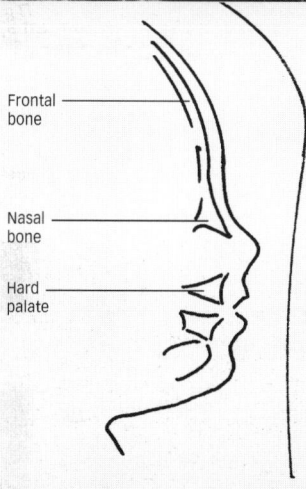

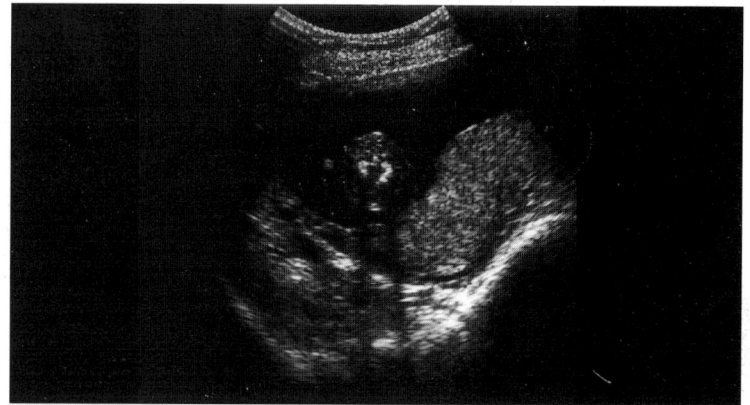

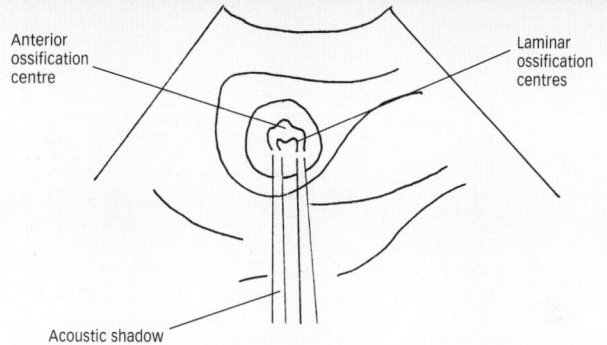

Frontal bone

Nasal bone

Hard palate

Fig. 15. below
Sagittal section of a fetus at 12 weeks of gestation to show detail of the nuchal fold. At 12 weeks this should measure less than 3 mm in diameter and at 14 weeks less than 6 mm in diameter.

12 WEEKS

Head

Nuchel lucency

Spine

Anterior ossification centre

Laminar ossification centres

Acoustic shadow

Fig. 16.
Transverse view of the fetal neck in the region of the larynx at 19–20 weeks gestation.

(the globular prominence), and one of the maxillary prominences will give rise to a unilateral cleft lip. The normal nose and lips are imaged regularly with ultrasound (Fig. 14).

Neck

The neck has a circular cross-section. The shape of the neck is examined, looking for the presence of masses such as cystic hygromas, or for nuchal oedema, which is a marker for trisomy 21 (Fig. 15). The cervical vertebrae are clearly visible. The larynx and thyroid are visible in later pregnancy (Fig. 16).

Trunk

The trunk is composed of the thorax and abdomen, separated by the diaphragm. The shoulder girdle and pelvis are also examined at the same time.

Chest

The clavicles are best seen in transverse (axial) section. The clavicle begins to ossify from two primary centres which fuse at about the forty-fifth day *in utero*. A secondary centre develops at the sternal end in late teens. The clavicles are easily seen at the routine 18-week scan, and mark the cranial boundary of the chest (Fig. 17). The lateral borders of the chest are demarcated by the ribs seen as reflective lines, although these are difficult to examine in detail (Figs. 18 and 19).

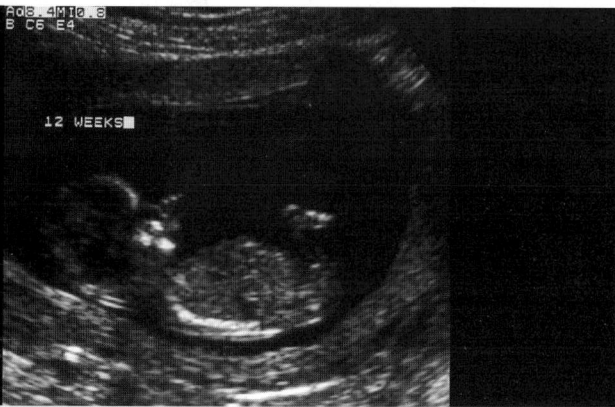

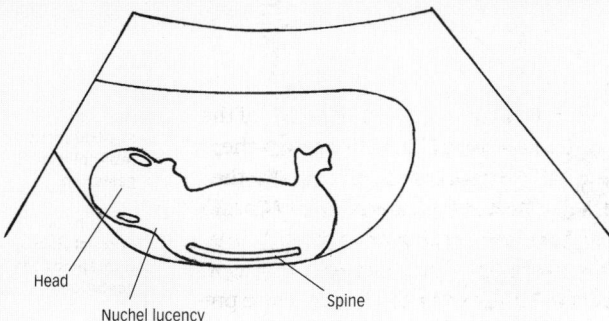

Spine

Clavicles

Scapula

Ribs

Femur

Part of head

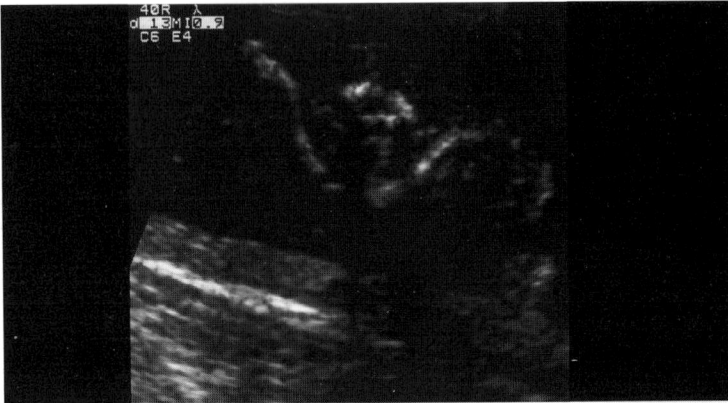

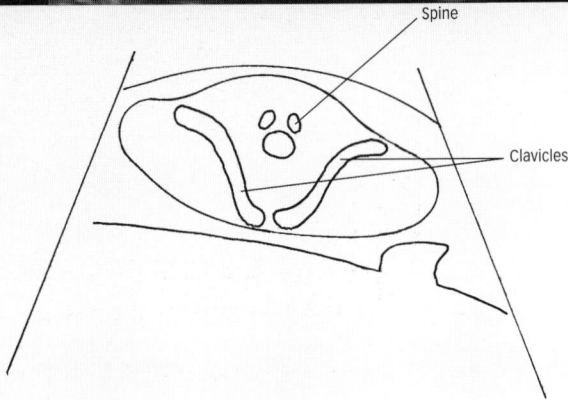

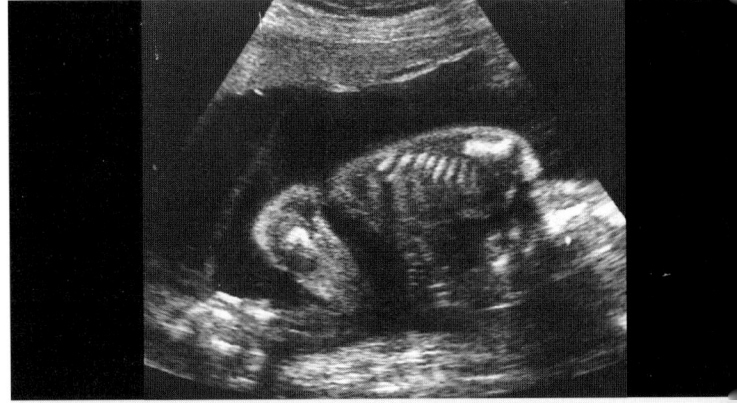

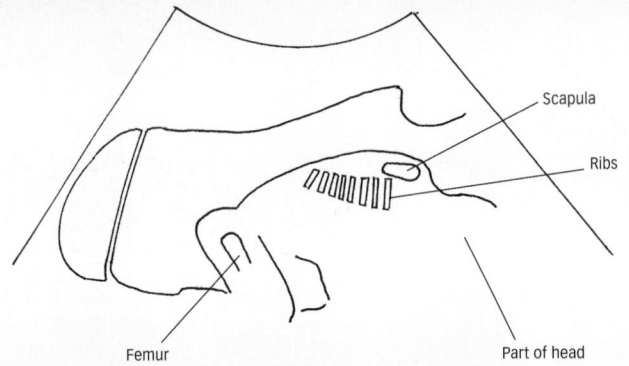

Fig. 17.
The root of the neck and the clavicles at 19 weeks gestation.

In the fetus the heart occupies about one-third of the chest. The majority of the heart lies to the left of the midline, with the left ventricle posterolaterally and the right ventricle anteromedially. The heart lies more horizontally than it does after birth. The four-chamber view is obtained in axial section just above the level of the diaphragm, and constitutes the principal screening view for cardiac abnormalities (Fig. 20). A more detailed search is indicated if hydrops fetalis or an arrythmia are present. The Eustachian valve of the inferior cava can be identified to show atrial situs, and the atrioventricular connections determined. The opening of the foramen ovale can be seen. The right ventricle may appear slightly larger than the left. The ascending and descending aorta and pulmonary artery are identified for a full assessment of the heart (Figs. 21 and 22).

Early in gestation the lungs are poorly reflective compared to liver, but become more reflective than liver as the pregnancy progresses and the alveoli develop (Fig. 23). The left lung is smaller than the right and lies behind the heart. The fetal diaphragm is seen as a smooth echo-poor band between the lungs and the liver and spleen (Fig. 24). Movements of the diaphragm and chest wall as part of breathing are evident from early in the second trimester.

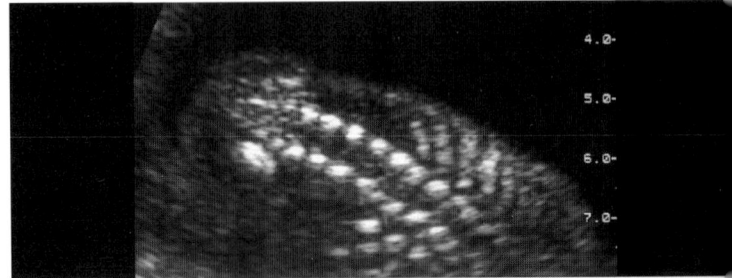

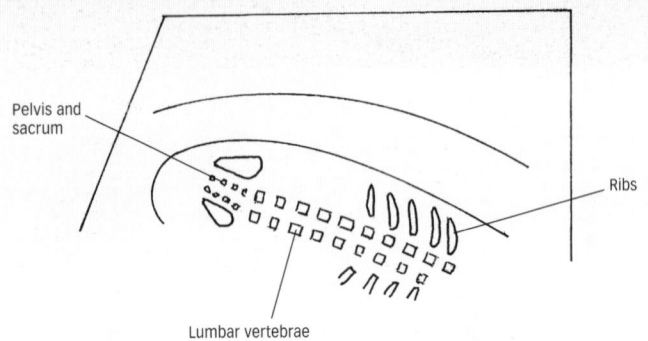

Pelvis and sacrum

Ribs

Lumbar vertebrae

Fig. 18. top
Longitudinal view of the fetal trunk to show the scapulae and portions of the ribs at 19–20 weeks gestation.

Fig. 19. above
Coronal view showing the spine and portions of the ribs on both sides at 19 weeks gestation.

22

Ventricles

Atrioventricular
valves

Atria

Thorax

Pulmonary trunk   Right ventricle

Ductus
arteriosus

Spine

Atria   Root of aorta   Descending aorta

23

Diaphragm

Left ventricle

Atria (inferior
vena cava and
pulmonary veins
are just visible)

Arch vessels

Ascending aorta   Descending aorta   Spine

Lungs

Head (out of picture)

Liver

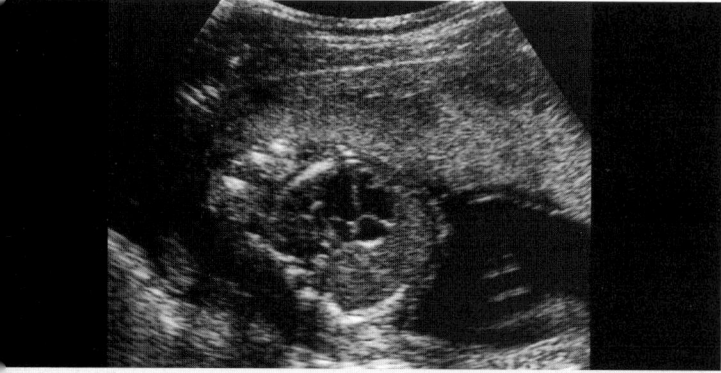

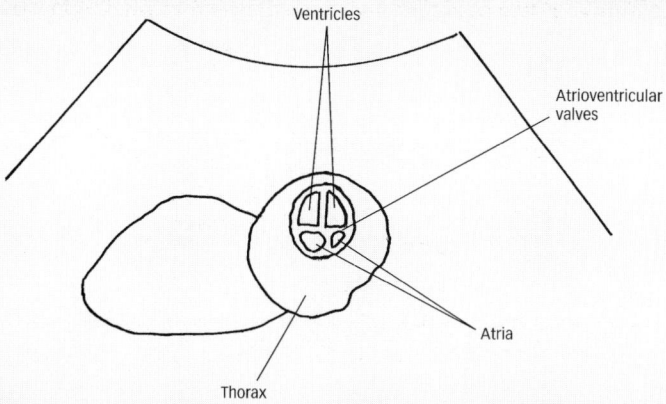

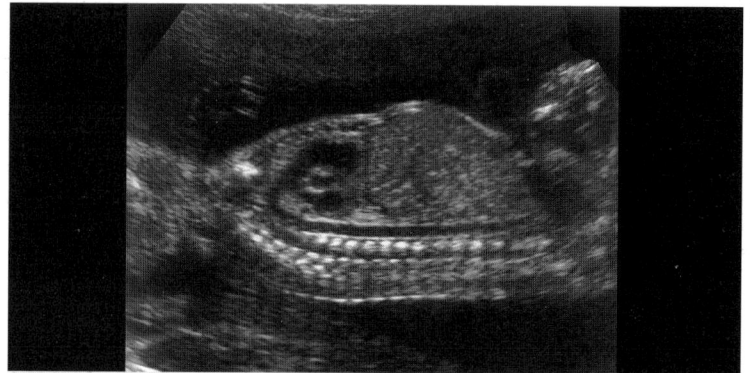

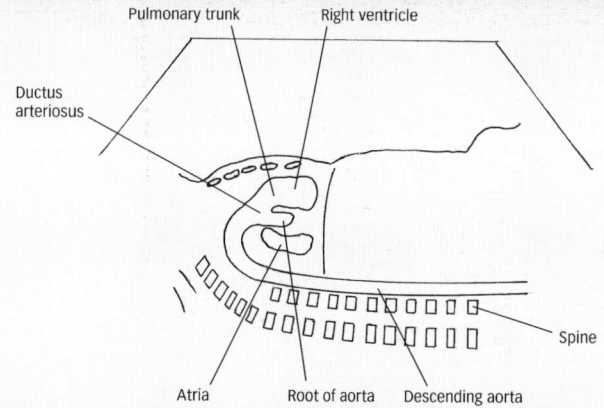

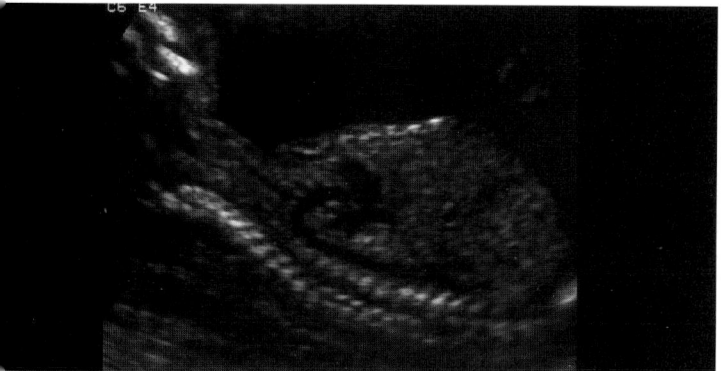

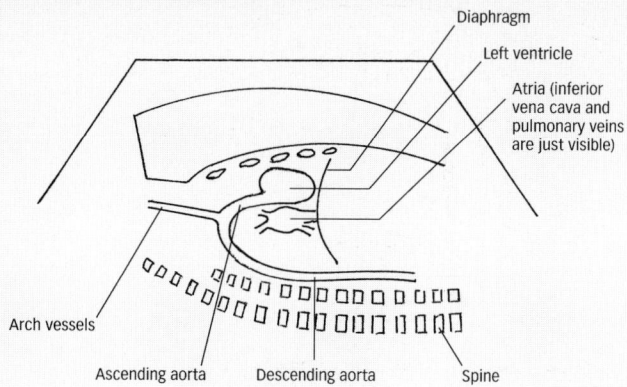

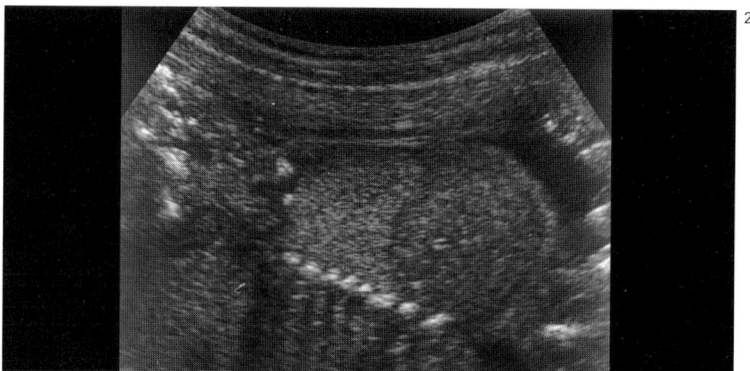

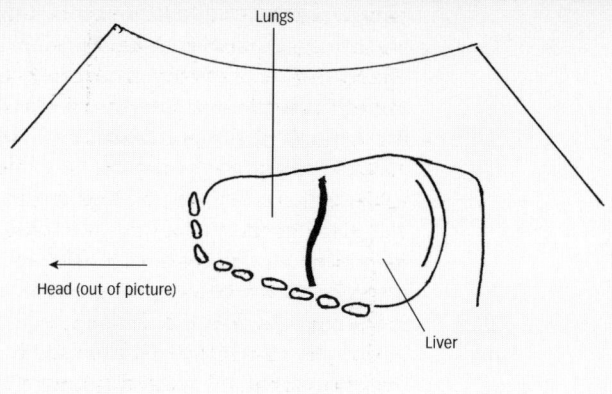

20. top left
r-chamber view of
heart at 19–20 weeks
tation. The two
tricles and atria are

of approximately equal size
and the centre of the heart
is formed by the offset crux
of the endoventricular
septum and the AV valves.

Fig. 21. above left
Sagittal section of the fetal
trunk at 19 weeks gestation
showing the aortic arch
arising from the (posterior)
left ventricle.

Fig. 22. top right
Similar section at same age
showing the pulmonary arch
arising from the (anterior)
right ventricle. The root of the
aorta is seen just tucked in
behind the pulmonary artery.

Fig. 23. above right
The lungs at about 22
weeks gestation. They
are now more reflective
than the liver.

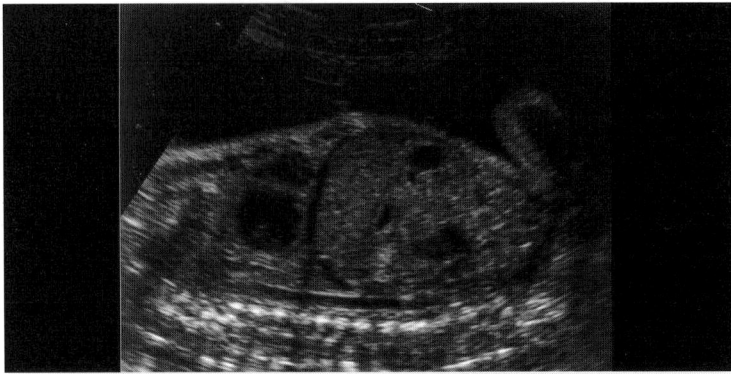

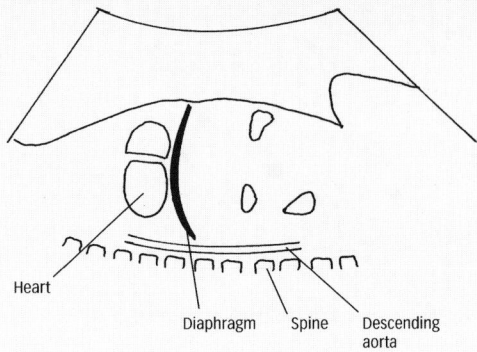

Fig. 24. above
22 weeks gestation. View of the fetal diaphragm which is shown as a poorly reflective band separating the liver from the chest.

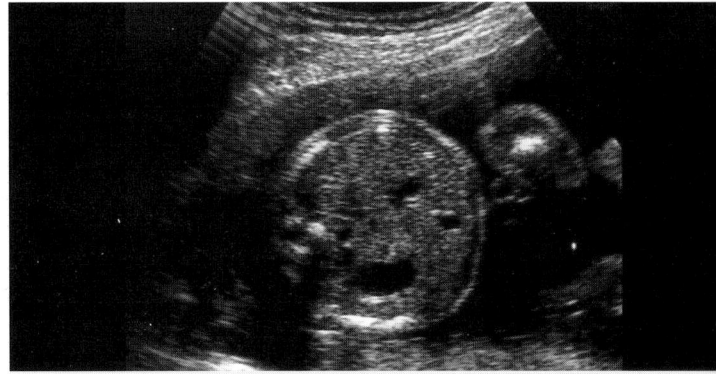

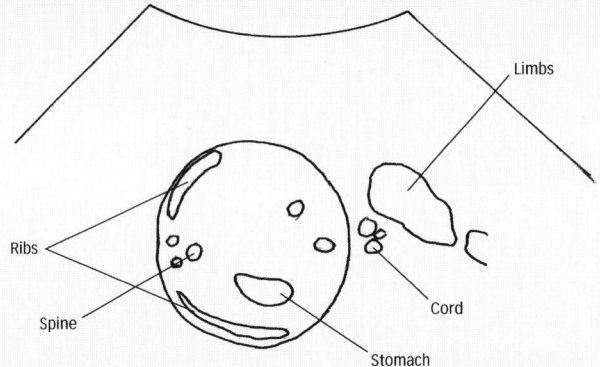

Fig. 25. top right
Transverse scan through the fetal abdomen at 20 weeks gestation, showing the fluid-filled stomach lying to the left of the midline.

Abdomen

The fluid-filled structures in the abdomen, the stomach and bladder, are easily identified. The stomach lies on the left, separated from the heart by the diaphragm and is seen as an anechoic crescent shape (Fig. 25). In many cases it can be seen from 14 weeks onwards and always on a routine 18–20 week scan. The stomach is remarkably constant in volume, despite the fact that peristalsis may be seen from the fourth to the fifth month.

Meconium, a combination of desquamated cells, bile pigment and mucoproteins, accumulates in the distal small intestine from the fifteenth to sixteenth week onwards. This makes the small intestine rather reflective in the second trimester, becoming increasingly less reflective as more amniotic fluid is swallowed later in pregnancy.

The colon is detected as an echo-poor well-defined tubular structure in the flanks and upper abdomen. It is visible on ultrasound from the second trimester and in virtually all cases after 28 weeks (Fig. 26). Low level echoes are often seen within it, believed to be from meconium. Colonic peristalsis cannot be detected *in utero*, although small bowel peristalsis is commonly seen in the third trimester.

Both small and large bowel are formed as part of the primitive intestinal loop. This herniates out of the abdominal cavity at about the sixth week of development. The intestine then twists about the central axis of the superior mesenteric artery, with a counterclockwise rotation of 270°, with the result that the caecum lies on the right of the abdomen. The small intestine increases markedly in length, coiling as it does so. The herniated loops begin to return to the abdominal cavity at about the

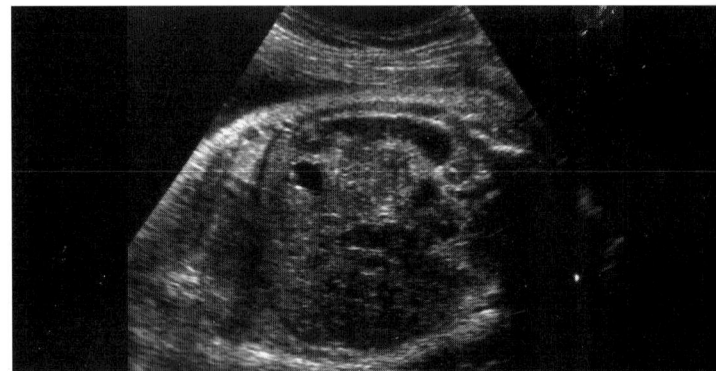

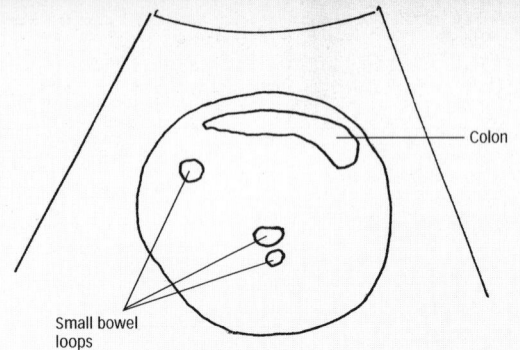

Fig. 26. above
View of the fetal abdomen at 32 weeks gestation, showing the peripheral location of a segment of colon

(b) Fig. 28. below left and top right
(a) and (b) Longitudinal and transverse sections of the normal umbilical cord at 30 weeks gestation in which two arteries and a vein can be identified.

Physiological umbilical hernia

Cord

Lung Liver/abdomen

Vein 2 arteries

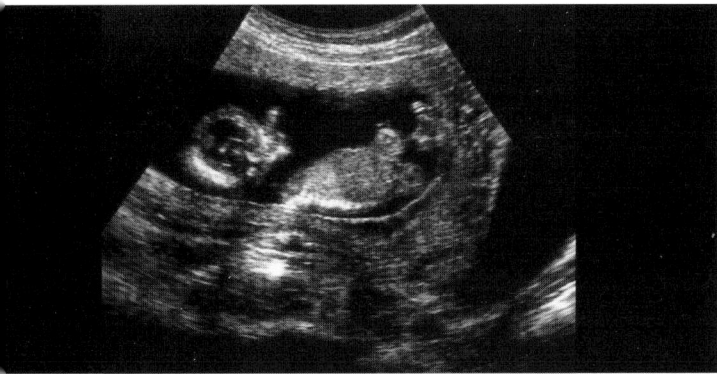

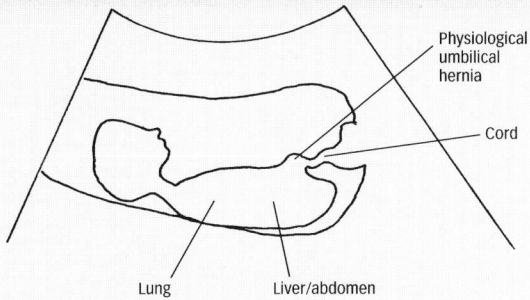

Fig. 27.
ngitudinal scan of a fetus
t 13 weeks gestation. The normal physiological umbilical hernia can be dentified projecting from the anterior part of the abdomen.

end of the third month, starting with the proximal part of the jejunum. The last part to re-enter is the caecum, which then descends to the right iliac fossa. Care must be taken to ensure that the abdominal wall is intact during ultrasound examination of the normal fetus in the middle trimester. The diagnosis of central abdominal wall defects can only be made after 14 weeks when the 'physiological umbilical hernia' has disappeared (Fig. 27).

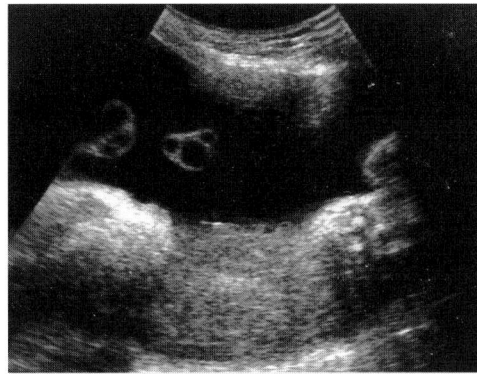

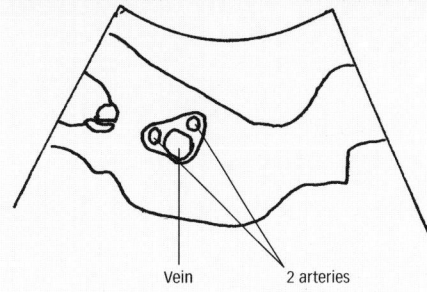

A single, thin-walled umbilical vein and two umbilical arteries can be identified in the umbilical cord (Fig. 28). The umbilical vein (UV) may be traced cephalad from the cord insertion to the left portal vein (Fig. 29). The UV has no branches, while the left portal vein does. Blood flows from the left portal vein via two channels, through the ductus venosus to systemic veins (inferior vena cava or left hepatic vein), or medially from the left portal

Fig. 29. below
Sagittal section of the fetus at 22 weeks gestation showing the umbilical vein passing through the anterior abdominal wall to enter the left portal vein and the ductus venosus.

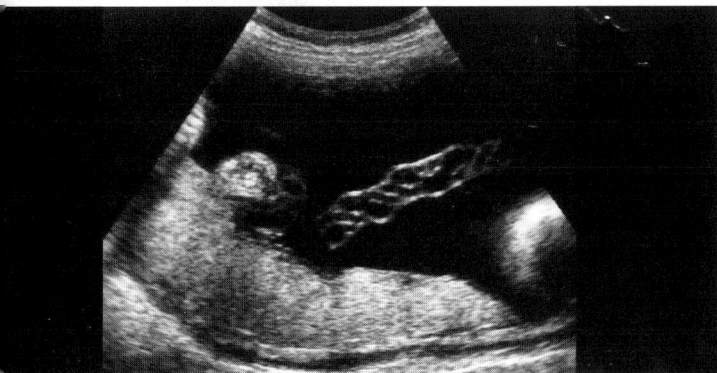

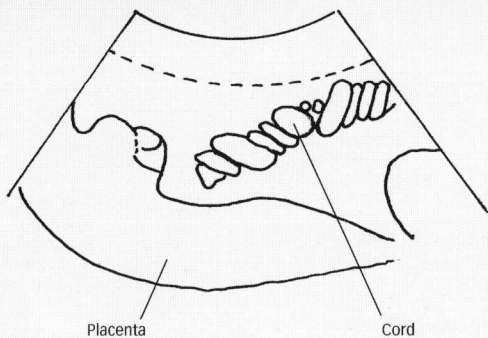

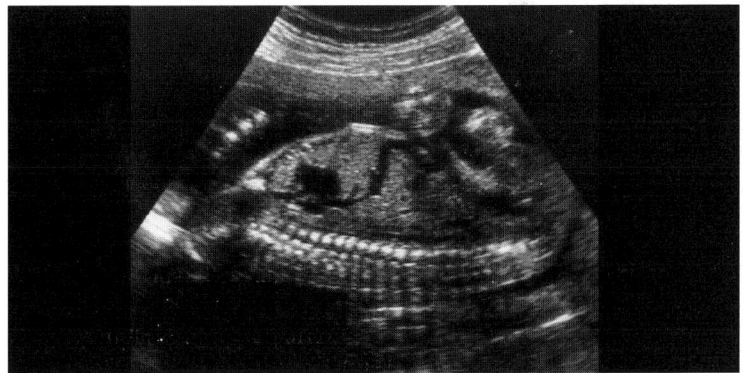

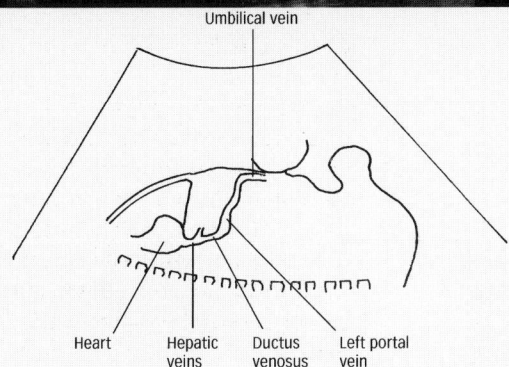

Placenta Cord

Umbilical vein

Heart Hepatic veins Ductus venosus Left portal vein

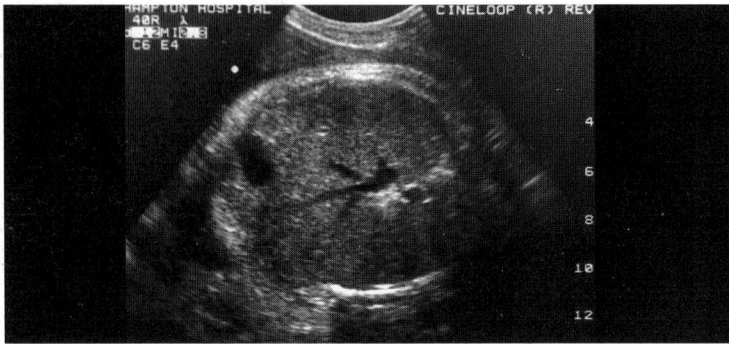

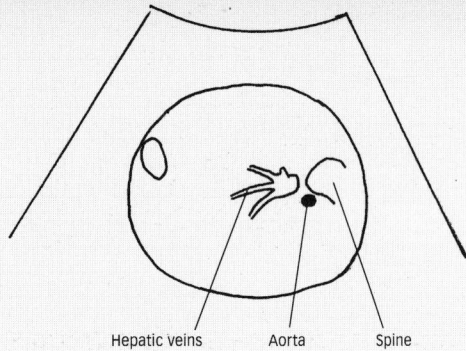

Fig. 30.
Transverse view of the fetal abdomen at 30 weeks gestation, showing normal hepatic veins running down to their confluence at the intrahepatic vena cava.

Fig. 31. top right
Oblique section of the fetal abdomen, showing detail of the fetal kidney at 30 weeks gestation. The poorly reflective medullary pyramids can be clearly distinguished from the renal cortex. The central collecting system echo is separated by no more than 3 mm, which is normal.

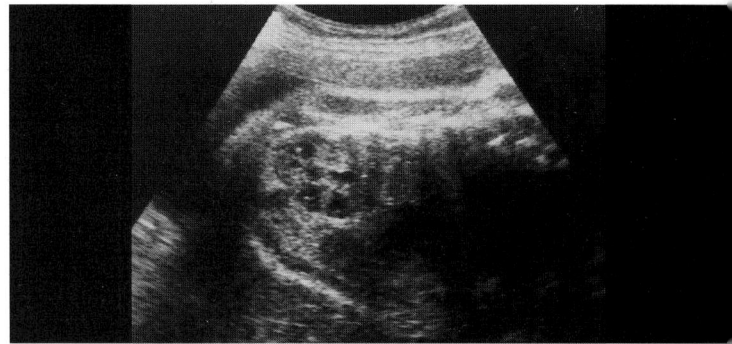

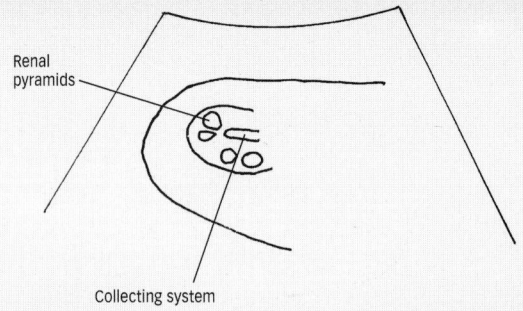

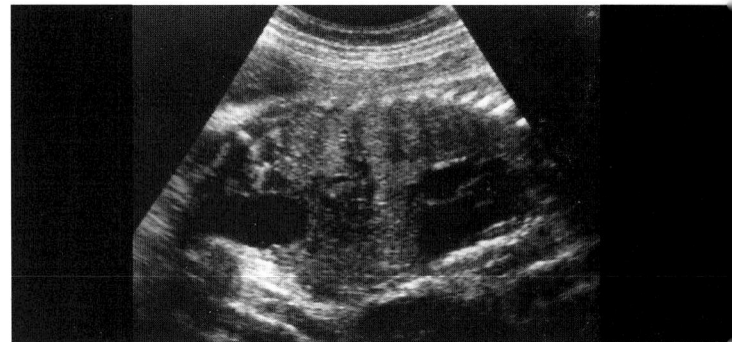

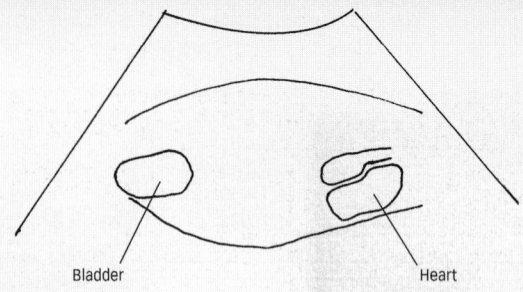

vein to the right portal vein to perfuse the liver. The ductus venosus is a muscular vein which is seen sonographically as a thin intrahepatic channel with echogenic walls. The ductus venosus is patent until shortly after birth, when the ductus transforms into the ligamentum venosum. The umbilical arteries may be followed caudad from the cord insertion to the internal iliac arteries close to the urinary bladder.

The liver occupies the upper third of the abdomen. It is low in reflectivity in contrast to highly reflective lung or bowel which lie adjacent to it. The hepatic veins can be traced to their confluence at the intrahepatic vena cava (Fig. 30). The right lobe is larger than the left.

The middle hepatic vein and the gall bladder mark the position of the main lobar fissure, which separates right and left lobes. The course of the ductus venosus marks the position of a fissure (fissure for the ligamentum venosum), which separates the left hepatic lobe and caudate lobe. The gall bladder is seen as an oblique anechoic structure at the right inferior border of the liver, seen to the right of the portal umbilical vein and separate from it.

The spleen lies in the upper left quadrant of the abdomen, above the kidney. It has a similar reflectivity to liver and may be difficult to distinguish in the fetus.

The kidneys are visible in their paraspinous location from 14 weeks and should be identified in all 18–20 week scans. In the first part of the second trimester they may be identified as rounded areas of low reflectivity with little visible internal architecture. The renal pelvis may be seen as a slit-like echo-free space in the centre of the kidney. The renal capsule becomes visible as a thin reflective rim from the nineteenth week. Fetal lobulation becomes apparent from the twenty-fourth week. In later pregnancy, the medullary pyramids may be distinguished as echo-poor areas with poorly defined margins arranged around the renal sinus, which is highly reflective due to multiple interfaces at the renal pelvis (Fig. 31).

Fig. 32. above
Coronal section of the fetal trunk at 32 weeks gestation, showing the urine-filled bladder in the pelvis.

(b)

Central part of right suprarenal gland (corresponds to the suprarenal medulla)

Outer zone of suprarenal gland (echopoor)

Spine

Aorta

Stomach

Testes

Penis

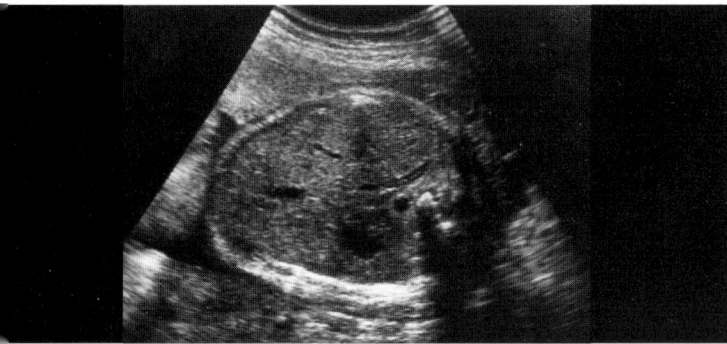

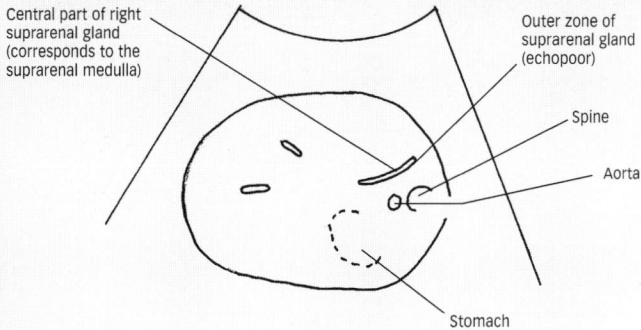

Fig. 33. above
Transverse view of the fetal upper abdomen at 32 weeks gestation, showing detail of the right suprarenal gland.

The accepted upper limit of normal for the size of the renal pelvis is 5 mm in AP diameter.

Normal ureters are not visualized. The bladder is seen as an echo-free structure arising out of the pelvis, which is visible after 14 weeks (Fig. 32). If the bladder is not seen, the patient should be rescanned after about 30 minutes, since the fetal bladder is emptied at least once an hour.

Fetal suprarenal glands are large, being 20 times the relative adult size at birth. The thick outer zone of the suprarenal is echo-poor and

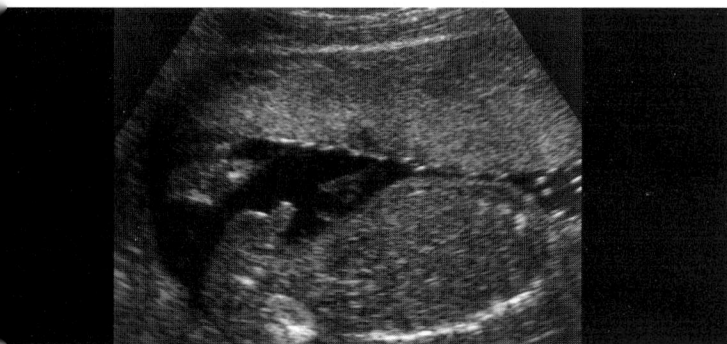

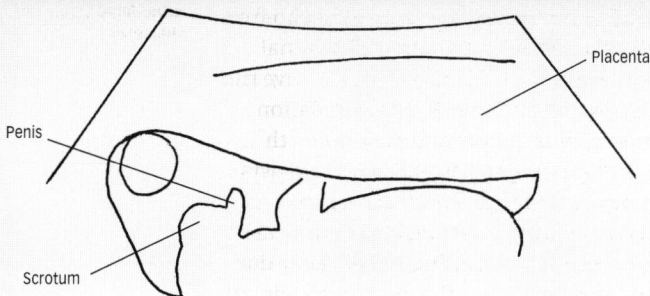

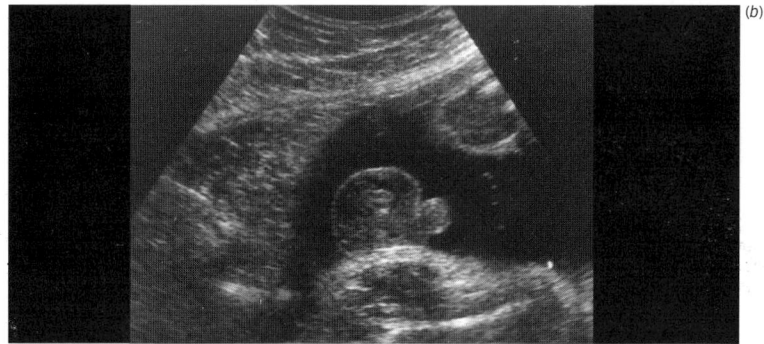

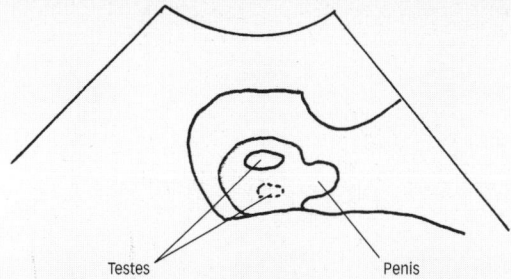

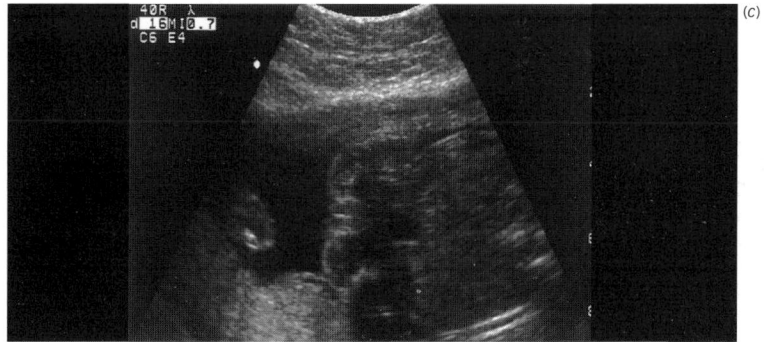

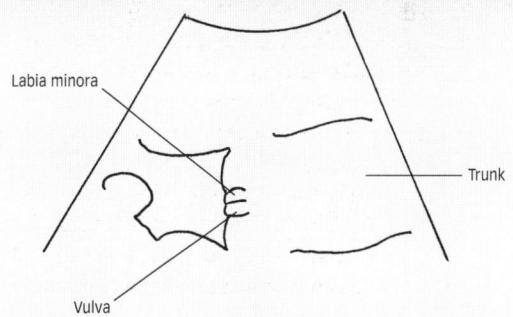

(c)

Labia minora

Trunk

Vulva

Placenta

Penis

Scrotum

is thought to represent an inner fetal zone of adrenal cortex and an outer zone of permanent cortex. The central part of the gland corresponds to the suprarenal medulla (Fig. 33). The left suprarenal lies superior to the upper pole of the left kidney and moves to its normal position anterior and medial to the kidney after birth. The suprarenal glands decrease rapidly in prominence on ultrasound after birth.

Measurement of abdominal circumference is part of the routine assessment to estimate gestational age in the middle trimester. A section is obtained at the level of the fetal liver.

Fig. 34.
Male genitalia, (a) sagittal view at 19 weeks; (b) coronal view at 30 weeks, scrotum and penis can be clearly identified, allowing a confident diagnosis of a male fetus, (c) perineal view of a female infant at 19 weeks gestation in which vulva and labia are identified.

35

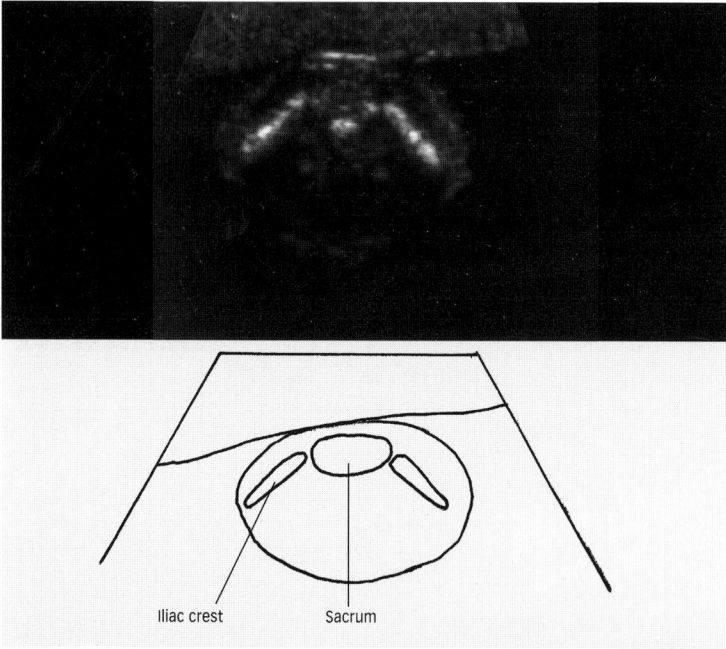

Iliac crest   Sacrum

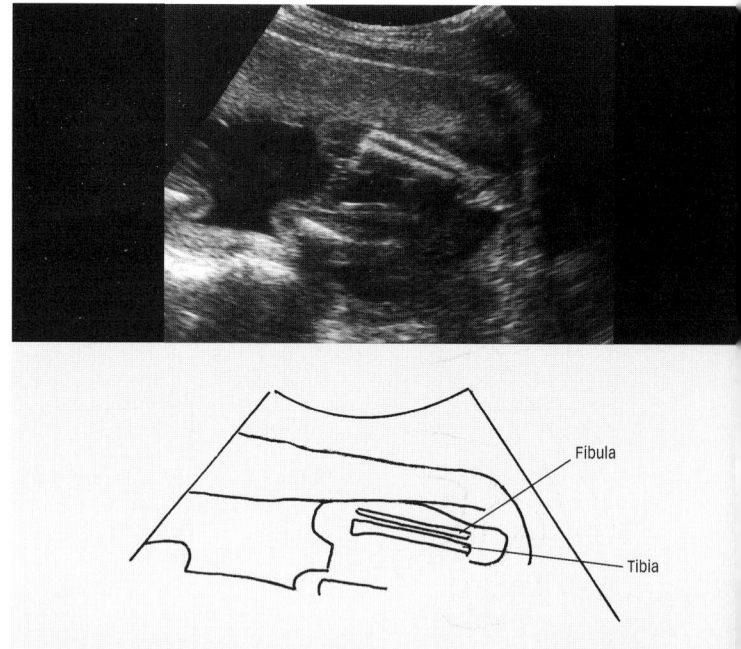

Fibula

Tibia

36

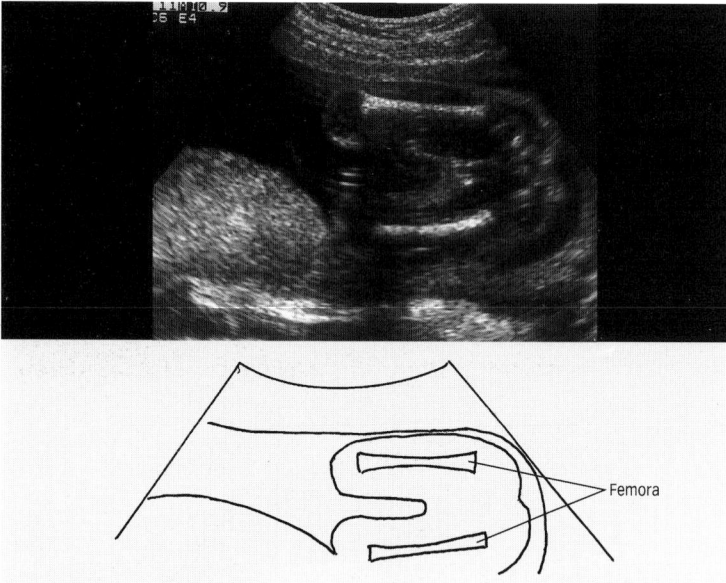

Femora

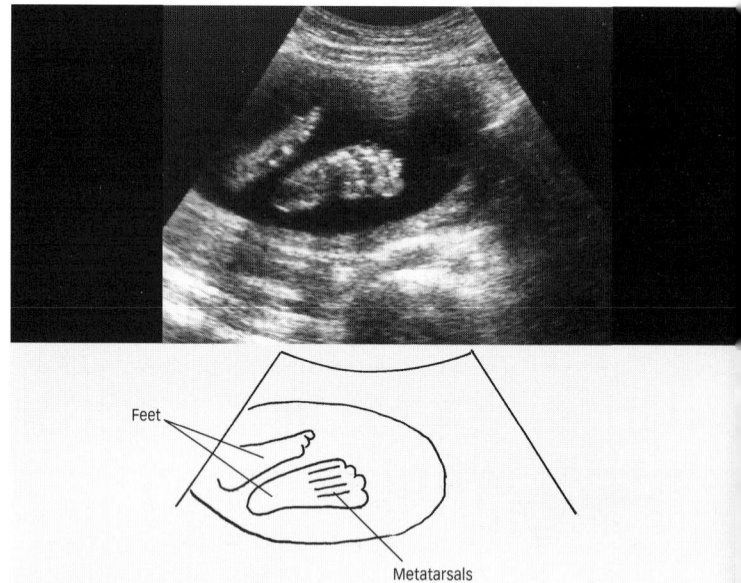

Feet

Metatarsals

Fig. 35. top
Axial view through the pelvis at 19 weeks gestation, showing the iliac crest and ischium on both sides.

Fig. 36. above
A view of both femora at 19 weeks gestation.

The umbilical part of the portal vein acts as a marker, and should be equidistant from both sides of the liver. Stomach and spine are also seen, and ribs on either side.

Assessment of fetal gender is of great interest to the parents, but may be fundamental in cases of X-linked conditions. The penis may be seen early in the second trimester, depending on the position of the fetus. Assignment of sex may be unreliable early in the pregnancy since the clitoris may be enlarged. In later pregnancy the presence of testes in the scrotum confirms a baby boy (Fig. 34(a)). In a girl the vulva may be seen, with fine lines (the labia minora) centrally (Fig. 34(c)).

Limbs

The iliac crest and ischium may be seen in two planes in the second trimester (Fig. 35). Routine assessment includes measurement of femur length at the 18–20 week scan, since this is as accurate a measure of gestational age as the BPD (Fig. 36). The probe should be aligned along the long axis of the diaphysis at a slight angle.

The femur begins to ossify at 6–12 weeks and is therefore strongly reflective at the time of routine assessment. Lower femoral epiphyses and upper tibial epiphyses appear later in the third trimester. The distal epiphysis of the femur ossifies at 36 weeks and its presence on a radiograph was previously used as a

Fig. 37. top
19 weeks gestation. View of the tibia and fibula.

Fig. 38. above
View of the feet at 19 weeks gestation.

Humerus

Head

Femur

41

Thumb

Fingers

Radius

Fetal hand

Ulna

42

Cord

Placenta

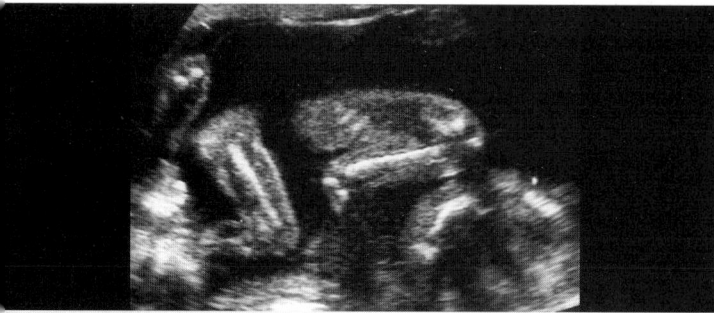

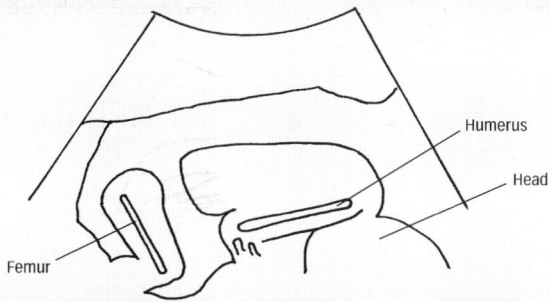

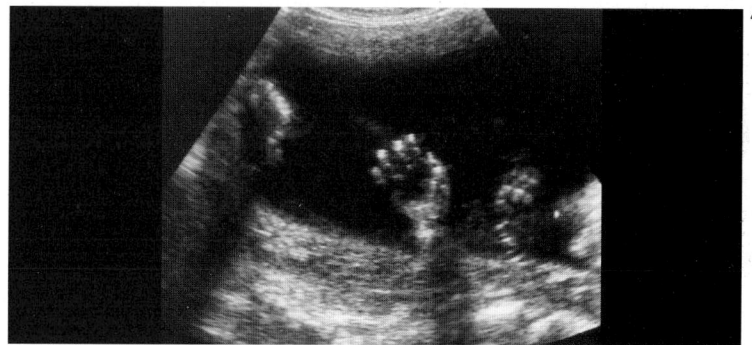

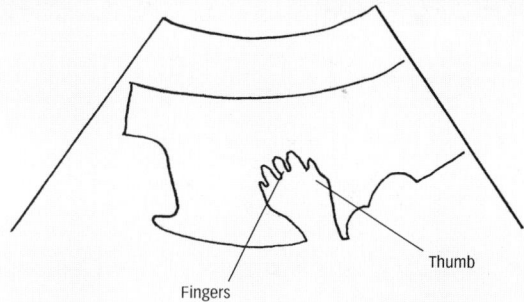

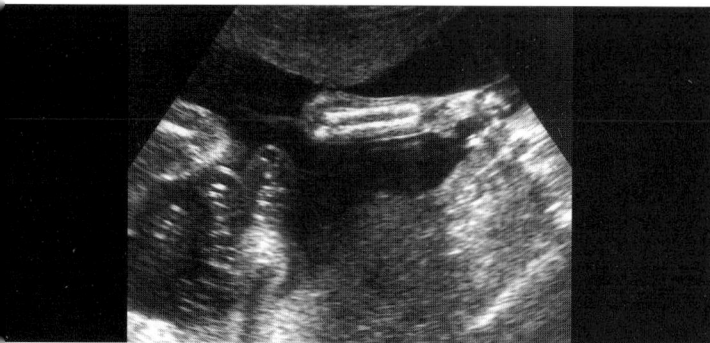

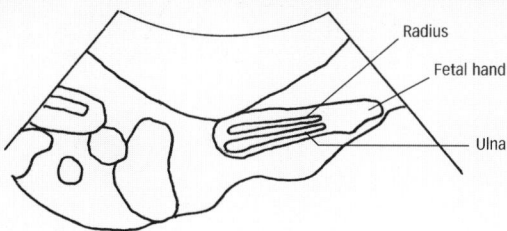

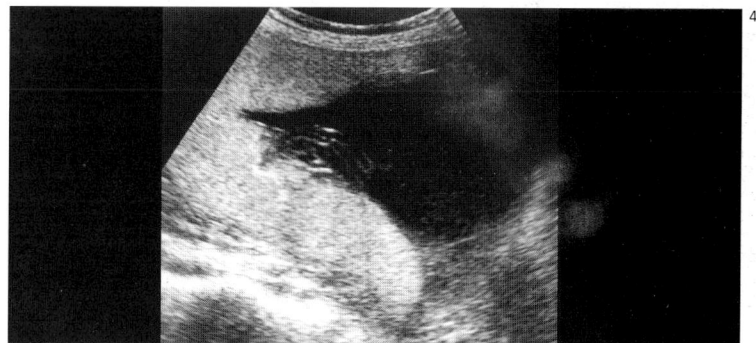

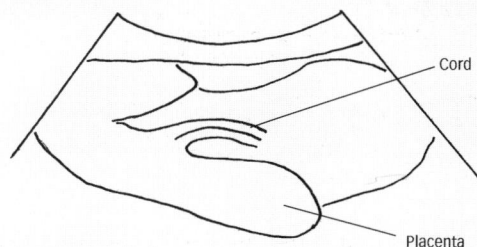

determinant of maturity. The tibia and fibula have similar lengths to each other (Fig. 37). The foot should be viewed in three planes to examine the relationship of the tarsal bones and the number of toes (Fig. 38).

The humerus is often held adducted against the thorax. Its length is not measured routinely, although the beginning of ossification in its proximal epiphyseal ossification centre is good evidence for the development of lung maturity (Fig. 39). The ulna extends more proximally than the radius at the elbow but the diaphysis of each bone extends to the same level at the wrist. The demonstration of this relationship is important since many bony anom-

alies foreshorten the distal radius (Fig. 40). The carpal bones are not ossified until after birth, while the metacarpals and phalanges are readily appreciated *in utero*, particularly if the fetus opens its hands (Fig. 41).

Placenta

The placenta may be seen as a focal thickening along the periphery of the gestational sac as early as 6–8 weeks of gestation. The placenta can be clearly identified as a discrete structure from 12 weeks, when the decidua capsularis and decidua parietalis fuse, with obliteration of the uterine cavity. The placenta is formed from a chorionic or fetal plate, the placental villous tissue of substance and the basal, or maternal, plate. The placenta is divided into 20 to 40 functional units (cotyledons). The maternal surface is divided into lobes by septae running from the basal plate to the chorionic plate, although the lobes have no physiological significance. As pregnancy progresses, the placental circulation is established. Ultrasound is used for placental localization and assessment of maturity (Fig. 42).

Further reading

Callen, P.W. (ed.). (1988). *Ultrasonography in Obstetrics and Gynaecology*, 2nd edn. Philadelphia: W.B. Saunders.

Demarel, P., Kendall, B. & Brunello, F. (1994). Techniques and indications in paediatric brain imaging. In *Imaging Children*, ed. H. Carty, F. Brunello, D. Shaw & B. Kendall, pp. 1370–4. Edinburgh: Churchill Livingstone.

Griffin, D.R. (1993). The normal fetus. In *Ultrasound in Obstetrics and Gynaecology*, ed. K. Dewbury, H. Meire & D. Cosgrove, pp. 187–209. Edinburgh: Churchill Livingstone.

Parkin, I.G. (1993). Embryology. In *Ultrasound in Obstetrics and Gynaecology*, ed. K. Dewbury, H. Meire & D. Cosgrove, pp. 125–143. Edinburgh: Churchill Livingstone.

20

Paediatric anatomy

R. A. L. BISSET, B. WILSON *and* N. WRIGHT

Introduction

Children are not simply small adults. They show a different spectrum of disease from adults, and congenital anatomical variants play a far more important role in disease pathogenesis. An appreciation of normal paediatric anatomy is crucial to the recognition of these variants. The main differences in radiological anatomy between adults and children are due to the following.

Differences in size

The average baby weighs between 3 and 4 kg at birth. Adults may weigh over 100 kg.

Differences in the proportion of many organs

The weight of the neonatal suprarenal gland, for example, may be 30% that of a normal kidney. A normal suprarenal gland may therefore be mistaken for a kidney, if the kidney is absent.

The imaging technique and projection used

Expediency demands that the most rapid and straightforward imaging techniques are used in young children. The projections may not be those used routinely in adult radiology and magnification, obliquity and movement artefact are more commonly encountered than in adult practice. The anteroposterior projection is used routinely for chest radiography in young children, which may result in significant cardiac magnification.

Ultrasonography is widely used in paediatrics, where its real-time and cine-loop playback facilities are of particular value when imaging a moving target. However, the appearances of organs, when scanning at high frequencies, do not always correspond directly with those seen at lower frequencies, and the presence of more acutely curved reflecting sur-faces in young children (such as the diaphragm and posterior bladder wall), increases the incidence of mirror image artefacts, which can give the false impression of the presence of a mass.

The distribution of fat in and around organs in children

This is not the same as in adults. Organ appearances may thus differ and the paucity of fat within the mediastinum and retroperitoneum, in particular, causes some difficulty in paediatric imaging.

The rate of maturation of normal structures and functions

This varies both in health and disease. Radiological appearances must therefore be considered in relation to the child's age and sex. Bony maturation, for example, shows a significant sex difference. Cardiac and respiratory rates are significantly higher in neonates and young children than in adults, and the swallowing pattern seen in babies is less advanced than that seen in older children and adults. Gastro-oesophageal and vesicoureteric reflux are so common in neonates that they are virtually physiological.

The MRI appearances of the neonatal brain differ from those of older children and adults owing to incomplete myelination. Myelination occurs in a sequential fashion and is reflected by the functional capabilities of the child. The stepwise progression of myelination allows brain development to be dated and a 'white matter' age to be ascribed. At term, the brain is largely non-myelinated but by the age of 2 years the pattern is similar to the adult brain (see Chapter 2).

The variable persistence of primitive tissues

Certain organs, notably the kidney, show variable persistence of primitive tissues for some time after birth, which can significantly alter anatomical appearances.

Congenital anatomical variants

These are common, being easily recognizable in at least 25% of the population. Those with pathological significance usually present in childhood.

Cranial ultrasonography

The anterior fontanelle provides an excellent acoustic window in the majority of children during the first year of life. The period varies during which the fontanelle is sufficiently large to allow scanning. It begins to close from around 9 months of age with complete closure at around 15 months. Thus cranial sonography is usually possible throughout the first year. At times, the posterior fontanelle and the cranial sutures can also serve as acoustic windows, particularly if they are widened and an ultrasound probe with a small 'footprint' is used. Cranial sonography is usually undertaken with a 5 MHz sector probe, as this gives good resolution but also allows sufficient depth of field to view the posterior cranial fossa. 7.5 and 10 MHz probes can also be useful to evaluate the surface of the brain. Unfortunately, scanning via the anterior fontanelle does result in significant blind spots under the convexity of the skull vault.

Cranial ultrasonography is usually performed in a standard manner. A series of coronal and sagittal and parasagittal images are taken, using specific anatomical landmarks to indicate the position of the section (Figs. 1 and 2). Finally, Doppler evaluation of the major intracranial arteries may be undertaken if clinically appropriate. The number of sections recorded will depend upon local preferences but generally midline sagittal and right and left parasagittal images are recorded, together with coronal sections at the following levels:

(a) the frontal lobes;
(b) the frontal horns of the lateral ventricles;
(c) the foramen of Monro;
(d) the thalami and the posterior aspect of the third ventricle;
(e) the trigones of the lateral ventricles;
(f) the posterior parietal and occipital cortex.

The anatomical detail seen at cranial sonography allows an accurate assessment of gross intracranial anatomy and also allows evaluation of major vessel flow and pulsatility.

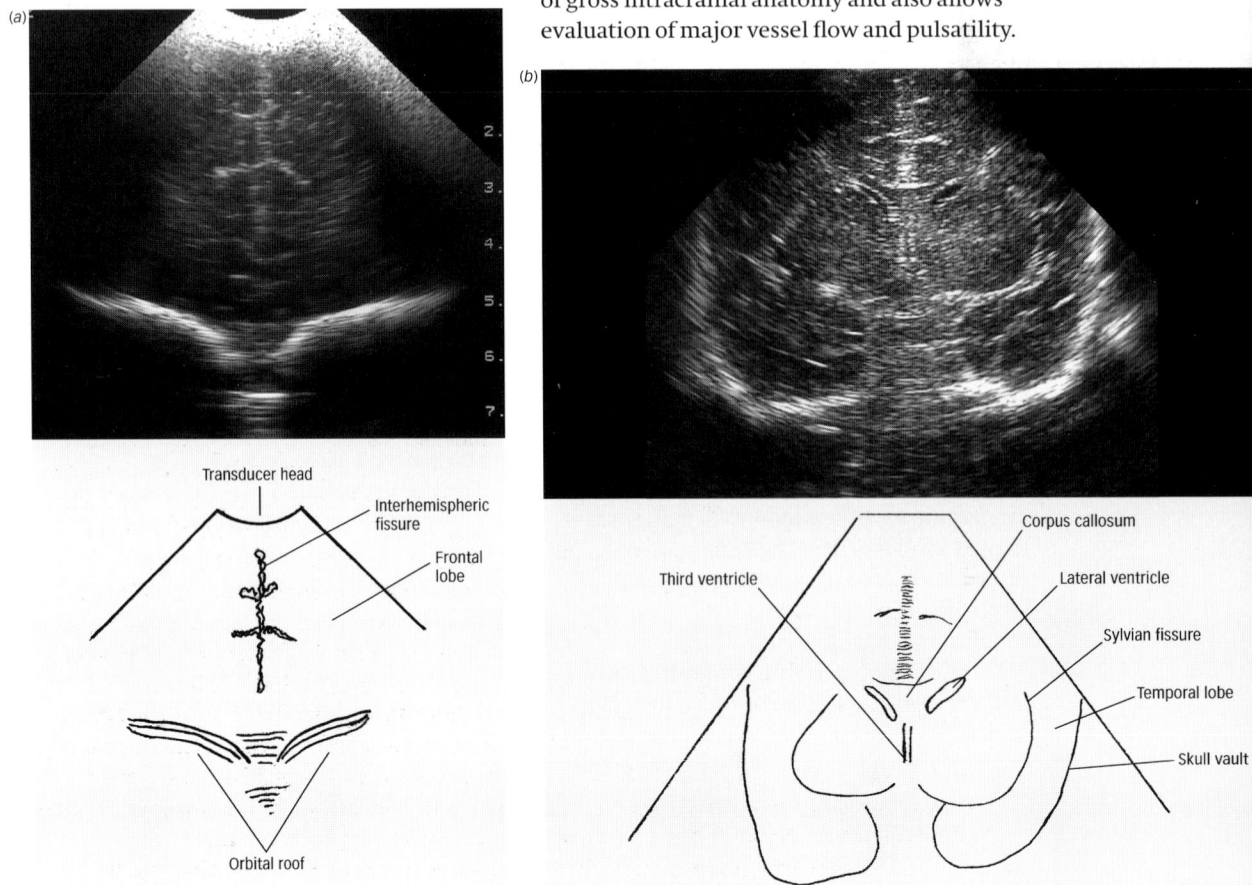

Fig. 1. Neonatal cranial ultrasound. Coronal scans ((a)–(d), anterior to posterior). Note in (d) the trigones of the lateral ventricles filled with echogenic choroid plexus.

416

Fig. 2.
Neonatal cranial ultrasound, midline sagittal section, showing the third and fourth ventricles and the cerebellum.
c, cerebellum; m, medulla; p, pons; Cl, clivus; csp, cavum septi pellucidi; cc, corpus callosum. * acoustic shadowing from the choroid plexuses.

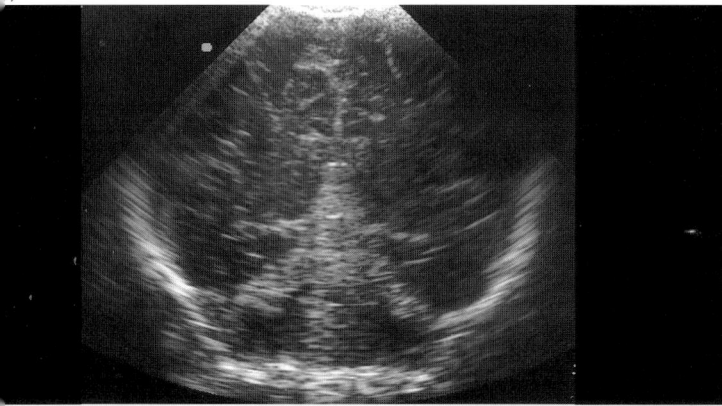

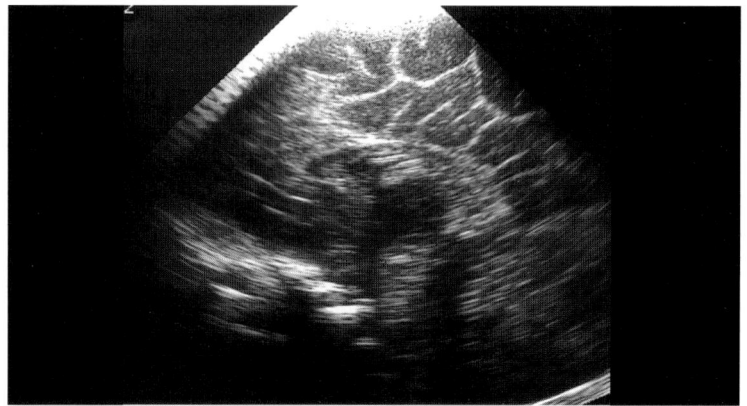

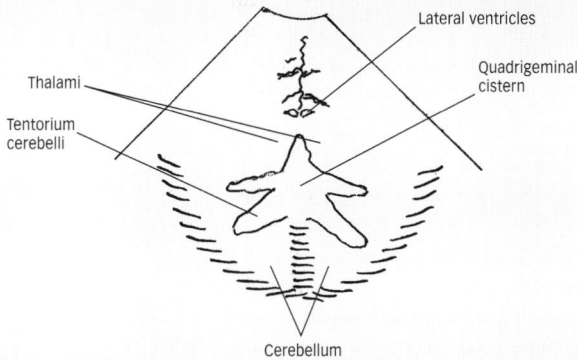

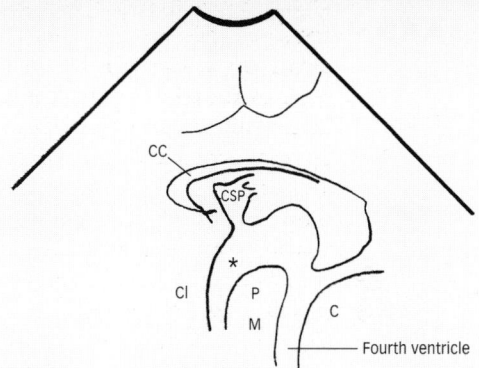

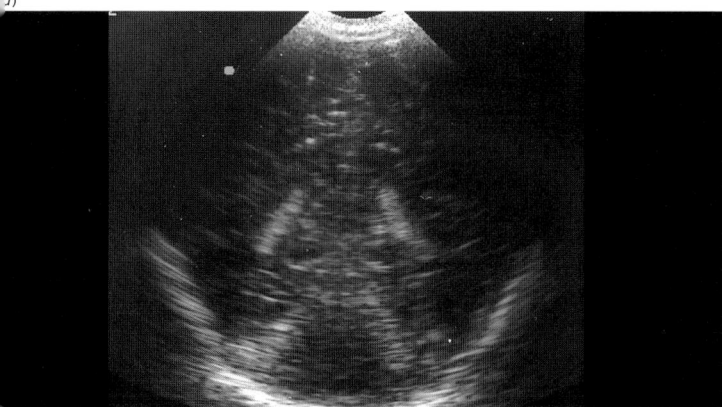

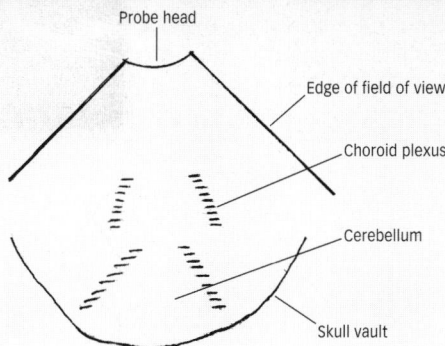

However, although sonography has advantages of cost, mobility and availability, it is becoming clear that neonatal MR scanning is more sensitive at detecting early ischaemic damage in the neonatal brain. The anatomical sections demonstrated at cranial sonography are similar to the sagittal and coronal images provided by MR scanning and correlation of the two can be very helpful when learning cranial sonographic anatomy.

Care must be taken to ensure correct probe positioning before assessing the position of the midline structures, as probe obliquity may give the impression that the ventricles and midline structures are displaced to one side. The lateral ventricles are the most widely used landmark when scanning. They are seen as triangular anechoic slits lying either side of the midline. Their walls are echogenic, whilst their roof is formed by the hypoechoic corpus callosum. Posteriorly, the lateral ventricles contain the echogenic choroid plexus which may fill the region of the trigones, in which case anechoic cerebrospinal fluid will not always be seen around the choroid.

An anterior coronal section will show the anechoic cavum septi pellucidi between the lateral ventricles which have a triangular or crescentic configuration. The heads of the caudate nuclei lie inferolateral to the lateral walls of the lateral ventricles. The cingulate gyri lie above the corpus callosum, which forms the ventricular roof. The Sylvian fissures are seen laterally as horizontal Y-shaped fissures containing the pulsating middle cerebral arteries (Fig. 1(b)).

At the level of the foramen of Monro, the third ventricle may just be visible beneath the cavum septi pellucidi. When the third ventricle is visible as an anechoic slit on sagittal sections, the interthalamic connection may be seen, but the ventricle is frequently too narrow to be seen clearly. Inferiorly, the slightly echogenic pons and medulla can also be identified.

Coronal scans taken through the posterior aspect of the third ventricle may show echogenic choroid within its roof. The choroid plexus within the adjacent lateral ventricles may also be seen, giving the appearance of three adjacent white dots. At this level, the bodies of the caudate nuclei lie lateral to the bodies of the lateral ventricles and the thalami lie inferiorly. The echogenic tentorium begins to come into view when the probe is directed more posteriorly, and is seen more completely beneath the central diamond- or star-shaped quadrigeminal cistern (Fig. 1(c)). The cistern is echogenic, although the reason for this is not fully understood. The most posterior sections show echogenic choroid within the trigones of the lateral ventricles, which diverge inferiorly (Fig. 1(d)). Slight asymmetry of the trigones is usually normal. Periventricular echogenicity may also be increased in this area. The splenium of the corpus callosum is seen between the trigones as a horizontal echogenic line. The number of sulci and gyri in the overlying brain increases with age.

The fourth ventricle and brainsten are most easily appreciated on sagittal sections (Fig. 2). The brain stem is of moderate echogenicity, but is less echogenic than the cerebellar vermis, which lies in the midline behind the fourth ventricle. The highly echogenic clivus lies anterior to the brainstem and the basilar artery can be seen pulsating between the clivus and brainstem. Parasagittal sections show the caudothalamic groove between the caudate nucleus anteriorly and thalamus posteriorly. When seen together, the caudate nucleus is slightly more echogenic than the thalamus. The germinal matrix, a site of haemorrhage in preterm infants, lies anterior to the caudothalamic groove. This very vascular tissue lines the floor of the lateral ventricles above the heads and bodies of the caudate nuclei. Further geminal matrix may be present in the grooves of the third and fourth ventricles. Germinal matrix involutes from the early stages of gestation and is not normally present at birth. Further lateral parasagittal sections allow the temporal horns of the lateral ventricles and temporal lobes to be visualized.

The appearances of the neonatal brain vary with age. Sulci and gyri are far less prominent in the very premature and increase with age. Primary sulci are present by the seventh month of gestation and begin to branch and convolute to form secondary sulci during the eighth and ninth months. The lateral ventricles appear larger in preterm infants than at term and their size decreases relative to the rest of the brain as the child grows. At term, the frontal horns of the lateral ventricles may be seen as narrow slits and can be hard to identify. Asymmetry in ventricular size also decreases with age, being present in up to 40% of premature infants but in less than 20% at term. Ventricular size can also be affected by position and this should be remembered when scanning ill babies who may have had their head on one side for some time before scanning. In these cases, the dependent ventricle is usually smaller. Premature babies may also show the presence of a cavum septum vergae. The cavum septum vergae is a normal midline cerebrospinal fluid space between the bodies of the lateral ventricles behind the cavum. The cavum vergae begins to close during the sixth month of gestation and is not normally present at birth. The cavum is present in around 60% of term infants but usually closes by 2 months of age.

Spinal sonography

Sonography of the spine is possible because the incompletely ossified posterior spinal arches leave an acoustic window, particularly in the lumbar region, for several months after birth. Sonography may also be undertaken after surgical intervention, if a laminectomy has been performed. A high frequency linear array probe is used until the posterior arches ossify, when a small footprint sector probe may be useful.

The spinal cord is seen as an hypoechoic tube with echogenic anterior and posterior

Fig. 3.
Longitudinal ultrasound scan of the lumbar region showing the cord termination.

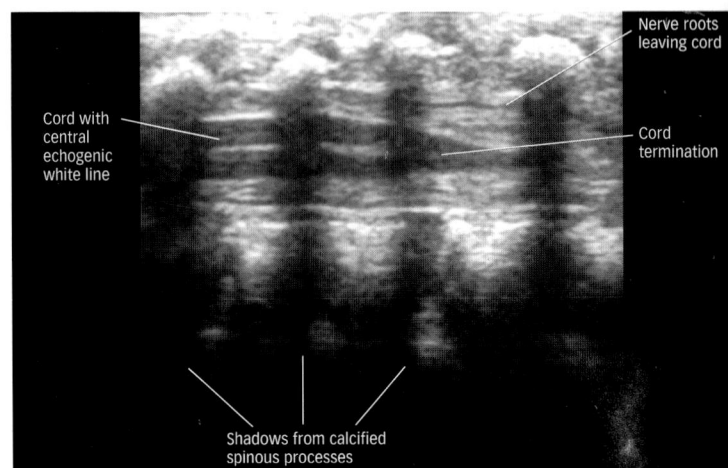

Nerve roots leaving cord

Cord with central echogenic white line

Cord termination

Shadows from calcified spinous processes

walls (Fig. 3). A central echogenic line is present due to the interface between the central part of the anterior median fissure and myelinated ventral white commissure. The spinal cord is surrounded by anechoic cerebrospinal fluid with peripheral echogenic bands representing the dura. Anteriorly, the vertebrae are seen as echogenic blocks separated by echo-poor intervertebral discs. On transverse sections the spinal cord is seen as an oval structure with a central echogenic dot. The cord tapers inferiorly to end at a level between the first and second lumbar vertebrae as the conus medullaris. This is continuous with the filum terminale, an echogenic band which extends through the lower spinal canal to the sacrum, surrounded by spinal nerve roots. Accurate measurement of the level of cord termination by sonography can be difficult. The lowest rib may be used as a landmark, but it is often necessary to place a metal marker at the level of the cord termination as shown by sonography and then take a radiograph to confirm the vertebral position. A tethered cord usually ends below the level of the upper end plate of the third lumbar vertebra.

One of the most remarkable features of spinal sonography is the mobility of the contents of the spinal canal. Both the spinal cord and nerve roots show a great deal of movement due to transmitted vascular pulsation.

Neonatal cord dimensions (term infants) are as follows:

- cervical cord diameter 0.53 cm;
- thoracic cord diameter 0.44 cm;
- lumbar cord diameter 0.58 cm.

The chest

With the exception of the size of the thymus gland, gross thoracic anatomy in the child is similar to that of the adult. However, the trachea and airways are much narrower than in adults, as a result of which bronchial obstruction by mucus is far more common and the classical appearances of lobar collapse and consolidation are seen frequently. The airways in children are far more pliable than in adults, and the trachea may be seen to bend through nearly 90 degrees on a lateral cervical film when a child makes a forced expiration when crying. The trachea is also prone to compression by a distended oesophagus in oesophageal atresia or severe reflux, and repeated or persistent compression may result in tracheomalacia in which the trachea becomes weak and flaccid tending to collapse and obstruct expiration.

The mediastinum in young children appears widened owing to the presence of the thymus gland. This is a bilobed lymphoid organ, which may protrude into either or both lung fields giving the 'sail' sign on a frontal chest radiograph (Fig. 4). The thymus gland may also be identified by sonography via the

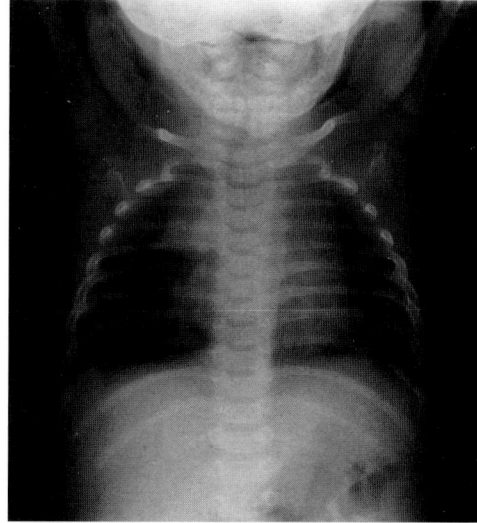

Fig. 4.
Chest radiograph showing the 'sail sign' of the thymus extending into the right lung.

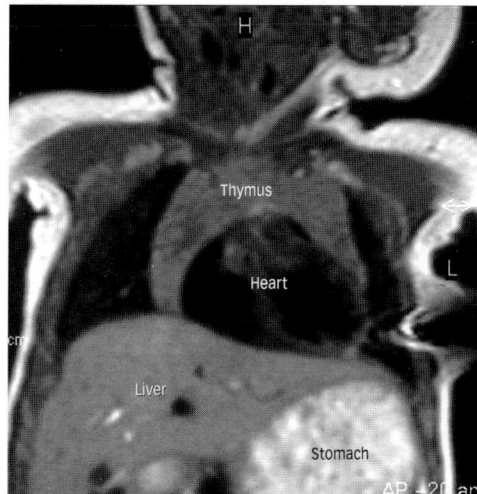

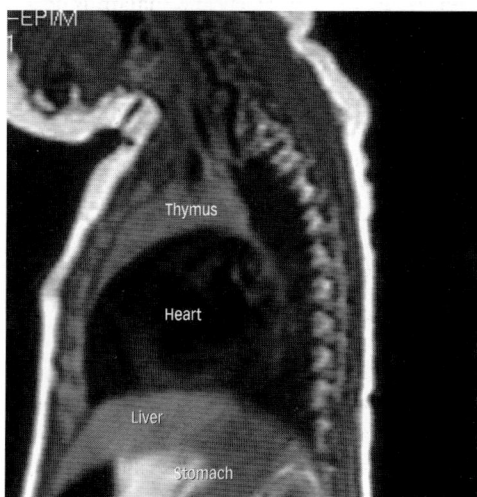

Fig. 5.
(a) Coronal and (b) sagittal T1W MR scans showing the bilobed thymus gland in the superior mediastinum.

suprasternal notch or a parasternal approach and is of moderate echogenicity (but generally less than the adjacent thyroid gland). The thymus lies anterior to the trachea in the superior mediastinum and thoracic inlet. Like many other organs it can appear quite mobile on ultrasound scanning, bulging into the lower neck with respiration particularly if respiration is rapid. MRI can demonstrate both lobes lying across the trachea (Fig. 5). The gland is fatty and of slightly low attenuation on CT, but, even so, the lack of fat within the mediastinum in young children makes it difficult to delineate the margins of the thymus from other mediastinal structures with CT (Fig. 6).

In younger children, the thymus has a quadrilateral shape with straight or convex borders. Over 5 years of age, the bilobed configuration is more obvious and the gland can appear triangular. It extends from the level of the brachiocephalic veins at the origin of the superior vena cava (SVC) to the most cranial aspect of the heart. As the gland is largely lymphoid, it shows a variation in size between health and disease. Ill health, 'stress' and steroids can cause the thymus to reduce in size. As the child recovers, the thymus regrows and may become visible on a chest radiograph, having previously not been prominent. This can lead to an erroneous diagnosis of thymic or mediastinal tumours as a cause for the child's ill health.

The thymus is commonly seen on chest radiographs of infants and young children, but it decreases in size with age and is encountered uncommonly on chest radiographs in children over 5 years. It remains visible on CT and MR scans in young adults, though it has, by then, undergone substantial involution.

Fig. 6. below
Axial CT scan of the infant chest showing the thymus gland lying anteriorly in the mediastinum. The relative paucity of fat planes in the paediatric mediastinum makes the mediastinal border of the thymus difficult to define.

Fig. 7. bottom
A bronchogram showing contrast medium injected into an accessory right upper lobe bronchus (pig bronchus). The pliability of the trachea during rigid bronchoscopy is also demonstrated.

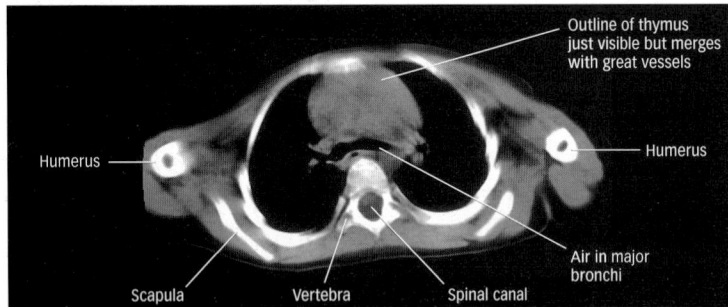

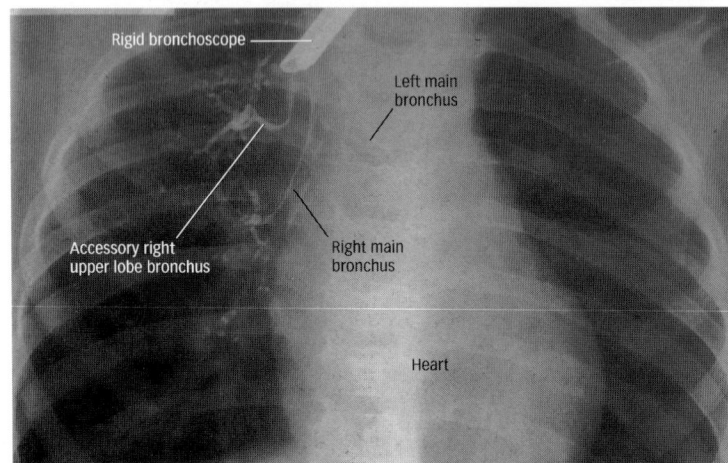

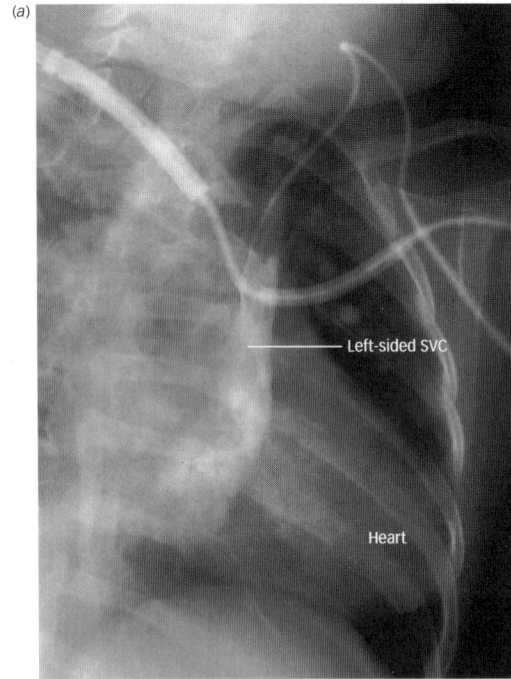

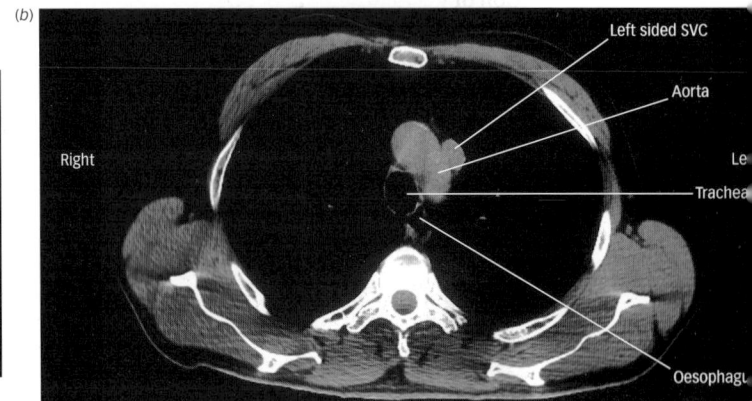

(a)

Fig. 6.

(b)

The heart size in children is very dependent upon the child's position and the radiographic projection used. There is little substitute for experience when assessing cardiac size but, though the rules used in adults apply, the normal paediatric heart appears smaller on a posteroanterior chest radiograph than its adult counterpart. If there is any doubt about heart size, the appearance of the pulmonary vasculature can be a helpful pointer.

The appearances of the lungs are also similar to those of an adult. However, on expiration, a neonate can almost 'white out' the chest radiograph, and it is therefore important

Fig. 8.
(a) Contrast medium injected via a central line demonstrates a left-sided superior vena cava draining to the coronary sinus.
(b) Axial section of the chest showing the left-sided superior vena cava the left of the aortic arch

to ensure that opaque lungs are not simply due to expiration. Obliquity may also result in an apparent difference in density of the lung fields. The fissures in young children are very thin and are not usually visible unless thickened by fluid or disease.

Accessory fissures and congenital variants of pulmonary anatomy are thus not usually visible unless rendered opaque or highlighted by an unusual pattern of lung consolidation (Fig. 7).

Congenital heart disease and abnormalities of the mediastinal vessels may be diagnosed *in utero* by ultrasonography or after birth by ultrasound or MRI. However, abnormalities may pass undetected until brought to light by disease elsewhere. The left-sided superior vena cava, for example, which is a common occurrence in congenital heart disease, can occur, albeit rarely, in isolation and may be encountered when placing central lines (Fig. 8). Despite this, apparently abnormally placed central lines are more likely to be due to the line being misplaced or lying in a small vessel in the posterior mediastinum than to a congenital vascular abnormality.

Abnormal vessels may form vascular rings around the oesophagus and thus give rise to symptoms referable to the upper gastrointestinal tract (Fig. 9). Chest and abdominal radiographs are frequently used to show the position of vascular lines in babies (Fig. 10). Umbilical artery lines can be differentiated from venous lines as the umbilical arteries are derived from the internal iliac arteries. Thus an umbilical arterial line turns down into the pelvis before running up into the aorta. The ductus arteriosus is a fetal vascular channel connecting the left pulmonary artery to the aorta. It normally closes at birth unless there is

cardiopulmonary compromise, in which case it may remain patent. Occasionally, the obliterated track is seen as focal calcification between the left pulmonary artery and aorta on a chest radiograph.

The diaphragm is usually visualized at ultrasonography during abdominal examination. In young children it is sharply curved, as a result of which mirror image artefacts are common. This may lead at times to the erro-

Fig. 10.
Radiograph of the thorax and abdomen of an infant showing umbilical arterial and venous lines. The arterial line descends into the pelvis to the iliac artery before ascending in the aorta over the left side of the spine.

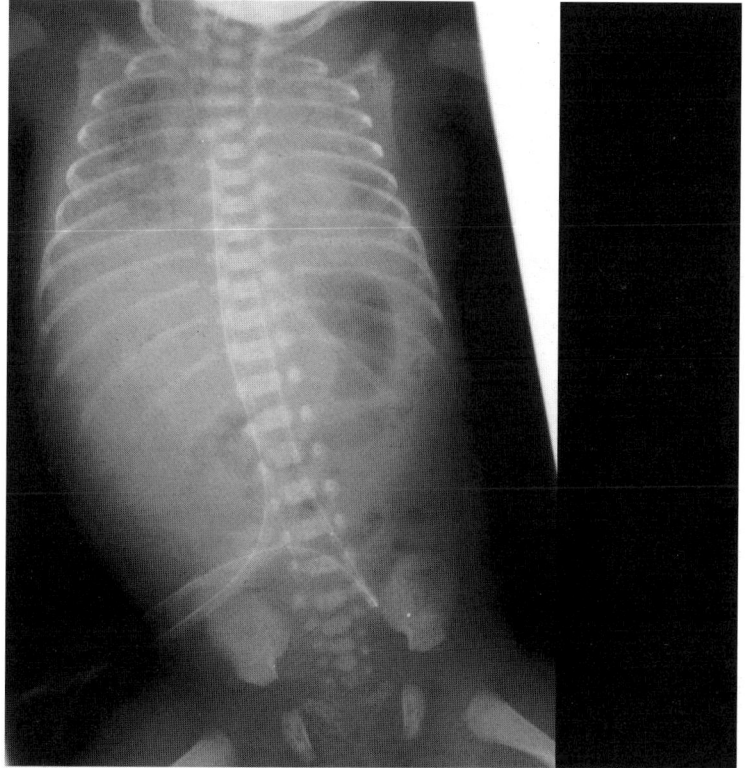

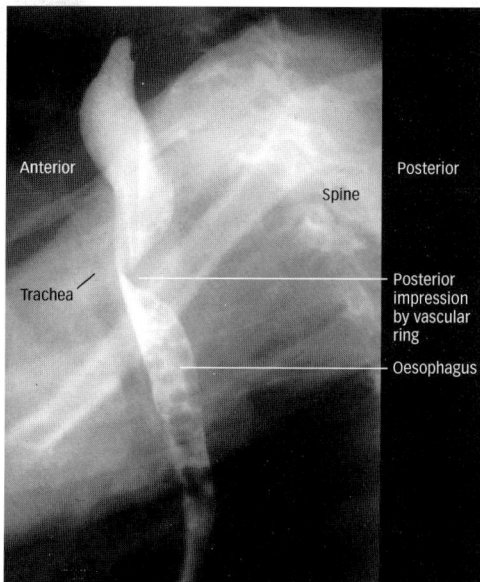

Endotracheal tube

Right

Left

Umbilical venous line

Umbilical artery line

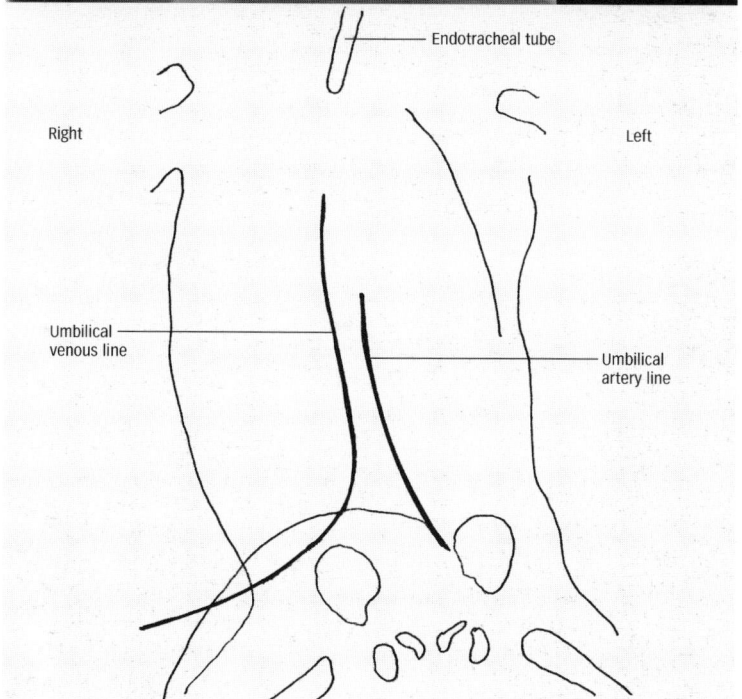

Fig. 9.
Barium swallow examination (lateral projection), showing a posterior impression on the oesophagus due to a vascular ring caused by a right-sided aortic arch.

Anterior

Posterior

Spine

Trachea

Posterior impression by vascular ring

Oesophagus

neous sonographic diagnosis of upper abdominal or lower thoracic pathology. As in adults, the posterior aspect of the diaphragm moves more than the anterior aspect. The degree of movement depends upon the depth and rate of respiration, but in infants movement in the longitudinal plane at the midpoint of the hemidiaphragm may be up to:

• anterior diaphragm   2.6 cm
• mid-diaphragm   3.6 cm
• posterior diaphragm 4.5 cm (Lang *et al.*, 1988).

The gastrointestinal tract, liver and biliary system, pancreas and spleen

The functional process of swallowing in the newborn and in young infants differs from that seen in adults and older children. Once mature, the swallowing process shows a rapid series of stages which merge to allow the smooth passage of a bolus from the mouth to the stomach. An oral bolus is propelled backwards by the whip-like action of the tongue pressing against the hard palate. As the bolus passes the anterior pillars of the fauces, the pharyngeal swallow reflex occurs with rapid pharyngeal elevation, closure of the larynx, depression of the epiglottis and relaxation and opening of cricopharyngeus. The bolus thus traverses the pharynx unimpeded, entering the oesophagus and being carried to the stomach by a primary peristaltic wave. Infants below the age of 18 months show a more primitive swallowing pattern, which is also seen in primates. A neonate will grasp the nipple within the mouth, forming an airtight seal with the lips. Rhythmical depression of the jaw creates a vacuum within the mouth, which sucks in milk. Each milk bolus is then propelled backwards into the pharynx, but three to five boluses may be held in the pharynx before a swallow reflex is triggered.

Coordination of breathing and swallowing is thus critical as the pharynx remains filled with fluids for a greater time during swallowing in infants than in older children.

The appearances of the oesophagus are the same as those seen in the adult, though congenital vascular rings may give rise to extrinsic compression (Fig. 9). The oesophagus is usually visible within the abdomen at ultrasonography, lying between the aorta and left lobe of liver before moving to the left to the gastro-oesophageal junction. Reflux may be seen as the retrograde movement of fluid containing densely echogenic microbubbles. Babies are usually most easily examined after a feed, when relaxed and sleepy. At this time the gas-

tric fundus is usually seen as a fluid-filled structure containing a great deal of solid milk curd. When milk curd predominates, the stomach may have a mass-like appearance and should not be confused with a pathological mass (Fig. 11). If there is doubt, the child should be scanned again after an interval or given dextrose to drink and rescanned during feeding when fluid will be seen entering the stomach.

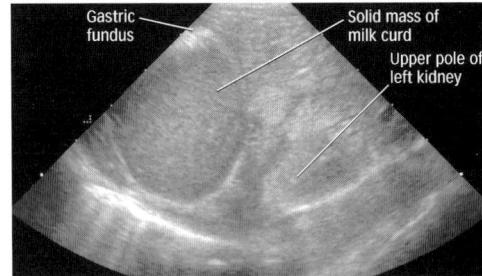

Fig. 11.
Longitudinal ultrasound scan of the left upper quadrant of the abdomen showing the mass-like appearance of the gastric fundus filled with milk curd.

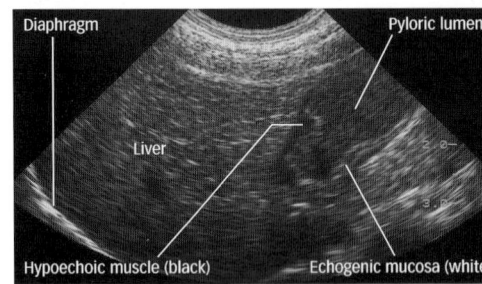

Fig. 12.
Transverse oblique ultrasound scan of the right upper quadrant showing the normal pyloric wall.

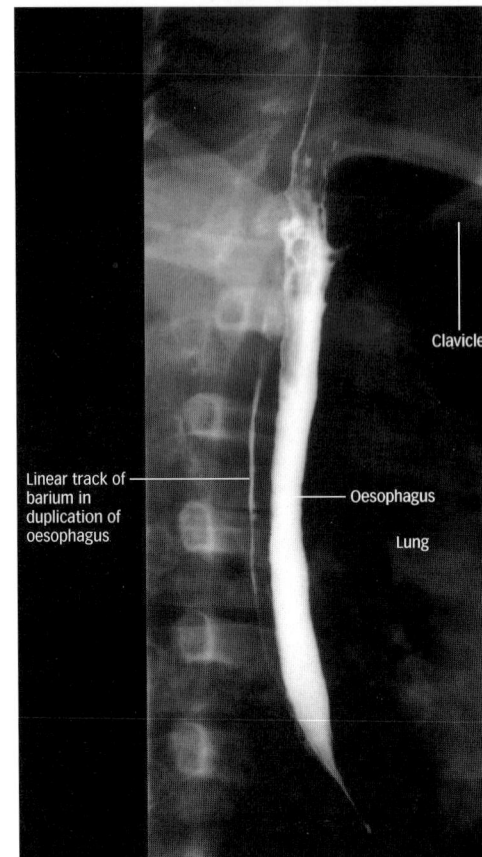

Fig. 13.
Barium swallow examination showing duplication of the oesophagus with a narrow second lumen.

A crying child swallows air and the upper gastrointestinal tract can rapidly distend with air. When distended with food and air, the infantile stomach may extend across the upper abdomen almost from one side to the other. Despite the size of a baby's stomach after feeding, it should contain only a small residue after four hours' fasting.

The small bowel may also rapidly fill with air when a baby is crying. The small bowel should not normally be dilated, but distension with air may cause colic and may make the child cry still further.

Ultrasonography is used to assess the gastric wall in children, particularly in cases of suspected hypertrophic pyloric stenosis. The gastric wall in children is normally less than

3 mm in thickness (including both the inner echogenic mucosa and outer hypoechoic muscle). Measurements should be taken with the stomach filled or partially filled with fluid but not when contracted (Fig. 12). Larger children have a greater normal muscle thickness than small preterm infants. The use of normal measurements must therefore be considered in relation to the child's size and age. The thickness of the normal pyloric muscle should be no more than 3 mm and the length of the pylorus should not exceed length 17 mm. Measurements are usually taken on longitudinal sections.

The intestine in children may also be assessed by ultrasonography. The small bowel in particular can be visualized when filled with fluid after a feed. The appendix can be seen in up to 90% of children with appendicitis. The small bowel shows inner echogenic mucosa and outer hypoechoic muscle similar to that seen in the stomach. Bowel duplication, which can occur anywhere from the oesophagus to the rectum may give rise to a cyst-like structure or a separate bowel tube (Figs. 13 and 14).

The position and configuration of the duodenal loop are of particular importance in children and should be demonstrated on every barium meal series undertaken in a child for any indication. The normal duodenal loop has a U-shaped configuration. The duodeno-jejunal (D/J) flexure should lie to the left of the upper lumbar spine at the level of the pylorus (Fig. 15). Any deviation from this configuration is a form of malrotation. Barium examinations have the drawback that barium shows only the bowel lumen from which the position of the D/J flexure must be assumed. Ultrasonography has the advantage that the position of the superior mesenteric artery and vein can be demonstrated. The vein normally lies on the right of the artery (see Chapter 12). Most cases of volvulus will show inversion of the vessel relationship, but malrotation can occur with apparently normally related vessels, particularly in malrotation with bowel obstruction due to Ladd's bands and not volvulus. Thus both barium meal examination and sonography may be necessary if malrotation is suspected. The position of the caecum in malrotation is also variable and as malrotation is associated with increased bowel mobility the position of the bowel can vary from day to day. Proximal small bowel obstruction may also occur from other anatomical variants such as annular pancreas, bowel atresia and stenosis (Fig. 16).

The liver is relatively larger in the neonate than in the adult and is relatively larger still

Fig. 14.
Barium enema (single contrast, 'filling' film) showing almost complete colonic duplication

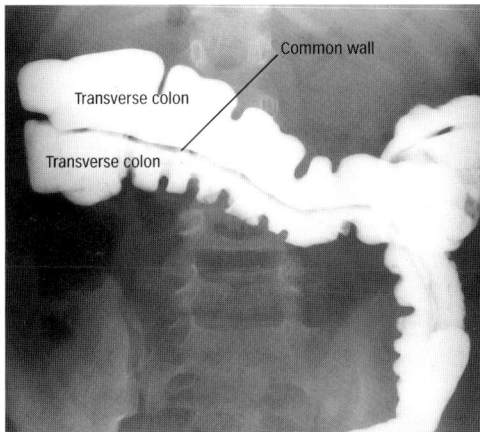

Fig. 15.
Barium meal examination showing a normal duodenal loop and the duodenal–jejunal flexure to the left of the spine at the level of the pylorus.

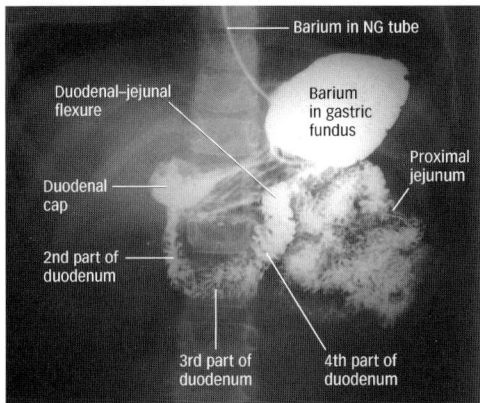

Fig. 16.
Barium study showing duodenal obstruction due to an annular pancreas.

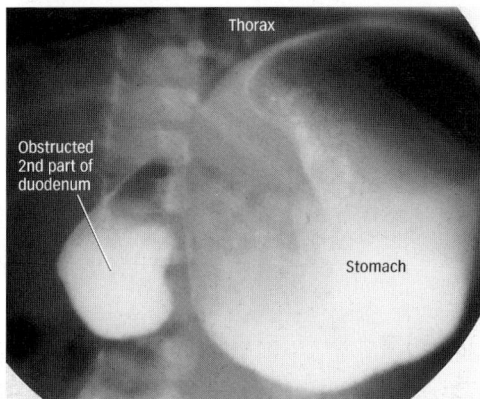

in utero. As a result, the left lobe of liver may extend to the left lateral abdominal wall anterior to the spleen. This does not normally cause confusion as the liver shows a branching portal venous pattern which the spleen does not. However, in cases of trauma with fluid in the abdomen, a trace of fluid between the spleen and the left lobe of liver may be mistaken for a splenic laceration. The umbilical vein extends from the umbilicus to the liver in the falciform ligament. The left portal vein receives the umbilical vein and gives rise to the ductus venosus, which drains into the hepatic veins as they enter the inferior vena cava (IVC). The ductus venosus is usually 1.5 cm long (range 1.1–1.9 cm) and 0.1–0.2 cm in diameter. Blood flow can usually be seen within it during the first 2 days of life and may be visible in up to 11% of infants at 18 days. The remnant of the ligamentum venosum separates the caudate lobe and the left lobe of liver.

Small portal veins may be difficult to identify in the liver in neonates, but become increasingly visible with age and with improved sonographic technology. The main portal vein trunk measures around 0.85 cm up to 10 years of age and around 1 cm in diameter from 10–20 years. The normal common bile duct measures up to 0.2 cm in infants, 0.4 cm in older children and 0.7 cm in adolescents. The normal gall bladder wall is less than 0.3 cm diameter when distended. The size of the gall bladder is variable and depends upon the rate of bile flow and the period of fasting prior to imaging (which may be short as infants like to feed at regular intervals). In infants the distended gall bladder is usually 1.5–3 cm long.

Visualization of the biliary system is important in neonates with possible biliary atresia. The diagnosis is one of exclusion, as imaging is directed at demonstrating biliary flow. HIDA isotope scanning shows normal biliary excretion, but severe cases of neonatal hepatitis may be associated with little bile flow. Liver biopsy may be equivocal, thus percutaneous transhepatic cholangiography may be attempted either by direct biliary puncture or gall bladder puncture. Percutaneous transhepatic cholangiography is successful in at least 50% of neonates with normal bile ducts (Fig. 17), but as the neonatal bile ducts are so narrow, failure to enter a bile duct does not always indicate biliary atresia. Laparotomy or laparoscopy may be necessary in these cases to make a final diagnosis.

The spleen is a lymphoid organ, and splenic size may vary with disease. However, normal splenic volume is roughly proportional to body length in childhood (Table 1). Accessory spleens or splenuncules are common, being visible in 15% of children as small, rounded structures usually adjacent to the splenic hilum. These are particularly obvious when the spleen is enlarged.

The pancreas lies in the anterior pararenal space of the retroperitoneum. It is more easily visualized at sonography in children as the larger left lobe of liver provides an acoustic window.

The pancrease is less echogenic in young children than it is in adults and echogenicity increases with age and in disease (such as cystic fibrosis). The size of the pancreas is less important in children than in adults but normal sizes have been documented (Table 2).

TABLE 1
Splenic dimensions

Age	Length (cm)
3 months	6
6 months	6.5
1 year	7
2 years	8
4 years	9
6 years	9.5
8 years	10
10 years	11
15 years	12–13

After Rosenberg *et al.* (1991)

TABLE 2
Pancreatic dimensions (cm)

Age	Head	Body	Tail
neonate	1.0	0.6	1.0
up to 1 year	1.5	0.8	1.2
1–5 years	1.7	1.0	1.8
5–10 years	1.8	1.0	1.8
10–19 years	2.0	1.1	2.0

After Siegel, Martin & Worthington (1987).

The genitourinary tract and suprarenal glands

The suprarenal glands are paired retroperitoneal glands lying antero-medial to the upper poles of the kidneys in the perirenal fascia. The right suprarenal gland lies between the right lobe of liver, right diaphragmatic crus, the inferior vena cava and the upper pole of the right kidney. The left lies lateral to the aorta and left diaphragmatic crus, medial to the spleen and behind the stomach. The suprarenal glands are large at birth and may

Fig. 17.
Percutaneous transhepatic cholangiogram (PTC) in an infant showing normal biliary drainage. Contrast medium has entered the bile ducts just within the porta hepatis.

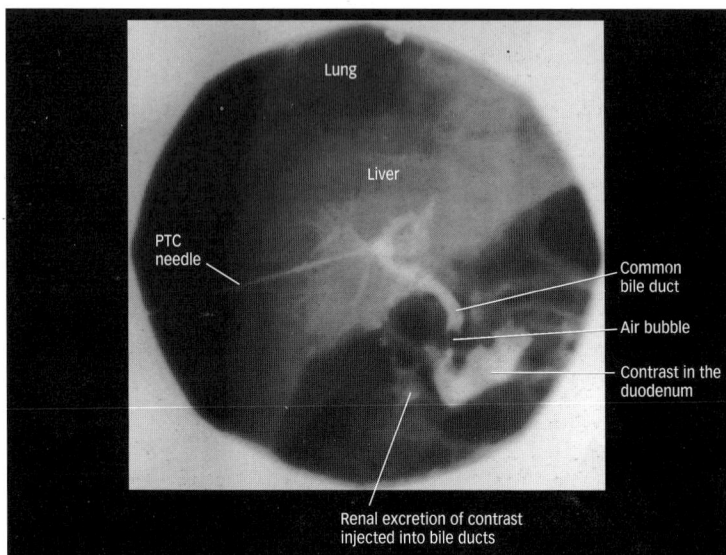

Lung

Liver

PTC needle

Common bile duct

Air bubble

Contrast in the duodenum

Renal excretion of contrast injected into bile ducts

be one-third the mass of the adjacent kidney. Of this mass 80% is fetal cortex, which rapidly undergoes haemorrhagic necrosis after birth, as a result of which the suprarenal glands lose 30% of their weight in the first 2–3 weeks after delivery. The glands have an echogenic centre and hypoechoic rim and have limbs giving a V- or Y-shape, depending upon the plane of imaging (Fig. 18).

The neonatal suprarenal gland is around 1.5 cm long (range 1–3.6 cm) and 0.3 cm thick (range 0.2–0.5). Adult glands may be 4–6 cm long and 0.2–0.6 cm thick (Kangarloo et al., 1986; Oppenheimer, Carroll & Yousem, 1983).

The ultrasound appearances of the neonatal and infant kidney differ from those of the older child in three unique respects. The echogenicity of the cortex is increased, being similar to liver or spleen. This is due to the cellular components of the glomerular tuft occupying a greater proportion of the cortex. The glomeruli form 20% of the neonatal cortex but only 9% of the adult cortex. Secondly, the medullary pyramids are larger and more hypoechoic than in older children. Thirdly, the renal sinus contains less fat than in older children and may not be visible at birth (Fig. 19). Neonatal kidneys may have a more lobulated contour due to the persistence of fetal lobulation after birth. Echogenic septa may also be seen within the neonatal kidney at the anterosuperior or posteroinferior margins, representing the points of fusion of metanephric elements. The majority of kidneys have an adult pattern by 6 months of age.

The lack of renal sinus fat in neonates, together with the prominent hypoechoic pyramids, may give rise to the erroneous diagnosis of hydronephrosis. Minor degrees of upper tract dilatation are more commonly seen in children than adults, particularly when the bladder is full. In these cases the distension will usually resolve after micturition and is of no real significance. The renal size is related to the child's age and build. The average renal length at birth is 4.5 cm. The range of normal sizes increases with age as does the incidence of asymmetry (Table 3).

TABLE 3
Renal dimensions

Age	Average renal length (cm)
birth	4.5
6 months	6.0
1 year	6.25
5 years	8.0
10 years	9.0
18 years	10.5

Congenital variations in renal anatomy are common and affect 3–4% of the population. Unilateral absence of a kidney occurs once in every 1000 births but inability to locate a kidney is a common clinical problem and, in most cases, the kidney is ectopic or small and scarred. Ectopic kidneys lie low in the abdomen or pelvis. They do not have a normal reniform shape as they have not been moulded by the upper abdominal organs. Bilateral renal agenesis occurs once in every 3300 births. These latter cases are usually diagnosed in utero due to the presence of oligohydramnios and other secondary features. Occasionally, an ectopic kidney may cross the midline as it ascends, giving rise to crossed renal ectopia (Fig. 20). Although the kidney lies on the wrong side of the abdomen, its ureter will cross the abdomen to enter the correct side of the bladder. Horseshoe kidney occurs when the kidneys fuse across the midline. The fusion is nearly always at the lower renal poles and has an incidence of 1 in 600. The horseshoe kidney cannot ascend through the abdomen completely as the bridge of renal tissue cannot pass the inferior mesenteric artery. Thus a horseshoe kidney is low in position and the renal axis is more vertical than normal as the lower poles are more medial than normal.

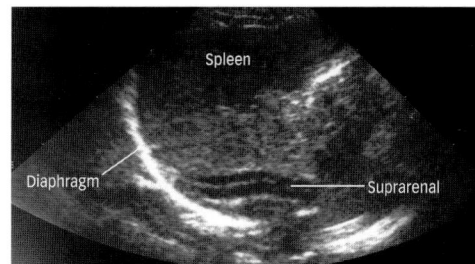

(a)

(b)

Fig. 18.
(a) Longitudinal ultrasound scan of the left upper quadrant of the abdomen showing a long prominent limb of the neonatal suprarenal gland with a thick hypoechoic exterior and an echogenic centre. (b) Longitudinal oblique ultrasound scan of a prominent neonatal suprarenal gland at the upper pole of the right kidney.

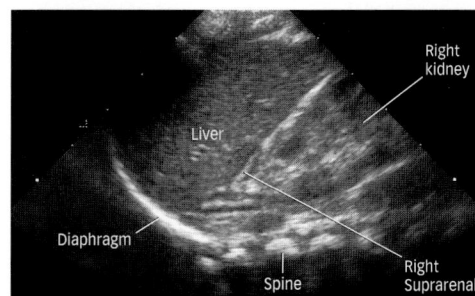

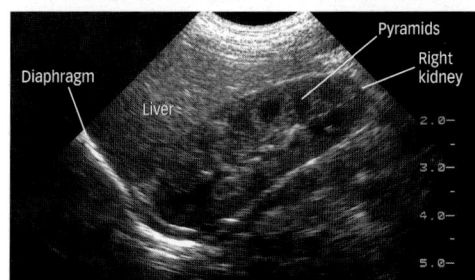

Fig. 19.
Neonatal renal ultrasound (longitudinal scan) showing prominent hypoechoic pyramids, echogenic cortex and a paucity of renal sinus fat.

Twenty-five per cent of kidneys are supplied by more than one renal artery, while only 10% have supernumerary veins. Accessory vessels can cause ureteric compression and are important at angiography. Duplication of the renal collecting system and ureter is common, being found in 1 in 70 people. The duplicated ureters often fuse before reaching the bladder (Fig. 21), but if they enter the bladder separately, the ureter from the lower renal moiety enters the bladder at the site of the normal ureteric orifice. The ureter from the upper moiety enters the bladder below this level at an ectopic site, occasionally entering the urethra below the sphincter causing persistent day and night time wetness.

The bladder in young children is an abdominal organ which rises out of the pelvis as it fills, since the pelvic cavity is too small to contain it. Occasionally, a narrow track persists at the dome of the bladder which represents the remnant of the urachus which extended to the umbilicus *in utero*. This may be visible at cystography or can give rise to midline cysts between the umbilicus and bladder. The female urethra is short and may be imaged at cystography in the anteroposterior projection as congenital abnormalities are rare. The most commonly seen variant at female cystography is reflux of urine into the vagina, which is a normal finding in a girl micturating when lying down. In boys, it is essential to visualize

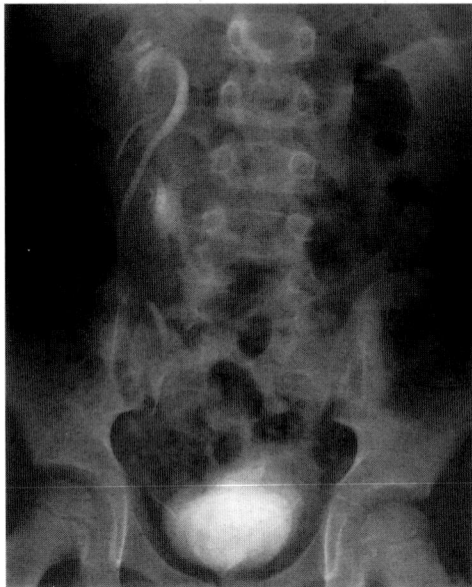

Fig. 20.
Intravenous urogram showing a duplex right kidney with crossed renal ectopia, the left kidney lying on the right.

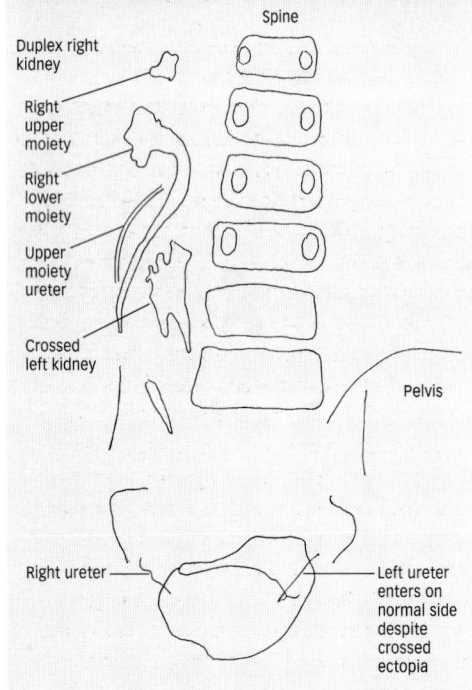

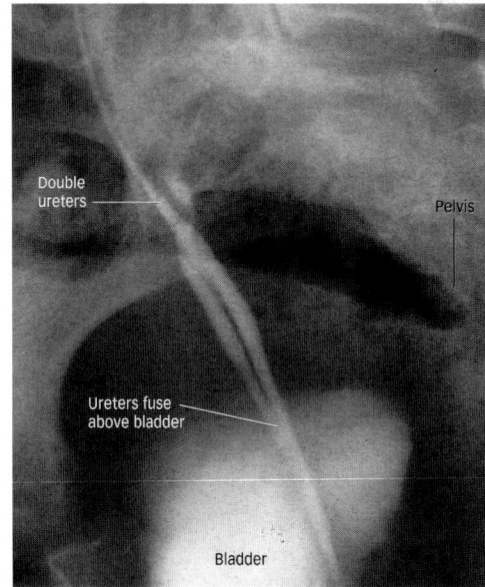

Fig. 21.
Retrograde pyelogram showing duplex ureters crossing then uniting distally before entering the bladder

the entire length of the urethra at micturating cystography as this remains the most reliable means of diagnosing posterior urethral valves (1 in 6000 boys), which may not be easily visible at cystoscopy. A true lateral or steep oblique projection is therefore necessary during forceful micturition (Fig. 22).

The testes arise in the abdomen and descend into the scrotum, where spermatogenesis occurs at a slightly lower temperature than exists in the abdomen. Thirty-three per cent of testes have not reached the scrotum in preterm babies less than 2.5 kg. The incidence of undescended testes at term is 3–4%, falling to 0.7% at 1 year. Between 80 and 90% of undescended testes lie within the inguinal canal just proximal to the internal inguinal ring and 10–20% lie within the abdomen. The testis is an ovoid structure of uniform low to medium echogenicity surrounded by an echogenic line due to the tunica. This becomes more echogenic with age. At 3 months the testis

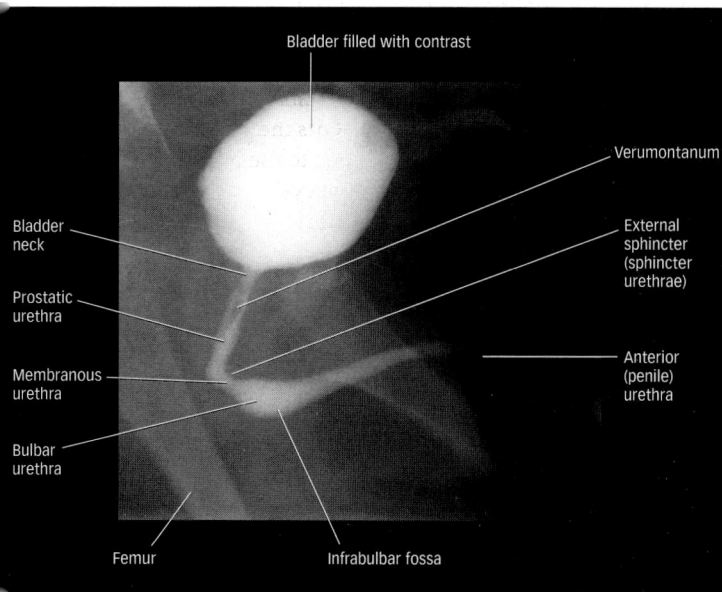

Bladder filled with contrast

Verumontanum

Bladder neck

External sphincter (sphincter urethrae)

Prostatic urethra

Membranous urethra

Anterior (penile) urethra

Bulbar urethra

Femur

Infrabulbar fossa

Fig. 22. Micturating cystourethrograms (oblique views) showing (*a*) the abdominal position of the distended urinary bladder in young children and (*b*) a normal posterior urethral calibre. (Courtesy of Dr S.T. Vinnicombe.)

(*b*)

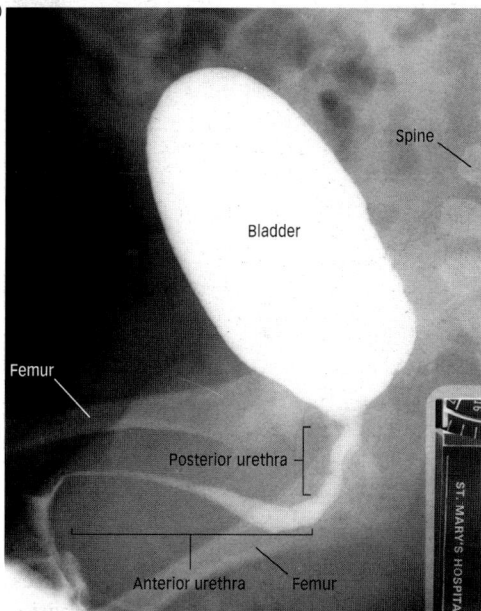

Spine

Bladder

Femur

Posterior urethra

Anterior urethra

Femur

ST. MARY'S HOSPITAL

Fig. 23. Longitudinal ultrasound scan of the female pelvis showing the slender calibre of a prepubertal uterus.

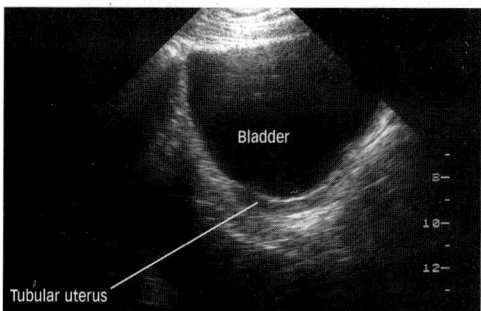

Bladder

Tubular uterus

The uterus and ovaries are of moderate size at birth, due to the effect of maternal hormones. The infantile uterus is seen as a tubular structure (Fig. 23), although unlike the mature uterus, the cervix has a slightly greater anteroposterior diameter than the fundus. The neonatal uterus measures 2.3–4.6 cm in length by 1.2 cm in width. The endometrial cavity is usually visible as an echogenic line with a slightly hypoechoic halo around it in 30% of female infants. The uterus reduces in size after birth, its size remaining relatively constant until 7 years. Slow growth then occurs, which becomes more rapid, leading up to the menarche. The uterus elongates and the fundus thickens to gain the adult pear shape (5–8 cm long, 1.5–3 cm thick and 3.5 cm wide.) The ovaries are usually found in the pelvis, but can lie anywhere from the inferior edge of the kidney to the broad ligament. They can easily be displaced from the infantile pelvis by a full bladder. Small follicles can be seen within many ovaries throughout childhood. These are a normal finding, which can be resolved by modern high resolution ultrasound scanners. The average neonatal ovary measures 1.5 cm in length, 0.3 cm in width and 0.25 cm in thickness. Ovarian volume is calculated by the formula, $0.5 \times length \times width \times thickness$. The average ovarian volume is 1 cm^3 at 1 year, 0.7 cm^3 at 2 years and up to 33.8 cm^3 at 12 years. After puberty, the ovary is 2.5–5 cm long, 1.5–3 cm wide and 0.6–1.5 cm thick with a volume of up to 18 cm^3.

Paediatric bones and joints

Ultrasonography is an excellent method of demonstrating the neonatal hip, which is a largely cartilaginous structure. It also allows dynamic evaluation of the hip during manipulation. Examination is initially undertaken in the coronal plane with the femur extended and using a high frequency linear array probe. The cartilaginous femoral head, labrum and bony acetabulum are demonstrated (Figs. 24 and 25). The femoral head is seen as a round, hypoechoic structure containing fine stippled echoes. As the hip matures, ossification becomes visible at the centre of the femoral head. The acetabulum is seen as an echogenic bony cup which has a V-shape on transverse sections. The V is formed by the ischium posteriorly and the pubis anteriorly. The central defect between these bones is the triradiate cartilage. At least 50% of the femoral head should be contained within the acetabulum. Measurements may be taken to assess the depth of the acetabulum and the position of

measures 2 cm in length by 1.2 cm in width. The length remains relatively constant until 6 years following which the testes grow, reaching 3–5 cm in length and 2–3 cm in width post-puberty. Testicular volume is 1.1 cm^3 in neonates and up to 30 cm^3 after puberty.

Head   Labrum   Foot
Gluteus
Femoral head
Calcified femoral neck
Ilium
Gap of triradiate cartilage
Acetabulum

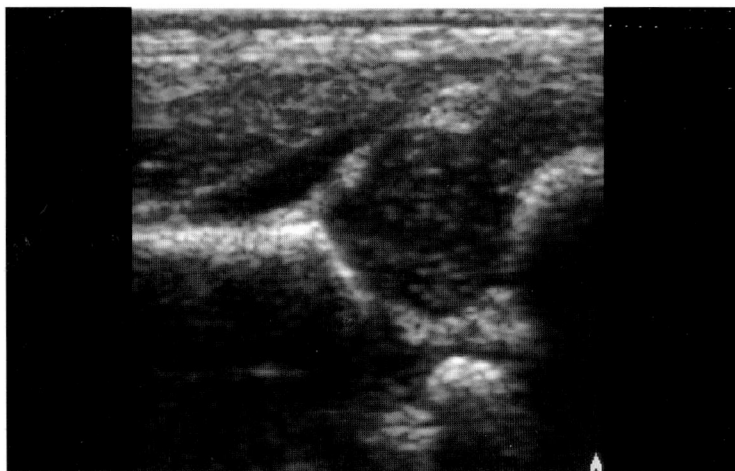

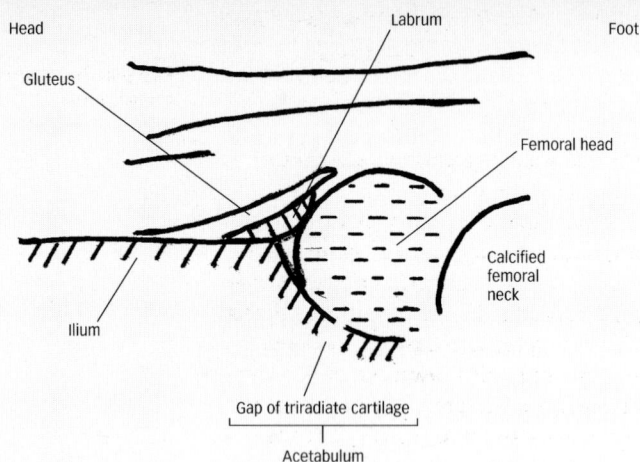

Fig. 24.
Ultrasound scan of the hip of an infant showing the stippled appearance of the femoral head.

ticularly of the hip, which is frequently scanned to demonstrate an effusion. In all cases, the normal side should be examined first to act as a reference.

Bony maturation and development are assessed on a single film of the left (non-dominant) hand and wrist, centred over the head of the third metacarpal. The appearances are compared with a set of standard radiographs (Greulich & Pyle, 1959). A more scientific approach which gives similar results is also available (Tanner *et al.*, 1984). It allows assessment of the maturation of individual bones, each of which is given a score. This is preferable in any case of endocrine disease which may affect differential bony maturation.

Bones form by the ossification of cartilage (e.g. long bones) or membrane (e.g. clavicle). The long bones have a cartilagenous growth plate or physis (Fig. 27). The ossified area distal to the physis is the epiphysis, whilst the area of bone closer to the centre of the shaft is the metaphysis. The central shaft of the long bone is termed the diaphysis, while the area where the metaphysis and diaphysis merge is termed the diametaphysis. An apophysis is an accessory area of ossification which occurs at the side of the bone and does not contribute to

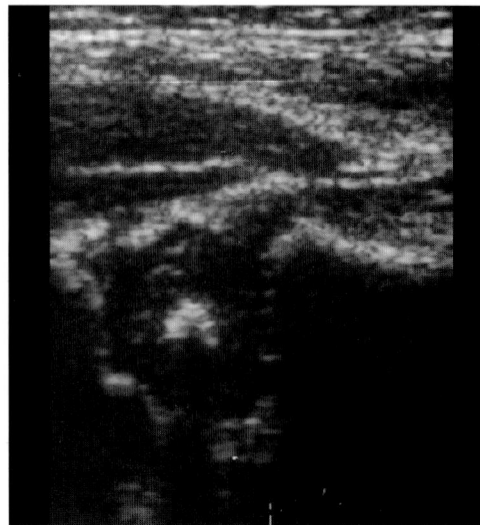

the labrum. A line is drawn parallel to the ilium (Fig. 26). A second line is then drawn from the bony edge of the acetabulum along the edge of the labrum and a third line is drawn from the outer edge of the bony acetabulum to the lowest part of the acetabulum deep within the joint. The alpha angle assesses the depth of the acetabulum. Dysplastic acetabulae have low alpha angles and high beta angles. The beta angle assesses the prominence of the labrum. Normally the alpha angle is above 60°.

In the dynamic assessment, the hip is examined with the child supine and the femur extended. The hip is then flexed as the examiner applies backward pressure and reviews femoral head position by constant sonographic monitoring. Abduction and adduction movements are then made as in the modified Ortolani test looking for evidence of subluxation or dislocation.

Sonography is gaining increasing acceptance as a means of evaluating growth plates and joints in children. The radiologist should therefore try to become accustomed to the normal appearances of bones and joints, par-

Fig. 25.
Longitudinal ultrasound scan of the infant hip showing femoral head calcification.

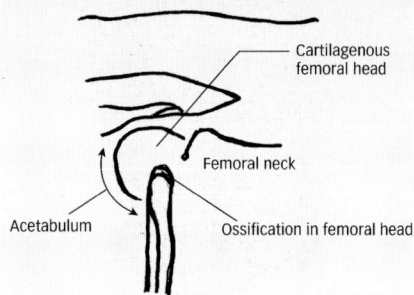

Cartilagenous femoral head
Femoral neck
Acetabulum
Ossification in femoral head

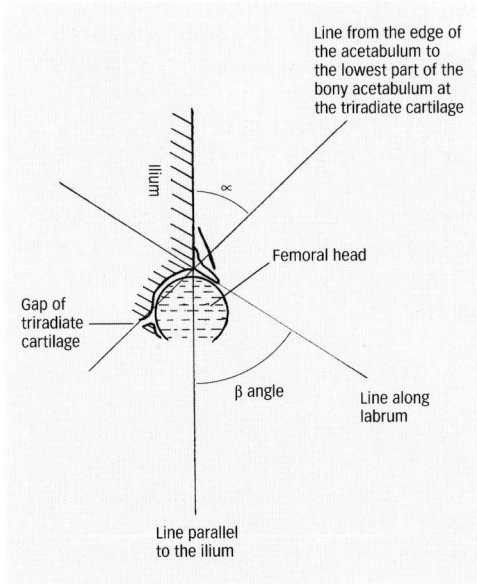

Fig. 26.
valuation of the infant hip.

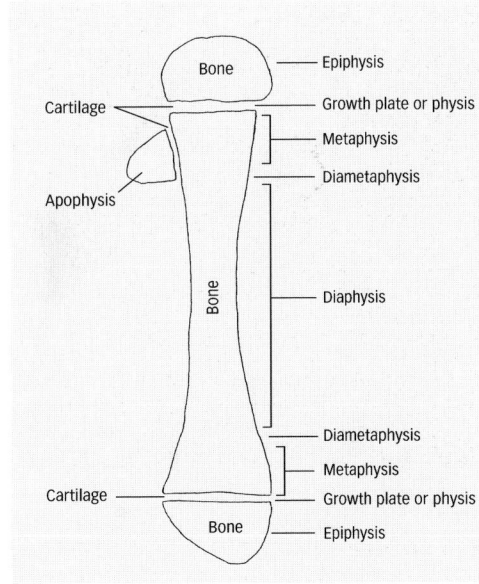

Fig. 27.
Anatomical nomenclature
of a long bone.

bone length, usually acting as a site for the insertion of ligaments and tendons.

The appearance of primary (shaft) and secondary (epiphyseal/apophyseal) ossification centres can give a rough estimation of the age of a child, although it should be remembered that there is significant variation between populations and girls show more rapid maturation than boys. The areas of greatest metabolic bone activity at the growth plates are seen as areas of increased activity on isotope bone scans (Fig. 28).

References

Kangarloo, H., Diament, M.J., Gold, R.H., Barrett, C., Lippe, B., Geffner, M., Boechat, M.I., Dietrich, R.B. & Amundson, G.M. (1986). Sonography of adrenal glands in neonates and children. *Journal of Clinical Ultrasound*, **14**, 43–7.

Lang, I.A., Teel, R.L. & Stark, A.R. (1988). Diaphragm movement in newborn infants. *Journal of Paediatrics*, **112**, 638–43.

Oppenheimer, D.A., Carroll, B.A. & Yousem, S. (1983). Sonography of normal neonatal adrenal gland. *Radiology*, **146**, 157–60.

Rosenberg, H.K., Markowitz, R.I., Kolberg, H., Park, C., Hubbard, A., Bellah, R.D. (1991). Normal splenic size in infants and children. *American Journal of Roentgenology*, **157**, 119–21.

Siegel, M.J., Martin, K.W. & Worthington, J.L. (1987). Normal and abnormal pancreas in children. Ultrasound studies. *Radiology*, **165**, 15–18.

Further reading

Greulich, W.W. & Pyle, S.I. (1959). *Radiographic Atlas of Skeletal Development of the Hand and Wrist*. 2nd edn. Stanford: Stanford University Press.

Tanner, J.M., Whitehouse, R.H., Marshall, W.A., Healy, M.J.R. & Goldstein, H. (1984). *Assessment of Skeletal Maturity and Prediction of Adult Height (TW2 method)*. 2nd edn. New York: Academic Press.

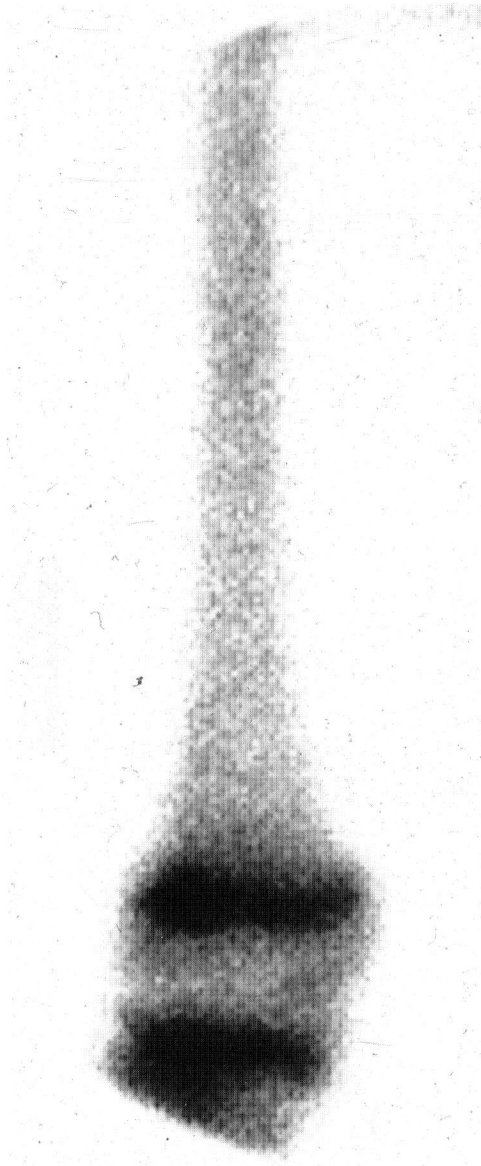

Fig. 28.
Isotope bone scan showing increased tracer uptake at the growth plates at the knee.

Index

Note: page numbers in *italics* refer to figures.

abdomen 7–8
  fetal circumference 411–12
  obstetric anatomy 408–12
  sympathetic plexuses 276–7
abdominal lymphatic system
  imaging 274
  nodes 274–6
abdominal radiography, plain 208
abdominal wall
  anterior
    anatomy 198–204, *205*
    fascia 280
    imaging 189
    muscles 198–203, *204*
    superfical fascia 198
  posterior 277–8
  veins 274
abducent nerve 36
abscess
  ischiorectal 281
  pericolic 219
  psoas 281
accessory nerve 32, 35
  cranial root 35
  jugular foramen 94
  lymph node chain 115
  tongue 107
acetabular labrum 358
acetabular ligament, transverse 358, 359
acetabulum 352, 358
  fibrofatty pad 358
  paediatric 427, *427*
Achilles tendon 370, 373
Achilles tendon *see* calcaneal tendon
acini 130, 132, *132*
acoustic neurinoma 93
acromioclavicular joint 9, 333–4, 337
acromioclavicular ligament 333
acromion 332, 333
  process 9, 337
acromiothoracic artery 385
Adam's apple see laryngeal prominence
adductor brevis muscle 362
adductor canal 387
adductor hiatus 392
adductor longus muscle 362
adductor magnus muscle 362
adductor tubercle 13, *14*
adenoids 109–10
aditus 87, *88, 89*

agger nasi cells 106
airways 128, *129*
Allen's test 382
alveolar process, inferior 99
alveolar recess 104
alveoli, development 122, 123
amastia 179
amazia 179
ambient cistern 50
Ammon's horn 46, 47
amnion 400, 401
amniotic volume 399
ampulla of Vater 252, 255
amygdala 40
anal canal 221–2
  development 187
anal columns 221
anal sphincters 221–2
anal valves 221
anatomical snuffbox 10, 11, 386
aneurysms, berry 50
angiography
  aorta 272
  brain 19
  cardiac circulation 154
  chest imaging 122
  renal tract 262–3
  small intestine 216
angle of Louis 4, 6
angular artery 55
ankle joint 371–3
  fibrous capsule 371
  imaging 377, *378, 380*
  movements 372
  relations 372–3
annular ligament 343
annulus fibrosus 304, *305*
annulus of Zinn 70
anococcygeal body 281
antecubital vein 383
anterior atlanto-dental interval (AADI) 314
anterior junction 144–5
aorta 167–8
  abdominal 8, 272
  angiography 272
  ascending 136, 167
  calcification 271
  CT 271
  descending 141–2, 167, 168
  divisions 386
  fixed points in thorax 169
  imaging 153, 271–2
  MRI 272

Index

oesophageal branches 209
pelvic 281
segmental branches 310
thoracic 153
ultrasound 271, 272
aortic arch 6, 142, 144, 167, 168
angiography 154
anomalies 17, 168
branches 145
development 155–6
fetal 407
right-sided 421
aortic coarctation 156
aortic hiatus 146, 150
diaphragm 168
aortic root 167, 168
aortic valve 160, 163
aortopulmonary window 143, 144–5
lymph nodes 147
apocrine sweat gland 173
appendices epiploicae 218
appendicoliths 217
appendicular artery 233
appendix 217, 219
appendix testis 292, 301
aqueous 68
arachnoid granulations 21
transverse sinus 56
arachnoid mater 26, 328
areae gastricae 212, 213
arc of Bühler 224–5
arc of Riolan 231, 232
arcuate eminence 90, 93
arcuate fibres 35
arcuate ligament, medial 278, 282
arcus epiploicus magnus of Barkow 227
areola 174
arteria pancreatica magna 226, 227, 255
arteria radicularis magna 329–30
arteriography, vertebral column 303
arteriovenous fistula, spinal cord
communicating veins 330
artery of Adamkiewicz 329–30
artery–bronchus ratio measurement 132
arthrography
double contrast 337
knee 367
aryepiglottic fold 112
arytenoid cartilage 112
atlantal ligament, transverse 314
atlanto-axial joints 314
atlanto-axial ligament, accessory 313
atlanto-occipital joint 313–14
atlanto-occipital membrane 312, 314
atlas 3, 311–12
transverse ligament 313
atrial cavity, development 154
atrioventricular node 162, 163
atrioventricular valve 157, 158–9
atrium
development 154
left 159–60
right 156–7
auditory canal, internal 91
auditory meatus
external 86, 100, 101
internal 89, 90–1, 93
auditory ossicles 87, 89
auditory pathways, imaging 85–6
auricular artery, posterior 117
autosomal recessive polycystic kidney
disease (ARPKD) 259
axilla 334–5
axillary artery 11, 334, 382, 385
axillary lymph nodes 334–5, 396

surgical levels 174
axillary nerve 349
axillary sheath 334
axillary vein 11, 334, 385, 391
axis 3, 311, 312–13
azygo-oesophageal line 145, 148, 149, 210
azygo-oesophageal recess 127, 144, 145, 149
azygos arch 137
azygos artery 55
azygos continuation of the inferior vena
cava 127
azygos fissure 136–7
azygos vein 6, 123, 127, 136–7, 169
aortic hiatus 146
embryology 394
oesophageal drainage 209

back, surface anatomy 8–9
Baker's cyst 364
Bartholin's duct 108
Bartholin's gland 280
basal ganglia 40–1
basal plate 414
basilar artery 52, 53, 59
basilic vein 11, 390, 391
basiocciput 311
basisphenoid synchondrosis 24, 25
basivertebral vein 310, 330
biceps femoris muscle 363
biceps muscle 341, 343
biceps tendon 343
bicipital aponeurosis 11, 343
bilaminar zone 101
bile duct
common 424
tributaries 251
biliary atresia 249, 424
biliary system imaging in children 424
biliary tree 241, 251–3
extrahepatic 253
biparietal diameter (BPD) 402
bladder 284–5
development 260–1
fetal 408, 411
paediatric 426
trigone 260–1, 285
wall 269
blastocyst 400
blood vessels of head and neck 3–4
Bohler's angle 377
bone marrow, vertebral 304
bones
age assessment 349
growth 331–2
growth plates 429
isotope scan 429
long 428–9
maturation 415
ossification 428–9
paediatric 415, 427–9, 427
bowel
atresia 187
stenosis 187
vascular supply 208
Bowman's capsule 265
brachial artery 11, 382, 384, 385–6
deep 177
brachial plexus 120, 334, 349
axillary artery relations 385
brachial vein 391
brachialis muscle 340, 343
brachiocephalic artery 6, 141
aortic arch 168
development 155
thyroid gland 115

brachiocephalic trunk 383
brachiocephalic vein 120, 127, 128, 142,
143, 168, 209
embryology 393
formation 391
interconnecting with superior vena
cava 144
left 169
right 3, 6, 169
brachium, superior 75
brain
angiography 19
child (4 years) 60
development 59–60
digital subtraction angiography 19
gyri 403, 418
imaging 17–19
intracranial circulation 50–2
MRI in children 415, 417
myelination in children 415
neonatal 59
normal development 28–30
sulci 403, 418
brainstem 31, 33, 35
osseous relationsip of spine 314
breasts
accessory 178, 179
adipose tissue 180, 181
benign change 176
development 173–4
ductography 181–2, 183
fat imaging 183
fatty replacement tissue 176
fibroglandular tissue 176–7, 180–1, 183
hypoplasia 179
imaging 173
intramammary lymph nodes 176
lymphatic drainage 174
male 177
malignancy risk 177
naevus 180
papilloma 179, 182
pathological calcification 179
pathophysiological changes 175
retroareolar ducts 182
sebaceous gland calcification 179, 180
ultrasound 179–81, 182
breathing coordination with swallowing
422
broad ligament 303, 304
bronchi 128, 129, 138
segmental 130, 132
bronchial arteries 138, 168
bronchial buds 123
bronchial tree 129
bronchial veins 127, 128, 140
bronchography, chest imaging 122
bronchopulmonary lymph nodes 137
bronchopulmonary segments 130, 133
bronchovascular bundle 130, 132
bronchus
apicoposterior 140
main-stem 130, 131
buccal cavity 106
Buck's fascia 302
Budd–Chiari syndrome 248
bulbospongiosus muscle 280
bulbourethral glands 281
bulbus cordis 155
bundle of His 163

caecal arteries 216
caecum 8, 216–17
anatomical relations 216
lymph drainage 217

paediatric 423
plain abdominal radiography 208
vascular supply 216–17
calcaneal pitch measurement 377
calcaneal tendon 12, 370, 371, 373, 374
calcaneocuboid joint 377
calcaneofibular ligament 372
calcaneonavicular coalition 378
calcaneonavicular ligament 372, 376–7
calcaneum 12–13, 373, 375, 376
congenital fusion with navicular 378
imaging 377
calcar avis 80
calcarine artery 60
callosal cistern 50
callosomarginal artery 53, 54
capitate bone, ossification 347, 348
capitulum 339, 341
capsulopalpebral muscle of Hessel 71
cardiac arrhythmia, fetal 406
cardiac circulation, angiography 154
cardiac notch 5
cardiac pulsation, fetal 400
cardiac valve calcification 153
cardiac vein 166, 167
anterior 157
cardiac vessel calcification 153
cardinal veins 393
cardio-oesophageal arteries 225
cardiophrenic angle, anterior 147
caroticocavernous fistula 52
carotid artery 3
aberrant 94
common 115, 141
aortic arch 168
bifurcation 116, 119
branches 116
Doppler flow studies 119
development 155
duplex sonography 118, 119
external 28, 72, 116
branches 116–17
duplex sonography 119
nasal cavity supply 104
thyroid gland 115
internal 50–2
branches 51–2
circle of Willis 52
course 50–1
duplex sonography 118
embryonic brain 28
nasal cavity supply 104
optic chiasm blood supply 77
optic nerve relationship 73
termination 52
carotid pulse 3
carotid sheath 115, 119
carotid siphon 50
carpal bones 10, 345, 346
fetal 413
carpal tunnel 346, 346
carpi radialis muscle tendon 346
carpi ulnaris muscle 346, 349
carpometacarpal joint, thumb 348
carpus 344–7
cauda equina 327, 328
caudate nucleus 40–1, 418
cavagram, inferior vena cava 273
cave of Retzius 286
cavernosography 302
cavernous nodules 56
cavernous sinus 28, 36, 40, 56, 57
cavernous veins 302
caviar sign of Kinmouth 396
cavum septum pellucidum 46, 48, 403, 4

vum septum vergae 418
vum vergae 48, 49
ntral nervous system, obstetric
    anatomy 402–4
phalic vein 11, 383, 390
rebellar artery 59
anterior inferior 59, 93
posterior 56–7, 60
posterior inferior 58–60
superior 59
rebellar hemispheres, fetal 414
rebellopontine angle 35
cistern 93
rebellum 34–5, 36, 37, 39
fetal 402, 403
paediatric 417
peduncles 34, 36, 39
rebral aqueduct 37
rebral artery
anterior 52, 53–5, 55, 73
middle 52, 53, 55, 78, 417
posterior 54, 55, 60, 77, 78, 79
rebral envelope 26–7
rebral hemispheres 42–3
visual cortex 83
rebral parenchyma 33, 34, 35–7, 38,
    39–47
brainstem 31, 33, 35
cranial nerves 35–6
rebral vein, middle 57
rebral ventricles 28, 47–50
rebrospinal fluid
CT 301
fourth ventricle 49
MRI 302
optic nerve 69
rvical artery 115–19
ascending 383
duplex sonography 117–19
transverse 383–4
rvical dorsal root ganglia 326
rvical fascia
deep 111, 114
superficial 111
rvical glands 301
rvical ligaments, transverse 303, 304
rvical lordosis 303
rvical lymph node chain, deep 115
rvical rib 316
rvical spine 308, 315–17, 320–1
alignment 316–17
canal 309
facet joints 307
movements 309
prevertebral soft tissue 316–17
rvical vertebrae 8, 315–16
rvix
paediatric 427
uterine 303
amberlain's line 314
emonucleolysis 303
est
imaging 121–2
obstetric anatomy 405–6, 407, 408
paediatric anatomy 419–21
plain radiography 121
est wall 125–8
blood supply 126–8
muscles 125–6
nerves 128
iasmatic cistern 50, 74
ilaiditi syndrome 218, 219
ildren
size 415
see also paediatric anatomy

cholangiography, intravenous/oral 241
chorda tympani nerve 92
chordae tendinae 158, 160
chorion 400, 401
chorionic membrane 400, 401
chorionic plate 414
chorionic villi 400
choroid 66
choroid plexus 47, 48, 403
    paediatric 417, 418
choroidal artery, anterior 51–2, 77
ciliary body 66
cingulate gyrus 44, 417
circle of Willis 3, 40, 50, 52
circumflex artery, left 166
circumvallate papillae 96
cisterna chyli 141, 276, 397
cisterna magna 49–50
    contrast medium injection 302–3
    fetal 403, 404
claustrum 40, 41
clavicle 9, 332–3
    fetal 405, 406
    ossification 333
clavipectoral fascia 391
cleft lip/palate 95, 405
clivus 24–5
cloaca 187, 260
coccygeal vertebrae 354
coccygeus muscle 280
coccyx 351, 353, 354
cochlear 89
    aqueduct 90
Cockett's point 393
coeliac arteriography 241
coeliac artery origins 224–5
coeliac axis 225, 227, 228
    dorsal pancreatic artery 231
    ultrasound 272
coeliac ganglion, liver nerve supply 249
coeliac nodes, abdominal lymphatics 274
coeliac plexus 276
coeliac trunk 223, 224, 225
    arteriography 213
    collateral circulation 225, 227
coeliacomesenteric trunk 224, 225
colic 423
colic artery 217, 231, 233
colic nodes, abdominal lymphatics 275
colic vein 235
Colles' fascia 280, 281
colliculus, superior 74–5
colon
    ascending 216, 217
    descending 218
    fetal 408
    mesentery development 187
    reversed rotation 187
    sigmoid 8, 218
        innominate grooves 219
    structure 218–19
    transverse 216, 217–18, 219
common bile duct 251–2
communicating artery
    anterior 53
    posterior 52, 77
computed tomographic arterio-
    portography (CTAP) 239
computed tomography (CT)
    abdominal lymphatic system 274
    anterior abdominal wall 189
    aorta 271
    axial scans 18
    bladder 285
    brain imaging 17–19
    chest imaging 121, 122

cisternography 85
female genital tract 305
foot 378–9
gastrointestinal tract 207
high resolution (HRCT) 85, 86, 121
hip joint 359
inferior vena cava 273
intracranial visual pathway 62
iodinated contrast medium 18
liver 242
lower limb 351
lymph nodes 395, 396
myelography 302
optic nerve 61
orbit 61
pelvimetry 356–7
peritoneum 189
prostate gland 288, 289
renal tract 260, 262
seminal vesicles 289
shoulder joint arthrography 337–8
suprarenal glands 269, 270
upper abdomen organs 239, 240
vertebral column 301–2
conchae 103
condyloid process 2
congenital anomalies 123–4
congenital heart disease, paediatric 420
coning 27
connective tissue, extraperitoneal 203
conoid ligament 333
conus artery 164, 165
conus medullaris 9, 328
Cooper's ligaments 181
coracoacromial arch 336
coracobrachialis muscle 341
coracoclavicular ligament 333
coracohumeral ligament 335
coracoid process 332, 333, 335
cord see umbilical cord
corona radiata 41
coronal suture 21
coronal venous plexus 330
coronary artery
    left 161, 166, 167
    right 164, 165, 166, 168
coronary circulation 164, 165, 166–7
coronary dominance 164
coronary ligament 194–5
    superior 250, 250
coronary sinus 144, 157, 159, 166–7
    anterior 168
    posterior 161
coronary veins 166–7
coronoid fossa 341, 342
coronoid process 2
corpora albicantia 305
corpora cavernosa 302
corpora lutea 305
corpora quadrigemina 75, 77
corpus callosum 42
    myelination 29–30
    paediatric 417, 418
corpus spongiosum 286, 302
corpus striatum 40
cortical gyri 42, 43
corticobulbar tracts 41–2
corticospinal tracts 41–2, 325
costal cartilage 6, 125, 198
costal elements 311
    vestigial 355
costal margin 4, 7
costocervical artery, left 384
costocervical trunk 310
costoclavicular ligament 333
costotransverse articulations 317

Cowper's glands 281
cranial fossa 22, 23–4
cranial nerves 28, 35–6
cranial ultrasonography, paediatric
    416–18
craniocervical lymphatic system 115
craniovertebral joints 313–14
craniovertebral junction 311–14
craniovertebral ligaments 313
cribriform plate 21, 22
cricoid cartilage 3, 112
cricopharyngeus 110, 422
cricothyroid ligament 2, 3
cricothyroid puncture 15
crista falciformis 91
crista galli 21
crista supraventricularis 157
crista terminalis 156, 162
CRITOL mnemonic 341
crown–rump length 400, 401
cruciate ligament 365, 366
    anterior 367
    posterior 365, 367
cubital vein, median 11, 343, 390–1
cuboid bone 374, 379
cuneiform bone 375, 379
cystic artery 228, 253
cystic duct 251, 253
cystic veins 253

dacryocystography 62, 70
decidua capsularis/parietalis 400, 401, 413
defaecation proctography 222
deglutition 208
deltoid collateral ligament 370
deltopectoral groove 391
deltopectoral triangle see infraclavicular
    fossa
Denonvillier's fascia 286
dentate gyrus 46, 47
denticulate ligament 325, 328
dentition 101–2
dermoids, inclusion 96
descending artery, posterior 164
diaphragm 124, 125–6, 150
    aortic hiatus 168
    congenital hernia 124
    fetal 406, 408
    oesophgeal hiatus 140
    paediatric 421–2
    posterior abdominal wall 278, 282
    see also pelvic diaphragm
diaphragma oris 106
diaphragma sellae 28
diaphragmatic crura 146, 282
diaphragmatic hernia, congenital 124
diencephalon 36, 39–40
digestive system 207–8
digital subtraction angiography (DSA)
    brain 19
    gastrointestinal tract 223
    limb arteries 381–3
    vascular imaging of orbit/visual
        pathway 62
digital veins, foot 392
diploic veins 21
discography 303, 305, 306
diverticulum 156
Doppler flow studies 118, 119
    paediatric intracranial arteries 416
Dorello's canal 36
dorsal nerve root ganglia 301, 326
dorsalis pedis
    artery 388
    pulse 14
dorsum sella 22

duct of Rivinius 108
duct of Santorini 255
duct of Wirsung 255
ductography 181–2, *183*
ductus arteriosus 155, 170, 421
ductus venosus 409, 410
duodenal cap 213, 214
duodenal loop, paediatric 423
duodenocolic ligament 196, *198*
duodenum 213–14
　ampulla of Vater 255
　development 186
　lymphatic drainage 214
duplex sonography, cervical arteries
　117–19
dura 27, 327–8
dura mater 26
　meningeal sheath of optic nerve 69
dural folds 27, 28
dural sac 328
　CT 301
　termination 9
　thoracic 309
dural venous sinuses 26, *27*, 55, 56–7

ear 86–7, 88, 89–94
　imaging 85–6
echocardiography *see* ultrasound, cardiac
ejaculatory duct 259, 260, 286, 287, 289,
　292
elbow, ossification *340*, 341
elbow joint *340*, 342–3
　radial nerve 349
embryo 400
emissary vein 21, 22, 26
endocardial cushion development 154
endolymph 90
endometrium 303, 305, 306–1
endoscopic retrograde
　cholecystopancreatography (ERCP)
　241
epicondyle 340
　lateral 10
epicranial aponeurosis 21
epididymis 259, 290–1
　imaging 292–301
epidural vein 320
epidural venous plexus 310–11, 330
epigastric artery 201, 204, 282, 283, 387
epigastric vein 201
epiglottis 111, *112*
epiphyseal line 375
epiploic artery 230
epiploic foramen 189, 191, 243
epithalamus 39
epitympanum 88, 89
erector spinae muscle 126, 308
ethmoid bone, perpendicular plate 97
ethmoid infundibulum 104
ethmoid sinus 103, 106
Eustachian tube 86, 87, 108
Eustachian valve 157
eventration, partial 150
extensor muscles 308–9
extradural space 327–8
extraocular muscles 70–1
extrapyramidal system 325
eye 61–2, 66–8

fabella 361
face 97
　development 95–6
　inclusion dermoids 96
　obstetric anatomy 404–5
facet joints 306–7

facial artery 116
facial canal, cochlear section 92, *94*
facial colliculi 35
facial musculature 98
facial nerve 36, 91–2, *94*
　cerebellopontine angle cistern 93
　facial muscle innervation 98
　labyrinthine segment 91–2, *94*
　parotid gland 107
　tongue 96
　tympanic segment 87, 88, 92, *94*
facial skeleton 97–8
facial veins 119
falciform ligament 195, *196*, 249, 250, *250*
falcotentorial junction 76
Fallopian tubes 279, 301, 304
falx cerebelli 28
falx cerebri 27
fascia lata 201
fasciculus cuneatus 35
fasciculus gracilis 35
fat, epidural 319–20
fat lines, properitoneal 208
faucial pillars 110
femoral artery 13, 14, 381–2, 387–8
　circumflex 361, 388
　common 387–8
　deep 361, 388
　　external pudendal branch 291
　superficial 388
femoral canal 381
femoral head, blood supply 361
femoral muscles, anterior 362–3
femoral nerve 281, 381, 382
femoral pulse 13
femoral vein 13, 389, 392
femur 12, 360–2
　condyles 360, 361
　fetal 412–13
　gluteal tuberosity 355
　greater trochanter 12
　head 357–8, 360
　　paediatric 427, *427*
　intercondylar fossa 367–8
　ossification 361–2
　trochanters 360
fertilization 400
fetal age assessment 402
fetal anomalies, structural 399
fetal development 399
fetal gender *411*, 412
fetal lie 399
fetal weight estimation 399
fibula 12, 369–70
　fetal *412*, 413
fibular collateral ligament 365
filum terminale 328
　paediatric 419
finger bones 347
flexor digitorum longus muscle 371
flexor digitorum profundus muscle 346
flexor digitorum superficialis muscle 346
fontanelle 20, 402, 416
foot 12–13, 372–6
　calcaneocuboid joint 377
　CT 378–9
　cuboid bone 374
　cuneiform bone 374
　fetal *412*, 413
　imaging 377–9, *380*
　longitudinal arches 13
　MRI 379
　navicular 374, 375
　ossification 375
　plain radiography 377–8

sesamoid bones 375, *375*
subtalar joint 376–7
superficial veins 14
tarsus 372
veins 392
see also calcaneum; metatarsal bones;
　phalanges; talus
foramen lacerum 23
foramen of Magendie 35, 49
foramen magnum 311, 328
foramen of Monro 46, 47, *48*, 49
　paediatric 418
foramen ovale 22, 155
foramen rotundum 22, 99
foramen secundum 154, *155*
foramen spinosum 22
foramen transversarium 312
foramen of Vesalius 22, 24
foramen of Winslow *see* epiploic foramen
foramina of Luschka 49
foraminal boundary, anterior 307
foraminal veins 308
forebrain, fetal development 402
foregut 207, 208
　development 185–6
fornix *46*, 47
fossa of Rosenmuller 109, 110
fovea capitis 357–8
frontal bone 21, 22
　orbit 64–5
　orbital plate 65
frontal lobe 42, 43
　frontal process, orbit 63
frontal recess 104
frontal sinus 103, 104, *105*
frontonasal process 95
frontonasal prominence fusion 404–5
frontopolar artery 53
frontozygomatic suture 1

galea aponeurotica 21
gall bladder 250, 252–3, *253*
　anomalies 253
　cystic artery 228
　fetal 410
　imaging 239, *240*, 241
　lymphatic drainage 253
　paediatric 424
gastric artery
　accessory left 227
　left 225–6, *228*
　　oesophageal branches 209
　right 225, 228–9, *228*
　short 227
gastric emptying, ^{111m}Indium DPTA
　212–13
gastric group of nodes, abdominal
　lymphatics 275
gastric vein, left 209
gastric vessels 257
gastro-oesophageal reflux, children 415
gastro-splenic ligament 257
gastrocnemius bursa 364
gastrocnemius muscle 361, 363, 370
gastrocnemius–semimembranosus bursa
　364
gastrocolic ligament 217
gastroduodenal artery 214, 226, 227, 228,
　229–30
gastroepiploic artery 225, 226, 227
gastrohepatic ligament *196*, 198
gastrointestinal tract
　arterial anatomy 224–34
　arteriography 223–4
　embryology 185–7, 207–8

endodermal lining proliferation 187
　imaging 207
　lumen recanalization 187
　paediatric 422–4
　regions 207
　vascular anatomy 223–35
　venous anatomy 234–5
gastrosplenic ligament 195, *196*
gemelli muscles 355
genicular anastomosis 388
geniculate body *31*, 39, 40
　lateral 74–5, 77
geniculate ganglion 91, 92
geniculocalcarine pathway 75–6
genioglossus muscles 107
genital tract
　female 302
　male 286–302
genitourinary tract, paediatric 424–7
germinal matrix of paediatric brain 418
Gerota's fascia 266, 267
gestational age 399
gestational sac 400
glabella 1
glenohumeral ligament 335
glenoid fossa 332, 335
glenoid labrum 335
globus pallidus 18, 41
glomerulus 265
glomus tympanicum tumour 94
glossoepiglottic fold 111
glossopharyngeal nerve 35, 93, 96
glottis *113*
gluteal artery 283, 284, 356, 361
gluteus maximus muscle 355
gluteus medius 355
gluteus minimus 355
goitre, retrosternal 96
gonadal vein 273, 394
gracilis muscle 362
great saphenous vein 12, 13, 14
great vessels
　anomalous origins 210
　thoracic 6
　see also aorta; brachiocephalic artery;
　　brachiocephalic vein; carotid artery
　　common; superior vena cava
gynaecomastia 177
gyrus rectus 47

habenula 39
habenular commissure 40
haemorrhoidal artery *see* rectal artery,
　superior
Haller's cells 106
hallucis brevis muscle, flexor 374–5
hallucis longus muscle
　extensor 370
　flexor 371, 379
hallux 375
hamate bone ossification 347, *348*
hamstrings 363
hand, fetal 413
Harris's ring 313
Hartmann's pouch 253
head
　fetal 402
　and neck surface anatomy 1–4
　venous drainage 119–20
heart
　chambers 156–62
　conducting system 161–4, *165*, 166
　development 154–5
　fetal 406, *407*
　imaging 153–4

paediatric 420
rate in children 415
surface anatomy 6
eel pad thickness 377
emiazygos vein 127, 128
  aortic hiatus 146
  embryology 394
  left azygos fissure 137
emidiaphragm 150, 422
epatic artery 214, 228, 242–3, 248, 251
  accessory 228, 235, 246, 247
  branches 243
  Doppler trace 245
  replaced 246
epatic duct 250–1, 253
epatic group of lymph nodes 275
epatic vein 242, 243, 248, 273
  access 241
  Doppler trace 245
  middle 410
epatoduodenal ligament 195–6, 197
epatorenal fossa 190
eubner's recurrent artery 28, 53
iatus semilunaris 103, 104
ilar lymph nodes 140, 147
ilar points 170
ilton's white line 221
ndbrain, fetal development 402
ndgut 187, 208, 260
p joint 357–60
  dislocation 428
  imaging 359–60
  movements 359
  neonatal 427, 427
  relations 358, 359
  subluxation 428
ppocampal gyrus 47
ppocampus 44–6, 46
ok of hamate 10
uman chorionic gonadotrophin (hCG) 400
umerus 9–10, 339, 341
  epicondyles 342
  fetal 413
  ossification 341
unter's canal 387
drocephalus 47–8
drops fetalis 406
oglossus muscles 107
oid bone 2, 3
pogastric plexus 277
poglossal condylar canal 25
poglossal nerve 35–6, 107
pothalamus 40
potympanum 94
sterosalpingography 279, 301, 302

eal arteries 232
eocaecal junction 217
eocaecal valve 216, 217
eocolic artery 217, 231, 232, 233
eum 215
ac artery
  common 272, 281, 282, 386, 387, 393
  deep circumflex 282, 387
  external 204, 282, 383, 386, 387
  internal 282, 283–4, 386, 387
  superficial circumflex 387
ac crest 9, 12, 352
  fetal 412
ac lymph nodes 276, 284, 397
ac spine 353
  anterior 12, 352, 362
  posterior superior 12
ac vein
  common 274, 281, 387, 391, 392–3

flow phenomena 393
external 282, 392
imaging 274
internal 387, 389, 392
left common 284
iliacus muscle 281, 282, 353
iliofemoral ligament 358
iliolingual nerve 202
iliolumbar artery 284
iliolumbar ligament 277, 319
iliopectineal line 352, 356
iliopsoas muscle 353
iliopsoas nerve 381
iliotibial tract 355, 363
ilium 352–3, 354–5
imaging
  ankle joint 377, 378, 380
  aorta 271–2
  auditory pathways 85–6
  biliary system of children 424
  bladder 285
  brain 17–19
  ear 85–6
  eye 61–2
  Fallopian tubes 301
  foot 377–9, 380
  gallbladder 239, 240, 241
  gastrointestinal tract 207
  hip joint 359–60
  intervertebral disc 305–6
  intracranial visual pathway 62
  lacrimal pathway 62
  limb vasculature
    arterial 381–3
    venous 389–90
  liver 239, 240, 241
  lower limb 351
  obstetric anatomy 399
  optic nerve 61
  orbit 61
  ovaries 301, 305–6
  paediatric anatomy 415
  pancreas 239, 240, 241
  penis 289–90, 302
  peroneal tendons 379
  prostate gland 287–9
  shoulder joint 336–8
  skull 17–19
  spleen 239, 240, 241
  subarachnoid space 302
  subtalar joint 378
  suprarenal glands 269–70
  thymus 420
  ureter 285
  urethra 286
  uterus 305–1
  vagina 305–6
incudomallear articulation 88, 89
incudostapedial joint 89
incus 89, 92
111mIndium DPTA, gastric emptying 212–13
indusium griseum 44
inferior vena cava 139, 144
  acquired thrombosis 274
  azygos continuation 127
  cavagram 273
  congenital absence 274
  congenital anomalies 393, 394–5
  course 273–4
  CT 273
  double 394, 395
  Eustachian valve 406
  hepatic segment 393
  hiatus 149
  imaging 273, 389

liver caudate lobe drainage 248
metastatic spread 274
MRI 273
pelvic venous plexus connection 274
posterior abdominal wall drainage 274
renal segment 393
right atrium 157
sacrocardinal segment 393
thoracic 170
tributaries 273
ultrasound 273
valve absence 391
infraclavicular fossa 9
inframesocolic compartment 193
inframesocolic space 193
infraorbital artery 72
infraorbital canal 63–4
infraorbital groove 63
infrapatellar fat pad 364, 364
infrapatellar fold 364
infraspinatus muscle 336
infraspinatus tendon 339
infratemporal fossa 98–9, 100–1
inguinal canal, paediatric 426
inguinal ligament 201, 203, 353, 381
inguinal lymph nodes 302, 396–7
inguinal ring
  deep 203, 204, 292
  superficial 201–2
inguinal triangle 392
inner ear 89–94
  bony labyrinth 88, 89
innominate bone 351, 352, 355
innominate grooves 219
innominate vein see brachiocephalic vein
insula 42, 43, 47, 55
inter-atrial septum 156–7
interclinoid ligament calcification 26
intercondylar fossa 363
intercostal artery 7, 126, 127, 168
  posterior 127
  right 310
intercostal muscles 126
intercostal nerves 126, 201
intercostal stripe 133
intercostal veins 7, 126–8, 137
intermediate nerve 91
internodal tract 162
interosseous artery 385–6
interpeduncular cistern 50
interspinous ligaments 306
intertransversalis muscle 277
intertransverse ligament 306
intertrochanteric crest 360
intertrochanteric line 360
interventricular septum 158, 160, 164
intervertebral canal 307–8
intervertebral disc 303, 304–6
  imaging 301, 302, 305–6
  see also discography
intestinal adnexae, development 185
intestinal loop, primitive 408
intestine
  development 187
  see also large intestine; small intestine
intracranial arteries 416
intracranial circulation 50–2
intralimbic gyri 44
intrasplenic arteries 227
intrasutural bones 26
iris 66
iron deposition, MRI 18
ischial ramus 353
ischial tuberosity 12, 353
ischiocavernosus muscle 280
ischiofemoral ligament 358–9

ischiopubic synchondrosis 352, 353
ischiorectal abscess 281
ischium 352, 353, 354, 412
isthmus 44

jejunal arteries 231–2
jejunum 215, 409
joints, paediatric 427–9, 427
jugular arch 119
jugular bulb
  high 94
  internal 119–20
jugular foramen 25, 93–4, 94
jugular lymph node chain, internal 115
jugular vein 93
  anterior 119
  external 3, 391
  internal 2, 3–4, 115, 119–20, 142
jugulo-omohyoid node 115
jugulosubclavian junction 397
junction line, anterior 148

Kasai procedure 249
kidney 263–5
  accessory vessels 426
  calyces 263–5
  capsule 266
  congenital variations 259, 426
  convoluted tubules 265
  cortex 263
  crossed fused ectopia 269, 425, 426
  development 259–60
  duplex 259, 264, 269, 425, 426
  ectopic 425
  fascial spaces 266–7
  fetal 410–11
  fetal lobulation 269
  horseshoe 259, 269, 425
  medulla 263
  microstructure 265
  nerve supply 266
  paediatric 425–6
  palpation 8
  pancake 269
  pelvic 269
  persistent pelvic 259
  polycystic 259
  primitive tissue persistence 416
  pyramid 263–4, 265
  relations 267
  stone impaction 267
  vascular anomalies 259
Killian's dehiscence 110
knee joint 12, 363–8
  arthrography 366
  bursae 364–5
  fibrous capsule 363, 364
  imaging 366–8
  ligaments 363, 364–5, 364
  menisci 365–6
  movements 366
  MRI 366
  plain radiography 366–7
  relations 365–6
  synovial membrane 364
Koerner's septum 88, 89

labia majora 302
labia minora 302
labyrinth, membranous 90
labyrinthine artery 59, 91
labyrinthine fistula 90
lacrimal artery 72
lacrimal gland 71
lacrimal pathway 62, 71
lactation 175

lactiferous ducts 173, 174
lacunar ligament 201
Ladd's bands 187, 423
lambda 2
lambdoid suture 20, 21, 24
lamina papyracea 63, 65
lamina terminalis cistern 50
large intestine 216–22
  double contrast barium enema 219
  fetal 408
  hepatodiaphragmatic interposition 219
  paediatric ultrasound 423
  radiographical examination 219
laryngeal aditus 110, 111
laryngeal nerve, recurrent 155–6
laryngeal prominence 2, 3
laryngeal sinus 113
laryngopharynx 108, 110
laryngotomy 15
larynx 111–13, 114
  fetal 405
leg see lower limb
lens 66–7, 68
lenticulostriate arteries 42
lentiform nucleus 40, 41
lesser sac 190–2
levator ani muscles 279–80, 303, 304
levator palpebrae superioris muscle 70
lienohepatomesenteric trunk 224
lienorenal ligament 255, 256, 257
ligament of Struthers 340
ligament of Treitz 214
ligamentum arteriosum 144, 155, 156, 170
ligamentum flavum 303, 306, 310
ligamentum nuchae 1, 306
ligamentum patellae 12, 364, 364, 365, 366
ligamentum teres 358, 360, 361
ligamentum venosum 424
limb
  buds 401
  obstetric anatomy 412–13
  see also lower limb; upper limb
limb vasculature
  arterial 381–9
  Seldinger technique 381–3
  venous 389–95
  see also lower limb; upper limb
limbic gyrus 44
limbic lobe 44, 45
limbic system 44–7
linea alba 200–1, 202, 203, 204
linea aspera 363
lingual artery 107, 116
lingual nerve 108
lingual vein 108
lip 95–6
  cleft 95, 405
  philtrum 95
lipiodol 243
lipohaemarthrosis 366
Little's area 104
liver
  anatomy 240, 241–3, 244–5, 246–50
  bare area 250, 250
  biliary drainage 251–2, 251
  blood supply 243, 245, 246–8
  caudate lobe 248
  CT scan 242
  development 186
  fetal 410
  imaging 239, 240, 241, 242
  lobes 250
  lymphatic drainage 248–9
  nerve supply 249
  paediatric 423–4

palpation 8
peritoneal attachments 249–51
principal plane 241, 243
Riedel's lobe 243
segments 243, 244
tumours 242–3
ultrasound 242
visceral relations 241–2
longitudinal ligament 303, 304, 306
longitudinal veins 310
longus capitis muscle 308
longus colli muscle 308, 313
loop of Henle 265, 266
lower limb 368–71
  arteries 13–14, 386–9
  imaging 351
  lymphatic drainage 396–7
  muscles 370–1
  surface anatomy 12–14
  veins 14, 391–3
    normal architecture 389–90
lumbar dorsal root ganglia 326
lumbar lordosis 268, 303
lumbar plexus 277
lumbar puncture 302
lumbar spine 318, 319
  facet joints 307
  lateral recess 309
  nerve roots 326, 327
  spinal canal 309
  vertebrae 318
lumbar trunks 397
lumbar veins 273, 274
lumbarization 320–1
lumbosacral junction 319–21
lumbosacral ligament 319
lumbosacral plexus 322–3
lunate bone 344, 346
lungs 129, 130
  buds 123
  development 123–4, 125
  fetal 406, 407
  fissures 5–6
  lobules 130, 132, 134
  lymphatics 132
  paediatric 420–1
  surface anatomy 5–6
  upper lobe pulmonary arteries 140
lymph node imaging 274, 395–6
lymphangiography 122, 397
lymphatic system, craniocervical 115
lymphography 274, 396
lymphoscintigraphy 396

McGregor line 314
macrostoma 95
macular area 79, 83
magnetic resonance angiography (MRA)
  limb veins 389
  upper abdomen organs 241
magnetic resonance imaging (MRI) 207, 395, 396
  abdominal lymphatic system 274
  anal sphincters 222
  anterior abdominal wall 189
  aorta 272
  axial scans 18
  bladder 285–6
  brain 17–19
    paediatric 415, 417
  chest imaging 122
  flow-related enhancement 18–19
  foot 379
  gadolinium DTPA contrast
    enhancement 18, 19

hip joint 359–60
inferior vena cava 273
intracranial visual pathway 62
inversion recovery (IR) images 28–30
knee joint 367–8
lower limb 351
mammography 183
obstetric anatomy 399
optic nerve 61
orbit 61
patellofemoral joint 368, 369
pelvis 356, 357
peritoneum 189
prostate gland 288–9
renal tract 261, 262
seminal vesicles 289, 292
shoulder joint 337, 338
suprarenal glands 270
upper abdomen organs 239, 241
vertebral column 302
malleolus 12–13, 370, 371
malleus 89, 92
Malpighian corpuscle 265
mamillary bodies 40
mammography
  anatomy 175–7
  magnetic resonance 183
mandible 2, 99, 101–2
mandibular condyle 101
mandibular foramen 99
mandibular nerve 99
mandibular processes 95
manubriosternal joint 333
manubrium 4, 6, 89, 92
marginal artery
  of (Drummond) large bowel 218, 234
  of (Dwight) small bowel 233
masseter muscle 98, 99, 101
mastication muscles 98, 99
mastoid 2, 87, 88, 89
maxillary artery 72, 99, 104, 117
maxillary processes 95
maxillary sinus 103, 104, 105
mean sac diameter (MSD) 400
Meckel's cave 22, 36, 57
Meckel's diverticulum 187, 215, 216, 232
meconium 408
median nerve 349
mediastinal blood vessels 141–4
mediastinal border 148
mediastinal contours 148–9
mediastinal lymph nodes 146–7
  anterior 146–7
  posterior 147
  regional nodal stations 146
  size 147
mediastinal spaces 143, 144–5
  junction areas 135, 144
mediastinum 140–1, 149, 419
medulla 33, 35
mendosal suture 24
meningeal artery 28, 117, 311
meningeal vein 311
meninges 26, 28
meningioma, skull base 22
menisci 365–6, 366, 367
  discoid 366
meniscofemoral ligaments 365, 366
mental foramen 2, 99
mental symphysis 99
mesencephalic sulcus, lateral 32–3, 37
mesencephalon 402
mesenteric arteriography 207
mesenteric artery
  inferior 218, 233–4

superior 215, 217, 230–3
  origins 224–5
  paediatric 423
  ultrasound 272
mesenteric lymph nodes 275
mesenteric vein
  inferior 218, 235, 247, 269
  superior 215, 217, 231, 235, 256
  paediatric 423
  portal vein 234
mesentery 196–7, 198, 199, 200
mesial temporal sclerosis 46
mesoappendix 197, 198, 217
mesocolon
  sigmoid 197, 200
  transverse 196–7, 198
mesonephros 259
mesosalpinx 304
mesovarium 304
metacarpal bones 347–8, 349
  fetal 413
metacarpal joints 348, 349
metanephric duct 259
metastases, inferior vena caval spread 2
metatarsal bones 370, 374–5
  fetal 412, 413
metatarsal veins 392
metatarsus adductus 375
metopic suture 21
Meyer's loop 76, 79
microstoma 95
micturating cystourethrogram (MCUG) 279, 285
micturition 426, 427
mid-carpal joint 345
mid-clavicular line 7, 8
midbrain 32, 37
middle ear 87, 88, 89
midgut 186–7, 207–8
milk line 173, 179
mini-tracheostomy tube 16
mitral valve 157, 158, 160–1
moderator band 158
Montgomery's tubercles 174
Morison's pouch 190, 193
morula 400
motor pathways 41–2
mouth, fusion of prominences 95
movement control, voluntary 41–2
mucociliary escalator 104, 106
Muller's muscle 71
musculophrenic artery 230
musculus submucosa ani 222
myelinated fibre tracts 17–18
myelination, cerebral 28–30
myelography, vertebral column 302–3
mylohyoid muscles 106
myometrium 303, 305, 306–1

nasal cavity 102–4
  blood supply 104
  sphenopalatine branch of maxillary artery 99
nasal cycle 103–4
nasal fibres 78
nasal mucosa 103–4
nasal septum 103
  bony 97
nasion 1
nasolacrimal duct 71, 95
nasopalatine nerve 103
nasopharyngeal carcinoma 109
nasopharynx 108, 109–10
navicular 374, 375
  bipartite 377

congenital fusion with calcaneum 378
fossa 286
[n]eck
anterior triangle 2
deep fascia 111
fascial layers 110–11
obstetric anatomy 405
posterior triangle 2
surface anatomy 2–3
venous drainage 119–20
[n]eural arch 303, 311
[n]eural plate 402
[n]eural tube 28, 402
[n]eurocentral joints of Luschka 315
[n]ipple
accessory 178, 179
anatomy 174
congenital anomalies 179
development 173, 174
duct orifice cannulation 181–2, 183
[n]on-coronary sinus 160, 161, 168
[n]uchal oedema 405
[n]uclear medicine
cardiac applications 154
gastrointestinal tract 207
lower limb 351
upper abdomen organs 241
[n]ucleus pulposus 303, 305

[ap]ex 33
[ob]lique muscle
external 201–2, 205, 353
internal 202, 203
[ob]stetric anatomy
abdomen 408–12
central nervous system 402–4
chest 405–6, 407, 408
developmental timetable 399
face 404–5
first trimester 400–1
imaging 399
limbs 412–13
neck 405
second trimester 401–6, 407, 408–14
skull 401–2
spine 404
trunk 405
see also pregnancy
[ob]turator artery 282, 283, 387
[ob]turator externus muscle 355
[ob]turator internus muscle 353, 355
[ob]turator membrane 353
[ob]turator nerve 281
[oc]cipital artery 28, 116–17
ascending 310
[oc]cipital bone 23–5
[oc]cipital horn 47
[oc]cipital lobe 42
[oc]cipital sinus 56
[oc]cipitofronal diameter (OFD) 402
[oc]ular globe 66
[oc]ulomotor nerve 37
[od]ontoid process 312
[o]esophageal atresia 419
[o]esophageal compression 421, 422
[o]esophageal hiatus 150
[o]esophageal reflux 419, 422
[o]esophageal sphincter, upper 110
[o]esophagogastric junction varices 257
[o]esophagus 141, 208–11
air 141
anatomy/anatomical relations 209
atresia 156
azygos vein relationship 127
lymphatic drainage 209–10
mucosal folds 209, 211

paediatric 422
radiological examination 210
vascular ring 421
vascular supply 209
vestibule 211
Z line 211
olecranon 10
foramen/fossa 339–40, 342
oleocolic lymph nodes 275
olfactory bulb 46, 47
olfactory pathways 46, 47
olfactory stria 46, 47
olfactory trigone 47
olive 33, 35
omental bursa 189
omentum 189
greater 196, 197–8
lesser 196, 197–8, 250
operculofrontal artery 53
operculum 43
ophthalmic artery 71–2
anterior 51, 52
ophthalmic vein 72
optic canal 64, 65, 69
optic chiasm 40, 73, 74, 75
blood supply 77
compression 79
optic disc 68
optic nerve 69–70
anterior cerebral artery relationship 73
CT 61
fibre organization 78
imaging 61
internal carotid artery relationship 73
meningeal sheath 65, 68, 69
MRI 61
segments 73
optic pathways 40
intracranial 72–7
retrochiasmal 79
optic radiations 75–6
blood supply 77–8
fibre organization 79, 84
myelination 29
optic tract 74, 76, 77, 79
oral cavity 106–7
floor 107
orbit 65, 66–9
arteries 71–2
computed tomography (CT) 61
frontal bone 64–5
imaging 61
lateral wall 64
magnetic resonance imaging (MRI) 61
medial wall 63–4
osseous anatomy 62–5
roof 64–5
soft tissues 66
veins 71–2
venous anastomoses 72
walls 97
orbital fat 66
orbital fissure, superior 64, 65
orbitofrontal artery 53, 55
organ of Corti 89
oropharynx 108, 110
Ortolani test 428
os acromiale 332
os odontoideum 311
os peroneum 375, 376
os subtibiale 376
os tibiale externum 375
os trigonum 375–6
os Vesalianum pedis 375
ossicular chain 87, 89
ostiomeatal complex 104, 105, 106

oval window 87, 88
ovarian artery 303, 305
ovarian ligament 304
ovary 304–5
follicles 304
imaging 301, 305–6
paediatric 427

paediatric anatomy
congenital anatomical variants 416
imaging 415
organs 415
primitive tissue persistence 416
ultrasound 415
cranial 416–18
palate
cleft 95
development 95–6
hard 97
palatoglossal fold 106, 110
palatoglossus muscles 107
palatopharyngeal fold 110
palmar arch, deep 386
pampiniform plexus 301, 305
pancreas 253, 256
blood supply 255–6
body 254
development 186, 255
head 254, 256
imaging 239, 240, 241
lymphatic drainage 256
neck 254
paediatric 424
tail 255
uncinate process 254
pancreatic artery 255
caudal 226
dorsal 226, 231
transverse 230
pancreatic duct 254, 255
pancreatico-duodenal arcade 225, 229, 230
pancreatico-duodenal artery 214, 226, 229
anterior superior 229, 230
inferior 229, 230, 231
superior 256
pancreatico-duodenal vein, posterior superior 235
pancreaticosplenic group of lymph nodes 275
papillary muscles 157, 160
para-aortic lymph nodes 284, 396, 397
paracolic gutter 193
paraglenoid sulcus 356, 356
paraglottic space 113
parahippocampal gyrus 44–5, 46
paranasal sinuses 104, 105, 106
paraoesophageal lymph nodes 147
parapharyngeal space 110, 111
parotid gland 107
pararenal space, posterior 267
paraspinal areas 145–6
paraspinal line 144, 149, 317
paraspinal space 317
paraspinal vein 330
paraspinous muscles 308–9
parathyroid gland 115
paratracheal lymph nodes 147
paratracheal space, right 143, 145
paraurethral glands 286
paravesical spaces 193–4
parietal artery
posterior 55
superior internal 54
parietal bone 21–2
parietal eminence 1
parietal foramina 26

parietal lobe 42, 43
parieto-occipital artery 60
parieto-occipital fissure 42
parotid duct 108
parotid gland 107–8
parotid sialogram 2
patella 12, 361, 363, 367
articular surface 363
variants 361, 361–2
patellar retinaculae 363
patellar tendon 366
patellar tracking 366
patellofemoral joint, MRI 366, 369
pectinate line 187
pectineus muscle 363
pectoralis major muscle 126
pelvic brim 353, 387
pelvic diaphragm 279
pelvic fascia 303, 304
pelvic floor anatomy 279–81
pelvic girdle muscles 355–8
pelvic inlet 353
pelvic kyphosis 303
pelvic outlet dimensions 356–7
pelvic vasculature 281–4, 389
pelvic veins 389
pelvic viscera 284–302
pelvic walls 351–3
pelvimetry 356–7
pelvis
bony 351–3
conjugate diameter 356–7
CT 356, 357
false 353
fetal 405
gender differences 353
hysterosalpingogram 279
imaging 279, 355–8
ligaments 353
lymphatics 284
MRI 356, 357
nerves 281
plain radiography 355–6, 357
pregnancy 356–7
true 353
pelviureteric junction 267
penis 302
fetal 411, 412
percutaneous transhepatic cholangiography (PTC) 241
perforating arteries 388
pericallosal artery 54
pericardial fat pads 156
pericardial recess, superior 144
pericardium 156
pericolic abscess 219
perihepatic space, left 192
perilymph 90
perimedullary venous plexus 330
perineal fascia, superficial 198
perineal muscles, superficial transverse 280
perineal pouch 280, 281
perineum 279, 280
perineural cysts of Tarlov 327
periosteum 26–7
periprostatic plexus 287
perirectal nodes, abdominal lymphatics 274
perirenal space 266
peritoneal cavity 189
peritoneal fluid 189, 249
peritoneal ligaments 189, 194–6
peritoneal reflections 194–8
peritoneal spaces 189–94
inframesocolic 193

pelvic 193–4
  posterior 190
  supramesocolic 190–3
peritoneum, anatomy 189–98
peroneal artery 388–9
peroneal nerve 370
peroneal tendon imaging 379
peroneal tubercle 13
peroneus brevis muscle 370
  tendon 375
peroneus longus muscle 370
  tendon 375
peroneus tertius muscle 370
petroclinoid ligament, calcification 26
petrosal sinus 57
petrosal vein of Dandy 93
phalangeal joints 347–8, 349
phalanges 348, 349, 375
  fetal 413
pharyngeal arches 96
pharyngeal artery, ascending 116, 310
pharyngeal pouch 110
pharyngeal swallow reflex 422
pharyngeal tonsils 109–10
pharyngobasilar fascia 109
pharyngotympanic tube see Eustachian
  tube
pharynx 108–10
  constrictor muscles 109
  mucosal layer 108, 109
  muscle layer 108–9
philtrum, upper lip 95
phrenic artery
  inferior 150, 226, 230, 271
  superior 169
phrenic nerve 150, 391
phrenic vein 150, 273
phrenicocolic ligament 193, 195, 196, 217
Phrygian cap 253
pia mater 26, 328
pial network, lateral 330
pineal gland 39, 40
piriform fossa 111–12
piriformis muscle 353, 355
pisiform bone 344
  ossification 347, 348
pituitary gland 37–9, 40
  ectopic tissue 40, 40
placenta 401, 413–14
plantar artery 388
plantar calcaneonavicular ligament 371,
  377
plantar ligament 373, 377
plantaris muscle 371
pleura 133–7
  fissures
    accessory 136, 137
    major 134–6, 136
    minor 136–7, 137
    junction lines 134, 135
  margin 5
  parietal 134
  reflection lines 5
  visceral 134, 140
pleuro-oesophageal line 148, 149, 210
plicae circulares 214, 215
Poland's syndrome 179
pollicis brevis muscle tendon 348
pollicis longus muscle tendon 345
polymastia 179
polythelia 179
pons 33, 36–7
pontine cistern 50
pontomedullary junction 35, 57
popliteal artery 13, 14, 388–9

retrograde 382
popliteal bursa 364
popliteal cyst 364
popliteal fossa 388
popliteal ligament, oblique 363, 364
popliteal pulse 13–14
popliteal vein 389
popliteus muscle 371
porta hepatis 235, 249, 250, 251
portal hypertension, umbilical vein 235
portal vein 234–5, 242, 243, 247–8, 250
  caudate lobe of liver 248
  Doppler trace 245
  formation 247
  left 409, 424
  pancreatic drainage 256
  right 410
  trunk 424
  umbilical part 412
portal–systemic anastomosis 257
porus acousticus 91
posterior fossa veins 59, 60
posterior junction 145, 146, 148–9
posterior sinus, left/right 161
pouch of Douglas 194, 195, 219, 220, 285
  imaging 305
  uterosacral ligaments 304
  uterus relationship 303
pre-aortic lymph nodes 274, 397
pre-auricular sulcus 356
pre-epiglottic space 113
pregnancy
  breasts 175
  intrauterine 399
  pelvic changes 357
  pelvimetry 356–7
  ureter compression 268
  see also obstetric anatomy
prepyloric vein 214
pretracheal space 143, 144
primitive tissue persistence 416
profunda brachii see brachial artery, deep
profunda femoris artery see femoral
  artery, deep
profunda femoris vein see femoral vein
promontory 87
pronator quadratus 344
pronator teres 344
pronephros 259
prosencephalon 402
prostate gland 286–9
  blood supply 287
  imaging 287–9
  lobes 287
  lymphatic drainage 287
  zones 287, 288–9
prostatic sinus 286
Prussak's space 89
psoas muscle 281, 308, 353
  abscess 281
  major 362
  ureter forward displacement 268
pterion 22
pterygoid muscle 98, 99, 101
pterygoid plate 22, 97
pterygoid plexus 119
pterygomaxillary fissure 99
pterygopalatine fossa 98–9, 100–1, 104
pterygopalatine ganglion 99
puberty, breasts 173
pubic arch 353
pubic crest 8, 353
pubic ramus 353
pubic symphysis 7, 351–3, 387
  instability 356

pubic tubercle 7
pubis 352, 353, 354
pubocervical ligament 303, 304
pubofemoral ligament 358
puborectal sling 221
pudendal artery
  deep external 387
  internal 281, 283
  superficial external 387
pudendal nerve 281
pudendal vein, internal 302
pulmonary agenesis 124
pulmonary arch, fetal 407
pulmonary artery 130, 131, 132, 139, 140,
  170
  interlobar 140
  left 140, 170, 171
    aberrant 210, 211
  right 140, 168, 170, 171
pulmonary hila 130, 131
pulmonary hypoplasia, unilateral 124
pulmonary ligament
  inferior 137
  lymph nodes 147
pulmonary lobules, secondary 130, 132, 134
pulmonary trunk 139, 140
  bifurcation 170
  relationships 168, 169–70, 171
  venous 155
pulmonary valve 158, 160
pulmonary vein 130, 131, 132, 170
  left atrium 160
  superior 170
putamen 41
pyloric stenosis, hypertrophic 423
pyramidalis muscle 201

quadratus femoris muscle 355
quadratus lumborum muscle 281
quadriceps femoris muscle 362
quadrigeminal cistern 50
quadrigeminal plate 78
  cistern 48, 56, 59

radial artery 11, 385, 386
  catheterization 382
radial collateral ligament 343
radial fossa 342
radial nerve 349
radicular arteries 328–9
radiculomedullary artery 329
radiculomedullary junction 329
radiocarpal joint 345
radiography
  elbow joint 343
  foot 377–8
  hip joint 359
  knee joint 366
  pelvis 355–6, 357
  shoulder joint 336–7
  skull 17, 21, 25–6
  vertebral column 301
radionuclide investigation
  small intestine 216
  vertebral column 303
radioulnar joint 345
radius 10, 343–4, 344
  distal 345
  fetal 413
  ossification 344
  styloid process 10
rectal ampulla 219–20
rectal artery
  inferior 220
  middle 220, 283

superior 220, 222, 233
rectal evacuation studies 222
rectal vein 220
recto-sigmoid junction 219
recto-vesical pouch 194
rectouterine pouch see pouch of Dougla
rectovesical fascia 285
rectum 219–21, 222
rectus abdominis muscle 199–201, 202,
  203, 308, 387
  sheath 204
rectus capitis muscle 308
rectus femoris muscle 352, 362
rectus muscles 70
  sheath 200, 201, 202, 203
red nucleus 37
  iron deposition 18, 19
renal agenesis 425
renal artery 265–6, 271
  development 259
  right 273
renal duct system development 259
renal ectopia, crossed 269, 425, 426
renal migration, abnormal 269
renal pelvis 264, 410–11
renal rudiment, metanephric 259
renal tract
  angiography 262–3
  CT 260, 262
  developmental abnormalities 269
  imaging 261–3
  intravenous urogram 261
  MRI 261, 262
  radiographs 261
  ultrasound 260, 262
  variants 269
  venography 263
renal vein 265–6, 273
  left 393, 395
  tributaries 266
  variants 266
respiratory diverticulum 123
respiratory rate in children 415
respiratory tract
  congenital anomalies 123–4
  development 122–4
retina 66
retinaculum muscle 358
  extensor 346, 370
  flexor 345
retroaortic lymph nodes 397
retrocrural area, lymph nodes 147
retrocrural space 144, 145, 146, 278, 282
retroduodenal artery 229
retromandibular vein 119
retropubic space 286
retrosternal line 150
retrotracheal area 149
rhombencephalon 402
rhomboid ligament 333
ribs 125
  cervical 316
  fetal 405, 406
  thoracic spine 317
  tubercles 317
Riedel's lobe 243
Rolandic fissure 28, 42
rotator cuff muscles 336
round window 87, 88
rubroreticulospinal tract 325

saccule 90
sacral artery
  lateral 284, 310
  median 220, 386

sacral canal 354
sacral crest 354
sacral dimple 9
sacral foramina 354
sacral nerves 354
sacral nodes, abdominal lymphatics 276
sacral plexus 281
sacralization 320
sacrocardinal veins 393
persistent 395
sacroiliac joint 9, 351, 354–5, 356
sacroiliac ligament 354–5
sacrospinous ligament 353
sacrotuberous ligament 353
sacrum 351, 353, 354, 355
sagittal sinus 55, 56, 57
sagittal suture 21
sail sign 419
salivary glands 107–8
saphenous nerve 12, 14
saphenous vein
long 390, 392
short 392
small 14
sartorius muscle 362
scaphoid bone 344, 346–7
ossification 347, 348
scapula 4–5, 9, 331, 332
scapular artery 384, 385
scapulothoracic joint 332
Scarpa's fascia 280
sciatic artery, persistent 283
sciatic foramen, greater/lesser 353
sciatic nerve 13
scintigraphy, renal tract 262, 263
sclera 66
scoliosis
idiopathic 309
physiological right lateral 303
scotoma 78, 84
scrotum 292
blood supply 291–2
fetal 411, 412
paediatric 426
scutum 86
Seldinger technique, arterial system 381–3
sella, partially empty 40
semicircular canals 89–90
semicircular ducts 90
semilunar cusps 158
semimembranosus muscle 363
seminal vesicles 284, 287–8, 289
imaging 301, 302
transrectal ultrasound 289, 292
semitendinosus muscle 363
septal vein 58
septum pellucidum 47, 48
fetal 403
septum primum/secundum 154, 155
serratus anterior muscle 126
sesamoid bone 347, 374–5, 376
Sharpey's fibres 305
Shenton's line 356
shoulder girdle 332
fetal 405
muscles 126
shoulder joint 335–8
coronal section 334
CT arthrography 337–8
double contrast arthrography 337
imaging 336–8
MRI 337, 338
plain radiography 336–7
Striker's view 337
ultrasound 338

sigmoid mesocolon 197, 200
sigmoid sinus 55, 56
sinus artery 164
sinus epididymis 291
sinus epithelium, cilia 104, 106
sinus of Morgagni 109
sinus node 162
sinus tarsi 373, 376
sinus of Valsalva 160, 164, 166, 167
sinus venosus 154, 155
sinusitis 104, 106
skull
base 18, 19–20
meningioma 22
fontanelle 402
imaging 17–19
obstetric anatomy 401–2
osteology 19–25
radiograph 17, 21, 25–6
submentovertical projection 24
sutures 20, 21, 97, 401–2
vault 19, 20, 21, 401
lucencies 26
small intestine 215–16
air distension 423
fetal 408
lymphatic drainage 215
malrotation 423
mesentery 196, 198, 199
anatomical relations 215
radiological examination 215–16
ultrasound in children 423
ascular supply 215
visceral angiography 216
snake's eyes 92, 94
soleal line 369
soleal pump 391
soleus muscle 370, 371
spermatic cord 291, 301
spheno-ethmoidal recess 106
sphenobregmatic sinus 25
sphenoid bone 22
greater wing 22, 64
lesser wing 64
pneumatization 106
sphenoid ridge 22
sphenoid sinus 106
sphenopalatine artery 117
sphenopalatine foramen 99, 103
sphenoparietal sinus 57
sphincter of Oddi 252
spina bifida 311
spinal accessory nerve see accessory nerve
spinal artery 169, 328–9, 330
spinal canal, tonsillar descent 314
spinal cord 320, 321–3
anterior horn 323–4
anterior median fissure 322
anterolateral tract 325
ascending tracts 323–5, 325
blood supply 328–30, 383
central canal 322–3
cervical expansion 322
CT 301
descending tracts 325
fetal 402, 404
grey matter 323
internal structure 323–5
lateral column 324
umbar expansion 322
paediatric 418–19
posterior column 323
posterior horn 324
spinal meningeal sheath 327
surface anatomy 9

terminal ventricle 323
venous drainage 330
white matter 323, 324
spinal fusion 303
spinal lemniscus 325
spinal meninges 301, 327–8
spinal nerve
cervical 325
rootlets 322
spinal nerve roots 325–8
conjoined 326
dorsal 326
dorsal nerve root ganglion 326
lumbar 326, 327
perineural cysts of Tarlov 327–8
ventral 325
spinal vein, posterior 330
spine see vertebral column
spinocerebellar tract 324–5, 325
spinolaminar line 316
spinothalamic tracts 325
spiral valve of Hiester 253
splanchnic nerve 127, 128
spleen 256–7
accessory 424
blood supply 257
development 186
fetal 410
hilum 192, 255
imaging 239, 240, 241
lympatic drainage 257
paediatric 424
pulp measurement 241
splenic artery 226–7, 255, 257
splenic vein 234, 235, 247, 256
splenoportography 241
splenorenal ligament 195, 197
splenuncles 424
stapedius muscle 87
stapes 89
sternoclavicular joint 9
sternocleidomastoid muscle 2, 4, 308
sternum 4, 6, 125
stomach 211–13
anatomical relations 211, 212
body 211
development 185–6
fetal 408
olds 212
fundus 211
lymphatic drainage 212
muscles 211–12
paediatric 423
pyloric antrum 211
pylorus 211
radiological investigation 212
regions 211
rotation 186
structure 211–12
vascular supply 212
Z line 211
stomodaeum 95
straight sinus 55, 56, 76
striate cortex see visual cortex
Striker's view of shoulder joint 337
styloglossus muscles 107
styloid process 23
stylomandibular ligament 108
stylomastoid foramen 23
subacromial subdeltoid bursa 334, 335–6
subarachnoid cisterns 49–50
subarachnoid haemorrhage 50
subarachnoid space 9, 26, 302, 328
subcallosal gyrus 44
subcardinal veins 393
subcarinal lymph nodes 147, 396

subcarinal space 143, 145
subclavian artery 11, 383–4
branches 383–4
inferor thyroid branch 209
internal thoracic branch 126
eft 141
aortic arch 168
right 141
aberrant 210
development 155
hyrocervical branch 328
variations 384
vertebral artery branch 117
subclavian vein 11–12, 120, 142, 391
left 397
subcostal arteries 169
subcostal muscles 126
subcostal plane of abdomen 7
subhepatic space, right 190, 193
sublingual gland 107, 108
submandibular duct 108
submandibular gland 107, 108
subphrenic space
left 192
right 190, 193
subpleural lymphatic vessels 132
subsartorial canal 387
subscapular artery 385
subscapularis muscle 336
subscapularis tendon 339
substantia nigra 37
iron deposition 18, 19
subtalar joint 376–7, 378
sulcus
calcanei 373, 376
central 44
artery 55
marginal 41
tali 373, 376
terminalis 106
superciliary arch 1
superior mesenteric arteriography 241
superior vena cava 6, 127, 143–4, 168, 170, 393
IV DSA 383
left-sided 421
neck region 3
persistent left 144
right 144
right atrium 157
supernumerary bones 349
supracardinal vein 393
supracondylar spur 341
supracristal plane of abdomen 7–8
supraduodenal artery of Wilkie 229
supramesocolic compartment 190–3
supramesocolic space
left 192–3
right 190–2
supraorbital notch 1
suprapatellar bursa 364, 364–5, 366
suprapatellar pouch 12
suprarenal artery 230, 271
suprarenal gland 261, 266, 270–1
abnormalities 269
blood supply 271
cortical bodies 271
CT 269, 270
fetal 411
imaging 269–70
microstructure 271
MRI 270
nerves 271
paediatric 424–5
relations 271
ultrasound 270

variants 271
venography 270
suprarenal vein 270
suprascapular artery 383–4
suprasellar cistern *see* chiasmatic cistern
supraspinatus muscle 336, 338
supraspinatus tendon 339
supraspinous ligament 306
suprasternal notch 2, 3, 4
supratentorial venous system 57–60
supratrochlear foramen 341
surface anatomy
  abdomen 7–8
  head and neck 1–4
  heart 6
  lungs 5–6
  spinal cord 9
  thorax 4–7
suspensory ligament
  of Cooper 176
  of ovary 304
sustenaculum tali 373
swallowing 208
  paediatric 415, 422
Sylvian fissure 43, 44, 55
  paediatric 417
sympathetic trunk 276
synchondroses 97

taeniae coli 218, 219
talocalcaneal coalition 378
talocalcaneal joint, posterior 377
talocalcaneal ligament, interosseous 377
talocalcaneonavicular joint 377
talofibular ligament 371
talonavicular joint 377
talonavicular ligament 377
talus 372–3, 375, 377
  imaging 378, 379
tarsal bones, fetal 412, 413
tarsal coalitions, congenital 378
tarsus 372
taste buds 106
tear ducts 71
tectorial membrane 306, 313
tectum 37
teeth 99, 101–2
tegmen tympani 87
tela choroidea 48
telencephalon, fetal 402–3
temporal artery 117
  anterior 55, 117
  superficial 72, 117
temporal bone 22, 23
  mandibular fossa 101
temporal fossa, articular eminence 101
temporal horn 46, 47
temporal lobe 43, 43, 46, 47
temporal sclerosis, mesial 46
temporalis muscle 98, 99, 101
temporo-occipital incisure 42
temporomandibular joint 99, 101–2
  articular disc 101
tendo Achilles *see* calcaneal tendon
tendo calcanea *see* calcaneal tendon
tendon reflexes 325
tenography 379
tensor fasciae latae muscle 362
tensor tympani muscle 87
tentorium cerebelli 27
teres minor muscle 336
  tendon 339
terminal duct lobular unit (TDLU) 174, 175
testicular artery 291
testicular vein 292

testis 290, 291
  appendix 304, 305
  blood supply 291–2
  fetal 411, 412
  imaging 292, 301
  paediatric 426–7
  ultrasound 292, 301
thalamostriate vein 58
thalamus 39, 40
Thebesian valve 157
thigh 360–2
  muscles 362–3
thoracic aortic plexus 128
thoracic artery 385
  internal 7, 126, 383
thoracic cage, muscular covering 125–6
thoracic duct 141, 146
thoracic ganglia 128
thoracic kyphosis 303, 317
thoracic lymph duct 397
thoracic nerve of Bell, long 385
thoracic spine 317
  facet joints 307
  ribs 317
  vertebrae 125, 317
thoracic vein, internal 7, 128
thoracic wall vessels 6–7
thoracolumbar fascia 202
thorax
  bony landmarks 4
  surface anatomy 4–7
thryocervical trunk 115
thumb joints 347, 348
thymus 146, 147–8, 419–20
thyrocervical trunk 310, 383
thyroglossal cyst 96
thyroglossal duct 96
thyroglossal sinus 96
thyroid artery
  inferior 383
  superior 116
thyroid cartilage 112
thyroid gland 114–15
  development 96–7
  embryonic descent 96–7
  fetal 405
  isthmus 2, 3
thyroidea ima 115
thyropharyngeus 110
tibia 12, 368–9
  fetal 412, 413
  ossification 369–70
  shaft 368–9
tibial artery 388
tibial collateral ligament 364, 365
tibial condyle 12
  lateral 368
tibial tuberosity 12, 368
tibial vein 389, 392
tibialis anterior muscle 370
tibialis posterior muscle 374
  tendon 376
tibiofemoral articulations 363
tibiofibular joints 370
toes, fetal 412, 413
tongue 106–7
  development 96
  innervation 96, 107
  lymphatic drainage 115
  muscle 96, 107
torus aorticus 156, 167
torus tubarius 109
trabeculae carnae 157
trachea 130, 149
  paediatric 419

tracheal space, posterior 145
tracheo-oesophageal fistula 123
tracheobronchial diverticulum 122
tracheobronchial groove 122, 156
tracheobronchial lymph nodes 146, 147
tracheomalacia 419
tracheostomy 15–16
transforaminal ligament 307
transpyloric plane of abdomen 7
transrectal ultrasound
  prostate gland 287, 288
  seminal vesicles 289, 292
transversalis fascia 203, 204
transverse sinus 56, 57
transversus abdominis muscle 203, 277, 282
  aponeurosis 202, 203
trapezium ossification 347, 348
trapezius muscle 126
trapezoid bone ossification 347, 348
trapezoid ligament 333
triangular ligaments 250
triceps muscle, tendon 341
tricuspid valve 157, 158
trigeminal artery 50
trigeminal ganglion 57
trigeminal nerve 36
  cerebellopontine angle cistern 93
  inferior alveolar branch 99
  nuclei 36
  sensory root 57
  tongue 96
triquetral bone 344, 345
  ossification 347, 348
triradiate cartilage 352, 354–5
trisomy 21 405
trochanteric anastomosis 361, 388
trochanteric fossa 355
trochlea 339, 341
trochlear nerve 37
trochlear notch 343
truncus arteriosus 154, 155
trunk, obstetric anatomy 405
tunica albuginea 292, 301, 302, 305
tunica vaginalis 301
tympanic cavity 87, 88
tympanic membrane 86, 87, 89
tympanic ring 86

ulna 10, 342, 343–4, 344
  distal 345
  fetal 413
  ossification 344
  styloid process 10
ulnar artery 11, 346, 385, 386
ulnar collateral ligament 343
ulnar nerve 10, 11, 346, 349
ultrasound
  abdominal lymphatic system 274
  aorta 271, 272
  appendix 219
  bladder 285
  cardiac 153–4
  endoscopic 207
  female genital tract 305
  gastrointestinal tract of children 423
  hip joint 359
  inferior vena cava 273
  limb veins 389
  liver 242
  lower limb 351
  obstetric anatomy 399
  paediatric anatomy 415
  placenta 414
  prostate gland 287, 288

renal tract 260, 262
shoulder joint 339
suprarenal glands 270
testis 292, 301
transabdominal 207
transoesophageal 154
upper abdomen organs 239
vertebral column 303
see also duplex sonography
umbilical artery 409, 410
  lines 421
  obliterated 283
umbilical cord 400, 409, 413
umbilical hernia, physiological 409
umbilical vein 235, 409
  paediatric 423, 424
umbilicus 186, 187
uncinate process 315
upper limb
  anatomy 331–2
  arterial supply 383–6
  lymphatic drainage 396
  nerve supply 349
  pulses 11
  surface anatomy 9–12
  veins 390–1
    superficial 11–12
upper respiratory obstruction, surgical access 15–16
urachal remnant 426
ureter 267–9, 285
  blood supply 268
  development 259–60
  duplex 269
  duplication 426
  imaging 285
  intravesical part 269
  lymphatic drainage 268
  microstructure 268
  nerve supply 268
  relations 268–9
  retrocaval 269
ureteric junction 267
ureterocele 269
urethra 284–5, 286, 287, 302
urinary tract
  development 259–60
  imaging 279
  see also bladder; kidney; ureter
urogenital diaphragm 286, 302
urogenital sinus 260
urogenital triangle 280
urogram, intravenous 261
uterine artery 283, 303
uterine cavity, imaging 279
uterine ligaments 303
uterine tubes 304
utero-vesical pouch 194
uterosacral ligament 303, 304
uterus 302, 303–4
  congenital anomalies 302
  imaging 305–1
  paediatric 427
utricle 90
uvula, bifid 95

vagal trunk, liver nerve supply 249
vagina 284, 302–3
  attachments 302, 303
  imaging 305–6
vaginal artery 283, 303
vaginal vein 303
vagus nerve 35
  carotid sheath 115
  development 155

jugular foramen 93–4
kidney supply 266
tongue 96, 107
valsalva manoeuvre 389
valvulae coniventes 214
vas deferens 259, 292, *301*, 302
vasa corona, arterial 330
vasa deferentia 284
vasa recta 266
vasography 302
vastus intermedius muscle 362
vastus lateralis muscle 362
tendon 363
vastus medialis muscle 362–3
tendon 363
vein of Galen 56, 58, 60
vein of Labbé 57, 58
vein of Rosenthal, basal 58, 59, 60
vein of Trolard 57
veins
embryology 393–5
limb 11–12, 14, 389–95
paired 390
valves 389–90, 391
velum interpositum 48–9
venae comitantes 390, 392
venae cordi minimae 167
venography
chest imaging 122
lower limb 389–90
renal tract 263
suprarenal glands 270
venous arch, dorsal 11, 14
ventricles
development 154
fourth 49
lateral 46, 47–8
fetal 402–3
paediatric 417, 418
left 160–2
paediatric *417*, 418
right 157–9
third 49
ventricular septum 157
ventricular vein, left posterior 166
vertebrae 304
abnormal segmentation 311
block 311
ossification 311
see also cervical spine; lumbar spine;
thoracic spine
vertebral arch 310
vertebral artery 117, *118*, 383
duplex sonography 119
occipital artery anastomoses 117
segmental branches 309
vertebral body 303, 304
epiphyses 311
vertebral canal 309
vertebral column
arteriography 303
blood supply 309–11
compartments 303
CT 301–2
curves 303
facet joints 306–7
fetal 404
imaging 301–3
joints 306–7
ligaments 306
movements 309
MRI 302
myelography 302–3
obstetric anatomy 404
paediatric sonography 418–19
radiography 301

radionuclide bone scanning 303
ultrasound 303
see also cervical spine; lumbar spine;
thoracic spine
vertebral levels
cervical region 3
thorax 4–5
vertebrobasilar arterial system 58–60
verumontanum 286
vesical artery
inferior 282
superior 283
vesicoureteric reflux, children 415
vestibular aqueduct 90
vestibular bulbs 302
vestibular folds 112–13
vestibular gland, greater 280, *281*
vestibulocochlear nerve 36
cerebellopontine angle cistern 93
vestibulospinal tract 325
Vidian canal 22
visceral angiography, small intestine 216
visceral layer of neck fascia 111
visual association areas 77, *83*
visual cortex 76–7, *79, 80, 81–2*
blood supply 78
visual pathways
blood supply 77–8, *83*
fibre organization 78–9, *84*
intracranial 62
vitelline duct 186, 187
vitelline vein, right 393
vitellointestinal artery, persistent 232–3
vitreous 68
vocal cords 112–13
volvulus 423
neonatorum 187
vomer 97
vulva, fetal *411*, 412

Wernicke's area 76
white matter, myelination 28, 30
Wilbrand's knee 78
Wormian bones 26
wrist 10, 344–7
fetal 413
median nerve 349
ossification 347, *348*

xiphisternal joint 4
xiphisternal plane of abdomen 7
xiphoid 7, 198
process 4

yolk sac, primary/secondary 400

Z line 211
Zenker's diverticulum 110
zona fasciculata 271
zona glomerulosa 271
zona reticularis 271
zygomatic arches 97
zygomatic bone 1, 64
zygomatic process 98

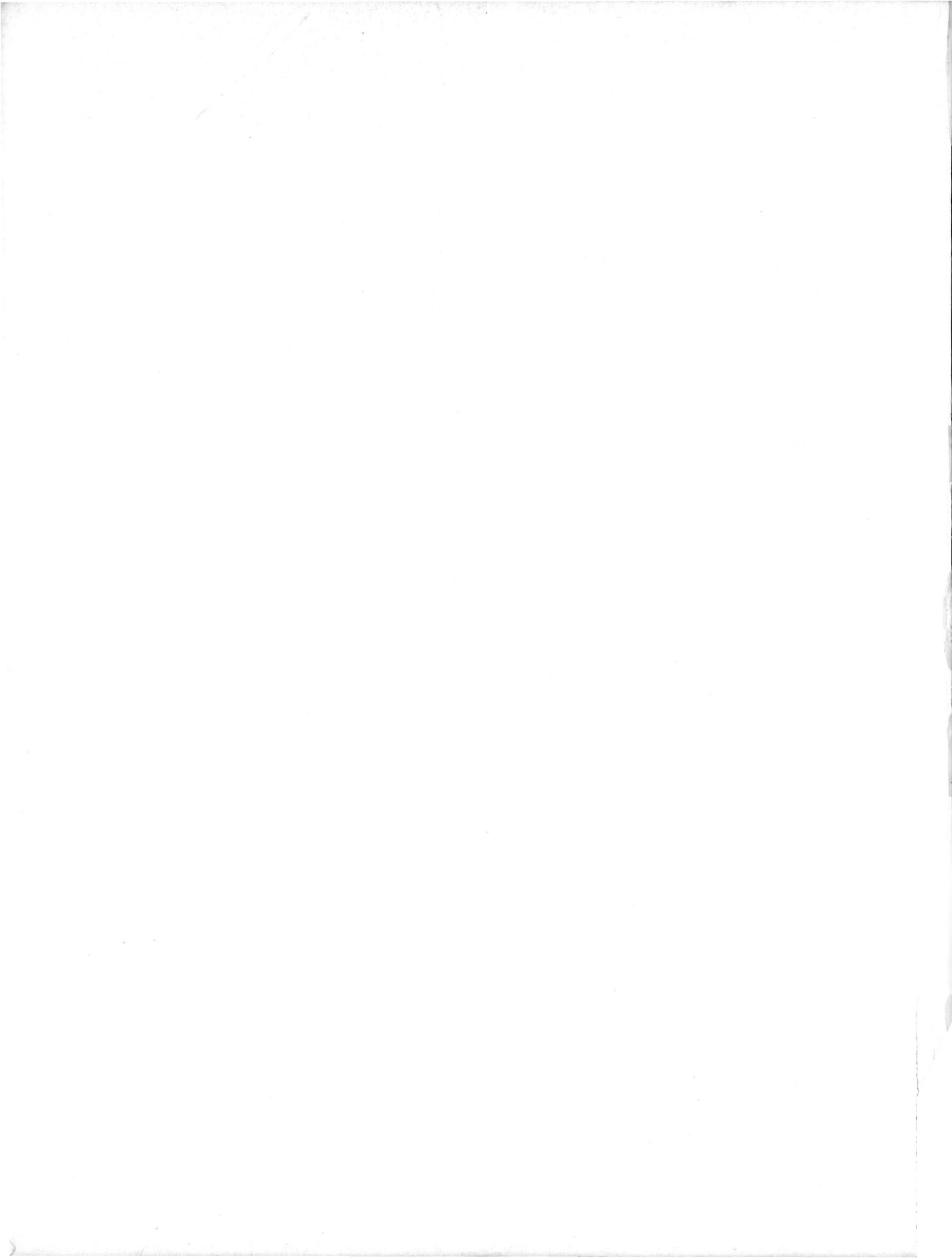